The Hippocampus Book

The Hippocampus Book

EDITED BY

Per Andersen, Richard Morris,
David Amaral, Tim Bliss, & John O'Keefe

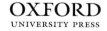

OXFORD
UNIVERSITY PRESS

2007

To

Kari Andersen
Hilary, Louise, and Josephine Morris
David Joseph and Jennie Amaral
Isabel Vasseur
Eileen O'Keefe

Preface

The hippocampus is one of the most widely studied regions of the brain and is of interest to a wide spectrum of neuroscientists, ranging from those who study its normal structure and function to others who study its malfunction in various diseases and pathological conditions. Information about it has accrued across a considerable span of time and is spread over a wide variety of publications. It seems all the more remarkable, therefore, given the explosion of texts on every conceivable topic in neuroscience, that there is no single, comprehensive source of information on the hippocampal formation. It would clearly be helpful to the community of hippocampologists to have the essential information about hippocampal neurobiology gathered together in one volume. This book is our attempt at a reasonably comprehensive survey of hippocampal research, as viewed through many eyes and collected with a wide variety of methods. We hope that the book will be useful at several levels. For those new to the arena of hippocampal research, we hope it will act as a primer pointing to the important advances of the past decades and suggesting important research paths to be pursued; for hippocampal veterans, we hope that by laying bare the many uncertainties and open questions that remain, it will provide ample stimulus to see old problems with new eyes and to pursue them with renewed vigor.

The hippocampus is a structure eminently worthy of study in its own right, but it has also been seen by many as a model structure for the study of cortical function and plasticity in general. The twin aims of the book therefore are to discuss hippocampal structure and function in its own terms and to highlight how study of the hippocampus has revealed ideas and advances that are of wider significance and generality for neuroscience.

The inception of *The Hippocampus Book* occurred many years ago, at the end of a symposium in the beautiful, stimulating city of Palermo in Sicily. We ended up at a street-side cafe, each with a glass of birra glowing in the setting Mediterranean sun. We were four old friends, all long-term card-carrying hippocampologists. Inevitably, our conversation turned to our favorite brain structure and in particular to the lack of reviews and surveys to which we could direct fledgling hippocampologists. Eventually, Per Andersen threw out the challenge: Could the four of us write a treatise on the hippocampal formation that captured the essentials, derived as they were from so many branches of neuroscience? He wondered whether, among us, we could cover the entire field from synapse to behavior by way of the cells and the nerve nets in between. The original crew had a not inconsiderable breadth of experience from physiology, psychology, and behavioral science, but we quickly realized the essential need for structural information as one of the foundations of such a book. We were happy to bring on board a neuroanatomist with great knowledge and experience of the hippocampus, and the gang of four became five.

Over the next 10 years, the Editors met in numerous delightful venues in the United States and Europe to read each other's work and to confer on the book. Although much writing was done during this phase, it gradually dawned on us that two formidable obstacles made our objective significantly more difficult than we had originally anticipated. First, the material on the hippocampus was even more extensive than we had expected and, with the explosion of neuroscience, was growing rapidly day by day. A recent PubMed search elicited more than 73,000 references to the target word "hippocampus." More daunting still, the breadth of the field had expanded with the introduction of new methods and information, not least from the rapidly developing fields of molecular biology, genetics, and development. To cover these important fields adequately, we decided to ask a set of colleagues with the appropriate specialist knowledge to join us in the effort. We were fortunate to attract a powerful team, and the Editors are extremely grateful to these colleagues for their important contributions.

We hope that *The Hippocampus Book* will prove useful to its readers. We are confident that many share our affection for this uniquely fascinating structure. If the book helps future neuroscientists in their planning and execution of hippocampal studies, our project will have been a success. If, in addition, the book facilitates new lines of thought and experimental approaches that challenge existing ideas and concepts, our reward will be even greater. With its important role in mem- ory and its involvement in a host of psychological and psychiatric conditions, the hippocampal formation will undoubtedly continue to be an active focus of energetic research. Our hope is that *The Hippocampus Book* will act as a springboard and a guide for some of that research.

Per Andersen
Richard Morris
David Amaral
Tim Bliss
John O' Keefe

Acknowledgments

Over the years, several individuals and institutions have helped us in various ways with the creation of this book. An important planning session took place at The Institute for Neuroscience, then at The Rockefeller University. We thank its Director Gerald Edelman and Research Director Einar Gall for their generous support. Twice we were accommodated for writing sessions at the Centre for Advanced Studies at the Academy of Science and Letters in Oslo, and we thank the director of the Centre Vigdis Ystad and the President of the Academy Bjarne Waaler for their hospitality. At other times we met in La Jolla, California, Overstrand, Norfolk and in London at the Royal Society and the Novartis Institute. We enjoyed several editorial meetings in Edinburgh at the Centre for Neuroscience. To all these institutions we express our gratitude.

Many dozens of our colleagues have been badgered with questions over the years and have replied with patience and dispatch. Per Andersen particularly thanks Theodor Blackstad, Gyorgyi Buzsaki, Leif Gjerstad, Vidar Jensen, Edward Jones, Bruce Piercey, Geoffrey Raisman, Eric Rinvik, Thomas Sears, and Jon Storm-Mathisen. Finally, we express our particular gratitude to Fiona Stevens, at Oxford University Press, New York for keeping faith with our project through too many fallow periods and, also at OUP to Joan Bossert and Mallory Jensen for the graceful pressure they applied during the final months while shepherding the book to publication. Finally, we are deeply grateful for the efficient, yet gracious manner, in which Berta Steiner at Bermedica Production helped us to bring the book to fruition.

Contents

Chapter 11

Hippocampal Neurophysiology in the Behaving Animal 475

John O'Keefe

Contributors

David Amaral, PhD
The M.I.N.D. Institute
Department of Psychiatry and Behavioral Sciences
University of California-Davis
Davis, California, United States

Per Andersen, MD PhD
Department of Neurophysiology
University of Oslo
Oslo, Norway

Tim Bliss, PhD
Division of Neurophysiology
MRC National Institute for Medical Research, London
London, United Kingdom

Eberhard Buhl, Dr Med*
School of Biomedical Sciences
Leeds University
Leeds, United Kingdom

Neil Burgess, PhD
Institute of Cognitive Neuroscience
University College London
London, United Kingdom

Dennis Chan, PhD MRCP
Dementia Research Group
Institute of Neurology
University College London
London, United Kingdom

Graham Collingridge, PhD
MRC Centre for Synaptic Plasticity
University of Bristol
Bristol, United Kingdom

Michael Frotscher, Dr Med
Institute of Anatomy
University of Freiburg
Freiburg, Germany

Elizabeth Gould, PhD
Department of Psychology
Princeton University
Princeton, New Jersey, United States

Dimitri Kullmann, MBBS DPhil FRCP
Institute of Neurology
University College London
London, United Kingdom

Pierre Lavenex, PhD
Institute of Physiology
Department of Medicine
University of Fribourg
Fribourg, Switzerland

Chris McBain, PhD
Laboratory of Cellular and Synaptic Neurophysiology
National Institute of Child Health and Human Development
Bethesda, Maryland, United States

Richard Morris, DPhil
Laboratory for Cognitive Neuroscience
College of Medicine and Veterinary Medicine
University of Edinburgh
Edinburgh, Scotland

John O'Keefe, PhD
Department of Anatomy & Developmental Biology
University College London
London, United Kingdom

*Deceased

Pavel Osten, PhD
Department of Molecular Neurobiology
Max-Planck-Institute for Medical Research
Heidelberg, Germany

László Seress, MD PhD
Central Electron Microscopic Laboratory, Faculty of Medicine
University of Pécs
Pécs, Hungary

Rolf Sprengel, PhD
Department of Molecular Neurobiology
Max-Planck-Institute for Medical Research
Heidelberg, Germany

Nelson Spruston, PhD
Department of Neurobiology and Physiology
Institute for Neuroscience
Northwestern University
Evanston, Illinois, United States

Craig Stark, PhD
Department of Psychology
Johns Hopkins University
Baltimore, Maryland, United States

Maria Thom, MRCPath
Department of Clinical and Experimental Epilepsy
Institute of Neurology
University College London
London, United Kingdom

Matthew Walker, PhD MRCP
Department of Clinical and Experimental Epilepsy
Institute of Neurology
University College London
London, United Kingdom

Miles Whittington, PhD
Department of Neuroscience
Newcastle University
Newcastle upon Tyne, United Kingdom

William Wisden, PhD
Department of Neuroscience
University of Aberdeen
Aberdeen, Scotland

The Hippocampus Book

1

Per Andersen, Richard Morris, David Amaral, Tim Bliss, and John O'Keefe

The Hippocampal Formation

1.1 Overview

Buried deep within the medial temporal lobe of the human brain lies a group of many millions of neurons organized into a network quite different from that found anywhere else in the nervous system. It is a structure whose bulb-like shape, protruding into the lateral ventricles, has captivated anatomists since the first dissections took place in classical Egypt. The hippocampal formation is a group of brain areas consisting of the dentate gyrus, hippocampus, subiculum, presubiculum, parasubiculum, and entorhinal cortex. The basic layout of cells and fiber pathways of the hippocampal formation is much the same in all mammals (Fig. 1–1).

There are several reasons the hippocampus has attracted the interest of scientists in the many disciplines that now characterize modern neuroscience—the hippocampus has something for everyone. Whether you are a psychologist interested in memory, a synaptic physiologist investigating neuronal and synaptic plasticity, or a computational neuroscientist wanting to build a neural network model, the hippocampus and its associated structures are an attractive set of brain structures on which to work. In parallel, clinicians concerned with the basis of neurological conditions such as epilepsy or Alzheimer's disease had their attention drawn to the hippocampal formation because of the pathological processes observed to occur there and the opportunities that scientific study of this area of the brain offers for novel therapeutics. The hippocampus has been a neural Rosetta Stone. The striking discovery, 50 years ago, that patient H.M. had a relatively pure memory deficit after surgical excision of the medial temporal lobe for the relief of epilepsy had a profound effect on the study of memory and, through that, on our understanding of the functions of the hippocampus itself.

During the last 30 years, the pyramid-shaped cells of the hippocampus have become the most intensively studied neurons in the brain. As a result, we now know a great deal about their development, synaptogenesis, neurotransmitter receptors and ion channels, micro-circuitry, and cell biological machinery. No less impressive has been the molecular analysis of neurotransmission in hippocampal cells; what has been learned from this has revealed general properties that seem to apply in other areas of the central nervous system. We also know something about why and when these cells are activated in the living brain. Recordings from freely moving animals as they navigate around a space with which they have become familiar have shown that individual hippocampal pyramidal cells fire in particular locations. This finding led to the development of new behavioral tools to study the neural mechanisms of memory in animals. Along the extensive dendritic arborizations of these pyramidal cells, there can be many thousands of miniature dendritic spines. These are the sites where most of the excitatory synapses are to be found. An important finding is that the efficiency with which these excitatory synapses transmit messages can vary as a function of neural activity. The circumstances bringing about this synaptic plasticity are now well understood, and we are beginning to understand some of the underlying biochemical mechanisms. Many suspect that synaptic plasticity is a key mechanism of memory. Another exciting feature of the hippocampal formation is that the dentate granule cell is one of the rare types of nerve cell that multiplies throughout life. Adult neurogenesis is likely to yield important lessons about neuronal growth and survival. This is an area of obvious potential importance for neuronal repair and therapeutic intervention.

These observations have emerged from the widespread fascination with this beautiful cortical structure that so attracted the early anatomists. As we shall see, certain structural principles that are characteristic of the hippocampal formation have greatly facilitated structural, physiological, and behavioral analyses.

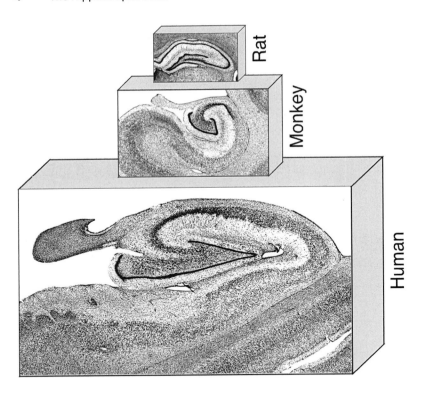

Rat

Monkey

Human

Figure 1–1. Nissl-stained coronal sections through the rat, monkey, and human hippocampal formation. Although there are obvious differences in certain regions, the most striking feature is the general similarity of this brain region across phylogeny.

1.2 Why Study the Hippocampal Formation on Its Own?

Can one profitably focus on one group of brain structures and appear to ignore the rest of the brain? The brain is so heavily interconnected that it is misleading to think about the function of one small part of it in isolation. What it does and how it does it might be understood better by comparing it with other brain areas and by thinking about how it works in conjunction with them to realize the seamless fabric of normal brain function. We have much sympathy with this view, not least because the general significance of the many exciting discoveries that have been made about the hippocampus can only become clear with a more inclusive approach in which it and other parts of the brain are considered together. We believe, nonetheless, that there is still value in our focused approach. There are two primary reasons for singling out the hippocampal formation as a brain area worthy of a book in its own right. They have to do with trying to understand its function(s) within the brain and the way in which work on hippocampal tissue has revealed general principles in neuroscience.

First, contemporary research points strongly to the hippocampus having a highly specific role in memory. There has been a great deal of debate about how that role should be characterized; and after the explosive period of research during the last quarter century, a consensus is beginning to emerge. It is now generally recognized that there are multiple types of memory and that the hippocampus plays a part in only some of them. There is also general agreement that some types of learning and memory are propositional—that is, they relate to memories that can be described as a series of propositional statements—whereas other types, such as the process of acquiring motor skills, are not. The hippocampus is engaged in remembering information that can be described in a propositional or declarative manner. That much is clear. Beyond that, there remain many areas of disagreement and debate that continue to fuel imaginative new research in behavioral and cognitive neuroscience. A striking feature of this strand of research has been the constructive convergence of both "top-down" and "bottom-up" approaches to the study of brain function. Work on the function of the hippocampal formation, arguably more than any other brain area, has led to the development of current concepts about the organization of memory systems in the brain.

Some traditionalists still hold that the various subjects that make up the biomedical sciences—such as psychology, physiology, biochemistry—each has a self-contained level of analysis that is logically independent of other levels of analysis. With this view, a psychological problem requires an answer in strictly psychological terms and a physiological problem a physiological approach. The emerging view at the start of the twenty-first century, however, is that many years of a strictly psychological analysis of learning and memory—beginning with the discovery of Pavlovian conditioning, the ensuing dark phase of behaviorism, and the subsequent enlightenment of the cognitive revolution—failed to unravel the existence of multiple memory systems. It was not until a different "brain-systems" approach was taken during the last part of the twentieth century, an approach that emerged from studies of the memory problems faced by patient H.M. and other amnesic patients, that the major breakthroughs in our understanding of the cerebral organization of memory came about. Such thinking led to research that married brain and behavior in single-unit recording and lesion studies in awake primates and freely moving rodents, as well as the development of new behavioral tests of learning and memory. There is a lesson here that we believe is generally applicable to other branches of functional neuroscience. Specifically, the brain-systems approach is one in which there is analytical value in juxtaposing the biomedical sciences with psychology and, in particular, in thinking carefully about what bits of the brain do what.

The second justification for writing this book is that the hippocampus has preeminently been the structure in which many of the general principles of modern neuroscience have been studied and established. Thirty years ago, the most widely studied cell in the nervous system was the alpha motoneuron of the ventral horn of the spinal cord. Today it is the pyramidal cell of the hippocampus. One reason for this development has been the peculiar anatomy of the hippocampus, with all principal cells in a single layer and synaptic inputs to well defined dendritic lamina. This simplified architecture facilitated the recording of both synaptic signals and population discharges. Field potential recording became possible because the well defined somatic and dendritic laminae allowed identification of current sources and sinks in extracellular recordings made in vivo. It was through these studies that the basic principle of unidirectional excitatory transmission was first described and the phenomenon of long-term potentiation was discovered. Of particular importance for the study of synaptic function in the context of learning and memory was the fact that field-potential recording of synaptic responses could be made as easily in the freely moving animal as in the hippocampal slice. The pyramidal cell also became a popular cell to study because of the analytical potential of the in vitro brain slice. The first brain slices were made from neocortex and piriform cortex with limited synaptic activation. With its better identification of cells and input fibers, the development of the transverse hippocampal slice revolutionized neurophysiology and neuropharmacology. Of course, many fundamental concepts had been worked out beforehand—in the axon of the giant squid, spinal cord, and cerebellum—but the hippocampal slice rendered analytical extra- and intracellular studies of mammalian cells and identified synapses feasible on an unprecedented scale. Work in the hippocampus has been a major contributor to our understanding of the actions and mechanisms of various types of synapse and the various classes of receptors for excitatory and inhibitory amino acids, the many transmitter uptake mechanisms, activity-dependent synaptic plasticity, and the deleterious consequences of excitotoxicity for brain cells. It is the two- or three-layered architecture of the hippocampus and its capacity to survive in vitro for long periods of time coupled with a strict layering of synapses in the dendritic tree that has rendered the design and analysis of electrophysiological and other experiments tractable in a manner that remains difficult in other brain areas and would be wholly impracticable in vivo.

Beyond its key role in the development of in vitro techniques, the hippocampus has also been the area of choice for many other types of brain research. It is involved in a number of disparate neurological disorders, including epilepsy, Alzheimer's disease, and cerebrovascular disease. Thus, the abnormal electrical activity that is at the root of seizures in epileptic patients is often easily detected in the hippocampus. Moreover, a hallmark feature of the neuropathology of temporal lobe epilepsy is loss of neurons in several hippocampal fields. For example, the characteristic pathological changes of Alzheimer's disease manifest initially in the entorhinal cortex—one of the components of the hippocampal formation—and the disease spreads from there to involve the hippocampus proper and ultimately the entire cerebral cortex. Such findings have led to the development of model systems in which pathophysiological events such as these may be studied and, hopefully, alleviated by treatment.

These two main reasons for writing the book therefore provide us with two intersecting themes that run through many of its chapters. One perspective is functional, the other heuristic.

- What does the hippocampus do?
- What can we learn about general principles of neuroscience from studying the hippocampus?

To achieve these twin aims, we have broken up our task into chapters that are largely organized along conventional disciplinary lines but where, when appropriate, both strands of thought are intertwined.

1.3 Defining the Contemporary Era

Our starting point when preparing this book was to define the contemporary era of research as beginning in the 1960s and to regard discoveries made before that as "modern" and those made afterward as "contemporary." Any division of this kind is arbitrary, but the period of the 1960s and 1970s was a watershed for both functional and mechanistic studies of the hippocampus. That decade saw the first intracellular analysis of synaptic, antidromic, and epileptiform activities of hippocampal neurons; the characterization and interpretation of field potentials signaling excitation and inhibition; and electron micrographs of synapse types and their distribution along the cell bodies and their extensions. It was also at this time that several of the new tract-tracing techniques became available to anatomists, replacing the classic degeneration techniques hitherto used to identify regional connectivity. These advances made it possible to map the extrinsic connections of the hippocampal formation at a previously unachievable level of sensitivity and detail. During the same decade, hippocampal place cells were discovered and the phenomenon of long-term potentiation was first described in detail. Methodological developments of the 1970s included the hippocampal slice, new tests of recognition memory for primates, and the open-field watermaze, a behavioral technique to study learning in rodents that has since been used extensively to analyze the role of the hippocampus in spatial navigation. Mathematicians also started thinking about the hippocampus as a neural network and so set in motion a theoretical neuroscience that has attracted increasing attention.

1.4 Organization and Content of the Book

During the discussions about when the contemporary era actually started, we recognized the enormous contributions made beforehand and upon which so much of modern research rests. Accordingly, we have devoted Chapter 2 to a historical discussion of the key discoveries and concepts of hippocampal neurobiology of the modern era up to about the 1970s. In it, we also identify some of the key figures whose work helped to usher in the contemporary era. In addition, we highlight key concepts in neurobiology that were first established through work on the hippocampal formation.

In Chapter 3, we outline the anatomy of the hippocampal formation, beginning with issues of nomenclature and definition. Here we present the three-dimensional organization of the rodent, monkey, and human hippocampal formation, the detailed architecture of each of its component structures, and the patterns of cellular interconnectivity. Straightaway, we found that we disagreed about certain conceptual issues, such as the status of the "lamella hypothesis" that was proposed nearly 30 years ago on the basis of electrophysiological data. Modern neuroanatomical tract-tracing studies are thought not to support this concept in its original form, although the electrophysiological data remain on the table. After long debate, we arrived at a description of the extent to which connectivity is primarily in the transverse plane and the extent to which longitudinal and other more diffuse projections are a characteristic feature of hippocampal anatomy. Similarly, although recognizing that the original concept of the "trisynaptic circuit" may be too narrow, we continue to stress the sense in which unidirectional connectivity is a distinctive feature of the hippocampus compared to the neocortex, including the parallel connections made from the entorhinal cortex to the dentate gyrus, and to areas CA3 and CA1 of the hippocampus proper.

Chapter 4 considers how this intricate structure develops both from the perspective of overall organization and from that of individual cells. Here the interplay moves from pure anatomy to genes and molecular biology. Modern studies of the development of the hippocampus are characterized by molecular studies in which the temporal expression of the genes responsible for migration, neuronal specification, and axonal guidance—and for major cellular constituents such as receptor subunits—are being mapped out.

Chapter 5 takes us forward to a detailed analysis of individual cells in which we present, side by side, both anatomical and physiological ideas. To understand the principal cell types of the hippocampal formation—pyramidal and granule cells—and the several types of interneuron, one must know what these cells look like, know about their inputs and outputs, and grapple with the biophysical principles that govern how current injected into the cell at a dendritic synapse contributes to cell firing. It is necessary to understand how synapses at various dendritic locations differ in their synaptic effects and how these individual effects sum to control the cell discharge pattern. The large group of after-hyperpolarizing responses is essential for cellular behavior. The important modulatory effects of a set of controlling systems comprise a major topic.

The intricacies of neurotransmission are considered in Chapters 6 and 7 from physiological, pharmacological, and molecular biological perspectives. Chapter 6 considers how the release of glutamate from presynaptic terminals in the hippocampus and its action on various glutamatergic receptors mediate excitatory synaptic transmission. It also discusses the essential role of inhibitory synaptic transmission at GABAergic synapses. Because the hippocampus is one of the few regions where it is possible to have experimental control over a large set of converging inputs to an individual cortical cell, most of our ideas on cellular integration are derived from studies on hippocampal tissue. This chapter describes the intricate molecular machinery responsible for the mobilization of glutamate-containing vesicles, the exocytotic release machinery for glutamate, and its postsynaptic actions. It also outlines the various ligand-binding and modulatory sites on these receptors, the insights coming from the relatively new work on receptor subunits afforded by molecular biology and the mechanisms responsible for transmitter uptake. In many of these studies, genetically altered animals have been essential tools. The chapter touches on the important and developing topic of neuromodulatory transmitters in the hippocampus, such as acetylcholine, norepinephrine, 5-hydroxytryptamine, dopamine, and peptides such as dynorphin and somatostatin. The transmitters influence hippocampal excitability and second-messenger effector mechanisms in an orchestrated cascade of formidable complexity. Chapter 6 also discusses how the many neuromodulatory systems influence the traditional synaptic processes and the mechanisms by which they are mediated. These studies often are models for the general neuronal activity seen in other parts of the nervous system. Chapter 7 discusses the molecular biology of hippocampal cells with particular emphasis on synaptic function. Here, much of the pioneering work on glutamate receptor categorization was made in the spinal cord, whereas the important discovery of the voltage-dependent magnesium block of the N-methyl-D-aspartate (NMDA) receptor channel was discovered in hippocampal tissue. Notably, the hippocampal slice has been of critical importance for developing the modern understanding of ionotropic and metabotropic glutamate receptors.

Having described the three-dimensional organization of the hippocampus, its cells, synapses, and their transmitters and receptors, we need next to consider the local circuits that these structures produce and the possible types of neuronal processing they make possible. Chapter 8 takes on this task and endeavors to explain how an impressive multitude of inhibitory interneurons shape the number and pattern of the participating cells in a near-physiological situation. These interactions between principal cells and interneurons are particularly evident during periods of rhythmical theta and gamma activity.

The chapter on local circuits also provides an introduction to Chapters 9 and 10, where we confront activity-dependent neuronal and synaptic plasticity. One of the more extraordinary discoveries of recent times has been that new neurons can be formed in the adult brain. This is contrary to established dogma but, interestingly, the dogma that had been challenged in hippocampal studies nearly 30 years ago but was unappreciated at the time. The dentate gyrus is one of two major sites of adult neurogenesis. In Chapter 9, we discuss the extent to which new cells and connections can be made, a field of acute interest for basic and practical neurobiology. Chapter 10 focuses on processes to explain the fact that, once formed, hippocampal circuits are not immutable, as synapses throughout the various components of the hippocampal formation show both short-term and long-term changes. The latter includes the intensively studied phenomenon of long-term potentiation (LTP). Research on this form of synaptic plasticity has revealed a range of properties that are highly suggestive of a potential cellular memory mechanism. The effort to understand LTP mechanistically led to passionate debates that have stimulated a host of ingenious experiments. Research on synaptic plasticity, perhaps more than any other area of hippocampal neurobiology, spans the twin themes of the book. What is the purpose of LTP? Are its underlying neural mechanisms applicable to other areas of cortex? Research on the induction of this phenomenon has helped unravel one of the most satisfyingly elegant biophysical mechanisms in the nervous system: the role of the NMDA receptor as a coincidence detector. Having detected the conjunction of presynaptic activity and postsynaptic depolarization, this receptor signals the conjunction by an influx of the divalent cation calcium (Ca^{2+}), which then sets in train a cascade of biochemical effects. The discussion of the NMDA receptor complements the earlier description of its molecular basis in Chapter 7. It activates signaling proteins associated with the receptor itself and calcium-dependent kinases. It may also help trigger the release of calcium from intracellular stores, thereby sustaining the synaptically evoked Ca^{2+} transient beyond the period that the NMDA receptor-associated ion channel remains open. The resulting biochemical cascade eventually results in an increase in synaptic strength. It should also be recognized that activity-dependent synaptic plasticity is not restricted to increases in synaptic efficacy—decreases can also be induced. This bidirectional feature of synaptic plasticity—that "what goes up must come down"—adds computational flexibility

and power. However, the extent to which bidirectional changes can be seen in the hippocampus in freely moving adult animals remains unclear. Chapter 10 also takes on the task of explaining the various behavioral studies that have attempted to identify the role LTP might play in learning, memory, or other cognitive processes. We outline studies that have examined correlations between the physiological properties of synaptic plasticity and behavioral learning and the effects of blocking it, saturating it, and erasing it. We offer no definitive answer to the question of the purpose of these various types of plasticity, but the tenor of our account is sympathetic to a role in the encoding and storage of certain kinds of memory.

Chapter 11 continues the behavioral theme with a survey of studies in which electrical activity in structures of the hippocampal formation has been recorded during various kinds of behavior. The pioneering work of this kind was conducted in rats and was heralded by the discovery of place cells noted earlier (neurons that fire when rats occupy particular positions in space). The further discovery of a different group of cells that fired during certain kinds of movement and in phase with slow-wave electroencephalographic activity was also important, as were findings of cells that code for the direction in which an animal's head is pointing or show grid-like patterns as an animal traverses a familiar space. These categories of cell are found in distinct areas of the hippocampal formation and in different cell classes within a single area. Work in nonhuman primates has also identified a class of cells that are responsive to the animal's view. The properties of these cells, their role in mapping space, and, according to some, other cognitive functions as well are gradually being unraveled. The process of discovery has been accompanied by the development of a new single-cell methodology that permits simultaneous recording from large numbers of neurons. This tetrode-recording technique enables the properties of several individual neurons in a population to be mapped simultaneously and has applications that extend well beyond hippocampal neurobiology.

Chapter 12 begins with the discovery, almost 50 years ago, that surgical damage to the hippocampal formation and related structures on both sides of the brain causes a profound, lasting global amnesia. Once this unexpected consequence had been observed, neurosurgeons took care not to perform bilateral medial temporal lobectomies. Such memory-impaired patients are therefore rare, but their very existence spurred the development of animal models through which, it is hoped, the role of the hippocampus in memory can be worked out. Modern functional imaging techniques are also providing new insights into the differential activation of various brain areas for different types of memory and different stages of memory processing. Such work has led to new concepts, such as the extent to which neuronal activation in a memory-related area reflects the effort devoted to encoding or retrieval or to the success of achieving either. Such conceptual dissociations are almost impossible to draw on the basis of lesion studies alone.

Chapter 13 takes up the theme set by these human studies to lay out a number of prominent theories of hippocampal function that have been developed from work on animals. One theory concerns the role of the hippocampus in remembering facts and events that can be consciously recalled, and another has to do with its role in mapping and navigating through space. Other theories have been developed to help address some of the issues and problems that have arisen in connection with these two ideas, particularly in situations of predictable ambiguity. We also outline current interest in the idea that the hippocampus plays a critical role in contextual encoding and retrieval, including episodic memory. This section attempts to link behavioral studies on rapidly learned forms of associative memory to the neurobiological observations on circuitry and synaptic plasticity outlined earlier in the book. Although one of the authors of this book is an architect of the second theory discussed, we attempt to present as objective an account of the state of the field as possible.

Chapter 14 takes us to computational models of hippocampal function. Some models focus on its global function, but even when they work they often involve assumptions that seem far removed from real neurobiology. These models are the artificial intelligence and idealized neural network models that can solve interesting cognitive problems—including navigation around the world or remembering associations in memory—but using processing units and learning algorithms that may not exist among real hippocampal cells. Other models incorporate more realistic assumptions about the hippocampal network and its neuronal components, the different classes of cells, and their phase relationships; but their processing tends to be more limited. Ultimately, the value of these models is to provide a predictive framework for understanding the mass of detail we have covered in other chapters of this book. To date, no model incorporates information realistically at each of the levels of the anatomical circuit, cellular architecture, and synaptic transmission. However, the pieces and patches that will eventually enable a comprehensive neural network account of hippocampal function to be woven together are beginning to become apparent.

Last come Chapters 15 and 16. The first of these chapters picks up from a set of intriguing observations suggesting that the hippocampus, together with the amygdala and prefrontal cortex, play a role in regulating the hypothalamic-pituitary-adrenal axis, which is responsible for the release of stress hormones. The hippocampus contains a particularly high density of corticosteroid receptors of two major types, and this neuroendocrine detection of mild or severe stress has a dramatic impact on hippocampal physiology and memory function, including effects on LTP. Glucocorticoid receptors act as transcription factors, and it has long been thought that the primary expression mechanism was an intracellular regulation of genes. However, it is now becoming clear that there are a variety of more rapid effects of corticosteroid action in the hippocampus. Chapter 16 considers hippocampal pathologies. This is, of course, a large subject in its own right, and we cannot here do justice to a vast field of clinical research. To exclude it, however, would be wrong because all of us have an interest in alleviating the impact of human neurological disease. The importance of these conditions is underscored by the prevalence of disease: Alzheimer's disease alone affects around 20 million people worldwide. Substantial advances have been made in understanding the involvement of various components of the hippocampal formation in epilepsy and Alzheimer's disease, on which we focus; and this information has underpinned improvements in diagnosis and treatment.

This book is our tribute to the thousands of scientists who have contributed to our understanding of this beautiful and enigmatic part of the brain. We hope that it will help design new, revealing experiments and thereby increase our insight into its cellular, molecular, physiological, and behavioral processes. Should it also facilitate clinical studies, our satisfaction will be so much the greater.

2 ▦ Per Andersen, Richard Morris, David Amaral, Tim Bliss, and John O'Keefe

Historical Perspective: Proposed Functions, Biological Characteristics, and Neurobiological Models of the Hippocampus

2.1 Overview

This chapter has two major sections. In the first, we provide a selective overview of some of the historically important proposals concerning the function of the hippocampus. The current view, that the hippocampus plays a prominent role in memory, is dealt with in detail in Chapters 12 and 13. In the second major section, we highlight the historically significant advances in neurobiology that have been made by using the unique structure of the hippocampus for studies ranging from defining the morphology of excitatory and inhibitory synapses to developing computational models of memory. This second section is itself divided into subsections that emphasize first the biological characteristics of the hippocampus and then the advantages of the hippocampus as a model system for neurobiological research. Many of the most recent advances are dealt with in appropriate chapters, as we intend this chapter to be primarily a historical overview.

2.2 The Dawn of Hippocampal Studies

From the very start of brain investigations, the hippocampus has played a central role. No doubt this is due to the striking appearance of the large, bulging structure impressing itself into the lateral ventricle and visible even to the ancient anatomists. Members of the Alexandrian school of medicine were impressed by the elegant, curved structure, which when seen with its contralateral half strongly resembles the coiled horns of a ram. Hence, the ancient scholars named the hippocampus cornu ammonis, Latin for horn of the ram. This terminology survives in the acronyms for the hippocampal subfields CA1 (cornu ammonis), CA2, and CA3. Over the centuries, this part of the brain has been proposed as the seat of

many functions, ranging from olfaction to motor function and even reason, stubbornness, and inventiveness. The Bolognese anatomist Giulio Cesare Aranzi (circa 1564) was the first to coin the name "hippocampus," undoubtedly because of its similarity to the tropical fish (Fig. 2–1).

After the advent of microscopy, the hippocampus was perhaps even more impressive, with its characteristic, neatly regimented cellular arrangement. Although the hippocampal formation is organized in a very different way from other cortical areas, it has still played an important role in unraveling some of the basic principles of cortical organization.

Its stunning structure, with cell populations apparently condensed into single layers, has attracted the attention of many investigators of the central nervous system. A striking example is Camillo Golgi's picture from 1886, where he used his revolutionary new technique to illustrate the unique organization of the hippocampus, here reproduced from Golgi et al. (2001) (Fig. 2–2).

As noted in Chapter 1, the two themes of this book—the overall functions of the hippocampus and how its study has shed light on a range of general principles in neuroscience—can be highlighted by reference to the history of research on the hippocampus. Early work inevitably focused on anatomical issues, whereas later research successively brought in physiological, behavioral, and other technologies in an effort to fathom the function of the hippocampus and through it the workings of the brain.

2.2.1 A Famous Dispute About the Significance of the Hippocampus

Interest in the hippocampus was particularly high during the eighteenth and nineteenth centuries, a notable example being its curious role in the famous debate between Richard Owen and Thomas Huxley at the British Association in Oxford in June 1860 following the publication of Charles Darwin's book *On the Origin of Species* in 1859 (Gross, 1993). The superin-

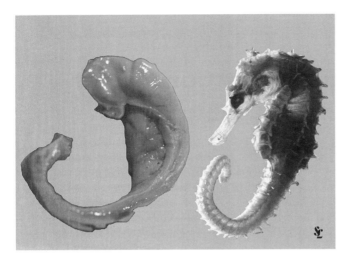

Figure 2–1. Human hippocampus dissected free (*left*) and compared to a specimen of *Hippocampus leria* (*right*). (*Source:* Courtesy of Professor Laszlo Seress, University of Pecs.)

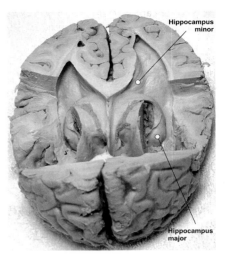

Figure 2–3. Hippocampus major and minor as seen in a human brain after the dorsal cortex and corpus callosum have been removed.

tendent of the natural history collections of the British Museum, Richard Owen, claimed that only human brains contain a structure he called hippocampus minor, this being one essential distinguishing feature between Man and Apes. This structure is a relatively small bulge on the medial wall of the posterior horn of the lateral ventricle (Fig. 2–3). Huxley

Figure 2–2. Section of a rabbit hippocampus stained with the original Golgi method (1886). (*Source*: Golgi et al., 2001).

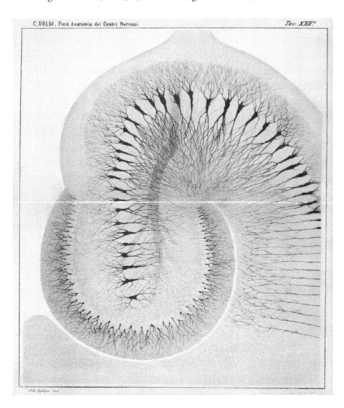

objected strongly, not least because of his own dissection results. Today, it is difficult to see how this particular bulge could have any bearing on the question of human evolution. The name hippocampus minor is really a misnomer because it has nothing to do with the hippocampal formation per se but is a fold of white matter around the calcarine fissure, in other words a visual cortical structure.

2.3 Early Ideas About Hippocampal Function

2.3.1 The Hippocampal Formation and Olfactory Function

Although the hippocampus had been casually implicated in a number of functions during the nineteenth and early twentieth centuries, until the 1930s the hippocampal formation was considered by neuroanatomists to be part of the olfactory system. Perhaps this was because macroscopic investigations left the impression that the hippocampus is especially large in macrosmatic animals (with large olfactory mucosa and bulbs) such as nocturnal insectivores and rodents. However, in these macrosmatic animals, the absolute sizes of the olfactory parts of the brain are quite small. In fact, it was claimed that the ratio of the volume of the hippocampus to the olfactory bulb is largest in humans (Rose, 1935). Indeed, as observed by Brodal (1947):

> From a functional point of view it is worth emphasizing that the development not only of the fornix, but also of the mammillary body, the mammillo-thalamic tract, the anterior (more particularly the antero-ventral) nucleus of the thalamus and the cingular gyrus runs roughly parallel with the degree of develop-

ment of the hippocampus. All these structures reach their peak of development in man.

A possible basis for the idea of an olfactory function for the hippocampus (an idea that was repeated in numerous textbooks during the first half of the twentieth century) is the appearance of a few early behavioral and clinical observations. For example, David Ferrier (1876) observed "movements of the lip and nostrils on stimulation of the hippocampal lobe in monkeys." John Hughlings Jackson and Charles Beevor (1890) reported a patient who had subjective olfactory sensations during seizures that originated in the olfactory cortex of the periamygdaloid gyrus. Later, Wilder Penfield and Theodore Erickson (1941) reported a patient who had "olfactory sensations as part of his epileptic seizure and where it seems to be the hippocampus which must be the site of the discharge" (p. 56).

In a scholarly and comprehensive review, Alf Brodal (1947) summarized the evidence for and against such a role for the hippocampal formation. He noted that phylogenetic and comparative neuroanatomical studies suggested that the hippocampus develops in parallel with the olfactory portions of the brain and that it is particularly prominent in macrosmatic mammals such as rodents and insectivores. Moreover, even in the gross brain or in normal histological preparations, fibers from the lateral olfactory tract can easily be traced to brain regions surrounding the hippocampal formation. Even so, Brodal raised a number of arguments against an olfactory role for the hippocampus, suggesting that the association of the hippocampal formation with olfactory function was largely based on circumstantial evidence.

Central to his thesis was the claim that fibers arising in the olfactory bulb did not, in fact, directly innervate any portion of the hippocampus. In particular, although he agreed that some olfactory fibers innervated the anterior portions of the parahippocampal gyrus, they did not extend back into the caudal portion of this gyrus where the entorhinal cortex resides. He did not entirely dismiss an olfactory role for the hippocampal formation and suggested that the entorhinal cortex "should be considered as concerned mainly with the association and integration of olfactory impulses . . . with other cortical influences" (p. 206). Among other negative evidence, Brodal cited several studies that attested to the fact that the hippocampal formation was present in anosmatic and microsmatic animals such as dolphins and whales (Ries and Langworthy, 1937) and that there was substantial regional differentiation in microsmatic humans. Furthermore, he cited the data of William F. Allen (1940) in which lesions of the temporal lobe had no effect on the ability of dogs to perform olfactory discrimination tasks. Brodal (1947) concluded, "No decisive evidence that the hippocampus is concerned in olfaction appears to have been brought forward" (p. 180).

Brodal's review was highly influential in raising doubts concerning the role of the hippocampus in olfaction. However, at least one of the pieces of evidence cited by Brodal—that there are no olfactory projections to the hip-

pocampal formation—has subsequently proven incorrect. More sensitive anatomical techniques have shown that in the rodent the entorhinal cortex receives a massive direct projection from the olfactory bulb as well as secondary olfactory inputs from the piriform and periamygdaloid cortices (Shipley and Adamek, 1984). Even in the monkey, the anterior portion of the entorhinal cortex is directly innervated by the lateral olfactory tract (Amaral et al., 1987). Thus, the olfactory system retains a privileged position in relation to the entorhinal cortex as none of the other sensory channels from which it receives information originates in primary or even higher order unimodal sensory cortices; rather, it comes from polysensory association cortices. Thus, although Brodal's review was a milestone in the evaluation of hippocampal function and is partially responsible for the currently held view that the hippocampal formation is not a major component of the olfactory system, olfactory information certainly must contribute to the functions in which the hippocampus is engaged. Interestingly, olfactory learning and memory tasks are now widely used in studies of hippocampal function in rodents.

2.3.2 The Hippocampal Formation and Emotion

Another influential neuroanatomical hypothesis was proposed by James W. Papez (1937), who suggested that the hippocampus was part of a circuit that provides the anatomical substrate of emotion. He was influenced by the work of Walter B. Cannon (1929) and Philip Bard (1934), which indicated that the hypothalamus was essential for evocation of the autonomic and visceral aspects of emotional behavior. He accepted the view of Cannon and Bard that emotion has two component processes: emotional behavior and the cognitive appreciation of emotion. In an attempt to explain certain aspects of emotion, he proposed a circuit that interconnected cortical and subcortical structures (Fig. 2–4). In this now famous circuit, which bears his name (Papez circuit), he viewed the hippocampus as a collector of sensory information; this information, in turn, would develop an emotive "state" that would be transferred to the mammillary nuclei. In addition to mediating the appropriate behavioral response to this emotive state, the mammillary nuclei would also relay information to the anterior cingulate cortex via the anterior thalamic nuclei where conscious appreciation of the emotion would be achieved.

The central emotive process of cortical origin may then be conceived as being built up in the hippocampal formation and as being transferred to the mammillary body and thence through the anterior thalamic nuclei to the cortex of the gyrus cinguli. The cortex of the cingular gyrus may be looked on as the receptive region for the experiencing of emotion as the result of impulses coming from the hypothalamic region, in the same way as the area striata is considered the receptive cortex for photic excitations coming from the retina. (Papez, 1937, pp. 725–743)

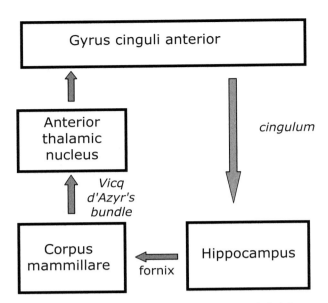

Figure 2–4. Original Papez circuit. Later versions included the amygdala, hypothalamus, prefrontal cortex, and some association cortices.

Again, a comment from Brodal (1981) is skeptical. After having scrutinized the anatomical literature, he stated: "There is no sound biological basis for selecting a few brain regions as being involved in these complex functions (emotions), and today the theory of Papez is of historical interest only" (p. 672).

However, we may conclude that the Papez circuit *was* important historically because it shifted emphasis away from the idea of olfactory functions of the hippocampus. Moreover, it was one of the early ideas about how the brain might have more autonomy from the environment than suggested by the then current stimulus–response behaviorism. As we shall see, there is only moderate evidence to support the specific idea that the hippocampus is involved in emotion, although the idea has occasionally been championed, most notably in recent years by Jeffrey Gray (1982, 2001).

Papez's speculations about the role of the hippocampus in emotion appeared to receive support from the experiments of Heinrich Klüver and Paul Bucy, which were carried out at the same time (1937). Klüver was a psychologist interested in the neural locus of action of psychotropic drugs such as mescaline. Together with Bucy, a neurologist, he searched for the locus of action by removing brain tissue from monkeys and looking for changes in their behavioral response to drugs. The changes that followed temporal lobe removal were interesting enough to warrant extensive description, and the constellation of changes is now known as the Klüver-Bucy syndrome. There are two important aspects to the syndrome: changes in visually guided behavior and changes in emotional expression. The lesioned monkeys appeared to have visual agnosia but would compulsively follow stimuli brought into their visual field; they continually placed all objects encountered in their mouths, perhaps owing to their failure to recognize the

objects by sight. In the emotional sphere, they were sexually aberrant and apparently without fear of stimuli that usually are frightening to them. It was this latter observation that appeared to confirm the role of the hippocampus in emotion predicted by Papez. However, it was subsequently shown that the loss of fear and other behavioral alterations could be attributed to damage to the amygdala and its connections with the visual regions of the inferotemporal cortex (Mishkin, 1954; Schreiner and Kling, 1956; Weiskrantz, 1956; Aggleton, 1993; Hayman et al., 1998). The hippocampus was again in search of a function.

Unbeknown to Papez, and probably also to Klüver and Bucy, a report appearing nearly a half century earlier by Sanger Brown and Hans Schäfer (1888) described the results of a large bilateral temporal lobe lesion on a "fine, large, active rhaesus" monkey. In addition to describing virtually all of the behavioral and emotional alterations of the Klüver-Bucy syndrome, they also reported disturbances in memory. They commented on the apparent forgetfulness of the monkey in the following way: "And even after having examined an object in this way with the utmost care and deliberation, he will, on again coming across the same object accidentally, even a few minutes afterwards, go through exactly the same process, as if he had entirely forgotten his previous experience" (p. 262). This little known observation of Brown and Schäfer presaged what has become the most enduring notion of hippocampal function—that it plays an essential role in memory.

2.3.3 The Hippocampal Formation and Attention Control

As early as 1938, Richard Jung and Alois Kornmüller had noted that desynchronization of the neocortical electroencephalogram (EEG) was temporally linked to a large-amplitude, sinusoidal wave pattern in the rabbit hippocampus at between 4 and 7 Hz, which they named "theta" activity. Later work suggested that this particular activity was related to enhanced attention (Green and Arduini, 1954). John Green and W. Ross Adey (1956) found that arousal caused an inverse relation between the electrocortical waves of the hippocampus and neocortex. Endre Grastyán and colleagues (1959) proposed that theta activity could be coupled to specific learning states (Fig. 2–13). Both hippocampal and entorhinal theta waves showed distinct changes during the acquisition of conditioned response (Holmes and Adey, 1960).

Other signs pointing to a role for the hippocampus in the control of attention came from electrical stimulation of the anterior part of the temporal lobe, including the hippocampus, which led to widespread and long-lasting desynchronization of the EEG in both anesthetized and awake cats (Kaada et al., 1949; Sloan and Jasper, 1950). Such responses were taken as evidence of a general activation of attention. Stimulation of the hippocampus in awake cats produced a peculiar reaction with pupillary dilatation and slow turning of the head and neck to the contralateral side, as if the animal experienced a weird sensory stimulus in the contralateral visual field (Kaada et al., 1953). The reaction was associated with enhanced respiration and blood pressure. Similar reactions were elicited from the anterior cingulate gyrus, later to be associated with higher analysis of emotional signals. Modern imaging methods have revealed that this latter area is deeply engaged in the analysis of emotional aspects of sensory stimuli, suggesting that it is a device for estimating potential conflicts between old and new experiences (Bush et al., 2000; Botvinick et al., 2001; Bishop et al., 2004; Kerns et al., 2004).

In summary, this evidence suggests that together with the anterior cingulate cortex some portion of the hippocampus takes part in a certain form of general attention control.

2.3.4 The Hippocampal Formation and Memory

An early effort to analyze memory functions was that by Théodule-Armand Ribot, a French philosopher and psychologist. He proposed that memory loss was a symptom of progressive brain disease. His *Les Maladies de la Mémoire* [*Diseases of Memory*] (1881) constitutes an influential early attempt to analyze abnormalities of memory in physiological terms. He even proposed that a plausible memory mechanism could be an alteration in the activity of engaged cells in the cortex. This seems to be the first hypothesis to suggest a direct role of nerve cells for memory functions. Strongly influenced by Paul Broca's reports on language localization (Broca, 1861a,b), Ribot's views on localization of function in general were further supported by the clinical evidence of John Hughlings Jackson (1865), which showed memory loss in selected lesions, and by the experimental evidence from David Ferrier (1876), who reported on lip and nostril movements upon stimulation of the hippocampal lobes in monkeys. Richard Semon, much influenced by Ribot but working in Berlin (1908), was responsible for coining the term "engram" to signify a memory "trace" in the form of a physical change in the participating nerve cells.

Remembering that the hippocampal efferent impulses influence many hypothalamic nuclei, including the mammillary bodies, the first link between memory functions and part of the hippocampal system was made by three scientists during the 1880s who sequentially and semi-independently described an affliction causing amnesia. This condition was commonly associated with heavy drinking of alcohol and was later to be named Wernicke-Korsakoff psychosis. Subsequently, this disorder was associated with thiamine deficiency, which is often a correlate of dietary lack in the presence of alcoholism. In 1881, Carl Wernicke first described three patients whose illnesses were characterized by paralysis of eye movements, ataxia, and mental confusion. All three patients, two men with alcoholism and a woman with persistent vomiting following sulfuric acid ingestion, developed coma and died. In all three patients at autopsy, Wernicke detected punctate hemorrhages affecting the gray matter around the third and fourth ventricles and near the aqueduct of Sylvius. He believed them to be inflammatory and therefore named the disease polioencephalitis hemorrhagica superioris (Fig. 2–5).

Independently, Sergei S. Korsakov (1889, 1890), a Russian psychiatrist, described a similar clinical picture he called psychosis polyneuritica and emphasized that the main symptoms were memory deficits. Finally, Johann Bernhard Aloys von Gudden (1896) associated the condition with pathology of the mammillary bodies and the mediodorsal nucleus of the thalamus, both important target stations for hippocampal efferent pathways (see Chapter 3). After the first description of the Wernicke-Korsakov syndrome, a similar condition with an emphasis on memory impairment was described by another Russian neurologist, Vladimir Bekhterev (1900). He reported two patients with a prominent memory deficit who were later found at autopsy to have softening of the hippocampus and neighboring cortical areas on both sides. This study appears to be the first hint of a hippocampal localization for memory.

2.3.5 More Direct Evidence for Hippocampal Involvement in Memory

The idea that the hippocampal formation is intimately associated with memory is due to observations made on brain-damaged patients by William Scoville and Brenda Milner in 1957. Scoville removed the mesial aspects of the temporal lobes from several patients in an attempt to relieve a variety of neurological and psychiatric conditions. The most famous of these, H.M., was a severely epileptic patient whose seizures were resistant to antiepileptic drug treatment. Following surgery, his seizures were reduced, but he was left with a profound global amnesia that has persisted to this day. H.M.'s memory deficit is observable as an inability to remember material or episodes experienced after the operation (anterograde amnesia); it also includes an inability to recall information experienced for some period of time prior to the operation (retrograde amnesia). H.M. can remember items for brief periods, provided he is allowed to rehearse and is not distracted. Upon distraction, however, H.M. rapidly forgets. Thus, he never remembers for any length of time the doctors who test him, his way around the hospital, or the story he has been reading. He reports his conscious existence as that of "constantly waking from a dream" and everything looking unfamiliar (see Chapter 12). The temporal characteristics of H.M.'s retrograde amnesia continue to be controversial. Originally it was thought by Milner to extend up to 2 years prior to the operation, with memories for events earlier than that remaining relatively intact. This duration of retrograde amnesia was later extended to 11 years (Sagar et al., 1985), with the recollection of more distant events preserved. The interpretation of the extent of retrograde amnesia is complicated by the fact that this length of time was approximately equivalent to the period of the preoperative epileptic condition. We shall return to a more detailed discussion of the subsequent work on H.M. and other amnesic patients in Chapter 12. Suffice it to say here that his memory disabilities are due to the removal of a large part of the hippocampal formation and surrounding cortical regions (Fig. 2–7).

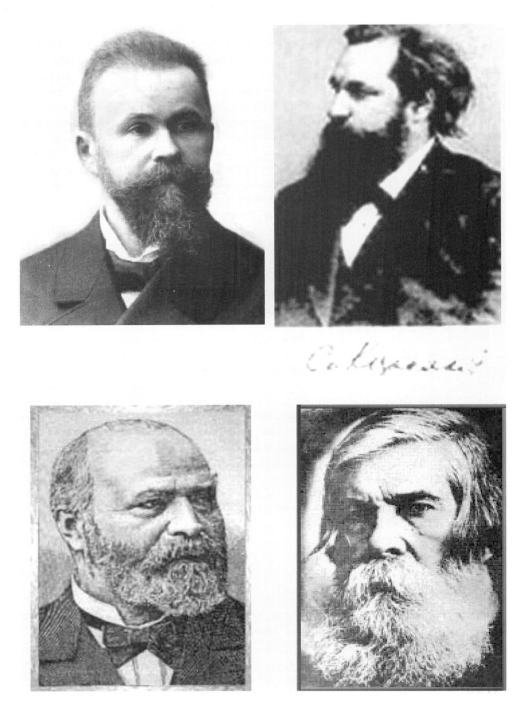

Figure 2–5. Cerebral localization and memory pioneers. Upper left: Carl Wernicke. Upper right: Sergei Korsakoff. Lower left: Bernard v. Gudden. Lower right: Vladimir Bekhterev. (*Source*: Courtesy of www.alzheimermed.com.br/)

The global amnesia reported in H.M. spurred efforts to find an animal model of amnesia. Early studies by Jack Orbach, Brenda Milner, and Theodore Rasmussen (1960) and by R.E. Correll and William Scoville (1967) looked at the effects, in primates, of various temporal lobe lesions on memory tasks such as delayed alternation and delayed response. Deficits were seen with combined lesions of the amygdala and hippocampal formation in the delayed alternation task (where animals are required to alternate their response from one trial to the next) but not the delayed response task (where animals choose a well learned response after a delay period). Even lengthening the delay failed to reveal a deficit in the delayed response task. Thus, these early attempts in the primate were viewed as falling short of developing an animal model of medial temporal lobe amnesia.

Work on rats also failed to find a convincing memory deficit following hippocampal damage. Lesioned rats had no difficulties learning simple sensory discriminations: to press

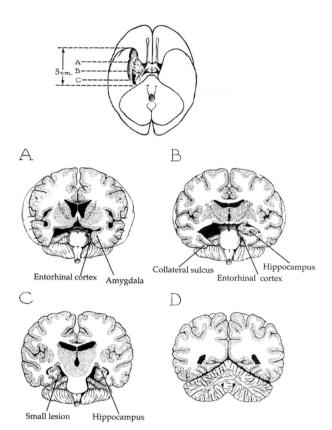

Figure 2–6. Drawings of the brain of patient H.M., made on the basis of an MRI examination performed 40 years after bilateral resection of the medial temporal lobe. Drawings are of transverse MRI sections from various anterior-posterior levels: A through the amygdala; D at the posterior tail of the hippocampus. (*Source*: Corkin et al., 1997.) The lesion was bilateral, but its right side is here left intact to show structures that were resected.

levers in a Skinner box or to run down alleys to obtain food or avoid punishment. What emerged, however, was a loose constellation of deficits, including changes in exploration and habituation to novelty. For example, hippocampus-lesioned rats placed in novel environments were hyperactive (i.e., they moved around more than control rats and failed to reduce their activity progressively over time). They also failed to alternate choices on two successive runs in a simple T-maze when no rewards were available (spontaneous alternation). Both changes in behavior were attributed to deficits in inhibitory processes; and consequently a role for the hippocampus in response inhibition or Pavlovian inhibition was postulated by Robert Isaacson and his colleagues Robert Douglas and Daniel Kimble (e.g., Kimble, 1963, 1968; Douglas and Isaacson 1964; Isaacson and Kimble, 1972). Another change was a striking deficit in the ability to withhold a prepotent behavioral response, a finding taken as support for the response inhibition hypothesis. Hippocampectomized rats learned to run down an alley or press a lever for food as quickly as normals but were deficient in changing this behavior when the circumstances altered (e.g., when food was withdrawn or when an alternate response was rewarded). Interestingly, they were consistently better at learning one particular type of avoidance task: two-way active avoidance. In this task, the animal must learn to run back and forth between two compartments of a shuttle box to escape punishment. This improved learning seemed particularly anomalous in light of the presumed role of the hippocampus in memory. A third deficit lay in complex maze learning. Whereas they had no trouble learning to make a turn in a simple T- or Y-maze, they failed miserably at more complex multichoice configurations (Kaada et al., 1961; Kimble, 1963; Kveim et al., 1964).

Figure 2–7. Brenda Milner (*left*) pioneered the analysis of the role of the medial temporal lobes in memory. Donald Hebb (*right*) influenced a generation of neuroscientists with his theories on memory mechanisms. (*Source*: Courtesy Brenda Milner and www.williamcalvin.com/.)

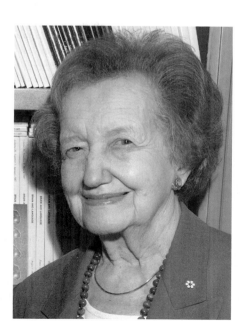
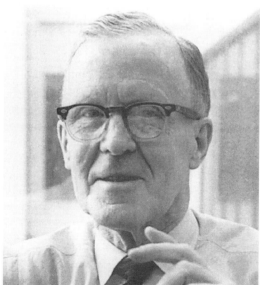

This confused state of affairs remained until around 1970 when several developments took place that together changed the approach to the hippocampal theory. The changes, which have continued to be influential, involved alterations in concepts about memory, the development of new tests for assessing memory, and the application of single-cell recording techniques to behaving animals.

Around this time, it was realized that there might be more than one type of memory, only one of which involved the hippocampus (Gaffan, 1974a; Hirsh, 1974; Nadel and O'Keefe, 1974; Olton et al., 1978). Two related ways of classifying human memory proved particularly influential. The first was Endel Tulving's contrast between memories for episodes set in a spatiotemporal context as distinguished from those for semantic items such as facts and other context-independent material (Tulving, 1972). The second was the related but different distinction between declarative and procedural memories, which was originally introduced by Terry Winograd (1975) in the field of artificial intelligence, subsequently applied to studies of amnesia by Cohen and Squire (1980), and extensively promulgated by Larry Squire and his colleagues (Squire, 1988, 2004). The former include both episodic and semantic memory, and the latter refers to skills and other stimulus-response habits. Both memory schemes have influenced research on amnesic patients and animal models of amnesia (see Chapters 12 and 13).

The second important development around 1970 flowed from the realization that the behavioral tests for animal memory available at that time were not optimal for testing hippocampal function. David Gaffan (1974b) introduced unique object recognition tasks. Mortimer Mishkin and Jean Delacour (1975) developed a version of this task that has become the standard test for recognition memory in the monkey (see Chapter 13). Following the introduction of these more powerful testing paradigms, efforts to establish memory systems became increasingly more fruitful.

2.3.6 The Hippocampus as a Cognitive Map

An important development in the analysis of hippocampal function was the use of implanted microelectrodes to monitor single-neuron activity in the hippocampus of the awake intact animal (Hirano et al., 1970; Vinogradova et al., 1970; O'Keefe and Dostrovsky, 1971; Ranck, 1973). These experimenters described the relations between cellular activity and a variety of sensory and behavioral parameters (Fig. 2–8). One correlate—that of the animal's location in the environment—gave rise to the cognitive map theory, which has fostered research into the spatial functions of the hippocampus (O'Keefe and Dostrovsky, 1971, see Chapters 11 and 13). This theory suggested that the hippocampus in animals was dedicated to spatial memory and allowed the animal to navigate in familiar environments. Extension of this theory to humans envisaged the addition of a temporal signal, allowing the hippocampus to act as a spatiotemporal context-dependent (episodic) memory. Lynn Nadel, John O'Keefe, and Abe Black (1975) proceeded to look carefully at the problems that rats with hippocampal

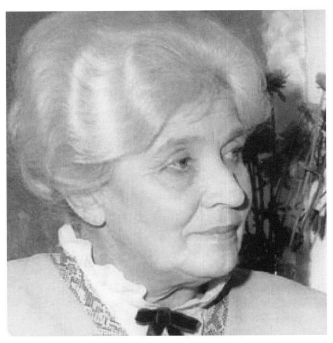

Figure 2–8. Olga Vinogradova was among the first who recorded single units from the hippocampus of awake animals (rabbits) while testing their behavioral responses to natural stimuli. She interpreted her recordings to mean that the hippocampus served as a novelty detector. (*Source*: Courtesy of Richard Morris.)

lesions had with avoidance learning. They concluded that deficits were found only when the animals had to learn to avoid places, not when they were given a clear prominent object or cue to avoid. Selective tests for the spatial functions of the hippocampus, including the Olton radial arm maze and the Morris watermaze, were subsequently developed (see Chapter 13).

2.3.7 Conclusions

We have provided a brief overview of some of the historical perspectives concerning the function of the hippocampal formation. Although there is widespread acceptance of the view that the hippocampal formation is involved in some aspects of memory, there may still be some surprises as to other potential functions of the hippocampal formation. As an important example, the hippocampus has been implicated in the modulation of stress responses through inhibitory projections to the hypothalamus. As described in Chapter 15, this putative role of the hippocampus has been implicated in a variety of normal and abnormal stress responses such as post-traumatic stress disorder.

2.4 Special Features of Hippocampal Anatomy and Neurobiology

We now turn to an overview of some of the early research on the hippocampal formation and the important historical figures associated with it. The outcome of some of this research led to general principles of neuroscience (e.g., the neuron doctrine), whereas others have established the existence of unique features of the hippocampal system (e.g., the largely unidirectional nature of the intrinsic excitatory connections). In some cases, the motivation for studying the hippocampal formation was not so much to understand its function but to capitalize on some unique aspect of its anatomical and physiological organization to carry out an experiment of more general interest more easily.

A number of features have attracted scientists to the hippocampus for studies of general neuronal and systems properties. A short list of the useful anatomical and neurobiological features of the hippocampus includes the following.

- A single cell layer and strictly laminated inputs
- Predominantly unidirectional connections between a series of cortical regions
- Extrinsic and intrinsic fibers making numerous *en passage* contacts with target neuronal dendrites, running orthogonal to the main dendritic axis
- Synapses that are highly plastic
- Tissue that can be used in transplantation studies
- Neurons that can be successfully grown in culture
- Acute or cultured slices surviving for prolonged periods in vitro

The most striking difference between hippocampal and neocortical cortices is the aggregation of the principal cells in a single layer. Another major difference between the two cortical types is the direction of the afferent fibers. In contrast to the input to neocortical areas where most afferent fibers are radially oriented, the extrinsic and intrinsic afferent nerve fibers of the hippocampal formation run in a horizontal direction (parallel to the pial surface) and orthogonal to the apical dendritic axis.

Hippocampal studies were important during the nineteenth century controversy between the *neuron doctrine* and the *reticular theory*. The neuron doctrine proposed that each neuron was an individual cell that contacted but did not merge with other target neurons. The reticular theory, on the other hand, posited that nerve cells form a syncytium where one cell emits a protrusion, or fibril, that continues into other cells, thus creating an interconnected network of fibers from a large number of neurons. This controversy continued for some time because microscopes at the time were not able to resolve the neuronal membranes and the spaces (e.g., the synaptic clefts) that separated individual neurons.

Camillo Golgi, who strongly supported the reticular theory, used observations of the hippocampal formation to bolster his arguments. Employing the *reazione nera* (black reaction), as he called the staining technique, later to be called the Golgi method, he repeatedly pointed to the convergence of fine axonal branches from a large number of dentate granule cells to form a dense bundle in the hilus of the dentate gyrus (vertical bundle in Fig. 2–2). Here, he believed filaments from various axons made a large intertwined feltwork, thus sup-

porting the reticular theory. He also pictured the dendrites of granule cells as being continuous with blood vessels that occupied the hippocampal fissure. Camillo Golgi's most outspoken adversary in the conflict over the neuron doctrine versus the reticular theory was Ramon y Cajal, whose support of the neuron doctrine came, ironically, from preparations made with Golgi's method. Although he also had many examples from the hippocampal formation, particularly in newborn rodents, his favorite preparation was the cerebellum. After examining thousands of preparations, he became convinced that individual neurons did not form a syncytial network. One particularly important piece of evidence was that he observed individual neurons that were in the process of dying. Neurons adjacent to these cells were entirely healthy. This was convincing evidence to Ramon y Cajal that neurons were individuals, not just members of interdependent groups. The debate lasted a number of years with a large number of participants, and was notable for the vigorous exchanges between the two factions.

The final resolution of this classic debate did not occur until the advent of electron microscopy, which conclusively supported the neuron doctrine by showing the neurons as individual entities with no connecting intercellular fibrils (Shepherd, 1972).

2.4.1 Early Neuroanatomical Studies of the Hippocampus

Hippocampal neuroanatomy benefited from the pioneering investigations of Camillo Golgi (1886), Luigi Sala (1891), and Karl Schaffer (1892). Santiago Ramon y Cajal (1893) described the stratification of the various afferent systems and drew a distinction between cells with long and short axons (Fig. 2–9). This observation made it clear that a hippocampal neuron could influence a large number of target cells and areas. Even before the formal definition of synapses by Charles Sherrington in 1897, Ramon y Cajal saw the functional implication of lamination. He suggested that there was a convergence of afferent input onto a single neuron, a notion that we take for granted today. His monumental effort, including an analysis of all portions of the hippocampal formation in a number of animal species, allowed him to propose a functional circuit diagram of this region. Following his principle of dynamic polarization—input to the dendrites, output through the axon—he placed arrows indicating his view of the direction of impulse flow through the hippocampal formation; many of these circuit characteristics have stood the test of time. He emphasized the size and variability of the various dendritic trees and gave a detailed description of dendritic spines and their distribution (structures that were dismissed by Golgi as artifacts of his staining method).

Simultaneous with Ramon y Cajal's first studies, the Hungarian anatomist Karl Schaffer, who gave his name (Schaffer collaterals) to the axons from CA3 cells that terminate in CA1 (1892), found by meticulous charting of well impregnated Golgi material not only that axons had short

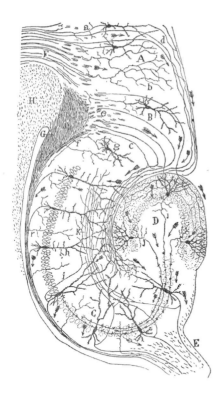

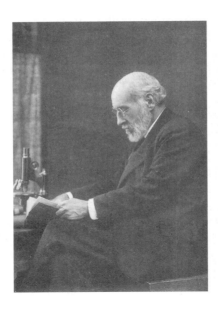

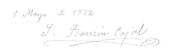

Figure 2–9. Santiago Ramon y Cajal and his famous drawing of the hippocampus in his 1911 book *Histologie de Système Nerveux.* in two volumes. The arrows give his interpretation of likely impulse direction. Later functional studies have vindicated his ideas on nearly all points. Portrait from Royal Society, London, gratefully acknowledged. Permission to reproduce drawing from Cajal (1911) from Istituto Cajal is gratefully acknowledged.

branches but that some axons could be very long, connecting neurons in neighboring cortical fields. Nearly 40 years later Rafael Lorente de Nó (1934), building upon the work of his compatriot Ramon y Cajal, greatly extended the analysis of the many hippocampal cell types and their axonal and dendritic patterns. He described many detailed networks of interconnected neurons (Fig. 2–10). On the basis of their dendritic tree and connections, he divided the hippocampal formation into a set of clearly defined divisions and coined the well known terms CA1 to CA4.

The pioneering neuroanatomists came impressively close to modern-day thinking in their proposed schemata for functional connectivity in the hippocampus. More often than not, the diagrams of Ramon y Cajal (1893, 1911) indicated the correct direction of information flow. Likewise, the detailed drawings of various neurons by Lorente de Nó (1934)—in which he used the number of dendritic spines to estimate the relative efficiency of afferents terminating at various positions on the dendrites—allowed him to formulate a general rule about summation. Even so, to understand the operational rules of the hippocampus, specific details beyond the major sources and trajectories of the main afferent and efferent pathways were needed.

2.4.2 New Fiber Tracing Methods

In parallel with the classic neuroanatomical studies with the Golgi method just described, much work was carried out to trace major afferent and efferent fiber systems in the central nervous system. The early studies exploited the fact that degenerating fibers could be stained better than intact fibers. Temporal myelinization gradients were also useful. Unfortunately, these methods initially met with limited success in the hippocampus. Although the hippocampus contains several fiber systems with moderately thick myelinated fibers, most of its axons are much thinner than in other parts of the central nervous system (Shepherd et al., 2002). These features are probably one reason why the first available methods for experimentally establishing pathways by degenerating fibers did not give satisfactory results. For example, even after appropriate lesions, Vittorio Marchi's original method (Marchi and Algeri, 1886) stains only a small number of degenerating fibers in the alveus and fimbria. In addition, the stained fibers are exclusively among the thicker of those present.

2.4.3 New Anatomical Techniques that Revolutionized Connectivity Studies

The situation improved greatly when certain variants of silver impregnation were applied to lesioned hippocampal pathways. Admittedly, the first silver degeneration method developed by Paul Glees (1946), was disappointing in the hippocampus despite the success it had in pathways of the brain stem. However, Nauta's 1950 method, soon followed by the Nauta and Gygax variant (1954) and Fink and Heimer's method (1967), were all remarkably effective.

Although similar in principle to other methods, Walle Nauta's methods turned out to be highly useful in hippocampal tissue. By employing the first variant of Nauta's tech-

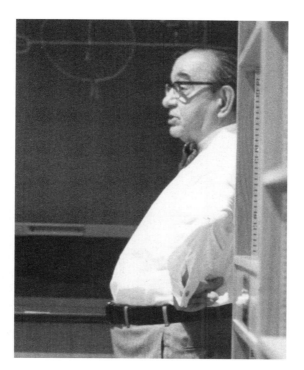

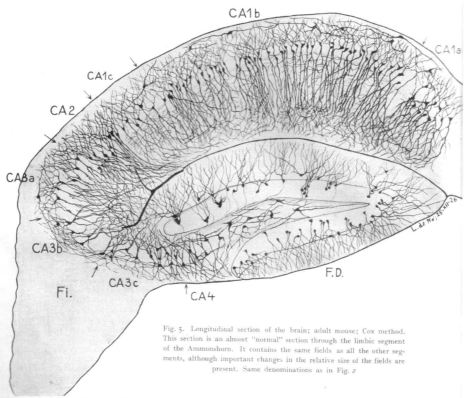

Fig. 5. Longitudinal section of the brain; adult mouse; Cox method. This section is an almost "normal" section through the limbic segment of the Ammonshorn. It contains the same fields as all the other segments, although important changes in the relative size of the fields are present. Same denominations as in Fig. 2

Figure 2–10. Top: a rare picture of the pioneer Lorente de Nó, who had every reason to be proud of his 1934 drawings shown below, signed along the margin. The diagram shows the cell types and divisions and the terminology in general use today: fascia or gyrus dentata, CA1 to 4, subiculum, pre- and parasubiculum and the entorhinal area. Acknowledgment to Larry Swanson for the portrait. Permission from Georg Thieme Verlag, Stuttgart to reproduce de Nó's drawing gratefully acknowledged.

niques, Theodor Blackstad (1956, 1958) (Fig. 2–11) showed how commissural and ipsilateral afferents to several parts of the hippocampus terminated in laminae oriented parallel to the cell layers (Fig. 2–11). These data not only verified the general principles established by Ramon y Cajal on stratification of afferent fibers but in addition showed astonishing density of presynaptic boutons in the innervated zone.

2.4.4 Predominantly Unidirectional Connectivity Between Cortical Strips

A key aspect of hippocampal connectivity was to emerge from these analyses: unidirectionality. Because the Golgi technique stains a relatively small proportion of the total number of neurons, this picture needed to be complemented by methods giving more quantitative data. Systematic study of each region of the hippocampal formation with suitable silver degeneration techniques, later supplemented by electron microscopic and anterograde and retrograde tracing methods, led to the realization that each component of the hippocampal formation projects to its neighboring region but generally does not receive a return pathway from this target (Hjorth-Simonsen, 1973). This was in good accord with previous physiological studies in which activation of the perforant path led to sequential activation of CA3 followed by CA1. A cut of CA3-to-CA1 fibers removed activity caudal to the section in CA1 and subiculum. On the other hand, stimulation in CA1 did not give synaptic activation in the CA3 region. These findings

Figure 2–11. Theodor Blackstad, often called the father of modern hippocampal histology because of his ground-breaking studies of its external and internal connectivity, with charting of degenerating fibers through silver staining and electron microscopy. (*Source*: Courtesy of Jon Storm-Mathisen.)

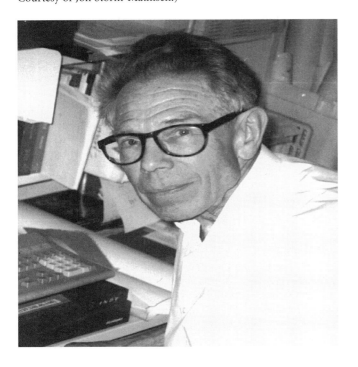

were the basis for the so-called trisynaptic circuit (Andersen et al., 1966). With this unidirectionality, the hippocampal system differs fundamentally from the reciprocal connectivity of nearly all neocortical areas. This principle of hippocampal neuroanatomy is discussed in detail in Chapter 3.

When a small fiber bundle of the Schaffer collaterals was stimulated, the amplitude of the synaptic potentials showed a characteristic distribution over the CA1 region. Signals were detected in the whole transverse extension of CA1. However, within the borders to CA3 and the subiculum, the largest potentials were detected along a strip oriented nearly transversely to the longitudinal axis of the hippocampus, with gradually reducing amplitudes on either side, the range spanning nearly half the length of the hippocampus. With stronger stimulation, the synaptic potentials generated a population spike (see Section 2.3), which had the same main orientation but with more restricted longitudinal distribution (Andersen et al., 1971b). This general arrangement was found for all four pathways studied—perforant path, mossy fibers, Schaffer collaterals, CA1 axons in the alveus—and the same orientation was found with orthodromic as with antidromic testing. This arrangement, which was named the lamellar organization, has received considerable opposition, mostly on anatomical grounds (see Chapter 3), probably because the name lamella invited vsualizing a set of thin slices with sharp borders, like a loaf of bread. Instead, the lamella should be seen as the main orientation of a set of overlapping fan-shaped fiber regions (Li et al., 1994), with most branches and their synaptic effect along the major orientation and gradually less influence on either side. The efficiency of the transverse slice is an illustration of this organization, although the spread of fiber orientation allows signals to be elicited in slices cut at a less than optimal angle.

2.4.5 New Tracing Studies Using Axonal Transport

In addition to the connectivity of single cells, it was necessary to determine how aggregations of neurons were connected so early researchers could gain insight into how larger systems could operate in concert. New anatomical techniques exploited intra-axonal transport. Maxwell Cowan (Fig. 2–12) and his colleagues introduced a new technique for fiber tracing based on the anterograde transport of injected radioactive amino acids (Cowan et al., 1972) (Fig. 2–12). Here, they exploited earlier information showing that radioactive proteins could be transported inside axons in both anterograde and retrograde directions (Grafstein, 1971; Lasek, 1975). Cowan had an impressive lineage: His doctoral (PhD) studies were carried out under the mentorship of Thomas Powell of Oxford University (Fig. 2–12). Powell, Cowan, and Geoffrey Raisman were responsible for many of the classic studies of hippocampal and fornix connections (Raisman et al., 1965, 1966). Max Cowan's laboratory, in turn, spawned a number of hippocampal researchers, including Larry Swanson, Brent Stanfield, and David Amaral, who among them conducted a

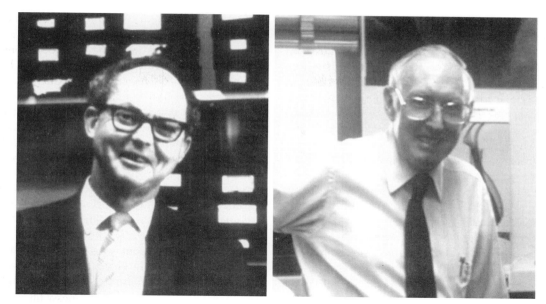

Figure 2–12. Thomas (Tom) Powell (*top left*) and W. Maxwell (Max) Cowan (*top right*), the former born in Britain and the latter in South Africa. They both had illustrious careers in neuroscience, starting their work by tracing fiber systems in the hippocampal formation. (*Source*: Courtesy of Geoffrey Raisman.)

substantial portion of the modern studies on hippocampal connectivity. The autoradiographic method had the merit of allowing extremely small and discrete injections to be placed, with the ³H-amino acids being taken up and transported by cells of origin, not fibers of passage. One important result of this study was that it became clear that direct hypothalamic projections of the hippocampal formation arose not from the hippocampus proper but from subicular regions (Swanson and Cowan, 1977). However, the hippocampal formation can influence a multitude of hypothalamic nuclei through multisynaptic pathways.

In addition to the autoradiographic method, new methods that depended on axonal transport of various proteins or plant lectins were developed (Kristensson and Olsson, 1971; Gerfen and Sawchenko, 1984).

Fibers containing monoamines were also found to innervate the hippocampus. The first reports described noradrenaline (norepinephrine)-containing axons from the locus coeruleus (Segal and Bloom, 1974a,b).

2.4.6 Electron Microscopy Offers New Opportunities

The first steps toward analysis of the number and types of synapses in the central nervous system also profited from work on the hippocampus. Following the pioneering work of Sanford Palay and George Palade in other brain regions (Palay and Palade, 1955), Lionel Hamlyn (1963) carried out the first electron microscopic analysis of the hippocampus. He provided the first comprehensive description of all synapses contacting the various portions of the dendritic tree in both CA3 and CA1 pyramidal cells. The introduction of electron

microscopy gave an unprecedented view of the details of individual cells and the contacts of neural circuits of the hippocampus and its main target nuclei (Raisman, 1969).

Moreover, the electron microscope also provided a new method for fiber tracing. When a fiber system was lesioned, the subsequent degeneration of both fibers and their associated boutons darkened within 1 to 2 days, a process that could be used for both synapse indentification and connectivity studies (Alksne et al., 1966).

2.4.7 Hippocampal Synapses Are Highly Plastic: Early Studies of Sprouting

The term *plasticity* is used to indicate several types of change. In addition to the well known activity-dependent alterations of synaptic efficiency (e.g., long-term potentiation, described in Chapter 10) there are numerous examples of anatomical changes in cell dimensions and number and in axonal length, branching and connections, and biochemical content in response to various stimuli or injury (see Chapter 9). The hippocampal formation was the first brain region in which axonal sprouting and reactive synaptogenesis were unequivocally demonstrated. Convincing experimental evidence of adult synaptic reorganization was described by Geoffrey Raisman (1969). He studied two sets of afferent fibers—one from the hypothalamus and the other from the hippocampus—that converged on cells of the septal nuclei. After long-term lesions of the fimbria, there was an increased number of multiple synapses (boutons in contact with several dendritic spines), interpreted as being the result of residual axons sprouting. Conversely, following removal of hypothalamic afferents, fimbrial fibers were found to contact somata of septal cells, which they rarely do normally. In another report, Raisman and Pauline Field (1973) exploited the fact that fimbria fibers innervate a segment of the lateral septal nucleus on both sides of the midline. A unilateral fimbrial lesion gave rise to remarkable sprouting from the contralateral fiber system such that the total number of fimbrioseptal synapses remained unchanged. Further work by the same group using transplantation of embryonic tissue for reinnervation of denervated hippocampal areas (Raisman and Field, 1990) sparked interest in the plasticity of hippocampal afferent and efferent fiber systems. However, the authors also warned that the reorganization was not necessarily adaptive or functionally important. A special case was the crossed entorhinal-dentate pathway, allowing a set of control experiments to determine factors of importance for reinnervation (Steward et al., 1974).

Nearly simultaneously, sprouting of hippocampal fiber systems was demonstrated with another approach by Gary Lynch and Carl Cotman and their associates (Lynch et al., 1972; Mosko et al., 1973; Matthews et al., 1976; Cotman et al., 1977; Goldwitz and Cotman, 1978). This group first showed that the acetylcholinesterase-containing septohippocampal fibers innervating the dentate gyrus increased in intensity and distribution if the perforant path fibers to the same region were removed. Electron microscopy confirmed that there was an early postlesion loss of synapses followed by a partial recovery. The remarkably efficient and fast regeneration is an impressive example of the plastic properties of hippocampal neurons. After lesions to the perforant path, for example, the maximal reduction of associated boutons in the molecular layer of the dentate gyrus was seen after about 5 days. However, after 2 weeks there was substantial recovery, and after 3 weeks the tissue had regained normal bouton density (Matthews et al., 1976).

2.4.8 Hippocampal Neurons: Transplantable with Retention of Many Basic Properties

Another remarkable example of neuronal plasticity is the ability of transplanted neuronal cells to emit axonal branches that grow and connect to existing neuronal target cells. The hippocampal formation was the testing ground for analysis of incorporation of embryonic transplants. After the work by Raisman's group, described above, Anders Björklund's group (Björklund et al., 1975, 1976) independently investigated the regenerative ability of transplanted monoaminergic tissue to reinnervate normal hippocampal tissue. They showed that transplanted tissue containing catecholamine- or acetylcholine-synthesizing neurons could extend axons and reinnervate the hippocampus in a normal fashion. When a graft of norepinephrine-containing neurons, whether from a peripheral source such as the sympathetic superior cervical gland or from a central location such as the locus coeruleus, was allowed to grow into a noradrenergic denervated hippocampus, grafted cells were observed to send out axons that entered the hippocampal formation but only if the cholinergic septo-hippocampal fibers were cut (Björklund and Stenevi,

1981, 1984). Lesions of the commissural or perforant path fibers did not induce such effects. The grafted sympathetic axons respected the lamination borders and formed typical norepinephrine-containing boutons with target neurons.

Similar results were obtained when cholinergically deafferented hippocampi received implants of acetycholine-containing cells placed in a cavity formed after the original septal region had been removed. Again, both peripherally and centrally located donor neurons were effective, and the reinnervation by transplanted cholinergic fibers displayed homotypic localization. Particularly impressive was the functional recovery of spatial learning ability and the partial restitution of hippocampal place cell activity (Shapiro et al., 1989), which paralleled the regrowth of cholinergic fibers (Dunnett et al., 1982).

Following these encouraging initial observations, transplantation research in the hippocampal formation flourished. Subsequent efforts were directed at determining if cerebellar neurons would survive when transplanted into the hippocampus and if hippocampal tissue might be electrophysiologically active when grafted into the cerebellum and vice versa. In the latter situations, the transplanted hippocampal tissue assumed its original cellular appearance and synaptic lamination, and the cells showed electrophysiological properties typical of hippocampal neurons (Hounsgaard and Yarom, 1985).

2.4.9 Hippocampal Cells Grow Well in Culture

The hippocampus has become a favorite source of neurons in several forms of tissue culture. Early successes at defining the parameters for successful survival and maturation of hippocampal neurons came from the work of Gary Banker in the laboratory of Max Cowan (Banker and Cowan, 1977; Banker and Goslin, 1991). In such cultures both neurons and glial cells are readily identifiable and may be manipulated or recorded as individual elements. A disadvantage, however, is that the original cytoarchitecture disappears, including such characteristic hippocampal features as the laminated input with synaptic segregation. This problem led to the development of the organotypic slice by Beat Gähwiler and colleagues (Gähwiler, 1981, 1988; Gähwiler and Brown, 1985). With this technique, thin slices of hippocampal tissue can be grown for several weeks with an impressive capacity for neuronal growth and differentiation (Zimmer and Gähwiler, 1984). With care, most neuronal phenomena seen in vivo or in acute slices can be demonstrated. In addition, the longevity of the preparation makes possible a number of experiments, including rehabilitation after injury and analysis of the long-lasting effects of growth factors.

2.4.10 Development of Hippocampal Slices: From Seahorse to Workhorse

A major technological advance for hippocampal research, and indeed for the field of neurobiology, was the development of the in vitro hippocampal slice preparation. The pioneer in this effort was the neurochemist Henry McIlwain. He set out to develop a reliable and functional in vitro preparation to investigate how various stimuli and compounds influenced the biochemistry of central nervous tissue (Li and McIlwain, 1957). He used a variety of preparations from the central nervous system. Despite considerable success, most of the horizontally cut neocortical slices did not allow a physiologically realistic afferent impulse pattern. More physiologically relevant data came when he employed slices from the piriform cortex. Here, stimulation of the lateral olfactory tract elicited synaptic and cell activity in neurons of the piriform cortex (Yamamoto and McIlwain, 1966a,b; Richards and McIlwain, 1967; McIlwain and Snyder, 1970). Tim Bliss and Chris Richards (1971) showed that field potentials similar to those found in the intact animal could be elicited in slices of the dentate gyrus cut along the septal-temporal axis of the hippocampus. With some technical modifications of the McIlwain procedure, Per Andersen, Knut Skrede, and Rolf Westgaard started to use transversally sectioned hippocampal slices from guinea pigs and demonstrated that intrinsic pathways could be successfully activated (Skrede and Westgaard, 1971). Single-cell activity could be recorded and showed short-term synaptic plasticity similar to that in intact, anesthetized preparations (Andersen et al., 1972). Rat and mouse hippocampal slices were useful as well, with the same type of signals as are seen in intact preparations. A distinct advantage was the great stability of the isolated slice preparation, which allowed long-lasting high-quality intracellular recordings to be made (Schwartzkroin, 1975). Important also was the precision with which electrodes could be placed and lesions created. The virtual lack of a blood-brain barrier is an experimenter's dream. A new opportunity arose when intracellular recording could be combined with iontophoretic delivery of transmitter candidates or blockers from multiple pipettes arranged to hit various parts of the dendritic tree (Schwartzkroin and Andersen, 1975). Fortunately, acute slices also supported well developed long-term potentiation (Schwartzkroin and Wester, 1975), a prerequisite for the wealth of analytical studies of this phenomenon (see Chapter 10).

2.5 Several Neurophysiological Principles Have Been Discovered in Hippocampal Studies

Although at first glance the hippocampal formation appears to be a special part of the brain with many features not seen elsewhere, it shares enough general features with other cortical regions to make it remarkably useful for studies of a general nature. Neurobiological principles that have been discovered from work on hippocampal preparations include:

- Identification of excitatory and inhibitory synapses and their localization, transmitters, and receptors
- Discovery of long-term potentiation and long-term depression

- Role of oscillations in neuronal networks
- Underlying mechanisms of epileptogenesis

2.5.1 Identification of Excitatory and Inhibitory Synapses

George Gray (1959) found that synapses in visual and frontal cortex could be divided into two distinct structural types, which he called type 1 and 2. Type 1 synapses were more heavily stained, and the synaptic specialization was asymmetrical in that the presynaptic density was less intensely stained than the postsynaptic density. Type 1 synapses were usually associated with dendritic spines. Type 2 synapses had pre- and postsynaptic densities with the same moderate staining intensity, and they were found mainly in association with dendritic shafts and neuronal somata. As to possible functional consequences of these differences, Gray (1959) concluded that, "At present there is no evidence to suggest that type 1 and type 2 synapses are functionally different" (p. 252).

When Gray's colleague Lionel Hamlyn (1963) studied the hippocampus, he found the same two synapse types and a similar distribution on dendritic spines and shafts. All synapses involving spines were of type 1, whereas synapses formed on the soma and thicker dendritic trunks or smooth branches were always type 2. A simultaneous report by Theodor Blackstad and Per Flood (1963) corroborated these data. It was comforting that the hippocampal cortex showed the same synaptic structures as those in neocortical areas. Conversely, this similarity made it possible that findings in hippocampal tissue also could be generalized to other cortical areas. What was needed for such a purpose was a correlation of functional and structural data from the same tissue. Such an opportunity arose with the advent of intracellular recordings from hippocampal neurons.

2.5.2 Gray Type 2 Synapses are Inhibitory and are Located on the Soma of Pyramidal and Granule Cells

In an influential intracellular study, Eric Kandel, W. Alden Spencer, and Floyd Brinley, Jr. (1961) reported on the ubiquitous and long-lasting inhibitory postsynaptic potentials (IPSPs) following both orthodromic and antidromic activation of cat CA2-CA3 pyramidal cells. Per Andersen, John Eccles, and Yngve Løyning (1964a) used a combination of intracellular recording of IPSPs and laminar analysis of the associated field potentials elicited by the same two activation modes. They showed that the initial phase of the IPSP in both CA1 and CA3 pyramidal cells and in dentate granule cells was associated with an extracellular positive field potential with a sharp maximum at the cell body layer, indicating a synaptic current leaving the somata of many principal neurons. This observation could be explained if the basket cell synapses, which terminate at the soma and initial axon, caused activated hyperpolarizing chloride conductances, and were in fact inhibitory interneurons. The basket cell synapses were exclusively Gray type 2 (Hamlyn, 1963). Andersen, Eccles, and Løyning (1964b) looked for cells that were not antidromically invaded from the alvear fibers and thus were not pyramidal cells. They discovered a subset of such neurons that discharged repetitively with a time course corresponding to the rise time of synaptically activated IPSPs found in pyramidal and dentate granule cells, respectively. The location of such cells corresponded to the basket cells described by Ramon y Cajal (1911) and Lorente de Nó (1934). Hippocampal IPSPs were found to be bicuculline-sensitive by David Curtis, John Felix, and Hugh McLennan (1970) and therefore were mediated by γ-aminobutyric acid ionotropic receptor type A (GABA$_A$) receptors.

Thus, the dentate and hippocampal basket cells were the first interneurons for which both the functional role and the identity of the effective synapses were revealed. Subsequently, findings from the hippocampal formation served as a template for similar searches in the cerebellum, thalamus, and other parts of the central nervous system.

However, the basket cell inhibition was far from exclusive. Later work in the cerebellum, hippocampus, and neocortex showed that many more types of inhibitory interneurons and synapses were present (Eccles et al., 1966).

2.5.3 Gray Type 1 Synapses are Excitatory and are Located on Dendritic Spines

Identification of the morphological and functional characteristics of excitatory synapses was also first carried out in the hippocampus. Kandel et al. (1961) saw examples of excitatory postsynaptic potentials (EPSPs) in cat CA3 and CA2 pyramidal cells in response to subiculum or fimbria stimulation, but they were surprised how relatively rare such responses were compared to the ubiquitous IPSPs. This relative rarity made them difficult to analyze in detail. In rabbits and rats, field potential recording allowed better identification of synaptically activated cells.

Identification of excitatory synapses and their localization were the result of a combination of extra- and intracellular responses to various excitatory afferent pathways and a new method for marking synapses. In the perforant path-to-dentate granule cells, the first association between a field EPSP (fEPSP) and an intracellular EPSP was made by Per Andersen, Birgitta Holmqvist, and Paul Voorhoeve (1966b), proving that the fEPSPs used were monosynaptic events and that the synapses in question were excitatory.

With a similar approach, several other excitatory synapses were identified including perforant path fibers activating dentate granule cells, mossy fibers activating CA3 cells, and commissural and local intrinsic fibers in the stratum oriens activating CA1 pyramidal cells. Using intracellular recordings of monosynaptic EPSPs in rabbits and cats, in response to stimulation of four independent afferent fiber systems to CA1 and the dentate granule cells, the activated synapses were identified as excitatory. In each system, synaptic activation

gave rise to a localized fEPSP carrying a population spike, proving the excitatory nature of the connection. Following specific surgical lesions to each of these monosynaptic excitatory pathways, the method of Alksne et al. (1966) showed that boutons belonging to all four pathways were electron-dense, closely associated with dendritic spines, and Gray type 1 (Andersen et al., 1966a). Thus, the widely accepted idea that cortical (and many other) excitatory synapses are Gray type 1 and are usually located on dendritic spines emerged from these studies of the hippocampal formation.

In conclusion, within a few years during the 1960s, both inhibitory and excitatory synapses of the hippocampus were identified with respect to location, anatomical type, and function. These findings turned out to be applicable to many, albeit not all, parts of the central nervous system.

2.5.4 Long-lasting Alterations of Synaptic Efficiency After Physiological Stimulation

Since the discovery of long term potentiation (LTP), hippocampal synapses have been the most studied exemplars of synaptic plasticity. These investigations are dealt with in detail in Chapter 10. Prior to the discovery of LTP, many other processes had been studied as potential models for learning. In particular, post-tetanic potentiation (PTP) was a common candidate for a number of years. Originally described by Martin Larrabee and Detlev Bronk in the sympathetic ganglia (1939), PTP appeared as enhanced synaptic responses following a period of high frequency tetanization of afferent fibers. The main weakness of PTP as an adequate mechanism for behavioral learning was its limited duration; in the spinal cord, PTP lasted only up to 7 minutes (Lloyd, 1949). The duration was increased to 30 minutes by Alden Spencer (Spencer et al., 1966) using long-lasting tetanization of polysynaptic spinal reflexes.

Limited duration was also an obstacle in the usefulness of the early studies of synaptic plasticity in the hippocampus. Several investigators had noted the remarkable growth of synaptic potentials during a period of high frequency stimulation (Cragg and Hamlyn, 1955; Kandel and Spencer, 1961b; Gloor et al., 1964). The critical question was: Would the enhanced excitability last for a significant period following cessation of the tetanic stimulation? Andersen (1960) noted that a period of enhanced synaptic response of commissural responses of CA3 and CA1 cells did indeed follow a short period of 10- to 20-Hz stimulation, but the duration was only up to 8 minutes and was initially regarded as an example of a special form of PTP. It soon became clear, however, that longer-lasting enhancement could be achieved when higher stimulation frequencies and, above all, repeated tetani were applied, as was first reported by Lømo (1966). This important discovery led the way to a description of truly long-term synaptic plasticity (hours and weeks), which is the basis for studies of LTP to this day (Bliss and Lomo, 1970, 1973). For a full description of the processes and mechanisms underlying LTP, see Chapter 10.

2.5.5 Hippocampal Systems: Exhibiting Several Types of Oscillatory Behavior

A few years after Hans Berger (1929) described the human EEG, Alois Kornmüller in Berlin began a search for possible electrical equivalents to the cytoarchitectonic parcellation of the cerebral cortex pioneered by Korbinian Brodmann (1909), as mentioned in Section 2.1.3.

Working with rats, Case Vanderwolf (1969) discovered that theta activity occurred each time the animal initiated a "voluntary" movement, in contrast to movements initiated more automatically or in a reflex-like manner. He also identified two types of theta activity—atropine-sensitive and atropine-insensitive—the former related to attention and the latter to movements (Kramis et al., 1975). Atropine is an alkaloid that blocks muscarinic cholinergic receptors. In elegant analytical studies, Abe Black obtained evidence that the higher-frequency hippocampal theta activity was related to motor activity rather than to learning as such (Dalton and Black, 1968; Black, 1972; Black and Young, 1972) (see also Chapter 11).

Theta activity is also of interest as a means of identifying hippocampal interneurons and their relation to behavior (see Chapters 8 and 11). In addition, other types of oscillation at different frequencies, including beta and gamma

2.5.6 Studies of Epileptiform Behavior

Richard Jung (1949) reported that electrical polarization (by long-lasting direct current) of the hippocampal formation readily gave rise to electrical after-discharges similar to those seen during epileptic seizures. By measuring the stimulus currents necessary to elicit such seizures in various tissues, he concluded that compared to other cortical areas the hippocampal formation needed considerably less current to elicit epileptiform seizures. This observation was in good accord with clinical experience gained from the EEG techniques introduced during the mid-1930s, suggesting that many epileptic conditions originated in medial temporal structures (Fig. 2-13).

Further progression of an electrographic seizure is often characterized by a set of depolarizing burst responses in which the extracellular responses are typically seen as a large local negative wave carrying a number of high frequency spikes of decreasing amplitude on its back, the so-called burst response (Ajmone-Marsan, 1961) at the onset of epileptiform discharges (von Euler et al., 1958; Kandel and Spencer, 1961b; Gloor et al., 1964). After a period with spontaneous high amplitude burst responses, the electrographic records diminish and all cells cease firing because of a depolarization block. Both in vivo and in vitro hippocampal preparations have been

Figure 2–13. Endre Grastyan (*left*), a Hungarian neuroscientist, was among the first to investigate the role of the hippocampus in conditioned learning. (*Source:* Courtesy of Gyorgyi Buzsaki.) Richard Jung (*right*) had a number of discoveries to his credit. He discovered and named theta waves, measured the low hippocampal threshold for epileptic seizures, and gave the first descriptions of visual cortical neuronal responses to contours, contrasts, and colors. (*Source:* Courtesy of Volker Dietz.)

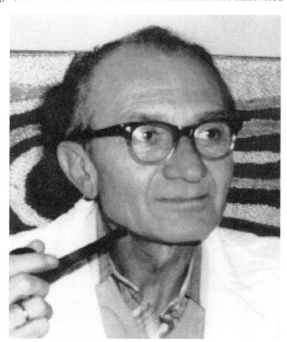
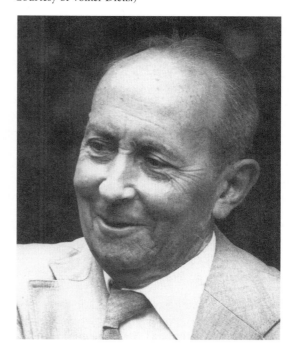

favorite tools in the search for cellular and network properties underlying the generation and spread of epileptiform activity (see Chapter 16). Among these preparations are the epileptiform activity provoked by kainic acid injections in CA3, GABA blockade by benzyl penicillin, and the effect of ouabain intoxication. An important model for epileptiform activity is the kindling phenomenon, described by Graham Goddard, D.C. McIntyre, and C.K. Leech (1969), who elicited seizures by repeated low-strength stimulation of the amygdala. Despite the ease with which electrographic seizures may be recorded from the hippocampus or the entorhinal area, these areas do not usually develop the kindling phenomenon. The role of the hippocampal formation in experimental and clinical epilepsy is discussed in Chapter 16.

2.6 Development of Methodological Procedures for General Use

The hippocampal cortex has served as a test bench for the development of a variety of general neuroscientific methodologies. In many instances this has led to the realization that the apparently special features of hippocampal tissue is also found in other central nervous structures. For example, the physiological properties of CA1 hippocampal pyramidal cells have much in common with those of neocortical pyramidal cells.

Below are listed some areas where hippocampal neurobiology has been instructive for neuroscience in general.

- First use of microelectrodes for extracellular neuronal studies
- Development of tetrodes for unit recording from behaving animals
- Interpretation of field synaptic potentials and population spikes as tools for analysis of extracellular signals
- Pioneering use of intracellular recording for central nervous system neurons
- Isolated slices of cortical tissue for neuroscience studies
- Development of histochemical methods for localization of neurotransmitters and receptor types
- Transplantation studies
- Pharmacological studies of central neurons and synapses
- Molecular biological analysis of synaptic function
- Formulation of computational models to explain ways in which neural networks can implement learning and memory

2.6.1 Hippocampus as a Test Bed for Microelectrode Work

Many of the standard methods used in neurobiology were developed in the peripheral or autonomous nervous systems or in muscular tissue. Recording from single nerve fibers was pioneered by Edgar Adrian and Yngve Zotterman working on the chorda tympani and lingual nerves (1926). Microelectrodes were developed during studies in cardiac and skeletal muscle by Ralph Gerard's group in Chicago (Ling and Gerard, 1949). In the spinal cord, Chandler McC. Brooks and John Eccles (1947) used microelectrodes to detect what they called a focal potential, a field potential generated by monosynaptic activation of motoneurons by volleys in muscle afferent fibers.

The first use of microelectrodes in the brain for extracellular recording of single nerve cell discharges was in the hippocampus by Birdsie Renshaw, Alexander Forbes and, Robert Morison (Renshaw et al., 1940). The researchers had greater success detecting activity of single nerve cells in the hippocampus than in neocortex, possibly because the latter tissue was more depressed at the levels of pentobarbital anesthesia used. In the hippocampus, these researchers recorded spontaneous and evoked discharges of what they called "axon-like spikes." Their description stated: "what is evidently the discharge of the same unit - they recur repeatedly with the same waveform" (p. 90). When describing the individual elements with a constant amplitude and predominantly negative polarity, they used what later became the classic critera for identifying individual nerve cell discharges. Renshaw et al. localized such discharges to elements in the pyramidal layer and concluded that the "axon-like spikes" were discharges of individual pyramidal cells.

2.6.2 Pioneers of Intracellular Recording

The same experimental advantages that facilitated the analysis of extracellular unit recording potentials also paved the way for using the hippocampus for intracellular recording. The first to succeed in this technically demanding enterprise were Denise Albe-Fessard and Pierre Buser in 1952. They were surprised by the fact that nearly all penetrated cells showed a large, long depolarizing signal. Both its large amplitude and long duration made interpretation difficult. Initially, they took the response to be an EPSP. Later, it turned out to be an artifactual recording of a large IPSP, which due to an electrode-induced chloride infusion went in the depolarizing direction. They did not record EPSPs with their technique, however.

The first satisfactory intracellular recordings from cortical neurons were made by Charles Phillips in 1956. He recorded from Betz' cells in the precentral gyrus of cats and characterized their response to both antidromic and orthodromic activation. This too proved a technically difficult task, not least because of the difficulty of finding monosynaptic afferent fibers to stimulate. Fortunately, the situation turned out to be easier in hippocampal preparations. As described in Section 2.3, Kandel, Spencer, and Brinley (1961) carried out the first comprehensive intracellular study of hippocampal pyramidal cells. In addition to their analysis of EPSPs and IPSPs (see above), they reported on prepotentials, which were short depolarizing deflections at the very start of the full action potential, interpreted as a sign of dendritically generated action potentials. They also recorded major features associated with the transition from normal behavior to epileptiform behavior in the form of slow depolarization waves and the occurrence of giant depolarizations with superimposed burst discharges (burst responses) (Kandel and Spencer, 1961a,b). This was an essential step in epilepsy research.

In contrast to the wealth of inhibitory synaptic data, there was a surprising paucity of excitatory synaptic signals. This may be related to the barbiturate anesthesia with its facilitating effect on IPSPs, an effect also discovered in the hippocampus by Roger Nicoll and Eccles (Nicoll et al., 1975). As mentioned above in the discussion of IPSP and EPSP identification (see Section 2.3.1), intracellular recording from hippocampal neurons was essential for the identification and localization of inhibitory synapses to the soma and of excitatory synapses to dendritic spines.

2.6.3 Tetrode Development

Following the recording of single-cell activity in awake, behaving animals (O'Keefe and Dostrovsky, 1971; Ranck, 1973) it became clear that hippocampal cells signaled differently from, say, visual cortical cells. The latter could be classified as sensitive to contrast or color and with specific and repeatable patterns to a standardized stimulus delivered to a restricted part of the visual field—the cell's receptive field. In contrast, hippocampal cells showed a much lower rate of discharge, more variability from one trial to the next, and a receptive field related to the aberrant concept of space (see Chapter 11). Subsequently, it became clear that hippocampal neurons operated in ensembles and deciphering the full code might receive simultaneous recording from a number of neighboring cells. This led to the development of recording techniques with double electrodes, or stereotrodes (McNaughton et al., 1983), and finally quadruple electrodes, or tetrodes (O'Keefe and Recce, 1993; Wilson and McNaughton, 1993). Such electrode assemblies allow simultaneous recording of a large number of cells in the freely moving and behaving animal by taking into account the constant shape and form of the potential generated by discharges of each of the active cells as seen by each of the four electrodes. The tetrode technique has revolutionized the study of hippcampal neuronal activity and spatial behavior. For a further account of this field, see Chapter 11.

2.6.4 Field Potential Analysis

After the pioneering use of microelectrodes during the 1940s, several years passed before further progress was made in studies of the hippocampal region using cell discharge recordings. During the mid-1950s, however, several groups started to use field potentials to understand the pattern of activation or inhibition of hippocampal systems.

In an early study of field potentials, Lorente de Nó (1947) studied the signal sequence when a nerve volley traveled antidromically into the hypoglossus motor nucleus. He offered the first theoretical explanation for the generation of such field potentials.

In the hippocampal formation, the histological arrangement is highly favorable for field potential studies of both orthodromic and antidromic activation (see Box 2–1). The dense packing of the cell bodies, the roughly parallel position of the apical dendrites of hippocampal neurons, and the ease with which they can be synchronously activated are three main reasons for the striking appearance of hippocampal field potentials.

The main advantage of using field potentials is that an extracellular potential recording may give an accurate index of synaptic activity with regard to amplitude, time, and polarity. First, the parallel orientation of a large number of principal cells may generate a field potential of considerable magnitude. The fEPSP has maximum negativity in the region with the highest concentration of activated excitatory synapses. Neighboring activated synapses add their effect largely linearly, justifying the use of the fEPSP amplitude as a measure of synaptic strength. Conversely, synchronous and local activation of inhibitory fibers also gives rise to large currents, but in the opposite direction. The usefulness of the recording procedure coupled with its simplicity lies at the heart of the popularity of field potential studies.

Brian Cragg and Lionel Hamlyn (1955) were the first to record significant elements of the hippocampal field potentials. However, because they placed their stimulation electrode very close to the recording site, the axonal conduction distance was very short. Consequently, their records of the synaptic component of the field potentials were brief and difficult to isolate from the rest of the compound signal ("action potential" in their nomenclature). Nevertheless, they were able to report the first evidence of conduction along the apical dendrites and found that the minimal latency was associated with the dendritic position of the activating synapses. With a commissural input, the shape and conduction of these action potentials were similar to those found with close-range stimulation (Cragg and Hamlyn, 1957).

The large compound action potential that followed stimulation at close range, later called the "population spike," was first noted by Cragg and Hamlyn (1955, 1957). Although claims to dendritic conduction had been made on the basis of neocortical surface stimulation, the specialized hippocampal histological arrangement made interpretation of the records much more convincing. Today, a new and much more detailed view on dendritic conduction has emerged, largely owing to whole cell patch recordings from dendrites. Again, much of the evidence for dendritic properties has been obtained from hippocampal preparations (Spruston et al., 1995; Johnston et al., 1996; Stuart et al., 1997) (see details in Chapter 5).

Several other groups exploited the laminated synaptic arrangement to identify the field potentials associated with restricted dendritic synapses. To make the hippocampus a useful preparation for studying synaptic activation, it was necessary to ascribe a standard extracellular signal to a standardized input. Recording from various dendritic positions, Andersen (1960) described how commissural fibers to CA1

Box 2–1
Field potentials and current source density analysis

Field potentials are extracellular potentials recorded from groups of nerve cells in response to synaptic or antidromic stimulation. In laminated structures such as the hippocampus, field potentials provide surprisingly detailed information on cellular activity.

A field potential is generated by extracellular current flowing across the tissue resistance between the recording electrode and, in general, the ground electrode. Although measurable extracellular voltages are generated by action potentials in a single neuron, and form the basis of single unit recording, synaptic currents generated by single neurons are generally too small to be detected. In the hippocampus, and other highly laminated structures such as the olfactory cortex, the synchronous and localized currents generated by synaptic activation of a population of pyramidal or granule cells gives rise to a characteristic and easily measured response called a population or field EPSP (fEPSP); with weak stimulation, the synaptic response is below threshold for the generation of action potentials in the target cells, and a pure fEPSP is generated. With stronger stimulation, the cells discharge synchronously, giving rise to a population spike which is superimposed on the rising phase of the fEPSP. Unlike the all-or-none action potential generated by a single neuron, the population spike is a graded response; as stimulus intensity increases, the number of neurons discharged becomes greater, and the population spike becomes correspondingly larger.

In Box Fig. 2–1 stimulation of medial perforant path fibers activates synapses in the middle third of the molecular layer of the dentate gyrus (shaded gray). The field responses recorded at various positions along the soma and dendritic tree are shown on the left. Synaptically generated current flows into the dendrites in the activated region; inside the cells, current flows proximally and distally away from the synaptic region, exiting where membrane area is greatest, notably in the region of the soma. The current loop is completed extracellularly, with current flowing radially from distal and proximal sources towards the sink in the synaptically active region. With a distal ground electrode, these synchronous extracellular currents give rise to field EPSPs that are negative in the region of current sinks and positive in regions of strong current sources. Note that the current sink generated by synaptic activation is in the molecular layer, while the passive source is in the cell body region and in distal dendrites; the converse situation obtains for the population spike; here, the active sink is in the cell body region while the passive source is in the dendrites. The polarity of the fEPSP and the population spike are, as a result, spatially out of phase.

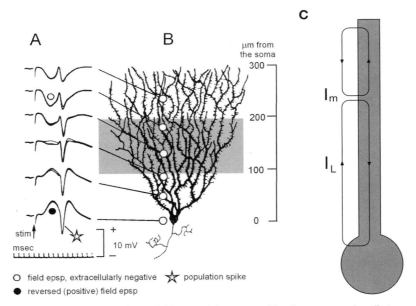

O field epsp, extracellularly negative ☆ population spike
● reversed (positive) field epsp

Box Fig. 2–1. Field potentials. A. Field potentials generated by dentate granule cells in response to stimulation of the medial perforant path. Activated synapses are located in the middle third of the dendritic tree (gray band in B). In this region the field potential (fEPSP) is negative, reversing to a positive polarity near the cell body layer. The population spike (star) is negative in the cell body layer, and positive in the dendritic region. (*Source*: Andersen et al., 1966a). C. The direction of intracellular, extracellular and transmembrane current flow generated by synaptic activation in an activated neuron.

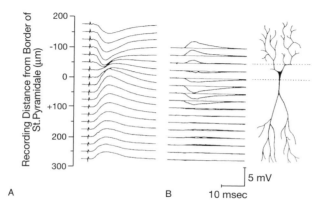

Box Fig. 2–2. Current source density analysis. A. Field potentials evoked by weak activation of fibers projecting to stratum oriens in area CA1, evoking a pure synaptic response without a superimposed population spike. B. CSD analysis reveals a sink (positive) in stratum oriens and a source (negative) in the cell body layer and proximal dendrites. Arbitrary units. (*Source*: Richardson et al., 1987).

A further refinement called current source density (CSD) analysis allows the precise regions of inward and outward current to be plotted. Box Fig 2–2A displays the fEPSPs recorded at different locations in area CA1 in vitro following weak synaptic activation. For a given latency, a depth profile can be generated, showing how the amplitude and polarity of the response changes with location.. By Ohm's law, the current flowing in the longitudinal direction, parallel to the dendrites, is proportional to the rate of change of voltage in that direction:

$$I_L = k.\partial V/\partial L$$

where I_L is the longitudinal current density at a given point L along the longitudinal axis of the cell, V is the potential at point L, and k is the conductivity of the extracellular space. Thus the first spatial derivative of the depth profile yields a plot of the longitudinal current as a function of location at the selected latency. Current flowing through the membrane at any point must be equal to the rate at which longitudinal current changes at that point, i.e.

$$I_M = -\partial I_L/\partial L = -k.\partial^2 V/\partial L^2$$

The second spatial derivative of the depth profile is thus proportional to the amplitude of the membrane current density, I_m. By repeating this analysis at a succession of latencies, the time course of current sinks and sources at each location can be calculated. A full CSD analysis, computed from the sequence of fEPSPs evoked at different locations along the dendritic tree by weak stimulation of Schaffer commissural fibers projecting to the basal dendrites of pyramidal cells in area CA1 is shown in Box Fig. 2–2B. The voltage responses are on the left, and the current source density analysis, revealing the development of sources and sinks over time, are plotted on the right.

Field EPSPs have the same time course as the synaptic current that generates them, and are therefore phase advanced with respect to intracellular EPSPs which are delayed by the time required for the membrane current to charge membrane capacitance (Box Fig 2–3). Further discussion of field potential theory can be found in Stevens (1966), Rall and Shepherd (1968), Nicholson and Freeman (1975) and Johnston and Wu (1994).

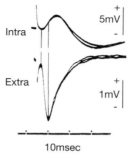

Box Fig. 2–3. The extracellular field EPSP reflects intracellular events, but is phase advanced with respect to the intracellular EPSP. Recordings were made from the dentate gyrus in vivo (*Source*: Lømo, 1971).

and CA3 gave a local negative field potential in exactly the same strata where Theodor Blackstad (1956) had found that the relevant fibers terminated. Such negative field potentials were taken as a sign of excitatory synaptic activity and was called a field excitatory postsynaptic potential (fEPSP). Above a given strength the fEPSP was interrupted by a compound action potential, called the population spike because it was interpreted as the synchronous discharge of a number of pyramidal cells. This interpretation was supported by the observation that most of the synaptically activated unitary cell discharges fell within the time envelope of the population spike (Andersen et al., 1971a).

Thus, the extracellular field potentials can be used as a sensitive, quantitative measure of the intensity of excitatory and inhibitory synaptic effects and the efficacy of postsynaptic activation. Final confirmation of the field potential interpretation given above came with intracellular recording of dentate granule cells (Andersen et al., 1966b; Lømo, 1971) and the use of isolated slices, where intracellularly recorded EPSPs were associated with excitatory field potentials in CA1 pyramidal cells (Schwarzkroin, 1975; Andersen et al., 1980).

2.6.5 Histochemistry: Pioneered in the Hippocampus

We have become used to the hippocampus as a favorite preparation for histological, electrophysiological, and behavioral studies. Less well known is its essential role in the development of neurochemical methodology and histochemistry. Once again, it was the packing of homogeneous cells into compact cell layers and the striking stratification of afferent fibers and synapses to specific parts of the dendritic tree of principal cells that appealed to the exploring scientist.

Until the middle of the twentieth century, virtually all neurochemical analyses were conducted on homogenized tissue of relatively large samples from various parts of the brain. This procedure was thought to be necessary because of the extreme complexity of central nervous tissue. In an attempt to perform analysis of more discrete CNS elements, Oliver Lowry exploited the synaptic lamination of the hippocampus to perform a detailed neurochemical dissection of cortical tissue. He noted the following:

> Ammon's horn is a region of the cerebral cortex which is organized in such a manner as to invite quantitative histochemical study.

Enzyme concentrations and lipid type and concentration were measured for individual strata of the hippocampal cortex. In a pioneering series of papers (Lowry et al. 1954a,b,c; 1964), Lowry and his colleagues made several fundamental advances. First, they introduced a number of methodological improvements. By dissecting freeze-dried tissue from thin slices of hippocampus under a microscope, they were able to reduce the sample size to 5 to 10 μg of tissue. Second, the accuracy of the enzymatic measurements greatly improved. The enzymes of interest spanned a large range from acid and alkaline phosphatases through adenosine triphosphatase,

cholinesterases, and aldolase to lactic, malic, and glutamic dehydrogenases. Lowry's group also determined the lipid content and type as related to cortical layers. Third, it was the first instance when a neurochemist explicitly exploited a special histological arrangement for localizing biochemical elements, initially in the hippocampus and then in the cerebellum. His group reported impressive homogeneity in a single stratum and often a considerable variation among various strata. In particular, he noted the much higher ATP concentration in the dendritic areas than in the cell body layer.

Using a microdissection method, Storm-Mathisen and Fonnum (1972) were able to attain quantitative data for GABA and glutamate concentrations in various hippocampal strata. The amount of GABA was particularly high in the pyramidal layer, in accord with the concentration of inhibitory boutons here. However, the high amount of GABA even in the stratum lacunosum-moleculare pointed to new challenges.

Peter Lewis and Charles Shute (1967) extended the chemical dissection by performing the histochemical analysis directly on sections from the hippocampus. They showed that the distribution of acetylcholinesterase was concentrated in certain lamina, an approach that heralded a new approach to chemical analysis of the CNS. This histochemical approach also provided the groundwork for many of the studies on synaptic sprouting that followed during the 1970s (see Chapter 9).

The later development of histochemical and immunohistochemical studies have largely concentrated on microscopic sections. For this approach, hippocampal tissue has also been a favorite choice. Among these developments, the electron microsopic identification of bouton contents with antibodies raised against an aggregate of amino acids and bovine globulin marked an entirely new, powerful approach (Storm-Mathisen et al., 1983). Thus, the hippocampus has played an important role in the development of histochemical techniques for both fresh and fixed tissue.

2.6.6 Pharmacological Analysis of Cellular Properties

The hippocampus has also been important for the development of ideas in the neuropharmacology of synaptic transmission in the CNS. Following the demonstration of glutamate sensitivity of spinal cord cells by David Curtis and Jeff Watkins (1960), Tim Biscoe and Donald Straughan (1966) found that hippocampal pyramidal cells were sensitive to iontophoretic application of glutamate. Together, these studies suggested the radical (at the time) possibility that glutamate was an excitatory neurotransmitter in the CNS. Support came from an ingenious study on hippocampal slices in which Nadler et al. (1976) measured Ca^{2+}-dependent release of aspartate and glutamate. Because the release of both compounds was grossly reduced after lesions of commissural or entorhinal fibers, the release is likely to have come from boutons of the two fiber systems, thus supporting the idea that aspartate or glutamate could be excitatory transmitters.

Postsynaptic inhibition produced by Purkinje cells in the lateral vestibular, and deep cerebellar nuclei was first shown to be mediated by GABA by Obaka and colleagues (1967). As mentioned above for hippocampal inhibition, David Curtis, John Felix, and Hugh McLellan (1970) showed that the large, ubiquitous IPSPs in all principal cells of the hippocampus could be blocked by localized application of bicuculline methochloride, establishing that these IPSPs were therefore mediated by $GABA_A$ receptors. Thus, the studies of Curtis and his colleagues extended the Obata et al. results to cortical inhibitory pathways.

2.6.7 Development of Computational Models of Neural Networks

In a remarkable set of three papers, David Marr (1969, 1970, 1971) developed a theoretical proposal for the mode of operation of three major components of the CNS. Arguably, the triad inaugurated modern computational neuroscience. Further description of this development is found in Chapter 14.

Marr started with the cerebellum, for which he proposed the main operation to be a comparison between an initial state of the motor system and the state after an elemental movement had taken place (Marr, 1969). The next article dealt with the neocortex and how the cortical matrix behaved during perception and attention (Marr, 1970). The third paper contained a description of the mode of operation of the archicortex (Marr, 1971), meaning the hippocampal formation. Basing his proposal on what was then known about its neural cytoarchitecture, he hypothesized that the hippocampus performed a simple memory function which allowed the animal to make use of previous experience to adapt its behavior. In the process, he described how elemental neurophysiological processes could perform certain basic mathematical procedures. For example, inhibition exerted at a dendritic level would cause relatively little enhancement of the resting membrane potential of the neuron, a procedure equivalent to subtraction. In contrast, inhibition at the soma level, produced by basket cells, would represent a much stronger change of the membrane potential, removing a substantial part of the synaptic drive, equivalent to mathematical division.

He also pointed to the recurrent axon collaterals of CA3 as a possible neural basis for attractor networks in which the excitatory interactions between networks of pyramidal cells could form the basis of content-addressable memories and support retrieval of a complete memory from partial information (see Section 5 in Chapter 14).

2.6.8 The Hippocampal Formation: A Test Bed for Several Types of Neural Dysfunction and Neuropathology

It is a well established clinical observation that epileptic patients exhibit a high frequency of temporal lobe foci, often coupled with the neuropathological finding of hippocampal sclerosis (Sommer, 1890; Gastaut, 1956). As a result, the hippocampus has been a focus of interest in epilepsy research (Schwartzkroin, 1997).

The hippocampal formation has proven to be particularly vulnerable to various traumatic insults. Spielmeyer (1925) noted that Sommer's sector, which corresponds to the CA1 field of the hippocampus, is a brain structure extremely vulnerable to ischemic or hypoxic insults. This may be related to a lower level of mitochondrial oxidative enzymes in CA1 pyramidal dendrites than in other hippocampal subregions (Davolio and Greenamyre, 1995; Kuroiwa et al., 1996). Early neuropathologists also noted that the hippocampal formation is a major target for pathological changes in patients suffering from senile dementia of the Alzheimer's type (Alzheimer, 1909). These issues continue to challenge modern neuroscience, as described in Chapter 16.

REFERENCES

Adrian ED, Zotterman Y (1926) The impulses produced by sensory nerve-endings. Part 2. The response of a single end-organ. *J Physiol (Lond)* 61:151–171.

Aggleton JP (1993) The contribution of the amygdala to normal and abnormal emotional states. *Trends Neurosci* 16:328–333.

Ajmone-Marsan C (1961) Electrographic aspects of "epileptic" neuronal aggregates. *Epilepsia* 2:22–38.

Albe-Fessard D, Buser P (1952) Étude de réponses neuroniques à l'aide de microélectrodes intrasomatiques. *Rev Neurol (Paris)* 87:455.

Alksne JF, Blackstad TW, Walberg F, White LE Jr (1966) Electron microscopy of axon degeneration: a valuable tool in experimental neuroanatomy. *Ergeb Anat Entwicklungsgesch* 39:3–32.

Allen WF (1940) Effect of ablating the frontal lobes, hippocampi and occipito-parieto-temporal (excepting pyriform areas) lobes on positive and negative olfactory conditioned reflexes. *Am J Physiol* 132:81–91.

Alzheimer A (1907) Über eine eigenartige Erkrankung der Hirnrinde. *Allg Z Psychiatr Psych Gerichtl Med (Berl)* 64: 146–148.

Amaral DG, Insausti R, Cowan WM (1987) The entorhinal cortex of the monkey. I. Cytoarchitectonic organization. *J Comp Neurol* 264:326–355.

Andersen P (1960) Interhippocampal impulses. II. Apical dendritic activation of CA1 neurons. *Acta Physiol Scand* 48:178–208.

Andersen P, Eccles JC, Løyning Y (1964a) Location of postsynaptic inhibitory synapses on hippocampal pyramids. *J Neurophysiol* 27:592–607.

Andersen P, Eccles JC, Løyning Y (1964b) Pathway of postsynaptic inhibition in the hippocampus. *J Neurophysiol* 27:608–619.

Andersen P, Blackstad TW, Lømo T (1966a) Location and identification of excitatory synapses on hippocampal pyramidal cells. *Exp Brain Res* 1:236–248.

Andersen P, Holmqvist B, Voorhoeve PE (1966b) Excitatory synapses on hippocampal apical dendrites activated by entorhinal stimulation. *Acta Physiol Scand* 66:461–472.

Andersen P, Bliss TVP, Skrede KK (1971a) Unit analysis of hippocampal population spikes. *Exp Brain Res* 13:208–221.

Andersen P, Bliss TVP, Skrede KK (1971b) Lamellar organization of hippocampal exitatory pathways. *Exp Brain Res* 13:222–238.

Andersen P, Bland BH, Skrede KK, Sveen O, Westgaard RH (1972)

Single unit discharges in brain slices maintained in vitro. *Acta Physiol Scand* 84:1A–2A.

Andersen P, Sundberg, SH, Sveen O, Wigström H (1977) Specific long-lasting potentiation of synaptic transmission in hippocampal slices. *Nature* 266:736–737.

Andersen P, Silfvenius H, Sundberg SH, Sveen O (1980) A comparison of distal and proximal dendritic synapses on CA1 pyramids in guinea-pig hippocampal slices in vitro. *J Physiol* 307:273–299.

Aranzi GC (1564) *De humano foetu opusculum.* Bologna: Rubrii.

Banker GA, Cowan WM (1977) Rat hippocampal neurons in dispersed cell culture. *Brain Res* 126:397–425.

Banker G, Goslin K (1991) Primary dissociated cell cultures of neural tissue. In: *Culturing nerve cells* (Banker G, Goslin K, eds), pp 1–71. Cambridge, MA:MIT Press.

Bard P (1934) On emotional expression after decortication with some remarks on certain theoretical views. Part 1. *Psychol Rev* 4:309–322; Part 2: 4:424–449.

Bekhterev V (1900) Demonstration eines Gehirns mit Zerstörung der vorderen und inneren Theile der Hirnrinde beider Schlafenlappen. *Neurol Zentralbl* 19:990–991.

Berger H (1929) Über das Elektroenkephalogramm des Menschen. *Arch Psychiatr Nervenkr* 87:527–570.

Biscoe T, Straughan D (1966) Micro-electrophoretic studies of neurones in the cat hippocampus. *J Physiol (Lond)* 183:341–359.

Bishop S, Duncan J, Brett M, Lawrence AD (2004) Prefrontal cortical function and anxiety: controlling attention to threat-related stimuli. *Nat Neurosci* 7:184–188.

Björklund A, Stenevi U (1981) In vivo evidence for a hippocampal adrenergic neuronotrophic factor specifically released on septal deafferentation. *Brain Res* 229:403–428.

Björklund A, Stenevi U (1984) Intracerebral neural implants: neurological replacement and reconstruction of damaged circuitries. *Annu Rev Neurosci* 7:279–308.

Bjorklund A, Johansson B, Stenevi U, Svendgaard NA (1975) Re-establishment of functional connections by regenerating central adrenergic and cholinergic axons. *Nature* 53:446–448.

Bjorklund A, Stenevi U, Svendgaard N (1976) Growth of transplanted monoaminergic neurones into the adult hippocampus along the perforant path. *Nature* 262:787–790.

Black AH (1972) The operant conditioning of central nervous system electrical activity. In: *The psychology of learning and motivation,* vol 6 (Bower G, ed), pp 47–95. San Diego: Academic Press.

Black AH, Young GA (1972) Electrical activity of the hippocampus and cortex in dogs operantly trained to move and to hold still. *J Comp Physiol Psychol* 79:128–141.

Blackstad TW (1956) Commissural connections of the hippocampal region in the rat, with special reference to their mode of termination. *J Comp Neurol* 105:417–537.

Blackstad TW (1958) On the termination of some afferents to the hippocampus and fascia dentata. *Acta Anat (Basel)* 35:202–214.

Blackstad TW, Flood PR (1963) Ultrastructure of hippocampal axosomatic synapses. *Nature* 198:542–543.

Bliss TVP, Lømo T (1970) Plasticity in a monosynaptic cortical pathway. *J Physiol (Lond)* 207:61P.

Bliss TVP, Lømo T (1973) Long-lasting potentiation of synaptic transmission in the dentate gyrus of the anaesthetized rabbit. *J Physiol (Lond)* 232:331–356.

Bliss TVP, Richards C (1971) Some experiments with in vitro hippocampal slices. *J Physiol (Lond)* 214:7–9P.

Botvinick MM, Braver TS, Barch DM, Carter CS, Cohen JD (2001) Conflict monitoring and cognitive control. *Psychol Rev* 108:624–652.

Broca P (1861a) Sur le principe des localisations cérébrales. *Bull Soc Anthropol* 2:190–204.

Broca P (1861b) Perte de la parole, ramollissement chronique et destruction partielle du lobe antérieur gauche [sur le siège de la faculté du langage]. *Bull Soc Anthropol* 2:235–238.

Brodal A (1947) Hippocampus and the sense of smell. *Brain* 70:179–222.

Brodal A (1981) *Neurological anatomy in relation to clinical medicine.* New York: Oxford University Press.

Brodmann K (1909) *Vergleichende Lokalisationslehre der Grosshirnrinde in ihren Prinzipien dargestellt auf Grund des Zellenbaues.* Leipzig: Johann Ambrosius Barth Verlag.

Brooks CMcC, Eccles JC (1947) Electrical investigations of the monosynaptic pathway through the spinal cord. *J Neurophysiol* 10:251–274.

Brown S, Schäfer EA (1888) An investigation into the function of the occipital and temporal lobes of the monkey's brain. *Philos Trans R Soc B* 179:303–327.

Bush G, Luu P, Posner MI (2000) Cognitive and emotional influences in anterior cingulate cortex. *Trends Cogn Sci* 4:215–222.

Cannon WB (1929) *Bodily changes in pain, hunger, fear and rage.* New York: Appleton-Century-Crofts.

Cohen NJ, Squire LR (1980) Preserved learning and retention of pattern-analyzing skill in amnesia: dissociation of knowing how and knowing that. *Science* 210:207–210.

Corkin S, Amaral DG, Gonzalez RG, Johnson KA, Hyman BT (1997) H.M.'s medial temporal lobe lesion: findings from magnetic resonance imaging. *J Neurosci* 17:3964–3979.

Correll RE, Scoville WB (1967) Significance of delay in the performance of monkeys with medial temporal lobe resections. *Exp Brain Res* 4:85–96.

Cotman C, Gentry C, Steward O (1977) Synaptic replacement in the dentate gyrus after unilateral entorhinal lesion: electron microscopic analysis of the extent of replacement of synapses by the remaining entorhinal cortex. *J Neurocytol* 6:455–464.

Cowan WM, Gottlieb DI, Hendrickson AE, Price JL, Woolsey TA (1972) The autoadiographic demonstration of axonal connections in the central nervous system. *Brain Res* 37:21–51.

Cragg B, Hamlyn LH (1955) Action potentials of the pyramidal neurons of the hippocampus of the rabbit. *J Physiol (Lond)* 129:608–627.

Cragg B, Hamlyn LH (1957) Some commissural and septal connections of the hippocampus in the rabbit: a combined histological and electrical study. *J Physiol (Lond)* 135:460–485.

Curtis DR, Watkins JC (1960) The chemical excitation of spinal neurones by certain acidic amino acids. *J Physiol (Lond)* 150:656–682.

Curtis DR, Felix D, McLellan H (1970) GABA and hippocampal inhibition. *Br J Pharmacol* 40:881–883.

Dalton AJ, Black AH (1968) Hippocampal electrical activity during the operant conditioning of movement and refraining from movement. *Commun Behav Biol* 2:267–273.

Davolio C, Greenamyre JT (1995) Selective vulnerability of the CA1 region of hippocampus to the indirect excitotoxic effects of malonic acid. *Neurosci Lett* 192:29–32.

Douglas RJ, Isaacson RL (1964) Hippocampal lesions and activity. *Psychon Sci* 1:187–188.

Dunnett SB, Low WC, Iversen SD, Stenevi U, Björklund A (1982) Septal transplants restore maze learning in rats with fornix-fimbria lesions. *Brain Res* 251:335–348.

Eccles JC, Llinás R, Sasaki K (1966) The inhibitory interneurones within the cerebellar cortex. *Exp Brain Res* 1:1–16.

Ferrier D (1876) *The functions of the brain.* London: Smith, Elder.

Fink RP, Heimer L (1967) Two methods for selective silver impregnation of degenerating axons and their synaptic endings in the central nervous system. *Brain Res* 4:369–374.

Gaffan D (1974a) Loss of recognition memory in rats with lesions of the fornix. *Neuropsychologia* 10:327–341.

Gaffan D (1974b) Recognition impaired and association intact in the memory of monkeys after transaction of the fornix. *J Comp Physiol Psychol* 86:1100–1109.

Gähwiler BH (1981) Organotypic monolayer cultures of nevous tissue. *J Neurosci* Methods 4:329–342.

Gähwiler BH (1988) Organotypic cultures of neural tissue. *Trends Neurosci* 11:484–489.

Gähwiler BH, Brown DA (1985) Functional innervation of cultured hippocampal neurons by cholinergic afferents from co-cultured septal explants. *Nature* 313:577–579.

Gastaut H (1956) Étude electroclinique des épisodes psychotiques survenant en dehors des crises clinique chez les épileptiques. *Rev Neurol (Paris)* 94:587–594.

Gerfen CR, Sawchenko PE (1984) An anterograde neuroanatomical tracing method that shows the detailed morphology of neurons, their axons and terminals: immunohistochemical localization of an axonally transported plant lectin Phaseolus vulgaris-leucoagglutinin. *Brain Res* 290:219–238.

Glees P (1946) Terminal degeneration within the central nervous system as studied by a new silver method. *J Neuropathol Exp Neurol* 5:54–59.

Gloor P, Vera CL, Sperti L (1964) Electrophysiological studies of hippocampal neurons. 3. Responses of hippocampal neurons to repetitive perforant path volleys. *Electroencephalogr Clin Neurophysiol* 17:353–370.

Goddard GV, McIntyre DC, Leech CK (1969) A permanent change in brain function resulting from daily electrical stimulation. *Exp Neurol* 25:295–330.

Goldwitz D, Cotman CW (1978) Induction of extensive fimbrial branching in the adult rat brain. *Nature* 275:64–67.

Golgi C (1886) *Sulla fina anatomia degli organi centrali del sistema nervosa.* Milan: Hoepli.

Golgi C, Bentivogli M, Swanson L (2001) On the fine structure of the pes hippocampi major. *Brain Res Bull* 54:461–483. Translated from Golgi C (1886)

Grafstein B (1971) Transneuronal transfer of radioactivity in the central nervous system. *Science* 172:177–179.

Grastyán E, Lissák K, Madarász I, Donhoffer H (1959) Hippocampal electrical activity during the development of conditioned reflexes. *Electroencephalogr Clin Neurophysiol* 11:409–430.

Gray EG (1959) Axo-somatic and axo-dendritic synapses of the cerebral cortex: an electron microscope study. *J Anat (Lond)* 93:420–433.

Gray JA (1982) *The neuropsychology of anxiety: an enquiry into the functions of the septo-hippocampal system.* New York: Oxford University Press.

Gray JA (2001) Emotional modulation of cognitive control: approach-withdrawal states double-dissociate spatial from verbal two-back task performance. *J Exp Psychol Gen* 130:436–452.

Green JD, Adey WR (1956) Electrophysiological studies of hippocampal connections and excitability. *Electroencephalogr Clin Neurophysiol* 8:245–263.

Green JD, Arduini AA (1954) Hippocampal electrical activity in arousal. *J Neurophysiol* 17:533–557.

Gross CG (1993) Huxley versus Owen: the hippocampus minor and evolution. *Trends Neurosci* 16:493–498.

Hamlyn LH (1963) An electron microscope study of pyramidal neurons in the Ammon's horn of the rabbit. *J Anat (Lond)* 97:189–201.

Hayman LA, Rexer JL, Pavol MA, Strite D, Meyers CA (1998) Klüver-Bucy syndrome after selective damage of the amygdala and its cortical connections. *J Neuropsychiatry Clin Neurosci* 10:354–358.

Hirano T, Best P, Olds J (1970) Units during habituation, discrimination learning, and extinction. *Electroencephalogr Clin Neurophysiol* 28:127–135.

Hirsh R (1974) The hippocampus and contextual retrieval of information from memory: a theory. *Behav Biol* 12:421–444.

Hjorth Simonsen A (1973) Some intrinsic connections of the hippocampus in the rat: an experimental analysis. *J Comp Neurol* 147:145–161.

Holmes JE, Adey WR (1960) Electrical activity of the entorhinal cortex during conditioned behavior. *Am J Physiol* 199:741–744.

Hounsgaard J, Yarom Y (1985) Intrinsic control of electroresponsive properties of transplanted mammalian brain neurons. *Brain Res* 335:372–376.

Isaacson RL, Kimble DP (1972) Lesions of the limbic system: their effects upon hypotheses and frustration. *Behav Bull* 7:767–793.

Jackson JH (1865) In: *Selected writings of John Hughlings Jackson* (2 vols). (Taylor J, ed). London: Hodder & Stoughton, 1932.

Jackson JH, Beevor CE (1890) Case of tumor of the right temporosphenoidal lobe bearing on the localization of the sense of smell and on the interpretation of a particular variety of epilepsy. *Brain* 12:346–357.

Johnston D, Wu M-S (1994) *Foundations of cellular neurophysiology.* Cambridge, MA: Bradford Books, MIT Press.

Johnston D, Magee JC, Colbert CM, Cristie BR (1996) Active properties of neuronal dendrites. *Annu Rev Neurosci* 19:165–186.

Jung R (1949) Hirnelektrische Untersuchungen über den Elektrokrampf: Die Erregungsabläufe in corticalen Hirnregionen bei Katze und Hund. *Arch Psychiatr Nervenkr* 183:206–244.

Jung R, Kornmüller AE (1938) Eine methodik der Ableitung lokalisierter Potentialschwankungen aus subcorticalen Hirngebieten. *Arch Psychiatr Nervenkr* 109:1–30.

Kaada BR, Pribram KH, Epstein JA (1949) Respiratory and vascular responses in monkeys from temporal pole, insula, orbital surface and cingulate. *Fed Proc* 8:83–84.

Kaada BR, Jansen J Jr, Andersen P (1953) Stimulation of the hippocampus and medial cortical areas in unanesthetized cats. *Neurology* 3:844–857.

Kaada BR, Rasmussen EW, Kveim O (1961) Effects of hippocampal lesions on maze learning and retention in rats. *Exp Neurol* 3:333–355.

Kandel ER, Spencer WA (1961a) Electrophysiology of hippocampal neurons. II. After-potentials and repetitive firing. *J Neurophysiol* 24:243–259.

Kandel ER, Spencer A (1961b) Excitation and inhibition of single pyramidal cells during hippocampal seizure. *Exp Neurol* 4:162–179.

Kandel ER, Spencer WA, Brinley FJ (1961) Electrophysiology of hippocampal neurons. I. Sequential invasion and synaptic organization. *J Neurophysiol* 24:225–242.

Kerns JG, Cohen JD, MacDonald AW, Cho RY, Stenger VA, Carter CS (2004) Anterior cingulate conflict monitoring and adjustments in control. *Science* 303:1023–1026.

Kimble DP (1963) The effects of bilateral hippocampal lesions in rats. *J Comp Physiol Psychol* 56:273–283.

Kimble DP (1968) Hippocampus and internal inhibition. *Psychol Bull* 70:285–295.

Klüver H, Bucy PC (1937) Psychic blindness and other symptoms following bilateral temporal lobectomy in rhesus monkeys. *Am J Physiol* 119:352–353.

Korsakov SS (1889) Étude médico-psychologique sur une forme des maladies de mémoire. *Rev Philos* 28:501–530.

Korsakov SS (1890) Eine psychische Störung kombiniert mit multiplen Neuritis. *Allg Z Psychiatr* 46:475–485.

Kramis R, Vanderwolf CH, Bland BH (1975) Two types of hippocampal rhythmical slow activity in both the rabbit and the rat: relations to behavior and effects of atropine, diethyl ether, urethane, and pentobarbital. *Exp Neurol* 49:58–85.

Kristensson K, Olsson Y (1971) Retrograde axonal transport of protein. *Brain Res* 29:43–47.

Kuroiwa T, Terakado M, Yamaguchi T, Endo S, Ueki M, Okeda R (1996) The pyramidal layer of sector CA1 shows the lowest hippocampal succinate dehydrogenase activity in normal and postischemic gerbils. *Neurosci Lett* 206:117–120.

Kveim O, Setekleiv J, Kaada BR (1964) Differential effects of hippocampal lesions on maze and passive avoidance learning in rats. *Exp Neurol* 9:59–72.

Larrabee MG, Bronk DW (1939) Prolonged facilitation of synaptic excitation in sympathetic ganglia. *J Neurophysiol* 10:139–154.

Lasek R (1975) Axonal transport and the use of intracellular markers in neuroanatomical investigations. *Fed Proc* 34:1603–1611.

Lewis PR, Shute CCD (1967) The cholinergic limbic system: projection to the hippocampal formation, medial cortex, nuclei of the ascending cholinergic reticular system and the subfornical organ and supra-optic crest. *Brain* 90:521–537.

Li C-L, McIlwain H (1957) Maintenance of resting membrane potentials in slices of mammalian cerebral cortex and other tissues in vitro. *J Physiol (Lond)* 139:178–190.

Li XG, Somogyi P, Ylinen A, Buzsaki G (1994) The hippocampal CA3 network: an in vivo intracellular labeling study. *J Comp Neurol* 339:181–208.

Ling G, Gerard RW (1949) The normal membrane potential of frog sartorius fibers. *J Cell Physiol* 34:383–396.

Lloyd DPC (1949) Post-tetanic potentiation of response in monosynaptic pathways of the spinal cord. *J Gen Physiol* 33:147–170.

Lømo T (1966) Frequency potentiation of excitatory synaptic activity in the dentate area of the hippocampal formation. *Acta Physiol Scand* 68(Suppl 277):128.

Lømo T (1971) Patterns of activation in a monosynaptic cortical pathway: the perforant path input to the dentate area of the hippocampal formation. *Exp Brain Res* 12:18–45.

Lorente de Nó R (1934) Studies on the structure of the cerebral cortex. II. Continuation of the study of the ammonic system. *J Psychol Neurol (Lpz)* 46:113–177.

Lorente de Nó (1947) Action potential of the motoneurons of the hypoglossus nucleus. *J Cell Comp Physiol* 29:207–288.

Lowry OH, Roberts NR, Leiner KY, Wu M-L, Farr AL (1954a) The quantitative histochemistry of brain. I. Chemical methods. *J Biol Chem* 207:1–17.

Lowry OH, Roberts NR, Wu M-L, Hixon WS, Crawford EJ (1954b) The quantitative histochemistry of brain. II. Enzyme measurements. *J Biol Chem* 207:19–27.

Lowry OH, Roberts NR, Leiner KY, Wu M-L, Farr AL, Albers RW (1954c) The quantitative histochemistry of brain. III. Ammon's horn. *J Biol Chem* 207:39–49.

Lowry O (1964) In: *Morphological and biochemical correlates of neural activity* (Cohen MM, Snider RS, eds), pp. 178–191. New York: Harper & Row.

Lynch G, Matthews DA, Mosko S, Parks T, Cotman C (1972) Induced acetylcholinesterase-rich layer in rat dentate gyrus following entorhinal lesions. *Brain Res* 42:311–318.

McIlwain H, Snyder SH (1970) Stimulation of piriform and neo-cortical tissues in an in vitro flow-system: metabolic properties and release of putative transmitters. *J Neurochem* 17:521–530.

McNaughton BL, O'Keefe J, Barnes CA (1983) The stereotrode: a new technique for simultaneous isolation of several single units in the central nervous system from multiple unit records. *J Neurosci Methods* 8:391–397.

Marchi V, Algeri EG (1886) Sulle degenerazioni discendenti consecutive a lesioni in diverse zone della corteccia cerebrale. *Riv Sper Freniatr Med Leg Alien Ment* 14:1–49.

Marr D (1969) A theory of cerebellum. *J Physiol (Lond)* 202:437–470.

Marr D (1970) A theory for cerebral neocortex. *Proc R Soc B* 176:161–234.

Marr D (1971) Simple memory: a theory for archicortex. *Philos Trans R Soc B* 262:23–81.

Matthews DA, Cotman C, Lynch G (1976) An electron microscopic study of lesion-induced synaptogenesis in the dentate gyrus of the adult rat. I. Magnitude and time course of degeneration. *Brain Res* 115:1–21.

Mishkin M (1954) Visual discrimination performance following partial ablations of the temporal lobe. II. Ventral surface vs. hippocampus. *J Comp Physiol Psychol* 47:187–193.

Mishkin M, Delacour J (1975) An analysis of short-term visual memory in the monkey. *J Exp Psychol Anim Behav Process* 1:326–334.

Mosko S, Lynch G, Cotman CW (1973) The distribution of septal projections to the hippocampus of the rat. *J Comp Neurol* 152:163–174.

Nadel L, O'Keefe J (1974) The hippocampus in pieces and patches: an essay on modes of explanation in physiological psychology. In: *Essays on the nervous system: a festschrift for Prof JZ Young* (Bellairs R, Gray EG, eds), pp 367–390. Oxford: Clarendon Press.

Nadel L, O'Keefe J, Black AH (1975) Slam on the brakes: a critique of Altmann, Brunner and Bayer's response inhibition model of hippocampal function. *Behav Biol* 14:151–162.

Nadler JV, Vaca KW, White WF, Lynch GS, Cotman CW (1976) Aspartate and glutamate as possible transmitters of excitatory hippocampal afferents. *Nature* 260:538–540.

Nauta WJH (1950) Über die sogenannte terminale Degeneration in der Zentralnervensystem und ihre Darstellung durch Silberimprägnation. *Schweiz Arch Neurol Psychiatr* 66:353–376.

Nauta WJH, Gygax PA (1954) Silver impregnation of degenerating axons in the central nervous system: a modified technic. *Stain Technol* 29:91–93.

Nicoll RA, Eccles JC, Oshima T, Rubia F (1975) Prolongation of hippocampal inhibitory postsynaptic potentials by barbiturates. *Nature* 258:625–627.

Obata K, Ito M, Ochi R, Sato N (1967) Pharmacological properties of the postsynaptic inhibition of the Purkinje cell axons and the action of γ-aminobutyric acid on Deiters neurons. *Exp Brain Res* 4:43–57.

O'Keefe J, Dostrovsky J (1971) The hippocampus as a spatial map: preliminary evidence from unit activity in the freely-moving rat. *Brain Res* 34:171–175.

O'Keefe J, Recce ML (1993) Phase relationship between hippocampal place units and the EEG theta rhythm. *Hippocampus* 3:317–330.

Olton DS, Walker JA, Gage FH (1978) Hippocampal connections and spatial discrimination. *Brain Res* 139:295–308.

Orbach J, Milner B, Rasmussen T (1960) Learning and retention in monkeys after amygdala-hippocampus resection. *Arch Neurol* 3:230–235.

Palay SL, Palade GE (1955) The fine structure of neurons. *J Biophys Biochem Cytol* 1:69–88.

Papez JW (1937) A proposed mechanism of emotion. *Arch Neurol Psychiatry* 38:725–743.

Penfield W, Erickson TC (1941) *Epilepsy and cerebral localization: a study of the mechanism, treatment, and prevention of epileptic seizures.* Springfield, IL: Charles C Thomas.

Phillips CG (1956) Intracellular records from Betz cells in the cat. *Q J Exp Physiol* 41:58–69.

Raisman G (1969) Neuronal plasticity in the septal nuclei of the adult rat. *Brain Res* 14:25–48.

Raisman G, Field PM (1973) A quantitative investigation of the development of collateral reinnervation after partial deafferentation of the septal nuclei. *Brain Res* 50:241–264.

Raisman G, Field P (1990) Synapse formation in the adult brain after lesions and after transplantation of embryonic tissue. *J Exp Biol* 153:277–287.

Raisman G, Cowan WM, Powell TPS (1965) The extrinsic, commissural and association fibres of the hippocampus. *Brain* 88:963–998.

Raisman G, Cowan WM, Powell TPS (1966) An experimental analysis of the efferent projection of the hippocampus. *Brain* 89:83–108.

Rall W, Shepherd GM (1968) Theoretical reconstruction of field potentials and dendrodendritic synaptic interactions in olfactory bulb. *J Neurophysiol* 31:884–915.

Ramon y Cajal S (1893) Estructura del asta de Ammon. *Anal Sociedad Español Historia Natural*, vol 22. Translated to German by von Kölliker A (1893). In *Zeitschr Wiss Zool* 56.

Ramon y Cajal S (1911) *Histologie du système nerveux de l'homme et des vertébrés.* Paris: A. Maloine. Reprinted (1955) Madrid: Instituto Ramon y Cajal.

Ranck JB Jr (1973) Studies on single neurons in dorsal hippocampal formation and septum in unrestrained rats. *Exp Neurol* 41:461–455.

Renshaw B, Forbes A, Morison BR (1940) Activity of isocortex and hippocampus: electrical studies with micro-electrodes. *J Neurophysiol* 3:74–105.

Ribot T (1881) *Les maladies de la mémoire.* Paris: Ballière.

Richards CD, McIlwain H (1967) Electrical responses in brain samples. *Nature* 215:704–707.

Richardson TL, Turner RW, Miller JJ (1987) Action-potential discharge in hippocampal CA1 pyramidal neuron: current source-density analysis. *J Neurophysiol* 58:981–996.

Ries FA, Langworthy OR (1937) A study of the surface structure of the brain of the whale (Balaenoptera physalus and Physeter catodon). *J Comp Neurol* 68:1–47.

Rose M (1935) Cytoarchitektonik und Myeloarchitektonik der Grosshirnrinde. In: *Handbuch der Neurologie* (Bumke O, Foerster O, eds), vol 1, pp 588–778. Berlin.

Sagar JH, Cohen NJ, Corkin S, Growdon JH (1985) Dissociations among processes in remote memory. *Ann NY Acad Sci* 444:533–535.

Sala L (1891) Zur Anatomie des grossen Seepferdfusses. *Zeitschr Wiss Zool* 52.

Schaffer K (1892) Beitrag zur Histologie der Ammonshorn-formation. *Arch Mikr Anat* 39:611–632.

Schreiner L, Kling A (1956) Rhinencephalon and behavior. *Am J Physiol* 184:486–490.

Schwartzkroin P (1975) Characteristics of CA1 neurons recorded intracellularly in the hippocampal in vitro slice preparation. *Brain Res* 85:423–436.

Schwartzkroin PA (1997) Origins of the epileptic state. *Epilepsia* 38:853–858.

Schwartzkroin P, Andersen P (1975) Glutamic acid sensitivity of dendrites in hippocampal slices in vitro. *Adv Neurol* 12:45–51.

Schwartzkroin P, Wester K (1975) Long-lasting facilitation of a synaptic potential following tetanization in the in vitro hippocampal slice. *Brain Res* 89:107–119.

Scoville W, Milner B (1957) Loss of recent memory after bilateral hippocampal lesions. *J Neurol Neurosurg Psychiatry* 20:11–21.

Segal M, Bloom FE (1974a) The action of norepinephrine in the rat hippocampus. I. Iontophoretic studies. *Brain Res* 72:79–97.

Segal M, Bloom FE (1974b) The action of norepinephrine in the rat hippocampus. II. Activation of the input pathway. *Brain Res* 72:99–114.

Semon R (1908) *The mneme.* English translation: London: 1908, 1911, and 1921. First German edition: 1904.

Shapiro ML, Simon DK, Olton DS, Gage FH III, Nilsson O, Bjorklund A (1989) Intrahippocampal grafts of fetal basal forebrain tissue alter place fields in the hippocampus of rats with fimbria-fornix lesions. *Neuroscience* 32:1–18.

Shepherd GM (1972) The neuron doctrine: a revision of functional concepts. *Yale J Biol Med* 45:584–599.

Shepherd MG, Raastad M, Andersen P (2002) General and variable features of varicosity spacing along unmyelinated axons in the hippocampus and cerebellum. *Proc Natl Acad Sci USA* 99:6340–6345

Sherrington CS (1897) The central nervous system. In: *A textbook of physiology* (Foster M, ed), vol 3, 7th ed. London: Macmillan.

Shipley MT, Adamek GD (1984) The connections of the mouse olfactory bulb: a study using orthograde and retrograde transport of wheat germ agglutinin conjugated to horseradish peroxidase. *Brain Res Bull* 12:669–688.

Skrede KK, Westgaard RH (1971) The transverse hippocampal slice: a well-defined cortical structure maintained in vitro. *Brain Res* 35:589–593.

Sloan N, Jasper H (1950) Studies of the regulatory functions of the limbic cortex. *Electroencephalogr Clin Neurophysiol* 2:317–327.

Sommer W (1890) Erkrankung des Ammonshorns als aetiologisches Moment der Epilepsie. *Arch Psychiatr Nervenkrank* 10:631–675.

Spencer WA, Thompson RF, Neilson DR Jr (1966) Response decrement of the flexion reflex in the acute spinal cat and transient restoration by strong stimuli. *J Neurophysiol* 29:221–239.

Spielmeyer W (1925) Zur Pathogenese örtlich elektiver Gehirnveränderungen. *Z Ges Neurol Psychiatr* 99:756–776.

Spruston N, Jonas P, Sakmann B (1995) Dendritic glutamate receptor channels in rat hippocampal CA3 and CA1 pyramidal neurons. *J Physiol (Lond)* 482:325–352.

Squire LR (1998) Memory systems. *C R Acad Sci III* 321:153–156.

Squire LR (2004) Memory systems of the brain: a brief history and current perspective. *Neurobiol Learn Mem* 82:171–177.

Stevens CF (1966) *Neurophysiology: a primer.* New York: Wlley.

Steward O, Cotman C, Lynch GS (1974) Growth of a new fiber projection in the brain of adult rats: reinnervation of the dentate gyrus by the contralateral entorhinal cortex following ipsilateral entorhinal lesions. *Exp Brain Res* 20:45–66.

Storm-Mathisen J, Fonnum F (1972) Localization of transmitter candidates in the hippocampal region. *Prog Brain Res* 36:41–58.

Storm-Mathisen J, Leknes AK, Bore AT, Vaaland JL, Edminson P, Haug FM, Ottersen OP (1983) First visualization of glutamate and GABA in neurones by immunocytochemistry. *Nature* 301: 517–520.

Stuart G, Spruston N, Sakmann B, Häusser M (1997) Action potential initiation and backpropagation in neurons of the mammalian CNS. *Trends Neurosci* 20:125–131.

Swanson LW, Cowan, WM (1977) An autoradiographic study of the organization of the efferent connections of the hippocampal formation in the rat. *J Comp Neurol* 172:49–84.

Tulving E (1972) Episodic and semantic memory. In: *Organization and memory* (Tulving E, Donaldson W, eds), pp 382–403. San Diego: Academic Press.

Vanderwolf CH (1969) Hippocampal electrical activity and voluntary movement in the rat. *Electroencephalogr Clin Neurophysiol* 26:407–418.

Vinogradova O, Semyonova TP, Konovalov VP (1970) Trace phenomena in single neurons of hippocampus and mammillary bodies. In: *Biology of memory* (Pribram KH, Broadbent DE, eds), pp 191–222. San Diego: Academic Press.

Von Euler C, Green JD, Ricci G (1958) The role of hippocampal dendrites in evoked responses and after-discharges. *Acta Physiol Scand* 42:87–111.

Von Gudden JBA (1896) Klinische und anatomische Beiträge zur Kenntniss der multiplen Alcoholneuritis nebst Bemerkungen über die Regenerationsvorgänge in peripheren Nervensystem. *Arch Psychiatr Nervenkr* 28:643–741.

Weiskrantz L (1956) Behavioral changes associated with ablation of the amygdaloid complex in monkeys. *J Comp Physiol Psychol* 49: 381–391.

Wernicke C (1881) *Lehrbuch der Gehirnkrankheiten,* vol 2. Berlin: Theodore Fischer.

Wilson MA, McNaughton BL (1993) Dynamics of the hippocampal ensemble code for space. *Science* 261:1055–1058.

Winograd T (1975) Frame representations and the declarative/procedural controversy. In: *Representation and understanding* (Bobrow DG, Collins A, eds), pp 185–210. San Diego: Academic Press.

Yamamoto C, McIlwain H (1966a) Potentials evoked in vitro in preparations from the mammalian brain. *Nature* 210: 1055–1056.

Yamamoto C, McIlwain H (1966b) Electrical activities in thin sections from the mammalian brain maintained in chemically defined media in vitro. *J Neurochem* 13:1333–1343.

Zimmer J, Gähwiler BH (1984) Cellular and connective organization of slice cultures of the rat hippocampus and fascia dentata. *J Comp Neurol* 228:432–446.

3

David Amaral and Pierre Lavenex

Hippocampal Neuroanatomy

3.1 Overview

Where is the hippocampal formation and what does it look like? What types of neurons are located in this group of structures, and what types of connections do they form? What is the difference between the hippocampus and the hippocampal formation? Does the hippocampus look similar in the rat, monkey, and human brains? Are other components of the hippocampal formation similar across species? Are the principles of neuroanatomical connectivity similar or different from those found in other brain regions? These are only some of the neuroanatomical issues that are explored in this chapter. The elegant neuronal architecture of the hippocampal formation and the simplicity and orderliness of its major connections have been seductive features to neuroscientists for decades. Yet, there are pragmatic reasons why a working knowledge of its neuroanatomy is important.

First, it is likely that certain peculiarities of the neural organization of the hippocampus, such as its highly associational intrinsic connections, provide important clues to its function(s). Second, the design of functional, electrophysiological, pharmacological, and behavioral studies require increasingly sophisticated knowledge of its boundaries, cell types, connections, and chemical neuroanatomy. This chapter lays the structural foundations for discussions of the functional organization of the hippocampal formation explored later in the book.

3.1.1 Hippocampus: Part of a Functional Brain System Called the Hippocampal Formation

One of the most captivating features of the hippocampus is its neuroanatomy. The relatively simple organization of its principal cell layers coupled with the highly organized laminar distribution of many of its inputs has encouraged its use as a model system for modern neurobiology. Despite more than a

century of neuroanatomical study and literally tens of thousands of research articles on the hippocampus, there is still no consensus concerning certain facets of its nomenclature. Hippocampal researchers tend to follow one of several implicit "views" about what the hippocampus is and what it is not. The view adopted in this book is that the hippocampus is one of several related brain regions that together comprise a functional system called the hippocampal formation.

The hippocampus proper has three subdivisions: CA3, CA2, and CA1. (CA comes from *cornu ammonis*; the derivation of these terms is discussed shortly.) The other regions of the hippocampal formation include the dentate gyrus, subiculum, presubiculum, parasubiculum, and entorhinal cortex. Thus, although the title for this book is *The Hippocampus Book*, a more correct, albeit less melodious, title would have been *The Hippocampal Formation Book*. The rationale for grouping these cytoarchitectonically distinct brain regions under the rubric hippocampal formation is developed throughout this chapter.

3.1.2 Similarities and Differences Between the Hippocampal Formation and other Cortical Areas

In some ways, such as the occurrence of large, pyramid-shaped projection neurons and smaller interneurons, the neural organization of some portions of the hippocampal formation resembles other cortical regions. Yet in important ways, such as the largely unidirectional passage of information through intrahippocampal circuits and the highly distributed three-dimensional organization of intrinsic associational connections, the neuroanatomy of the hippocampal formation is unique. It has often been touted as a heuristically simple model of neocortical organization, but this perspective demeans both the hippocampal formation and the neocortex. It is more profitable to highlight and investigate the distinctive neuroanatomical features of the hippocampal formation as potential clues to its particular function(s) and the mechanisms by which these functions are realized.

Our understanding of hippocampal neuroanatomy leads to the prediction that whatever processes this group of structures carries out they are likely to be quite different from those performed in other cortical regions. The hippocampal formation, for example, is one of only a few brain regions that receive highly processed, multimodal sensory information from a variety of neocortical sources. Moreover, its own system of widely distributed intrinsic neuronal networks is ideally suited for further mixing or comparing this information. This ability to integrate information from all sensory modalities may thus be a unique attribute of the hippocampus conferred by the highly convergent-divergent organization of its connections.

3.1.3 Hippocampal Formation: With A Unique Set of Unidirectional, Excitatory Pathways

A common organizational feature of connections between regions of the neocortex is that they are largely reciprocal (Felleman and Van Essen, 1991). If cortical region A projects to cortical region B, region B often sends a return projection back to region A. As first described by Ramón y Cajal (1893), this is clearly not the case for the connections that link the various parts of the hippocampal formation (Fig. 3–1). The entorhinal cortex can, for convenience, be considered the first step in the intrinsic hippocampal circuit. The logic behind this is developed later in the chapter, but the priority afforded to the entorhinal cortex is based on the fact that much of the neocortical input reaching the hippocampal formation does so through the entorhinal cortex. Cells in the superficial layers of the entorhinal cortex give rise to axons that project, among other destinations, to the dentate gyrus. The projections from the entorhinal cortex to the dentate gyrus form part of the major hippocampal input pathway called the perforant path. Although the entorhinal cortex provides the major input to the dentate gyrus, the dentate gyrus does not project back to the entorhinal cortex. This pathway is therefore nonreciprocated, or unidirectional.

Likewise, the principal cells of the dentate gyrus, the granule cells, give rise to axons called mossy fibers that connect with pyramidal cells of the CA3 field of the hippocampus. The CA3 cells, however, do not project back to the granule cells. The pyramidal cells of CA3, in turn, are the source of the major input to the CA1 hippocampal field (the Schaffer col-

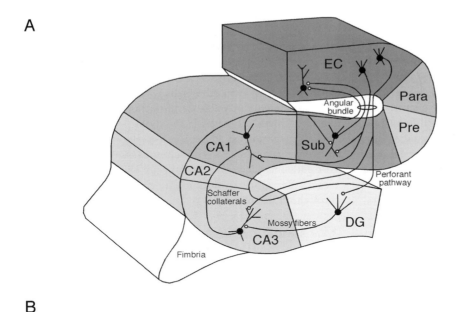

Figure 3–1. The hippocampal formation. *A.* Neurons in layer II of the entorhinal cortex project to the dentate gyrus and the CA3 field of the hippocampus proper via the perforant pathway. Neurons in layer III of the entorhinal cortex project to the CA1 field of the hippocampus and the subiculum via the perforant and alvear pathways (see text for a detailed description). The granule cells of the dentate gyrus project to the CA3 field of the hippocampus via mossy fiber projections. Pyramidal neurons in the CA3 field of the hippocampus project to CA1 via Schaffer collaterals. Pyramidal cells in CA1 project to the subiculum. Both CA1 and the subiculum project back to the deep layers of the entorhinal cortex. *B.* Projections along the transverse axis of the hippocampal formation; the dentate gyrus is located proximally and the entorhinal cortex distally.

lateral axons). Following the pattern of its predecessors, CA1 does not project back to CA3. The CA1 field of the hippocampus then projects unidirectionally to the subiculum, providing its major excitatory input. Again, the subiculum does not project back to CA1.

Once one reaches CA1 and the subiculum, the pattern of intrinsic connections begins to become somewhat more elaborate. CA1, for example, projects not only to the subiculum but also to the entorhinal cortex. Furthermore, whereas the subiculum does project to the presubiculum and the parasubiculum, its more prominent cortical projection is directed to the entorhinal cortex. Through these connections both CA1 and the subiculum close the hippocampal processing loop that begins in the superficial layers of the entorhinal cortex and ends in its deep layers. Although this cursory survey of the intrinsic connections of the hippocampal formation leaves out many of the facts that make the system somewhat more complex, it does serve to emphasize that the hippocampal formation is organized in a fashion that is distinctly different from most other cortical areas.

3.1.4 Hippocampus of Humans and Animals: Same or Different?

Once one has gained a familiarity with the neuroanatomical appearance of the rat hippocampal formation, it is not difficult to identify each of the major subdivisions in the monkey or human hippocampal formation (Fig. 3–2). Although the volume of the hippocampus is about 10 times larger in monkeys than in rats and 100 times larger in humans than in rats, the basic hippocampal architecture is common to all three species. Yet there are some striking species differences. The compact pyramidal cell layer in the CA1 region of the rat, for example, becomes thicker and more heterogeneous in the monkey and human. Whereas this layer is only about 5 cells thick in the rat, it can be more than 30 cells thick in the human. The other region that demonstrates striking species differences is the entorhinal cortex. In the rat, the entorhinal cortex is typically divided into two main, cytoarchitectonically distinct subdivisions. In the monkey there are seven subdivisions, and in the human brain the classical cytoarchitectonicists defined as many as 27 subdivisions (although recent descriptions recognize only 8 subdivisions, similar to what is observed in monkeys). Thus, despite the fact that the hippocampal formation is often portrayed as a phylogenetically primitive brain region, it nonetheless demonstrates substantial species differences.

Although the patterns of connectivity appear to be generally similar in the rodent and primate brains, there are again striking species differences. One example is the organization of the commissural connections of the dentate gyrus. In the rat, there is a massive commissural system that provides nearly one-sixth of the excitatory input to the dentate gyrus (Raisman, 1965; Gottlieb and Cowan, 1973). In the macaque monkey and presumably in humans, however, commissural connections in the dentate gyrus are almost entirely absent (Amaral et al., 1984). Another example is the more complex organization of the primate entorhinal cortex, which appears to be associated with stronger interconnections with the associational areas of the neocortex, which are more developed in primates. Myriad other subtle species differences (e.g., the chemical neuroanatomy of the hippocampal formation) have been noted in the literature. Certain neuroanatomical differences have even been described in different strains of mice that seem too subtle to be worthy of note yet could be of enormous practical importance given the current interest in the use of transgenic techniques. A major future challenge is to determine whether and how these structural and neurochemical alterations affect the functioning of the hippocampal formation.

Thus, to address the question posed in the title of this section—is the hippocampus of humans and animals same or different—the answer is both.

3.1.5 Synopsis of the Chapter

Our rationale for focusing on the rodent (mainly the rat) hippocampal formation in the first half of this chapter is that much of the available neuroanatomical data have been derived from studies carried out in this animal and because of the prominent role the rat plays in current functional analyses of the hippocampal formation. Unfortunately, far less work has been carried out in the mouse, the clear choice for molecular biology studies. It is widely presumed that the neuroanatomy of the mouse hippocampal formation is similar to that of the rat—though some additional confirmation would certainly be welcome. We next compare and contrast the picture of hippocampal anatomy obtained from studies of the rat with that of the monkey. We also describe the extensive cortical connections of the entorhinal cortex in the macaque monkey and the emerging prominence of adjacent related brain regions, such as the perirhinal and parahippocampal cortices. We then move on to compare information on the monkey hippocampal formation with what is known about the human hippocampal formation. The chapter concludes with a summary of the principles of hippocampal intrinsic circuitry and a discussion of how they may govern the flow of information through the hippocampal formation.

3.2 Historical Overview of Hippocampal Nomenclature—What's in a Name?

The hippocampal formation has been prodded and sliced and stained by anatomists for nearly 400 years. Like many brain regions, it has fallen victim to the imposition of various and often confusing terminologies to describe its gross anatomical and histological structure. The term hippocampus (derived from the Greek word for sea horse) was first coined during the sixteenth century by the anatomist Arantius (1587), who considered the three-dimensional form of the human hip-

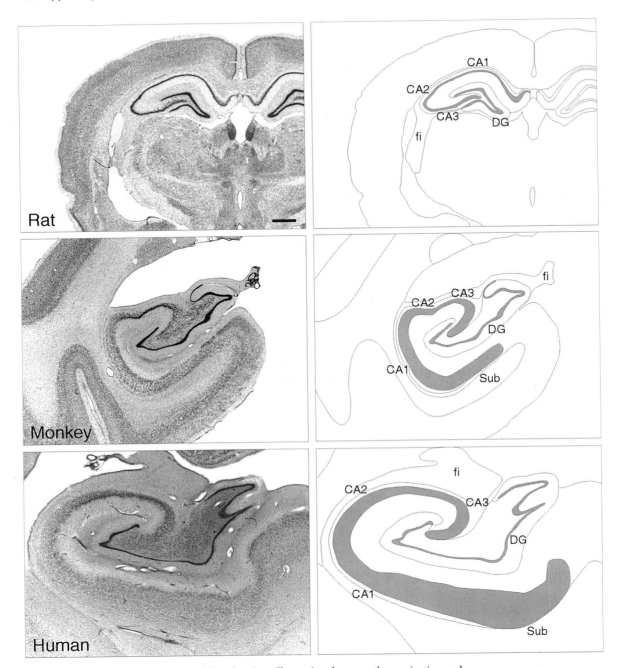

Figure 3–2. Nissl-stained sections and line drawings illustrating the general organization and similarities of the subdivisions of the hippocampal formation in the rat, monkey, and human. Note the differences in the relative position of the fimbria in the rat (located lateroventrally) and in the monkey and human (located mediodorsally). Bar in *A* = 1 mm and applies to all panels.

pocampus, lying in the floor of the inferior horn of the lateral ventricle, to be reminiscent of this sea creature (Fig. 3–3). Arantius also likened the shape of the hippocampus to a silk worm, but his term "bombycini or bombyx" never caught on. Because Arantius did not take the trouble to stake claim to the hippocampus by illustrating its location and structure, other anatomists felt free to devise their own terms. The main, or intraventricular, portion of the human hippocampus was first illustrated by Duvernoy in 1729, and he continued to assign

both the names sea horse and silk worm to this region. Others likened the arched structure of the hippocampus to a ram's horn, and De Garengeot (1742) named the hippocampus "cornu ammonis" or "Ammon's horn" after the mythological Egyptian god Amun Kneph, whose symbol was a ram. According to the Nomina Anatomica, the term hippocampus is currently acknowledged to be the standard term for the bulge occupying the floor of the lateral ventricle in the human brain. The term Ammon's horn is now only rarely used,

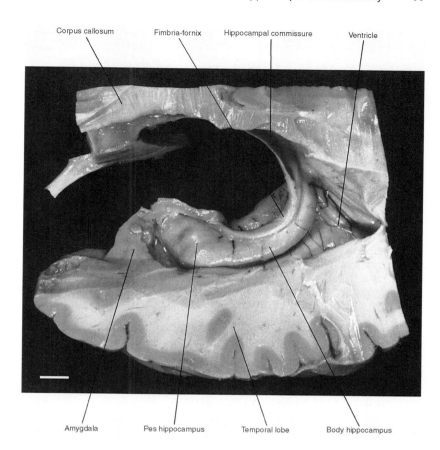

Corpus callosum   Fimbria-fornix   Hippocampal commissure   Ventricle

Amygdala   Pes hippocampus   Temporal lobe   Body hippocampus

Figure 3–3. Dorsolateral view of the human hippocampus after removing the overlying structures. The lateral ventricle has been opened, exposing the shape of the hippocampus. Bar = 1 cm.

although a curious irony of current terminology is that, although hippocampus has become the standard term, subdivisions of this structure are referred to using abbreviations of cornu ammonis (CA3, CA2, CA1). Some of the terms mentioned above, as well as many others, have found their way into descriptions of the histological structure of the hippocampal formation; hence it is helpful, at the start, to discuss neuroanatomical terms currently associated with the hippocampus.

A few terms are now of only historical interest. The hippocampus was for some time considered to be a prominent part of the rhinencephalon, which, loosely speaking, referred to a group of forebrain structures thought to be related especially to the sense of smell. In a classic article published in 1947, however, Alf Brodal concluded that the hippocampus could not be functioning solely as an olfactory structure because anosmic mammals such as dolphins had a substantial hippocampal formation (Brodal, 1947). It seemed unreasonable to Brodal that the hippocampus would be so robust in a nonsmelling creature if it functioned solely as a component of the olfactory system (see Chapter 2).

During the 1930s, the neurologist James Papez considered the hippocampus to be a central component of a system for emotional expression, and in many textbooks the hippocampus is still claimed to be the central component of the so-called Papez circuit. In Papez's view, the hippocampus was a conduit by which perceptions of emotionally salient situations could be collected and channeled to the hypothalamus where

they could recruit or effect appropriate emotional responses (Papez, 1937). Despite the admirable job done by Papez in marshaling largely circumstantial evidence in support of his view, there has been little modern substantiation of Papez's theory. The role of orchestrator of emotional expression is now more closely linked with another prominent medial temporal lobe structure, the amygdaloid complex.

The hippocampus is also associated with the term "limbic system." The origin of this term stems from the description by the neurologist Broca (1878) of "le grande lobe limbique," which comprised a series of contiguous cortical and subcortical structures located on the medial surface of the brain and surrounding the ventricle at the border (limbus) of the cortical mantle. The limbic lobe was described initially as including such circumventricular structures as the subcallosal, cingulate, and parahippocampal gyri, as well as the underlying hippocampal formation. The number of structures included under the rubric "limbic system" has escalated dramatically since the 1950s, however, and has included such diverse structures as the amygdala, septal nuclei, and midbrain periaqueductal gray matter. The proliferation of brain regions encompassed by the term limbic system has fueled a long-lasting debate about the utility of this term either as a neuroanatomical or functional entity. Suffice it to say that in this book the hippocampal formation is viewed as an independent functional system rather than part of the larger, ill-defined group of structures collectively referred to as the limbic system. That said, the hippocampal formation obviously does not function in isolation. Even as a functionally defined, independent system, it relies on interconnections with many other brain systems to do its job effectively.

3.2.1 Definition of Hippocampal Areas: Definition of Terms

When a histological section through the hippocampus is prepared and stained for cell bodies by a Nissl method, it is immediately obvious that a number of cytoarchitectonically distinct structures are encompassed in the region grossly defined as the "hippocampus." A number of terminologies have been applied to some of these regions, and several synonymous terms are still commonly employed. Beyond the problem of different terms being applied to the same region, the borders between several regions of the hippocampal formation have not yet been firmly established. The terms adopted in this book are based, in part, on converging evidence from cytoarchitectonic, histochemical, connectional, and functional data and in part on personal preference.

The term hippocampus has historically been plagued by the fact that it is used as a term both for a gross anatomical region of the brain (the bulge or protuberance in the floor of the human lateral ventricle) and for one of the cytoarchitectonically distinct entities that make up the region. As a result, the meaning of the word hippocampus is context-dependent and may be ambiguous. We reserve the term hippocampus for the region of the hippocampal formation that comprises the CA fields (CA3, CA2, CA1) identified by the neuroanatomist Rafael Lorente de Nó (Lorente de Nó, 1934). The term hippocampal formation, in contrast, is applied to a group of cytoarchitectonically distinct adjoining regions including the dentate gyrus, hippocampus, subiculum, presubiculum, parasubiculum, and entorhinal cortex (Fig. 3–1). The adjective hippocampal, by necessity, remains somewhat vague and context-dependent. In general, it is used to refer to the larger area (as in "hippocampal lesions") rather than to the cytoarchitectonic region. If this seems confusing, the terminological definitions of the next few paragraphs may provide clarification.

The main justification for including the six regions named above under the rubric hippocampal formation is that they are linked, one to the next, by unique and largely unidirectional (functional) neuronal pathways. The early literature on the hippocampal formation emphasized the first three links in the hippocampal circuitry that were highlighted by applying the term "trisynaptic circuit" to the ensemble of pathways (Andersen et al., 1971).

$$EC \rightarrow DG \text{ (synapse 1)}, DG \rightarrow CA3 \text{ (synapse 2)},$$
$$CA3 \rightarrow CA1 \text{ (synapse 3)}$$

The definition of this powerful excitatory circuit was produced by a collaboration between early neuroanatomical and electrophysiological studies. It should be borne in mind, however, that the term trisynaptic circuit was coined during an era when it was assumed that the hippocampus proper generated

the main output projections and that these projections were directed subcortically. With the discovery of robust projections from CA1 to the subiculum and entorhinal cortex, and the major projections from the entorhinal cortex to the neocortex, the trisynaptic circuit is now considered to be only a portion of the functional circuitry of the hippocampal formation. As it is now clear that the subiculum is the main source of subcortical projections and the entorhinal cortex is the main source of projections to the neocortex, the concept of the trisynaptic circuit, although of great significance in the history of hippocampal research, is currently less influential on theories of hippocampal function.

The reader who ventures from the relative safety of this book into the primary hippocampal literature should be aware that our usage of the term "hippocampal formation" is widely, though not universally, accepted. Some authors include only the allocortical (a term applied to cortical regions having fewer than six layers) regions as parts of the hippocampal formation. Three-layered cortical regions typically have a single neuronal cell layer with fiber-rich plexiform layers above and below the cell layer. In articles employing this usage, the hippocampal formation comprises the dentate gyrus, hippocampus, and subiculum. The remaining fields—presubiculum, parasubiculum, and entorhinal cortex—are then typically grouped together on the basis of their multilaminate structure under the term retrohippocampal (retro = behind) or parahippocampal (para = alongside or near) cortex. In yet other variants, the terms hippocampus or hippocampal complex are sometimes applied to the combination of the dentate gyrus and hippocampus proper. Clarification of the nomenclature is typically the first sign of maturity for a scientific enterprise, and we scrupulously adhere to the nomenclature in which the hippocampal formation comprises the six structures listed above.

Having outlined the major regions of the hippocampal formation, we now delve more deeply into the subdivisions of each of these regions. Before doing so, however, it is important to note that the terminology we apply to these regions is a hybrid derived from the analyses of classical and modern hippocampal neuroanatomists. The two main contributors to the surviving hippocampal terminologies are Santiago Ramon y Cajal (Ramón y Cajal, 1893) and his student Raphael Lorente de Nó (Lorente de Nó, 1933, 1934). Some of their subdivisions, based solely on the analysis of Golgi-stained material, have not stood the test of time or the introduction of modern neuroanatomical methods. Many revisions of their nomenclature have been made as information has become available concerning the connections and chemical architecture of the hippocampal formation.

3.2.2 Subdivisions of Hippocampal Areas

The dentate gyrus is a trilaminate cortical region with a characteristic V or U shape. The dentate gyrus has a relatively similar structure at all levels of the hippocampal formation and is not typically divided into subregions. When discussing features of the dentate gyrus, however, it is often useful to refer to a particular portion of the V- or U-shaped structure. The portion of the granule cell layer that is located between the CA3 field and the CA1 field (separated by the hippocampal fissure) is called the suprapyramidal blade; and the portion opposite this is the infrapyramidal blade. The region bridging the two blades (at the apex of the V or U) is the crest.

The hippocampus, especially in rodents, can easily be divided into two major regions: a large-celled region that abuts the dentate gyrus and a smaller-celled region that follows from it. Ramon y Cajal called these two regions regio inferior and regio superior, respectively. The terminology of Lorente de Nó has achieved more common usage and is employed here. He divided the hippocampus into three fields: CA3, CA2, and CA1. His CA3 and CA2 fields are equivalent to the large-celled regio inferior of Ramon y Cajal, and his CA1 field is equivalent to the regio superior. In addition to the greater size of the pyramidal cells in CA3 and CA2 compared to CA1, the inputs and outputs of these areas are also different. The pyramidal cells of CA3, for example, receive the mossy fiber input from the dentate gyrus, whereas the CA1 pyramidal cells do not.

The CA2 field has been the subject of substantial controversy. As originally defined by Lorente de Nó, it is a narrow zone of cells interposed between CA3 and CA1. CA2 has large pyramidal cell bodies similar to those in CA3 but, like CA1, it is not innervated by the mossy fibers from the dentate gyrus. Although the existence of CA2 has often been questioned, the bulk of available evidence indicates that there is indeed a narrow CA2 field that can be distinguished from the other hippocampal fields using a variety of criteria, including neurochemical markers. Lorente de Nó also defined a CA4 field. As originally clarified by Theodor Blackstad (1956) and then by David Amaral (1978), the region that Lorente de Nó called CA4 is actually the deep, or polymorphic, layer of the dentate gyrus.

The subiculum, presubiculum, and parasubiculum are sometimes grouped under the term "subicular complex." Because each of these regions has distinct neuroanatomical features, they are better thought of as independent cortical areas. The border between CA1 and the subiculum occurs precisely at the point where the Schaffer collateral projection from the CA3 field ends. In the rodent, this occurs approximately where the condensed pyramidal cell layer of CA1 begins to broaden into the thicker layer of the subiculum.

The presubiculum lies adjacent to the subiculum and is typically thought to have more than the three layers that characterize the dentate gyrus, hippocampus, and subiculum. However, the exact delimitation of the deep layers of the presubiculum and the differentiation of cells belonging to the presubiculum from those that belong to the deep layers of the entorhinal cortex has never been clearly established. The most distinctive feature of the presubiculum is the densely packed external cellular layer, which is populated by relatively small, tightly packed pyramidal cells. The parasubiculum is characterized by a wedge-shaped layer II with cells that resemble but

are somewhat larger and less compact than those in the presubiculum.

The entorhinal cortex is the only hippocampal region that unambiguously demonstrates a multilaminate appearance. Based on differences in the organization of these layers and more recently on differences in connectional attributes, the entorhinal cortex has been divided into two or more subregions depending on the species. We shall return to a description of the subdivisions of the entorhinal cortex later in the chapter.

Before moving on to descriptions of the three-dimensional organization of the hippocampal formation in the rat, monkey, and human brains, we must say a few more words concerning nomenclature. We often want to refer to a specific portion of one of the hippocampal regions. Given the complex shape of the hippocampal formation, no reference system is wholly adequate, and any description inevitably involves arbitrary decisions about where to start or finish, which direction is up or down, and so on. We have adopted a reference system in which the dentate gyrus is considered to be the proximal pole of the hippocampal formation and the entorhinal cortex is the distal pole (Fig. 3–1). A portion of any hippocampal field can therefore be defined in relation to this proximo-distal axis. For example, the proximal portion of CA3 is located closer to the dentate gyrus, and the distal portion is located closer to CA2.

We also often need to specify subregions within the thickness of a particular hippocampal region. As in most other cortical areas, this radial dimension is usually described along a superficial-to-deep axis. In six-layer structures, layer I is close to the pial surface, and layer VI is located close to the subcortical white matter. Consistent with this convention, regions closer to the pia or hippocampal fissure are considered superficial and those in the opposite direction—closer to the alveus or ventricle where applicable) are considered deep. The molecular layer of the dentate gyrus, for example, is superficial to the granule cell layer. This superficial–deep nomenclature has the merit of being applicable to all portions of the hippocampal formation and to all of its cytoarchitectonic fields. It has the drawback, however, of being somewhat counterintuitive to neuroscientists, especially electrophysiologists, whose electrodes approach the hippocampus from the alveus in the septal (or dorsal) portion of the hippocampus. As an electrophysiologist advances an electrode from the dorsal surface of the brain toward the hippocampus, it would first hit the alveus and then the pyramidal cell layer. Although the alveus might seem like the "superficial" portion of the hippocampus because it is closer to the surface of the brain, it is actually its deep portion. As the electrode continues its advance toward the hippocampal fissure, it enters the superficial portion of the hippocampus. Crossing the hippocampal fissure, it then enters the superficial portion of the molecular layer of the dentate gyrus, and a further advance would bring it to the deep portion of the molecular layer, the suprapyramidal granule cell layer, the hilus, and finally the infrapyramidal granule cell and molecular layers.

3.2.3 Major Fiber Bundles of the Hippocampal Formation

Three major fiber systems are associated with the hippocampal formation (Fig. 3–4, see color insert). The first is the angular bundle, which carries fibers between the entorhinal cortex and the other fields of the hippocampal formation. The second is the fimbria-fornix pathway through which the hippocampal formation is interconnected with the basal forebrain, hypothalamic, and brain stem regions. The third comprises the dorsal and ventral commissures, through which the hippocampal formation of one hemisphere is connected with the hippocampal formation of the contralateral hemisphere. We deal with these in greater detail in Section 3.3.2.

3.3 Three-dimensional Organization and Major Fiber Systems of the Hippocampal Formation

The hippocampal formation is positioned quite differently in the rodent and primate brains (Figs. 3–5 through 3–7, see color insert). This is due in part to the more developed cerebral cortex in primates, which tends to "force" the dentate gyrus and hippocampus into the temporal lobe. Whereas many of the fields of the rodent hippocampal formation are grossly C-shaped and vertically oriented, they tend to be much more linear and horizontally oriented in primates.

3.3.1 Rat Hippocampal Formation

The rat hippocampal formation is an elongated, banana-shaped structure with its long axis extending in a C-shaped manner from the midline of the brain near the septal nuclei (rostrodorsally) over and behind the thalamus into the incipient temporal lobe (caudoventrally). The long axis of the hippocampal formation is referred to as the septotemporal axis and the orthogonal axis as the transverse axis (Fig. 3–8). What is not obvious from a surface view of the hippocampal formation is that different regions make up the structure at different septotemporal levels. At extreme septal levels, for example, only the dentate gyrus and the CA3–CA1 fields of the hippocampus are present. About a third of the way along the septotemporal axis the subiculum first appears, and the presubiculum and parasubiculum are seen at progressively more temporal levels. The entorhinal cortex is located even farther caudally and ventrally. The dorsolateral limit of the entorhinal cortex occurs approximately at the rhinal sulcus, which forms a prominent, rostrocaudally/horizontally oriented indentation on the ventrolateral surface of the rat brain. This sulcus nominally separates the entorhinal cortex ventrally

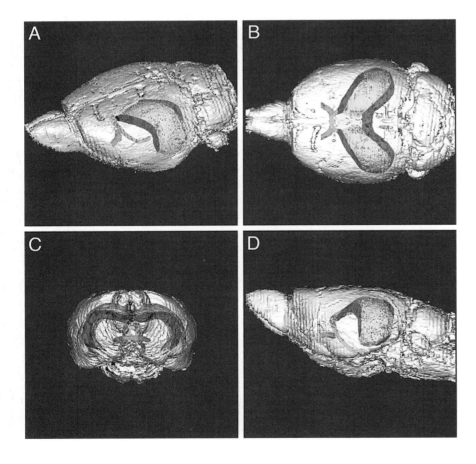

Figure 3–4. Major fiber systems of the rat hippocampal formation: angular bundle; fimbria-fornix; dorsal and central commissures.

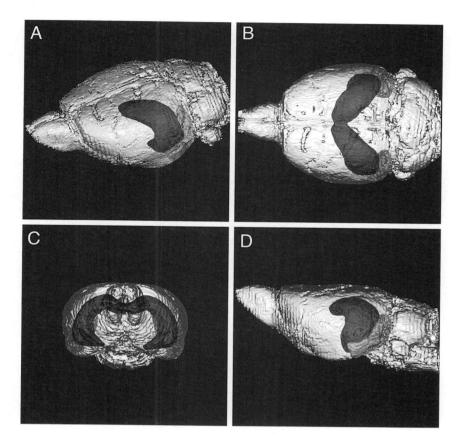

Figure 3–5. Magnetic resonance imaging of the rat brain shows the position of the hippocampus (dentate gyrus + hippocampus proper + subiculum) in red and the entorhinal cortex in green. *A.* Oblique view. *B.* Dorsal view. *C.* Frontal view. *D.* Lateral view. (*Source*: Courtesy of Dr. G. Allan Johnson, Center for In Vivo Microscopy, Duke University.)

Figure 3–6. Magnetic resonance imaging of the monkey brain shows the position of the hippocampus (dentate gyrus + hippocampus proper + subiculum) in red and the entorhinal cortex in green. *A.* Oblique view. *B.* Dorsal view. *C.* Frontal view. *D.* Lateral view.

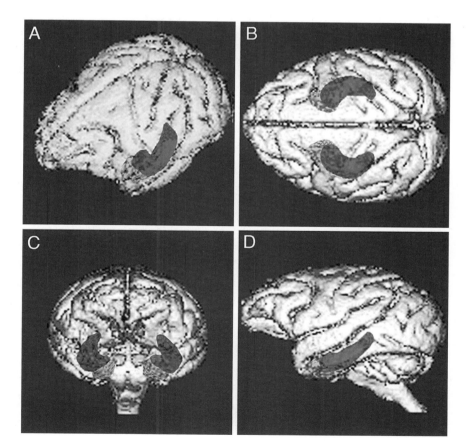

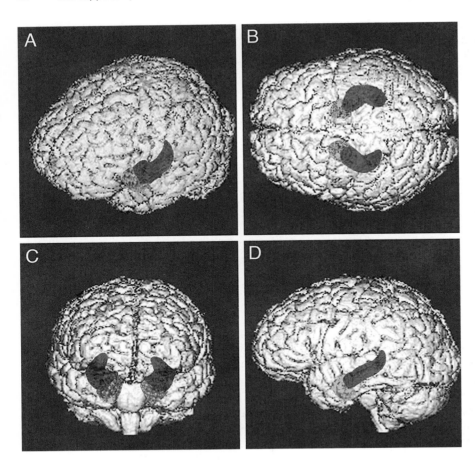

Figure 3–7. Magnetic resonance imaging of the human brain shows the position of the hippocampus (dentate gyrus + hippocampus proper + subiculum) in red and the entorhinal cortex in green. *A.* Oblique view. *B.* Dorsal view. *C.* Frontal view. *D.* Lateral view.

Figure 3–8. Line drawing of the rat brain shows the septotemporal and transverse axes of the hippocampal formation.

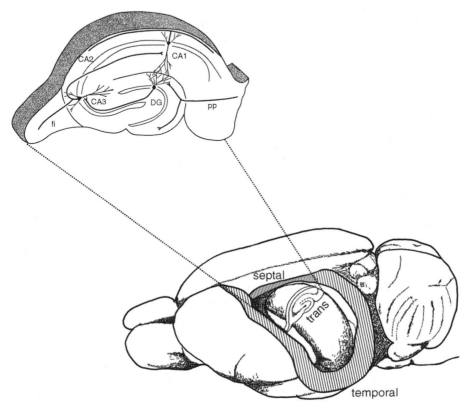

from the perirhinal and postrhinal cortices dorsally. At rostral levels, however, the perirhinal cortex extends somewhat ventral to the rhinal sulcus, and at caudal levels the entorhinal cortex extends just slightly dorsal to the rhinal sulcus.

3.3.2 Major Fiber Systems of the Rat Hippocampal Formation

Angular Bundle

A major fiber pathway associated with the hippocampal formation is the angular bundle, a fiber bundle interposed between the entorhinal cortex and the presubiculum and parasubiculum. The angular bundle is the main route taken by fibers originating from the ventrally situated entorhinal cortex as they travel to all septotemporal levels of the other hippocampal fields, particularly the dentate gyrus, hippocampus, and subiculum. In addition, the angular bundle contains commissural fibers of entorhinal and presubicular origin and fibers to and from a variety of cortical and subcortical structures that are interconnected with the entorhinal cortex.

The perforant path comprises the efferent entorhinal projections that traverse, or perforate, the subiculum on their way to the dentate gyrus and the hippocampus. This is the main route by which neocortical inputs reach the dentate gyrus and the hippocampus. We present a more detailed description of the perforant path in the discussion of the inputs to the dentate gyrus and the connectivity of the entorhinal cortex.

Entorhinal fibers also reach the hippocampus via the alveus, the temporoammonic alvear pathway first described by Cajal. At temporal levels, most of the entorhinal fibers reach the CA1 field of the hippocampus after perforating the subiculum (via the classic perforant pathway). At more septal levels, the number of entorhinal fibers that take the alvear pathway increases (Deller et al., 1996). In fact, in the septal portion of the hippocampal formation, most of the entorhinal fibers to CA1 reach this subfield via the alveus. These fibers make sharp right-angle turns in the alveus, perforate the pyramidal cell layer, and finally terminate in the stratum lacunosum-moleculare. The alveus is therefore also a major route by which entorhinal fibers reach their targets in CA1.

Fimbria-Fornix Pathway

The fimbria-fornix fiber system provides the major conduit for subcortical afferent and efferent connections (Daitz and Powell, 1954; Powell et al., 1957). It is perhaps easiest to understand the fimbria-fornix system by analogy with the corticospinal fiber system. The corticospinal fibers are given different names at different points on their journey from the motor cortex to the spinal cord. Similarly, the subcortical afferent and efferent fibers of the hippocampal formation are given different names at different points in their trajectory from or toward the forebrain or brain stem. Because of this, and because the exact transition between fimbria and fornix is difficult to define, some hippocampal researchers use the term fimbria-fornix to emphasize the continuity of fibers in these bundles.

The ventricular, or deep, surface of the hippocampus is covered by a thin sheet of myelinated fibers called the alveus. These fibers form a white sheet overlying the hippocampus that can be clearly seen when the overlying neocortex is aspirated. The alveus is a complex fiber system with both extrinsic afferent and efferent fibers, and fibers forming part of the intrahippocampal network travel within it (i.e., the entorhinal–CA1 alvear pathway, the CA1–subiculum projection, and the CA1–entorhinal projection). Some alvear fibers originate from the pyramidal cells of the hippocampus and subiculum and are en route to subcortical termination sites (Meibach and Siegel, 1975). At temporal levels of the hippocampal formation, the subcortically directed output fibers extend obliquely in the alveus, from medial to lateral, over the surface of the hippocampus and collect in a bundle called the fimbria (from the Latin word for fringe), which becomes progressively thicker as it progresses from the temporal to the septal level (i.e., as axons from more septally located pyramidal cells are added to the bundle). The rat fimbria has a flattened appearance, contains approximately 900,000 axons, and is situated along the lateral and rostral aspects of the hippocampus. The fibers of the fimbria are not randomly distributed but are organized in a topographic fashion (Wyss et al., 1980). Axons located medially in the fimbria (i.e., those closest to the hippocampus) tend to arise from more septal levels, whereas those located laterally arise from more temporal levels. Fibers from the subiculum are situated deeper to those from the hippocampus.

The fornix is the continuation of this bundle of hippocampal output fibers to the subcortical target structures; it forms a flattened bundle located just below the corpus callosum very close to the midline (fornix is the Latin word for arch, which is the shape of this tract over the diencephalon). Both fimbria and fornix carry fibers from the hippocampus and subiculum; the fornix, however, carries fibers primarily from the septal third of these structures. As the fibers of the fimbria leave the hippocampus and descend into the forebrain, they are referred to as the columns of the fornix. The fornix splits around the anterior commissure to form a rostrally directed precommissural fornix, which innervates the septal nuclei and nucleus accumbens, and a caudally directed postcommissural fornix, which extends toward the diencephalon. As the postcommissural fornix begins its course into the diencephalon (ultimately reaching the mammillary nuclei of the posterior hypothalamus), two smaller bundles split off. One, the medial corticohypothalamic tract, innervates a number of anterior hypothalamic areas. The other, called the subiculothalamic tract, carries fibers to the anterior thalamic nuclei (Swanson and Cowan 1975; Canteras and Swanson, 1992).

The fimbria and fornix also carry fibers that are traveling to the hippocampal formation. Many of the subcortical inputs to the hippocampal formation, including those from the septal nuclei (to the septal portion of the hippocampal formation), the locus coeruleus, and the raphe nuclei enter via the fimbria-fornix pathway. Some subcortical structures have projections that follow other pathways into the hippocampal formation. Fibers from the anterior thalamus, for example, travel through the thalamic radiations and supracallosal stria to innervate the presubiculum. Still other subcortical projections, particularly those from the amygdala, travel to the hippocampal formation via the external capsule.

Dorsal and Ventral Hippocampal Commissures

A third major fiber system associated with the hippocampal formation is the commissural system (Blackstad, 1956; Raisman et al., 1965; Laatsch and Cowan, 1967; Laurberg, 1979). In the rat, there are both dorsal and ventral commissures. Some 350,000 fibers cross the midline in the ventral hippocampal commissure, which is located just caudal to the septal area and dorsocaudal to the anterior commissure. Many of these fibers are true commissural fibers and are directed to both homotopic and heterotopic fields in the contralateral hippocampal formation. A much smaller number of fibers are directed into the contralateral descending column of the fornix and ultimately innervate the same structures on the contralateral side of the brain that receive the ipsilateral pre- and postcommissural fornix. The dorsal hippocampal commissure crosses the midline just rostral to the splenium (posterior part) of the corpus callosum and carries fibers mainly originating from or projecting to the presubiculum and entorhinal cortex. The dorsal hippocampal commissure is the route by which the presubiculum contributes a major projection to the contralateral entorhinal cortex.

3.3.3 Monkey Hippocampal Formation

The first point we address in this section is how the appearance and position of the nonhuman primate hippocampal formation differs from that of the rat. Much of the work on the monkey hippocampal formation has been carried out in Old World monkeys, primarily the macaque monkey. The description we provide here is for the hippocampal formation of typical research monkeys, such as *Macaca fascicularis* and *Macaca mulatta* (cynomolgus and rhesus macaque monkeys, respectively). The hippocampal formation in the macaque monkey is not nearly as C-shaped in its long axis as it is in the rat. It lies almost horizontally in the temporal lobe; and, as in the human, it makes up the major portion of the floor of the temporal horn of the fourth ventricle. The major determinant of the change in position of the primate hippocampal formation is the massive development of the associational cortices of the frontal and temporal lobes. As a result of the caudal and ventral transposition of the temporal lobes that takes place developmentally to accommodate the larger cortical surface, the primate hippocampal formation comes to lie almost entirely within the medial temporal lobe. Because of the ventrorostral rotation of the monkey hippocampal formation, the homologue of the temporal pole of the rat hippocampal formation is located rostrally in the monkey brain, and the equivalent of the septal pole of the rat hippocampal formation

is located caudally. Because the term septotemporal is not appropriate for the monkey hippocampal formation (no portion of it approaches the septal area), it is more common to refer to the long axis in the primate as the rostrocaudal axis. The orthogonal axis, however, is still referred to as the transverse axis.

Two additional points should be made about the position of the monkey hippocampal formation. First, at the rostral limit of the lateral ventricle, some fields of the monkey hippocampal formation flex medially and then caudally. This is the monkey homologue of the pes hippocampi that is so prominent in the human brain. At the rostral levels where this flexure occurs, there are two representations of the hippocampal formation in standard coronal views of the brain. It is difficult in this flexed region of the monkey hippocampal formation, when viewed in standard coronal, Nissl-stained sections, to specify the identity and borders of the subdivisions of the hippocampal formation. The most medial and caudal portion of the hippocampal formation (i.e., the part that is bent backward) is the actual "rostral" pole of the monkey hippocampal formation, even though it is physically located somewhat caudal to the rostral extreme of the hippocampal formation. To make reference to different portions of the monkey hippocampal formation, we call the medial portion of the hippocampal formation the uncal region (because it forms much of the medially situated bulge that in the human would be called the uncus). The flexed, rostrally located portion that runs mediolaterally is called the genu; and the laterally situated, main portion of the hippocampus is the body.

The second point to note is that the monkey entorhinal cortex is physically associated with only the rostral portion of the other hippocampal fields. The entorhinal cortex extends caudally just to the level of the lateral geniculate nucleus, whereas the dentate gyrus, hippocampus, and subiculum extend well caudal to this level. It is equally important to point out that the rostral half of the entorhinal cortex extends beyond the rostral limit of the other hippocampal fields, where it is located ventromedial to the amygdaloid complex. Throughout virtually all of its rostrocaudal extent, the lateral border of the entorhinal cortex is at the rhinal sulcus, as in the rat.

The fiber bundles of the monkey hippocampal formation are fundamentally similar to those in the rat, although there are a number of minor differences. First, the fimbria is located dorsomedially in the monkey rather than ventrolaterally as in the rat (Fig. 3–2). Second, the fimbria leaves the substance of the hippocampal formation at a point near the splenium of the corpus callosum. Thus, the compact bundle of fibers that is called the body of the fornix travels rostrally as a pendulous, flattened cable hanging under the corpus callosum. Upon reaching the level of the anterior commissure, the bundle descends as the columns of the fornix and follows the same trajectories outlined for the rat. Third, the ventral and dorsal hippocampal commissures are relatively less prominent in the monkey than in the rat, reflecting the more restricted commissural connections observed in the monkey brain (Amaral et al., 1984; Demeter et al., 1985). The more prominent of the two commissures in the monkey is the dorsal hippocampal commissure. It carries fibers from the presubiculum and entorhinal cortex to the contralateral side; it also carries fibers originating in the parahippocampal cortex.

The subdivision of the hippocampal formation into various regions is fundamentally the same in rat and monkey brains. There are, however, substantial species differences in certain subregions, especially CA1 and the entorhinal cortex, which are addressed in greater detail later in the chapter.

3.3.4 Human Hippocampal Formation

The three-dimensional position of the human hippocampal formation is similar to that in the macaque monkey brain (Figs. 3–6 and 3–7, respectively). However, owing to the larger development of the temporal association cortex, in particular that of the entorhinal and perirhinal cortices, the structure of the ventromedial surface of the brain, including the gyral patterns, is substantially different in the human and monkey brains. After a brief summary of the gross anatomical attributes of the main or intraventricular portions of the human hippocampal formation, we review some of the differences of the associated cortical regions.

The classic gross anatomical image of the human hippocampal formation is of a prominent bulge in the floor of the temporal horn of the lateral ventricle (Fig. 3–3). As in the monkey, this portion of the hippocampal formation is widest at its rostral extent where the structure bends toward the medial surface of the brain. In this area, two to five subtle gyri, or digitationes hippocampi, form the pes hippocampi (Gertz et al., 1972). The substance of the pes hippocampi is formed by several of the hippocampal fields, and the constituents differ at different rostrocaudal levels (see below). Continuing caudally from the pes hippocampi, the main body of the hippocampus gets progressively thinner as it bends dorsally toward the splenium of the corpus callosum.

The fimbria is situated on the medial surface of the human hippocampus, as in the monkey (Fig. 3–2). At rostral levels, the fimbria is thin and flat but becomes progressively thicker caudally as fibers are continually added to it. As the fimbria leaves the caudal extent of the hippocampus, it fuses with the ventral surface of the corpus callosum and travels rostrally in the lateral ventricle. The portion of these fimbrial fibers located between the caudal limit of the hippocampal formation and the fusion with the corpus callosum is called the crus of the fornix, whereas the major portion of the rostrally directed fiber bundle is, as in the monkey, called the body of the fornix. At the end of its rostral trajectory, the body of the fornix descends as the columns of the fornix. At about the point where the fimbria fuses with the posterior portion of the corpus callosum, fibers extend across the midline to form the hippocampal commissure. A variety of gross anatomical terms have been applied to this commissure, but the term psalterium (alluding to a harp-like stringed instrument) is most common. As noted previously, the primate hippocampal commissural connections are much more limited than in the rodent; and as suggested by stereotaxic depth

encephalography, there is almost no commissural interaction between the hippocampal formations located on each side of the human brain (Wilson et al., 1987).

The ventral surface of the human temporal lobe is demarcated into mediolateral strips by two prominent rostrocaudally oriented sulci (Figs. 3–9 and 3–10). The more lateral of the two is the occipitotemporal sulcus, which is often broken by small, transverse gyri. The more medial of the sulci, and the one that is more closely associated with the hippocampal formation, is the collateral sulcus. The collateral sulcus is often continuous with the rostrally situated rhinal sulcus. Unlike the situation in the rat and the monkey, however, the rhinal sulcus is relatively insignificant in the human brain and is associated only with the most rostral portion of the entorhinal cortex. It is thus not a useful border for the lateral boundary of the entorhinal cortex.

The collateral sulcus forms most of the lateral border of what has classically been termed the parahippocampal gyrus. The parahippocampal gyrus is a complex region that contains a number of distinct cytoarchitectonic fields and has been defined in different ways by different authors. In recent years, the parahippocampal gyrus has often been broken up into an anterior part, which comprises mainly the entorhinal cortex and associated perirhinal cortex, and a posterior part, which includes the areas TF and TH of Von Economo (1929).

Unlike the situation in the monkey, where the rhinal sulcus forms a reasonably reliable lateral border for the entorhinal cortex, the collateral sulcus does not provide a discrete lateral boundary for the human entorhinal cortex. The entorhinal cortex actually ends approximately midway along the medial bank of the collateral sulcus. The two fields of the perirhinal cortex, areas 35 and 36 of Brodmann (1909), form the remainder of the medial bank, fundus, and a portion of the lateral bank of the collateral sulcus. The perirhinal cortex is massively enlarged in the human brain and may account, in part, for the prominence of the collateral sulcus. The border zone between the entorhinal cortex and the perirhinal cortex was called the trans-entorhinal zone by Braak (1972, 1980). In this region, neuroanatomical markers that label layer II of the entorhinal cortex demonstrate an oblique band of labeled cells, which makes it appear that layer II is diving underneath the layers of the perirhinal cortex. Because the perirhinal cortex terminates at a variable point along the lateral bank of the collateral sulcus, it is extremely difficult to define the borders of the entorhinal and perirhinal cortices using imaging modalities such as magnetic resonance imaging. The only way it is currently possible to define the border of these fields accurately is through histological analysis.

Interestingly, much of the areal extent of the human entorhinal cortex (at least the rostral portions) can be visually identified on the surface of the brain by the conspicuous bumps, named verrucae (latin for warts), that mark its pial surface. These bumps mark the islands of cells that constitute layer II of the entorhinal cortex. The dorsomedial aspect of the entorhinal cortex is marked by a conspicuous mound, or secondary gyrus, referred to as the gyrus ambiens (Fig. 3–10). The dorsomedial limit of the entorhinal cortex with the amyg-

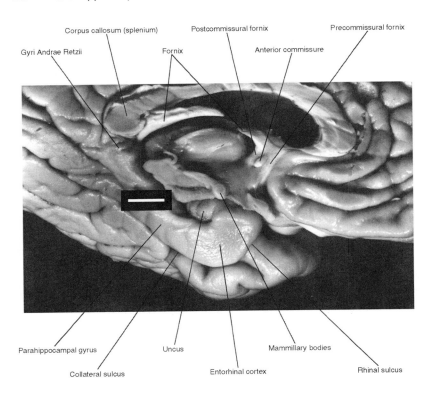

Corpus callosum (splenium)   Postcommissural fornix   Precommissural fornix
Gyri Andrae Retzii   Fornix   Anterior commissure

Parahippocampal gyrus   Uncus   Mammillary bodies
Collateral sulcus   Entorhinal cortex   Rhinal sulcus

Figure 3–9. Ventromedial view of the human temporal lobe. Bar = 1 cm.

daloid complex is marked by the shallow sulcus semiannularis, which is located dorsal to the gyrus ambiens.

There is a series of prominent bulges on the medial surface of the hemisphere just caudal to the dorsomedial portion of the entorhinal cortex; this is generally labeled the uncus

(or hook) in gross anatomical descriptions (Fig. 3–9). The most rostral of the uncal bulges is often separately labeled the gyrus uncinatus. Histological sections through the gyrus uncinatus indicate that it is made up of the amygdalohippocampal region (of the amygdaloid complex) and the

Figure 3–10. Ventral surface of the human brain after the brain stem and cerebellum have been removed. Bar = 1 cm.

Uncus   Mammillary bodies   Collateral sulcus
Parahippocampal gyrus   Corpus callosum (splenium)   Intrarhinal sulcus

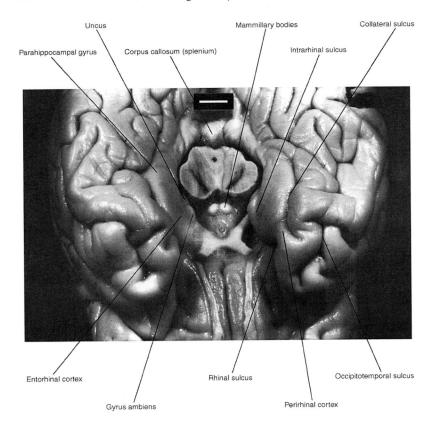

Entorhinal cortex   Rhinal sulcus   Occipitotemporal sulcus
Gyrus ambiens   Perirhinal cortex

transition zone between the amygdala and hippocampus. The middle bulge, called the band of Giacomini, is generally composed of the most medial part of the dentate gyrus. The most caudal of the uncal bulges, called the intralimbic gyrus, is composed mainly of a portion of the CA3 field of the hippocampus.

As the parahippocampal gyrus meets the retrosplenial region caudally, a group of small bumps known as the gyri Andreae Retzii are seen on the medial surface of the brain (Fig. 3–9). This irregular region of human cortex marks the caudal limit of the hippocampal formation and is composed principally of CA1 and the subiculum. Two obliquely oriented small gyri located deep to the gyri Andreae Retzii are called the fasciola cinerea (which corresponds to the caudalmost part of the dentate gyrus) and the gyrus fasciolaris (which corresponds to the caudal pole of the CA3 field). A thin remnant of the hippocampal formation surrounds the splenium of the corpus callosum and ascends dorsally over the corpus callosum to form the induseum griseum (or supracommissural hippocampal formation), which comprises remnants of the subiculum and other fields of the hippocampal formation.

3.4 Neuroanatomy of the Rat Hippocampal Formation

We have now concluded our overview of the gross or three-dimensional organization of the rat, monkey, and human hippocampal formations. In the sections that follow, we review the neuroanatomical organization of each of the fields of the hippocampal formation of the rat, beginning with the dentate gyrus and ending with the entorhinal cortex. In each section, we describe the cytoarchitectonic organization followed by a summary of the resident neurons and finally a survey of the pattern of intrinsic and extrinsic connections. The amount of information available for each of the cytoarchitectonic fields of the hippocampal formation varies substantially. The most detailed anatomical information is available for the dentate gyrus, perhaps because it is the simplest of the hippocampal fields. For this reason and because the dentate gyrus is the first structure to receive direct entorhinal input and does not project outside the hippocampal formation, we begin our description here. We then progress through the hippocampus and other hippocampal fields.

We have prepared a series of illustrations to demonstrate the cytoarchitectonic organization of the rat hippocampal formation (Figs. 3–11 through 3–14). The first figure (Fig. 3–11) is a photomicrograph of a section cut in the horizontal plane. This plane has the advantage of illustrating all components of the rat hippocampal formation. A Nissl-stained section is shown at the top, and a Timm's sulfide silver section is shown at the bottom. The latter has been used extensively for highlighting various fiber and terminal systems in the hippocampal formation. After Figure 3–11, we provide images of

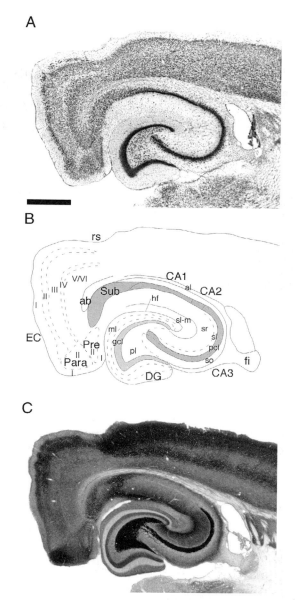

Figure 3–11. Horizontal section through the rat hippocampal formation. *A.* Nissl-stained section. *B.* Line drawing shows the various regions, layers, and fiber pathways. *C.* Timm's sulfide silver-stained section. Note the three bands of the molecular layer of the dentate gyrus in *C.* The outer band corresponds to the terminal zone of the lateral perforant pathway; the middle unstained region corresponds to the terminal zone of the medial peforant pathway; the inner band corresponds to the zone of termination of the associational and commissural pathways of the dentate gyrus. ab, angular bundle; al, alveus; CA1, CA1 field of the hippocampus; CA2, CA2 field of the hippocampus; CA3, CA3 field of the hippocampus; DG, dentate gyrus; EC, entorhinal cortex; fi, fimbria; gcl, granule cell layer of the dentate gyrus; hf, hippocampal fissure; ml, molecular layer of the dentate gyrus; Para, parasubiculum; pcl, pyramidal cell layer of the hippocampus; pl, polymorphic layer of the dentate gyrus; Pre, presubiculum; sl, stratum lucidum of CA3; sr, stratum radiatum of the hippocampus; sl-m, stratum lacunosum moleculare of the hippocampus. Roman numerals: cortical layers. Bar in A = 500 μm and applies to all panels.

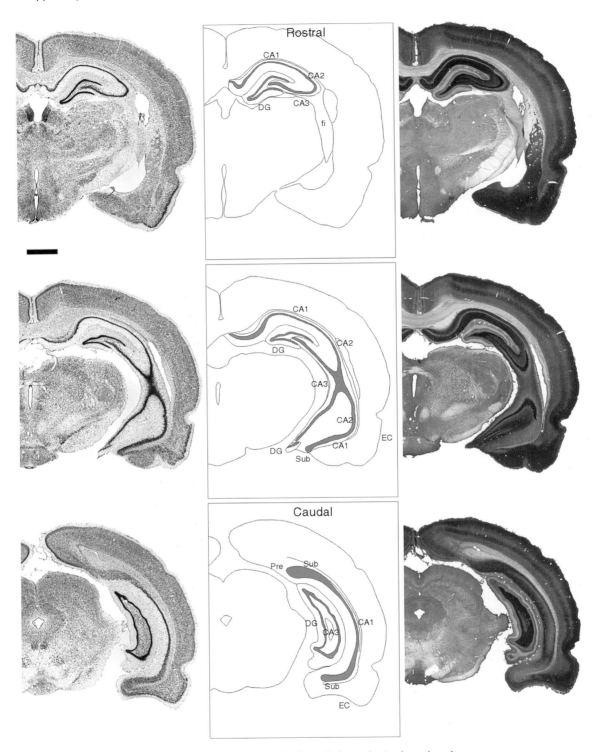

Figure 3–12. Coronal sections at three rostrocaudal levels through the rat brain show the relative position of the hippocampal formation. The three panels on the left are Nissl-stained sections; the three panels on the right are adjacent sections stained with Timm's sulfide silver stain; the line drawings (middle column) highlight the regions of the rat hippocampal formation seen in the stained sections. For abbreviations see Figure 3–11. Bar = 1 mm.

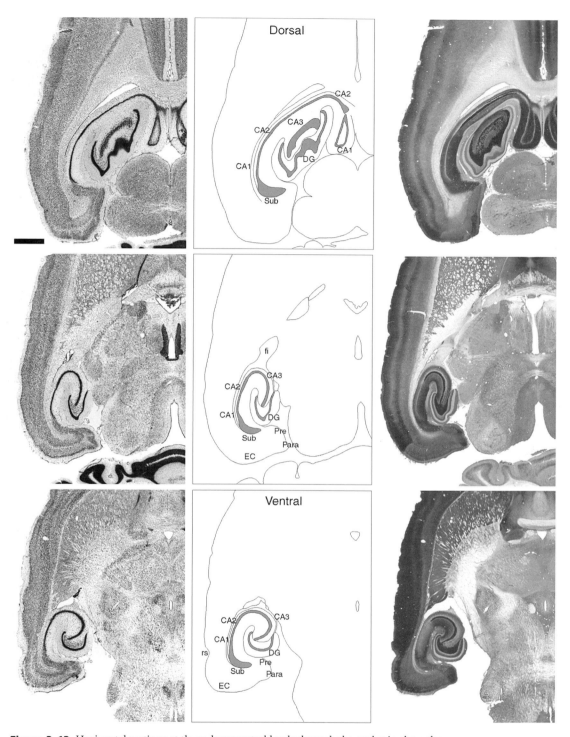

Figure 3–13. Horizontal sections at three dorsoventral levels through the rat brain show the relative position of the hippocampal formation. The three panels on the left are Nissl-stained sections; the three panels on the right are adjacent sections stained with Timm's sulfide silver stain; the line drawings (middle column) highlight the regions of the rat hippocampal formation seen in the stained sections. For abbreviations see Figure 3–11. Bar = 1 mm.

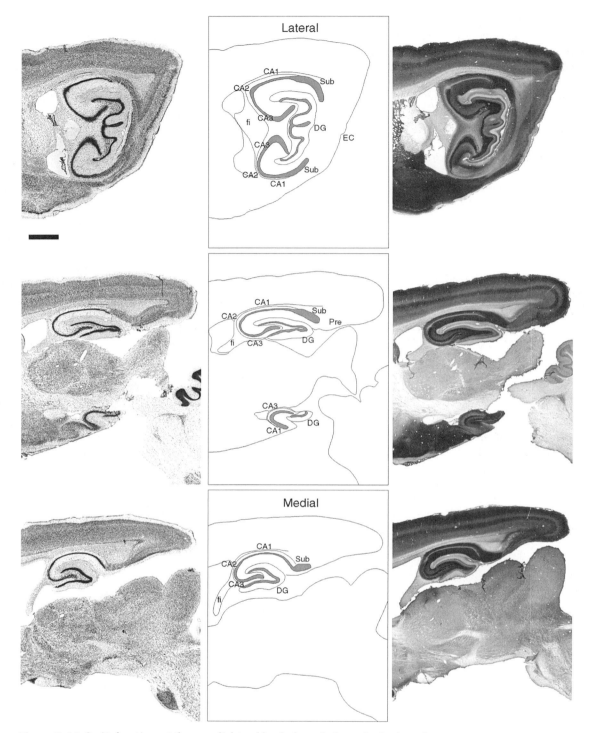

Figure 3–14. Sagittal sections at three mediolateral levels through the rat brain show the relative position of the hippocampal formation. The three panels on the left are Nissl-stained sections; the three panels on the right are adjacent sections stained with Timm's sulfide silver stain; the line drawings (middle column) highlight the regions of the rat hippocampal formation seen in the stained sections. For abbreviations see Figure 3–11. Bar = 1 mm.

similar stains of coronal (Figure 3–12), horizontal (Fig. 3–13), and sagittal (Fig. 3–14) sections through different levels of the hippocampal formation. Finally, we must point out that to keep this chapter readable we have used citations sparingly. Detailed references for the information provided in this chapter can be found in Witter and Amaral (2004).

3.4.1 Dentate Gyrus

Cytoarchitectonic Organization

The dentate gyrus is comprised of three layers. Superficially, closest to the hippocampal fissure is a relatively cell-free layer called the molecular layer. In the rat, this layer has an average thickness of approximately 250 μm. The principal cell layer (granule cell layer) lies deep to the molecular layer and is made up of a densely packed layer that is four to eight granule cells thick. The granule cell and molecular layers (which together are sometimes referred to as the fascia dentata) form a V- or U-shaped structure (depending on the septotemporal position) that encloses a cellular region, the polymorphic cell layer, which constitutes the third layer of the dentate gyrus (Fig. 3–11).

Neuron Types

Dentate Granule Cell

The principal cell type of the dentate gyrus is the granule cell (Figs. 3–15 and 3–16) The dentate granule cell has an elliptical cell body with a width of approximately 10 μm and a height of 18 μm (Claiborne et al., 1990). Each cell is closely apposed to other granule cells, and in most cases there is no glial sheath intervening between the cells. The granule cell has a characteristic cone-shaped tree of spiny dendrites with all the branches directed toward the superficial portion of the molecular layer; most of the distal tips of the dendritic tree end just at the hippocampal fissure or at the ventricular surface. The dendritic trees of granule cells located in the suprapyramidal blade tend, on average, to be larger than those of cells located in the infrapyramidal blade (3500 μm vs. 2800 μm). Desmond and colleagues (Desmond and Levy, 1985) provided estimates for the number of dendritic spines on the granule cell dendrites. They found that cells in the suprapyramidal blade have 1.6 spines/μm, whereas cells in the infrapyramidal blade have 1.3 spines/μm. With these numbers and the mean dendritic lengths given above, an estimate of the number of spines on the average suprapyramidal granule cell would be 5600 and for an infrapyramidal cell 3640.

The total number of granule cells in one dentate gyrus of the rat is about 1.2×10^6 (West et al., 1991; Rapp and Gallagher, 1996). Although cell proliferation and neurogenesis in the dentate gyrus persist into adulthood and appear to be under environmental control, modern stereological studies have shown that the total number of granule cells does not vary in adult animals (Rapp and Gallagher, 1996). Only infant and juvenile mice exposed to running wheels or socially complex, "enriched" environments demonstrate a larger dentate gyrus and a greater number of granule cells that persist into adulthood than animals raised in standard laboratory cages (Kempermann et al., 1997). Similar manipulations performed in adult animals can affect cell proliferation and/or survival of newly generated neurons, but they have no significant impact on the volume of the dentate gyrus or the total number of granule cells (Kempermann et al., 1998).

Before leaving the topic of granule cell number, we should note that the packing density and thickness of the granule cell layers varies somewhat along the septotemporal axis of the dentate gyrus (Gaarskjaer, 1978a). The packing density of

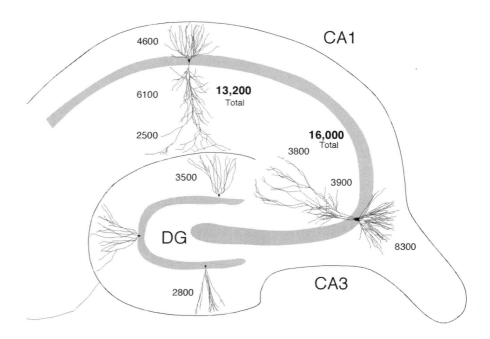

Figure 3–15. Dendritic arborization of the principal cells in the rat dentate gyrus (granule cells) and hippocampus proper (pyramidal cells). See the text for details.

Granule cell

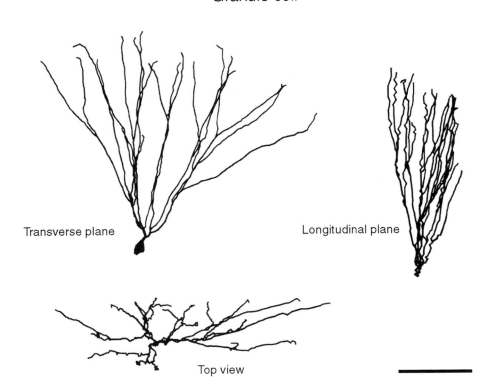

Transverse plane

Longitudinal plane

Top view

Figure 3–16. Dendritic organization of dentate granule cells. Computer-generated reconstructions of horseradish peroxidase (HRP)-filled granule cells from the suprapyramidal blade. Bar = 100 μm. (*Source*: Adapted from Claiborne et al., 1990.)

granule cells is higher septally than temporally. Because the packing density of CA3 pyramidal cells follows an inverse gradient, the net result is that at septal levels of the hippocampal formation the ratio of granule cells to CA3 pyramidal cells is something on the order of 12:1, whereas at the temporal pole the ratio drops to 2:3. Because the CA3 pyramidal cells are the major recipients of granule cell innervation and the number of mossy fiber synapses is roughly the same along the septotemporal axis, contact probability is much lower septally than temporally.

The granule cell is the only "principal" cell of the dentate gyrus; that is, it is the only cell type that gives rise to axons that leave the dentate gyrus to innervate another hippocampal field (i.e., CA3). There is one type of neuron, called the mossy cell, whose axon leaves the dentate gyrus of one side of the brain only to innervate the dentate gyrus of the other side. There are numerous other types of neuron, most of which are inhibitory interneurons. We describe them in turn.

Pyramidal Basket Cell
The most intensively studied interneuron is the pyramidal basket cell (Fig. 3–17). These cells are generally located along the deep surface of the granule cell layer. They have pyramid-shaped cell bodies 25 to 35 μm in diameter and are wedged slightly into the granule cell layer. The basket portion of the name refers to the fact that the axon of these cells forms pericellular plexuses that surround and form synapses with the cell bodies of granule cells. Ramon y Cajal first described the pyramidal basket cells as having a single, principal aspiny api-

cal dendrite directed into the molecular layer (where it divides into several aspiny branches) and several principal basal dendrites that ramify and extend into the polymorphic cell layer. Most of these cells contain biochemical markers for the inhibitory transmitter γ-aminobutyric acid (GABA) and are thus presumably inhibitory (Ribak et al., 1978; Ribak and Seress, 1983). The number of basket cells is not constant throughout the transverse or septotemporal extents of the dentate gyrus (Seress and Pokorny, 1981). At septal levels, the ratio of basket cells to granule cells is 1:100 in the suprapyramidal blade and 1:180 in the infrapyramidal blade. At temporal levels, the number is 1:150 for the suprapyramidal blade and 1:300 for the infrapyramidal blade. These data raise a theme that is repeated throughout the chapter: that despite the apparent cytoarchitectonic homogeneity of the hippocampal fields, there are several differences (especially regarding neurochemical innervation) at different septotemporal levels of the hippocampal formation.

Other Interneurons
There has been an explosion in the number of interneurons identified in the rat hippocampal formation. A detailed overview of the characteristics of the various hippocampal interneurons has been published by Freund and Buzsaki (1996). Hippocampal interneurons, which form a heterogeneous population, are designed to carry out different functions. Many of the cell types can be distinguished on the basis of the distribution of their axonal plexus. Some have axons that terminate on cell bodies, whereas others have axons that

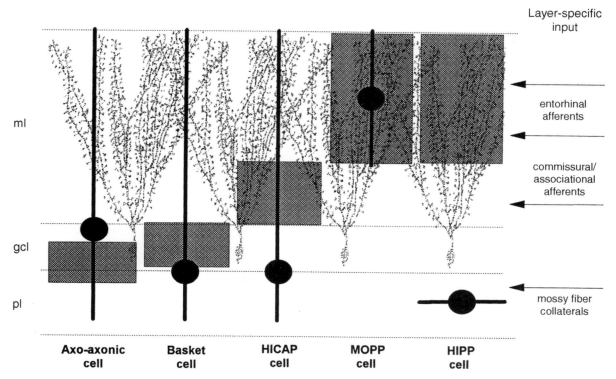

Layer-specific
input

ml

→ entorhinal
afferents

→ commissural/
associational
afferents

gcl

pl

→ mossy fiber
collaterals

| **Axo-axonic cell** | **Basket cell** | **HICAP cell** | **MOPP cell** | **HIPP cell** |

Figure 3–17. Morphological classification of the interneurons of the rat dentate gyrus. Filled circles indicate the location of the cell bodies, and thick lines indicate the predominant orientation and laminar distribution of the dendritic tree. The dentate granule cells (principal neurons) are illustrated in the background, providing an indication of which domain is innervated by which interneuron groups. The laminar distribution of various inputs, often showing correspondence with the interneuron type or axon distribution, is also indicated. (*Source*: Adapted from Freund and Buzsaki, 1996.)

terminate exclusively on the initial segments of other axons. Interneurons have also been distinguished on the basis of their inputs. Some are preferentially innervated (e.g., by the serotonergic fibers originating from the raphe nuclei). Interneurons can also be differentiated from principal cells on the basis of their electrophysiological characteristics. At least some interneurons have high rates of spontaneous activity and fire in relation to the theta rhythm. For this reason, interneurons are often called theta cells (see Chapter 11). A major challenge is to determine if different classes of interneurons demonstrate distinct electrophysiological response profiles.

Within the same subgranular region occupied by the cell bodies of the pyramidal basket cells are several other cell types with distinctly different somal shapes, as well as different dendritic and axonal configurations (Amaral, 1978). Some of these cells are multipolar with several aspiny dendrites entering the molecular and polymorphic layers, whereas others tend to be more fusiform-shaped with a similar dendritic distribution. As Ribak and colleagues pointed out, many of these cells share fine structural characteristics such as infolded nuclei, extensive perikaryal cytoplasm with large Nissl bodies, and intranuclear rods. Moreover, it appears that all of these cells give rise to axons that contribute to the basket plexus in the granule cell layer. Many of these neurons are immunore-

active for GABA. They form symmetrical synaptic contacts with the cell bodies, proximal dendrites, and occasionally axon initial segments of granule cells and therefore function as inhibitory interneurons. These cells are not neurochemically homogeneous, however, as subsets appear to colocalize distinct categories of other neuroactive substances.

Neurons of the Molecular Layer

The molecular layer is occupied primarily by dendrites of the granule, basket, and polymorphic cells as well as axons and terminal axonal arbors from the entorhinal cortex and other sources. At least two neuron types are also present in the molecular layer. The first is located deep in the molecular layer, has a multipolar or triangular cell body, and gives rise to an axon that produces a substantial terminal plexus largely limited to the outer two-thirds of the molecular layer. This neuron, which has aspiny dendrites that remain mainly within the molecular layer, has been called the MOPP cell (molecular layer perforant path-associated cell). This terminology was proposed by Han et al. (1993) to bring some order to naming interneurons in the hippocampal formation. The lettering system refers to the location of the cell body and to the region where the axon is distributed.

Frotscher and colleagues described a second type of neuron in the molecular layer that resembles the so-called chandelier, or axo-axonic, cell originally found in the neocortex (Soriano and Frotscher, 1989). These cells are generally located immediately adjacent to or even within the superficial portion of the granule cell layer. The axo-axonic cell is named for the fact that its axon descends from the molecular layer into the granule cell layer, collateralizes profusely, and then terminates, with symmetrical synaptic contacts, exclusively on the axon initial segments of granule cells. Thus, their shape resembles that of a chandelier. Each axo-axonic cell may innervate the axon initial segments of as many as 1000 granule cells. Because these cells are immunoreactive for markers of GABAergic neurons and make symmetrical synapses, it is likely that they provide a second means of inhibitory control of granule cell output. The inputs to the axo-axonic cells are currently unknown although their dendrites remain mainly in the molecular layer, where they are likely to receive perforant path input from the entorhinal cortex.

Other neurons with cell bodies located in the molecular layer are members of the IS (interneuron-specific) class of interneuron, which are specialized for termination on other interneurons. These IS neurons are demonstrated using immunohistochemistry for vasoactive intestinal peptide (VIP), and their axons overlap with the dendrites of the O-LM and HIPP cells (these cell types are defined shortly).

Neurons of the Polymorphic Cell Layer

The polymorphic layer harbors a variety of neuron types, but little is known about many of them (Amaral, 1978). The most common type, and certainly the most impressive, is the mossy cell (Fig. 3–18). This cell type is probably what Ramon y Cajal referred to as the "stellate or triangular" cells located in his subzone of fusiform cells; and it is undoubtedly what Lorente de Nó referred to as "modified pyramids." The cell bodies of the mossy cells are large (25–35 μm) and are often triangular or multipolar in shape. Three or more thick dendrites originate from the cell body and extend for long distances in the polymorphic layer. Each principal dendrite bifurcates once or twice and generally gives rise to a few side branches. Although most of the daughter dendritic branches remain within the polymorphic layer, an occasional dendrite pierces the granule cell layer and enters the molecular layer. The mossy cell dendrites virtually never enter the adjacent CA3 field.

The most distinctive feature of the mossy cell is that all of its proximal dendrites are covered by large, complex spines evocatively called thorny excrescences. These spines are the distinctive sites of termination of the mossy fiber axons (i.e., axons of the dentate granule cells). Although thorny excrescences are also observed on the proximal dendrites of pyramidal cells in CA3, they are never as dense as the ones on the mossy cells. The distal dendrites of the mossy cell have typical pedunculate spines that appear to be less densely distributed than those on the distal dendrites of the pyramidal cells in the hippocampus. The mossy cells are immunoreactive for glutamate and give rise to axons that project to the inner third of the molecular layer of the ipsilateral and contralateral dentate gyrus, making asymmetrical terminations on the dendrites of granule cells. The mossy cells thus appear to be the major source of the excitatory associational/commissural projection to the dentate gyrus. For this reason, the mossy cell does not fit the classic description of an interneuron.

There are also a number of fusiform cells in the polymorphic layer. The main difference between the fusiform cell types is whether they have spines. One type, the long-spined multipolar cell first described by Amaral (1978), has recently been called the HIPP cell (hilar perforant path-associated cell). This cell type has two or three principal dendrites that originate from the poles of the cell, run mainly parallel to the granule cell layer, and can extend for nearly the entire transverse length of one blade of the granule cell layer. The conspicuous feature of this cell is the distribution of copious, long, often branched spines over its cell body and dendrites. Intracellular staining techniques demonstrate that these cells have axons that ascend into the outer two-thirds of the molecular layer (i.e., the perforant path zone) and terminate with symmetrical and presumably inhibitory synapses on the dendrites of granule cells. An amazing feature of these neurons is that their

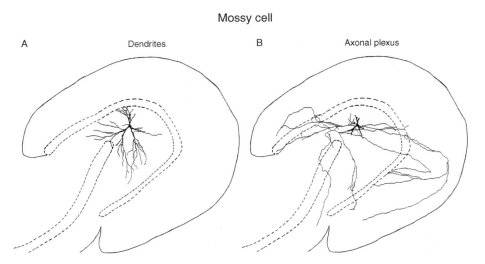

Mossy cell

A   Dendrites   B   Axonal plexus

Figure 3–18. Mossy cell of the polymorphic layer of the rat dentate gyrus. *A.* Camera lucida drawing of the soma and dendritic arbor. Note that the dendrites extend widely in the polymorphic layer but do not penetrate the granule cell layer. *B.* Camera lucida drawing of the soma and axonal plexus. The axon ramifies throughout the polymorphic layer and enters the dentate granule cell layer at considerable distances from the soma. A single collateral projects through the CA3 cell body layer and toward the fimbria. Bar = 100 μm. (*Source:* Adapted from Buckmaster et al., 1992.)

axonal plexus can extend for as much as 3.5 mm along the septotemporal axis of the dentate gyrus (the entire length of the dentate gyrus in the rat is only about 10 mm) and may generate as many as 100,000 synaptic terminals. Because inhibitory interneurons typically have aspiny dendrites and relatively local axonal plexuses, this long-spined multipolar HIPP cell is a highly atypical interneuron. At least some of these HIPP cells appear to correspond to the somatostatin/GABA cells that give rise to the somatostatin innervation of the outer portion of the molecular layer.

There are also multipolar or triangular cells in the polymorphic layer with thin, aspiny dendrites that extend within both the hilus and the molecular layer. The axons of these HICAP cells (hilar commissural-associational pathway-related cells) extend through the granule cell layer and branch profusely in the inner third of the molecular layer. A variety of other neuron types exist in the polymorphic layer of the dentate gyrus whose axonal plexus has not yet been well described.

Before leaving the typing of interneurons in the dentate gyrus, it is perhaps worth noting that the field has come a long way from believing that interneurons merely damp down neuronal activity. Rather, most current hippocampologists highlight the heterogeneity of interneurons and see them as integral components of normal information processing in the hippocampal formation.

Extrinsic Connections

Entorhinal Cortex Projection to the Dentate Gyrus

The dentate gyrus receives its major input from the entorhinal cortex via the so-called perforant pathway (Ramón y Cajal, 1893). The projection to the dentate gyrus arises mainly from cells located in layer II of the entorhinal cortex, although a minor component of the projection also comes from layers V and VI (Steward and Scoville, 1976). In the molecular layer of the dentate gyrus, the entorhinal terminals are strictly confined to the superficial (outer) two-thirds, where they form asymmetrical synapses that account for nearly 85% of the total axospinous terminations (Nafstad, 1967; Hjorth-Simonsen and Jeune, 1972). These contacts occur primarily on the dendritic spines of granule cells, although a small number of perforant path fibers also form asymmetrical synapses on the shafts of GABA-positive interneurons. The organization of the perforant path projection in the mouse is similar to that in the rat, although there are some detectable species differences, such as a paucity of commissural connections in the mouse (van Groen et al., 2002, 2003).

The perforant pathway can be divided into two parts based on the region of origin, pattern of termination, and appearance in histochemical and immunohistochemical preparations. In the rat, the two divisions have been called the lateral and medial perforant paths because they originate from the lateral and medial entorhinal areas, respectively. Perforant path fibers originating in the lateral entorhinal area terminate in the most superficial third of the molecular layer, whereas

the perforant path fibers originating from the medial entorhinal area terminate in the middle third of the molecular layer. These terminal zones are readily distinguished by the classic Timm's staining method for visualizing heavy metals; this method demonstrates dense staining in the outer third of the molecular layer, a near absence of staining in the middle third, and dark staining in the inner third that is associated with the commissural/associational connection (Fig. 3–11). Projections from both areas of the entorhinal cortex innervate the entire transverse extent of the molecular layer. The thin axon branches (0.1 μm) in the molecular layer of the dentate gyrus show periodic varicosities with a thickness of 0.5 to 1.0 μm. Most of entorhinal cortex layer II spiny stellate cells project up to 2 mm in the septotemporal direction, forming a sheet-like axon arbor in the molecular layer (Fig. 3–19) (Tamamaki and Nojyo, 1993). There is surprisingly little quantitative information about the termination of the perforant path projections.

Because the perforant path fibers terminate exclusively in the molecular layer, certain neurons of the dentate gyrus are not innervated by this input. Cells with dendrites confined to the polymorphic layer do not receive entorhinal input. The mossy cells, for example, are thus likely to receive little or no direct perforant path input.

It has often been assumed that the perforant path fibers from the entorhinal cortex are the only hippocampal input reaching the dentate gyrus, but it is now clear that at least a minor projection also arises in the presubiculum and parasubiculum (Kohler, 1985). These fibers enter the molecular layer of the dentate gyrus and ramify in a zone that is interspersed between the lateral and medial perforant path projections. The presubicular axons tend to be thicker than those from the entorhinal cortex and give rise to collaterals that take

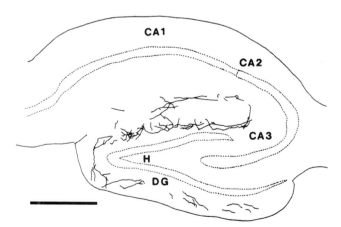

Figure 3–19. Perforant path projections. Distribution of labeled axon branches of a layer II spiny stellate neuron in the molecular layer of the dentate gyrus and the stratum lacunosum-moleculare of the CA2-CA3 fields of the hippocampus observed in a parasagittal section. Bar = 500 μm. (*Source:* Tamamaki and Nojyo, 1993. With permission of Wiley-Liss, a subsidiary of John Wiley & Sons.

a radial course in the molecular layer, in contrast to the predominantly transverse orientation of the entorhinal perforant pathway fibers. Virtually nothing is currently known about which cells these fibers innervate or what type of transmitter they use. Because the presubiculum receives the only direct input from the anterior thalamic nucleus, these fibers provide a potential link by which thalamic information could reach the dentate gyrus.

Basal Forebrain Inputs: Projections from the Septal Nuclei

The dentate gyrus receives relatively few inputs from subcortical structures. Certainly the most robust and longest studied is the projection from the septal nuclei (Mosko et al., 1973; Swanson, 1978a; Baisden et al., 1984; Amaral and Kurz, 1985; Wainer et al., 1985; Nyakas et al., 1987). The septal projection arises from cells of the medial septal nucleus and the nucleus of the diagonal band of Broca, and it travels to the hippocampal formation via four routes: the fimbria, dorsal fornix, supracallosal stria, and a ventral route through and around the amygdaloid complex. Septal fibers heavily innervate cells of the polymorphic layer, particularly in a narrow region just subjacent to the granule cell layer. The large mossy cells are innervated by cholinergic fibers (Lubke et al., 1997). Septal fibers are lightly distributed throughout the molecular layer (Fig. 3–20a).

A large portion of the fibers of the septal projection to the dentate gyrus are cholinergic. Altogether, 30% to 50% of the cells in the medial septal nucleus and 50% to 75% of the cells in the nucleus of the diagonal band that project to the hippocampal formation are cholinergic. Although it had long been assumed that the septal projection to the hippocampal formation was entirely cholinergic, it is now clear that many of the septal cells that project to the dentate gyrus are actually GABAergic. The most interesting facet of this heterogeneous septal projection is that the cholinergic and GABAergic components target different cell types. Fibers of the septal GABAergic projections terminate preferentially on other GABAergic nonpyramidal cells, such as the basket pyramidal cells of the dentate gyrus, and form symmetrical, presumably inhibitory, contacts. The heaviest GABAergic septal termination is on interneurons located in the polymorphic layer. The cholinergic septal projection to the dentate gyrus, in contrast, terminates mainly on granule cells, making asymmetrical, presumably excitatory, contacts on dendritic spines, chiefly in the inner third of the molecular layer; only 5% to 10% of the cholinergic synapses are on interneurons.

The septal projection to the dentate gyrus and to the remainder of the hippocampal formation is topographically organized. Cells located medially in the medial septal nucleus tend to project preferentially to septal or dorsal levels of the dentate gyrus, whereas cells located laterally in the medial septal nucleus tend to project to temporal levels. Because the medially situated neurons in the medial septal nucleus tend to be GABAergic rather than cholinergic, septal levels of the dentate gyrus receive most of their cholinergic input from the nucleus of the diagonal band. In contrast, temporal levels of the dentate gyrus receive their cholinergic innervation primarily from the medial septal nucleus. The ventral septal pathway

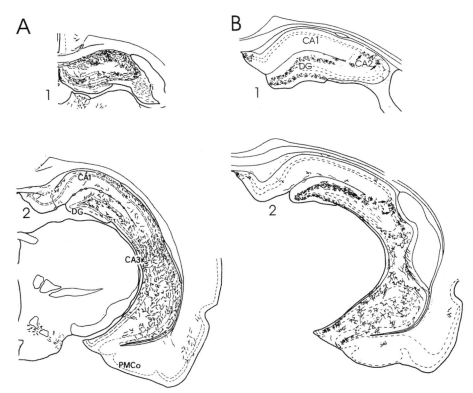

Figure 3–20. Septal and hypothalamic inputs to the rat hippocampal formation. *A.* Distribution of PHA-L-labeled fibers in the hippocampal formation resulting from an injection focused in the medial portion of the medial septal nucleus. *B.* Distribution of PHA-L-labeled fibers resulting from an injection in the supramammillary nucleus. Note the dense plexus of fibers located just superficial to the granule cell layer and in the CA2 region of the hippocampus (between the small arrows). (*Sources: A.* From Gaykema et al., 1990. *B.* Adapted from Haglund et al., 1984.)

appears to arise mainly from the nucleus of the diagonal band of Broca.

Supramammillary and Other Hypothalamic Inputs

The major hypothalamic projection to the dentate gyrus arises from a population of large cells, the supramammillary area, which caps and partially surrounds the medial mammillary nuclei (Wyss et al., 1979; Dent et al., 1983; Vertes, 1993; Magloczky et al., 1994). The supramammillary projection terminates heavily in a narrow zone of the molecular layer located just superficial to the granule cell layer and only lightly in the polymorphic layer or the rest of the molecular layer (Fig. 3–20b). Most of the supramammillary fibers terminate on the proximal dendrites of granule cells. There has been some controversy about the neurotransmitter of the supramammillary projection. There is substantial evidence that this projection is excitatory and is likely using glutamate as a primary neurotransmitter (Kiss et al., 2000). Most, but not all, of the glutamatergic suprammamillary neurons that project to the dentate gyrus also colocalize calretinin; some of these cells also colocalize substance P (Borhegyi and Leranth, 1997).

In addition to the supramammillary cells, there are cells scattered in several hypothalamic nuclei (many of which are in a perifornical position or in the lateral hypothalamic area) that project to the dentate gyrus. Although taken together these cells constitute a sizable input to the hippocampal formation, their diffuseness and lack of any distinguishing biochemical marker has made it difficult to study their patterns of termination in the hippocampal formation.

Brain Stem Inputs

The dentate gyrus receives a particularly prominent noradrenergic input from the pontine nucleus locus coeruleus (Pickel et al., 1974; Swanson and Hartman, 1975; Loughlin et al., 1986). The noradrenergic fibers terminate mainly in the polymorphic layer of the dentate gyrus and extend into the stratum lucidum of CA3, as if preferentially terminating in the zones occupied by mossy fibers (Fig. 3-21).

The dentate gyrus receives a minor, diffusely distributed dopaminergic projection that arises mainly from cells located in the ventral tegmental area. The dopaminergic fibers terminate mainly in the polymorphic layer.

The serotonergic projection that originates from median and dorsal divisions of the raphe nuclei also terminates most heavily in the polymorphic layer in an immediately subgranular portion of the layer (Conrad et al., 1974; Moore and Halaris, 1975; Köhler and Steinbusch, 1982; Vertes et al., 1999). A number of GABAergic interneurons appear to be

Figure 3–21. Line drawing of horizontal sections through the rat hippocampal formation shows the distribution of *A.* noradrenergic, *B.* serotonergic, and *C.* dopaminergic fibers. (*Source*: Adapted from Swanson et al., 1987.

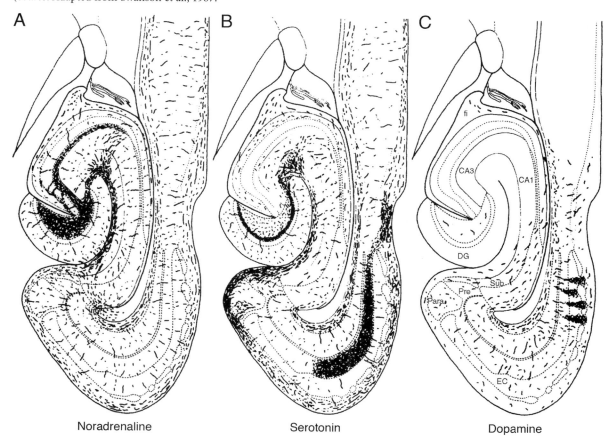

Noradrenaline   Serotonin   Dopamine

preferentially innervated by the serotonergic fibers. The targets are often the pyramidal basket cells. Fusiform neurons in the region, particularly those that stain for the calcium-binding protein calbindin, are also heavily innervated. As with the cholinergic projection from the septum, many of the cells in the raphe nuclei that project to the hippocampal formation appear to be nonserotonergic, but their transmitter is not known.

Intrinsic Connections

Basket Cell and Axo-axonic Cell Innervation of the Granule Cell Layer

As already noted, a variety of basket cells are located just below the granule cell layer and appear to contribute to a extremely dense terminal plexus that is confined to the granule cell layer (Struble et al., 1978; Sik et al., 1997). The terminals in this basket plexus are GABAergic and form symmetrical, inhibitory contacts located primarily on the cell bodies and proximal dendritic shafts of apical dendrites of the granule cells. GABAergic neurons in the polymorphic layer are themselves innervated by other GABAergic terminals, some of which arise from extrinsic sources, such as the GABAergic septal input. This polysynaptic cascade of inhibitory interconnections indicates that the hippocampal circuitry provides intricate inhibitory and disinhibitory control of cell excitability, an issue discussed in Chapters 5 and 6.

Given the small number of basket cells relative to granule cells, the question arises as to how widespread the influence of a single basket cell is. Analysis of Golgi-stained axonal plexuses from single basket cells indicates that they extend for distances of more than 900 μm in the transverse axis and about 1.5 mm in the septotemporal axis. This widely distributed axonal plexus would allow a single basket cell to influence as many as 10,000 granule cells (about 1%). The other inhibitory input to granule cells originates with the chandelier (axo-axonic) cells located in the molecular layer. These cells form symmetrical contacts exclusively with the axon's initial segment of granule cells.

Granule Cell Projection to the Polymorphic Layer

The granule cells give rise to distinctive unmyelinated axons that Ramon y Cajal called mossy fibers. The mossy fibers have unusually large boutons that form en passant synapses with the CA3 pyramidal cells; we describe this projection in more detail shortly. What is not generally appreciated is that the mossy fiber axons form a distinctive set of collaterals that also innervate cells in the polymorphic layer of the dentate gyrus (Fig. 3–22). Each principal mossy fiber (which is on the order of 0.2–0.5 μm in diameter) gives rise to about seven thinner collaterals in the polymorphic layer before entering the CA3 field of the hippocampus. As much as 2300 μm of the collateral axonal plexus is generated by a single mossy fiber in the polymorphic layer (Claiborne et al., 1986). In the polymorphic layer, the mossy fiber collaterals branch extensively, and

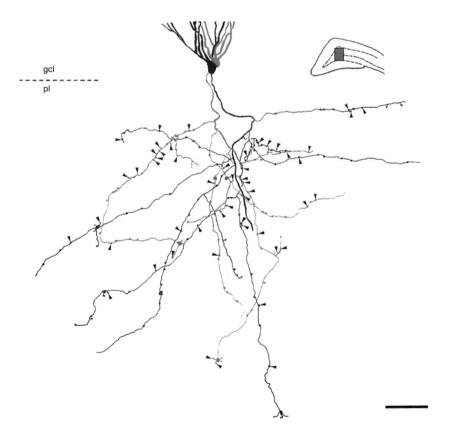

gcl

- - - - - - - - - - -

pl

Figure 3–22. Granule cell projections to the polymorphic cell layer. Axon arbors of two adjacent granule cells (gray and black) and their mGluR1a immunoreactive targets reconstructed from three neighboring 60 μm thick sections. Of the 175 small terminals and filopodiae (arrowheads) 52 innervated mGluR1a immunoreactive targets, whereas large mossy terminals contacted none. gcl, granule cell layer; pl, polymorphic layer. Bar = 50 μm. (*Source*: Adapted from Acsady et al., 1998.)

the daughter branches bear two types of synaptic varicosity. Numerous small (approximately 2 μm) spherical synaptic varicosities are distributed unevenly along these collaterals. There are about 160 to 200 of these varicosities distributed throughout the axonal collateral plexus of a single granule cell, and they form contacts on dendrites located in the polymorphic layer. At the end of each of the collateral branches there are also larger (3–5 μm diameter), irregularly shaped varicosities that resemble, although are smaller than, the mossy fiber boutons found in CA3. The mossy fiber terminals in the polymorphic layer establish contacts with the proximal dendrites of the mossy cells (Ribak et al., 1985), the basal dendrites of the pyramidal basket cells, and other, unidentified cells. Acsady et al. (1998) made the surprising discovery that most of the granule cell collaterals in the polymorphic cell layer terminate on GABAergic interneurons. Because there are 160 to 200 such varicosities (compared with about 20 of the larger thorny expansions), mossy fiber axons synapse on a larger number of interneurons than do mossy cells or CA3 pyramidal cells. Mossy fiber collaterals may enter the granule cell layer, but they virtually never enter the molecular layer. The collaterals that enter the granule cell layer appear to terminate preferentially on the apical dendritic shafts of pyramidal basket cells. This lack of mossy fiber innervation of the molecular layer is of some importance because in the presence of kindling and some pathological conditions, such as epilepsy, mossy fibers can be induced to sprout into the molecular layer.

Mossy Cell Projection to the Associational/Commissural Zone

The inner third of the molecular layer receives a projection that originates exclusively from neurons in the polymorphic layer (Laurberg and Sorensen, 1981; Buckmaster et al., 1992, 1996; Frotscher, 1992). Because in the rat this projection originates in both the ipsilateral and contralateral sides of the hippocampus, it has been called the associational/commissural projection. This projection was initially thought to arise from both the cells of the polymorphic layer and the CA3 pyramidal cells located within the confines of the dentate gyrus. If this were true, it would mean that at least one of the intrinsic hippocampal connections would be bidirectional. It is now clear, however, that the associational/commissural projection arises exclusively from cells in the polymorphic layer, and CA3 cells do not project to the molecular layer. Although this statement is generally true, it appears that at least some CA3 neurons in the most temporal extreme of the hippocampal formation might send collaterals into the molecular layer of the dentate gyrus. Aside from the existence of this projection, almost nothing is known concerning its magnitude. Nor is it known why this projection is observed only in the temporal portion of the hippocampal formation. Thus, the principle of unidirectionality, although generally true, may have exceptions to the rule. For all practical purposes, the organization of the commissural projection is similar to that of the ipsilateral associational connection.

Most of the synaptic terminals of the associational/commissural pathway form asymmetrical, presumably excitatory synaptic terminals on the spines of proximal dendrites of granule cells. Many, perhaps all, of the axons contributing to these synaptic terminals originate from the mossy cells of the polymorphic layer, and individual mossy cells contribute a projection to both the ipsilateral associational and commissural projections. The fact that the mossy cells are immunoreactive for glutamate adds credence to the notion that the associational/commissural projection is excitatory.

There are a number of interesting features of this "feedback" projection from the mossy cells to the granule cells. First, the projection from mossy cells located at any particular level of the dentate gyrus is distributed widely along the longitudinal axis, both septally and temporally from the point of origin. Axons from any particular septotemporal point in the dentate gyrus may innervate as much as 75% of the long axis of the dentate gyrus (Amaral and Witter, 1989). Second, the projection to the molecular layer at the septotemporal level of origin is extremely weak but becomes increasingly stronger at levels that are progressively more distant from the cells of origin. Remembering that mossy cells are the recipients of massive innervation from the granule cells at their same level (via the mossy fiber collaterals into the polymorphic layer), it appears that the mossy cells pass on the collective output of granule cells from one septotemporal level to granule cells located at distant levels of the dentate gyrus.

The full impact of this longitudinal organization of the associational projection cannot be fully appreciated without one further piece of information: The associational fibers contact not only the spines of the granule cell dendrites but also the dendritic shafts of the GABAergic basket cells, which in turn innervate the granule cells. Thus, the associational projection may function both as a feedforward excitatory pathway to distant granule cells and as a disynaptic feedforward inhibitory pathway, with the pyramidal basket cell as the intermediary.

GABA/Somatostatin Projection from the Polymorphic Layer to the Outer Molecular Layer

Although the neuroanatomy of the hippocampal formation has been analyzed for many years, new components of its intrinsic circuitry continue to be discovered. This is often the result of applying new neuroanatomical techniques. One example is the discovery of a second projection from the polymorphic layer to the molecular layer. Antibodies directed against the peptide somatostatin have revealed that neurons scattered throughout the polymorphic layer are immunoreactive for this peptide and account for approximately 16% of the GABAergic cells in the dentate gyrus (Morrison et al., 1982; Bakst et al., 1986; Freund and Buzsaki, 1996; Sik et al., 1997; Boyett and Buckmaster, 2001). As noted earlier, the somatostatin immunoreactive cells may correspond, in part, to the HIPP cells. The somatostatin-positive cells all colocalize with GABA and are the source of the somatostatin immunoreactive fibers and terminals in the outer two-thirds of the molecular layer. This system of fibers, which forms contacts on the distal dendrites of the granule cells, provides a third means of releasing inhibitory control of granule cell activity (in addition to the basket cell plexus and the axo-axonic terminals provided by the chandelier cells). Because electron microscopic studies have demonstrated that somatostatin cells are contacted by mossy fiber terminals, the projection to the outer molecular layer thus constitutes a local feedback inhibitory circuit.

Interestingly, unlike the mossy cell associational projection, which terminates more heavily at distant levels of the dentate gyrus, the GABA/somatostatin projection terminates most heavily at the level of the cells of origin; moreover, termination rapidly decreases within approximately 1.5 mm septally and temporally to the cells of origin. Thus, the mossy cell projection and the somatostatin/GABA cell projection have terminal fields that are spatially complementary in both radial and horizontal axes; the distribution suggests that the two cell types mediate distal excitation and local inhibition, respectively.

Dentate Gyrus Efferent Projection: Mossy Fibers

The dentate gyrus does not project to any brain region other than the CA3 field of the hippocampus. The axons that project to CA3, the mossy fibers, arise exclusively from the granule cells and terminate in a relatively narrow zone mainly located just above the CA3 pyramidal cell layer (Blackstad et al., 1970; Gaarskjaer, 1978b; Swanson et al., 1978; Claiborne et al., 1986). In the proximal portion of CA3, mossy fibers are also located below and within the pyramidal cell layer. The layer of mossy fiber termination located just above the pyramidal cell layer is called the stratum lucidum because the lack of myelin on the mossy fibers gives the layer a relatively clear appearance in fresh tissue (as one might visualize in a hippocampal slice experiment). There is no indication that dentate neurons other than the granule cells project to CA3; in particular, cells in the polymorphic layer do not project to the hippocampus, at least in the rodent. The dentate projection to CA3 stops precisely at the border of CA3 with CA2, and the lack of granule cell input is one of the main features that distinguishes CA3 from CA2 pyramidal cells.

All dentate granule cells project to CA3, and the axon trajectory is partially correlated with the position of the parent cell body. Before describing features of the mossy fiber projection, it is worth making a few points concerning the organization of the terminal regions in CA3. In the proximal portion of CA3 (close to the dentate gyrus), mossy fibers are distributed below, within, and above the pyramidal cell layer. The fibers located below the layer (i.e., those that are in the area occupied primarily by basal dendrites) are generally called the infrapyramidal bundle. The fibers located in the pyramidal cell layer are called the intrapyramidal bundle, and those located above the pyramidal cell layer (i.e., in the area occupied mainly by proximal apical dendrites) are called the suprapyramidal bundle; the suprapyramidal bundle occupies the stratum lucidum. At mid and distal portions of CA3, the

intra- and infrapyramidal bundles are largely eliminated, and virtually all mossy fibers travel in the stratum lucidum. Although our focus is primarily on human, monkey, and rat hippocampus in this chapter, it is worth noting in passing that variations in the relative size of the infrapyramidal mossy fibers have been noted across different strains of mice, including mouse strains used widely in transgenic experiments; this variation sometimes correlates with different behavioral profiles (Lipp et al., 1987; Hausheer-Zarmakupi et al., 1996).

Granule cells at all transverse positions in the granule cell layer generate mossy fibers that extend for the full proximo-distal distance of CA3 (Fig. 3–23). Cells located in the infrapyramidal blade of the granule cell layer have axons that tend to enter CA3 in the infrapyramidal bundle but ultimately cross the pyramidal cell layer to enter the deep portion of the stratum lucidum. The axons of granule cells located in the crest of the dentate gyrus tend to enter CA3 in the intrapyramidal bundle and also ultimately ascend into the stratum lucidum. Cells located in the suprapyramidal blade of the dentate gyrus give rise to axons that enter CA3 in the stratum lucidum and continue within the most superficial portion of the stratum lucidum (Claiborne et al., 1986).

The mossy fibers give rise to unique, complex en passant presynaptic terminals called mossy fiber expansions (Amaral and Dent, 1981). Part of the uniqueness of these terminals is their size; they can be as large as 8 μm in diameter but more typically range from 3 to 5 μm in greatest dimension. Their large size has attracted the attention of physiologists interested in using them for patch-clamp studies of transmitter release (Henze et al., 2000). The mossy fiber expansions form highly irregular, complex, interdigitated attachments with the intricately branched spines called thorny excrescences that are located on the proximal dendrites of the CA3 pyramidal cells. The thorny excrescences are so distinctive they clearly mark the location of mossy fiber synaptic termination. In the proximal portion of CA3, for example, thorny excrescences are located on both the basal and apical proximal dendrites of pyramidal cells, which are therefore in contact with both the infra- and suprapyramidal mossy fiber bundles. In the mid and distal portions of CA3, however, thorny excrescences are almost entirely restricted to the apical dendritic processes that traverse the stratum lucidum (Fig. 3–24). The CA2 pyramidal cells, which do not receive any mossy fiber input, are devoid of thorny excrescences (Fig. 3–25).

Another distinctive feature of the mossy fiber expansion is the number of active synaptic zones they demonstrate. A single mossy fiber expansion can make as many as 37 synaptic contacts with a single CA3 pyramidal cell dendrite. Three-dimensional analysis of serial sections through these synapses indicates that although a mossy fiber expansion may be in synaptic contact with more than one complex spine originating from the same parent dendrite it does not typically contact spines on two different dendrites. Thus, one mossy fiber expansion does not typically contact two pyramidal cells.

The large mossy fiber expansions occur approximately every 135 μm along the parent axon (Fig. 3–23), and each mossy fiber axon forms about 15 of these complex boutons.

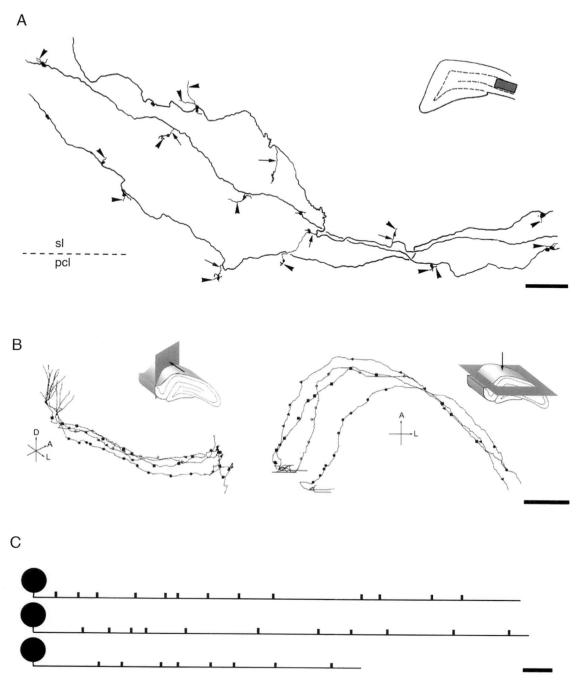

Figure 3–23. Topography of the mossy fibers in the CA3 region. *A.* Camera lucida drawing of mossy fibers of three adjacent granule cells (truncated). Note the numerous filopodial extensions of the large mossy terminals in *A* (arrowheads) and thin stalks of large mossy terminals (arrows). Boxed area in the inset in *A* shows the position of the fibers in CA3. *B.* Neurolucida reconstruction of the same three axons shown in *A* and an additional mossy fiber of a fourth granule cell located posteriorly. The original coronal images are rotated to emphasize the spatial characteristics of the fibers. *C.* Wire diagram of the three mossy fibers shown in *A*, depicting the distribution of mossy terminals. Note that a shorter interbouton distance prevails in the proximal portion of CA3. sl, stratum lucidum; pcl, pyramidal cell layer. Bars: *A*, 50 μm; *B*, 400 μm; *C*, 200 μm. (*Source*: Adapted from Acsady et al., 1998.)

CA3 pyramidal cell

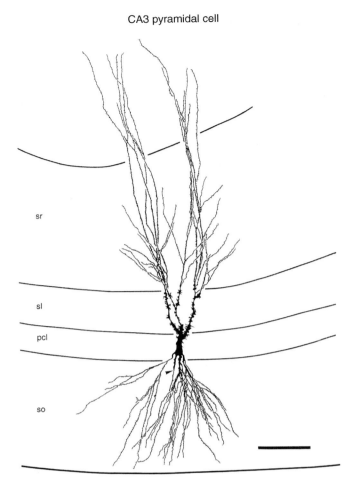

sr

sl

pcl

so

Figure 3–24. Camera lucida drawing of a CA3 pyramidal neuron located in the midportion of the field. As this neuron lies outside the zone of the infrapyramidal mossy fiber bundle, most of the thorny excrescences are located on the proximal apical dendrites. The axon of this neuron is indicated by an arrowhead. pcl, pyramidal cell layer; sl, stratum lucidum; so, stratum oriens; sr, stratum radiatum. Bar = 100 μm. (*Source*: Adapted from Ishizuka et al., 1995.)

Thus, each granule cell communicates with only 15 CA3 pyramidal cells. It is important to point out, however, that these 15 pyramidal cells are distributed throughout the full proximo-distal length (transverse axis) of CA3. Because there are approximately 2.5×10^5 CA3 pyramidal cells and approximately 1.2×10^6 granule cells, each pyramidal cell is expected to receive input from about 72 granule cells. That is, an individual dentate granule cell has the potential to activate about 15 CA3 pyramidal cells, whereas an individual pyramidal cell receives input from about 72 granule cells. This pattern, not seen elsewhere in the brain, has attracted considerable interest among computational neuroscientists. The fact that each of the mossy fiber expansions has many release sites might ensure highly efficient depolarization of the innervated pyramidal cells. This is, however, currently controversial (see Chapters 5 and 6).

Early Golgi anatomists indicated that the mossy fiber axons were mainly oriented perpendicular to the long axis of the hippocampus. Theodor Blackstad and colleagues confirmed the largely transverse trajectory of the mossy fibers using degeneration track tracing methods, and Andersen and colleagues demonstrated this electrophysiologically. Modern studies, such as those carried out by Claiborne and colleagues, also indicate that mossy fibers do not collateralize once they enter the hippocampus; they stay largely within the same septotemporal level as their cells of origin. There is one peculiarity of the mossy fiber projection, however, that has eluded explanation. Lorente de Nó (1934) and McLardy (McLardy and Kilmer, 1970) indicated that the mossy fibers actually do change their course and take a longitudinal direction but not until they reach the distal portion of CA3. The extent of this distal longitudinal projection was further clarified by Swanson and colleagues using the autoradiographic method of neural tract tracing (Swanson et al., 1978). They showed that granule cells located at septal levels give rise to mossy fibers that travel throughout most of the transverse extent of CA3 at the same septotemporal level. Just at the CA3/CA2 border, however, they abruptly change course and travel toward the temporal pole for nearly 2 mm. The extent of this longitudinal component appears to depend on the septotemporal location of the cells of origin. Granule cells in the mid to temporal portions of the dentate gyrus have mossy fibers that exhibit only a slight temporal inclination at their distal extremity; mossy fibers that originate at the extreme temporal pole of the dentate gyrus barely extend to the CA3/CA2 border and have little or no longitudinal component. Thus, in the septal half of the hippocampus, there appears to be some overlap of mossy fibers originating from different septotemporal levels, but it occurs only at a restricted distal portion of the CA3 field. On the face of it, this indicates that some CA3 pyramidal cells located extremely close to the border with CA2 may be contacted by mossy fiber axons from granule cells spread out over a much broader septotemporal extent of the dentate gyrus. They might therefore form a special class of integrator CA3 cells. Elegant neuroanatomical verification of this has come from the work of Acsady and colleagues (1998), who stained dentate granule cells using in vivo intracellular techniques. Not only do mossy fibers travel 2 to 3 mm in the longitudinal direction, they demonstrate typical mossy fiber expansions along this portion of their trajectory; these terminals do, in fact, make contact with thorny excrescences.

Before leaving this description of the mossy fibers, it should be noted that in addition to the mossy fiber expansions there are infrequent thin collaterals that emanate from the parent axon or from the mossy fiber expansions. These collaterals appear to terminate preferentially on cells other than the pyramidal cells, such as the GABAergic pyramidal basket cells in CA3.

There is substantial evidence indicating that the granule cells use glutamate as their primary transmitter, and the asymmetrical contacts made between the mossy fiber expansions and the thorny excrescences tend to confirm this notion.

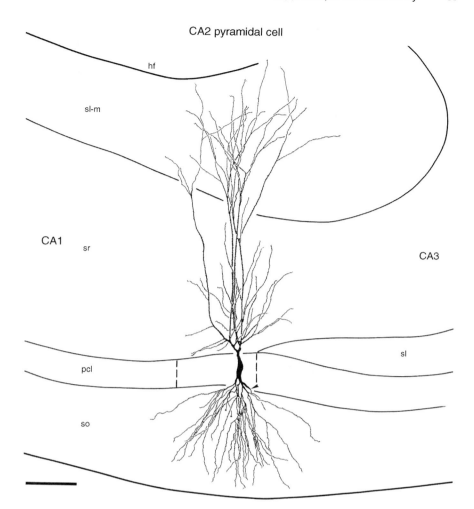

CA2 pyramidal cell

hf

sl-m

CA1   sr

CA3

sl

pcl

so

Figure 3–25. Camera lucida drawing of a CA2 pyramidal neuron. Note that although the size and general characteristics of this neuron are similar to those in CA3, there are no thorny excrescences on the proximal apical dendrites. Two basal dendrites cut at the surface of the slice are indicated by asterisks. The axon of this neuron is indicated by an arrowhead. CA1, CA1 field of the hippocampus; CA3, CA3 field of the hippocampus; hf, hippocampal fissure; pcl, pyramidal cell layer; sl, stratum lucidum; sl-m, stratum lacunosum-moleculare; so, stratum oriens; sr, stratum radiatum. Bar = 100 μm. (*Source*: Adapted from Ishizuka et al., 1995.)

Nonetheless, the mossy fibers are also immunoreactive for several other neuroactive substances. At least some of the mossy fibers demonstrate immunoreactivity for the opioid peptide dynorphin and are also immunoreactive for GABA (Walker et al., 2002). Interestingly, although the granule cells do not normally demonstrate mRNA for the synthetic enzymes GAD65 or GAD67, prolonged stimulation of the perforant path can induce GAD messenger expression in rat granule cells. The possible role of GABA or opioid peptides in the synaptic economy of the mossy fibers is discussed in relation to synaptic plasticity at these synapses in Chapter 10.

3.4.2 Hippocampus

Cytoarchitectonic Organization

An overview of the major fields of the hippocampus was given earlier in the chapter. We now go into more detail about its laminar organization, which is generally similar for all the fields of the hippocampus. The principal cellular layer is called the pyramidal cell layer. The pyramidal cell layer is tightly packed in CA1 and more loosely packed in CA2 and CA3. The narrow, relatively cell-free layer located deep to the pyramidal cell layer is called the stratum oriens. This layer contains the basal dendrites of the pyramidal cells and several classes of interneurons. Stratum oriens can be defined as the infrapyramidal region in which some of the CA3 to CA3 associational connections and the CA3 to CA1 Schaffer collateral connections are located. Deep to the stratum oriens is the thin, fiber-containing alveus. In the CA3 field, but not in CA2 or CA1, a narrow acellular zone, the stratum lucidum, is located just above the pyramidal cell layer and is occupied by the mossy fibers. There is a slight thickening of the stratum lucidum at its distal end, where, at least at septal levels of the hippocampus, the mossy fibers bend temporally and travel longitudinally. This zone, called the end bulb, is more prominent in species such as the guinea pig than in the rat; it marks the CA3/CA2 border. The stratum radiatum is located superficial to the stratum lucidum in CA3 and immediately above the pyramidal cell layer in CA2 and CA1. The stratum radiatum can be defined as the suprapyramidal region in which the CA3 to CA3 associational connections and the CA3 to CA1 Schaffer collateral connections are located. The most superficial layer of the hippocampus is called the stratum lacunosum-molecular. It is in this layer that fibers from the entorhinal cortex terminate. Afferents from other regions, such as the nucleus reuniens of the midline thalamus, also terminate in the stratum lacunosum-moleculare. Both the stratum radiatum and the stratum lacunosum-moleculare contain a variety of interneurons.

In the following sections, we sometimes deal with the organization of the CA3 and CA2 fields of the hippocampus first and then move on to the CA1 field. For other topics, such as the interneurons of the hippocampus, there is not enough known to warrant discussing CA3, CA2, and CA1 separately. For these topics, we discuss data for the entire hippocampus. Moving on from the dentate gyrus, we begin our discussion with the CA3 field.

Pyramidal Cells of CA3 and CA2

The principal neuronal cell type of the hippocampus is the pyramidal cell, which makes up most of the neurons in the pyramidal cell layer. Pyramidal cells have a basal dendritic tree that extends into the stratum oriens and an apical dendritic tree that extends to the hippocampal fissure.

Ishizuka and colleagues (Ishizuka et al., 1995) demonstrated that the dendritic length and organization of CA3 pyramidal cells are quite variable (Figs. 3–24 and 3–27). The smallest cells (with a soma size of about 300 μm^2 or 20 μm in diameter) are located in the limbs of the dentate gyrus and have a total dendritic length of 8 to 10 mm. The largest cells (with a soma size of about 700 μm^2 or 30 μm in diameter), which are located distally in the field, have total dendritic lengths of 16 to 18 mm. The distribution of the dendritic trees of CA3 pyramidal cells also varies depending on where the cell body is located. Cells located in the limbs of the dentate gyrus, for example, have few or none of their dendrites extending into the stratum lacunosum-moleculare, and thus these cells receive little or no direct input from the entorhinal cortex. The cells, however, receive a larger number of mossy fiber terminals on their apical and basal dendritic trees and are thus under greater influence of the granule cells than distally located CA3 cells, which receive only apical mossy fiber input.

Pyramidal Cells of CA1

In contrast to the substantial heterogeneity of dendritic organization characteristic of CA3 pyramidal cells, investigators such as Norio Ishizuka and Dennis Turner and colleagues (Pyapali et al., 1998) demonstrated that the CA1 pyramidal cells show remarkable homogeneity of their dendritic trees (Figs. 3–26 and 3–27). As well as being more homogeneous, they are also, on average, smaller than CA3 cells. The total dendritic length averages approximately 13.5 mm, and the average size of CA1 cell somata is about 193 μm^2 or 15 μm in diameter. Regardless of where a pyramidal cell is located in CA1, it has about the same total dendritic length and the same dendritic configuration. Some pyramidal cells have one apical

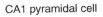

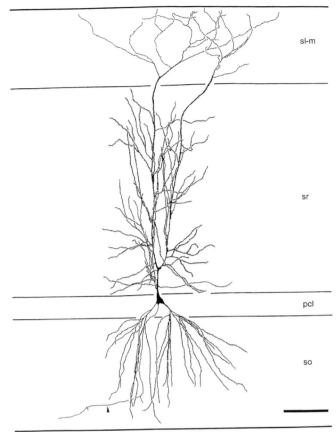

Figure 3–26. Camera lucida drawing of a CA1 pyramidal neuron from the midportion of the field. Note that side branches originate from the primary dendrites throughout the full extent of the stratum radiatum. Note also the curved and irregular trajectories of dendritic branches in the stratum lacunosum-moleculare. The axon of this neuron is indicated by an arrowhead. pcl, pyramidal cell layer; sl-m, stratum lacunosum-moleculare; so, stratum oriens; sr, stratum radiatum. Bar = 100 μm. (*Source:* Adapted from Ishizuka et al., 1995.)

dendrite, and others have two. Cells with two apical dendrites tend to have slightly greater total dendritic length in the apical direction. Neurons with a single apical dendrite, however, tend to have slightly larger basal dendritic trees; thus, overall, the dendritic tree in all CA1 neurons have about the same total length. This anatomical homogeneity, however, cannot reflect functional homogeneity because, as we shall see shortly, there are differences in the entorhinal cortex inputs received at different locations along the transverse axis of CA1.

Interneurons

Pyramidal neurons are by far the most numerous neurons in the hippocampus. As in the dentate gyrus, however, there is a fairly heterogeneous group of interneurons that are scattered through all layers (Fig. 3–28) (Freund and Buzsaki, 1996).

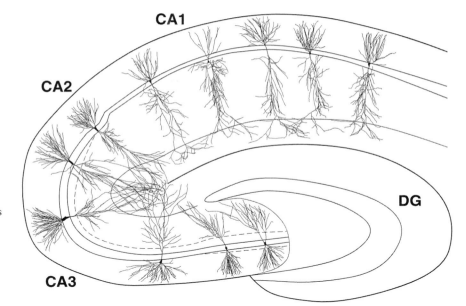

Figure 3–27. Summary of the organization of hippocampal pyramidal cells produced as a composite of computer-generated line drawings of neurons from CA3, CA2, and CA1. Dashed line in CA3 marks the region occupied by the infrapyramidal and suprapyramidal mossy fibers. *Source*: (Adapted from Ishizuka et al., 1995.)

Figure 3–28. Morphological classification of the interneurons in the hippocampus proper. Filled circles indicate the location of the cell bodies, and thick lines indicate the predominant orientation and laminar distribution of the dendritic tree. The pyramidal cells (principal neurons) are illustrated in the background, providing an indication of which domain is innervated by the various interneu-

ron groups. The laminar distribution of the inputs, which often show correspondence with the interneuron type or axon distribution, is also indicated. pcl, pyramidal cell layer; sl-m, stratum lacunosum-moleculare; so, stratum oriens; sr, stratum radiatum. (*Source*: Adapted from Freund and Buzsaki, 1996.)

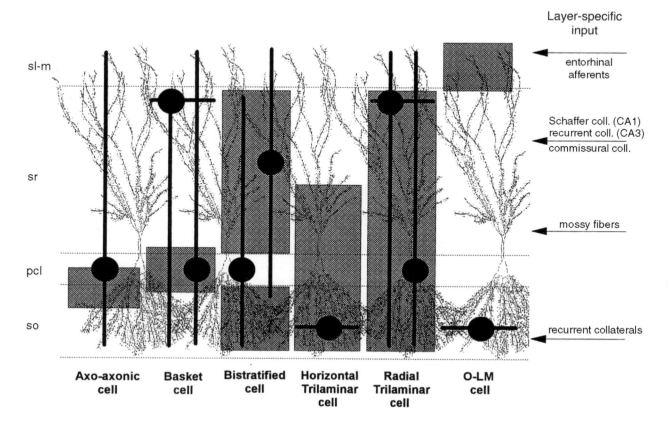

Most types of interneuron are found in all the hippocampal subfields. The pyramidal basket cell resides in or close to the pyramidal cell layer, and its dendrites extend into the stratum oriens, stratum radiatum, and stratum lacunosum-moleculare. The dendrites are beaded and aspiny, and they receive both asymmetrical and symmetrical synapses. Most of the excitatory inputs are known to arise from hippocampal pyramidal cells. In fact, the dendritic tree of a pyramidal basket cell receives at least 2000 excitatory inputs. Because each pyramidal cell contributes only a single synapse to a particular basket cell, the degree of pyramidal cell convergence on an individual basket cell is enormous. Neurons with basket cell-like axons have a variety of morphologies. There are fusiform-shaped basket cells in the stratum oriens and stellate-shaped basket cells in the stratum radiatum. In all cases, the axons of these cell types innervate the soma and proximal dendrites of the pyramidal cells. The transverse extent of the basket cell axonal plexus (in a 400-μm in vitro slice preparation) is between 900 and 1300 μm. Within this plexus, there are as many as 10,000 synaptic varicosities; and because a basket cell makes only 2 to 10 synapses on each pyramidal cell, a typical basket cell innervates as many as 1000-plus pyramidal cells. A single basket cell could thus have substantial inhibitory influence over a large population of pyramidal cells.

A second type of hippocampal interneuron is the chandelier, or axo-axonic, cell. The axo-axonic cells found in the hippocampus are similar to the ones described in the dentate gyrus. Their cell bodies, like those of the basket cells, are located in or adjacent to the pyramidal cell layer, and their dendrites span all the hippocampal strata. The axons of the chandelier cells have a transverse spread of approximately 1 mm. They travel just superficial to the pyramidal cell layer and periodically give rise to collaterals that enter the pyramidal cell layer and terminate on the proximal axons of the pyramidal neurons. Each axo-axonic cell terminates on approximately 1200 pyramidal cell axon initial segments, and each initial segment is innervated by 4 to 10 axo-axonic cells.

The early Golgi studies of Ramon y Cajal and Lorente de Nó made it abundantly clear that there are a variety of non-pyramidal cell types in the stratum oriens, stratum radiatum, and stratum lacunosum-moleculare of the hippocampus. Ribak and colleagues (1978) were the first to discover that most of these neurons are immunoreactive for GABAergic markers, and most are thought to be interneurons. Freund and Buzsaki (1996) described the location, dendritic organization, and axonal distribution of these cells based on a classification system that is dependent on the region of innervation. One class of cells (Lacaille et al., 1987) has been called the O-LM cell (oriens lacunosum-moleclare(associated cell) and has as its defining feature a dense axonal arbor that is confined to the stratum lacunosum-moleclare (also known as cells terminating in conjunction with entorhinal afferents). The location of the cell body of this class of interneuron varies depending on which hippocampal field it inhabits. The principle seems to be that the cell body and dendritic tree are

located in the zones occupied by recurrent pyramidal cell collaterals. In CA3 this includes all strata except the stratum lacunosum-moleculare, but in CA1 it includes only the stratum oriens. The axons of the O-LM cell leave the stratum oriens (or in whichever layer the cell body is located) and rise directly to the stratum lacunosum-moleculare, ramifying there to form a dense plexus. These axons form symmetrical synapses with the distal apical dendrites of pyramidal neurons. Because most of the excitatory input to the O-LM cells appears to arise from recurrent collaterals of the pyramidal cells, this class of interneuron inhibits activity in the distal dendrites of pyramidal cells in a disynaptic, feedback manner.

Another class of hippocampal interneuron, the bistratified cell, also has its cell body located close to the pyramidal cell layer. The dendritic trees of these neurons are multipolar but do not reach the stratum lacunosum-moleculare. The axon of the bistratified cell sends collaterals into the stratum oriens and the deep portion of the stratum radiatum, where a dense terminal plexus is produced. These neurons generate an enormous axonal plexus, on the order of 80 mm in total length and generating up to 16,000 synaptic varicosities. The bistratified cells have axons that terminate on both the dendritic shafts and the dendritic spines of pyramidal cells. Although the inputs to these cells have not been thoroughly investigated, their dendrites reside in the zone of associational connections in CA3 and the Schaffer collateral fibers in CA1. It is likely, therefore, that they are driven in both a feedforward and feedback manner.

There are other interneurons located in the stratum radiatum, and their stellate or multipolar dendritic plexus is confined to the layer. The axons of these cells tend to ramify locally in the stratum radiatum and terminate primarily on the dendrites of pyramidal cells.

A fairly sizable population of interneurons is located in the stratum lacunosum-moleculare or at the border between the stratum lacunosum-moleculare and the stratum radiatum (Lacaille and Schwartzkroin, 1988). These LM neurons (stratum lacunosum-moleculare interneurons) have dendrites that are oriented horizontally (i.e., within the layer) but occasionally have branches that extend into the pyramidal cell layer. The axon also takes a predominantly horizontal orientation and ramifies mainly in the stratum lacunosum-moleculare or the superficial portion of the stratum radiatum. Although the connectivity of this class of neurons is not well worked out, their axons do form symmetrical synapses on the distal dendrites of pyramidal cells.

An additional type of interneuron in the hippocampus is the IS neuron (interneuron-selective). The IS neurons' cell bodies are located in all layers and can be identified by staining with antibodies to the calcium-binding protein calretinin. The IS cells have a number of notable features, including the propensity for their dendrites to form bundles with dendrites of other IS neurons. The major unifying feature, however, is that their axons terminate exclusively on other interneurons. Little is yet known concerning their input/output characteristics. Their dendrites, however, are disposed so they could be innervated by all major afferent and intrinsic connections of the hippocampus, and their axons could potentially innervate all of the interneurons described above.

All of the interneurons we have described are immunopositive for markers of GABA. As in other cortical regions, the interneurons of the hippocampus colocalize a number of other neuroactive substances. Thus, many of these neurons can be visualized with antibodies to peptides such as somatostatin, VIP, cholecystokinin, neuropeptide Y (NPY), and calcium-binding proteins such as parvalbumin, calbindin, and calretinin. It remains something of a mystery what these neuroactive substances are doing in GABAergic neurons, but at the very least they provide useful markers for establishing subcategories of the large population of GABAergic interneurons.

Extrinsic Connections

One of the distinguishing features of the connectivity of the hippocampus is that most of its synaptic input arises from within its own boundaries. CA3 and CA2 are heavily innervated by collaterals of their own axons (i.e., associational connections) and from axons of the contralateral CA3 and CA2 (i.e., commissural connections). CA1, in turn, receives its heaviest input from CA3. A relatively lighter projection arises from the entorhinal cortex and terminates on the most distal dendrites of the pyramidal cells as well as on interneurons with dendrites in the stratum lacunosum-moleculare. There are relatively few other "extrinsic" inputs to the hippocampus, and the ones that do exist generally account for a relatively small number of synapses.

Entorhinal Cortex Projection to CA3/CA2

Although the entorhinal innervation of CA3 is mentioned in most studies of the perforant path projection, the organization of this component of the projection is generally not dealt with in much detail. Indeed, there has been little in-depth research on the entorhinal projections to the hippocampus despite the fact that its prominence suggests that it is extremely important. The perforant path takes its name from the observation that it perforates the subiculum and hippocampal fissure en route to the dentate gyrus, but it is now quite clear that collaterals of fibers that project to the dentate gyrus also project to the hippocampus. In fact, the origin and laminar terminal distribution of the perforant path projection to CA3 are similar to those to the dentate gyrus (Witter, 1993). Entorhinal terminals are distributed throughout the width of the stratum lacunosum-moleculare. As with the projection to the molecular layer of the dentate gyrus, projections from the lateral entorhinal area terminate superficially in the stratum lacunosum-moleculare, and those from the medial entorhinal area terminate in the deep half of the layer. The laminar origin, types, and numbers of synaptic contacts of this projection are similar to those to the dentate gyrus. The entorhinal projections to CA3/CA2

originate from cells in layer II, and collaterals of the same layer II cells reach both the dentate gyrus and CA3/CA2, implying that similar information reaches these structures.

Entorhinal Cortex Projection to CA1

Although the entorhinal cortex also projects to the CA1 field of the hippocampus, the organization of this projection is fundamentally different from the projection to CA3/CA2. First, the cells of origin are in layer III rather than in layer II. Second, the pattern of terminal distribution is organized in a topographical fashion rather than in a laminar fashion (Fig. 3–29). As in CA3/CA2, the entorhinal fibers terminate throughout the full width of the stratum lacunosum-moleculare of CA1. However, fibers originating in the lateral entorhinal area terminate in the distal portion of CA1 (close to the subiculum), whereas fibers originating in the medial entorhinal area terminate in the proximal portion of CA1 (close to CA2). Thus, depending on where a CA1 pyramidal cell is located in the transverse axis of the hippocampus, it receives inputs from a different portion of the entorhinal cortex. We noted earlier that CA1 cells are remarkably homogeneous in their dendritic length; the inputs they receive, however, differ as a function of their location along the proximodistal axis.

Hippocampal Projections to the Entorhinal Cortex

Early studies using autoradiographic tract-tracing techniques suggested that all fields of the hippocampus send a return projection to the entorhinal cortex, but it is now clear that only cells located in CA1 give rise to this projection (Naber et al., 2001). The projecting cells appear to send their axons to roughly the same region of the entorhinal cortex from which they receive their input (Fig. 3–29). Thus, proximal CA1 cells project to the medial entorhinal cortex, whereas distal CA1 cells project to the lateral entorhinal area. We return to a more detailed description of these projections in Section 3.4.5.

Hippocampal Connections with the Neocortex and Amygdaloid Complex

Although this book focuses on the hippocampal formation, we repeatedly emphasize that no brain structure can be seen in isolation. The hippocampus sends projections to and receives projections from numerous other brain regions, and these interconnections are vital to understanding its function. Having said that, and notwithstanding the extremely important functional relationship between hippocampus and neocortex, it turns out that only selected parts of the hippocampal formation have discrete, monosynaptic connections with the neocortex. The CA3 and CA2 fields of the hippocampus, for example, have no known connections with the neocortex.

Sensitive tracing methods have recently shown that CA3, in particular its temporal parts, receives input from the amygdaloid complex, which was previously thought to send projections only to CA1 and the subiculum (Pikkarainen et al., 1999; Pitkanen et al., 2000). These inputs originate mainly from the

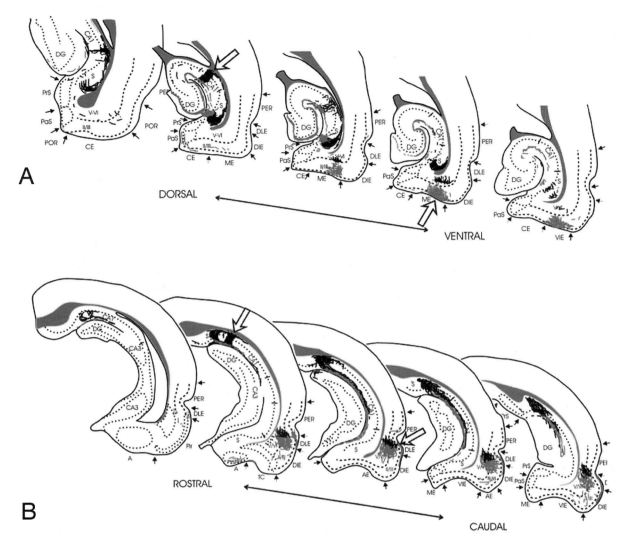

A

DORSAL

VENTRAL

B

ROSTRAL

CAUDAL

Figure 3–29. Reciprocal entorhinal–hippocampal connections. *A.* Distribution of labeled fibers in the hippocampus and entorhinal cortex after combined anterograde tracer injections into the medial portion of the entorhinal cortex and the proximal portion of the CA1 field of the hippocampus. The terminal fibers originating in the entorhinal cortex overlap with the injection site in CA1, and the terminal fibers originating in CA1 overlap with the injection site in the entorhinal cortex. *B.* Distribution of labeled fibers in the hippocampus and entorhinal cortex after combined anterograde tracer injections into the lateral entorhinal cortex and the distal portion of the CA1 field of the hippocampus. The terminal fibers originating in the entorhinal cortex overlap with the injection site in CA1, and the terminal fibers originating in CA1 overlap with the injection site in the entorhinal cortex. The subdivisions of the entorhinal cortex follow the nomenclature of Insausti et al. (1997). Areas CE and ME constitute the medial entorhinal cortex, whereas DLE, DIE, VIE, and AE constitute the lateral entorhinal cortex. (*Source*: Adapted from Naber et al., 2001.)

caudomedial portion of the parvicellular division of the basal nucleus and terminate heavily in the stratum oriens and stratum radiatum. The best-documented cortical connection, other than with the entorhinal cortex, which we have defined as part of the hippocampal formation, is with the perirhinal (areas 35 and 36) and postrhinal cortices. Cells in the perirhinal cortex give rise to a relatively selective projection to the most distal CA1 pyramidal cells (i.e., those located at the border with the subiculum). This projection terminates in the stratum lacunosum-moleculare and overlaps the projection arising from the lateral entorhinal area. The same CA1 cells give rise to a return projection to the perirhinal cortex. CA1 cells located in the septal portion of the hippocampus have also been reported to project to the retrosplenial cortex, and those located at mid-septotemporal levels provide a fairly substantial projection to the medial frontal lobe.

The temporal two-thirds of the distal portion of CA1 is reciprocally connected with the amygdaloid complex.

Projections from the basal nucleus of the amygdala terminate in the stratum oriens and stratum radiatum of the CA1/subiculum border region. In addition, the accessory basal and cortical nuclei projects to the stratum lacunosum-moleculare. CA1 cells in the same region give rise to a return projection to the basal nucleus of the amygdala.

Basal Forebrain Connections

The septum provides the major subcortical input to CA3. As with the dentate gyrus, the septal projection originates mainly in the medial septal nucleus and the nucleus of the diagonal band of Broca. The projection terminates most heavily in the stratum oriens and to a lesser extent in the stratum radiatum (Fig. 3–20). The CA1 field receives a substantially lighter septal projection than CA3, but the fibers are also most densely distributed in the stratum oriens.

Until the mid-1970s, it was commonly assumed that the hippocampal fields gave rise to both the precommissural and postcommissural projections to the basal forebrain and diencephalon. Indeed, Ramon y Cajal's classic diagram of the hippocampus shows fibers from CA1 coursing toward the fimbria. Swanson and Cowan demonstrated, however, that most of these projections originate from the subiculum (Swanson and Cowan, 1975). It is now quite clear that the only sizable subcortical projection from CA3 is to the lateral septal nucleus. The CA3 projection to the lateral septal nucleus travels via the fimbria and precommissural fornix. The CA3 projection to the septal complex is bilateral; and some CA3 fibers cross in the ventral hippocampal commissure to innervate the homologous region of the contralateral lateral septal nucleus. This pathway is topographically organized such that septal portions of CA3 project dorsally in the lateral septal nucleus, and progressively more temporal portions of CA3 project more ventrally; proximal CA3 cells tend to project medially in the lateral septal nucleus, and distally situated CA3 cells terminate more laterally. Interestingly, virtually all CA3 cells give rise to projections to both CA1 and the lateral septal nucleus.

Essentially all CA1 pyramidal cells also project to the lateral septal nucleus. However, the CA1 projection is strictly ipsilateral, and some of the fibers travel to the septal nuclei via the dorsal fornix rather than through the fimbria.

Hypothalamic Connections

There has been little work dealing specifically with the extrinsic inputs and outputs of CA2. In general, CA2 appears to have the same connections as CA3. However, the CA2 field receives particularly prominent innervation from the posterior hypothalamus, in particular from the supramammillary area (Fig. 3–20B) and the tuberomammillary nucleus. These projections terminate mainly in and around the pyramidal cell layer and mainly on principal cells (Magloczky et al., 1994). There is no evidence that CA2 returns the projection to the supramammillary region. In fact, none of the hippocampal fields appears to project into the postcommissural fornix.

The supramammillary region projects weakly, if at all, to CA3 and CA1.

Thalamic Connections: Nucleus Reuniens and Other Midline Nuclei

The thalamic inputs to the hippocampal formation have received relatively little attention. It has been known for some time that the anterior thalamic complex is intimately interconnected with the presubiculum. However, Herkenham and others demonstrated fairly prominent projections from midline ("nonspecific") regions of the thalamus to several fields of the hippocampal formation (Herkenham, 1978; Wouterlood et al., 1990; Dolleman-Van der Weel and Witter, 2000). The nucleus reuniens, located on the midline, gives rise to a prominent projection to the stratum lacunosum-moleculare of CA1, where it overlaps with fibers from the entorhinal cortex. The nucleus reuniens projection travels to CA1 via the internal capsule and cingulum bundle rather than through the fornix and fimbria. This projection innervates all septotemporal levels of CA1, with a preference for the mid-septotemporal levels. The nucleus reuniens fibers terminate with asymmetrical synapses on spines and thin dendritic shafts in the stratum lacunosum-moleculare on both principal neurons and GABAergic interneurons.

Brain Stem Inputs

The hippocampus, like the dentate gyrus, receives noradrenergic and serotonergic inputs from brain stem nuclei (Fig. 3–21). Noradrenergic fibers and terminals arising from the locus coeruleus are most densely distributed in the stratum lucidum and the most superficial portion of stratum lacunosum-moleculare. A much thinner plexus of axons is distributed throughout the other layers of CA3. Serotonergic fibers are distributed more diffusely and sparsely in CA3 than in the noradrenergic fibers. Despite the rather low number of fibers, the serotonergic innervation of the hippocampus demonstrates several interesting features. First, there are two calibers of axon, thick and thin, arising from the raphe nuclei that innervate the hippocampus. Most of the serotonergic varicosities, which are located on the thin fibers, do not appear to have standard synaptic junctions and may release transmitter into the extracellular space. The varicosities on the thicker fibers, in contrast, form standard asymmetrical synapses that preferentially terminate on GABAergic inhibitory neurons, specifically on the classes of interneuron that project to the dendrites of hippocampal neurons. Thus, even the relatively few serotonergic fibers that innervate the hippocampus may have a profound action by enhancing the GABAergic inhibitory activity of the hippocampal interneurons. There are few, if any, dopaminergic fibers in CA3. In general, CA1 receives much lighter monoaminergic innervation than CA3. The functional implications of monoaminergic inputs to the hippocampus, particularly in relation to long-term potentiation (LTP), is considered in more detail in Chapters 5, 6 and 7.

Intrinsic Connections: CA3 Associational Connections and Schaffer Collaterals

As mentioned earlier, the major source of input to the hippocampus is the hippocampus itself. The CA3 to CA3 associational connections and the CA3 to CA1 Schaffer collateral connections are unique in many respects. Perhaps the major distinguishing feature of these projections, however, is their extensive spatial distribution. Through these connections a particular pyramidal cell in CA3 can, in theory, interact with other hippocampal neurons distributed throughout much of the ipsilateral and contralateral hippocampus. The massive potential for association in the hippocampus is undoubtedly linked to its function. The hippocampal connections, although widely distributed, are nonetheless systematically organized. These projections have been studied by Ishizuka and colleagues (Ishizuka et al., 1990) and Buzsaki and colleagues (Li et al., 1994).

All CA3 and CA2 pyramidal cells give rise to highly divergent projections to all portions of the hippocampus. CA3 pyramidal cells give rise to highly collateralized axons that distribute fibers both within the ipsilateral hippocampus (to CA3, CA2, and CA1), to the same fields in the contralateral hippocampus (the commissural projections), and subcortically to the lateral septal nucleus. Some CA3 (especially those located proximally) and CA2 cells contribute a small number of collaterals that innervate the polymorphic layer of the dentate gyrus. Although claims of other hippocampal connections are found in the literature, it is now quite clear that CA3 does not project to the subiculum, presubiculum, parasubiculum, or entorhinal cortex.

The CA3 projections to CA3 and CA2 are typically called the associational connections, and the CA3 projections to the CA1 field are typically called the Schaffer collaterals. This terminology, however, may be misleading, as one should remember that these two projections are true collaterals and thus potentially carry the same information. Both the CA3 to CA3 associational projections and the CA3 to CA1 Schaffer collaterals demonstrate a systematic gradient-like projection pattern. Although it is somewhat out of sequence to discuss the CA3 to CA1 projections first, we do so because they have been worked out in somewhat better detail and provide a clear model for understanding CA3 projections. Moreover, the organization of the CA3 to CA1 projection shares many organizational similarities with the CA3 to CA3 projection.

CA3 to CA1 Connections: Schaffer Collaterals

All portions of CA3 and CA2 project to CA1. The pattern of terminal distribution, however, depends on the location of the CA3/CA2 cells of origin. The older notion that a typical CA3 pyramidal cell sends a single axon to CA1, traveling linearly through the field with equal contact probability at all regions in CA1 is clearly incorrect. In fact, each CA3 pyramidal cell gives rise to highly collateralized axons that follow both transverse and oblique orientations through CA1 (Ishizuka et al., 1990). Although Schaffer collaterals are typically illustrated

as extending only through the stratum radiatum, it should be emphasized that both the stratum radiatum and stratum oriens of CA1 are heavily innervated by CA3 axons. Thus, the Schaffer collaterals are as highly associated with the apical dendrites of CA1 cells in the stratum radiatum as they are with the basal dendrites in the stratum oriens. Moreover, CA3 cells located at any particular septotemporal level distribute some of their collaterals to much of the full septotemporal extent of CA1. This projection is not chaotic, however, and its topographical organization develops a network in which certain CA3 cells are more likely to contact certain CA1 cells.

The major organizational features of this projection are as follows: CA3 cells located close to the dentate gyrus (proximal CA3), although projecting both septally and temporally, project more heavily to levels of CA1 located septal to their location. CA3 cells located closer to CA1, in contrast, project more heavily to the levels of CA1 located temporally (Fig. 3–30). At or close to the septotemporal level of the cells of origin, those cells located proximally in CA3 give rise to collaterals that tend to terminate superficially in the stratum radiatum. Conversely, cells located more distally in CA3 give rise to projections that terminate deeper in the stratum radiatum and stratum oriens. At or close to the septotemporal level of origin, CA3 pyramidal cells located near the dentate gyrus tend to project somewhat more heavily to distal portions of CA1 (near the subiculum), whereas CA3 projections arising from cells located distally in CA3 terminate more heavily in portions of CA1 located closer to CA2. The truly thick Schaffer collaterals (those that Schaffer originally described) originate only from the proximal CA3 cells. These cells give rise to a thick axon that ascends from the stratum oriens into the most superficial portion of the stratum radiatum and travels to the distal part of CA1, where it contributes many collaterals.

Figure 3–30. Organization of the projections from the CA3 field to the CA1 field of the hippocampus—the Schaffer collaterals. The location of the cells of origin is indicated by small triangles in the middle coronal section. Terminals from these cells are indicated by different shades of gray similar to those in the triangles.

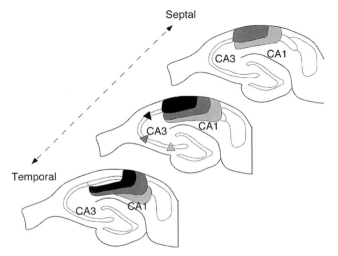

The axons of distal CA3 cells tend to be much thinner and to project directly to CA1, either within the stratum oriens or through the deep portion of the stratum radiatum.

The position of the terminal field in CA1 varies in a systematic fashion relative to the distance from the cells of origin. Regardless of the septotemporal or transverse origin of a projection, the highest density of terminal and fiber labeling in CA1 shifts to deeper parts of the stratum radiatum and stratum oriens at levels septal to the cells of origin and shifts away from the stratum oriens and into superficial parts of the stratum radiatum at levels temporal to the cells of origin. Moreover, the highest density of fiber and terminal labeling in CA1 shifts proximally (toward CA3) at levels septal to the origin and distally (toward the subiculum) at levels temporal to the origin.

The entire axonal plexus of several CA3 pyramidal cells have been labeled by intracellular staining techniques devised by Buzsaki and colleagues (Li et al., 1994). These studies provide convincing evidence that the axons of individual CA3 cells can distribute to as much as two-thirds of the septotemporal extent of the ipsilateral and contralateral CA1 fields. The plexus from a single CA3 neuron comprises as much as 150 to 300 mm of total axonal length, on which 30,000 to 60,000 synaptic varicosities are formed. Although single neurons have not been evaluated at all septotemporal levels, it appears that the extent of the CA3 connections is more restricted at temporal levels. Here neurons may give rise to axonal plexuses that innervate only the temporal third of the CA1 field.

A number of pieces of fundamental information concerning the CA3 projection to CA1 are still unknown. For example, it is not clear how many synapses a single CA3 cell makes on a typical CA1 cell. To answer this question using neuroanatomical procedures would be a monumental task. First, a CA3 and CA1 neuron would have to be impaled with dye-bearing pipettes, and the two cells would have to be tested for connectivity by electrophysiological methods. The two cells would then have to be filled and processed histologically for visualization. That is the easy part. The neurons would then have to be sectioned serially for electron microscopy and all putative synapses evaluated. Only in this way would one be able to determine how many synapses are made by all of the collaterals of a particular CA3 neuron on an identified CA1 pyramidal cell. A number of laboratories have estimated the extent of connectivity between CA3 and CA1 cells, and the numbers are always quite low. Work from Harris and colleagues (Sorra and Harris, 1993), which has been replicated by Trommaid et al. (1996), indicates that there are perhaps as few as two to four contacts between a single axon in the stratum radiatum and a particular dendritic tree and certainly no more than 10 synapses between typical CA3 and CA1 neurons. The surprising state of affairs, however, is that we simply do not know with certainty how many contacts a single CA3 neuron makes with a single CA1 cell. These data are critical for interpreting some of the quantal analysis studies described in Chapter 10.

To summarize, the CA3 to CA1 projection is the major input to CA1 pyramidal cells. The projection terminates on the basal dendrites in the stratum oriens and the apical dendrites in the stratum radiatum. Individual CA3 axons distribute extensively and may innervate neurons throughout as much as two-thirds of the entire septotemporal extent of the hippocampus. The probability that a particular CA1 cell is contacted by a particular CA3 cell depends, in part, on the transverse positions of the two cell bodies and their septotemporal distance. At one particular septotemporal level, a distal CA3 cell is more likely to interact with a proximal CA1 cell, whereas a proximal CA3 cells is more likely to interact with a distal CA1 cell. The proximal CA3 cells are the only ones with classic thick Schaffer collaterals, and the thickness of these initial axons is likely to reflect the longer distance the axon must travel to innervate distal CA1 cells.

CA3 to CA3 Associational Connections

The associational projections from CA3 to CA3 are also organized in a highly systematic fashion. One somewhat idiosyncratic facet of this projection is that cells located proximally in CA3 communicate only with other proximally located CA3 cells. Associational projections arising from mid and distal portions of CA3, however, project throughout much of the transverse extent of CA3 and also project much more extensively along the septotemporal axis. The density of CA3 associational projections also shifts along the septotemporal axis. The radial gradient of termination (superficial to deep in the stratum radiatum and stratum oriens) is similar to that described for the CA3 to CA1 projection. The transverse gradient, however, is the reverse; CA3 projections shift proximally in CA3 at levels located temporal to the cells of origin and shift distally in CA3 at more septal levels.

Commissural Connections of the Hippocampus

In the rat, the CA3 pyramidal cells give rise to commissural projections to the CA3, CA2, and CA1 fields of the contralateral hippocampal formation (Blackstad, 1956; Fricke and Cowan, 1978). In fact, the same CA3 cells give rise to both the ipsilateral and commissural projections. Although the commissural projections follow roughly the same topographical organization as the ipsilateral projections and generally terminate in homologous regions on both sides, there are minor differences in the distribution of terminals. If a projection is heavier to the stratum oriens on the ipsilateral side, for example, it may be heavier in the stratum radiatum on the contralateral side. The detailed topography of the commissural connections has not been as thoroughly investigated as the ipsilateral connections. As with the commissural projections from the dentate gyrus, CA3 fibers to the contralateral hippocampus form asymmetrical synapses on the spines of pyramidal cells in CA3 and CA1 but also terminate on the smooth dendrites of interneurons. As noted earlier, hippocampal commissural connections are much less abundant in the monkey and are likely to be absent in humans.

CA1 Lacks Associational Connections

Unlike CA3, pyramidal cells in CA1 give rise to a much more limited associational projection. As the CA1 axons travel in the alveus or the stratum oriens toward the subiculum (see below), occasional collaterals are generated that enter the stratum oriens and the pyramidal cell layer, most likely contacting interneurons such as basket cells in the stratum oriens and in turn inhibiting CA1 pyramidal cells. It is also conceivable that these collaterals might contact the basal dendrites of other CA1 cells. What is clear, however, is that the massive associational network, which is so apparent in CA3, is largely missing in CA1. Similarly, although a weak commissural projection to the contralateral CA1 appears to be present, there is no extensive commissural projection originating in CA1, as is the case in CA3.

CA1 Projection to the Subiculum

The CA1 field gives rise to two intrahippocampal projections. The first is a topographically organized projection to the adjacent subiculum. The second is to the deep layers of the entorhinal cortex. The latter projection is discussed in Section 3.4.5.

Axons of CA1 pyramidal cells descend into the stratum oriens or the alveus and bend sharply toward the subiculum (Amaral et al., 1991). The fibers reenter the pyramidal cell layer of the subiculum and ramify profusely in the pyramidal cell layer and the deep portion of the molecular layer. Unlike the CA3 to CA1 projection, which distributes throughout CA1 in a gradient fashion, the CA1 projection ends in a topographical fashion in the subiculum. Proximally located CA1 cells project to the distal portion of the subiculum, whereas distally located CA1 cells project just across the border into the proximal portion of the subiculum; the midportion of CA1 projects to the midportion of the subiculum (Fig. 3–31). Nobuaki Tamamaki (Tamamaki et al., 1987) injected horseradish peroxidase into single CA1 pyramidal cells and demonstrated that individual axonal plexuses distribute to about one-third of the transverse extent of the subicular pyramidal cell layer and for approximately one-third of the septotemporal length. It appears, therefore, that the CA1 to subiculum projection segments these structures roughly into thirds. The CA1 to subiculum projection, like the CA3 to CA1 projection, is organized in a divergent fashion, as even a small portion of CA1 projects to about a third of the septotemporal extent of the subiculum.

3.4.3 Subiculum

Cytoarchitectonic Organization

The cytoarchitectonic characteristics of the rat subiculum have been studied to a limited extent (O'Mara et al., 2001). The CA1/subiculum border is marked by abrupt widening of the pyramidal cell layer and an increased staining intensity with the Timm stain (Fig. 3–11). The stratum radiatum of

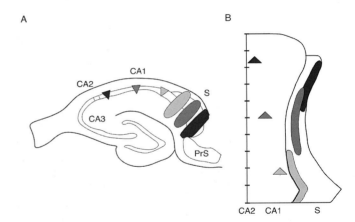

Figure 3–31. Organization of the projections from the CA1 field of the hippocampus to the subiculum. *A.* Coronal section shows the cells of origin (triangles) and their respective terminal fields, indicated by similar shades of gray. *B.* Two-dimensional unfolded map of CA1 and the subiculum. The septal portion of these fields is at the top of the figure, and the temporal pole is at the bottom; the border between CA2 and CA1 is on the left.

CA1 (defined as the region that receives CA3 projections) also ends at this border and is replaced with the molecular layer of the subiculum. This layer can be subdivided into a deep portion that is continuous with the stratum radiatum of CA1 and a superficial portion that is continuous with the stratum lacunosum-moleculare of CA1 and the molecular layer of the presubiculum. The deep portion receives fibers from CA1, whereas the superficial portion receives fibers from the entorhinal cortex. The stratum oriens of CA1 is no longer present in the subiculum.

Neuron Types

Research on the cytology and connectivity of the subiculum has lagged behind the research on other areas of the hippocampal formation; and until recently (Funahashi and Stewart, 1997a,b; Harris et al., 2001) much of the information on subicular cell types came from the classic Golgi studies of Ramon y Cajal and Lorente de Nó in young mice. The principal cell layer of the subiculum is populated by large pyramidal neurons (Fig. 3–32). This layer starts just underneath the distal end of CA1 and continues in a position deep to layer II of the presubiculum. These cells are relatively uniform in shape and size, and they extend their apical dendrites into the molecular layer and their basal dendrites into deeper portions of the pyramidal cell layer. A subdivision into at least two cell types has been proposed based on their firing characteristics: regular spiking cells and intrinsically bursting cells (Greene and Totterdell, 1997). Although these two cell types do not exhibit distinct morphological characteristics (but see below), they show a differential distribution in the pyramidal cell layer. Bursting cells are more numerous deep in the pyramidal cell layer, whereas regular spiking cells are more common superficially. The two populations can also be distinguished by

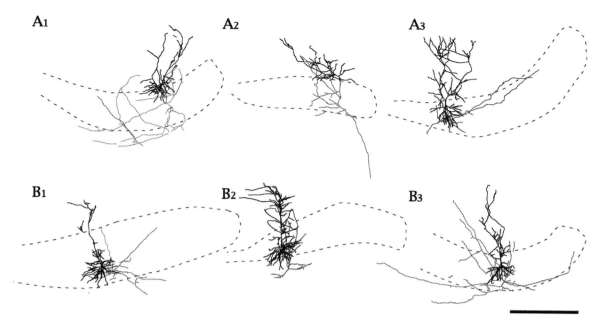

Figure 3–32. Neurolucida reconstructions of superficial and deep subicular cells. Somata and dendrites are shown in black. Axons are shown in gray. Local collaterals tend to be longer in the cell layer for superficially located cells; deep cells tend to have axon collaterals that ascend close to the primary dendrite. CA1 is at the left, and the presubiculum is at the right. Bar = 500 μm. (*Source*: Adapted from Harris et al., 2001.)

preferential staining for either NADPH-diaphorase/nitric oxide synthetase (regular spiking neurons) or somatostatin (bursting cells). Both cell types are projection neurons, but they might differ with respect to their connectivity because there is evidence suggesting that only bursting cells project to the entorhinal cortex. Intermingled among the pyramidal cells are many smaller neurons, presumably representing the interneurons of the subiculum. Little is known, however, about whether the interneurons seen in the subiculum are similar to those observed in the hippocampus. Subpopulations of these neurons appear to have characteristics similar to those described for CA1; among these subpopulations are GABAergic cells that stain for the calcium-binding protein parvalbumin.

Intrinsic Connections

The subiculum gives rise to a longitudinal associational projection that extends from the level of the cells of origin to much of the subiculum lying temporally (or ventrally). Interestingly, this projection seems to be largely unidirectional, as few if any associational projections course septally or dorsally from their point of origin (Harris et al., 2001). The associational fibers terminate diffusely in all layers of the subiculum. Recent studies have consistently found that the rat subiculum neither gives rise to nor receives commissural connections.

Subicular pyramidal cells provide a strong local input in the pyramidal cell layer and just superficial to it, targeting proximal portions of the apical dendrites. Interestingly, the density of this local intrinsic connection, as estimated by the number of varicosities on locally distributed axon collaterals, is much higher than in CA1. In addition, the two types of subicular pyramidal neurons differ with respect to their local connectivity. Intracellular labeling of electrophysiologically identified bursting cells generally show an axonal distribution that remains in the region circumscribed by their apical dendrites (i.e., a columnar organization), whereas the regular spiking cells generally give rise to an axon that shows more widespread distribution along the transverse axis (Fig. 3–33). It is not known whether differences exist with respect to possible septotemporal spread. Although much work remains to be done, available data indicate that the organization of the intrinsic connectivity of the subiculum is different from that of CA3 and CA1. There is both crude columnar and laminar organization, such that the bursting cells form a set of columns and the regular spiking neurons integrate columnar activity along the transverse axis.

Extrinsic Connections: Subiculum, a Major Output Structure

The subiculum is a major source of efferent projections from the hippocampal formation. Following the discovery by Swanson and Cowan that the subiculum, rather than the hippocampus, is the origin of the major subcortical connections to the diencephalon and brain stem (via the postcommissural fornix), evidence has mounted that the subiculum is one of the two primary output structures of the hippocampal formation (Swanson and Cowan, 1975; Swanson et al., 1981;

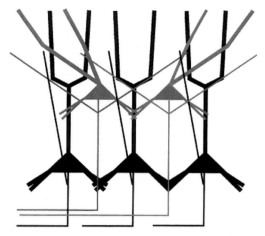

Figure 3–33. Model of intrinsic organization of the subiculum. Deep cells have ascending axon collaterals that remain in close proximity to their apical dendrites, giving rise to a columnar pattern for the deep cells. Superficial cells have axon collaterals that can run long distances in the cell layer perhaps serving to integrate activity between columns. (*Source*: Adapted from Harris et al., 2001.)

Donovan and Wyss, 1983; Groenewegen et al., 1987; Witter and Groenewegen, 1990; Witter et al., 1990; Canteras and Swanson, 1992; Naber and Witter, 1998; Ishizuka, 2001; Kloosterman et al., 2003).

Subiculum Projects to the Presubiculum and Parasubiculum

The subiculum projects to the presubiculum, but this projection is not of the magnitude of other intrinsic hippocampal formation projections. It is probably better to think of the subiculum projection to the presubiculum as one of a series of pathways that distributes information processed in the dentate gyrus, hippocampus, and subiculum to a series of cortical and subcortical structures. The subiculum can be viewed, therefore, as the last step in the large loop of processing through the hippocampal formation.

Subicular fibers terminate mainly in layer I of the presubiculum. The projection to the dorsal part of the presubiculum, however, terminates deep to the prominent layer II, with weaker projections to layers I and II. The projections from the subiculum to the parasubiculum mainly terminate in layer I and the superficial portion of layer II. These projections are topographically organized. Septal (or dorsal) portions of the subiculum project to dorsal and caudal aspects of both the presubiculum and the parasubiculum, and temporal (or ventral) portions of the subiculum project to ventral and rostral aspects of the pre- and parasubiculum.

Subiculum Reciprocally Connected with the Entorhinal Cortex

Because the perforant path fibers traverse the subiculum on their way to the dentate gyrus and hippocampus, the question of whether some of these fibers might terminate in the subiculum has long been a matter of controversy. Until recently, the collective hunch was that fibers simply passed through the subiculum and probably did not terminate in it. Earlier anterograde tracer studies indicated that perforant path fibers are directed toward the molecular layer of the subiculum, but proof that these fibers formed a terminal plexus among the subicular pyramidal cells was lacking. Witter and colleagues, however, have provided evidence, at both light and electron microscopic levels, that the subiculum receives a strong projection from the entorhinal cortex. The topography of the projection is similar to that described for CA1. Fibers are directed toward restricted transverse portions of the subiculum and terminate in the outer two-thirds of the molecular layer. The lateral component of the perforant pathway preferentially projects to the proximal part of the subiculum (i.e., the part of the subiculum that borders CA1), and the medial component distributes to more distal portions of the subiculum (i.e., closer to the presubiculum). The projection originates mainly from layer III, although some of the axons of layer II cells that cross the subiculum on their way to the dentate gyrus and CA3 may also give off collaterals that terminate in the subiculum. Entorhinal fibers target dendritic spines of presumed principal neurons with asymmetrical synapses (80%), whereas 5% to 10% of the asymmetrical synapses terminate on dendritic shafts, most likely belonging to interneurons. Subicular interneurons may also receive a minor inhibitory perforant path input in view of the symmetrical synapses onto dendritic shafts.

The subiculum reciprocates the entorhinal input (Fig. 3–34). Projections from the subiculum reach all parts of the entorhinal cortex and terminate in the deep layers; termination is particularly dense in layer V. A minor component of the subicular projection also extends superficial to the lamina dissecans, predominantly to layer III. Subicular fibers generally form asymmetrical synapses with spines and dendrites located in these layers. A small number of these fibers form symmetrical synapses, suggesting small inhibitory input from the subiculum to layer V. Therefore, the overall organization of the subiculo-entorhinal projection mimics that of the CA1-entorhinal projection. The presence of asymmetrical synapses at the termination of this pathway is consistent with its reported excitatory influences on the entorhinal cortex.

Subicular Connections with the Neocortex and Amygdaloid Complex

The subiculum gives rise to prominent projections to the medial and ventral orbitofrontal cortices and to the prelimbic and infralimbic cortices (Verwer et al., 1997). In the orbitofrontal and prelimbic cortices subicular fibers mainly innervate the deep layers, whereas in the infralimbic cortex the projection extends into the superficial layers. Subicular projections also reach medial portions of the anterior olfactory nucleus.

The subiculum provides a meager projection to the anterior cingulate cortex, whereas the projection to the retrosplenial cortex is substantial (Wyss and Van Groen, 1992). The

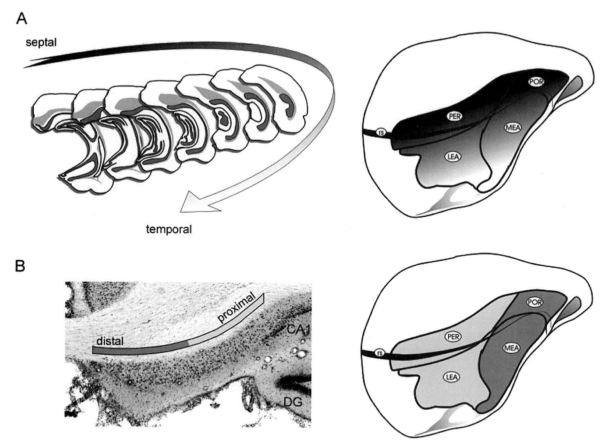

Figure 3–34. Topographical organization of the subicular projections to the parahippocampal region (entorhinal, perirhinal, and postrhinal cortices). *A*. Relation between the septotemporal origin in the subiculum with a lateral-to-medial termination in the parahippocampal region. The septal portion of the subiculum projects to the perirhinal and postrhinal cortices and the lateral portion of both the lateral and medial entorhinal cortex. The temporal portion of the subiculum projects to medial portions of the lateral and medial entorhinal cortex. *B*. Relation between the proximo-distal origin in the subiculum with a rostrocaudal termination in the parahippocampal region. The proximal subiculum projects to the perirhinal and lateral entorhinal cortex; the distal subiculum projects to the postrhinal and medial entorhinal cortex. (*Source*: Adapted from Kloosterman et al., 2003.)

subiculo-retrosplenial projection terminates predominantly in layers II and III. The projections to the retrosplenial cortex originate predominantly from the septal two-thirds of the subiculum. The perirhinal cortex receives a strong input from the subiculum, which terminates in both superficial and deep layers.

In the rat, there is a paucity of detailed information regarding direct cortical inputs to the subiculum. Many of the cortical regions that project fairly heavily to the entorhinal cortex (see below) do not project to the subiculum. No inputs, for example, have been reported from the pre- and infralimbic cortices. Similarly, no portion of the retrosplenial cortex projects to the subiculum. Reports of projections from the cingulate cortex have been somewhat contradictory. In a combined electrophysiological and neuroanatomical study, White et al. (1990) reported a projection from the anterior cingulate cortex to the subiculum. However, this projection has not been observed consistently. The perirhinal cortex projects to the subiculum, but this projection terminates only in the proximal third of the field (i.e., at the border region with CA1).

The proximal portion of the subiculum also receives an input from the parvicellular portion of the basal nucleus of the amygdaloid complex, the posterior cortical nucleus, and the adjacent amygdalohippocampal area. These amygdaloid inputs terminate mainly at the CA1/subiculum border region, where they preferentially innervate the molecular layer of the subiculum and stratum lacunosum-moleculare of CA1 (Pitkanen et al., 2000).

The temporal one-third of the subiculum gives rise to return projections to the amygdaloid complex. The major component of this projection terminates in the accessory basal nucleus, with more moderate projections reaching several other nuclei but not the lateral nucleus. The ventral subiculum also projects heavily to the bed nucleus of the stria terminalis and moderately to the ventral part of the claustrum or endopiriform nucleus.

Basal Forebrain Connections: Septal Nucleus and Nucleus Accumbens

The most prominent subcortical subicular projections are those to the septal complex, the adjacent nucleus accumbens, and the mammillary nuclei. The projection to the septal area terminates predominantly in the lateral septal nuclei. Closely associated with the septal projection is the equally robust projection to the nucleus accumbens and adjacent portions of the olfactory tubercle. Subicular fibers terminate throughout the nucleus accumbens, with the projection to its caudomedial part being most dense. As with other striatal structures, the subicular projection to the nucleus accumbens is unidirectional. Whereas the subicular projections to the lateral septal nucleus are almost entirely confined to the ipsilateral side, those to the nucleus accumbens show a weak contralateral component. The subiculum receives a relatively weak cholinergic projection from the septal complex; fibers originating from the medial septal nucleus and the nucleus of the diagonal band terminate in the pyramidal cell and molecular layers.

Hypothalamic Connections: Mammillary Nuclei

The subiculum provides the major input to the mammillary nuclei. The projection is heavy and is distributed bilaterally in nearly equal density. The subiculomammillary fibers originate mainly from the septal two-thirds of the subiculum. Although the temporal one-third of the subiculum also contributes to the mammillary projection, the major hypothalamic target of this portion of the subiculum is the ventromedial nucleus of the hypothalamus. The subicular projections to the mammillary nuclei reach all portions of the medial nucleus but are topographically organized; the lateral mammillary nucleus is only sparsely innervated by the subiculum. Subicular fibers also project to the lateral hypothalamic region located adjacent to the lateral mammillary nucleus.

Whereas the subiculum does not receive a return projection from the medial or lateral mammillary nuclei, the supramammillary region projects heavily to the subiculum, particularly to its temporal levels. This portion of the subiculum also receives an input from the premammillary nucleus. It is not clear whether there are any local connections between the medial mammillary nucleus and the supramammillary area or the premammillary nucleus that might complete the subiculohypothalamic loop.

Thalamic Connections: Nucleus Reuniens and Other Midline Nuclei

The thalamic inputs to the subiculum are similar to those to CA1. Thalamic inputs originate mainly in the nucleus reuniens, the paraventricular nucleus, and the parataenial nucleus. The septal and temporal extremes of the subiculum appear to be devoid of input from the nucleus reuniens. The midline thalamic projections terminate mainly in the molecular layer of the subiculum, whereas in CA1 they are coextensive with the projections from the entorhinal cortex.

Interestingly, the projections to the subiculum and to CA1 originate from different but intermingled populations of neurons in the nucleus reuniens. Although earlier studies had indicated that the subiculum was interconnected with the anterior nuclear complex, it is now clear that the anterior nucleus projects almost exclusively to the pre- and parasubiculum.

Some of the thalamic regions that project to the subiculum receive a return projection from the subiculum. Subicular fibers terminate bilaterally in the nucleus reuniens, the nucleus interanteromedialis, the paraventricular nucleus, and the nucleus gelatinosus. Although subicular projections to parts of the anterior thalamic complex have been described in the literature, more recent retrograde tracing studies have shown that these projections arise from the presubiculum.

Brain Stem Inputs

Monoaminergic ascending pathways from the noradrenergic locus coeruleus, the dopaminergic ventral tegmental area, and the serotonergic median and dorsal raphe nuclei reach the subiculum, but they do not show preferential innervation of this region. Few details are available concerning the regional localization of these pathways in the subiculum.

Topography of Subicular Efferent Projections

As with the projections from CA3 to CA1 and from CA1 to the subiculum, the subicular efferent projections are topographically organized. In large part, the subicular projections preserve the transverse topography established by the CA1 to subiculum projection. It is clear that different projections originate from at least the proximal and distal halves of the subiculum. The subiculum also demonstrates marked septotemporal topography, such that the projections that arise from the septal or dorsal two-thirds of the subiculum are different from those that arise from the temporal or ventral third (Witter and Amaral, 2004).

Turning first to the septotemporal topography, it appears that the projections to the entorhinal cortex, the lateral septal complex, the nucleus accumbens, and the medial mammillary nucleus originate from the entire septotemporal extent of the subiculum (Witter and Groenewegen, 1990; Ishizuka, 2001). Different septotemporal levels of the subiculum, however, project to different portions of these fields. In the entorhinal cortex, for example, the septal-to-temporal origin in the subiculum is related to a lateral-to-medial termination in the entorhinal cortex. Septal levels of the subiculum project preferentially to lateral and caudal parts of the entorhinal cortex (i.e., the parts that lie adjacent to the rhinal sulcus). Progressively more temporal levels of the subiculum project to more medially located parts of the entorhinal cortex. Although addressed in more detail below, it is important to point out that this topography is completely in register (i.e., they are point-to-point reciprocal) with the projections from the entorhinal cortex to the subiculum. Thus, cells in the subiculum that receive input from a subregion in the entorhinal cortex give rise to a return projection to the same region in the entorhinal cortex. In some respect this breaks the rule that all structures in the hippocampal formation have unidirectional connectivity, but other aspects of the neuroanatomy of these areas completely justify their inclusion in the functionally defined hippocampal formation.

In the nucleus accumbens, the septotemporal axis of origin in the subiculum determines a caudomedial to rostrolateral axis of termination. Dorsomedial portions of the lateral septal complex receive inputs from septal levels of the subiculum, and ventral portions of the lateral septal complex are innervated by fibers originating in more temporal parts of the subiculum.

Similar septotemporal topography has also been described for the subicular projections to the presubiculum and the medial mammillary nuclei. The latter projection arises mainly from the septal two-thirds of the subiculum, whereas the ventral one-third gives rise to projections to other hypothalamic regions such as the ventromedial nucleus.

This dichotomy between the septal two-thirds and the temporal one-third of the subiculum is reflected in the organization of other projections. Projections to the amygdala and the bed nucleus of the stria terminalis, for example, originate exclusively from the temporal one-third of the subiculum, whereas projections to the retrosplenial and perirhinal cortices originate predominantly from the septal two-thirds. The subicular projections to the midline thalamus demonstrate even greater septotemporal topography. The most septal part of the subiculum projects preferentially to the interanteromedial nucleus; mid-septotemporal levels of the subiculum preferentially project to the nucleus reuniens; and the temporal third of the subiculum projects most heavily to the paraventricular nucleus.

Whereas the septotemporal topography appears to be organized in a gradient, or gradual, fashion, the transverse organization of subicular efferents is remarkably discrete. Along the transverse axis of the subiculum, two essentially nonoverlapping populations of cells can be differentiated that give rise to projections to specific sets of brain structures. This transverse organization of the outputs of the subiculum is consistently observed along its entire septotemporal axis, although it is clearer septally than temporally.

Neurons in the proximal half of the subiculum (closest to CA1) project to the infralimbic and prelimbic cortices, the perirhinal cortex, the nucleus accumbens, the lateral septum, the amygdaloid complex, and the core of the ventromedial nucleus of the hypothalamus. Cells in the distal half of the subiculum project mainly to the retrosplenial cortex and the presubiculum. Cells projecting to the midline thalamic nuclei are mainly located in the midportion of the subiculum.

The subicular projections to the entorhinal cortex and to the medial mammillary nucleus do not follow a strictly transverse organization, as cells in all proximo-distal portions of the subiculum project to these areas. However, the topography of these projections indicates a more subtle transverse organ-

ization. Thus, the proximal portions of the subiculum project to rostral medial mammillary nuclei, and distal portions of the subiculum project more caudally. A similar situation exists for the subicular projections to the entorhinal cortex. The proximal half of the subiculum projects to the lateral entorhinal area, and the distal half of the subiculum projects to the medial entorhinal area.

Because the proximal third of the subiculum gives rise to projections to at least several cortical and subcortical regions, the question arises as to whether it is the same or different populations of subicular cells that innervate each structure. The answer initially appeared to be that projections to the septal complex, entorhinal cortex and mammillary complex arise, at least in part, as collaterals from single subicular neurons; but it now appears that largely independent populations of intermixed neurons in the subiculum project to each of its terminal regions (Naber and Witter, 1998). Given our earlier assertion that the subiculum is the last staging post of hippocampal processing, this state of affairs seems to create the possibility that the outputs destined for different target structures can be carrying distinctly different information.

3.4.4 Presubiculum and Parasubiculum

Cytoarchitectonic Organization and Neuron Types

The presubiculum, Brodmann's area 27, is relatively easily differentiated from the subiculum in standard Nissl-stained material. It has a distinct, densely packed external cell layer that consists mainly of darkly stained, small pyramidal cells. The most superficial cells are the most densely packed (layer II), whereas the deeper cells have a somewhat looser arrangement (layer III). The differentiation between layers II and III is more clear-cut at dorsal levels of the presubiculum.

The dorsal presubiculum (sometimes called the postsubiculum) has clearly distinguishable superficial and deep cell layers. In the ventral portion of the presubiculum, however, the deep layers are difficult to distinguish from the deep layers of the entorhinal cortex or from the principal cell layer of the subiculum. Deep to the lamina dissecans there are one or two layers of large, darkly stained pyramidal cells; and deep to these cells is a rather heterogeneous collection of pyramidal and polymorphic cells. The latter cells have not been studied anatomically in great detail (Fig. 3–35), although electrophysiological discoveries about their receptive field characteristics are important to one prominent theory of hippocampal function (see Chapter 8).

The parasubiculum (Brodmann's area 49) lies adjacent to the presubiculum. Layers II and III of the parasubiculum consist of rather densely packed, lightly stained, large pyramidal cells. This and other characteristics, such as the distinctive staining for heavy metals observable with the Timm's stain method, are the major features that differentiate the parasubiculum from the presubiculum (Fig. 3–11). There is no clear differentiation between layers II and III; and as with the

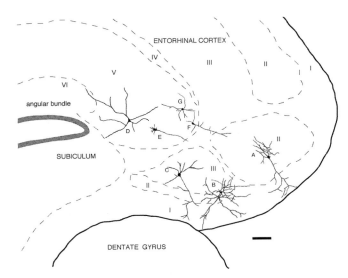

Figure 3–35. Cell types of the presubiculum and parasubiculum. Camera lucida drawings of neurobiotin-filled cells in a horizontal section through the hippocampal formation. *A.* Pyramidal cell in layer II of the parasubiculum. *B.* Stellate cell in layer II of the presubiculum. *C.* Pyramidal cell in layer III of the presubiculum. *D.* Stellate cell in layer V of the presubiculum. *E.* Pyramidal cell in layer V of the presubiculum. *F.* Pyramidal cell in layer V of the parasubiculum. *G.* Stellate cell in layer V of the parasubiculum. Bar = 100 μm. (*Source:* Adapted from Funahashi and Stewart, 1997a.)

presubiculum, the deep layers are continuous with those of the entorhinal cortex.

Intrinsic Connections

There are well developed associational connections in the presubiculum that interconnect all dorsoventral levels in a highly directional manner. Layer II cells in ventral portions of the presubiculum project to more dorsal levels of the presubiculum. Projections in the opposite direction (dorsal to ventral), however, arise preferentially from cells in the deep layers.

The parasubiculum also gives rise to associational connections that distribute both dorsally and ventrally from the cells of origin. The dorsally directed projections extend for short distances and are quite weak. The ventrally directed projections are substantially denser and extend for long distances along the long axis of the parasubiculum. The parasubiculum gives rise to a particularly dense projection to the dorsally located area 29e. This small wedge-shaped region was initially described by Blackstad (1956) and later characterized in more detail by Haug (1976). Although the neuroanatomy of area 29e remains sketchy, it might be part of the parasubiculum.

Commissural Connections

The presubiculum gives rise to strong commissural projections to layers I and III of the homotopic part of the contralateral presubiculum (Van Groen and Wyss, 1990).

Commissural projections from the dorsal portion of the presubiculum are relatively sparse. The parasubiculum also gives rise to a commissural projection that terminates most densely in layers I and III.

Extrinsic Connections

Presubiculum and Parasubiculum Reciprocally Connected with Anterior Thalamic Nuclei

The presubiculum and parasubiculum receive a number of subcortical inputs, but the one that is unique to these portions of the hippocampal formation is their interconnection with the anterior thalamic nuclear complex, primarily the anteroventral and anterodorsal nuclei and the closely related laterodorsal nucleus (Kaitz and Robertson, 1981; Robertson and Kaitz, 1981). Although earlier studies had suggested that the presubiculum also receives inputs from the anteromedial nucleus, the principal projections of this nucleus appear to be directed to the anterior parts of the cingulate cortex rather than to the presubiculum or parasubiculum.

There are topographical differences in the thalamic connections of the ventral and dorsal portions of the presubiculum. The ventral portion receives most of its input from the laterodorsal and anteroventral nuclei, whereas the dorsal part receives projections mainly from the laterodorsal and anterodorsal nuclei. The thalamic projections mainly terminate in layers I, III, and IV. The nucleus reuniens also projects to layer I of the presubiculum, but this is a much lighter projection.

Like most other thalamocortical connections, the presubiculum sends a return projection back to the thalamus. The presubiculum projects massively and bilaterally to the anterior nuclear complex. The presubicular projections arise mainly from cells located deep to the lamina dissecans (layer VI). The fact that these deep cells are related to the anterior nuclei of the thalamus lends some credibility to the idea that they are, in fact, deep layers of the pre- and parasubiculum rather than of the entorhinal cortex.

Presubiculum Projection to Layer III of the Entorhinal Cortex

The most prominent intrahippocampal projection from the presubiculum is to the entorhinal cortex (Shipley, 1975; Caballero-Bleda and Witter, 1993). This projection has a number of interesting features. First, the presubicular projection is directed only to the medial entorhinal area. Second, the projection terminates almost exclusively in layer III and to a much lesser extent in the deep part of layer I. Third, the crossed homotopic projection from the presubiculum to the contralateral entorhinal cortex is every bit as dense as the ipsilateral projection. The projection to the entorhinal cortex is topographically organized. The location of the presubicular terminal field in the entorhinal cortex is determined by both the proximo-distal and dorsoventral location of the presubicular cells of origin.

The parasubiculum selectively innervates layer II of the entorhinal cortex. In contrast to the presubiculum, the parasubiculum projects to both the medial and lateral entorhinal areas, although the projection to the lateral entorhinal area is less robust. The parasubiculum projects to the contralateral entorhinal cortex, but these projections are much weaker than the ipsilateral ones. The topographical organization of the parasubicular projection to the entorhinal cortex is comparable to that of the presubiculo-entorhinal projection.

Presubiculum and Parasubiculum Connected with Some Neocortical Regions

The presubiculum receives relatively few extrahippocampal cortical inputs. The most prominent one originates in the retrosplenial cortex (Van Groen and Wyss, 1990; Wyss and Van Groen, 1992). Cells located in layer V of the retrosplenial cortex give rise to projections that terminate in layers I and III/V of the presubiculum. A second cortical input originates from layer V of the visual area 18b. This projection mainly distributes to the dorsal half of the presubiculum and terminates in layers I and III. Minor cortical inputs originate in the prelimbic cortex and in a dorsal portion of the medial prefrontal cortex.

Extrahippocampal projections from layer V of the presubiculum reach the granular retrosplenial cortex, where they terminate preferentially in layers I and II. These projections are topographically organized, such that the ventral presubiculum projects mainly to the ventral part of the granular retrosplenial cortex, and the dorsal part of the presubiculum projects more dorsally. These projections also exhibit a rostro-caudal organization, such that rostral portions of the presubiculum project to rostral parts of the retrosplenial cortex, and caudal portions of the presubiculum project to caudal parts of the retrosplenial cortex. It has been suggested that the dorsal presubiculum projects to the deep layers of the most caudal portion of the perirhinal cortex, although an alternative interpretation is that this projection is directed to the most caudodorsal portion of the medial entorhinal cortex, which is difficult to differentiate from the caudal perirhinal cortex. The work of Burwell et al. (1998a,b) supports the latter idea.

With the exception of the relatively light projections from the retrosplenial cortex and the occipital visual cortex, there are no other known extrahippocampal cortical inputs to the parasubiculum. The laminar distribution of these inputs is similar to that described for the presubiculum.

Other Intrahippocampal Connections

The presubiculum projects to layers I and II of the parasubiculum bilaterally. Anterograde tracing studies with the lectin tracer PHA-L have demonstrated that the presubiculum and perhaps to a greater extent the parasubiculum contribute projections, albeit modest ones, to many of the other regions of the hippocampal formation. For example, there is a modest bilateral projection from the presubiculum to the subiculum. There is also a weak projection to all fields of the hippocampus and to the molecular layer of the dentate gyrus. The presubicular fibers to the dentate molecular layer are arranged in a radial manner, which is quite distinct from the predominantly transverse orientation of the entorhinal perforant pathway fibers.

A fact that has not been generally appreciated is that the parasubiculum gives rise to a fairly substantial projection to the molecular layer of the dentate gyrus (Kohler, 1985). Like the lighter projection from the presubiculum, this projection occupies the superficial two-thirds of the molecular layer (with a preference for the midportion of the molecular layer), and the fibers have a predominantly radial orientation. Because the parasubiculum receives a projection from the anterior thalamic nuclei, its projection to the molecular layer provides a route by which thalamic input might influence the very early stages of hippocampal information processing. The parasubiculum projects weakly to the stratum lacunosum-moleculare of the hippocampus and to the molecular layer of the subiculum. The parasubiculum also projects bilaterally to layers I and III of the presubiculum.

Basal Forebrain Connections

The presubiculum and parasubiculum receive heavy cholinergic input. The medial septal nucleus and the vertical limb of the diagonal band of Broca mainly innervate layer II of the presubiculum.

Hypothalamic Connections: Mammillary Nuclei

The deep layers of the presubiculum project bilaterally to the medial and lateral mammillary nuclei. The projections to the medial mammillary nuclei are topographically organized in a manner similar to those that originate in the subiculum (Thompson and Robertson, 1987; Allen and Hopkins, 1989; Van Groen and Wyss, 1990).

The presubiculum receives input from the area surrounding the mammillary nuclei. Fibers from the supramammillary nucleus terminate preferentially in the deeper cell layers of the presubiculum, although those characterized as being positive for α-melanocyte-stimulating hormone (an opiate peptide expressed in neurons whose somata are located in the lateral hypothalamic area) terminate in the molecular layer.

Brain Stem Inputs

The presubiculum receives input from various nuclei in the brain stem. A particularly dense innervation arises from the dorsal and ventral raphe nuclei; at least a component of this projection is serotonergic and innervates layer I. The noradrenergic locus coeruleus innervates the plexiform layer.

3.4.5 Entorhinal Cortex

The entorhinal cortex plays an extraordinarily important role in the flow of information through the hippocampal formation. It is not only the main entry point for much of the sensory information processed by the hippocampal formation, it provides the main conduit for processed information to be relayed back to the neocortex. As portrayed in this chapter, the entorhinal cortex is the beginning and the end point of an extensive loop of information processing that takes place in the hippocampal formation. Although neuroanatomical investigation of the entorhinal cortex has historically lagged behind the work conducted in other fields of the hippocampal formation, many new findings have been forthcoming in recent years. This progress has been spurred on, in part, by the appreciation, initially by van Hoesen et al. (1991), that the entorhinal cortex is a site of early, devastating pathology in degenerative diseases such as Alzheimer's disease. It has also been fostered by the reemergence of the notion first put forth by Ramon y Cajal that (to paraphrase) whatever the rest of the hippocampal formation is doing depends on what the entorhinal cortex has done. We begin our description of the entorhinal cortex with a discussion of some lingering controversies concerning its laminar and regional organization.

Cytoarchitectonic Organization

Laminar Organization

There are currently two schemes of cortical lamination applied to the entorhinal cortex. As one might expect, this causes substantial confusion, especially to the neophyte hippocampologist. One nomenclature, which divided the entorhinal cortex into seven layers, was first suggested by Ramón y Cajal and later modified to more closely resemble the standard six-layer scheme applied to the isocortex. According to this scheme, there are four cellular layers (II, III, V, VI) and two acellular or plexiform layers (I, IV). The acellular layer IV is also called lamina dissecans. Ramon y Cajal's scheme with slight modification has been employed by Amaral and colleagues in several primate studies. The other commonly used scheme was proposed by Lorente de Nó, who also differentiated six layers. Five of Lorente de Nó's layers were cellular (II, III, IV, V, VI) with a cell-free lamina dissecans (layer IIIb) between layers III and IV. This scheme was used in most of the older studies of the entorhinal cortex. It is still used in rodent studies and in at least some studies of the human entorhinal cortex, particularly those of Van Hoesen and colleagues.

Primarily to emphasize the lack of an internal granular cell layer in the entorhinal cortex, we have decided to adopt Ramon y Cajal's nomenclature and have labeled the cell-poor layer IV lamina dissecans. Starting from the pial surface, the layers include layer I, the most superficial plexiform or molecular layer, which is cell-poor but rich in transversely oriented fibers; layer II, containing mainly medium-sized to large stellate cells and a population of small pyramidal cells that tend to be grouped in clusters (cell islands) particularly in the lateral entorhinal area; layer III, containing cells of various sizes and shapes but predominantly pyramidal cells; layer IV (or lamina dissecans), a cell-free layer located between layers III and V that is most apparent in those portions of the entorhinal cortex that lie close to the rhinal fissure, particularly at the caudal levels of the entorhinal cortex. In the remainder of the entorhinal cortex, groups of cells invade this layer so it has an incomplete or patchy appearance. Next are layer V, a cellular

layer that can be subdivided into bands, and layer Va, which forms a band of large, darkly stained pyramidal neurons and is most conspicuous in the central parts of the entorhinal cortex. At other levels, the packing density of cells is not high, and the smaller cells of the deeper part of this layer (Vb) intermingle with it. Finally there is layer VI, containing a highly heterogeneous population of cell sizes and shapes. This cell density decreases toward the border with the white matter. The cells of layer VI appear to blend gradually into the subjacent subcortical white matter and the overlying layer V.

Regional Organization

There have been several attempts to subdivide the rat entorhinal cortex, and unfortunately there have been almost an equal number of differing opinions concerning the number and terminology of the subfields. The subject has been discussed and reviewed by Menno Witter, Ricardo Insausti, and their colleagues (Witter, 1993; Insausti et al., 1997; Witter et al., 2000; Burwell and Witter, 2002). Nevertheless, it is now generally accepted that the entorhinal cortex can be subdivided into two general areas: the lateral entorhinal area (LEA) and the medial entorhinal area (MEA) (Fig. 3–36). Layer II is more clearly demarcated in the LEA than in the MEA, and the cells are extremely densely packed and tend to be clustered in islands. The cells in layer II of the MEA are somewhat larger and do not show a distinct clustering into islands; the border between layers II and III is not as sharp as in the LEA. In both entorhinal areas, however, the overall differences in cell size between layers II and III facilitate the delineation of the two layers. The other cell layers, particularly layers IV to VI, can be better differentiated from each other in the MEA than in the LEA, and cells in the MEA generally show a more radial or columnar arrangement. The lamina dissecans of the MEA is sharply delineated but is less clear in the LEA.

It should also be stressed that the terms lateral and medial entorhinal areas do not relate in a simple manner to the cardinal transverse plane of the rat brain (Fig. 3–37). Both the LEA and the MEA have a more or less triangular shape. The LEA occupies the rostrolateral part of the entorhinal cortex; its base is oriented rostrally and its tip caudolaterally, next to the rhinal fissure. The MEA occupies the remaining triangular area, which has its base caudally and its tip rostromedially such that the tip lies medial to the LEA. A different nomenclature has recently been proposed by Insausti and colleagues to accommodate the oblique orientation of the rat entorhinal cortex and to address the need for subdemarcation of the LEA and MEA (Insausti et al., 1997).

Neuron Types

Our current knowledge of the cytology of the entorhinal cortex is based largely on the classic Golgi studies of Ramon y Cajal and Lorente de Nó in young mice. A few intracellular labeling studies have also been conducted in rats, and they have contributed important new information concerning entorhinal cell types (Hamam et al., 2000, 2002). It is proba-

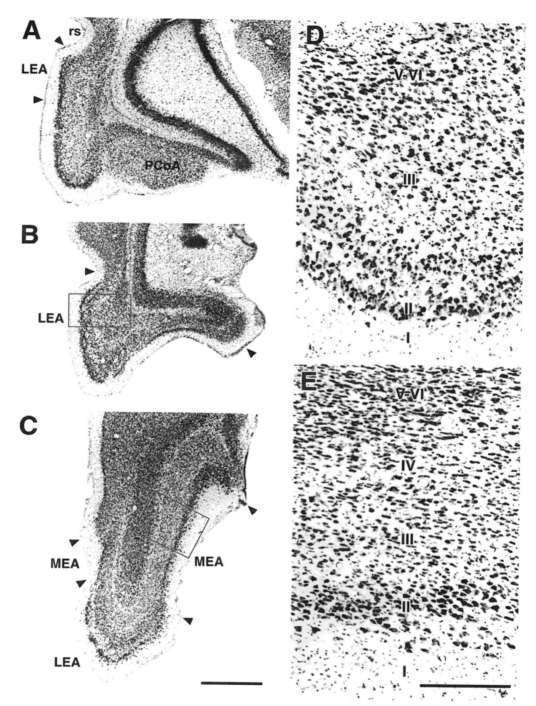

Figure 3–36. Cytoarchitectonic characteristics of the rat entorhinal cortex. *A–C.* Photomicrographs of Nissl-stained coronal sections through three selected rostrocaudal levels of the entorhinal cortex, arranged from rostral (*A*) to caudal (*C*), showing the lateral (LEA) and medial (MEA) entorhinal area subdivisions. Arrowheads indicate LEA and MEA boundaries. *D, E.* High magnification photomi- crographs of LEA (*D*) and MEA (*E*) taken from portions of the entorhinal cortex enclosed by boxes in *B* and *C*, respectively. The layers of the entorhinal cortex are indicated with roman numerals. PcoA, posterior cortical nucleus of the amygdala. Bars: *A–C,* 1 mm; *D* and *E,* 250 μm (*Source*: Dolorfo and Amaral, 1998b.)

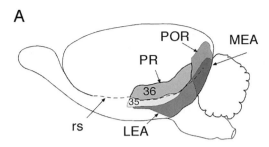

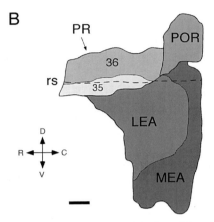

Figure 3–37. Relative positions of the lateral (LEA) and medial (MEA) entorhinal cortex and the perirhinal and postrhinal cortices. *A.* Lateral view of the rat brain. *B.* Unfolded map of the entorhinal, perirhinal, and postrhinal cortices. Bar = 1 mm. (*Source:* Adapted from Burwell and Amaral, 1998b.)

bly safe to predict that a number of new entorhinal cell types will be discovered as these techniques are applied more intensively to analysis of the entorhinal cortex. Other recent studies have focused on determining which particular neuron types project to the dentate gyrus, hippocampus, and subiculum. These studies have employed retrograde tracing techniques either alone or in conjunction with intracellular filling. The following description provides a short overview of the various cell types of each of the entorhinal layers and a brief comment on the major characteristics of their dendritic and axonal organization.

Layer I is populated by a small number of widely dispersed neurons that have been further differentiated using various criteria. There are stellate and horizontal GABAergic neurons that have been shown electrophysiologically to terminate on the dendrites of layer II cells that project to the dentate gyrus.

Layer II is populated by stellate and pyramidal cells (Fig. 3–38), both of which project to the dentate gyrus and CA3. These cells give rise to extensive associational projections to layer II of other regions of the entorhinal cortex, and they contribute a few collaterals to deeper layers of the entorhinal cortex. Although there are some exceptions, most layer II cells have a dendritic tree that is confined to superficial layers I and II. A class of axo-axonic cells, similar to the cortical chandelier cell, is also located in layer II; although some of these cells are present in layer III, they have not been observed in the deep layers.

In layer III, the most numerous neurons are the pyramidal cells (Fig. 3–39), which give rise to the perforant and alvear

Figure 3–38. Morphological characteristics of entorhinal cortex layer II neurons. *A.* Camera lucida drawing of a typical layer II pyramidal cell. Note the thick apical dendrite branching above the border with layer I, the thin basal dendrites arising radially from the soma, and the limited extent of the upper dendritic tree. The axon (arrow) emerges from the base of the soma and branches in layer III. *B.* Camera lucida drawing of a typical layer II stellate cell. Note the multiple thick primary dendrites and the widely diverging upper and lower dendritic trees, with superficially directed dendrites reaching the topmost portion of layer I. The axon (truncated) emerges from the base of the soma. Bar = 100 μm. (*Source:* Adapted from Klink and Alonso, 1997.)

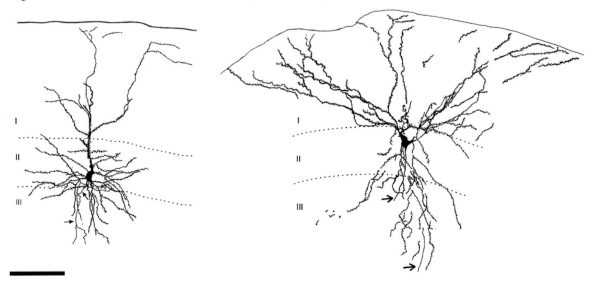

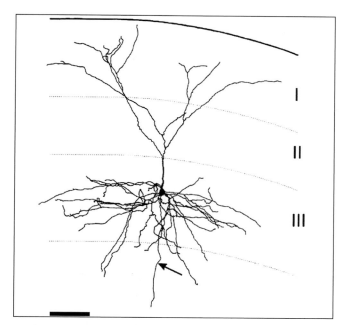

Figure 3–39. Morphological characteristics of entorhinal cortex layer III neurons. Camera lucida of a typical layer III pyramidal cell. The axon is indicated by an arrow. Bar = 100 μm. (*Source*: Adapted from Gloveli et al., 1997.)

path projections to CA1 and the subiculum. Their axons give rise to collaterals that distribute mainly to layers I to III. The apical dendrites of layer III pyramidal cells ascend, give off branches to layer II, and ultimately form a terminal tuft in layer I. Layer III also contains multipolar, stellate, fusiform, horizontal, and bipolar cells, all of which appear to contribute to the perforant pathway. This large, heterogeneous group of cells undoubtedly coincides with what Lorente de Nó described as atypical layer III neurons.

Layer IV, the lamina dissecans, although generally referred to as a cell-free layer, does contain scattered cell bodies described as fusiform or pyramidal cells that have apical dendrites reaching up to layer I and an axon reaching the deep white matter, a characteristic of projection neurons. Some of the cells in the lamina dissecans stain positively with antibodies against GABA, NPY, calretinin, calbindin, or somatostatin.

Layer V contains three main classes of neuron—pyramidal cells, small spherical cells, and fusiform neurons—according to the Golgi-based description of Lorente de Nó. Layer Va is characterized by its large, darkly staining pyramidal cells. These cells have large apical dendrites that ascend toward the superficial portion of layer II and into layer I. The axons of these cells run into the deep white matter and the angular bundle, and additional collaterals innervate the superficial layers of the entorhinal cortex. According to Lorente de Nó, the collaterals of such cells form a column-like plexus situated close to the location of the parent cell body and span the entire thickness of the entorhinal cortex. These collaterals mainly distribute to the deep cell layers (V/VI), although occasional collaterals reach layer II. Layer Va also contains various small neurons that have been characterized as horizontal, stellate, and multipolar cells. Golgi studies indicate that the axonal plexus of the latter group either remains in layer Va or extends to the superficial layers I to III. Angel Alonso and colleagues have used intracellular staining techniques to study the morphology of layer V neurons, particularly in the deeper portion of layer V, or layer Vb (Fig. 3–40). They also found that there are three main types of neuron. Large and small pyramidal cells, neurons with dendrites oriented horizontally and mainly confined to layer V, and an atypical form of multipolar neuron with long wavy dendrites. A surprising aspect of the latter neurons is that some of their dendrites meander from the entorhinal cortex, through the angular bundle, and

Figure 3–40. Morphological characteristics of entorhinal cortex layer V neurons. Computer-aided reconstructions of pyramidal, horizontal, and polymorphic cells. Dashed lines represent the borders of the indicated layers. Bar = 100 μm. (*Source*: Adapted from Hamam et al., 2002.)

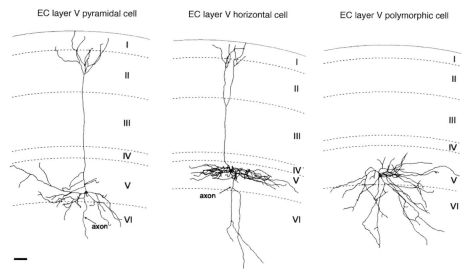

EC layer V pyramidal cell   EC layer V horizontal cell   EC layer V polymorphic cell

into the subiculum. Some of these cells may thus contribute to the projections to the dentate gyrus and the hippocampus. The overall picture emerging from these recent studies is that all three types of layer V neuron should be considered projection neurons in that they send an axon to the white matter. They also may function as local circuit neurons, connecting the deep layers to the superficial layers.

Layer VI contains a wide variety of neuron types. Based on the predominant distribution of their axonal plexus, these cells can be grouped into three categories: cells that mainly influence other cells in layer VI or Vb; cells that by means of their highly collateralized axons can influence a vertical column of cells in layers I to III; and cells whose axons are directed toward the deep white matter and are therefore likely to be projection neurons. Some of these cells contribute to the projections to the dentate gyrus and the hippocampus.

On the basis of their restricted axonal distribution, several of the smaller cell types in the entorhinal cortex have been classified as interneurons. Most of these interneurons are likely GABAergic. GABAergic neurons are found in all layers of the entorhinal cortex, although they are most abundant in the superficial layers. GABAergic interneurons can be subcategorized on the basis of their colocalization with various neuroactive substances (e.g., peptides) or their expression of one or more of the various calcium-binding proteins. The superficial layers contain a large number of cells that are immunoreactive for parvalbumin, whereas the number of calbindin-D28-positive neurons is much lower. Although most of the GABAergic neurons are undoubtedly interneurons, at least some of the GABAergic neurons in layers II and III project to the dentate gyrus.

Intrinsic/Associational Connections

The entorhinal cortex contains a substantial system of associational connections. Intraentorhinal fibers are organized in three rostrocaudally oriented bands, and connections that link different transverse (or mediolateral) regions of the entorhinal cortex are rather restricted (Dolorfo and Amaral, 1998b). Associational connections originate in both superficial and deep layers. Projections originating from layers II and III tend to terminate mainly in the superficial layers, whereas projections originating from the deep layers terminate in both the deep and superficial layers.

The global organization of the associational connections in the entorhinal cortex can be best understood in relation to the topography of the entorhinal projections to other fields of the hippocampal formation (Fig. 3–41). As we describe shortly, different parts of the entorhinal cortex project to different septotemporal levels of the dentate gyrus. The portions of the lateral and medial entorhinal areas that project to the septal half of the dentate gyrus, for example, are located laterally and caudally in the entorhinal cortex, close to the rhinal sulcus. Cells located in this region give rise to associational connections to other cells in the same region but not in any substan-

tial way to the portions of the entorhinal cortex that project to other levels of the dentate gyrus. Thus, the associational connections seem to be organized to integrate all of the information that comes into a particular portion of the entorhinal cortex and are relayed to a particular septotemporal level of the dentate gyrus.

Not much is known about the detailed microcircuitry of the entorhinal associational connections. Presumably, the layer II cells that project to other portions of layer II terminate on the same stellate and pyramidal cells that give rise to the perforant path projection. It is not known, however, if associational connections also terminate on interneurons in layer II. Of even greater functional significance is the issue of whether the deep layer cells project to the cells of layers II and III that give rise to the perforant pathway. This is a critical missing piece of information. Because the deep layer neurons receive feedback projections from CA1 and the subiculum, an associational connection from deep cells to superficial cells would provide the link for completing the loop through the hippocampal formation. Another issue is whether these associational connections are excitatory or inhibitory. If a substantial portion of the deep to superficial pathway originates from GABAergic neurons, or if the pathway is excitatory but terminates preferentially on inhibitory cells located in layer II, the output of the hippocampal formation from CA1 and the subiculum could inhibit layer II or III neurons that project to the dentate gyrus, hippocampus, and subiculum.

Commissural Connections

Relatively strong commissural connections, arising from all portions of the entorhinal cortex, terminate predominantly in layers I and II of the homotopic area of the entorhinal cortex (Goldowitz et al., 1975; Hjorth-Simonsen and Zimmer, 1975; Deller, 1998). The entorhinal cortex also gives rise to a commissural projection to other components of the contralateral hippocampal formation. The largest component of this projection is directed toward the dentate gyrus, but fields CA3 and CA1 of the hippocampus and the subiculum also receive a contralateral input. The crossed entorhinal projection is heaviest to septal portions of the hippocampal subfields and rapidly diminishes in strength at more temporal levels. This crossed projection apparently arises exclusively from layer III cells.

Organization of the Perforant and Alvear Pathway Projections

As a reminder of our earlier description of the perforant path input to the dentate gyrus, hippocampus, and subiculum, both the lateral and medial entorhinal areas project to all three areas. The lateral and medial components of the perforant path terminate along the superficial-to-deep gradient in the molecular layer of the dentate gyrus and the stratum lacunosum-moleculare of CA3 and along the transverse axis of CA1 and the subiculum (Fig. 3–42). Layer II cells give rise to the

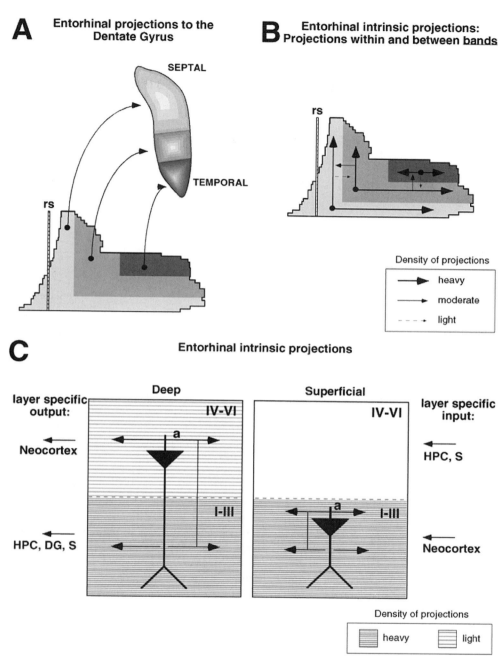

Figure 3–41. Summary of the intrinsic connections of the entorhinal cortex and the association of the entorhinal cortex with the hippocampal formation and neocortex. *A.* Organization of entorhinal projections to the dentate gyrus. A "band" of layer II cells located in the lateral and caudomedial portion of the entorhinal cortex (light gray) projects to the septal half of the dentate gyrus; a band in the mid-mediolateral entorhinal cortex (medium gray) projects to the third quarter of the dentate gyrus; and a band located in the most rostromedial entorhinal cortex (dark gray) projects to the temporal pole of the dentate gyrus. *B.* Organization of entorhinal intrinsic projections: projections within and between bands. Each of these projection zones has substantial associational connections (large arrows) that remain largely in the zone of origin. Projections between each band are less prominent (small arrows). *C.* Entorhinal intrinsic projections and entorhinal afferent and efferent projections. Entorhinal associational connections arise from both the deep and superficial layers of the entorhinal cortex (arrows in the boxes) and terminate mainly in the superficial layers. A less prominent associational connection in the deep layers is apparent primarily in lateral portions of the entorhinal cortex. (*Source*: Adapted from Dolorfo and Amaral, 1998b.)

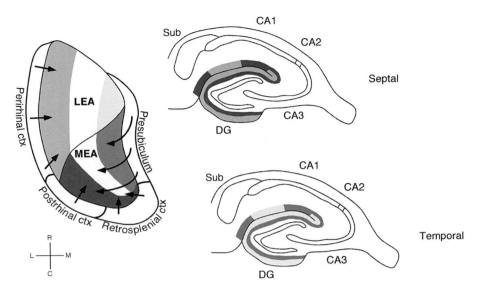

Figure 3–42. Laminar and topographical organization of the entorhinal projection to the dentate gyrus, the hippocampus, and the subiculum. The surface of the entorhinal cortex is represented on the left (the rhinal sulcus is to the left). Layer II entorhinal cortex projections to the dentate gyrus and the CA3 and CA2 fields of the hippocampus terminate in a laminar fashion; the LEA projects superficially in the molecular layer and the stratum lacunosum-moleculare, and the MEA projects deeper. In contrast in CA1 and the subiculum, layer III entorhinal cortex projections are organized topographically; the LEA projects to the distal CA1 and proximal subiculum (i.e., at the CA1/subiculum border), and the MEA projects to the proximal CA1 and distal subiculum. Laterally situated portions of the entorhinal cortex project to septal levels of the hippocampal formation, whereas progressively more medial portions of the entorhinal cortex project to more temporal levels of the hippocampal formation.

projection to the dentate gyrus and CA3, and layer III cells project to CA1 and the subiculum. Although current usage applies the term perforant path to all entorhino-hippocampal projections, entorhinal fibers also reach CA1 via the alveus (i.e., the alvear pathway originally described by Ramon y Cajal). In the temporal portion of the hippocampus, most of the entorhinal fibers reach CA1 after perforating the subiculum (classic perforant pathway). At more septal levels, however, the number of entorhinal fibers that take the alvear pathway increases; and in the septal portion of the hippocampus, most of the entorhinal fibers reach CA1 via the alvear pathway. These fibers make a sharp turn in the alveus, perforate the pyramidal cell layer, and terminate in the stratum lacunosum-moleculare. Both pathways demonstrate the same septotemporal organization of their projections. Thus, certain portions of the entorhinal cortex project to certain septotemporal levels of the other hippocampal fields. Following this brief overview, we now delve more deeply into the topographical organization of the perforant path projection.

Dolorfo and Amaral (1998a) have shown that cells located laterally and caudally in the entorhinal cortex project to septal levels of the hippocampal fields, whereas cells located progressively more medially and rostrally (in the medial entorhinal cortex) project to more temporal levels of the hippocampal subfields (Fig. 3–41). It now appears that there may be three largely nonoverlapping domains of the entorhinal cortex that project to three distinct levels of the dentate gyrus. The laterally situated domain (encompassing cells of both the lateral

and medial entorhinal areas) projects to the septal half of the dentate gyrus. Most of the cells in this domain project to all portions of the septal half of the dentate gyrus; thus, the projection is both divergent and convergent. The next domain is more medially situated and projects to the third quarter of the dentate gyrus. The last domain is medially and rostrally situated and projects to the temporal quarter of the dentate gyrus.

There are a number of functional implications of the organization of these projections. First and foremost, because the associational connections of the entorhinal cortex seem to respect this tripartite organization, it is reasonable to think of three functional, parallel systems encompassed within the entorhino-hippocampal system. Second, when conducting stimulation or lesion experiments designed to evaluate the contributions of the medial and lateral perforant paths to hippocampal function, one must be careful to bear in mind that the cells giving rise to the medial perforant path are located caudal (not medial) to the cells that give rise to the lateral perforant path.

One final comment must be made on the medial and lateral perforant path projections. Although the cellular characteristics of layers II and III of the medial and lateral entorhinal areas are similar, the lateral and medial perforant path projections demonstrate a number of differential features. Both components of the perforant path use glutamate as their primary transmitter, but they exhibit differential distributions of glutamate receptors. The medial perforant path fibers, for example, are immunoreactive for the metabotropic glutamate receptor mGLUR 2/3, whereas the lateral fibers are not. In contrast, the lateral perforant path demonstrates dynorphin immunoreactivity, whereas the medial perforant path does not. One would have thought that some of these differences would show up more clearly in the cells of origin, but thus far there is no distinctive marker at the level of the entorhinal cortex for cells that give rise to the lateral and medial perforant path projections.

Feedback Projections from the Hippocampus and Subiculum

We already mentioned that the dentate gyrus and the CA3 field of the hippocampus do not project back to the entorhinal cortex. Thus, the recipients of the layer II projection do not have any direct influence over the activities of the entorhinal cortex. It is only after the layer II and layer III projection systems are combined in CA1 and the subiculum that return projections to the entorhinal cortex are generated. The return projections mainly terminate in the deep layers (V and VI), although some fibers ascend into layer I (Witter et al., 1988; Naber et al., 2001; Kloosterman et al., 2003). It is not known which entorhinal neurons are the recipients of these return projections. What is clear, however, is that the projections from CA1 and the subiculum to the entorhinal cortex are also topographically organized (Figs. 3–29 and 3–34). Septal portions of CA1 and the subiculum project chiefly to lateral parts of the entorhinal cortex, and more temporal parts of CA1 and the subiculum project to more medial parts of the entorhinal cortex. Moreover, the transverse location of the cells of origin in CA1 and the subiculum also determines whether these projections terminate in the medial or lateral entorhinal cortex. The projections from the proximal part of CA1 and the distal part of the subiculum distribute exclusively to the medial entorhinal cortex, whereas cells located in the distal part of CA1 and the proximal part of the subiculum project mainly to the lateral entorhinal cortex.

The important point about these return projections is that they are exactly in register (i.e., they are point-to-point reciprocal) with the entorhinal inputs to these areas. Thus, at the global level, all of the circuitry is available for reverberatory circuits to be established through the loop, starting and ending at the entorhinal cortex. This remarkable topography confirms the critical role of the entorhinal cortex with respect to the input to and output from the hippocampal formation.

Extrinsic Connections

Interconnections of the Entorhinal Cortex with Neocortical Regions

If the entorhinal cortex is viewed as the first step of processing in the hippocampal formation, it is reasonable to wonder what types of information it receives. In other words, what is the "raw material" the hippocampal formation uses to accomplish its purported function(s). This is an area in which there are substantial species differences. Keeping to the format that we have followed so far, we give an overview of the inputs to the rat entorhinal cortex. However, doing so does a disservice to the significance of the connections between the entorhinal cortex and the neocortex, as these connections are so much more prominent in the monkey brain. Thus, when we provide our comparison of the organization of the hippocampal formation in the rat, monkey, and human in a later portion of the chapter, we return to a detailed overview of the cortical inputs of the monkey entorhinal cortex.

Burwell has carried out a thorough quantitative analysis of the organization of cortical inputs to the rat entorhinal cortex and compared the results with inputs to the perirhinal and postrhinal cortices (Fig. 3–43) (Burwell and Amaral, 1998a). She found many similarities in the complement of cortical inputs to the lateral and medial entorhinal areas. Each receive about one-third of its total input from the piriform cortex (LEA 34%, MEA 31%). These areas also receive roughly equal proportions from temporal (LEA 26%, MEA 21%) and frontal (LEA 11%, MEA 10%) regions. Some differences are observed in the proportions of insular, cingular, parietal, and occipital inputs. The lateral entorhinal area receives more input from insular cortex (LEA 21%, MEA 6%). In contrast, the medial entorhinal area receives more input from cingulate (LEA 3%, MEA 11%), parietal (LEA 3%, MEA 9%), and occipital (LEA 2%, MEA 12%) regions. Not all portions of the rat entorhinal cortex receive substantial cortical input. In fact, it is only the lateral and caudal parts of the entorhinal cortex (those projecting to septal levels of the dentate gyrus) that are heavily innervated by the neocortex. This neuroanatomical organization has strong functional implications and likely underlies the behavioral dissociations observed with dorsal (septal) versus ventral (temporal) hippocampal lesions.

The neocortical inputs to the entorhinal cortex of the rat comprise two groups: those that terminate in the superficial layers (I–III) and those that terminate in the deep layers (IV–VI). The first category delivers information to the superficially located entorhinal neurons, which are the source of the projections to the dentate gyrus, hippocampus, and subiculum. The second group has greater influence on the deeply located cells of the entorhinal cortex, which receive processed information from the other hippocampal fields and give rise to feedback projections to certain cortical regions. In general, the cortical afferents that reach the deep layers terminate rather diffusely, whereas those that terminate superficially have a more restricted mediolateral and/or rostrocaudal distribution. Although speculative, the first group may constitute a set of information-bearing inputs, whereas the second group may have more of a modulatory influence on the output of the hippocampal formation.

A substantial input to the superficial layers of the entorhinal cortex originates from olfactory structures such as the olfactory bulb, the anterior olfactory nucleus, and the piri-

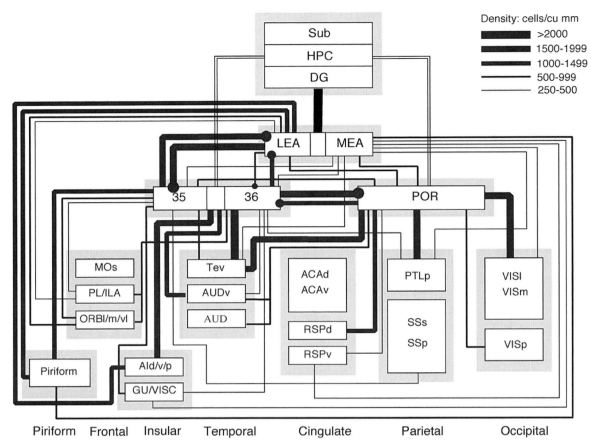

Figure 3–43. Pattern and strength of cortical and intrinsic connectivity of the rat parahippocampal region (entorhinal, perirhinal, and parahippocampal cortices). The thickness of the solid lines represents the relative strength of the connections based on the densities of retrogradely labeled neurons. Open lines represent reported connections for which no comparable quantitative data are available. The weakest projections ($<$ 250 labeled cells/mm³) are not shown here. ACAd and ACAv, dorsal and ventral anterior cingulate cortex; AId/v/p, dorsal, ventral, and posterior agranular insular cortices; AUD, primary auditory cortex; MOs, secondary motor area; Pir, piriform cortex; PTLp, posterior parietal cortex; RSPd and RSPv, retrosplenial cortex, dorsal and ventral; SSp and SSs, primary and supplementary somatosensory areas; Te$_v$, ventral temporal area; VISC, visceral granular insular cortex; VIS1 and VISm, lateral and medial visual association cortex; VISp, primary visual cortex. (*Source*: Adapted from Burwell and Amaral, 1998b.)

form cortex. These olfactory projections terminate throughout most of the rostrocaudal extent of the entorhinal cortex, mainly in layer I and the superficial portion of layer II. Only the most caudal portion of the rat medial entorhinal area does not receive any olfactory input. In addition to terminating on the principal cells of these layers, olfactory fibers also terminate on layer I GABAergic neurons, which presumably interact with the principal cells in layers II and III.

A second prominent cortical input to the superficial layers of the entorhinal cortex arises from the laterally adjacent perirhinal and postrhinal cortices. The perirhinal and postrhinal cortices are polysensory convergence areas that receive inputs from a variety of unimodal and polymodal sensory cortices. The perirhinal cortex terminates mainly in the lateral entorhinal area, and the postrhinal cortex terminates heavily, though not exclusively, in the medial entorhinal area. In both cases, the projections terminate preferentially in layers I and III of the entorhinal cortex.

We address the issue of the perirhinal cortex more exten-

sively in our discussion of the monkey entorhinal cortex, but it is important to give an overview of this area because it provides major input to the rat entorhinal cortex. The perirhinal cortex in the rat is made up of two areas, 35 and 36, which appear to receive slightly different complements of neocortical inputs (Fig. 3–43) (Burwell et al., 1995; Burwell, 2001). Area 36 of the perirhinal cortex receives more, higher-level cortical input than does area 35. Most of this input comes from the ventral temporal associational area (Te$_v$), which is located dorsally adjacent to area 36. Other major inputs are from the postrhinal cortex and the entorhinal cortex. The predominant inputs to area 35 arise from the piriform, entorhinal, and insular cortices. Area 35 receives more than one-fourth of its input from the piriform cortex and only slightly less from the lateral entorhinal area. About one-fifth of the total input arises from insular cortices. Interestingly, the perirhinal projections to the entorhinal cortex arise preferentially from area 35, and the intrinsic projections of the perirhinal cortex seem to be organized to funnel information into area 35, which in turn gives rise to the main perirhinal projections to the entorhinal cortex.

Cortical afferents to the deep layers of the entorhinal cortex arise from a variety of cortical areas. These areas include projections from the agranular insular cortex, the medial prefrontal region (particularly the infralimbic, prelimbic, and anterior cingulate cortices and the retrosplenial cortex (Insausti et al., 1997).

Efferents of the entorhinal cortex return projections to many of the cortical areas that provide input to the entorhinal cortex. There are projections to olfactory areas, originating predominantly from layers II, III, and Va. An important issue is whether the entorhinal cortex of the rat, like that of the monkey (see below), gives rise to prominent, widespread projections to multimodal association cortices. Initial studies in the rat indicated that the entorhinal cortex projects mainly to adjacent, limited portions of the temporal cortex. Swanson and Köhler (1986), however, suggested that the rat entorhinal cortex gives rise to projections that reach a much larger domain of the cortical surface. Whether one believes that the entorhinal cortex has widespread neocortical connections seems to hinge on the demarcation of the entorhinal cortex from the adjacent perirhinal cortex. Insausti and colleagues confirmed the report by Sarter and Markowitsch (1985) that the only cells that give rise to the extensive connections reported by Swanson and Köhler are located in the most dorsolateral region of the entorhinal cortex (i.e., on the border of the entorhinal and perirhinal cortices). Whether these cells indeed belong to the deep layers of the entorhinal cortex or form a population of perirhinal cells is not yet clearly established. Based on the distribution of immunoreactivity for parvalbumin or for certain glutamate receptor subunits, the border between the entorhinal and perirhinal cortex appears to be oblique and perhaps intermixed in this critical region. Thus, it remains unresolved at this point whether it is the entorhinal cortex or the perirhinal cortex that projects widely to the neocortex. One can safely conclude, however, that the major portion of the entorhinal cortex does not contribute projections to the unimodal areas of the neocortex, and that the bulk of neocortically directed projections are to higher-order associational and polysensory cortices and not to sensory or motor regions. In this respect, the situation in the rat closely resembles the connectivity observed in the monkey. Among the cortical areas that do receive entorhinal input are the infralimbic, prelimbic, orbitofrontal, agranular insular, perirhinal, and postrhinal cortices; these projections originate mainly from cells in layer Va. Only weak projections have been reported to the retrosplenial cortex.

Other Telencephalic Connections: Amygdala, Claustrum, Striatum

In addition to the cortical inputs just described, the entorhinal cortex receives a number of subcortical inputs. Whereas some of them, such as the monoaminergic and cholinergic inputs, may be viewed as largely modulatory, others, such as the input from the amygdaloid complex, might also provide additional sources of information. The substantial input from the amygdaloid complex, which originates mainly from the lateral and basal nuclei, is presumably conveying information about the emotional state of the organism (Pikkaraisen et al., 1999a). The densest termination of the amygdaloid fibers is in the ventrolateral part of the entorhinal cortex (Fig. 3–44). Efferents from the lateral amygdaloid nucleus distribute most intensely to the deep portion of layer III but end also between the cell islands of layer II and in layer I. The fibers from the basal nucleus terminate diffusely in layers III to V, whereas those from the cortical nuclei and the periamygdaloid cortex preferentially project to layers I and II. The entorhinal cortex sends feedback projections to the amygdala that terminate mainly in the basal nucleus. These projections originate from cells in layer V, although a few cells in more superficial layers may also contribute to the projection. Dense inputs also originate from the ventral part of the claustrum or endopiriform nucleus, but the topographical and laminar organization of these inputs is not well understood.

The entorhinal cortex projects bilaterally to the striatum, particularly to the nucleus accumbens and adjacent parts of the olfactory tubercle. These projections originate mainly from layer V and are topographically organized; medial parts of the entorhinal cortex project to the caudomedial portion of the nucleus accumbens, and more lateral portions of the entorhinal cortex project to more lateral parts of the nucleus.

Basal Forebrain and Hypothalamic Connections

The entorhinal cortex receives its cholinergic innervation mainly from the septum. This projection is topographically organized such that cells in the horizontal limb of the nucleus of the diagonal band preferentially project to the most lateral part of the entorhinal cortex, whereas the medial septal nucleus and the vertical limb of the nucleus of the diagonal band project to more medial parts of the entorhinal cortex. Septal projections terminate densely in the cell-sparse lamina dissecans and less densely in layer II.

Like the hippocampus and the subiculum but unlike the pre- and parasubiculum, the entorhinal cortex projects back to the septal region. The projection originates from cells in layer Va, although some layer II cells also contribute to these projections. The fibers from the entorhinal cortex preferentially terminate in the lateral septal complex.

The entorhinal cortex receives diffuse inputs from various structures in the hypothalamus. They include inputs from the supramammillary nucleus that terminate rather diffusely with some preference for layers III to VI, from the tuberomammillary nucleus distributing diffusely throughout the entorhinal cortex, and from the lateral hypothalamic area reaching the deep layers of the entorhinal cortex.

Thalamic Connections: Nucleus Reuniens and Other Midline Nuclei

The major thalamic inputs to the entorhinal cortex originate in the nucleus reuniens and the nucleus centralis medialis (Van der Werf et al., 2002). The rhomboid, paraventricular,

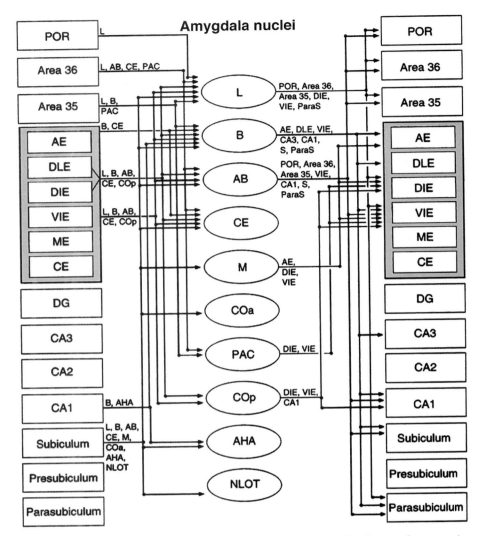

Figure 3–44. Summary of the reciprocal connections between the amygdala and the hippocampal formation and the perirhinal and parahippocampal cortices. The subdivisions of the entorhinal cortex follow the nomenclature of Insausti et al. (1997). Areas CE and ME of the medial entorhinal cortex do not receive amygdala inputs. Areas DLE, DIE, VIE, and AE of the lateral entorhinal cortex receive inputs from the various amygdala nuclei. (*Source*: Pitkänen et al., 2000.)

and parataenial nuclei contribute minor projections. The nucleus reuniens fibers densely innervate the deep portion of layers I and III and give rise to a few collaterals that extend into layer II. Separate populations of nucleus reuniens cells project to the entorhinal cortex, CA1, and the subiculum. There is no evidence that the entorhinal cortex projects back to the thalamus.

Brain Stem Inputs

The entorhinal cortex receives dopaminergic input from cells located in the ventral tegmental area. The projection preferentially terminates in a restricted rostrolateral part of the lateral entorhinal area, where fibers are arranged in dense, columnar patches in layers I to III. The serotonergic innervation arises from the central and dorsal raphe nuclei and terminates diffusely in all layers but with a preference for the superficial layers. The noradrenergic locus coeruleus sup-

plies the entorhinal cortex with a diffusely organized noradrenergic input that exhibits slightly more dense termination in layer I.

3.5 Chemical Neuroanatomy

3.5.1 Transmitters and Receptors

Detailed, comprehensive treatment of the chemical neuroanatomy of the hippocampal formation would demand a lengthy chapter of its own. We have already described the distribution of systems defined by their neurotransmitter content—noradrenaline (norepinephrine), serotonin, acetylcholine, GABA—and a variety of reviews are available on the chemical neuroanatomy of the hippocampus (Swanson et al.,

1987; Kobayashi and Amaral, 1998). We thus restrict ourselves here to providing an overview of the diversity of neurochemical substances in the hippocampal formation.

A variety of peptides and other chemical markers have been shown to subdivide the population of GABAergic interneurons. Among the peptides that colocalize with particular populations of GABAergic interneurons are VIP, somatostatin, NPY, corticotropin-releasing factor (CRF), substance P, cholecystokinin, galanin, and the opioid peptides dynorphin and enkephalin. It is worth commenting further on the distribution of the opioid peptides because, in addition to being localized to certain populations of interneurons, they are observed in intrinsic excitatory pathways of the hippocampal formation. The fibers of the lateral perforant path, for example, are immunoreactive for Leu-enkephalin, whereas the mossy fibers of the dentate gyrus are positive for dynorphin.

Another class of substances that appear to mark certain subsets of GABAergic neurons selectively is the family of calcium-binding proteins, including parvalbumin, calbindin, and calretinin. Whereas parvalbumin immunoreactivity appears to be exclusively confined to a subset of GABAergic interneurons, the other calcium-binding proteins can be found in both interneurons and principal neurons. Although the precise function of the various calcium-binding proteins has not been well established, their existence has provided a useful anatomical tool. Although standard immunohistochemistry of GABAergic neurons with antibodies to glutamic acid decarboxylase (GAD) or to GABA does not label dendrites very well, parvalbumin-immunoreactive neurons are fully labeled in a Golgi-like fashion. Thus, even though parvalbumin does not label all GABAergic neurons, those that are labeled can be subjected to precise analyses of their inputs.

3.5.2 Steroids

Neurons in the hippocampal formation have been shown to concentrate glucocorticoids and mineralcorticoids (McEwen and Wallach, 1973). Studies using uptake of ^{3}H-corticosterone show that cells in CA2 and CA1 exhibit the greatest uptake. There is slightly less uptake in CA3 cells and cells of the polymorphic layer of the dentate gyrus; dentate granule cells also demonstrate some ^{3}H-corticosterone uptake. The amount of uptake in other fields of the hippocampal formation has not yet been described. What is perhaps most surprising is the fact that, in the rat, the hippocampus demonstrates the highest level of uptake of any brain region. The distribution of glucocorticoid receptor mRNA has also been evaluated in the tree shrew. Here the highest density of mRNA was observed in the pyramidal cells of the subiculum and in the granule cells of the dentate gyrus. In the hippocampus, higher densities of mRNA were observed in CA1 than in CA3. Mineralcorticoid receptor mRNA is also expressed in the tree shrew hippocampus. It is expressed most strongly in CA1 and less strongly in CA3; this contrasts with the pattern in the rat, where mineralcorticoid expression is higher in CA3.

In situ hybridization has also been used in postmortem humans to study the distribution of glucocorticoid and min-

eralcorticoid receptors. Receptors for both steroids were highly expressed in cells of the dentate gyrus, CA3, and CA2. Lower levels of expression were observed in CA1. This is the opposite of the distribution observed in the rat and the tree shrew.

3.6 Comparative Neuroanatomy of the Rat, Monkey, and Human Hippocampal Formation

When one views Nissl-stained sections of the hippocampus from the rat, monkey, and human, it is immediately apparent that one is looking at the same brain region (Figs. 3–2 and 3–45). The densely packed granule cell layer is obvious in all three species, as is the progressively more complex lamination when one progresses from the dentate gyrus to the entorhinal cortex. On closer inspection, however, a number of differences make it clear that the hippocampal formation of the monkey or human is not simply a scaled-up version of the rat hippocampal formation. Some of the hippocampal fields, such as CA1 and the entorhinal cortex, are disproportionately larger in the primate. The entorhinal cortex has many more subdivisions in the monkey and human than in the rat; and the laminar organization is much more distinct in the primate brain. In the following sections, we review some of the similarities and differences in the organization and connections of the

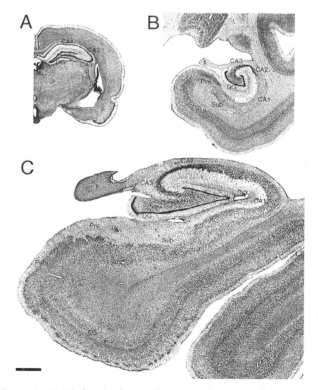

Figure 3–45. Nissl-stained coronal sections through the hippocampal formation of the rat (*A*), monkey (*B*), and human (*C*) presented at the same magnification. Bar in *C* = 2 mm and applies to all panels.

hippocampal formation in these three species. Of course, although we can address certain issues concerning cell number and distribution in the human brain, we are unable to say anything about patterns of connectivity in the human hippocampal formation.

3.6.1 Neuron Numbers

The number of neurons present in the various subdivisions of the hippocampal formation have been counted by several investigators, but rarely has the same author analyzed the rat, monkey, and human hippocampal formations. Moreover, there is a lot of variability in the estimates published in the literature, and few investigators have used modern stereological techniques to carry out these assessments. We have compiled a summary of current estimates of neuron number obtained with modern stereological techniques. The data presented here are derived from published and unpublished work from three laboratories: Mark West at Aarhus University, Peter Rapp at New York University, and our own at the University of California Davis (Table 3-1).

In our initial comparison of the hippocampal formation in the rat, monkey, and human, the volume of the hippocampal complex (dentate gyrus + hippocampus) was said to be about 10 times larger in monkeys than in rats and 100 times larger in humans than in rats (rat 32 mm^3, monkey 340 mm^3; human 3300 mm^3). If, however, we compare the total number of neurons in the various hippocampal areas, we observe that certain regions are comparatively more developed than others in the monkey and human brain. In the dentate gyrus, there are approximately 10 times more granule cells in the monkey than in the rat, a ratio that parallels the overall volume differences. However, there are only 15 times more dentate granule cells in humans compared to rats, whereas the volume of the dentate gyrus plus the hippocampus is about 100 times larger in humans than in rats. In CA1, however, there are only three times more pyramidal cells in the monkey than in the rat, whereas there are 35 times more cells in humans than in rats. We must add, however, that some of these estimates are still provisional and need to be replicated before drawing solid inferences on the relative development of the various hippocampal regions in rats, monkeys, and humans.

3.6.2 Comparison of Rat and Monkey Hippocampal Formation

In monkeys, the hippocampal formation lies entirely within the temporal lobe (Figs. 3–46 through 3–48) and lacks the pronounced C shape along its septotemporal axis that is so characteristic in the rat. The region equivalent to the septal pole of the rat hippocampus is located caudally in the monkey, and the equivalent of the temporal pole is located rostrally (Figs. 3–5 and 3–6). Much of the entorhinal cortex is located rostral to the remainder of the hippocampal formation. In fact, the rostral half of the entorhinal cortex lies ventral to the amygdaloid complex rather than the hippocampus.

Cytoarchitectonic Organization

There are several cytoarchitectonic differences between the rat and monkey hippocampal formation. The polymorphic layer of the dentate gyrus is relatively smaller in the monkey, and much of the territory located enclosed within the blades of the granule cell layers is occupied by the CA3 field. This "hilar" portion of the CA3 region is so expansive that some researchers have confused it for an enlarged polymorphic layer. Cells in this region bear the gold standard of inclusion in CA3, however, as they give rise to Schaffer collaterals to CA1.

The other obvious difference between the rat and monkey hippocampal formation is the much thicker pyramidal cell layer in the monkey CA1 (Fig. 3–49). In the rat, this layer is tightly packed and is typically about 5 cells thick. In the monkey, the cell layer is much more diffusely organized and is 10 to 15 cells thick. As a result, not only is the boundary between the pyramidal cell layer and the stratum radiatum less clear, so is the boundary between CA1 and the subiculum. In the monkey, at least some of the Schaffer collaterals from CA3 terminate in the pyramidal cell layer, presumably on the apical dendrites of cells located deep in the layer or on the basal dendrites of neurons located superficially in the layer.

The entorhinal cortex exhibits major cytoarchitectonic differences between the rat and the monkey. The laminar organization of the monkey entorhinal cortex is much clearer than that in the rat. Throughout much of the entorhinal cortex, for example, there is a clear distinction between layers V and VI in the monkey, whereas these layers tend to blur together in the rat. The monkey entorhinal cortex is also much more differentiated than in the rat. As noted previously, Amaral and colleagues typically divided the rat entorhinal cortex into only lateral and medial areas, whereas they divided the monkey entorhinal cortex into seven distinct subdivisions.

Neuron Types

Until recently, there has been little direct comparison of the morphology of similar neurons in the rat and monkey hippocampus. A few studies, using either the Golgi technique or intracellular staining techniques, have compared easily identified cell types.

The granule cells of the monkey dentate gyrus have been examined with both the Golgi technique and intracellular filling techniques in the in vitro slice preparation (Duffy and Rakic, 1983; Seress and Mrzljak, 1987, 1992). Depending on which aspects of these studies one wishes to emphasize, it could be concluded that granule cells are basically similar in rats and monkeys or that there have been substantial modifications of at least some granule cells. In general, dentate granule cells have the same unipolar apical dendritic tree in the monkey as in the rat. The total dendritic length of each granule cell is also relatively similar in the rat and the monkey. Seress and colleagues were the first to point out that at least some monkey granule cells have basal dendrites (Fig. 3–50),

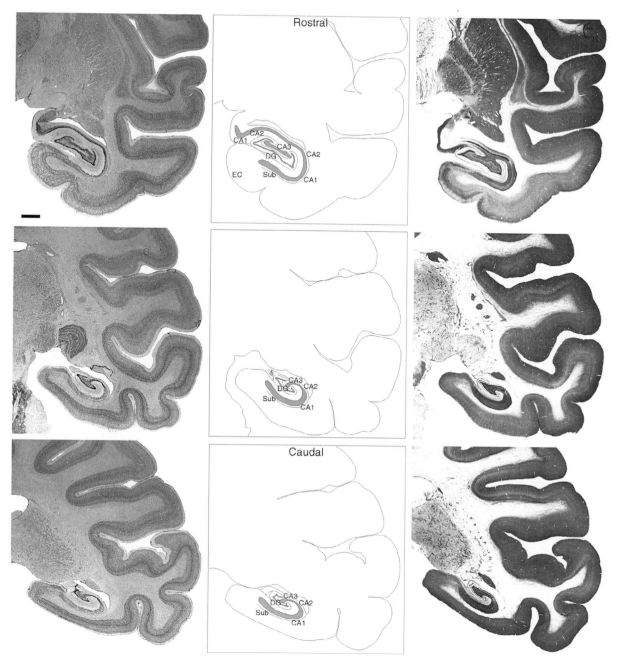

Figure 3–46. Coronal sections at three rostrocaudal levels through the monkey brain show the relative position of the hippocampal formation. The three panels on the left are Nissl-stained sections; the three panels on the right are adjacent sections stained with Timm's sulfide silver stain. The line drawings (middle column) highlight the regions of the monkey hippocampal formation seen in the stained sections. Bar = 2 mm.

and a similar observation has been made by Scheibel and colleagues. This feature has never been reported for normal rat granule cells. Thus, it appears that there are some species differences in dentate granule cell morphology, but the functional significance of these differences is yet unclear.

Another example of differences in an ostensibly similar cell type in the rat and the monkey has emerged from intracellular staining of mossy cells of the polymorphic region of

the dentate gyrus (Buckmaster et al., 1992; Buckmaster and Amaral, 2001). In the rat, these cells give rise to the associational-commissural connections to the inner portion of the molecular layer, and its dendrites are generally confined to the polymorphic area (i.e., the dendrites extend neither into the molecular layer nor into the adjacent CA3 field). The mossy cell in the monkey is quite different. First, there appear to be at least two forms. One is very much like the rat mossy cell,

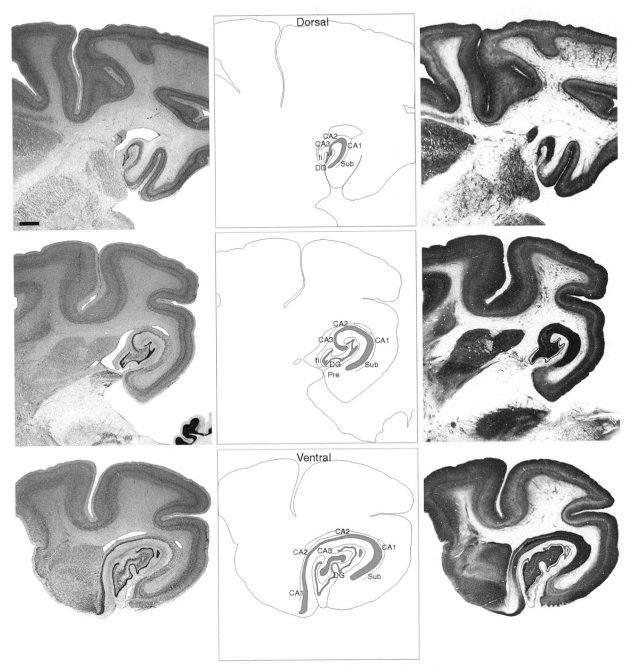

Figure 3–47. Horizontal sections at three dorsoventral levels through the monkey brain show the relative position of the hippocampal formation. The three panels on the left are Nissl-stained sections; the three panels on the right are adjacent sections stained with Timm's sulfide silver stain. The line drawings (middle column) highlight the regions of the monkey hippocampal formation seen in the stained sections. Bar = 2 mm.

with dendrites confined to the polymorphic cell layer and axons directed to the molecular layer. There is a second type, however, that extends much of its dendritic arbor into the molecular layer (Fig. 3–51). Moreover, many of these cells give rise to projections into the adjacent CA3 region. The implication of this altered morphology in the monkey is that these mossy cells are capable of receiving perforant path innerva-

tion in the molecular layer of the dentate gyrus, whereas standard mossy cells are not (because the perforant path does not enter the polymorphic layer). Moreover, in rats the granule cells are the only input to CA3, whereas in the monkey the mossy cells appear to contribute an additional projection. Although these structural alterations must be confirmed by functional studies, they suggest that there are fundamental

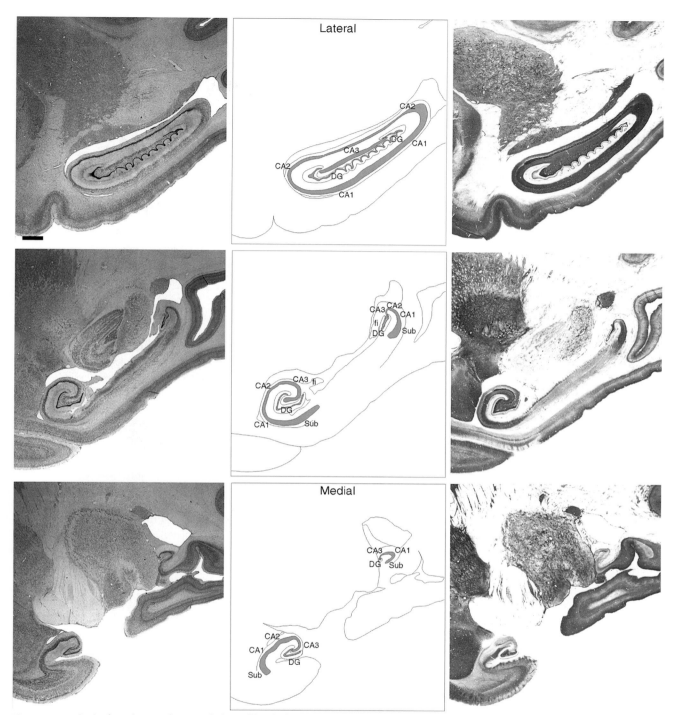

Figure 3–48. Sagittal sections at three mediolateral levels through the monkey brain show the relative position of the hippocampal formation. The three panels on the left are Nissl-stained sections; the three panels on the right are adjacent sections stained with Timm's sulfide silver stain. The line drawings (middle column) highlight the regions of the monkey hippocampal formation seen in the stained sections. Bar = 2 mm.

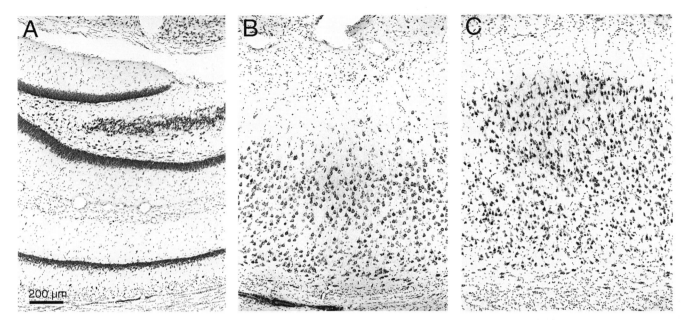

Figure 3–49. High magnification photomicrographs of Nissl-stained coronal sections through the CA1 field of the hippocampus in the rat (*A*), monkey (*B*), and human (*C*). Note that the CA1 pyramidal cell layer in the rat (which is the darkly stained layer at the bottom of panel *A*) is about 5 cells thick. The monkey pyrami-dal cell layer is approximately 15 cells thick and shows some sub-lamination, with the top half of the layer having a slightly higher density of neurons. The pyramidal cell layer in the human CA1 is even thicker and has a more laminated structure. Bar in *A* = 200 μm and applies to all panels.

differences regarding the circuit characteristics of the dentate gyrus between the rat and the monkey.

Connections

Basic Organization of the Intrinsic Hippocampal Circuitry
To the extent that it has been examined, the basic principles of organization of the intrinsic circuitry of the monkey hippocampal formation resemble those observed in the rat. Too little work has been carried out in the monkey, however, to know if the topographical organization of intrinsic circuits is the same in the two species. So far, minor differences have been observed. In the monkey, for example, perforant path fibers arising from the rostral entorhinal area (the equivalent of the rat lateral entorhinal area) terminate, as in the rat, mainly in the outer third of the molecular layer of the dentate gyrus. Some terminations, however, also continue in a decreasing gradient fashion into the middle third of the molecular layer.

Table 3–1.
Number of principal neurons in the subdivisions of the rat, monkey, and human hippocampal formation (in millions)

Cells	Rat	Monkey	Human
Gcl DG	1.20[a,b]	12[c]	18[d]
Hilus	0.05[b]	0.23[e]	1.72[d]
CA3	0.25[a,b]	1.27[e]	2.83[d]
CA1	0.39[a,b]	1.30[e]	14[d]
Subiculum	0.29[b]	0.75[e]	5.95[d]
Pre/parasubiculum	0.70[f]	2.08[e]	–
EC II	0.11[f]	0.26[e]	0.66[g]
EC III	0.25[f]	–	3.66[g]
EC V + VI	0.33[f]	–	3.78[g]
EC total	0.69[f]	2.16[e]	8.1[g]

Sources: [a]Rapp and Gallagher (1996); [b]West et al. (1991); [c]Lavenex et al. unpublished data; [d]West et al. (1994); [e]Rapp et al. unpublished data; [f]Mulders et al. (1997); [g]West and Slomianka (1998).

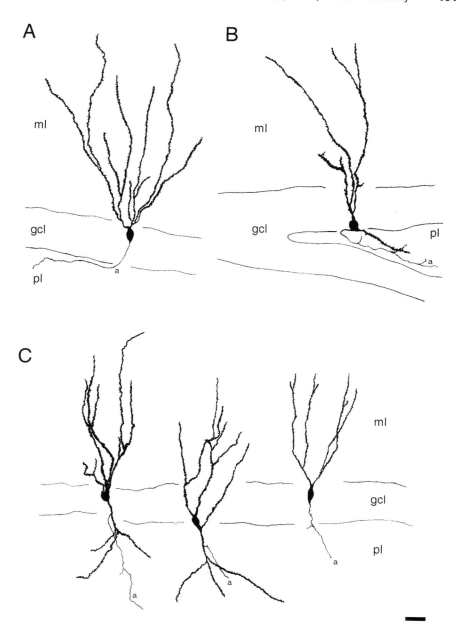

Figure 3–50. Camera lucida drawings of primate granule cells. *A.* Monkey granule cell in the upper part of the granule cell layer (gcl). The dendrites are cone-shaped in the molecular layer (ml); the axon (a) originates from the base of the soma and extends into the polymorphic layer (pl). *B.* Monkey granule cell in the deep part of the granule cell layer with a basal dendrite. Both apical and basal dendrites are fully covered with spines. The apical dendrites extend through the molecular layer, and the basal dendrites extend into the polymorphic layer. The axon originates from the base of the soma and extends into the polymorphic layer. *C.* Three types of human granule cell in the human dentate gyrus. The neuron on the right has dendrites in the molecular layer only, whereas the other two neurons have both apical dendrites extending into the molecular layer and basal dendrites extending into the polymorphic layer. Bar in *C* = 20 μm and applies to all panels. (*Source*: Adapted from Seress and Mrzljak, 1987.)

Projections from the caudal entorhinal cortex (the region equivalent to the rat medial entorhinal area) terminate in a similar fashion: heaviest in the middle third and gradually decreasing in the outer third of the molecular layer. Thus, the border between the lateral and medial entorhinal terminations is much less distinct in the monkey than in the rat.

Lack of Commissural Connections in the Monkey Hippocampal Formation

One of the most striking connectional differences between the rat and the monkey relates to the organization of the commissural connections (Amaral et al., 1984; Demeter et al., 1985). In the rat, there are extensive commissural projections from the polymorphic layer of the dentate gyrus to the contralateral molecular layer of the dentate gyrus and from the CA3 field of the hippocampus to the contralateral CA3 and CA1 fields. In the monkey, these connections are virtually absent. Only the most rostral part of the dentate gyrus and hippocampus (corresponding to the most temporal portion in the rat) demonstrates any commissural connections, and they are limited to the homotopic regions on the contralateral side. Interestingly, whereas the commissural connections of the dentate gyrus and hippocampus are largely absent, the connection originating in the presubiculum and terminating in layer III of the contralateral entorhinal cortex appears to be as robust in the monkey as in the rat.

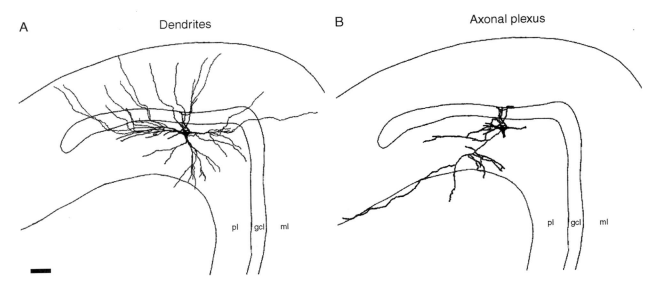

A   Dendrites

B   Axonal plexus

pl   gcl   ml

pl   gcl   ml

Figure 3–51. Mossy cell of the polymorphic layer of the monkey dentate gyrus. *A.* Camera lucida drawing of the soma and dendritic arbor. Note that the dendrites extend widely in the polymorphic layer and extend into the molecular layer, in contrast to what is observed in the rat. *B.* Camera lucida drawing of the soma and axonal plexus. Bar = 100 μm. (*Source*: Adapted from Buckmaster and Amaral, 2001.)

Increased Cortical Interconnectivity of the Monkey Hippocampal Formation

The big difference between the rat and monkey brain is the much greater amount of neocortex in the primate. Much of this neocortex is dedicated to visual processing, but there is also a substantial increase in the amount of association cortex, particularly in the frontal and temporal lobes. A substantial portion of this association cortex is polysensory, and most of the polysensory cortical regions are interconnected with the hippocampal formation via connections with the entorhinal cortex. The more robust neocortical connectivity has given rise to the suggestion that processing in the primate hippocampal formation is more highly dependent on and integrated with processing of sensory information in the neocortex.

In the monkey temporal lobe, there is massive expansion of the perirhinal and parahippocampal regions that border the hippocampal formation. Rostrally, this region includes the perirhinal cortex, which comprises areas 35 and 36 of Brodmann. The perirhinal cortex starts at a level through the rostral hippocampal formation and extends rostrally to form the medial portion of the temporal polar cortex. The caudal continuation of the perirhinal cortex is the parahippocampal cortex, which includes areas TF and TH of von Bonin and Bailey, both of which are bordered laterally by the unimodal visual areas TE or TEO. The perirhinal and parahippocampal cortices are important players in the economy of the neocortical innervation of the hippocampal formation, as they provide nearly two-thirds of the neocortical inputs to the entorhinal cortex.

The major inputs to the monkey entorhinal cortex are summarized in Figures 3–52 and 3–53. In both rats and monkeys, the entorhinal cortex provides the major interface for communication with the neocortex (Insausti et al., 1987). For essentially all cortical regions, the return projections from the entorhinal cortex originate in layers V and VI and terminate both deeply and superficially in a manner typical of other cortical feedback projections. The laminar organization of the inputs to the entorhinal cortex varies according to the cortical area of origin. Projections from some regions, such as the perirhinal and parahippocampal cortices, terminate preferentially in layers I to III, which give rise to the perforant path projections. Projections from other cortical areas, such as the orbitofrontal and insular cortices, project to the deep layers of the entorhinal cortex, which generate the major output pathways to the neocortex and other regions. These latter connections, therefore, might preferentially be involved in modulating the output of the hippocampal formation. However, they may also contribute to the perforant pathway via some of the few layer V and VI neurons that contribute to this pathway or through intrinsic deep to superficial connections in the entorhinal cortex.

Whereas the perirhinal and parahippocampal cortices provide the major input to the hippocampal formation, other substantial inputs originate in the retrosplenial cortex (area 29 in the caudal cingulate gyrus), the polysensory region of the superior temporal gyrus (along the dorsal bank of the superior temporal gyrus), and the orbitofrontal cortex (mainly caudal area 13). The general rule is that the entorhinal cortex receives input only from cortical regions with demonstrated polysensory convergence. Thus, only olfactory input (which originates from all levels of the olfactory system including the olfactory bulb in the primate) has direct access to the hippocampal formation. The olfactory connection, however, provides another example of a difference between the rat and

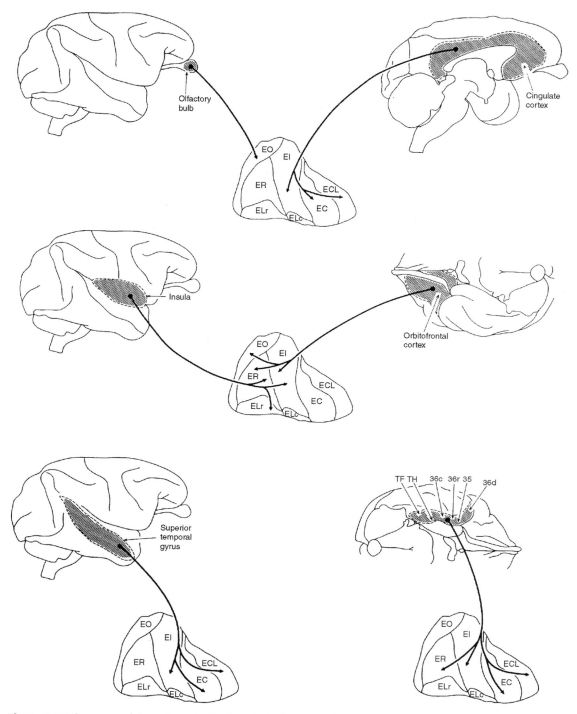

Figure 3–52. Summary of the major entorhinal cortical afferents in the macaque monkey. (*Source*: Adapted from Insausti et al., 1987.)

monkey hippocampal formations. Whereas in the rat almost the entire entorhinal cortex receives direct input from the olfactory bulb, in the monkey this is restricted to about 10% of the surface area of the entorhinal cortex.

Given this pattern of neocortical inputs to the monkey entorhinal cortex, the hippocampal formation can be viewed as the final stage in a cascade of neocortical sensory process-

ing. From the unimodal association cortices, information converges on a few polysensory cortical regions, which in turn project in a convergent fashion on the entorhinal cortex (Lavenex and Amaral, 2000). The entorhinal cortex relays this information to the other hippocampal fields via the perforant path projection. Once the information processed by the hippocampal formation is returned to the deep layers of the

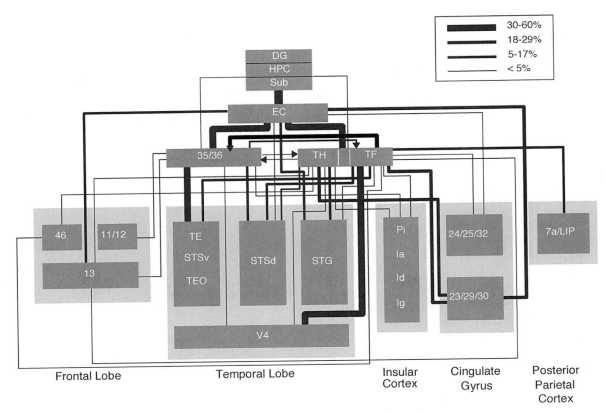

Figure 3–53. Summary of the organization and strength of cortical inputs to the monkey entorhinal, perirhinal (areas 35 and 36), and parahippocampal (areas TF and TH) cortices. (*Source*: Adapted from Suzuki and Amaral, 1994.)

entorhinal cortex, they return this highly processed information to many of the polysensory cortical regions that provide feedback projections to the unimodal sensory regions.

There are a number of implications of this cascade of projections into the entorhinal cortex and the organization of the entorhinal projections to the other hippocampal fields. One is that the information the hippocampal formation is using has been highly preprocessed and integrated. Except for the olfactory input, little elemental or unimodal sensory information is directed to the hippocampal formation. A second, related implication is that it is unlikely that there is appreciable segregation of sensory information processing in the hippocampal formation (i.e., visual information is not processed separately from auditory information). In fact, the pattern of neuroanatomical connectivity predicts that the hippocampal formation carries out whatever functions it accomplishes with high level, multimodal representations of sensory experiences.

3.6.3 Comparison of Monkey and Human Hippocampal Formation

At the risk of making points that may seem obvious, our understanding of the human hippocampus is necessarily primitive compared to that of the rat or the monkey. Because standard experimental tract-tracing studies cannot be done, novel approaches for mapping connections in the human brain do need to be developed. Perhaps the combination of transcranial electromagnetic stimulation during functional magnetic resonance imaging (fMRI) can provide some information on pathways in the human brain, and one can only hope that the wizardry of molecular biology will someday provide new pathway-selective markers that allow comparative studies of the rat, monkey, and human hippocampal formation. That being said, we next provide a short overview of the neuroanatomy of the human hippocampal formation.

Cytoarchitectonic Organization

The general appearance of the human hippocampal formation is reminiscent of the monkey hippocampal formation (Figs. 3–2, 3–45, 3–54). Yet, differences are also apparent. For example, the CA1 field of the hippocampus is even thicker in humans than in monkeys (Fig. 3–49); in some regions, it is as much as 30 cells thick. In addition to being thicker, the CA1 pyramidal cell layer takes on a distinctly multilaminate appearance, with cells of different size and shape predominating at different depths of the layer. Unfortunately, there is little information concerning the exact morphological or neurochemical characteristics of these neurons; there is not even a comprehensive Golgi analysis of the neurons of the human dentate gyrus and hippocampus.

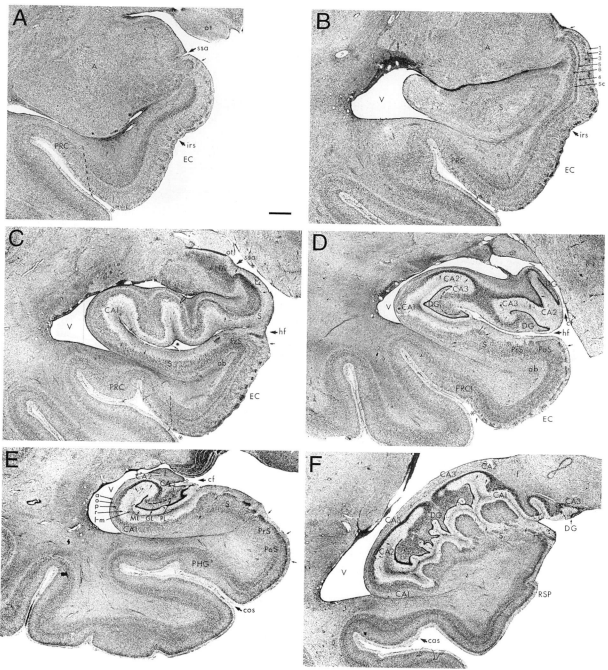

Figure 3–54. Nissl-stained coronal sections through the human hippocampal formation, arranged from rostral (*A*) to caudal (*F*). A, amygdaloid complex; a, alveus; ab, angular bundle; ac, anterior commissure; AHA, amygdalo-hippocampal area; CA1, CA1 field of the hippocampus; CA2, CA2 field of the hippocampus; CA3, CA3 field of the hippocampus; cas, calcarine sulcus; cf, choroidal fissure; cos, collateral sulcus; DG, dentate gyrus; EC, entorhinal cortex; f, fimbria; GL, granule cell layer of the dentate gyrus; hc, hippocampal commissure; hf, hippocampal fissure; irs, intrarhinal sulcus; LGN, lateral geniculate nucleus: l-m: stratum lacunosum-moleculare of the hippocampus; ML, molecular layer of the dentate gyrus; o, stratum oriens of the hippocampus; ot, optic tract; p, pyramidal cell layer of the hippocampus; PaS, parasubiculum; PHG, parahippocampal gyrus (areas TF and TH); pl, polymorphic layer of the dentate gyrus; PRC, perirhinal cortex (areas 35 and 36); PrS, presubiculum; r, stratum radiatum of the hippocampus; RSP, retrosplenial cortex; S, subiculum; ssa, sulcus semiannularis; V, temporal horn of the lateral ventricle. The numbers in *B* indicate the layers of the entorhinal cortex. Bar in *A* = 2 mm and applies to all panels.

Another obvious difference is the cellular composition of the region enclosed within the limbs of the granule cell layer. There are obviously far more cells in this region, and most appear to be cells of the CA3 field. The polymorphic layer of the dentate gyrus (the hilus) forms a narrow band that lies just subjacent to the granule cell layer. Little is known about the morphology of cells in the human dentate gyrus. As indicated in the comparison between the rat and the monkey, however, there are clear differences in the morphology of certain cell types. As many as 30% of granule cells in the human dentate gyrus have basal dendrites (Fig. 3–50); this number may be even larger than in the monkey.

Even less is known about the human subiculum, presubiculum, and parasubiculum. Although the distribution of various neurochemicals or receptors has been incidentally illustrated during the course of large survey studies, almost nothing has been written on the cellular morphology of these regions. The human entorhinal cortex has attracted considerably more attention because of its vulnerability in Alzheimer's disease. Although the same general regions identified in the monkey can be identified in the human, there is evidence for additional fields in the human entorhinal cortex. Classic cytoarchitectonicists, for example, have defined as many as 27 divisions.

Connections

There is little information concerning the organization of connections in the human hippocampal formation owing to the fact that most neuroanatomical tracing techniques require injection of tracers into the living brain. Some investigators have relied instead on techniques such as local application of the lipophilic dye DiI to map short pathways in human postmortem material. Clifford Saper and colleagues have used this technique to study the connections of the granule cells and the projections of the enclosed portion of CA3 (Lim et al.,

1997a,b). They found that both the mossy fiber projection and the Schaffer collateral system (from CA3 to CA1) can be labeled over short distances by DiI and that these projections resemble those observed in the monkey. As important as these limited observations are, they highlight the fact that we do not currently know whether the neuroanatomical connections that have been described for the rat and the monkey are applicable to the human brain.

Magnetic Resonance Imaging of the Human Hippocampal Formation

With the emergence of MRI studies of the human brain, there have been numerous structural (Jack et al., 2003) and functional (Maguire et al., 2003) studies of the human hippocampal formation. Studies have used both manual tracing techniques as well as algorithms for automated segmentation. Of course, without the benefit of cytoarchitectonic guidance, it has generally proven difficult if not impossible to differentiate the component parts of the hippocampal formation. It has even been complicated to define accurately the boundaries of regions, such as the entorhinal cortex (Insausti et al., 1998).

Figure 3–55 presents a coronal section stained by the Nissl method. To get a sense of the dimensions of this region and what can be distinguished during a standard functional imaging study, we have placed a grid of 4-mm square boxes over the medial temporal lobe. With resolution at this level (which might be typical for a standard functional imaging study), one might expect to have one voxel focused over the subiculum or perhaps two voxels over the entorhinal cortex. Other voxels, however, would clearly overlap adjacent fields, such as the dentate gyrus and CA3. Positron emission tomography studies have even poorer spatial resolution. Thus, given current functional imaging technologies, it is difficult to define specific activations for defined subfields of the hippocampal formation.

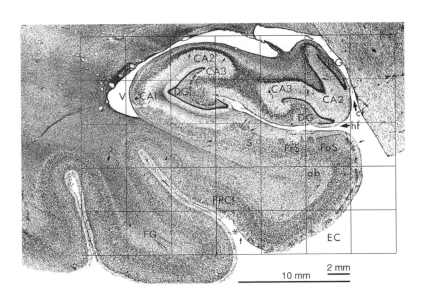

Figure 3–55. Nissl-stained coronal sections through the human hippocampal formation at the caudal aspect of the uncus. The grid overlay consists of squares that are 4 mm on edge. For abbreviations, see Figure 3–11. (*Source*: Adapted from Amaral, 1999.)

Critical Comparison of Neuroanatomy of Rat, Monkey, and Human Hippocampal Formation Must Await Comparable Quantitative Data for Each Species

This chapter has dealt primarily with the rat hippocampal formation because, as we pointed out at the beginning, much of the neuroanatomical information available has been gained from studies of the rat. Furthermore, much of the electrophysiological and behavioral literature discussed throughout the rest of the book is based on studies in the rat. With the dramatic increase in the use of noninvasive imaging of the human hippocampal formation, particularly in studies of memory, the need has grown for more detailed information about the neuroanatomical organization of the human hippocampal formation. This is also important as increasingly sophisticated models of hippocampus-related pathology are introduced based primarily on rodent studies. A variety of models for temporal lobe epilepsy, for example, have been advanced based on cell degeneration and fiber sprouting in the rat hippocampus. However, if the fundamental circuit diagram of the rat hippocampal formation is different from that of humans, models based on the rat may be misleading.

Unfortunately, the extent of the similarities and differences in the hippocampal formation of the rat, monkey, and human cannot yet be accurately gauged. Based on the few examples of established species differences described previously, it would not be surprising if substantial differences exist in the cellular morphology, connectivity, and chemical neuroanatomy of the hippocampal formation across species. The relevance of these differences to the normal function and the pathology of the hippocampal function will be an interesting area of comparative neuroanatomy in the future.

3.7 Principles of Hippocampal Connectivity and Implications for Information Processing

Neuroanatomy has the unfortunate characteristic of being detail-oriented, and it is easy to lose sight of the forest for the trees when absorbing and recounting information on the cells and connections of the hippocampal formation. In the following sections, we take a somewhat more integrative approach and attempt to draw implications from what we have described so far. These implications are generally quite speculative at this point, but they concern the important issue of the functional correlates of the known hippocampal neuroanatomy.

3.7.1 Highly Distributed Three-Dimensional Network of Intrinsic Connections

What is the hallmark of hippocampal connectivity? Beyond the defining aspect of unidirectional connectivity between individual components, perhaps the facet that is most striking is that each of the intrinsic connections of the hippocampal formation is both massively divergent and convergent. Cells located in a focused point in the entorhinal cortex, for example, can influence neurons in as much as 50% of the entire septotemporal axis of the dentate gyrus. Cells in the polymorphic layer of the dentate gyrus, in turn, can interconnect different levels of the dentate gyrus, providing further spread of information to as much as 75% of the septotemporal axis. Similarly, divergent projections have been described for the CA3 to CA1 connections and for the CA1 to subiculum connections. Thus, a perspective most consistent with the known neuroanatomy is that the hippocampal formation contains a series of three-dimensional networks of connections. Depending on the synaptic interactions of these connections (excitatory versus inhibitory), as well as the setting of the myriad physiological parameters described in Chapter 5 (e.g., density and efficiency of synapses, transmitter release, synaptic plasticity), they might focus information processing to a specific level, recruit neurons at distant levels into the ongoing processing, or have no effect at all. Presumably, the role of this distributed network will become better understood as increasingly massive parallel electrophysiological recording procedures are employed.

3.7.2 Functional Implications of the Septotemporal Topography of Connections

Given the septotemporal topography observed throughout the hippocampal formation, there may still be some segregation of functional divisions in this system. Although the massively divergent/convergent nature of hippocampal connections is inconsistent with a high degree of spatially restricted information processing, the possibility remains that there are a few septotemporally positioned domains of relatively restricted information processing, at least at early stages, through the hippocampal circuitry. It appears that there are at least three separable domains of neurons in the entorhinal cortex: a lateral region, a mid region and a medial region. The most laterally situated domain of neurons innervates the septal half of the dentate gyrus and other innervated hippocampal fields; the mid region innervates the next quarter; and the medial domain innervates the temporal quarter of the dentate gyrus (Fig. 3–41). Because the lateral portion of the rat entorhinal cortex receives the bulk of the input from other neocortical areas, it is reasonable to assume that septal levels of the hippocampal formation are more highly involved with processing exteroceptive sensory information. Because the medial portions of the rat entorhinal cortex are preferentially innervated by structures such as the amygdaloid complex, the temporal portion of the hippocampal formation may preferentially deal with interoceptive or emotional information. Because virtually all of the in vivo electrophysiological analysis of the rat hippocampal formation has been carried out in the septal portion (and most of the in vitro work was carried out to give slices from the rostral and mid-septotemporal levels), it is of interest to determine whether fundamentally different types of response patterns are observed when temporally situated neurons are probed. Several lines of behavioral data from lesioned animals are already consistent with this idea (see Chapter 14).

3.7.3 Functional Implications of the Transverse Topography of Connections

Despite the fact that intrinsic hippocampal connections have an extensive septotemporal distribution, they are not uniformly distributed along the transverse axis. This organization raises the possibility of partially independent channels of information flow through and out of the hippocampal formation (Fig. 3–56). As we mentioned previously, it is not the case that every CA1 cell has equal probability of input from every CA3 cell. The intrinsic circuitry of the hippocampal formation appears to be organized such that cells located at a particular transverse position in a field are much more likely to be connected with cells located at a particular transverse position of the innervated field. This allows the possibility, therefore, that there is some channeling of information processing through the various hippocampal fields. As described fully above, cells located proximally in CA3 tend to project to the most distal CA1 cells. Projections from the distal portion of CA3, in contrast, terminate mainly in the proximal portion of CA1. The midportion of CA3 fills in the spaces between these two projections. The CA1 projection to the subiculum demonstrates even more striking transverse topography. The proximal portion of CA1 projects discretely to the distal third of the subiculum; the distal portion of CA1 projects just across the border into the proximal third of the subiculum; and the middle portion of CA1 projects to the midregion of the subiculum.

The tripartite transverse organization in CA1 and the subiculum also appears to be respected by the entorhinal projections to these fields. The lateral entorhinal cortex projects to the border region of CA1 and the subiculum, whereas the medial entorhinal cortex projects either more proximally in CA1 or more distally in the subiculum. Layer III neurons of the medial entorhinal cortex are heavily influenced by presubicular input and thus by the thalamus, whereas layer III neurons in the lateral entorhinal area are heavily innervated by the amygdaloid complex.

Taken together, this organization suggests that CA1 cells located close to the CA3 field receive information from a subset of CA3 cells located close to CA2 and a subset of layer III cells located in the medial entorhinal cortex. CA1 cells located closer to the subiculum, in contrast, receive preferential input from CA3 cells located close to the dentate gyrus and from layer III cells in the lateral entorhinal cortex. A prediction would be, therefore, that the response properties of CA1 cells at different transverse positions, at a particular septotemporal level, should be different.

The notion of transverse topography of hippocampal connections is made all the more compelling when it is appreciated that the subicular output is also organized in a columnar fashion, with projections to different brain regions, or different parts of the same brain region, originating from the proximal, middle, and distal thirds of the subiculum. Neurons in the proximal third of the subiculum project to the infralimbic and prelimbic cortices, the nucleus accumbens, and the lateral septal region. Projections from this portion of the ventral part of the subiculum also project to the ventromedial nucleus of the hypothalamus and to the amygdala. The midtransverse portion of the subiculum projects mainly to the midline thalamic nuclei, and neurons in the distal portion of the subiculum project to the retrosplenial portion of the cingulate cortex and the presubiculum. Although all portions of the subiculum project to the entorhinal cortex, the pattern of projections

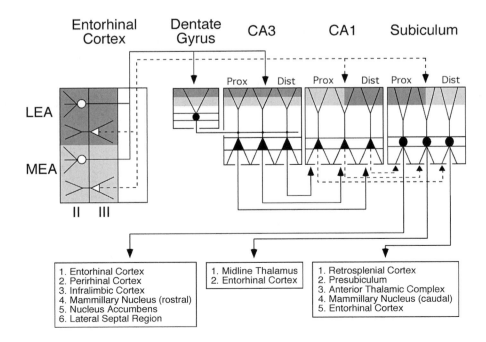

Figure 3–56. Summary of the transverse organization of the connections through the hippocampal formation. This figure highlights the possibility that information is segregated, or "channeled," through the hippocampal formation and ultimately reaches different recipients of hippocampal output.

reciprocates the topography of the perforant path projections to the subiculum. Thus, the proximal portion of the subiculum projects to the lateral entorhinal area, and more distal portions of the subiculum project to the medial entorhinal area. Thus, from CA3 on through the entorhinal cortex, there exists the potential for information that arrives at the earliest point in this chain of connections to maintain some uniquess from information that arrives at different portions of CA3. The functional significance of this neuroanatomical pathway segregation is unknown at present.

To summarize, although the intrinsic connectivity of the hippocampal formation is highly divergent, the network that is formed is not without some topography. The septotemporal and transverse components of this topography provide the increased probability of communication between certain neurons in each field and thus the possibility of some form of channeling or segregation of information processing in the hippocampal formation.

3.7.4 Serial and Parallel Processing in the Hippocampal Formation

A unique feature of the intrinsic hippocampal circuitry is the largely unidirectional organization of the projections that interconnect the various hippocampal regions. A popular notion is that these unidirectional projections also imply an exclusively serial or sequential flow of information—first from the entorhinal cortex to the dentate gyrus, then to the CA3 field of the hippocampus, and so on. However, the data summarized in the body of this chapter clearly indicate that the intrinsic hippocampal circuitry has both serial and parallel projections (Fig. 3–57).

The entorhinal cortex, in particular, contributes many parallel projections to several fields of the hippocampal formation. The same layer II entorhinal cells probably give rise to projections that terminate in both the dentate gyrus and the CA3 field of the hippocampus. Thus, whatever the information conveyed by layer II entorhinal cells, it arrives both monosynaptically and disynaptically (through mossy fiber intermediaries) at CA3. It is not known, of course, whether information from a single entorhinal cell reaches a particular CA3 cell both monosynaptically and disynaptically. This is an important question to resolve in future studies.

The existence of prominent associational connections in the dentate gyrus, hippocampus, and entorhinal cortex also provides the substrate for polysynaptic activation in hippocampal circuits. The functional implication of this more complex circuitry is that each hippocampal region is not entirely dependent on the preceding region for input, which raises the prospect that each region may be acting semi-independently from, as well as in concert with, other hippocampal fields. Hippocampal neuroanatomy is thus consistent with the electrophysiological findings—for example, that CA1 place fields are apparently normal even after pharmacological inactivation of the dentate gyrus.

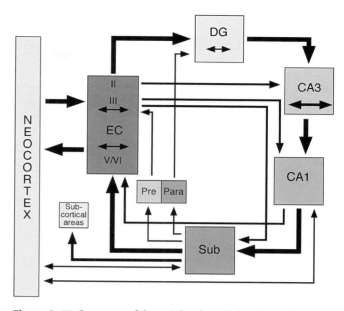

Figure 3–57. Summary of the serial and parallel pathways through the hippocampal formation. Although the intrinsic hippocampal circuitry is largely unidirectional, it contains both serial and parallel projections. See text for details.

3.8 Conclusions

Although this chapter has presented a substantial amount of neuroanatomical information, it has only begun to scratch the surface of what is available in the primary literature. However, beause we have focused on general features and principles of organization, it should be more than adequate for delving into the molecular and cellular aspects of hippocampal organization (see Chapters 5 and 7) as well as the function of the hippocampal formation in the living organism. The neuroanatomy of the hippocampal formation is unique and predicts that the behavioral functions it subserves are undoubtedly unique as well.

ACKNOWLEDGMENTS

The authors are indebted to the many colleagues who have worked in our laboratory over the years. Much of the knowledge they have uncovered has gone into the pages of this chapter. We are grateful particularly to Dr. Menno Witter and Dr. Ricardo Insausti, who not only co-authored earlier comprehensive summaries on the neuroanatomy of the rat and human hippocampal formation, but also reviewed the current chapter to help ensure its accuracy. We also thank Dr. Lazlo Seress for additional comments on the manuscript. The original research summarized in this chapter has been supported by the National Institutes of Health and the Human Frontier Science Program. Finally, we are grateful to our families who understand that science requires some sacrifice of time with them. Their support has made this chapter possible.

REFERENCES

Acsady L, Kamondi A, Sik A, Freund T, Buzsaki G (1998) GABAergic cells are the major postsynaptic targets of mossy fibers in the rat hippocampus. *J Neurosci* 18:3386–3403.

Allen GV, Hopkins DA (1989) Mamillary body in the rat: topography and synaptology of projections from the subicular complex, prefrontal cortex, and midbrain tegmentum. *J Comp Neurol* 286:311–336.

Amaral DG (1978) A Golgi study of cell types in the hilar region of the hippocampus in the rat. *J Comp Neurol* 182:851–914.

Amaral DG (1999) Introduction: what is where in the medial temporal lobe? *Hippocampus* 9:1–6.

Amaral DG, Dent JA (1981) Development of the mossy fibers of the dentate gyrus. I. A light and electron microscopic study of the mossy fibers and their expansions. *J Comp Neurol* 195:51–86.

Amaral DG, Kurz J (1985) An analysis of the origins of the cholinergic and noncholinergic septal projections to the hippocampal formation of the rat. *J Comp Neurol* 240:37–59.

Amaral DG, Witter MP (1989) The three dimensional organization of the hippocampal formation: a review of anatomical data. *Neuroscience* 31:571–591.

Amaral DG, Insausti R, Cowan WM (1984) The commissural connections of the monkey hippocampal formation. *J Comp Neurol* 224:307–336.

Amaral DG, Dolorfo C, Alvarez-Royo P (1991) Organization of CA1 projections to the subiculum: a PHA-L analysis in the rat. *Hippocampus* 1:415–436.

Andersen P, Bliss TVP, Skrede KK (1971) Lamellar organization of hippocampal excitatory pathways. *Exp Brain Res* 13:222–238.

Arantius G (1587) *De humano foetu . . . Ejusdem anatomicorum observationum liber*. Venice.

Baisden RH, Woodruff ML, Hoover DB (1984) Cholinergic and noncholinergic septo-hippocampal projections: a double-label horseradish peroxidase-acetylcholinesterase study in the rabbit. *Brain Res* 290:146–151.

Bakst I, Avendaño C, Morrison JH, Amaral DG (1986) An experimental analysis of the origins of the somatostatin immunoreactive fibers in the dentate gyrus of the rat. *J Neurosci* 6:1452–1462.

Blackstad TW (1956) Commissural connections of the hippocampal region in the rat, with special reference to their mode of termination. *J Comp Neurol* 105:417–537.

Blackstad TW, Brink K, Hem J, Jeune B (1970) Distribution of hippocampal mossy fibers in the rat: an experimental study with silver impregnation methods. *J Comp Neurol* 138:433–450.

Borhegyi Z, Leranth C (1997) Distinct substance P- and calretinin-containing projections from the supramammillary area to the hippocampus in rats: a species difference between rats and monkeys. *Exp Brain Res* 115:369–374.

Boyett JM, Buckmaster PS (2001) Somatostatin-immunoreactive interneurons contribute to lateral inhibitory circuits in the dentate gyrus of control and epileptic rats. *Hippocampus* 11:418–422.

Braak H (1972) Zur Pigmentarchitektonic der Grosshirnrinde des Menschen. I. Regio entorhinalis. *Z Zellforsch Mikrosk Anat* 127:407–438.

Braak H (1980) *Architectonics of the human telencephalic cortex*. New York: Springer.

Broca P (1878) Anatomie comparée des circonvolutions cérébrales: le grand lobe limbique. *Rev. Anthropol* 1:385–498.

Brodal A (1947) The hippocampus and the sense of smell: a review. *Brain* 70:179–222.

Brodmann K (1909) *Vergleichende Lokalisationslehre der Grosshirnrinde in ihren Prinzipien dargestellt auf Grund des Zellenbaues*. Leipzig.

Buckmaster PS, Amaral DG (2001) Intracellular recording and labeling of mossy cells and proximal CA3 pyramidal cells in macaque monkeys. *J Comp Neurol* 430:264–281.

Buckmaster PS, Strowbridge BW, Kunkel DD, Schmiege DL, Schwartzkroin PA (1992) Mossy cell axonal projections to the dentate gyrus molecular layer in the rat hippocampal slice. *Hippocampus* 2:349–362.

Buckmaster PS, Wenzel HJ, Kunkel DD, Schwartzkroin PA (1996) Axon arbors and synaptic connections of hippocampal mossy cells in the rat in vivo. *J Comp Neurol* 366:271–292.

Burwell RD (2001) Borders and cytoarchitecture of the perirhinal and postrhinal cortices in the rat. *J Comp Neurol* 437:17–41.

Burwell RD, Amaral DG (1998a) Perirhinal and postrhinal cortices of the rat: interconnectivity and connections with the entorhinal cortex. *J Comp Neurol* 391:293–321.

Burwell RD, Amaral DG (1998b) Cortical afferents of the perirhinal, postrhinal, and entorhinal cortices of the rat. *J Comp Neurol* 398:179–205.

Burwell RD, Witter MP (2002) *Basic anatomy of the parahippocampal region in monkeys and rats*. Oxford: Oxford University Press.

Burwell RD, Witter MP, Amaral DG (1995) Perirhinal and postrhinal cortices of the rat: a review of the neuroanatomical literature and comparison with findings from the monkey brain. *Hippocampus* 5:390–408.

Caballero-Bleda M, Witter MP (1993) Regional and laminar organization of projections from the presubiculum and parasubiculum to the entorhinal cortex: an anterograde tracing study in the rat. *J Comp Neurol* 328:115–129.

Canteras N, Swanson L (1992) Projections of the ventral subiculum to the amygdala, septum, and hypothalamus: a PHAL anterograde tract-tracing study in the rat. *J Comp Neurol* 324:180–194.

Claiborne BJ, Amaral DG, Cowan WM (1986) A light and electron microscopic analysis of the mossy fibers of the rat dentate gyrus. *J Comp Neurol* 246:435–458.

Claiborne BJ, Amaral DG, Cowan WM (1990) A quantitative three-dimensional analysis of granule cell dendrites in the rat dentate gyrus. *J Comp Neurol* 302:206–219.

Conrad LCA, Leonard CM, Pfaff DW (1974) Connections of the median and dorsal raphe nuclei in the rat: an autoradiographic and degeneration study. *J Comp Neurol* 156:179–206.

Daitz HM, Powell TPS (1954) Studies of the connexions of the fornix system. *J Neurol Neurosurg Psychiatry* 17:75–82.

De Garengeot RJC (1742) *Splanchnologie ou l'anatomie des visceres*, 2nd ed, pp 250–251. Paris: C. Osmond.

Deller T (1998) The anatomical organization of the rat fascia dentata: new aspects of laminar organization as revealed by anterograde tracing with Phaseolus vulgaris-Leucoagglutinin (PHAL). *Anat Embryol (Berl)* 197:89–103.

Deller T, Adelmann G, Nitsch R, Frotscher M (1996) The alvear pathway of the rat hippocampus. *Cell Tissue Res* 286:293–303.

Demeter S, Rosene DL, Van Hoesen GW (1985) Interhemispheric pathways of the hippocampal formation, presubiculum and entorhinal and posterior parahippocampal cortices in the rhesus monkey: the structure and organization of the hippocampal commissures. *J Comp Neurol* 233:30–47.

Dent JA, Galvin NJ, Stanfield BB, Cowan WM (1983) The mode of temination of the hypothalamic projection to the dentate gyrus: an EM autoradiographic study. *Brain Res* 258:1–10.

Desmond NL, Levy WB (1985) Granule cell dendritic spine density in the rat hippocampus varies with spine shape and location. *Neurosci Lett* 54:219–224.

Dolleman-Van der Weel MJ, Witter MP (2000) Nucleus reuniens thalami innervates gamma aminobutyric acid positive cells in hippocampal field CA1 of the rat. *Neurosci Lett* 278:145–148.

Dolorfo CL, Amaral DG (1998a) Entorhinal cortex of the rat: topographic organization of the cells of origin of the perforant path projection to the dentate gyrus. *J Comp Neurol* 398:25–48.

Dolorfo CL, Amaral DG (1998b) Entorhinal cortex of the rat: organization of intrinsic connerctions. *J Comp Neurol* 398:49–82.

Donovan MK, Wyss JM (1983) Evidence for some collateralization between cortical and diencephalic efferent axons of the rat subicular cortex. *Brain Res* 259:181–192.

Duffy CJ, Rakic P (1983) Differentiation of granule cell dendrites in the dentate gyrus of the rhesus monkey: a quantitative Golgi study. *J Comp Neurol* 214:224–237.

Felleman DJ, Van Essen DC (1991) Distributed hierarchical processing in the primate cerebral cortex. *Cereb Cortex* 1:1–47.

Freund TF, Buzsaki G (1996) Interneurons of the hippocampus. *Hippocampus* 6:347–470.

Fricke R, Cowan WM (1978) An autoradiographic study of the commissural and ipsilateral hippocampo-dentate projections in the adult rat. *J Comp Neurol* 181:253–269.

Frotscher M (1992) Application of the Golgi/electron microscopy technique for cell identification in immunocytochemical, retrograde labeling, and developmental studies of hippocampal neurons. *Microsc Res Tech* 23:306–323.

Funahashi M, Stewart M (1997a) Presubicular and parasubicular cortical neurons of the rat: electrophysiological and morphological properties. *Hippocampus* 7:117–129.

Funahashi M, Stewart M (1997b) Presubicular and parasubicular cortical neurons of the rat: functional separation of deep and superficial neurons in vitro. *J Physiol (Lond)* 501:387–403.

Gaarskjaer FB (1978a) Organization of the mossy fiber system of the rat studied in extended hippocampi. I. Terminal area related to number of granule and pyramidal cells. *J Comp Neurol* 178:49–72.

Gaarskjaer FB (1978b) Organization of the mossy fiber system of the rat studied in extended hippocampi. II. Experimental analysis of fiber distribution with silver impregnation methods. *J Comp Neurol* 178:73–88.

Gaykema RPA, Luiten PGM, Nyakas C, Traber J (1990) Cortical projection patterns of the medial septum-diagonal band complex. *J Comp Neurol* 293:103–124.

Gertz SD, Lindenberg R, Piavis GW (1972) Structural variations in the rostral human hippocampus. *Johns Hopkins Med J* 130: 367–376.

Gloveli T, Schmitz D, Empson RM, Dugladze T, Heinemann U (1997) Morphological and electrophysiological characterization of layer III cells of the medial entorhinal cortex of the rat. *Neuroscience* 77:629–648.

Goldowitz D, White WF, Steward O, Lynch G, Cotman C (1975) Anatomical evidence for a projection from the entorhinal cortex to the contralateral dentate gyrus of the rat. *Exp Neurol* 47:433–441.

Gottlieb DI, Cowan WM (1973) Autoradiographic studies of the commissural and ipsilateral association connections of the hippocampus and dentate gyrus of the rat. *J Comp Neurol* 149:393–420.

Greene JRT, Totterdell S (1997) Morphology and distribution of electrophysiologically defined classes of pyramidal and nonpyramidal neurons in rat ventral subiculum in vitro. *J Comp Neurol* 380:395–408.

Groenewegen HJ, Vermeulen-Van Der Zee E, Te Kortschot A, Witter M (1987) Organization of the projections from the subiculum to the ventral striatum in the rat: a study using anterograde transport of Phaseolus vulgaris leucoagglutinin. *Neuroscience* 23:103–120.

Haglund L, Swanson LW, Köhler C (1984) The projection of the supramammillary nucleus to the hippocampal formation: an immunohistochemical and anterograde transport study with the lectin PHA-L in the rat. *J Comp Neurol* 229:171–185.

Hamam BN, Amaral DG, Alonso AA (2002) Morphological and electrophysiological characteristics of layer V neurons of the rat lateral entorhinal cortex. *J Comp Neurol* 451:45–61.

Hamam BN, Kennedy TE, Alonso A, Amaral DG (2000) Morphological and electrophysiological characteristics of layer V neurons of the rat medial entorhinal cortex. *J Comp Neurol* 418:457–472.

Han ZS, Buhl EH, Lorinczi Z, Somogyi P (1993) A high degree of spatial selectivity in the axonal and dendritic domains of physiologically identified local-circuit neurons in the dentate gyrus of the rat hippocampus. *Eur J Neurosci* 5:395–410.

Harris E, Witter MP, Weinstein G, Stewart M (2001) Intrinsic connectivity of the rat subiculum. I. Dendritic morphology and patterns of axonal arborization by pyramidal neurons. *J Comp Neurol* 435:490–505.

Haug FM (1976) Sulphide silver pattern and cytoarchitectonics of parahippocampal areas in the rat. Special reference to the subdivision of area entorhinalis (area 28) and its demarcation from the pyriform cortex. *Adv Anat Embryol Cell Biol* 52:3–73.

Hausheer-Zarmakupi Z, Wolfer DP, Leisinger-Trigona MC, Lipp HP (1996) Selective breeding for extremes in open-field activity of mice entails a differentiation of hippocampal mossy fibers. *Behav Genet* 26:167–176.

Henze DA, Urban NN, Barrioneuvo G (2000) The multifarious hippocampal mossy fleer pathway: a review. *Neuroscience* 98: 407–427.

Herkenham M (1978) The connections of the nucleus reuniens thalami: evidence for a direct thalamo-hippocampal pathway in the rat. *J Comp Neurol* 177:589–610.

Hjorth-Simonsen A, Jeune B (1972) Origin and termination of the hippocampal perforant path in the rat studied by silver impregnation. *J Comp Neurol* 144:215–232.

Hjorth-Simonsen A, Zimmer J (1975) Crossed pathways from the entorhinal area to the fascia dentata. *J Comp Neurol* 161: 57–70.

Insausti R, Amaral DG, Cowan WM (1987) The entorhinal cortex of the monkey. II. Cortical afferents. *J Comp Neurol* 264:356–395.

Insausti R, Herrero MT, Witter MP (1997) Entorhinal cortex of the rat: cytoarchitectonic subdivisions and the origin and distribution of cortical efferents. *Hippocampus* 7:146–183.

Insausti R, Juottonen K, Soininen H, Insausti AM, Partanen K, Vainio P, Laakso MP, Pitkanen A (1998) MR volumetric analysis of the human entorhinal, perirhinal, and temporopolar cortices. *AJNR Am J Neuroradiol* 19:659–671.

Ishizuka N (2001) Laminar organization of the pyramidal cell layer of the subiculum in the rat. *J Comp Neurol* 435:89–110.

Ishizuka N, Weber J, Amaral DG (1990) Organization of intrahippocampal projections originating from CA3 pyramidal cells in the rat. *J Comp Neurol* 295:580–623.

Ishizuka N, Cowan WM, Amaral DG (1995) A quantitative analysis of the dendritic organization of pyramidal cells in the rat hippocampus. *J Comp Neurol* 362:17–45.

Jack CR Jr, Slomkowski M, Gracon S, Hoover TM, Felmlee JP, Stewart K, Xu Y, Shiung M, O'Brien PC, Cha R, Knopman D, Petersen RC (2003) MRI as a biomarker of disease progression in a therapeutic trial of milameline for AD. *Neurology* 60:253–260.

Kaitz SS, Robertson RT (1981) Thalamic connections with limbic cortex. II. Corticothalamic projections. *J Comp Neurol* 195:527–545.

Kempermann G, Kuhn G, Gage FH (1997) More hippocampal neurons in adult mice living in an enriched environment. *Nature* 386:493–495.

Kempermann G, Kuhn HG, Gage FH (1998) Experienced-induced neurogenesis in the senescent dentate gyrus. *J Neurosci* 18:3206–3212.

Kiss J, Csaki A, Bokor H, Shanabrough M, Leranth C (2000) The supramamillo-hippocampal and supramammillo-septal glutamatergic/aspartatergic projections in the rat: a combined [³H]D-aspartate autoradiographic and immunohistochemical study. *Neuroscience* 97:657–669.

Klink R, Alonso A (1997) Morphological characteristics of layer II projection neurons in the rat medial entorhinal cortex. *Hippocampus* 7:571–583.

Kloosterman F, Witter Menno P, van Haeften T (2003) Topographical and laminar organization of subicular projections to the parahippocampal region of the rat. *J Comp Neurol* 455:156–171.

Kohler C (1985) Intrinsic projections of the retrohippocampal region in the rat brain. I. The subicular complex. *J Comp Neurol* 236:504–522.

Köhler C, Steinbusch H (1982) Identification of serotonin and non-serotonin-containing neurons of the mid-brain raphe projecting to the entorhinal area and the hippocampal formation: a combined immunohistochemical and fluorescent retrograde tracing study in the rat brain. *Neuroscience* 7:951–975.

Laatsch RH, Cowan WM (1967) Electron microscopic studies of the dentate gyrus of the rat. II. Degeneration of commissural afferents. *J Comp Neurol* 130:241–262.

Lacaille JC, Schwartzkroin PA (1988) Stratum lacunosum-moleculare interneurons of hippocampal CA1 region. I. Intracellular response characteristics, synaptic responses, and morphology. *J Neurosci* 8:1400–1410.

Lacaille JC, Mueller AL, Kunkel DD, Schwartzkroin PA (1987) Local circuit interactions between oriens/alveus interneurons and CA1 pyramidal cells in hippocampal slices: electrophysiology and morphology. *J Neurosci* 7:1979–1993.

Laurberg S (1979) Commissural and intrinsic connections of the rat hippocampus. *J Comp Neurol* 184:685–708.

Laurberg S, Sorensen KE (1981) Associational and commissural collaterals of neurons in the hippocampal formation (hilus fasciae dentatae and subfield CA3). *Brain Res* 212:287–300.

Lavenex P, Amaral DG (2000) Hippocampal-neocortical interaction: a hierarchy of associativity. *Hippocampus* 10:420–430.

Li X-G, Somogyi P, Ylinen A, Buzsaki G (1994) The hippocampal CA3 network: an in vivo intracellular labeling study. *J Comp Neurol* 339:181–208.

Lim C, Blume HW, Madsen JR, Saper CB (1997a) Connections of the hippocampal formation in humans. I. The mossy fiber pathway. *J Comp Neurol* 385:325–351.

Lim C, Mufson EJ, Kordower JH, Blume HW, Madsen JR, Saper CB (1997b) Connections of the hippocampal formation in humans. II. The endfolial fiber pathway. *J Comp Neurol* 385:352–371.

Lipp HP, Schwegler H, Heimrich B, Cerbone A, Sadile AG (1987) Strain-specific correlations between hippocampal structural traits and habituation in a spatial novelty situation. *Behav Brain Res* 24:111–123.

Lorente de Nó R (1933) Studies on the structure of the cerebral cortex. I. The area entorhinalis. *J Psychol Neurol* 45:381–438.

Lorente de Nó R (1934) Studies on the structure of the cerebral cortex. II. Continuation of the study of the ammonic system. *J Psychol Neurol* 46:113–177.

Loughlin SE, Foote SL, Grzanna R (1986) Efferent projections of nucleus locus coeruleus: morphologic subpopulations have different efferent targets. *Neuroscience* 18:307–319.

Lubke J, Deller T, Frotscher M (1997) Septal innervation of mossy cells in the hilus of the rat dentate gyrus: an anterograde tracing and intracellular labeling study. *Exp Brain Res* 114:423–432.

Magloczky Z, Acsady L, Freund TF (1994) Principal cells are the postsynaptic targets of supramammillary afferents in the hippocampus of the rat. *Hippocampus* 4:322–334.

Maguire EA, Spiers HJ, Good CD, Hartley T, Frackowiak RS, Burgess N (2003) Navigation expertise and the human hippocampus: a structural brain imaging analysis. *Hippocampus* 13:250–259.

McEwen BS, Wallach G (1973) Corticosterone binding to hippocampus: nuclear and cytosol binding in vitro. *Brain Res* 57:373–386.

McLardy T, Kilmer WL (1970) Hippocampal circuitry. *Am Psychol* 25:563–566.

Meibach RC, Siegel A (1975) The origin of fornix fibers which project to the mammillary bodies in the rat: a horseradish peroxidase study. *Brain Res* 88:508–512.

Moore RY, Halaris AE (1975) Hippocampal innervation by serotonin neurons of the midbrain raphe in the rat. *J Comp Neurol* 164:171–184.

Morrison JH, Benoit, R., Magistretti PJ, Ling N, Bloom FE (1982) Immunohistochemical distribution of prosomatostatin-related peptides in hippocampus. *Neurosci Lett* 34:137–142.

Mosko S, Lynch G, Cotman CW (1973) The distribution of septal projections to the hippocampus of the rat. *J Comp Neurol* 152:163–174.

Naber PA, Witter MP (1998) Subicular efferents are organized mostly as parallel projections: a double-labeling, retrograde-tracing study in the rat. *J Comp Neurol* 393:284–297.

Naber PA, da Silva FHL, Witter MP (2001) Reciprocal connections between the entorhinal cortex and hippocampal fields CA1 and the subiculum are in register with the projections from CA1 to the subiculum. *Hippocampus* 11:99–104.

Nafstad PHJ (1967) An electron microscope study on the termination of the perforant path fibres in the hippocampus and the fascia dentata. *Z Zellforsch Und Mikrosk Anat* 76:532–542.

Nyakas C, Luiten PGM, Spencer DG, Traber J (1987) Detailed projection patterns of septal and diagonal band efferents to the hippocampus in the rat with emphasis on innervation of CA1 and dentate gyrus. *Brain Res Bull* 18:533–545.

O'Mara SM, Commins S, Anderson M, Gigg J (2001) The subiculum: a review of form, physiology and function. *Prog Neurobiol* 64:129–155.

Papez JW (1937) A proposed mechanism of emotion. *Arch Neurol Psychiatry* 38:725–743.

Pickel VM, Segal M, Bloom FE (1974) A radioautographic study of the efferent pathways of the nucleus locus coeruleus. *J Comp Neurol* 155:15–42.

Pikkarainen M, Ronkko S, Savander V, Insausti R, Pitkanen A (1999) Projections from the lateral, basal, and accessory basal nuclei of the amygdala to the hippocampal formation in rat. *J Comp Neurol* 403:229–260.

Pitkanen A, Pikkarainen M, Nurminen N, Ylinen A (2000) Reciprocal connections between the amygdala and the hippocampal formation, perirhinal cortex and postrhinal cortex in the rat. *Ann NY Acad Sci* 911:369–391.

Powell TPS, Guillery RW, Cowan WM (1957) A quantitative study of the fornix-mamillo-thalamic system. *J Anat* 91:419–437.

Pyapali GK, Sik A, Penttonen M, Buzsaki G, Turner DA (1998) Dendritic properties of hippocampal CA1 pyramidal neurons in the rat: intracellular staining in vivo and in vitro. *J Comp Neurol* 391:335–352.

Raisman G, Cowan WM, Powell TPS (1965) The extrinsic afferent, commissural and association fibres of the hippocampus. *Brain* 88:963–997.

Ramón y Cajal S (1893) Estructura del asta de Ammon y fascia dentata. *Ann Soc Esp Hist Nat* 22.

Rapp PR, Gallagher M (1996) Preserved neuron number in the hippocampus of aged rats with spatial learning deficits. *Proc Natl Acad Sci USA* 93:9926–9930.

Ribak CE, Seress L (1983) Five types of basket cell in the hippocampal dentate gyrus: a combined Golgi and electron microscopic study. *J Neurocytol* 12:577–597.

Ribak CE, Vaughn JE, Saito K (1978) Immunocytochemical localization of glutamic acid decarboxylase in neuronal somata following colchicine inhibition of axonal transport. *Brain Res* 140:315–332.

Ribak CE, Seress L, Amaral DG (1985) The development, ultrastructure and synaptic connections of the mossy cells of the dentate gyrus. *J Neurocytol* 14:835–857.

Robertson RT, Kaitz SS (1981) Thalamic connections with limbic cortex. I. Thalamocortical projections. *J Comp Neurol* 195:501–525.

Sarter M, Markowitsch HJ (1985) Convergence of intra- and inter-hemispheric cortical afferents: lack of collateralization and evidence for subrhinal cell group projecting heterotopically. *J Comp Neurol* 236:283–296.

Seress L (1992) Morphological variability and developmental aspects of monkey and human granule cells: differences between the rodent and primate dentate gyrus. *Epilepsy Res Suppl* 7:3–28.

Seress L, Mrzljak L (1987) Basal dendrites of granule cells are normal features of the fetal and adult dentate gyrus of both monkey and human hippocampal formations. *Brain Res* 405:169–174.

Seress L, Pokorny J (1981) Structure of the granular layer of the rat dentate gyrus: a light microscopic and Golgi study. *J Anat* 133:181–195.

Shipley MT (1975) The topographical and laminar organization of the presubiculum's projection to the ipsi- and contralateral entorhinal cortex in the guinea pig. *J Comp Neurol* 160:127–146.

Sik A, Penttonen M, Buzsaki G (1997) Interneurons in the hippocampal dentate gyrus: an in vivo intracellular study. *Eur J Neurosci* 9:573–588.

Soriano E, Frotscher M (1989) A GABAergic axo-axonic cell in the fascia dentata controls the main excitatory hippocampal pathway. *Brain Res* 503:170–174.

Sorra KE, Harris KM (1993) Occurrence and three-dimensional structure of multiple synapses between individual radiatum axons and their target pyramidal cells in hippocampal area CA1. *J Neurosci* 13:3736–3748.

Steward O, Scoville SA (1976) Cells of origin of entorhinal cortical afferents to the hippocampus and fascia dentata of the rat. *J Comp Neurol* 169:347–370.

Struble RG, Desmond NL, Levy WB (1978) Anatomical evidence for interlamellar inhibition in the fascia dentata. *Brain Res* 152:580–585.

Suzuki WA, Amaral DG (1994) Perirhinal and parahippocampal cortices of the macaque monkey: cortical afferents. *J Comp Neurol* 350:497–533.

Swanson LW (1978a) The anatomical organization of septo-hippocampal projections. In: *Functions of the septo-hippocampal system*, pp 25–48. Amsterdam: Elsevier North Holland.

Swanson LW, Cowan, WM (1975) Hippocampo-hypothalamic connections: origin in subicular cortex, not Ammon's horn. *Science* 189:303–304.

Swanson LW, Hartman BK (1975) The central adrenergic system: an immunofluorescence study of the location of cell bodies and their efferent connections in the rat utilizing dopamine-β-hydroxylase as a marker. *J Comp Neurol* 163:467–506.

Swanson LW, Köhler C (1986) Anatomical evidence for direct projections from the entorhinal area to the entire cortical mantle in the rat. *J Neurosci* 6:3010–3023.

Swanson LW, Wyss JM, Cowan WM (1978) An autoradiographic study of the organization of intrahippocampal association pathways in the rat. *J Comp Neurol* 181:681–716.

Swanson LW, Sawchenko PE, Cowan WM (1981) Evidence for collateral projections by neurons in ammon's horn, the dentate gyrus, and the subiculum: a multiple retrograde labeling study in the rat. *J Neurosci* 1:548–559.

Swanson LW, Köhler C, Bjorklund A (1987) The limbic region. I. The septohippocampal system. In: *Handbook of chemical neuroanatomy* (Bjorklund A, Hökfelt T, Swanson LW, eds), pp 125–227. Amsterdam: Elsevier.

Tamamaki N, Nojyo Y (1993) Projection of the entorhinal layer II neurons in the rat as revealed by intracellular pressure-injection of neurobiotin. *Hippocampus* 3:471–480.

Tamamaki N, Abe K, Nojyo Y (1987) Columnar organization in the subiculum formed by axon branches originating from single CA1 pyramidal neurons in the rat hippocampus. *Brain Res* 412:156–160.

Thompson SM, Robertson RT (1987) Organization of subcortical pathways for sensory projections to the limbic cortex. I. Subcortical projections to the medial limbic cortex in the rat. *J Comp Neurol* 265:175–188.

Trommald M, Hulleberg G, Andersen P (1996) Long-term potentiation is associated with new excitatory spine synapses on rat dentata granule cells. *Learn Mem* 3:218–228.

Van der Werf YD, Witter MP, Groenewegen HJ (2002) The intralaminar and midline nuclei of the thalamus: anatomical and functional evidence for participation in processes of arousal and awareness. *Brain Res Brain Res Rev* 39:107–140.

Van Groen T, Wyss JM (1990) The connections of presubiculum and parasubiculum in the rat. *Brain Res* 518:227–243.

Van Groen T, Kadish I, Wyss JM (2002) Species differences in the projections from the entorhinal cortex to the hippocampus. *Brain Res Bull* 57:553-556.

Van Hoesen GW, Hyman BT, Damasio AR (1991) Entorhinal cortex pathology in Alzheimer's disease. *Hippocampus* 1:1–8.

Van Groen T, Miettinen P, Kadish I (2003) The entorhinal cortex of the mouse: organization of the projection to the hippocampal formation. *Hippocampus* 13:133–149.

Vertes RP (1993) PHA-L analysis of projections from the supramammillary nucleus in the rat. *J Comp Neurol* 326:595–622.

Vertes RP, Fortin WJ, Crane AM (1999) Projections of the median raphe nucleus in the rat. *J Comp Neurol* 407:555–582.

Verwer RWH, Meijer RJ, Vanuum HFM, Witter MP (1997) Collateral projections from the rat hippocampal formation to the lateral and medial prefrontal cortex. *Hippocampus* 7:397–402.

Von Economo C (1929) *The cytoarchitectonics of the human cerebral cortex.* New York: Oxford University Press.

Wainer BH, Levey AI, Rye DB, Mesulam MM, Mufson EJ (1985) Cholinergic and non-cholinergic septohippocampal pathways. *Neurosci Lett* 54:45–52.

Walker MC, Ruiz A, Kullmann DM (2002) Do mossy fibers release GABA? *Epilepsia* 43:196–202.

West MJ, Slomianka L, Gundersen HJG (1991) Unbiased stereological estimation of the total number of neurons in the subdivisions of the rat hippocampus using the optical fractionator. *Anat Rec* 231:482–497.

White TD, Tan AM, Finch DM (1990) Functional reciprocal connections of the rat entorhinal cortex and subicular complex with the medial frontal cortex: an in vivo intracellular study. *Brain Res* 533:95–106.

Wilson CO, Isokawa-Akesson M, Babb TL, Engel J Jr, Cahan L D, Crandall PH (1987) Comparative view of local and interhemispheric limbic pathways in humans: an evoked potential analysis. In: *Fundamental mechanisms of human brain function* (Engel J Jr, Ojemann GA, Lüders HO, Williamson PD, eds), pp 23–38. New York: Raven Press.

Witter MP (1993) Organization of the entorhinal-hippocampal system: a review of current anatomical data. *Hippocampus* 3: 33–44.

Witter MP, Amaral DG (2004) The hippocampal region. In: *The rat brain* (Paxinos G, ed, 3rd ed), pp 637–670. San Diego, CA, London: Elsevier Academic Press.

Witter MP, Groenewegen HJ (1990) The subiculum: cytoarchitectonically a simple structure, but hodologically complex. In: *Understanding the brain through the hippocampus* (Storm-Mathisen J, Zimmer J, Ottersen OP, eds). Amsterdam: Elsevier.

Witter MP, Griffioen AW, Jorritsma-Byham B, Krijnen JLM (1988) Entorhinal projections to the hippocampal CA1 region in the rat: an underestimated pathway. *Neurosci Lett* 85:193–198.

Witter MP, Ostendorf RH, Groenewegen HJ (1990) Heterogeneity in the dorsal subiculum of the rat: distinct neuronal zones project to different cortical and subcortical targets. *Eur J Neurosci* 2:718–725.

Witter MP, Wouterlood FG, Naber PA, van Haeften T (2000) Structural organization of the parahippocampal-hippocampal network. *Ann NY Acad Sci* 911:1–25.

Wouterlood FG, Saldana E, Witter MP (1990) Projection from the nucleus reuniens thalami to the hippocampal region: light and electron microscopic tracing study in the rat with the anterograde tracer Phaseolus vulgaris-leucoagglutinin. *J Comp Neurol* 296:179–203.

Wyss JM, Van Groen T (1992) Connections between the retrosplenial cortex and the hippocampal formation in the rat: a review. *Hippocampus* 2:1–12.

Wyss JM, Swanson LW, Cowan WM (1979) Evidence for an input to the molecular layer and the stratum granulosum of the dentate gyrus from the supramammillary region of the hypothalamus. *Anat Embryol (Berl)* 156:165–176.

Wyss JM, Swanson LW, Cowan WM (1980) The organization of the fimbria, dorsal fornix and ventral hippocampal commissure in the rat. *Anat Embryol (Berl)* 158:303–316.

4

Michael Frotscher and László Seress

Morphological Development of the Hippocampus

4.1 Overview

A fundamental question in neurobiology is how the various brain structures and the enormous number of specific interneuronal connections that serve the complex functions of the mature CNS are formed during development. Work on the hippocampal formation has shed light on the principles underlying this process. With the advent of modern genetic approaches, including mutant mice lacking or overexpressing genes important for developmental processes, new insights into the development of the hippocampal formation are in the process of being obtained.

Not all aspects of hippocampal development are covered in this chapter. Traditionally, developmental processes are studied in a descriptive manner by monitoring the formation of mature structures from simpler, undifferentiated stages. Major contributions have also come from studies of the phylogenetic development of the hippocampal formation and have demonstrated that it is a form of phylogenetically old cortex, the archicortex, that develops in the medial wall of the telencephalic vesicle. Owing to the expansion of the cerebral cortex in higher vertebrates, the hippocampal formation is translocated medially and ventrally into the inferior portion of the lateral ventricle. In rodents, the primary focus of this chapter, much of the hippocampus is located dorsally, the curved structure of the hippocampus reflecting this rotation of the telencephalon (see Chapter 3). Phylogenetic development is not dealt with in detail here, although we do present some information on species other than rodents where appropriate. For a fuller treatment of phylogenetic differences, the reader is referred to the exhaustive coverage by Stephan (Stephan, 1975).

What are the fundamental issues regarding the development of the hippocampus? As in other organs, it is important to understand the signals governing cell proliferation. Once

neurons are formed, what molecules and mechanisms determine the fate of newly generated cells? For example, postmitotic neurons migrate to their final destination. How does this happen? Upon arrival in their appropriate structure or layer, the postmigratory neuroblasts start to develop their processes. Why does only one axon originate from the cell body, whereas many dendrites emerge from it? Moreover, as these processes emerge, they do so in an organized manner. For example, in the various hippocampal fields, principal neurons display a rather uniform structure. What are the molecules and mechanisms controlling this uniform differentiation? Why do the nonprincipal cells that invade the hippocampus from the ganglionic eminence (Pleasure et al., 2000) form such a heterogeneous population of neurons? Finally, what are the determinants of synapse formation? The hippocampus is a laminated structure in which all fibers originating from a particular afferent source terminate at identical dendritic segments. How is this layer-specific termination of hippocampal afferents to be explained? To what extent is neuronal activity involved in the differentiation of dendrites, dendritic spines, and synaptic contacts?

An attempt is first made to summarize our present knowledge on neuronal generation and migration in the hippocampus. We then address the development of major hippocampal connections by describing determinants of pathfinding, target layer recognition, and synapse formation of hippocampal afferents.

4.2 Neurogenesis and Cell Migration

Most of our knowledge about cell formation in the rodent hippocampal formation dates back to the seminal studies by Angevine (1965) and Altman and coworkers (Altman, 1966; Altman and Das, 1966; Altman and Bayer, 1975; Bayer, 1980).

These important papers provided the first descriptions of the origin, the time course of the generation, and the laminar distribution of principal neurons, pyramidal neurons, and granule cells.

4.2.1 Pyramidal Neurons

Stem cells of both pyramidal neurons and granule cells originate from the ventricular germinal layers (or ventricular neuroepithelial layers) that are located below the ventricular wall along the CA1 area. In contrast to the neocortical ventricular germinal layers, there is no subventricular zone at the hippocampal germinal area. Therefore the multiplying neurons directly migrate from the ventricular zone to their final target region (Altman and Bayer, 1990b). Pyramidal neurons of the rodent hippocampus are generated between embryonic days (E) 10 and E 18 in the mouse (Angevine, 1965) and between E 16 and E 21 in the rat brain (Bayer, 1980). Pregnancy lasts 19 days in mice and 21 days in rats. CA3 pyramidal cells are generated with a peak of generation on E 17, whereas the peak of cell generation of CA1 pyramidal cells is on E 18 and E 19 (Bayer, 1980).

Except for the CA3 pyramidal cells, the route of migration is short because the hippocampus closely follows the curve of the ventricle (Fig. 4–1). Future CA1 neurons form cell rows oriented perpendicular to the ventricular area that end in the incipient CA1 pyramidal layer. From the ventricular germinal layer, the early-generated CA3 pyramidal cells migrate 3 to 4 days longer (than the CA1 cells) along the ventricular wall in the only prenatally existing intermediate zone (Altman and Bayer, 1990b). As a consequence, the later-generated CA1 pyramidal cells establish a distinct layer earlier than the CA3 cells. It remains an open question whether the pyramidal neurons in CA1 and CA3 originate from the same segment of the hippocampal neuroepithelium. A separate ori-

gin might explain their characteristic morphological differences. On E 14.5 and E 15.5, the newly formed pyramidal cells already show field-specific genetic markers characteristic for the CA1 or CA3 area of the mouse hippocampus (Tole et al., 1997).

At birth, the pyramidal layer in the rat is thick and composed of 6 to 10 rows of neuronal somata. As the hippocampus gets larger postnatally, the pyramidal layer becomes thinner; and in adult rats it comprises two or three cell layers. This process of pyramidal cell rearrangement is unlikely to be a passive one due, for example, to the volumetric increase of the hippocampal formation. Postnatally generated glial cells might contribute to the reorganization. In fact, neonatal X-ray irradiation, which has its greatest impact on glial cells, prevents formation of the mature pyramidal cell layer (Czurkó et al., 1997). However, early-generated reelin-synthesizing Cajal-Retzius cells also appear to play a role in the formation of the pyramidal cell layer (see below).

It is worth noting that the pyramidal cell layer of the hippocampus also forms quite early in the human brain. The pyramidal layer is formed during the first half of pregnancy (Arnold and Trojanowsky, 1996). In addition, the CA1 to C3 subregions of the hippocampus can be differentiated as early as during the 16th embryonic week. Regional differentiation of the hippocampal formation thus substantially precedes that of the neocortex (Kostovic et al., 1989).

4.2.2 Granule Cells

The formation of the granule cell layer of the dentate gyrus differs in many respects from that of the pyramidal cell layer of the hippocampus. The first granule cells of the mouse dentate gyrus appear at approximately the same time as the first pyramidal cells (i.e., on E 10) (Angevine, 1965). There is a suprapyramidal to infrapyramidal, or medial to lateral, gradient in the formation of the two blades of the granule cell layer; that is, granule cells at the tip of the suprapyramidal blade are the first to be generated. The generation of granule cells lasts a much longer time than that of pyramidal neurons. There is substantial evidence that it continues long into the postnatal period and, at a reduced level, into adulthood. In the rat dentate gyrus, first granule cells are generated 1 day later than the first pyramidal neurons (i.e., on E 17) (Bayer, 1980). In rats, 15% of the granule cells are generated before birth (Altman and Bayer, 1975). Therefore, the time span of granule cell generation is approximately three times longer than that of pyramidal neurons and is likely to continue for the rest of the animal's life (for adult neurogenesis, see Chapter 9). Interestingly, adult granule cell formation does not follow the suprapyramidal to infrapyramidal sequence observed during the embryonic and early postnatal period. Granule cells are generated with no obvious pattern in both blades (Kempermann et al., 1997a,b).

The prolonged postnatal formation of granule cells is not a unique feature of rodents. In humans, granule cell formation lasts more than 30 weeks, beginning at approximately the 13th

Figure 4–1. Route of migration (arrows) of pyramidal cells from the ventricular germinative layer to the subiculum and to areas CA1 to CA3. DG, dentate gyrus; H, hilus.

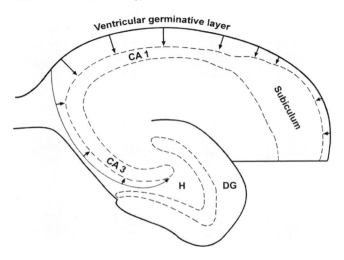

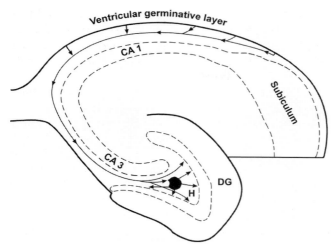

Figure 4–2. Route of migration of dentate granule cells. There are two possible ways for granule cells to reach the suprapyramidal or infrapyramidal blade of the dentate gyrus. 1, Granule cells formed in the germinative layer move along the pyramidal layer of Ammon's horn directly to the granule cell layer (arrows); 2, after migration from the ventricular germinative layer, stem cells form a secondary germinative layer (black spot) in the hilus (H) and, following further proliferation, move to the granule cell layer (arrows) of the dentate gyrus (DG). During the embryonic period both routes are used, whereas the latter route prevails during the postnatal period.

embryonic week (Humphrey, 1967; Seress et al., 2001). There is also evidence for adult neurogenesis in the human dentate gyrus (Eriksson et al., 1998).

The route of migration of the postmitotic granule cells is much longer than that of pyramidal neurons. Postmitotic cells must migrate from the ventricular germinal layer along the already formed hippocampus through the narrow intermediate zone between the alveus and future stratum oriens toward the hippocampus, where they form the cup-shaped dentate gyrus that surrounds the tip of CA3 (Fig. 4–2).

The two blades of dentate granule cells and the tip of the CA3 area border the hilus of the dentate gyrus (see Chapter 3). During postnatal ontogenesis, the hilus (Fig. 4–3A, see color insert) contains large numbers of mitotic cells (Bayer, 1980). Large hilar neurons, such as the mossy cells, are generated between E 15 and E 21 (Bayer, 1980). In addition, virtually all hilar interneurons, representing approximately half of the hilar cells (Seress and Ribak, 1983), are of subcortical origin and invade the hilus from the lateral and medial ganglionic eminence (Pleasure et al., 2000). Thus, the enduring cell proliferation in the hilar region (Fig. 4–2) mainly represents local generation of granule cells (Altman and Bayer, 1990c). In fact, the rate of postnatal cell formation in the hilus is similar to that in the periventricular germinal layer of the telencephalon (Seress, 1978). It is therefore reasonable to assume that the hilar region is a "displaced" secondary germinal layer of the dentate gyrus (Altman and Bayer, 1975; Seress, 1977). Proliferating cells persist in the hilar region during the entire

period of granule cell neurogenesis, and persisting hilar stem cells may also form new neurons during adulthood (Altman and Bayer, 1975, 1990a; Seress, 1978). In rodents, the total number of hilar cells rapidly decreases between postnatal days 10 and 25, with a parallel increase in the number of granule cells in the granule cell layer, suggesting that newly formed cells from the hilus move to the granule cell layer (Seress, 1977). During the entire period of postnatal development, labeled granule cells are always observed inside the granule cell layer as early as 1 hour following the injection of bromodeoxyuridine (BrdU) or thymidine (Fig. 4–3, see color insert). It is likely that stem cells from the hippocampal ventricular zone move to the hilar region and form a secondary germinal zone (Fig. 4–2). This possibility is supported by the fact that a single neonatal X-ray irradiation prevents further cell formation in both the ventricular zone and hilus without affecting the already formed neuronal subpopulations (Czurko et al., 1997).

To the extent that it has been studied, the developmental characteristics of the rodent hilar region are also observed in humans. In human fetuses, a large number of mitotic cells (indicated by the presence of Ki-67) are present in the hilar region from the 13th week onward (Fig. 4–4A, see color insert). These proliferating cells account for a large percentage of the total hilar cell population in 16- to 18-week-old fetuses (Seress, unpublished observations). Proliferating cells can also be found in the hilus during the late gestational period and after birth (Seress et al., 2001) (Fig. 4–4B, see color insert). Persisting stem cells have also been found in the hilus of the adult human hippocampal formation (Eriksson et al., 1998). However, proliferative activity drops off considerably during the postnatal period (Seress et al., 2001).

There is little morphological variability among granule cells even though they may be located at different places in the granule cell layer and may be born at different time points. This morphological uniformity leads one to assume that all granule cells originate from the same stem cell population. However, granule cells may originate from different germinal sources (Altman and Bayer, 1990a), and precursors of the perinatally and postnatally forming granule cells can be distinguished (Altman and Bayer, 1990c). A newly discovered gene (*Lef1*) has been found to distinguish granule cell precursors. This gene is expressed in the proliferating precursors of granule cells in the ventricular zone as well as in those of the secondary germinal zone. *Lef1*-deficient mice fail to form dentate granule cells (Galceran et al., 2000).

Most of the granule cells display similar features in the rodent and primate dentate gyrus. However, a subpopulation of granule cells in the primate dentate gyrus is characterized by the formation of basal dendrites (Seress and Mrzljak, 1987). It is likely that local environmental factors, such as available space for dendritic expansion, may play an important role in the formation of basal dendrites on granule cells (Seress and Frotscher, 1990). Basal dendrites have also been regarded as a pathological phenomenon. For example, increased activity of the granule cells may evoke the formation of basal dendrites in epileptic rats (Spigelman et al., 1998).

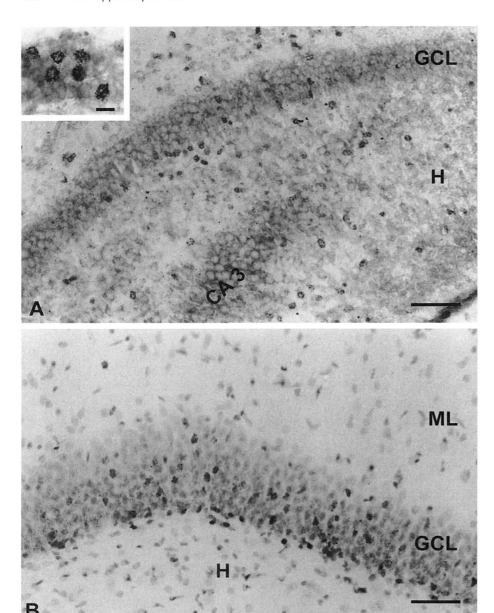

Figure 4–3. *A.* Photomicrograph showing ³H-thymidine-labeled cells (black) in the hilus (H) and granule cell layer (GCL) of the dentate gyrus of a 5-day-old rat that received a single injection of thymidine 1 hour before sacrifice. At this age, the infrapyramidal blade is still very short and hardly reaches the tip of the CA3 pyramidal layer. The large number of labeled cells above the granule cell layer suggests that glial cells are also formed at this age because the molecular layer contains only a few interneurons, which are born prenatally. Note the lack of labeling in the CA3 area of Ammon's horn where pyramidal cells are generated prenatally. *Inset.* Labeled cells in the granule cell layer of this animal at higher magnification. Section is 10 μm thick and stained with toluidine blue. *B.* BrdU-labeled cells (brown) in the suprapyramidal blade of the dentate gyrus of a 3-month-old rat that received daily injections of BrdU from P4 to P6. Bars: *A, B,* 50 μm; *inset,* 10 μm.

Epileptic seizures also appear to lead to an increased number of granule cells with basal dendrites in the human dentate gyrus (von Campe et al., 1997).

In summary, dentate granule cells in different mammalian species form a largely homogeneous neuronal population. Their dendritic morphology, however, may be modified to some extent depending on the local environmental or pathological factors.

4.2.3 Local Circuit Neurons and Hilar Neurons

Local circuit neurons of the hippocampal formation differ from the principal cells in both their morphological and developmental features. In contrast to the morphologically uniform granule cells and pyramidal neurons, local circuit neurons of the hippocampal formation form a heterogeneous population (Freund and Buzsáki, 1996) (see Chapters 3 and 8). Even the classic basket cell can be subdivided into five types based on differences in location and dendritic arborization (Ribak and Seress, 1983). Neurochemical studies have confirmed the existence of at least two basket cell types, which display different receptors and co-transmitters (Hájos et al., 1998; Katona et al., 1999). In addition to dendritic morphology, differences in axonal projections also distinguish subpopulations of local circuit neurons in both the dentate gyrus (Halasy and Somogyi, 1993a,b) and the hippocampus proper (Soriano and Frotscher, 1989, 1993; Halasy et al., 1996; Spruston et al., 1997; Vida et al., 1998; Vida and Frotscher, 2000).

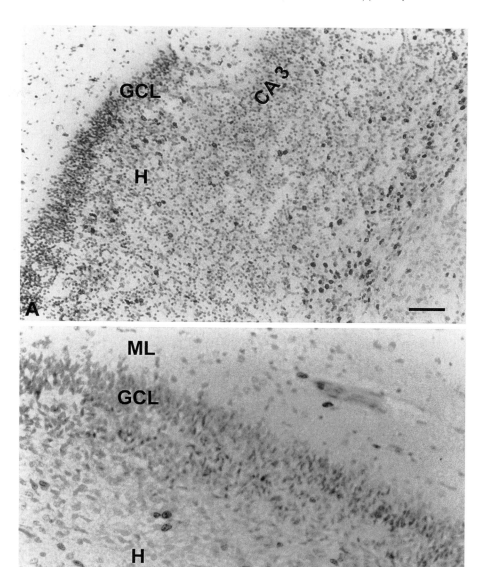

Figure 4–4. *A*. MIB-1 (Ki-67)-labeled cells (brown) in the dentate gyrus of a 16-week-old human fetus. A large number of labeled cells are seen in the hilus (H) underneath the granule cell layer (GCL). Note the absence of labeled cells in the CA3 area of Ammon's horn. In contrast, numerous labeled cells, migrating from the ventricular germinative layer along the pyramidal layer toward the hilus, are seen in the intermediate zone. *B*. MIB-1 (Ki-67)-labeled cells are still frequent in the hilus (H) of a 28-week-old fetus. The granule cell layer and molecular layer (ML) contain only a few labeled cells. Sections are 10 μm thick and are stained with cresyl violet. Bars: *A*, 50 μm; *B*, 20 μm.

In contrast to the heterogeneity of the local circuit neuron phenotype, their neurogenetic profile seems much more homogeneous; that is, there are no developmental events that would allow one to predict the large diversity among γ-aminobutyric acid (GABA)ergic cells. GABAergic interneurons are generated early in both the dentate gyrus and the hippocampus (Bayer, 1980). This conclusion was based on the observation that neurons in the molecular layer and hilus of the dentate gyrus as well as in the strata oriens, radiatum, and lacunosum-moleculare appear earlier than the neurons in the principal cell layers (Bayer, 1980). The peak cell formation in both the hilus and the molecular layer precedes the onset of granule cell generation. Similarly, in the CA1 to C3 areas, the peak cell generation in the strata oriens and radiatum pre-

cedes formation of the first pyramidal cells by 1 day (Bayer, 1980). Cell formation of the cells destined to reside in the dendritic layers ceases relatively early. It is reasonable to suggest that this exquisite timing may play some role in pyramidal and granule cell morphogenesis, although there is no evidence for this at this time.

Double-labeling studies have confirmed that GABAergic neurons are generated earlier than the principal cells of the hippocampal formation (Amaral and Kurz, 1985; Lübbers et al., 1985; Soriano et al., 1989a,b; Dupuy and Houser, 1997, 1999). The site of origin of hippocampal local circuit neurons is in the ventricular/subventricular zone of the medial and lateral ganglionic eminence. Available data do not allow one to correlate the site of generation with the diverse morphological features of the local circuit neurons (Pleasure et al., 2000).

Although GABAergic neurons are generated and positioned before their target cells, some of them change their position later on in development (Dupuy and Houser, 1999). Moreover, the differentiation of axonal collaterals and the arborization of dendrites takes place relatively late in postnatal life (Seress et al., 1989; Lang and Frotscher, 1990; Seress and Ribak, 1990). This raises the possibility that the maturation of local circuit neurons is influenced by interactions with their synaptic partners.

4.2.4 Determinants of Neuronal Migration in the Hippocampus

In the neocortex, cell layers are formed in an inside-out manner; that is, early-generated neurons form deep layers, whereas superficial layers are established by cells born late in ontogenetic development. As in the neocortex, the hippocampus follows a similar inside-out migration. The dentate gyrus, in contrast, has an outside-in migration pattern; that is, early-generated granule cells populate superficial portions of the granule cell layer and later-formed granule cells are located progressively deeper.

What are the signals controlling neuronal migration that lead to such well defined cell layers of principal neurons? It has been known for some time that these migrational processes are under fairly strict genetic control. In 1951, a mouse mutant, the reeler mouse, was described (Falconer, 1951) in which neocortical lamination was reversed. Recently, the gene missing in reeler mice was discovered (d'Arcangelo et al., 1995; Hirotsune et al., 1995). The gene product, reelin, was found to be synthesized by a well known group of neurons in the marginal zone, originally described by Cajal and Retzius more than 100 years ago (Retzius, 1893, 1894; Ramón y Cajal, 1911). These Cajal-Retzius cells are remarkable neurons. They extend long dendrites horizontally in the marginal zone, parallel to the pial surface. Cajal-Retzius cells synthesize and secrete reelin, so it forms a component of the extracellular matrix in the marginal zone (d'Arcangelo et al., 1997).

Available data are compatible with the proposal that reelin acts as a stop signal for migrating neurons. Early-generated neurons are stopped as they approach the marginal zone, which has a high concentration of reelin. For later neurons to reach this same stop signal, they must migrate past the early-generated neurons and approach the reelin-containing marginal zone. In this way the characteristic inside-out lamination of the cortex is formed (Frotscher, 1997, 1998). Because the marginal zone ultimately becomes layer I of the cortex, it remains an almost cell-free layer in normally developing mice. In reeler mice, in contrast, layer I (which does not have the stop signal) is densely filled with neurons. Early-generated neurons migrate until they reach the pial surface, and later-generated neurons accumulate underneath. The normal inside-out lamination is reversed (Fig. 4–5).

Although this scenario is certainly an oversimplification, it can be employed to explain the unusual lamination in the reeler hippocampus and dentate gyrus. In the hippocampus, a double pyramidal cell layer is formed in reeler mice. As in the neocortex, the marginal zone is located directly underneath the pial surface, which in the hippocampus proper corresponds to the stratum lacunosum-moleculare. The stratum lacunosum-moleculare contains Cajal-Retzius cells, and its extracellular matrix is enriched in reelin. The absence of the stop signal reelin in reeler mutants may allow some pyramidal cells to migrate deep into the stratum radiatum, forming there a second pyramidal layer (Stanfield and Cowan, 1979; Deller et al., 1999b).

The marginal zone of the dentate gyrus corresponds to the outer portion of the molecular layer. Assuming that reelin acts as a stop signal, one would expect that many granule cells would invade the molecular layer in reeler mice because they would not be stopped earlier. However, in the reeler dentate gyrus, the granule cells do not invade the molecular layer, whereas many granule cells are found in the hilar region with their dendrites oriented in all directions (Stanfield and Cowan, 1979; Drakew et al., 2002). What might be the explanation of the hilar location of the granule cells? Förster et al. (2002) found that the radial glial fibers required for neuronal migration are dramatically altered in the dentate gyrus of reeler mice. Thus, it has been proposed that the granule cell migration defect seen in the reeler mutant is due to a malformation of the radial glial scaffold required for proper neuronal migration (Förster et al., 2002; Frotscher et al., 2003; Zhao et al., 2004).

4.3 Development of Hippocampal Connections

When describing the development of neuronal connections, it is useful to distinguish at least three processes. First, there is the way an axon navigates to the target region, called axonal pathfinding. During this process, both soluble and membrane-bound molecules and attractant and repellent signals are involved (see Tessier-Lavigne and Goodman, 1996, for review). Next, the axon must recognize the appropriate target region and target cell, called target recognition. As far as the hippocampus is concerned, the segregated fiber systems must recognize their appropriate layers. Finally, there is the process of synapse formation.

There is substantial and increasing evidence that a variety of molecules are involved in these three processes. In principle, membrane-bound molecules that attract or repel the growing tip of an axon, diffusible factors building up a gradient, and components of the extracellular matrix are likely to play a role. The involvement of various ligand/receptor families in the formation of hippocampal connections has been summarized by Skutella and Nitsch (2001). Thus, the various

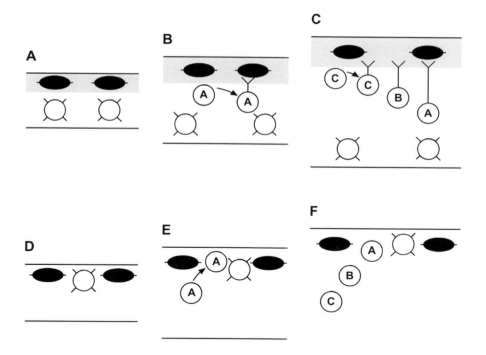

Figure 4–5. Hypothetical function of reelin in cortical lamination. *A.* In wild-type mice, the preplate splits into the marginal zone, largely containing Cajal-Retzius cells (black cells), and the subplate (white cells). Cajal-Retzius cells synthesize and secrete reelin (stippled zone). *B.* The cortical plate develops between the marginal zone and the subplate. An early-generated cell (A) migrates from the ventricular zone toward the marginal zone, where its migration is stopped by reelin. *C.* With increasing cortical thickness, the reelin-containing marginal zone is moved further outward, allowing later-generated neurons (B, C) to migrate farther than their predecessors before their migration is stopped by reelin. This way the characteristic inside-out pattern of cortical lamination is formed. Apical dendrites, branching in the reelin-containing marginal zone, are extended by the increase in cortical thickness. *D.* In reeler mice lacking reelin, the separation of the subplate from the marginal zone does not take place. *E.* In the absence of reelin, migrating cells (A) are not stopped and reach the pial surface. *F.* Later-generated neurons (B, C) accumulate underneath the early-generated neurons (A). As a result, the normal inside-out pattern of cortical lamination is reversed, and apical dendrites are not anchored in the marginal zone. (*Source*: Frotscher, 1997.)

semaphorins and their receptors neuropilin 1 and 2 and the plexins netrin 1 and its receptor DCC (deleted in colon cancer), the ephrin (Eph) family of tyrosine kinases and their ligands, the ephrins, and Slit and Robo were found to contribute to establishment of the hippocampal circuitry.

In the following paragraphs, we deal with the development of some of the main hippocampal afferent connections: those from the entorhinal cortex, the septum, and the contralateral hippocampus. Whereas the fibers from both the entorhinal cortex and the contralateral hippocampus are examples of a strictly laminated termination of hippocampal afferents, fibers from the septum have a more diffuse distribution.

4.3.1 Entorhinal Connections

Neuroanatomists have been intrigued by the unique course of the entorhino-hippocampal projection, which perforates the subiculum and hippocampal fissure en route to the dentate gyrus. From a developmental point of view, one would expect that the perforant path would utilize robust guidance signals for axonal pathfinding and target layer recognition. The entorhinal fibers terminating in the outer two-thirds of the dentate molecular layer and in stratum lacunosum-moleculare of the hippocampus proper form a sharp boundary toward the adjacent commissural/associational fibers in the inner molecular layer of the dentate gyrus and in the stratum radiatum of the hippocampus (see Chapter 3).

Recent studies have shed some light on the mechanisms underlying the pathfinding of entorhinal axons (del Rio et al., 1997; Chedotal et al., 1998; Förster et al., 1998; Frotscher, 1998; Ceranik et al., 1999; Deller et al., 1999a,b; Savaskan et al., 1999; Skutella et al., 1999; Steup et al., 1999). Investigators have focused on repulsive molecules expressed in the hippocampus that would prevent the entorhinal afferents from terminating in proximal layers close to the cell bodies of principal neurons. Similarly, molecules specifically expressed in the entorhinal cortex were studied for their capacity to repel entorhinal axons, thereby directing them toward the hippocampus. In particular, repulsive effects of semaphorins (Sema3A) on entorhinal fibers have been observed (Steup et al., 1999), an effect that can be blocked by antibodies against the semaphorin receptor neuropilin 1 (Chedotal et al., 1998). As Sema3A is expressed by granule cells, it has been speculated that this expression may be involved in the termination of entorhinal fibers on distal granule cell dendrites. Neuropilin 2, the receptor for Sema3F, is strongly expressed in the hippocampus, whereas the ligand is expressed in the developing entorhinal cortex. As Sema3F is repulsive for growing axons bearing its receptor, this particular pattern may be responsible for the lack of ingrowth of hippocampal and dentate axons into the entorhinal cortex (Chedotal et al., 1998; Steup et al., 1999; Skutella and Nitsch, 2001). Similarly, Slit 1 and Slit 2, being expressed in the entorhinal cortex, can repel axons of hippocampal neurons expressing their receptors Robo 1 and Robo 2 (Nguyen-Ba-Charvet et al., 1999). Also ephrins were found to be involved in repulsive effects on entorhinal axons, restricting their termination to distal dendritic portions of hippocampal neurons (Stein et al., 1999). In addition to these repulsive effects, neurotrophic factors with an attractive *neurotropic* effect, components of the extracellular matrix, and a guiding scaffold provided by pioneer neurons have been found to navigate the axons of entorhinal neurons to their hippocampal target structures.

What could be the sequence of events underlying this complex process? Probably as a first step, a guiding scaffold supporting the directed growth of entorhinal axons toward the hippocampus is formed. In fact, Ceranik et al. (1999) have shown that early-generated Cajal-Retzius cells, located in the marginal zones of the dentate gyrus (outer molecular layer) and hippocampus proper (stratum lacunosum-moleculare), give rise to a heavy projection to the entorhinal cortex that is established before the entorhino-hippocampal projection. Thus, Cajal-Retzius cells in the outer molecular layer of the rat dentate gyrus are retrogradely labeled from the entorhinal cortex as early as on E 17, whereas the first entorhino-hippocampal fibers were found to arrive in the dentate outer molecular layer only thereafter. Moreover, with combined injections of two tracers, DiI and DiO, into the entorhinal cortex and hippocampus, respectively, entorhinal axons were found to grow along axons of Cajal-Retzius cells. These findings suggest that the early-formed projection of hippocampal Cajal-Retzius cells to the entorhinal cortex provides a template for outgrowing entorhinal axons Fig. 4–6A(C). A role of Cajal-Retzius cells in the pathfinding of entorhinal axons is strongly supported by experiments in slice cultures, in which Cajal-Retzius cells had been caused to degenerate by excitotoxic lesions (del Rio et al., 1997). In the absence of Cajal-Retzius cells, entorhinal axons were unable to find their way to the hippocampus, whereas commissural fibers invaded their termination fields as normal.

Because the entorhino-hippocampal projection develops almost normally in reeler mice, it does not appear that reelin synthesized by Cajal-Retzius cells is essential to this process. In

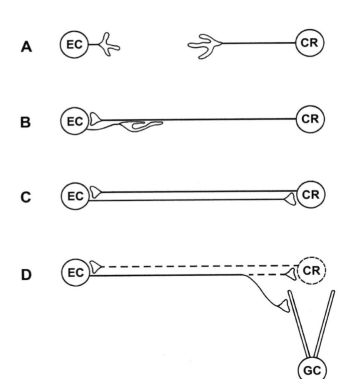

Figure 4–6. *A–C.* Early-generated hippocampal Cajal-Retzius (CR) cells form a template for outgrowing axons of projection neurons in the entorhinal cortex (EC). *D.* Later on in development when many CR cells have disappeared, the axons of projection cells in the entorhinal cortex establish definitive connections with distal dendrites of dentate granule cells (GC).

fact, Cajal-Retzius cells and their projections to the entorhinal cortex are also present in these mutants and may thus serve their normal function as a template for entorhinal axons. In normal mice, reelin affects the branching pattern of entorhinal terminals. In the absence of reelin, entorhinal axons give rise to fewer collaterals and synapses (del Rio et al., 1997; Borrell et al., 1999). The growth of entorhinal fibers along Cajal-Retzius cell axons is likely to be controlled by a variety of repulsive and attractive molecules (see above).

How do the entorhinal fibers recognize their target layer? Current evidence strongly suggests that components of the extracellular matrix play an important part in the segregation of hippocampal afferents. Förster et al. (1998), for example, demonstrated that fluorescent beads coated with entorhinal membranes precisely adhered to the correct entorhinal termination zone of the hippocampus. They then used this pattern as an assay to study the role of extracellular matrix components in this layer-specific adhesion. When slice cultures of hippocampus were treated with hyaluronidase, the membrane-coated beads no longer adhered with layer specificity, indicating that hyaluronic acid and proteoglycans bound to it may contribute to the layer-specific adhesion. Such adhesion seems also to be an important factor for target layer recognition of entorhinal fibers. When hippocampal slices were treated with hyaluronidase and then cocultured with entorhinal cortex, entorhinal fibers invaded the molecular layer but were no longer restricted to its outer two-thirds (Förster et al., 2001). It appears that hyaluronic acid and proteoglycans are essential for the formation of boundaries between afferent terminal zones in the hippocampus. Interestingly enough, no similar role of extracellular matrix components was found for the laminar specificity of commissural/associational fibers (Zhao et al., 2003). In conclusion, secreted molecules such as the semaphorins, membrane-bound receptors, extracellular matrix components, and a template formed by Cajal-Retzius cell axons are likely to be involved in the directed growth and layer-specific termination of entorhinal fibers.

What is the role of the postsynaptic target cell in the layer-specific termination of entorhinal afferents? In the rodent brain, entorhinal axons innervate the hippocampus proper at E 15 and the dentate gyrus at E 18/E 19 (Super and Soriano, 1994; Ceranik et al., 1999). The entorhinal fibers arrive much earlier than the commissural fibers from the contralateral hippocampus (see below). At this early stage, pyramidal neurons and granule cells have not yet grown their distal dendritic tips to the stratum lacunosum-moleculare and the outer molecular layer of the dentate gyrus. Most of the granule cells have not even been generated yet. Interestingly, the entorhinal fibers recognize their appropriate target layers from the very beginning despite the absence of their appropriate target dendrites at the stage of fiber ingrowth. Evidently, the target cells are unlikely to be involved in pathfinding of entorhinal axons and target layer recognition. The early-generated Cajal-Retzius cells, located in the termination zones of entorhinal fibers, may serve as primary targets. In fact, entorhinal fibers were found to establish synaptic contacts with cell bodies and dendrites of Cajal-Retzius cells (del Rio et al., 1997; Frotscher et al., 2001). A role of Cajal-Retzius cells as primary target neurons of entorhinal fibers is supported by X-irradiation experiments. Irradiation of newborn rats, which eliminates most of the postnatally generated granule cells but not the early-born Cajal-Retzius cells, does not alter the layer-specific termination of entorhinal fibers (Laurberg and Hjorth-Simonsen, 1977; Frotscher et al., 2001). Conversely, ablation of Cajal-Retzius cells prevented layer-specific ingrowth (del Rio et al., 1997).

Many Cajal-Retzius cells degenerate later during postnatal development (i.e., after the entorhino-hippocampal projection has been formed and pyramidal cells and granule cells have grown their distal dendrites into the entorhinal termination fields). At that time, the contacts of entorhinal fibers are reorganized, and definitive synapses with distal dendritic portions of pyramidal cells and granule cells are made (Fig. 4–6D). Although pathfinding and target recognition are not affected by the absence of neuronal activity, there is an effect on the maturation of synaptic structures. Drakew and colleagues (Drakew et al., 1999; Frotscher et al., 2000b) observed normal formation of the entorhino-hippocampal projection in cocultures of entorhinal cortex and hippocampus incubated in the presence of tetrodotoxin (TTX), which blocks fast sodium channels. However, they observed an increased num-

ber of long, immature spines, indicating that neuronal activity may be required for the maturation of spines.

Many questions concerning the layer-specific termination of entorhinal fibers remain open at present. As an example, the development of the fiber lamination in the infrapyramidal blade of the dentate gyrus is different from that in the suprapyramidal blade. Whereas the entorhinal fibers arrive before the commissural axons in the suprapyramidal blade, this sequence is reversed in the infrapyramidal blade (Tamamaki, 1999). Do the fibers to these different blades originate from the same cells of origin in the entorhinal cortex? If so, what causes the delay in the ingrowth into the infrapyramidal blade?

4.3.2 Commissural Connections

Commissural fibers, originating from CA3 pyramidal neurons and hilar mossy cells, project via the hippocampal commissure to the contralateral hippocampus and dentate gyrus. In the mouse hippocampus, the first commissural axons arrive in the contralateral hippocampus at E 18 and in the dentate gyrus at P 2. This is considerably later than the arrival of the entorhinal axons. The sequential generation of the entorhinal neurons and commissurally projecting hippocampal cells and their sequential ingrowth into their target fields has led to a hypothesis concerning their laminated termination in both the hippocampus proper and the dentate gyrus: The later the fibers invade their target zones, the more proximally do they terminate on their target cell dendrites (Bayer and Altman, 1987). Entorhinal axons, arriving early in development, contact distal dendrites of pyramidal cells and granule cells, whereas later-arriving commissural fibers establish synapses in the stratum radiatum of the hippocampus proper and in the inner molecular layer of the dentate gyrus. One of the last projections to be formed, the ipsilateral mossy fiber projection, accordingly terminates on the most proximal dendritic segments of CA3 pyramidal neurons.

This hypothesis is not easy to test in vivo. However, it can be addressed in slice culture experiments in which the time of arrival of growing axons can be brought under precise experimental control. Frotscher and Heimrich (1993) cocultured a hippocampal target culture first with an entorhinal culture and then with a second hippocampal culture, thus imitating the normal developmental sequence in this sequential culture system. They then traced the entorhinal and "commissural" connections to the hippocampal target culture and observed, as one would expect, that the entorhinal fibers terminated on the distal dendritic segments of their target neurons, as normal. Next, they reversed this sequence: First, the two hippocampal cultures were cocultivated; then, with a delay of a couple of days, an entorhinal slice culture was added. Despite the reversal of the sequence of fiber ingrowth, the commissural and entorhinal fibers still terminated in their appropriate layers, indicating that the sequence of fiber arrival in the target region is not responsible for the laminated, proximodistal termination of these two afferents.

As the time of arrival is not the factor governing lamination, the question arises as to potential cellular and molecular factors determining the layer specificity of commissural fibers. Soriano and colleagues (Super et al., 1998) have suggested that there are pioneer neurons, early-generated GABAergic cells, that serve as primary targets for the commissural fibers. Their role is comparable to that of the Cajal-Retzius cells as primary targets of the entorhinal afferents. This idea became testable with the possibility of depleting the hippocampus of GABAergic neurons during development (Pleasure et al., 2000). Contrary to Soriano's idea, commissural fibers still innervated their proper target areas in the absence of GABAergic neurons.

As the commissural fibers arrive relatively late in the hippocampus and dentate gyrus, an alternative proposal was that pioneer neurons are not required. This is because the target cells, the principal neurons, are already present at that time and have already grown a dendritic arbor (Deller et al., 1999a). Evidence relevant to this idea has come from studies in reeler mice. In this mutant, the granule cells are loosely distributed throughout the hilar region (Stanfield and Cowan, 1979; Deller et al., 1999a; Drakew et al., 2002) and the commissural fibers do not form a compact layer but are, instead, distributed all over the hilar region (Deller et al., 1999a). This target-dependent termination of commissural fibers is nicely seen when commissural axons from a wild-type culture are traced to both a second wild-type culture and a reeler culture: Whereas the commissural axons terminating in the wild-type culture form their normal compact projection to the inner molecular layer of the dentate, the commissural fibers that innervate the reeler culture terminate diffusely, corresponding to the scattered distribution of their target granule cells (Fig. 4–7, see color insert). This is in striking contrast to the entorhino-dentate projection, which forms a compact termination zone with sharp borders in the outer molecular layer of the reeler mutant (Deller et al., 1999a); moreover, this characteristic layer-specific projection is nicely preserved in slice cultures from wild-type animals and reeler mutants (Zhao et al., 2003) (Fig. 4–8, see color insert). Together, these findings support the hypothesis that entorhinal fibers, because of their early arrival in the dentate gyrus at a time when their definitive target cells, the granule cells, have not yet been generated, do require pioneer target neurons. These neurons are likely to be the Cajal-Retzius cells, which are, as normal, located in the outer molecular layer of reeler mice (see above). One is tempted to speculate that whereas the entorhinal fibers require pioneer neurons the commissural afferents establish contacts directly with principal cell dendrites, which is reflected in reeler mice by the irregular, loose distribution of both commissural fibers and granule cells (Fig. 4–9). In fact, when commissural fibers from a reeler culture are traced to a wild-type culture, they are found to form a normal, compact projection to the inner molecular layer, precluding a cell-autonomous effect of the reeler mutation on commissural neurons (Zhao et al., 2003).

Little is known about the molecules involved in pathfinding and target recognition of commissural fibers. As with other commissures, Netrin 1 and its receptor DCC are important for formation of the hippocampal commissure. Thus, a hippocampal commissure does not form in Netrin 1-deficient animals. Along this line, neurites of hippocampal neurons are attracted by Netrin 1 in the stripe choice assay (Steup et al., 2000). The molecules governing the laminar specificity of the commissural fibers in their target zones remain to be determined.

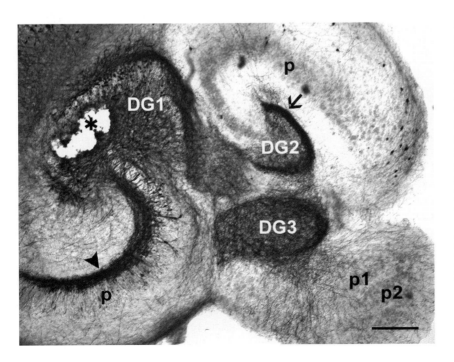

Figure 4–7. Triplet cocultures of two wild-type slices of hippocampus together with a reeler hippocampal slice. The biocytin injection site into the dentate gyrus of one of the wild-type cultures (DG1) is marked with an asterisk. Labeled commissural fibers invade the two other cultures, but only in the dentate gyrus of the second wild-type culture (DG2) do they show their characteristic compact termination in the inner molecular layer (arrow). In the reeler hippocampal culture, the commissural fibers arising from the same cells of origin have lost their laminar specificity and terminate throughout the hilar region of the dentate gyrus (DG3). Arrowhead points to the mossy fiber projection in the wild-type culture that was also labeled by the tracer injection into the hilus. p, pyramidal layer; p1, p2 two pyramidal layers in the reeler culture. Bar = 100 μm. (*Source*: Zhao et al., 2003, © 2003 by the Society for Neuroscience.)

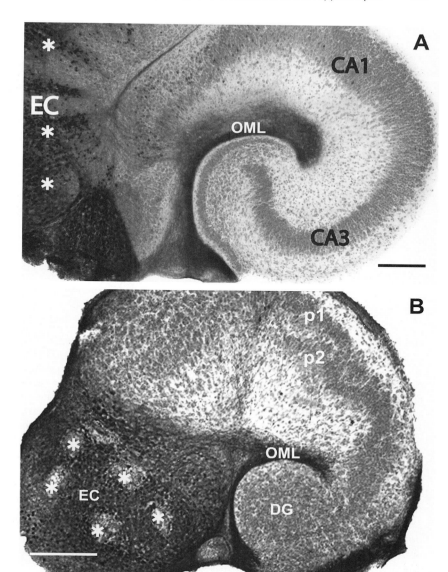

Figure 4–8. *A.* Entorhino-hippocampal projection in a complex culture of entorhinal cortex (EC) and hippocampus. Biocytin injection sites are labeled by asterisks. Note the layer-specific termination of the entorhinal fibers in the outer molecular layer (OML) of the dentate gyrus. *B.* In a slice culture of reeler hippocampus and entorhinal cortex, entorhinal fibers labeled by biocytin injection into the entorhinal cortex (asterisks) form a sharply segregated projection to the outer portion of the molecular layer of the dentate gyrus (DG) despite the malpositioned granule cells, demonstrating that the trajectory of entorhinal fibers is not influenced by the position of their target neurons. p1, p2, two pyramidal layers in the reeler hippocampus. Bar = 100 μm. (*Source*: Zhao et al., 2003; © 2003 by the Society for Neuroscience.)

4.3.3 Septal Connections

The septohippocampal projection consists of two parts: a cholinergic one and a GABAergic one. The cells of origin for both parts are located in the medial septal nucleus/diagonal band complex (MSDB) (see Chapter 3). The development of the septohippocampal projection can be understood only by taking into account the hippocampo-septal projection. The latter develops relatively early and surprisingly terminates in the medial septum during development as early as on E 15. In adults, hippocampo-septal fibers project to the lateral septum (Linke and Frotscher, 1993; Super and Soriano, 1994; Linke et al., 1995). This early termination in the medial septal nucleus has led to the hypothesis that the early formed hippocampo-septal projection serves as a template by which septohip-

pocampal fibers can find their way to the hippocampus. It has in fact been shown that growth cones of septohippocampal fibers grow along hippocampo-septal axons (Linke and Frotscher, 1993). The molecular mechanisms underlying the change of hippocampo-septal fibers from the medial to the lateral septum remain to be elucidated.

Unlike the entorhino-hippocampal and commissural projections to the hippocampus, septohippocampal cholinergic fibers do not terminate in clearly demarcated layers. They are found in all layers of the hippocampal formation but are certainly more concentrated in the cell body layers. In contrast, the septohippocampal GABAergic projection cells display a high target cell specificity terminating almost exclusively on GABAergic interneurons in the hippocampus. Inhibitory neurons afferent to inhibitory neurons serve a disinhibitory role

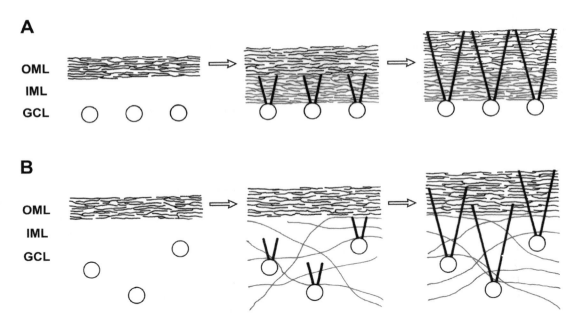

Figure 4–9. Different signals control the laminar specificity of entorhinal fibers (black) and commissural fibers (gray) to the dentate gyrus. *A.* In wild-type mice, entorhinal fibers, guided by Cajal-Retzius cell axons, reach the outer molecular layer (OML) of the dentate gyrus before the granule cells in the granule cell layer (GCL) have grown their distal dendritic tips to the OML. Molecules of the extracellular matrix control the laminar specificity of entorhinal axons. In contrast, later-arriving commissural fibers, terminating in the inner molecular layer (IML), meet the outgrowing granule cell dendrites. *B.* Findings in the reeler mutant, where the granule cells are not aligned but scattered over the dentate gyrus, confirm that the entorhinal axons are not guided by their target granule cells. As for the wild-type fibers, entorhinal fibers terminate with laminar specificity in the OML. In contrast, commissural fibers are loosely distributed over the dentate gyrus, thus following their scattered target cells. (*Source*: Adapted from Frotscher, 1998).

with respect to the principal neurons (Freund and Antal, 1988). The septal cholinergic fibers establish contacts with both principal neurons and interneurons, and their contacts are on cell bodies, dendritic shafts, and spines. Two types of contact are established: symmetrical and asymmetrical (Frotscher and Leranth, 1985, 1986). It remains to be established whether one of these types derives from the few intrahippocampal cholinergic cells (Frotscher et al., 1986, 2000a) that are found in the rat hippocampus but not in the monkey hippocampus.

The first septohippocampal fibers arrive in the hippocampus at E 17 (i.e., 2 days after the hippocampo-septal projection is established) (Linke and Frotscher, 1993; Super and Soriano, 1994). Little is known about the molecules involved in pathfinding and target recognition of septohippocampal fibers. Cholinergic fibers are known to bear the p75 neurotrophin receptor (p75^{NTR}), suggesting that neurotrophins play a role. Nerve growth factor (NGF), one of the ligands for the p75 receptor, is synthesized by GABAergic hippocampal neurons, which are distributed over all hippocampal layers, compatible with the diffuse termination of septohippocampal fibers. Moreover, NGF-synthesizing hippocampal nonprincipal neurons project to the septum (Acsady et al., 2000), thus providing both a neurotrophic source and a template

for axonal orientation (see above). A *neurotropic* effect of NGF was demonstrated some time ago (Gundersen and Barrett, 1979; see Tessier-Lavigne and Goodman, 1996, for review), but it needs to be confirmed that the ingrowth of septohippocampal fibers is controlled by neurotrophins. One of the semaphorins, Sema3C, was found to repel septal fibers (Steup et al., 2000); and neuropilin 2, its receptor, is present along the pathway of septal fibers (Chedotal et al., 1998; Steup et al., 2000), suggesting involvement of this ligand–receptor system in the formation of the septohippocampal projection.

4.3.4 General Principles Underlying the Formation of Synaptic Connections in the Hippocampus

We are now beginning to understand at least some of the principles underlying pathway formation in the hippocampus. Different cellular and molecular factors, probably being effective only during certain developmental time windows, are involved in the formation of the different projections to the hippocampus. When describing the formation of a pathway, we found it useful to distinguish between *axonal pathfinding*, *target recognition*, and *synapse formation*. For pathfinding and target recognition, pioneer neurons provide a template by an early-formed projection. Membrane-bound and soluble molecules and components of the extracellular matrix also seem to play a role at different times of development. A variety of ligand–receptor interactions has been elucidated that, by their repulsive or attractive effects, may guide the growth cone of a growing axon to the target region. Undoubtedly, new molecules or families of molecules of this kind will be discovered in the future. Extracellular matrix molecules, proteoglycans such as neurocan, may be essential for the segregation of fiber systems in the hippocampus (Förster et al., 2001; Zhao et al., 2003).

Synapse formation is dealt with only briefly here, and the reader is referred to quantitative electron microscopic analyses and Golgi studies on the development of synapses and dendritic spines (e.g., Crain et al., 1973; Minkwitz 1976; Frotscher et al., 1977). This is a rapidly developing field, and more recent studies have provided evidence that the mechanisms leading to new contacts or changes in the shape of synapses or spines may not only be effective during development but may also underlie plastic processes in the adult organism. A striking example is Engert and Bonhoeffer's (1999) in vitro observation of new spines formed during the development of long-term potentiation (LTP). Similarly, Woolley and McEwen (1993) have shown that estrogen application to ovariectomized adult rats induces new spines on CA1 pyramidal cell dendrites, an effect likely caused by estrogen acting primarily on CA3 pyramidal cells and inducing the sprouting of their Schaffer collaterals to CA1 pyramidal neurons (Rune et al., 2002). Interestingly, recent studies have shown that estrogens synthesized in the hippocampus are important for hippocampal synaptic plasticity (Kretz et al., 2004). Future studies will help us establish whether these plastic changes at spine synapses are specific for hippocampal neurons or are a more general phenomenon occurring at many synapses in the central nervous system.

4.4 Development of the Primate Hippocampal Formation

As in the previous chapter (see Chapter 3), one may raise the question of how hippocampal development varies across phylogenetically distant species such as rats, monkeys, and humans. What is similar and what is different? Do the steps of hippocampal development change proportionally with an extended life-span, or are there some fundamental differences in the mechanisms and the timing of cell formation, cell migration, dendritic development, and formation of neuronal connectivity? We provide a short comparative analysis of hippocampal development in primates. For details the reader should consult a review on monkey and human hippocampal development (Seress, 2001).

4.4.1 Neurogenesis

The duration of embryonic development is 19 to 21 days in mice and rats (life-span 1.5–3.0 years), 165 days in rhesus monkeys (life span 25–30 years), and 280 days in humans. As we have already noted, cell formation is a relatively late event in rodents: Pyramidal cells are generated during the second half of the embryonic period, and granule cell formation starts only a few days before birth. Furthermore, 85% of the dentate granule cells are formed postnatally. In contrast, neurogenesis in the primate hippocampal formation takes place relatively early. In rhesus monkeys, the first neurons appear almost simultaneously in the various subregions of the hippocampal formation, from the entorhinal cortex to the dentate gyrus, between E 36 and E 38 (Rakic and Nowakowski, 1981). Except for the dentate gyrus, cell formation ceases during the first half of pregnancy, between E 62 and E 65. Granule cell formation lasts until the end of the first postnatal month, with only 15% of the granule cells forming postnatally (Rakic and Nowakowski, 1981). Granule cell formation has also been found in the dentate gyrus of adult monkeys (Kornack and Rakic, 1999).

In humans, the time of pyramidal cell neurogenesis is not known and must be extrapolated from the time of the appearance of the cytoarchitectonic layers. Subfields of the hippocampal formation, such as the entorhinal cortex, subiculum, and hippocampus, are discernible between E 70 and E 80, whereas the dentate granular layer appears around E 90 (Humphrey, 1967). Between E 160 and E 170, the cytoarchitectonic characteristics of all of the divisions of the hippocampal formation are similar to what is observed in adults (Humphrey, 1967; Arnold and Trojanowski, 1996). With the aid of the mitotic marker MIB-1 (Ki-67), we have directly shown that the ventricular zone and hilus contain a large number of proliferating cells at E 100 (Fig. 4–4). The number of labeled cells decreases rapidly from E 170 onward (24th week), but MIB-1 (Ki-67)-positive cells are still observed in the hilus and granule cell layer during the first 6 months postnatally (Seress et al., 2001).

4.4.2 Neuronal Differentiation

Differentiation of pyramidal neurons and granule cells continues for a relatively long period in rodents and primates. Spine density increases until the time of sexual maturation, and total dendritic length is not reached before P 90 in the rat CA1 area (Pokorny and Yamamoto, 1981). In the monkey, the spine density of CA3 and CA1 pyramidal cells does not reach adult levels before sexual maturation (i.e., during the fourth year in rhesus monkeys) (Seress and Ribak, 1995b, unpublished observation). In humans, spine density and total dendritic length of CA1 pyramidal neurons increase until at least the third postnatal year (Simic et al., 2001). In contrast to the long-term differentiation of principal cells, local circuit neurons in the primate hippocampal formation mature fast, as indicated by the early fetal appearance of neurochemical markers of these neurons (Del Fiacco and Quartu, 1989; Berger et al., 1993, 1999).

Arrival of afferents at the rat hippocampal formation coincides with the development of their target cells. Thus, it takes place during the perinatal and early postnatal period, as previously noted. In both the monkey and human, however, afferent projections from the hypothalamus as well as from the entorhinal cortex arrive early during the fetal period (Kostovic et al., 1989; Hevner and Kinney, 1996; Berger et al., 2001). In contrast to extrinsic afferents, intrinsic associational connections of the rodent hippocampus develop relatively late, partly owing to the late formation of granule cells. Connections between dentate granule cells and CA3 pyramidal neurons as well as between dentate granule cells and hilar mossy cells develop postnatally (Ribak et al., 1985). This late development coincides with the prolonged postnatal development of hippocampal functions (Nadel and Willner, 1989). In contrast, the development of associational connections is relatively fast in rhesus monkeys, and the mainly prenatally formed granule cells establish a well developed synaptic network by the fifth to seventh postnatal month (Seress and Ribak, 1995a,b). Surprisingly, this is not the case in humans, where the prenatally formed granule cells appear to form the first connections with hilar mossy cells and CA3 pyramidal neurons as late as during the 33rd gestational week, as indicated by the late appearance of excrescences on hilar mossy cells and CA3 pyramidal neurons (Purpura, 1975). In fact, there are almost no light microscopic signs of such connections at birth (Seress and Mrzljak, 1992; Seress, 2001).

Taken together, developmental events of the hippocampal formation are different in rodents and primates. However, there are also common traits. In both rodents and humans the late development of intrahippocampal associational connections may influence the maturation of the entire hippocampal network. The factors contributing to this late development are likely to be different in rodents and primates. In rodents, the late formation of granule cells may play a role. It remains to be elucidated why the early-formed granule cells in humans do not immediately form synapses with their target cells as is the case in nonhuman primates.

ACKNOWLEDGMENTS

This work was supported by Deutscher Akademischer Austauschdienst (DAAD) with grants 323/2000 and 324/jo-H/2002, the Hungarian Ministry of Education (FKFP) with grant 0515/2000, and the Deutsche Forschungsgemeinschaft (SFB 505 and Transregio SFB TR-3).

REFERENCES

Acsady L, Pascual M, Rocamora N, Soriano E, Freund TF (2000) Nerve growth factor but not neurotrophin-3 is synthesized by hippocampal GABAergic neurons that project to the medial septum. *Neuroscience* 98:23–31.

Altman J (1966) Autoradiographic and histological studies of postnatal neurogenesis. II. A longitudinal investigation of kinetics, migration and transformation of cells incorporating tritiated thymidine in infant rats, with special reference to postnatal neurogenesis of some brain regions. *J Comp Neurol* 128:431–474.

Altman J, Bayer SA (1975) Postnatal development of the hippocampal dentate gyrus under normal and experimental conditions. In: *The hippocampus*, vol 2 (Isaacson RL, Pribram KH, eds), pp. 95–122. New York: Plenum Press.

Altman J, Bayer SA (1990a) Mosaic organization of the hippocampal neuroepithelium and the multiple germinal sources of dentate granule cells. *J Comp Neurol* 301:325–342.

Altman J, Bayer SA (1990b) Prolonged sojourn of developing pyramidal cells in the intermediate zone of the hippocampus and their settling in the stratum pyramidale. *J Comp Neurol* 301:343–364.

Altman J, Bayer SA (1990c) Migration and distribution of two populations of hippocampal granule cell precursors during the perinatal and postnatal periods. *J Comp Neurol* 301:365–381.

Altman J, Das DG (1966) Autoradiographic and histological studies of postnatal neurogenesis. I. A longitudinal investigation of the kinetics, migration and transformation of cells incorporating tritiated thymidine in neonate rats, with special reference to postnatal neurogenesis in some brain regions. *J Comp Neurol* 126:337–390.

Amaral DG, Kurz J (1985) The time of origin of cells demonstrating glutamic acid-like immunoreactivity in the hippocampal formation of the rat. *Neurosci Lett* 59:33–39.

Angevine JB (1965) Time of neuron origin in the hippocampal region: an autoradiographic study in the mouse. *Exp Neurol Suppl* 2:1–70.

Arnold SE, Trojanowski JQ (1996) Human fetal hippocampal development. I. Cytoarchitecture, myeloarchitecture and neuronal morphologic features. *J Comp Neurol* 367:274–292.

Bayer SA (1980) Development of the hippocampal region in the rat. I. Neurogenesis examined with ³H-thymidine autoradiography. *J Comp Neurol* 190:87–114.

Bayer SA, Altman J (1987) Directions in neurogenetic gradients and patterns of anatomical connections in the telencephalon. *Prog Neurobiol* 29:57–106.

Berger B, Alvarez C, Goldman-Rakic PS (1993) Neurochemical development of the hippocampal region in the fetal rhesus monkey. I. Early appearance of peptides, calcium binding proteins, DARPP-32 and the monoamine innervation in the entorhinal cortex during the first half of gestation (E47 to E90). *Hippocampus* 3:279–305.

Berger B, DeGrissac N, Alvarez C (1999) Precocious development of parvalbumin-like immunoreactive interneurons in the hippocampal formation and entorhinal cortex of the fetal cynamolgus monkey. *J Comp Neurol* 403:309–331.

Berger B, Esclapez M, Alvarez C, Meyer G, Catala M (2001) Human and monkey fetal brain development of the supramammillary-hippocampal projections: a system involved in the regulation of theta activity. *J Comp Neurol* 429:515–529.

Borrell V, Del Rio JA, Alcantara S, Derer M, Martinez A, D'Arcangelo G, Nakajima K, Mikoshiba K, Derer P, Curran T, Soriano E (1999) Reelin regulates the development and synaptogenesis of the layer-specific entorhino-hippocampal connections. *J Neurosci* 19:1345–1358.

Ceranik K, Deng J, Heimrich B, Lübke J, Zhao S, Förster E, Frotscher M (1999) Hippocampal Cajal-Retzius cells project to the entorhinal cortex: retrograde tracing and intracellular labelling studies. *Eur J Neurosci* 11:4278–4290.

Chedotal A, del Rio JA, Ruiz M He Z, Borrell V, de Castro F, Ezan F, Goodman CS, Tessier-Lavigne M, Sotelo C, Soriano E (1998) Semaphorins III and IV repel hippocampal axons via two distinct receptors. *Development* 125:4313–4323.

Crain B, Cotman C, Taylor D, Lynch G (1973) A quantitative electron microscopic study of synaptogenesis in the dentate gyrus of the rat. *Brain Res* 63:195–204.

Czurkó A, Czeh B, Seress L, Nadel L, Bures J (1997) Severe spatial navigation deficit in the Morris watermaze after single high dose of neonatal X-ray irradiation in the rat. *Proc Natl Acad Sci USA* 94:2766–2771.

D'Arcangelo G, Miao GG, Chen S-C, Soares HD, Morgan JI, Curran T (1995) A protein related to extracellular matrix proteins deleted in the mouse mutant reeler. *Nature* 374: 719–723.

D'Arcangelo G, Nakajima K, Miyata T, Ogawa M, Mikoshiba K, Curran T (1997) Reelin is a secreted glycoprotein recognized by the CR-50 monoclonal antibody. *J Neurosci* 17:23–31.

Del Fiacco M, Quartu M (1989) Ontogenetic variance of substance P in the human hippocampus. In: *The hippocampus: new vistas* (Chan Palay V, Kohler C, eds), pp 131–144. New York: Alan R. Liss.

Deller T, Drakew A, Frotscher M (1999a) Different primary target cells are important for fiber lamination in the fascia dentata: a lesson from reeler mutant mice. *Exp Neurol* 156:239–253.

Deller T, Drakew A, Heimrich B, Förster E, Tielsch A, Frotscher M (1999b) The hippocampus of the reeler mutant mouse: fiber segregation in area CA1 depends on the position of the postsynaptic target cells. *Exp Neurol* 156:254–267.

Del Rio JA, Heimrich B, Borrell V, Förster E, Drakew A, Alcántara S, Nakajima K, Miyata T, Ogawa M, Mikoshiba K, Derer P, Frotscher M, Soriano E (1997) A role for Cajal-Retzius cells and reelin in the development of hippocampal connections. *Nature* 385:70–74.

Drakew A, Frotscher M, Heimrich B (1999) Blockade of neuronal activity alters spine maturation of dentate granule cells but not their dendritic arborization. *Neuroscience* 94:767–774.

Drakew A, Deller T, Heimrich B, Gebhardt C, Del Turco D, Tielsch A, Förster E, Herz J, Frotscher M (2002) Dentate granule cells in reeler mutants and VLDLR and ApoER2 knockout mice. *Exp Neurol* 176:12–24.

Dupuy ST, Houser CR (1997) Developmental changes in GABAergic neurons of the rat dentate gyrus: an in situ hybridization and birth dating study. *J Comp Neurol* 389:402–418.

Dupuy ST, Houser CR (1999) Evidence for changing positions of GABA neurons in the developing rat dentate gyrus. *Hippocampus* 9:186–199.

Engert F, Bonhoeffer T (1999) Dendritic spine changes associated with hippocampal long-term synaptic plasticity. *Nature* 399:66–70.

Eriksson PS, Perfilieva E, Björk-Eriksson T, Alborn A, Nordborg C, Peterson DA, Gage FH (1998) Neurogenesis in the adult human hippocampus. *Nat Med* 4:1313–1317.

Falconer DS (1951) Two new mutants, "trembler" and "reeler," with neurological actions in the house mouse (Mus musculus L.). *J Genet (Paris)* 50:192–201.

Förster E, Kaltschmidt C, Deng J, Cremer H, Deller T, Frotscher M (1998) Lamina-specific cell adhesion on living slices of hippocampus. *Development* 125:3399–3410.

Förster E, Zhao S, Frotscher M (2001) Hyaluronan-associated adhesive cues control fiber segregation in the hippocampus. *Development* 128:3029–3039.

Förster E, Tielsch A, Saum B, Weiss KH, Johanssen C, Graus-Porta D, Müller U, Frotscher M (2002) Reelin, disabled 1 and beta1-integrins are required for the formation of the radial glial scaffold in the hippocampus. *Proc Natl Acad Sci USA* 99: 13178–13183.

Freund TF, Antal M (1988) GABA-containing neurons in the septum control inhibitory interneurons in the hippocampus. *Nature* 336:170–173.

Freund TF, Buzsáki G (1996) Interneurons of the hippocampus. *Hippocampus* 6:347–470.

Frotscher M (1997) Dual role of Cajal-Retzius cells and reelin in cortical development. *Cell Tissue Res* 290:315–322.

Frotscher M (1998) Cajal-Retzius cells, reelin, and the formation of layers. *Curr Opin Neurobiol* 8:570–575.

Frotscher M, Heimrich B (1993) Formation of layer-specific fiber projections to the hippocampus in vitro. *Proc Natl Acad Sci USA* 90:10400–10403.

Frotscher M, Leranth C (1985) Cholinergic innervation of the rat hippocampus as revealed by choline acetyltransferase immunocytochemistry: a combined light and electron microscopic study. *J Comp Neurol* 239:237–246.

Frotscher M, Leranth C (1986) The cholinergic innervation of the rat fascia dentata: identification of target structures on granule cells by combining choline acetyltransferase immunocytochemistry and Golgi impregnation. *J Comp Neurol* 243:181–190.

Frotscher M, Hámori J, Wenzel J (1977) Transneuronal effects of entorhinal lesions in the early postnatal period on synaptogenesis in the hippocampus of the rat. *Exp Brain Res* 30: 549–560.

Frotscher M, Schlander M, Leranth C (1986) Cholinergic neurons in the hippocampus: a combined light and electron microscopic immunocytochemical study in the rat. *Cell Tissue Res* 246: 293–301.

Frotscher M, Vida I, Bender R (2000a) Evidence for the existence of non-GABAergic, cholinergic interneurons in the rodent hippocampus. *Neuroscience* 96:27–31.

Frotscher M, Drakew A, Heimrich B (2000b) Role of afferent innervation and neuronal activity in dendritic development and spine maturation of fascia dentata granule cells. *Cereb Cortex* 10:946–951.

Frotscher M, Seress L, Abraham H, Heimrich B (2001) Early generated Cajal-Retzius cells have different functions in cortical development. In: *Brain stem cells* (Miyan J, Thorndyke M, Beesley PW, Bannister C, eds), pp. 43–49. Oxford: BIOS Scientific Publishers.

Frotscher M, Haas CA, Förster E (2003) Reelin controls granule cell migration in the dentate gyrus by acting on the radial glial scaffold. *Cereb Cortex* 13:634–640.

Galceran J, Miyashita-Lin EM, Devaney E, Rubenstein JLR, Grosschedl R (2000) Hippocampus development and generation of dentate gyrus granule cells is regulated by LEF1. *Development* 127:469–482.

Gundersen RW, Barrett JN (1979) Neuronal chemotaxis: chick dorsal-root axons turn toward high concentrations of nerve growth factor. *Science* 206:1079–1080.

Hájos N, Papp E, Acsády L, Levey AI, Freund TF (1998) Distinct interneuron types express m2 muscarinic receptor immunoreactivity on their dendrites or axon terminals in the hippocampus. *Neuroscience* 82:355–376.

Halasy K, Somogyi P (1993a) Distribution of GABAergic synapses and their targets in the dentate gyrus of rat: a quantitative immunoelectron microscopic analysis. *J Hirnforsch* 34:299–308.

Halasy K, Somogyi P (1993b) Subdivisions in the multiple GABAergic innervation of granule cells in the dentate gyrus of the rat hippocampus. *Eur J Neurosci* 5:411–429.

Halasy K, Buhl EH, Lorinczi Z, Tamás G, Somogyi P (1996) Synaptic target selectivity and input of GABAergic basket and bistratified interneurons in the CA1 area of the rat hippocampus. *Hippocampus* 6:306–329.

Hevner RF, Kinney HC (1996) Reciprocal entorhinal-hippocampal connections established by human fetal midgestation. J Comp Neurol 372:384–394.

Hirotsune S, Takahare T, Sasaki N, Hirose K, Yoshiki A, Ohashi T, Kusakabe M, Murakami Y, Muramatsu M, Watanabe S, Nakao K, Katsuki M, Hayashizaki Y (1995) The reeler gene encodes a protein with an EGF-like motif expressed by pioneer neurons. *Nat Genet* 10:77–83.

Humphrey T (1967) The development of the human hippocampal fissure. *J Anat* 101:655–676.

Katona I, Sperlágh B, Sík A, Kofalvi A, Vizi ES, Freund TF (1999) Presynaptically located CB1 cannabinoid receptors regulate GABA release from axon terminals of specific hippocampal interneurons. *J Neurosci* 19:4544–4558.

Kempermann G, Kuhn HG, Gage FH (1997a) More hippocampal neurons in adult mice living in an enriched environment. *Nature* 386:493–495.

Kempermann G, Kuhn HG, Gage FH (1997b) Genetic influence on neurogenesis in the dentate gyrus of adult mice. *Proc Natl Acad Sci USA* 94:10409–10414.

Kornack DR, Rakic P (1999) Continuation of neurogenesis in the hippocampus of the adult macaque monkey. *Proc Natl Acad Sci USA* 96:5768–5773.

Kostovic I, Seress L, Mrzljak L, Judas M (1989) Early onset of synapse formation in the human hippocampus: a correlation with Nissl-Golgi architectonics in 15 and 16.5-week-old fetuses. *Neuroscience* 30:105–116.

Kretz O, Fester L, Wehrenberg U, Zhou L, Brauckmann S, Zhao S, Prange-Kiel J, Naumann T, Jarry H, Frotscher M, Rune GM (2004) Hippocampal synapses depend on hippocampal estrogen synthesis. *J Neurosci* 24:5913–5921.

Lang U, Frotscher M (1990) Postnatal development of nonpyramidal neurons in the rat hippocampus (areas CA1 and CA3): a combined Golgi/electron microscope study. *Anat Embryol* 181: 533–545.

Laurberg S, Hjorth-Simonsen A (1977) Growing central axons deprived of normal target neurones by neonatal X-ray irradiation still terminate in a precisely laminated fashion. *Nature* 269:158–160.

Linke R, Frotscher M (1993) Development of the rat septohippocampal projection: tracing with DiI and electron microscopy of identified growth cones. *J Comp Neurol* 332:69–88.

Linke R, Pabst T, Frotscher M (1995) Development of the hippocamposeptal projection in the rat. *J Comp Neurol* 351:602–616.

Lübbers K, Wolff JR, Frotscher M (1985) Neurogenesis of GABAergic neurons in the rat dentate gyrus: a combined autoradiographic and immunocytochemical study. *Neurosci Lett* 62:317–322.

Minkwitz H-G (1976) Zur Entwicklung der Neuronenstruktur des Hippocampus während der prä- und postnatalen Ontogenese der Albinoratte. III. Mitteilung: Morphometrische Erfassung der ontogenetischen Veränderungen in Dendritenstruktur und Spinebesatz an Pyramidenneuronen (CA1) des Hippocampus. *J Hirnforsch* 17:255–275.

Nadel L, Willner J (1989) Some implications of postnatal maturation of the hippocampus. In: *The hippocampus: new vistas* (Chan-Palay V, Kohler C, eds), pp. 17–31. New York: Alan R Liss.

Nguyen-Ba-Charvet KT, Brose K, Marillat V, Kidd T, Goodman CS, Tessier-Lavigne M, Sotelo C, Chedotal A (1999) Slit2-mediated chemorepulsion and collapse of developing forebrain axons. *Neuron* 22:463–473.

Pleasure SJ, Anderson S, Hevner R, Bagri A, Lowenstein DH, Rubenstein JLR (2000) Cell migration from the ganglionic eminences is required for the development of hippocampal GABAergic interneurons. *Neuron* 26:727–740.

Pokorny J, Yamamoto Y (1981) Postnatal ontogenesis of hippocampal CA1 area in rats. I. Development of dendritic arborization in pyramidal neurons. *Brain Res Bull* 7:113–120.

Purpura DS (1975) Normal and aberrant neuronal development in the cerebral cortex of human fetus and young infant. In: *Brain mechanisms in mental retardation: UCLA forum in medical sciences* pp. 141–169. San Diego: Academic Press.

Rakic P, Nowakowski RS (1981) The time of origin of neurons in the hippocampal region of the rhesus monkey. *J Comp Neurol* 196:99–128.

Ramón y Cajal S (1911) *Histologie du système nerveux de l'homme et des vertébrés*, vol 2. Paris: Maloine.

Retzius G (1893) Die Cajalschen Zellen der Grosshirnrinde beim Menschen und bei Säugetieren. *Biol Unters* 5:1–9.

Retzius G (1894) Weitere Beiträge zur Kenntnis der Cajalschen Zellen der Grosshirnrinde des Menschen. *Biol Unters* 6:29–34.

Ribak CE, Seress L (1983) Five types of basket cell in the hippocampal dentate gyrus. *J Neurocytol* 12:577–597.

Ribak CE, Seress L, Amaral DG (1985) The development, ultrastructure and synaptic connections of the mossy cells of the dentate gyrus. *J Neurocytol* 14:717–730.

Rune GM, Wehrenberg U, Prange-Kiel J, Zhou L, Adelmann G, Frotscher M (2002) Estrogen up-regulates estrogen receptor alpha and synaptophysin in slice cultures of rat hippocampus. *Neuroscience* 113:167–175.

Savaskan NE, Plaschke M, Ninnemann O, Spillmann AA, Schwab ME, Nitsch R, Skutella T (1999) Myelin does not influence the choice behaviour of entorhinal axons but strongly inhibits their outgrowth length in vitro. *Eur J Neurosci* 11:316–326.

Seress L (1977) The postnatal development of rat dentate gyrus and the effect of early thyroid hormone treatment. *Anat Embryol* 151:335–339.

Seress L (1978) Divergent responses to thyroid hormone treatment of the different secondary germinal layers in the postnatal rat brain. *J Hirnforsch* 19:395–403.

Seress L (2001) Morphological changes in the human hippocampal formation from midgestation to early childhood. In: *Handbook of developmental cognitive neuroscience* (Nelson CA, Luciana M, eds), pp. 45–58. Cambridge, MA: MIT Press.

Seress L, Frotscher M (1990) Morphological variability is a characteristic feature of granule cells in the primate fascia dentata: a combined Golgi-electron microscopic study. *J Comp Neurol* 293:253–267.

Seress L, Mrzljak L (1987) Basal dendrites of granule cells are normal features of the fetal and adult dentate gyrus of both monkey and human hippocampal formations. *Brain Res* 405:169–174.

Seress L, Mrzljak L (1992) Postnatal development of mossy cells in the human dentate gyrus: a light microscopic Golgi study. *Hippocampus* 2:127–142.

Seress L, Ribak CE (1983) GABAergic neurons in the dentate gyrus appear to be local circuit and projection neurons. *Exp Brain Res* 50:173–182.

Seress L, Ribak CE (1990) Postnatal development of the light and electron microscopic features of basket cells in the hippocampal dentate gyrus of the rat. *Anat Embryol* 181:547–566.

Seress L, Ribak CE (1995a) Postnatal development and synaptic connections of hilar mossy cells in the hippocampal dentate gyrus of rhesus monkeys. *J Comp Neurol* 355:93–110.

Seress L, Ribak CE (1995b) The postnatal development of CA3 pyramidal neurons and their afferents in the Ammon's horn of rhesus monkeys. *Hippocampus* 5:217–231.

Seress L, Frotscher M, Ribak CE (1989) Local circuit neurons in both the dentate gyrus and Ammon's horn establish synaptic connections with principal neurons in five day-old rats: a morphological basis for inhibition in early development. *Exp Brain Res* 78:1–9.

Seress L, Ábrahám H, Tornóczky T, Kosztolányi GY (2001) Cell formation in the human hippocampal formation from midgestation to the late postnatal period. *Neuroscience* 105:39–51.

Simic G, Bjelos M, Rasin MR, Seress L, Kostovic I (2001) Postnatal development of human CA1 pyramidal neurons. *Soc Neurosci Abstr* 27:Program 250.2.

Skutella T, Nitsch R (2001) New molecules for hippocampal development. *Trends Neurosci* 24:107–113.

Skutella T, Savaskan NE, Ninnemann O, Nitsch R (1999) Target- and maturation-specific membrane-associated molecules determine the ingrowth of entorhinal fibers into the hippocampus. *Dev Biol* 211:277–292.

Soriano E, Frotscher M (1989) A GABAergic axo-axonic cell in the fascia dentata controls the main excitatory hippocampal pathway. *Brain Res* 503:170–174.

Soriano E, Frotscher M (1993) GABAergic innervation of the rat fascia dentate: a novel type of interneuron in the granule cell layer with extensive axonal arborization in the molecular layer. *J Comp Neurol* 334:385–396.

Soriano E, Cobas A, Fairén A (1989a) Neurogenesis of glutamic acid decarboxylase-immunoreactive cells in the hippocampus of the mouse. I. Regio superior and regio inferior. *J Comp Neurol* 281:586–602.

Soriano E, Cobas A, Fairen A (1989b) Neurogenesis of glutamic acid decarboxylase-immunoreactive cells in the hippocampus of the mouse. II. Area dentata. *J Comp Neurol* 281:603–611.

Spigelman I, Yan XX, Obenaus A, Lee EY-S, Wasterlain CG, Ribak CE (1998) Dentate granule cells form novel basal dendrites in a rat model of temporal lobe epilepsy. *Neuroscience* 86:109–120.

Spruston N, Lübke J, Frotscher M (1997) Interneurons in the stratum lucidum of the rat hippocampus: an anatomical and electrophysiological characterization. *J Comp Neurol* 385:427–440.

Stanfield BB, Cowan WM (1979) The morphology of the hippocampus and dentate gyrus in normal and reeler mice. *J Comp Neurol* 185:393–422.

Stein E, Savaskan NE, Ninnemann O, Nitsch R, Zhou R, Skutella T (1999) A role for the Eph ligand ephrin-A3 in entorhino-hippocampal axon targeting. *J Neurosci* 15:8885–8893.

Stephan, H (1975) *Allocortex: Handbuch der mikroskopischen Anatomie des Menschen*, vol IV/9. Berlin: Springer.

Steup A, Ninnemann O, Savaskan NE, Nitsch R, Püschel AW, Skutella T (1999) Semaphorin D acts as a repulsive factor for entorhinal and hippocampal neurons. *Eur J Neurosci* 11:729–734.

Steup A, Lohrum M, Hamscho N, Savaskan NE, Ninnemann O, Nitsch R, Fujisawa H, Püschel AW, Skutella T (2000) Sema3C and netrin-1 differentially affect axon growth in the hippocampal formation. *Mol Cell Neurosci* 15:141–155.

Super H, Soriano E (1994) The organization of the embryonic and early postnatal murine hippocampus. II. Development of entorhinal, commissural and septal connections studied with the lipophilic tracer DiI. *J Comp Neurol* 344:101–120.

Super H, Martinez A, del Rio JA, Soriano E (1998) Involvement of distinct pioneer neurons in the formation of layer-specific connections in the hippocampus. *J Neurosci* 18:4616–4626.

Tamamaki N (1999) Development of afferent fiber lamination in the infrapyramidal blade of the rat dentate gyrus. *J Comp Neurol* 411:257–266.

Tessier-Lavigne M, Goodman CS (1996) The molecular biology of axon guidance. *Science* 274:1123–1132.

Tole S, Christian C, Grove EA (1997) Early specification and autonomous development of cortical fields in the mouse hippocampus. *Development* 124:4959–4670.

Vida I, Frotscher M (2000) A hippocampal interneuron associated with the mossy fiber system. *Proc Natl Acad Sci USA* 97:1275–1280.

Vida I, Halasy K, Szinyei C, Somogyi P, Buhl EH (1998) Unitary IPSPs evoked by interneurons at the stratum radiatum/lacunosum-moleculare border in the CA1 area of the rat hippocampus in vitro. *J Physiol (Lond)* 503:755–773.

Von Campe G, Spencer DD, de Lanerolle NC (1997) Morphology of dentate granule cells in the human epileptogenic hippocampus. *Hippocampus* 7:472–488.

Woolley CS, McEwen BS (1993) Roles of estradiol and progesterone in regulation of hippocampal spine density during the estrous cycle in the rat. *J Comp Neurol* 336:293–306.

Zhao S, Förster E, Chai X, Frotscher M (2003) Different signals control laminar specificity of commissural and entorhinal fibers to the dentate gyrus. *J Neurosci* 23:7351–7357.

Zhao S, Chai X, Förster E, Frotscher M (2004) Reelin is a positional signal for the lamination of dentate granule cells. *Development* 131:5117–5125.

5

Nelson Spruston and Chris McBain

Structural and Functional Properties of Hippocampal Neurons

5.1 Overview

One of the most striking qualities of Cajal's drawings is the great diversity of form exhibited by neurons in the central nervous system (CNS). Looking at these drawings, it is difficult to escape the conclusion that neurons with different morphologies are likely to function differently. Indeed a plethora of anatomical, histological, and physiological studies support the view that diversity in form is mirrored by diversity of function. The hippocampus presents, in many ways, a microcosm of the cellular diversity exhibited on a larger scale throughout the CNS. An important step on the path to understanding the function of the hippocampus is to reveal the unique morphological and physiological properties of the great variety of neurons it comprises.

Much can be learned by examining neuronal structure. The dendritic tree defines which inputs can be received, and the axonal arborization indicates the targets of the output (although dendro-dendritic and axo-axonal communication should not be forgotten). Electron microscopy provides details about the nature of each neuron's inputs and output. It allows us to infer which synapses are inhibitory (symmetrical) and which are excitatory (asymmetrical) and where modulatory machinery resides (e.g., endoplasmic reticulum for calcium release, ribosomes for protein synthesis, vesicles for neurotransmitter release or insertion of membrane proteins). Histological studies (antibody or cDNA binding, histochemical assays) provide further information, ranging from which neurotransmitters are used to which voltage-gated channels are present and where. Physiological studies, using electrodes and imaging both in vitro and in vivo, reveal the dynamic function of each neuron.

A detailed picture of the function of each neuron can only emerge by bringing together information from this variety of techniques. Ultimately, complete understanding of the function of each type of neuron may be encapsulated by detailed models that can reproduce or explain virtually any aspect of neuronal function. The purpose of such models, of course, is to offer insight into the neuron's function within a network and provide experimentally testable predictions.

In this chapter, our aim is to summarize the wealth of structural, histological, and physiological information that is available for hippocampal neurons. Most of the available data on this topic come from studies of the rat hippocampal formation. Accordingly, we mention species primarily when referring to data from species other than rat. We begin with the CA1 pyramidal neuron because it is arguably the most studied class of neuron in the brain and probably better understood from both structural and functional points of view than any other type of neuron in the hippocampus. From there we proceed by comparing the function of the other pyramidal neurons in the hippocampus: those in CA3 and the subiculum. We next cover two nonpyramidal excitatory neurons in the hippocampus: granule cells of the dentate gyrus and mossy cells of the hilus. Finally, we conclude by describing the properties of a variety of neurons in other regions comprising the hippocampal formation: the entorhinal cortex, presubiculum, and parasubiculum. In the final section, we consider the many types of interneurons found in the hippocampus.

5.2 CA1 Pyramidal Neurons

The vastness of the literature on CA1 pyramidal neurons is largely attributable to a combination of structural considerations, cell viability, and historical accidents. Although long-term potentiation was first described in the dentate gyrus, most of the studies in the decades that followed its original description have focused on the CA1 region. This is because of the relative ease of obtaining field potential recordings and intracellular recordings in this region. Also, the Schaffer collateral axons from CA3 form a homogeneous pathway that is easily activated to study synaptic transmission and plasticity. Studies of CA1 are more numerous than adjacent CA3 because it is generally easier to keep cells in this region alive and healthy in slice preparations. Recently, CA1 pyramidal neurons have been the focus of several studies of dendritic integration because of the large primary apical dendrite, from which dendritic patch-clamp recordings can be obtained routinely. These factors have contributed to tremendous advances in understanding synaptic transmission, integration, and plasticity in the CNS.

5.2.1 Dendritic Morphology

Two elaborately branching dendritic trees emerge from the pyramid-shaped soma of CA1 neurons (Fig. 5–1A). The basal dendrites occupy the stratum oriens, and the apical dendrites occupy the stratum radiatum (proximal apical) and stratum lacunosum-moleculare (distal apical). [Note: in this context the terms "proximal" and "distal" refer to the relative distance from the soma and should not be confused with the "proximo-distal" axis of the hippocampal circuit (dentate-CA3-CA1-subiculum-entorhinal cortex) introduced in Chapter 3.] Both the apical and basal dendritic trees occupy a roughly conical (sometimes ovoid) volume (Pyapali et al., 1998). The size of the CA1 dendritic tree depends on species and age, but the best available data are from adult rats. The distance from the stratum pyramidale to the hippocampal fissure is about 600 μm, and the distance from the stratum pyramidale to the alveus is about 300 μm, yielding a distance of just under 1 mm from the tips of the basal dendrites to the tips of the apical dendrites. The combined length of all CA1 dendritic branches is 12.0 to 13.5 mm: basal dendrites contribute about 36% of the total length, apical dendrites in the stratum radiatum contribute about 40%, and apical dendrites in the stratum lacunosum-moleculare contribute the remaining 24% (Bannister and Larkman, 1995a; Ishizuka et al., 1995; Trommald et al., 1995; Megias et al., 2001). CA1 dendites are studded with spines (Fig. 5–1B), the sites of most excitatory synaptic contacts throughout the dendritic tree (Ramon y Cajal, 1904; Lorente de No, 1934; Bannister and Larkman, 1995b; Megias et al., 2001).

Studies of dendritic morphology in adult rats suggest that CA1 pyramidal neurons can be broadly classified into two groups on the basis of dendritic morphology. In one group of neurons, the primary apical dendrite extends all the way through the stratum radiatum before bifurcating in the stratum lacunosum-moleculare. The other group of CA1 neurons has apical dendrites that bifurcate in the stratum radiatum (Bannister and Larkman, 1995a). Most other features of these two classes of CA1 neurons are similar, so most structural studies consider CA1 pyramidal neurons as a single morphological class (Fig. 5–1C).

Along the length of the primary apical dendrite, several dendritic branches emerge obliquely in the stratum radiatum.

The number of these oblique branches varies from 9 to 30, with a mean of 17 (Bannister and Larkman, 1995a; Pyapali et al., 1998) (Fig. 5–1C). Oblique dendrites branch no more than a few times, with a typical branch bifurcating just once at a location close to its origin from the apical trunk. Despite their limited branching, however, oblique dendrites constitute most of the dendritic length in the stratum radiatum (Bannister and Larkman, 1995a; Megias et al., 2001). After the primary apical trunk enters the stratum lacunosum-moleculare the apical dendrites continue to branch, forming a structure referred to as the apical tuft, which has an average of about 15 terminal branches (Bannister and Larkman, 1995a; Trommald et al., 1995).

Emerging from the base of the pyramidal soma are two to eight dendrites (a mean of five). Most of these dendrites branch several times (maximum 15 branch points), forming a basal dendritic tree with about 40 terminal segments (Bannister and Larkman, 1995; Pyapali et al., 1998). Most branches in the basal dendrites occur rather close to the soma, so the terminal segments are quite long, constituting about 80% of the total dendritic length (Bannister and Larkman, 1995a; Trommald et al., 1995). CA1 neurons differ considerably in the position of the cell body, with some cells located in the stratum oriens as far as 100 μm from the border between the stratum pyramidale and the stratum radiatum. Cells with somata farther from this border tend to have more terminal dendrites in the stratum oriens (basal dendrites) and fewer terminal dendrites in the stratum radiatum (apical oblique dendrites) (Bannister and Larkman, 1995a).

Many of the organelles found in the cell body extend into the proximal apical dendrites of CA1 neurons (Harris and Stevens, 1989; Spacek and Harris, 1997). These include structures such as the smooth endoplasmic reticulum (SER) and the Golgi apparatus. At greater distances from the soma, however, a more limited set of organelles is found in dendrites. Microtubules, neurofilaments, and actin are prominent and serve transport and motility functions, and they are likely to be important in synaptic plasticity. A network of SER is also present in dendrites, where it is likely to serve important functions in calcium buffering and release. The SER forms a continuous reticulum, which can extend into dendritic spines (Spacek and Harris, 1997). Mitochondria are also numerous in dendrites and are often associated with the SER, but glycogen granules are largely absent, except in sliced tissue, where they probably represent a response to stress (Fiala et al., 2003). Dendritic mitochondria likely contribute to calcium handling in addition to serving as the primary energy source. In apical dendrites of CA1 pyramidal neurons, mitochondria fill about 2% of the area of the main apical dendrite but 13% of smaller-diameter branches (Nafstad and Blackstad, 1966). Sorting endosomes and multivesicular bodies form the endosomal pathway, which is responsible for sorting and recycling proteins in dendrites as well as packaging them for transport to the soma for degradation. This endosomal compartment forms a network that spans as many as 20 spines in CA1 den-

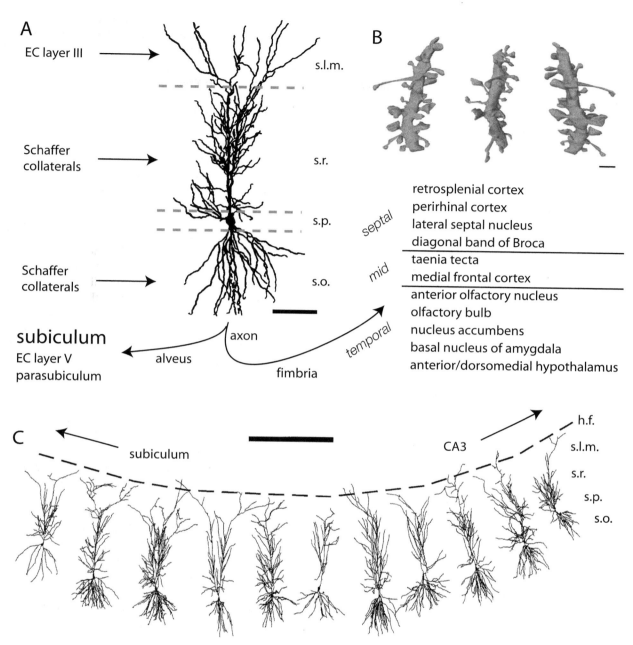

A

EC layer III ⟶ s.l.m.

Schaffer collaterals ⟶ s.r.

s.p.

Schaffer collaterals ⟶ s.o.

septal

mid

temporal

retrosplenial cortex
perirhinal cortex
lateral septal nucleus
diagonal band of Broca
_____
taenia tecta
medial frontal cortex
_____
anterior olfactory nucleus
olfactory bulb
nucleus accumbens
basal nucleus of amygdala
anterior/dorsomedial hypothalamus

subiculum
EC layer V
parasubiculum

axon

alveus

fimbria

B

C

subiculum

CA3

h.f.
s.l.m.
s.r.
s.p.
s.o.

Figure 5–1. CA1 dendritic morphology, spines, and synaptic inputs and outputs. *A.* Camera lucida drawing of a CA1 pyramidal neuron from an adult rat, showing the cell body in the stratum pyramidale (s.p.), basal dendrites in the stratum oriens (s.o.), and apical dendrites in the stratum radiatum (s.r.) and stratum lacunosum-molecu-lare (s.l.m.). The major excitatory inputs in each layer and the major outputs are also indicated. For the fimbrial projection, the septo-temporal positions noted indicate the source of CA1 cells projecting to different target regions. For the alveus projection, the subiculum is the major target. Bar = 100 μm. (*Source*: Adapted from Bannister and Larkman, 1995a.) *B.* Three views of a three-dimensional reconstruction of a stretch of dendrite from the s.r., illustrating the density of dendritic spines and their diverse structure on CA1 pyramidal neuron dendrites. Bar = 1 μm. (*Source*: Adapted from Synapse Web, by Kristen Harris (http://synapses.mcg. edu/anatomy/ca1pyrmd/radiatum/K18/K18.stm). *C.* Line drawings of several CA1 pyramidal neurons illustrating their diversity of dendritic structure. Dashed line represents the hippocampal fissure (h.f.). Bar = 500 μm. (*Source*: Adapted from Pyapali et al., 1998.)

drites (Cooney et al., 2002). Clathrin-coated pits and vesicles are also present in CA1 dendrites, often near the ends of tubular endosomal compartments. Ribosomes are present in CA1 dendrites, where they are usually clustered in the form of polyribosomes (Steward et al., 1996; Steward and Worley, 2002).

5.2.2 Dendritic Spines and Synapses

CA1 pyramidal neurons are covered with about 30,000 dendritic spines. Electron microscopic, immunocytochemical, and physiological analyses have all converged on the conclusion that most dendritic spines receive excitatory synaptic inputs, indicating that spine density can be used as a reasonable measure of excitatory synapse density (Gray, 1959; Andersen et al., 1966; Megias et al., 2001). The distribution of spines on different dendritic domains has been carefully quantified (Andersen et al., 1980; Bannister and Larkman, 1995b; Megias et al., 2001). The density of dendritic spines and synapses on CA1 pyramidal neurons is highest in the stratum radiatum and stratum oriens but lower in the stratum lacunosum-moleculare. The soma and the first 100 μm of the main apical dendrite (1.8–2.5 μm diameter) are almost completely devoid of spines. The next 150 μm of the apical dendrite (1.6–2.2 μm diameter) has a very low spine density, but the final 150 μm of the main apical dendrite (1.0–1.5 μm diameter) has a high spine density (about seven spines per linear micrometer). Spine density is lower in the oblique apical branches (0.5–0.6 μm diameter; about three spines per micrometer); but because these dendrites constitute a large fraction of the total dendritic length, about 47% of all CA1 spines are located on these branches. Together with the spines on the main apical dendrite, about 54% of all excitatory synapses contact spines in the apical dendrites in the stratum radiatum. Spine density is considerably lower in the apical tuft (0.2–1.2 μm diameter). Although these dendrites contribute about 20% of the total dendritic length, they contain only about 6% of the dendritic spines. Asymmetrical synapses, however, are also found on dendritic shafts in this region. If these synapses are excitatory, as is usually presumed, about 10% of all excitatory synapses are located in the apical tuft. The first 30 to 50 μm of the basal dendrites (0.5–0.9 μm diameter) have a low spine density, whereas the distal basal dendrites (0.3–0.5 μm diameter) have a spine density comparable to that of the apical oblique dendrites. Accordingly, about 36% of all excitatory synapses on CA1 neurons contact spines in the basal dendrites.

The distribution of symmetrical, GABA-positive synapses has also been quantified in CA1 neurons (Megias et al., 2001). About 24% of these synapses contact the soma and spine-free proximal dendrites (apical and basal). Somewhat surprisingly, the sparsely spiny and densely spiny regions of the main apical dendrite (in the stratum radiatum) receive similar numbers of inhibitory synapses, at about 3% of the total each. About 26% of the inhibitory synapses contact oblique apical branches. About 20% of all inhibitory synapses contact dendrites of the apical tuft. These dendrites therefore receive roughly twice as many inhibitory synapses as excitatory synapses. The remaining 24% of inhibitory synapses contact the distal basal dendrites. These dendrites are therefore similar to the apical obliques in terms of diameter, spine density, and numbers of excitatory versus inhibitory synapses.

The dendritic spines studding the surface of CA1 dendrites exhibit a broad range of size and morphological complexity (Fig. 5–1B). Although quantitative analysis of spine shapes does not indicate clear groups of spines (Trommald and Hulleberg, 1997), several investigators have used a variety of names to describe spines of different shapes (Laatsch and Cowan, 1966; Peters and Kaiserman-Abramof, 1970; Harris and Kater, 1994; Sorra and Harris, 2000). Thin spines are long, narrow protrusions terminating in a small, bulbous head. Sessile spines are long, narrow protrusions that do not terminate in a head. Stubby spines are small protrusions lacking a clearly distinguishable neck and a head. Mushroom spines have a narrow neck and a large, bulbous head. Branched spines consist of a neck that branches and terminates in two bulbous heads, each of which receives synaptic input from different axons. These five types of spines are not specifically localized to any particular region of the CA1 dendritic tree but can be found in close apposition on virtually any dendritic branch.

Spine structure is not static but may change in response to neurotransmitter receptor activation or environmental and hormonal signals (Hering and Sheng 2001; Bonhoeffer and Yuste, 2002; Nikonenko et al., 2002; Nimchinsky et al., 2002). Growth of new spines and changes in the structure of existing spines are possible substrates of synaptic plasticity in the hippocampus (Geinisman, 2000; Popov et al., 2004). Although the plasticity of spine structure in vivo is a matter of some controversy (Grutzendler et al., 2002; Trachtenberg et al., 2002), imaging studies of hippocampal neurons in vitro have revealed a rather dynamic picture of spine morphology (Hosokawa et al., 1995; Dailey and Smith, 1996; Engert and Bonhoeffer, 1999; Maletic-Savatic et al., 1999; Matsuzaki et al., 2004). One particularly noticeable feature of time-lapse movies of hippocampal dendrites is the continuous extension and retraction of filopodia. Occasionally, these filopodia extend without retracting fully, leading to the hypothesis that they form the precursors for mature, stable spines, which eventually establish functional synaptic connections with presynaptic boutons (Dailey and Smith, 1996; Fiala et. al. 1998; Parnass et al., 2000). The motility of dendritic filopodia and spines, which notably lack microtubules and neurofilaments, is facilitated by a network of filamentous actin (Sorra and Harris, 2000).

CA1 neurons have been the target of numerous studies of the mechanisms of calcium entry, buffering, and extrusion in dendritic spines (Yuste and Denk, 1995; Yuste et al., 1999; Majewska et al., 2000). Such studies have contributed to important advances in our understanding not only of calcium handling in spines but the mechanisms of synaptic transmission at single synapses and a variety of forms of morphological and functional plasticity (Emptage et al., 1999; Matsuzaki et al., 2001; Nimchinsky et al., 2002; Oertner et al., 2002; Sabatini et al., 2002; Yasuda et al., 2003; Matsuzaki et al., 2004; Nimchinsky et al., 2004).

Spines also contain numerous organelles, including smooth endoplasmic reticulum (SER). SER is found in about half of the spines in CA1 but is present in most of the largest, morphologically complex spines (Spacek and Harris, 1997; Cooney et. al. 2002). SER is occasionally associated with a spine apparatus, which consists of stacks of SER associated with other electron-dense material including polyribosomes. CA1 spines also contain free polyribosomes and mRNA, leading to the hypothesis that proteins can be synthesized on demand in individual dendritic spines (Steward et al., 1996). Endosomal organelles and coated vesicles are found in about one-third of CA1 spines (Cooney et al., 2002). Interestingly, mitochondria are absent from most spines (Sorra and Harris, 2000). The presence of a large number of molecules and organelles in spines, together with the separation that the spine neck provides from the dendritic shaft and other spines, has led to the hypothesis that spines function as isolated molecular compartments (Wickens, 1988; Koch and Zador, 1993; Harris and Kater, 1994; Sorra and Harris, 2000) and that such compartmentalization is necessary for synapse-specific changes in synaptic strength (Wickens, 1988; Harris and Kater, 1994).

A prominent feature of almost all CA1 spines (and spines throughout the nervous system) is a postsynaptic density (PSD), an electron-dense thickening of the postsynaptic membrane. The PSD is located adjacent to the presynaptic bouton(s) associated with the spine. Structurally, the size and shape of the PSD defines two classes of axo-spinous synapses: perforated synapses, which have large PSDs with complex shapes, and nonperforated synapses, which have smaller, disk-like PSDs (Harris et al., 1992). Functionally, the PSD is a biochemical specialization that allows numerous molecules (e.g., receptors, kinases, cytoskeletal elements) to be associated in a structured array at the synapse (Sheng, 2001). Perforated PSDs on CA1 pyramidal neurons have more α-amino-3-hydroxy-5-methyl-4-isoxazolepropionate (AMPA) and N-methyl-D-aspartate (NMDA) receptors than their nonperforated counterparts, suggesting that they may constitute a population of relatively powerful synapses (Ganeshina et al., 2004a,b).

A picture is now emerging concerning the organization of the glutamate receptors in the PSD found in excitatory synapses on CA1 spines (see Chapters 6 and 7). These synapses contain three types of glutamate receptors: NMDA, AMPA, and metabotropic glutamate (mGluR). NMDA receptors, which mediate a slow synaptic current blocked in a voltage-dependent manner by Mg^{2+} (see Chapter 6), occupy a disk-like space near the center of the PSD. AMPA receptors, which mediate a fast synaptic current, are distributed more evenly throughout the PSD (Lujan et al., 1996; Racca et al., 2000). The presence of the edited form of the GluR2 subunit, which is expressed abundantly in CA1 neurons under normal conditions, renders most of these AMPA receptors impermeable to Ca^{2+}, whereas NMDA receptors have a considerable Ca^{2+} per-

meability (Verdoorn et al., 1991; Burnashev et al., 1992; Vissavajjhala et al., 1996; Wenthold et al., 1996). mGluRs are located predominantly on the periphery of the PSD (Lujan et al., 1996). These receptors are coupled directly to the SER via a molecule called Homer, which may be coupled to mechanisms for releasing calcium from the SER (Xiao et al., 2000).

Individual excitatory synapses on CA1 neurons vary considerably in their expression of AMPA and NMDA receptors, even within particular dendritic domains. Indeed, silent synapses, which are thought to contain NMDA receptors but few or no functional AMPA receptors, were first discovered and most extensively studied at SC synapses on CA1 neurons (Isaac et al., 1995; Liao et al., 1995; Isaac, 2003). Immunocytochemical analysis suggests that whereas the number of NMDA receptors is relatively invariant, a tremendous range exists in the number of AMPA receptors at individual synapses (Nusser et al., 1998; Racca et al., 2000). Quantitative immunogold data suggest a correlation between synapse size and AMPA receptor number (Nusser et al., 1998; Takumi et al., 1999; Ganeshina et al., 2004a,b) and recent physiological data indicate that there are correlations between spine morphology and glutamate receptor distribution, with mushroom-shaped spines containing the most AMPA receptors and thinner spines and filopodia containing only NMDA receptors (Matsuzaki et al., 2001).

5.2.3 Excitatory and Inhibitory Synaptic Inputs

Like most neurons in the CNS, CA1 neurons receive input from both excitatory and inhibitory presynaptic neurons. The principle excitatory inputs arrive from the entorhinal cortex (EC) and CA3 pyramidal neurons. Direct inputs from layer III pyramidal neurons in the EC project to CA1 neurons via the perforant path (PP), so named because the fibers leaving the angular bundle perforate the subiculum (Cajal, 1911). The PP input from the EC to CA1 (also referred to as the temporo-ammonic path) selectively innervates the distal apical dendrites in the stratum lacunosum-moleculare (Blackstad, 1958). Some of the PP fibers forming synapses on CA1 pyramidal neurons reach their targets in the stratum lacunosum-moleculare via the temporo-alvear pathway (Deller et al., 1996a). Additional inputs from the nucleus reuniens of the thalamus and the basolateral nucleus of the amygdala also innervate CA1 neurons via synapses on the distal apical dendrites (Krettek and Price, 1977; Amaral and Witter, 1995; Dolleman-Van der Weel and Witter, 1996, 1997; Kemppainen et al., 2002). Inputs from CA3 pyramidal neurons on both sides of the brain form the Schaffer collateral/commissural system (SC), which form synapses on the apical dendrites in the stratum radiatum and on the basal dendrites in the stratum oriens (Schaffer, 1892; Blackstad, 1956; Storm-Mathisen and Fonnum, 1972; Hjort-Simonsen, 1973).

A few notable differences between PP and SC synaptic inputs have been identified. First, the PP synapses are located farther from the soma. Without a mechanism for compensating for this dendritic disadvantage, these synapses would be expected to have a weaker influence on action-potential initiation in the axon than the SC synapses (see Sections 5.2.8 and 5.2.9). A second difference is that, relative to the stratum radiatum, a greater proportion of synapses in the stratum lacunosum-moleculare are formed on dendritic shafts, rather than spines (Megías et al., 2001). Thus, any functions normally attributed to spines (e.g., biochemical compartmentalization) must be absent at many of these synapses (but see Goldberg et al., 2003a). The functional significance of the shaft synapses in the stratum lacunosum-moleculare is not known, but approximately equal numbers of these synapses are formed by the perforant path and thalamic nucleus reuniens projections (Wouterlood et al., 1990). Another possible difference between PP and SC synapses is that there appears to be more NMDA receptor activation at stratum lacunosum-moleculare synapses (Otmakhova and Lisman, 1999), although immunogold EM studies do not reveal increased NMDA receptor density in the stratum lacunosum-moleculare (Nicholson et al., 2006). Finally, PP synapses are inhibited by dopamine, serotonin, and noradrenaline (norepinephrine) to a much greater degree than SC synapses (Otmakhova and Lisman, 2000).

Numerous inhibitory neurons also target CA1 pyramidal neurons. Some of these interneurons target the soma and axon, and others target the dendrites. This selective targeting suggests that the PP and SC synapses are under differential control of different populations of interneurons. For example, the oriens-alveus/lacunosum-moleculare (O-LM) interneurons project a single axon to the stratum lacunosum-moleculare region of CA1, where the axon collateralizes extensively and forms synapses on the same dendritic branches as the PP synapses from entorhinal cortex. (For more details on interneuron targeting, see Section 5.9 and Chapter 8.) Despite the differential targeting of the various interneurons in CA1, a common feature is that they all use γ-aminobutyric acid (GABA) as the principal neurotransmitter. GABA activates GABA$_A$ (ionotropic Cl$^-$ channels) and GABA$_B$ receptors (G protein receptors coupled to K$^+$ channel activation). GABA$_A$ receptor function, however, is inhomogeneous, with more rapid kinetics associated with proximal GABA$_A$ receptors and slower kinetics associated with more distal GABA$_A$ receptors (Pearce, 1993).

CA1 pyramidal neurons also receive neuromodulatory inputs from a number of subcortical nuclei. A large input arriving from the septum contains cholinergic afferents (Swanson et al., 1987). Projections from the locus coeruleus contain noradrenergic inputs; the raphe nuclei projections contain serotonergic inputs; and the ventral tegmental area sends dopaminergic afferents to the hippocampus (Storm-Mathisen, 1977). CA1 pyramidal neurons express numerous receptor subtypes for each of these neuromodulators, but their distribution is not always uniform throughout various subcellular domains. For example, dopamine receptors are localized preferentially in the stratum lacunosum-moleculare (Swanson et al., 1987; Goldsmith and Joyce, 1994), suggesting that neuromodulation via this pathway is selectively positioned to influence PP synapses to a greater extent than SC

synapses (Otmakhova and Lisman, 1999). Similarly, the noradrenergic fibers from the locus coeruleus project preferentially to the stratum lacunosum-moleculare region of CA1 (Pasquier and Reinoso-Suarez, 1978).

5.2.4 Axon Morphology and Synaptic Targets

A single axon emanates from the pyramidal soma of CA1 pyramidal neurons and projects through the stratum oriens and into the alveus. CA1 axons branch extensively, forming collaterals with several targets, both within and beyond the hippocampus. In the CA1 subfield, CA1 axons form a limited arbor restricted primarily to the stratum oriens; very few collaterals enter the stratum radiatum (Amaral et al., 1991). Anatomical and physiological analyses indicate that CA1 neurons show a remarkably low connection probability of about 1% (Knowles and Schwartzkroin, 1981; Deuchars and Thomson, 1996). Thus, unlike CA3 pyramidal neurons, CA1 cells do not make many connections among themselves, except in the developing hippocampus (Tamamaki et al., 1987; Amaral et al., 1991; Aniksztejn et al., 2001). By contrast, CA1-interneuron connectivity is much higher, and the strength of excitatory postsynaptic potentials (EPSPs) on interneurons is powerful (Gulyás et al., 1993a; Ali et al., 1998; Csicsvari et al., 1998; Marshall et al., 2002). Because the CA1 axon does not enter the stratum radiatum, local synaptic connections onto other CA1 neurons occur on basal dendrites. Interneurons outside the stratum oriens are not significantly contacted by CA1 axons.

The most significant intrahippocampal connection of CA1 neurons is to pyramidal neurons in the subiculum (Tamamaki et al., 1987; Tamamaki and Nojyo, 1990; Amaral et al., 1991). This connection is likely to be especially important because the subiculum forms a powerful output of the hippocampus (see Section 5.4). CA1 axons collateralize extensively in the subiculum but form a topographical projection. CA1 neurons closest to the subiculum contact their nearest neighbors in the proximal subiculum, whereas CA1 neurons farther from the subiculum project to the most distal regions of the subiculum (see Chapter 3). Collaterals from individual CA1 axons form a column extending the full height of the subiculum (500 μm in the rat) occupying about one-third the width of the subiculum (250–300 μm) and extending about 2 mm along the septo-temporal length of the hippocampus (Tamamaki et al., 1987; Tamamaki and Nojyo, 1990).

The extrahippocampal projections of CA1 neurons via the fimbria depend on their position along the septo-temporal axis (Fig. 5–1A). Septal CA1 neurons project to retrosplenial and perirhinal cortex as well as to the lateral septal nucleus and the diagonal band of Broca. Midsepto-temporal CA1 neurons project to the taenia tecta and medial frontal cortex. Temporal CA1 neurons project to the taenia tecta, medial frontal cortex, anterior olfactory nucleus, olfactory bulb, nucleus accumbens, basal nucleus of the amygdala, and anterior and dorsomedial hypothalamus (Jay et al., 1989; van Groen and Wyss, 1990; Amaral and Witter, 1995). Importantly, however, not all CA1 neurons project to each of these regions. For example, only a subset of CA1 pyramidal neurons, along with a population of giant, nonpyramidal principal neurons, project to the olfactory bulb (van Groen and Wyss, 1990; Gulyás et al., 1998).

No studies have explicitly quantified the total axonal length or number of synapses formed by CA1 axon collaterals. More extensive data are available for the CA3 axon, which is discussed in Section 5.3.4. Light microscopic studies indicate, however, that the CA1 axon, which has a diameter of less than 1 μm, has numerous en passant and terminal synaptic specializations along its length (Tamamaki and Nojyo, 1990). The total number of synaptic connections is likely on the order of several thousand.

5.2.5 Resting Potential and Action Potential Firing Properties

CA1 pyramidal neurons have resting potentials, recorded in slice preparations, in the range of −60 to −70 mV. Similar values have been recorded using either sharp microelectrodes or patch pipettes (e.g., Storm, 1987; Spruston and Johnston, 1992; Staff et al., 2000). At birth, resting potentials are 5 to 10 mV depolarized from this value but gradually hyperpolarize to their adult value by 2 to 3 weeks of age (Spiegelman et al., 1992). In response to depolarizing current injections, action potentials typically have a threshold in the range of −40 to −50 mV (Spruston and Johnston, 1992; Staff et al., 2000; but see Fricker et al., 1999). Thus, CA1 neurons must be depolarized by about 20 mV before action potentials are triggered in vitro. The resulting action potentials have amplitudes of about 100 mV.

The data discussed above are from recordings made in hippocampal slices. Such measurements provide good estimates of the intrinsic properties of CA1 neurons, but the values may be slightly different in an active network. In vivo the ongoing synaptic activity causes action potentials at a rate of 1 to 10 Hz, and the average membrane potential between spikes is sometimes as much as 10 mV depolarized from the in vitro measurements (Henze and Buzsáki, 2001). During locomotion through a place field, action potential firing transiently increases to rates of around 8 Hz (theta frequency), with occasional bursts of high-frequency action potential firing (> 100 Hz) (Frank et. al. 2001) (see Chapter 11).

Action potential firing patterns in vivo are determined in part by the timing of synaptic inputs and in part by the intrinsic firing properties of CA1 neurons. The intrinsic firing properties of CA1 neurons have been studied extensively in the slice preparation, in which it is relatively easy to obtain recordings and to isolate the effects of intrinsic properties on spike firing due to the low rate of spontaneous background synaptic input. Under these conditions, brief depolarizing current injections typically elicit a single action potential followed by four after-potentials (Storm, 1987, 1990): (1) a fast afterhyperpolarization (AHP); (2) an after-depolarization (ADP); (3) a medium AHP; and (4) a slow AHP (Fig. 5–2A). A fast K^+ conductance gated by voltage and Ca^{2+} (named I_C or BK)

contributes to the fast AHP, whereas a slow, Ca^{2+}-activated K^+ conductance contributes to the slow AHP (I_{AHP}, mediated by SK channels). A K^+ conductance reduced by muscarinic receptor activation (I_M) and I_C contribute to the medium AHP (Storm, 1990) (Fig. 5–2B). The ADP is mediated in part by a Ca^{2+} tail current mediated by R-type Ca^{2+} channels (Metz et al., 2005) and may also have a contribution from persistent Na^+ current (Yue et al., 2005).

Action potentials in CA1 pyramidal neurons typically have a half-width of about 1 ms (Staff et al., 2000). In mature rats, repolarization is slowed by application of either tetraethylammonium (TEA) or 4-aminopyridine (4-AP) at concentrations that block the delayed rectifier K^+ current, the inactivating A-type and D-type K^+ currents, and fast voltage- and Ca^{2+}-gated K^+ currents (Storm, 1987; Golding et al., 1999). Such results suggest that a variety of voltage-gated and Ca^{2+}-sensitive K^+ currents contribute to action-potential repolarization as well as the various phases of the AHP (Storm, 1990) (Fig. 5–2B).

Longer depolarizing current injections via somatic recording electrodes typically elicit continuous action potential firing at a rate that is roughly proportional to the amount of current injected. These spike trains usually exhibit spike-frequency accommodation: a high frequency of action potentials at the beginning of a step current injection followed by a gradual reduction in spike frequency later in the current injection (Madison and Nicoll, 1984) (Fig. 5–2C$_1$). Spike-frequency accommodation is caused by gradual activation of K^+ conductances such as I_M and I_{AHP} (Lancaster and Adams, 1986; Lancaster and Nicoll, 1987). These K^+ currents increase cumulatively during the action potential train because they do not inactivate and also deactivate slowly, resulting in a larger AHP and longer times to repolarize back to threshold for the next spike. Trains of action potentials are followed by an after-hyperpolarization (AHP) lasting more than a second (Fig. 5–2C$_2$); and the amplitude of each of these AHPs increases with the number of action potentials in the preceding train (Hotson and Prince, 1980; Madison and Nicoll, 1984) owing to increased Ca^{2+} entry and activation of SK-type Ca^{2+}-activated K^+ channels (Marrion and Tavalin, 1998; Bowden et al., 2001).

K^+ currents that are activated below threshold for action potentials can also affect spike-firing patterns. The best example of this is the delay to firing of the first action potential observed with current injections just above threshold. K^+ conductances, such as A-type and D-type K^+ currents, can be activated by subthreshold depolarizations, thus keeping the membrane potential from reaching the action potential threshold. As these conductances inactivate, however, their hyperpolarizing influence is removed, allowing the membrane to reach threshold. The delay to first spike is partly determined, therefore, by the activation and inactivation rates of subthreshold K^+ currents (Storm, 1990).

A common feature of action-potential firing patterns in vivo is bursting (Kandel and Spencer, 1961; Ranck, 1973; Fox and Ranck, 1975; Suzuki and Smith, 1985; Frank et al., 2001),

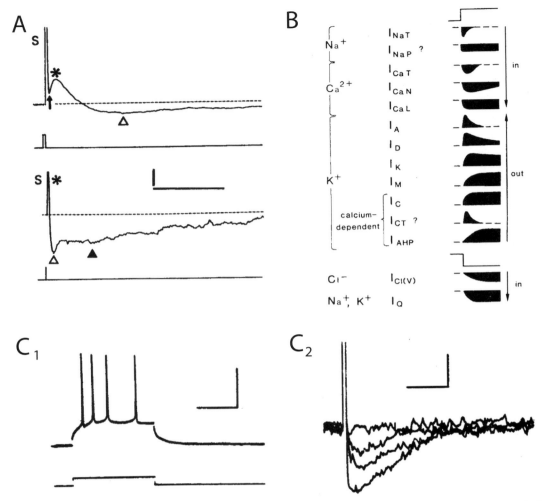

Figure 5–2. CA1 spike frequency adaptation and slow after-hyperpolarization (AHP). *A.* Four after-potentials following single spikes (S) in CA1 pyramidal neurons: (1) fast AHP (↑); (2) after-depolarization (ADP) (∗); (3) medium AHP (Δ); and (4) slow AHP (▲). The lower trace is on a slower time scale. Bar = 5 mV, 50 ms (top) or 5 mV, 500 ms (bottom). Spikes are truncated. (*Source:* Adapted from Storm, 1987.) *B.* Overview of a variety of voltage- and Ca²⁺-dependent currents in hippocampal pyramidal neurons: transient Na⁺ current (I_{NaT}); persistent Na⁺ current (I_{NaP}); T-type Ca²⁺ current (I_{CaT}); N-type Ca²⁺ current (I_{CaN}); L-type Ca²⁺ current (I_{CaL}); fast transient K⁺ current (I_A); delay K⁺ current (I_D); delayed rectifier K⁺ current (I_K); M current (I_M); fast Ca²⁺-dependent K⁺ current (I_C); transient Ca²⁺-dependent K⁺ current (I_{CT}); slow Ca²⁺-dependent K⁺ current (I_{AHP}); voltage-dependent Cl⁻ current ($I_{Cl(V)}$); hyperpolarization-activated mixed cation current ($I_Q = I_H$). (*Source:* Adapted from Storm, 1990.) *C.* Spike-frequency adaptation and the slow AHP in CA1 pyramidal neurons. C_1 shows a train of adapting action potentials in response to a step current injection. Bar = 40 mV and 2 nA vertical and 40 ms horizontal. C_2 shows the slow AHP corresponding to 1, 4, 5, and 7 action potentials. Bar = 5 mV, 1 second. (*Source:* Adapted from Madison and Nicoll, 1984.

defined broadly as a brief period of high-frequency spiking (> 100 Hz) followed by a longer period of inactivity. The relative contributions of synaptic drive and intrinsic membrane properties to the burst firing of CA1 neurons in vivo are unclear. Although CA1 cells exhibit some intrinsic bursting under normal in vitro conditions (Wong and Prince, 1981; Masukawa et al., 1982), it is modest compared to other neurons, such as pyramidal neurons of subiculum, which burst much more robustly (see Section 5.4.4). In the absence of a strong intrinsic burst mechanism, bursting may occur as a consequence of large synaptic inputs, which could transiently increase the action potential firing rate. The intrinsic properties of CA1 neurons may, however, provide an additional contribution to bursting in vivo.

In vitro studies have identified two types of intrinsic bursting in CA1 neurons: Low-threshold bursting occurs in response to somatic current injections just above action potential threshold; they are generated when the ADP that follows an action potential is large enough to trigger additional action potentials (Jensen et al., 1994; Metz et al., 2005; Yue et al., 2005). High-threshold bursting occurs in response to strong dendritic current injection or synaptic activation and is caused by the generation of Ca^{2+} spikes in CA1 dendrites (Wong and Prince, 1978; Golding et al., 1999; Magee and Carruth, 1999) (see Section 5.2.11).

A variety of factors influence the spike-firing mode of CA1 pyramidal neurons. Increasing extracellular K^+, decreasing extracellular Ca^{2+}, and decreasing osmolarity all enhance bursting through different mechanisms (Jensen et al., 1994; Azouz et al., 1997; Su et al., 2002). Bursting is also likely to be a target of modulation by neurotransmitters. For example, cholinergic activation facilitates the induction of plateau potentials, which may be associated with some kinds of burst firing in vivo (Fraser and MacVicar, 1996). Because so many factors influence bursting, it is important to determine the mechanism of bursting under conditions mimicking in vivo states as closely as possible. Intrinsic burst-firing mechanisms have also been implicated as targets of epileptogenesis in the hippocampus (Wong et al., 1986), so understanding the pathophysiology of bursting may lead to new treatments of epilepsy.

A number of aspects of pyramidal cell physiology are also under modulatory control. Activation of muscarinic receptors causes depolarization and a reduction in spike-frequency accommodation due to inhibition of I_M, I_{AHP}, and voltage-insensitive K^+ conductances (Benardo and Prince, 1982a,b,c; Madison et al., 1987; Benson et al., 1988). Norepinephrine also reduces spike-frequency accommodation due to inhibition of I_{AHP} (Madison and Nicoll, 1982; Pedarzani and Storm, 1996). Dopamine causes hyperpolarization and elevated action-potential threshold owing in part to activation of Ca^{2+}-sensitive K^+ conductances; it also raises the action-potential threshold in CA1 neurons (Benardo and Prince, 1982d,e; Stanzione et al., 1984). Serotonin has biphasic effects on CA1 neurons, initially causing hyperpolarization owing to activation of a K^+ current, but later causing depolarization

and inhibition of the AHP (Andrade and Nicoll, 1987; Ropert, 1988). Numerous other modulatory effects have been reported in CA1 neurons, indicating that the resting and active properties of these neurons in vivo are likely to depend on behavioral states.

5.2.6 Resting Membrane Properties

One key to understanding neurons at the cellular level is to be able to predict action potential output in response to a given spatiotemporal pattern of synaptic inputs. In addition to the properties of the synapses themselves, a neuron's response to a synaptic input depends on three things: its dendritic geometry and the location of the synapse(s), its passive membrane properties, and its active membrane properties. Passive membrane properties are those that do not depend on membrane potential (i.e., they are linear). Active membrane properties, by contrast, do depend on membrane potential (e.g., the voltage-gated Na^+ and K^+ channels that mediate the action potential, which are highly nonlinear). These properties are very much interdependent, but physiologists attempt to treat them separately, as we do in our discussion here. One justification for doing this is that detailed neuronal simulations require a description of the passive membrane properties, which constitute a foundation on which active membrane properties are superimposed.

CA1 pyramidal neurons, like most neurons in the brain, have long and extensively branching dendrites. A quantitative understanding of how membrane potential changes (such as EPSPs) spread through these structures requires a theoretical treatment of dendrites combined with experimental measurements. Wilfrid Rall provided the theoretical framework with his seminal work on the "cable theory" (Box 5–1). Hippocam-

---

Box 5–1
Cable Theory

During the 1950s and 60s, Wilfrid Rall developed a theory for treating the flow of current in passive dendrites. The seminal articles comprising this theory have been compiled and republished in book form (Segev et al., 1995). Because the theory was based on a theory similar to that for trans-Atlantic telegraph cables, it is referred to as the "cable theory." With this mathematical treatment, neurons are considered to be long, leaky cables immersed in a conductive medium (cerebrospinal fluid). A synaptic current propagating along a passive dendrite is influenced by three factors: membrane resistance, membrane capacitance, and axial (or intracellular) resistance. These properties depend in part on geometry (narrower dendrites have higher membrane resistance, smaller capacitance, and higher axial resistance) and in part on the composition of the membrane and cytoplasm. In his theory, Rall defined three geometry-independent variables: membrane resistivity (R_m), specific membrane capacitance (C_m), and intracellular resistivity (R_i). He also used two useful measures. The first is called the "space constant" (λ), which is equal to the length, in an infinitely long cable, over which the membrane potential decays to $1/e$ of its original value. The second is the "electrotonic length" ($L = l/\lambda$), which is the ratio of the physical length to the space constant, a measure of the total electrical length of a finite cable.

(Continued)

Box 5–1
Cable Theory *(Continued)*

Rall also showed that a class of branching dendritic trees with certain characteristics could be collapsed to an "equivalent cylinder" with a characteristic L. He also described methods for estimating L experimentally. Because most neurons deviate from the assumptions necessary to collapse them to a single cable, however, the lasting impact of Rall's cable theory is that it provides the foundation for modern computational analysis of neurons. Properties such as dendritic structure and R_m (and possibly R_i, but less so C_m) differ across different types of neurons and influence their integrative properties, which can be predicted using computer models.

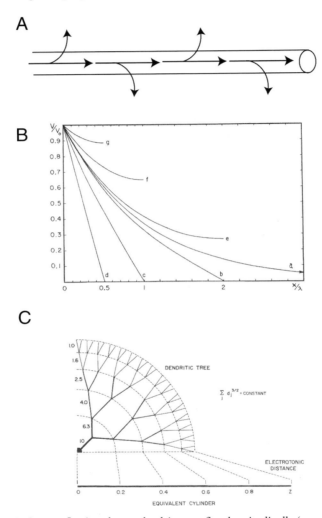

Box Fig. 5–1. *A.* Current flowing along a dendrite may flow longitudinally (e.g., toward the soma), or it may leak out across the dendritic membrane. *B.* Voltage attenuates with distance along a dendritic cable in a way that depends on R_m, R_i, and dendritic geometry. Curve a shows the decay of voltage in a semi-infinite cylinder. Curves b–d show attenuation in finite, open-ended cylinders of decreasing length. Curves e–g show attenuation in finite, closed-end cylinders of decreasing length. All curves are for dendritic cylinders with R_m, R_i and diameter yielding a space constant of 1. (*Source*: Adapted from Rall, 1959.) *C.* Dendritic trees with particular geometries can be collapsed to an equivalent cylinder representation. Two criteria must be met: At each branch point, the diameter of the parent dendrite, raised to the 3/2 power, must equal the sum of the daughter-dendrite diameters, each raised to the 3/2 power. In addition, each dendritic branch must terminate at the same electrotonic length.
(*Source*: Adapted from Rall, 1964.)

pal neurons were among the first to have their cable properties determined experimentally. Initially, microelectrode recordings were used to estimate the electrotonic length (L) of CA1 pyramidal neurons (Brown et al., 1981; Johnston, 1981). These estimates proved to be of limited value, however, because CA1 dendrites clearly violate the conditions required to collapse them to a single cylinder (Mainen et al., 1996). For example, basal, apical, and oblique dendritic branches terminate at different electrotonic distances (Turner, 1984; Pyapali et al., 1998). Furthermore, there are indications that the membrane properties that contribute to L are not uniform over the surface of the dendritic tree (Golding et al., 2005). For these reasons, a more accurate picture of the passive behavior of the CA1 dendritic tree is best achieved by computer simulation methods, which facilitate the characterization based on the measured geometry and membrane properties of CA1 pyramidal neurons.

The most reliable measures of the parameters affecting cable properties—R_m, C_m, R_i—come from patch-clamp recordings made in hippocampal slices. Earlier estimates of these parameters using microelectrodes were affected by the leak that is introduced by microelectrode penetration (Spruston and Johnston, 1992; Staley et al., 1992). Patch-clamp recordings are not without their own problems, namely the possible complications introduced by dialysis of the cytoplasm. There is good evidence, however, that this problem does not affect passive membrane properties substantially (Spruston and Johnston, 1992; Staff et al., 2000). More serious problems are posed by the voltage-gated channels that are active near the resting potential, as well as differences between in vitro and in vivo conditions (see below).

Passive membrane properties are typically estimated by measuring the response of a neuron to a step current injection. Two features define the response: the steady-state amplitude and the time course of the voltage change. Theoretically, this time course can be described by the sum of several exponentials, with the slowest component having a time constant equal to the membrane time constant (τ_m), given by the product $R_m C_m$. The steady-state voltage response (ΔV) is determined by the neuron's input resistance (R_N) in a way that depends on R_m and geometry (large neurons with many dendrites and low R_m have the lowest R_N). Input resistance can be measured directly using Ohm's law ($R_N = \Delta V / \Delta I$), but determination of R_m (from τ_m) requires a value of C_m. Because C_m is largely dependent on the lipid composition of the membrane, its value has long been assumed to be nearly constant at 1 $\mu F/cm^2$, an assumption that was validated by experimental measurements of capacitance in cells with simple geometry (Gentet et al., 2000). Estimates of C_m from neurons with more complex geometry are often close to this value; in instances where substantial deviations are reported, however, it is difficult to know if these reflect real variability in C_m or the extreme difficulty of accurately reconstructing the surface area of neurons with branching dendrites studded with spines. Most estimates of R_m have therefore been derived by measuring τ_m and assuming a value for C_m of 1 $\mu F/cm^2$.

Another complication when determining R_m is the presence of voltage-gated channels that are open at the resting membrane potential. Investigators typically seek to minimize the contribution from activation or deactivation of these channels by making the evoked voltage change small (e.g., 1–5 mV). In CA1 pyramidal neurons, however, this problem cannot be avoided entirely because of the presence of a powerful hyperpolarization-activated, nonspecific-cation current (I_h) that is active at rest (Halliwell and Adams, 1982; Spruston and Johnston, 1992). This conductance introduces a noticeable "sag" in the voltage response. Hyperpolarizing voltage responses activate I_h, resulting in a gradual return of V_m toward the resting potential during the current injection (hyperpolarizing "sag"). Depolarizing voltage responses deactivate I_h, similarly resulting in a gradual return of V_m toward the resting potential (depolarizing "sag"). The presence of I_h-mediated sag makes it difficult or impossible to determine τ_m. To solve this problem, τ_m is usually measured with I_h blocked by bath application of 2 to 5 mM CsCl or 50 to 100 μM ZD7288. Under these conditions, CA1 pyramidal neurons from adult rats and guinea pigs have an R_N of about 120 to 150 MΩ and τ_m of about 35 to 40 ms (Spruston and Johnston, 1992; Staff et al., 2000; Golding et al., 2005) (Fig. 5–3). Assuming a C_m of 1 $\mu F/cm^2$, this corresponds to an R_m of about 40,000 Ωcm^2 (to understand the units of R_m, it may help to understand that the units of its inverse are conductance per unit area). It is important to realize, however, that these values are strongly affected by blocking I_h. In the absence of its blockers, R_N is 38% to 54% lower, and the membrane potential changes decay accordingly faster (Spruston and Johnston, 1992; Staff et al., 2000; Golding et al., 2005).

In guinea pig CA1 neurons, hyperpolarizations or depolarizations of about 5 mV from rest result in about a 20% decrease and increase in R_N, respectively (Hotson et al., 1979; Spruston and Johnston, 1992). Even after block of I_h, estimates of R_m and R_N are sensitive to small changes in the resting membrane potential, but in the opposite direction of the voltage dependence caused by I_h. These findings indicate that the experimental estimates of these parameters are influenced by multiple voltage-gated conductances; therefore, these parameters may never be truly passive. Thus, it may be more appropriate to refer to the "resting membrane properties" of CA1 neurons, which should be regarded as approximations of the theoretical "passive" membrane properties.

Despite the voltage dependence of these parameters, estimates of their values near rest are essential because they provide important parameters for computer models of neurons. One of the purposes of constructing such models, using methods originally developed by Rall (Segev et al., 1995) and currently incorporated into user-friendly programs such as NEURON (http://www.yale.edu) and GENESIS (http://www.genesis-sim.org/GENESIS/), is to estimate how synaptic potentials attenuate between the dendrites and the soma. Such estimates, however, are highly dependent on the intracellular resistivity, R_i. This parameter is best estimated using computer models of carefully reconstructed neurons along with a meas-

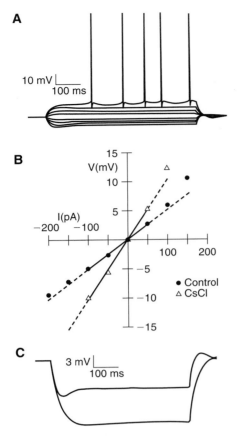

Figure 5–3. CA1 passive properties and sag. *A.* Voltage responses to step current injections from –200 to +200 pA in 50-pA increments. *B.* Voltage–current plot of the steady-state responses shown in *A*, as well as similar responses following the addition of 5 mM CsCl to the bath. Solid lines are the points used for linear fits to the data. Dashed lines are extrapolations of the fits. *C.* Effect of 5 mM CsCl on the hyperpolarizing voltage response to a current step of –150 pA. Note the block of the sag in the voltage response. (*Source:* Adapted from Staff et al., 2000.)

ure of voltage attenuation. Modeling of neurons from which attenuation was measured with simultaneous somatic and dendritic patch-clamp electrodes yielded a value for R_i of about 180 Ωcm for CA1 pyramidal neurons (Golding et al., 2005). This study also revealed that the membrane resistivity of CA1 neurons is nonuniform, with the dendritic membrane increasingly leaky at greater distances from the soma. Similarly, I_h, which is activated at rest and therefore increases voltage attenuation in dendrites, also increases with distance from the soma (Magee, 1998; Golding et al., 2005) (see Section 5.2.13).

5.2.7 Implications for Voltage-Clamp Experiments in CA1 Neurons

Knowledge of the structure and membrane properties of CA1 neurons allows predictions regarding the functional coupling of the soma and dendrites. Detailed compartmental modeling of CA1 neurons suggests that functional coupling between the

soma and distal dendrites is limited. One of the interesting consequences of this is that it makes it extremely difficult to study synaptic or voltage-gated conductances in dendrites using electrodes placed at the soma. Space-clamp errors are likely to be enormous for distal conductances and substantial even for relatively proximal conductances (Spruston et al., 1993, 1994; Major et al., 1994; Mainen et al., 1996). These errors are greatest for transient conductance changes; and even when measures of steady-state voltage control (such as reversal potential measurements) indicate reasonable voltage control, errors can be very large for the transient case. The presence of voltage-gated conductances in dendrites, though presumably advantageous for the normal function of the neuron, makes it still more difficult to control dendritic membrane potential using somatic electrodes. Thus, other methods are needed to complement somatic recordings to determine the functional properties of dendrites. Fortunately, several such methods are now available (see Sections 5.2.11 through 5.2.13).

5.2.8 Attenuation of Synaptic Potentials in CA1 Dendrites

The functional significance of the dendritic tree, with these nonuniform membrane properties and high R_i, is perhaps best understood by considering the extent to which synaptic potentials attenuate as they propagate from the dendrite to the soma. Compartmental models constrained by simultaneous recordings have been used to predict synaptic attenuation, and the results are striking. Distal synaptic inputs are expected to attenuate many times 10-fold from the most distal sites to the soma (Mainen et al., 1996; Andreasen and Lambert, 1998; Golding et al., 2005) (Fig. 5–4). Most of this enormous attenuation occurs between the synapse and the primary apical dendrite, but direct dendritic recordings indicate an additional three- to fourfold attenuation between dendritic sites at about 300 μm and the soma. The structure of the CA1 dendritic tree appears to maximize synaptic attenuation (Jaffe and Carnevale, 1999), a point that is considered in more detail below by way of comparison to dentate granule cells (see Section 5.5.5).

The severe synaptic attenuation predicted on the basis of in vitro studies and modeling might even be an underestimate of the attenuation that could occur in passive dendrites in vivo. Because dendrites are constantly receiving synaptic inputs, attenuation may be enhanced by the increased conductance produced at active synapses (Destexhe and Pare, 1999). The magnitude of this effect, however, has not been directly determined in the hippocampus.

5.2.9 Mechanisms of Compensation for Synaptic Attenuation in CA1 Dendrites

Faced with this much attenuation, it seems almost pointless for a CA1 neuron to have synapses on its distal dendrites. Yet a large number of axons (primarily the perforant path input from the entorhinal cortex) do synapse on distal apical

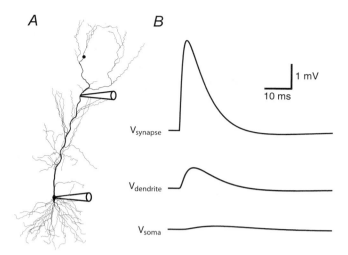

Figure 5–4. CA1 dendritic attenuation of synaptic potentials. Simulations of excitatory postsynaptic potential (EPSP) attenuation from the apical tuft to the soma. A model with nonuniform R_m and G_h was used in the simulation. The synaptic conductance was 1 nS with a rise time constant of 0.5 ms and a decay time constant of 5 ms. *A.* The synapse location is indicated by the black dot in the apical dendrite, 583 μm from the soma. The somatic and dendritic recording sites are indicated by the electrode cartoons (dendritic recording electrode at 365 μm). *B.* Example of simulated EPSPs in response to activation of the distal apical synapse (black dot in *A*) and measured at the synapse, the dendritic recording site, and the soma. In this example the EPSP attenuates 26-fold between the synapse and the soma. (*Source:* Adapted from Golding et al., 2005.)

dendrites. Even Schaffer collaterals, the excitatory axons from CA3, form many synapses on relatively distal dendritic regions. Two mechanisms are likely to overcome this problem of "dendritic disadvantage." First, there is now evidence that the average synaptic conductance in the stratum radiatum increases as a function of distance from the soma (Magee and Cook, 2000). The synapses at distal sites may have larger conductances as a result of an increased abundance of large, perforated synapses and a higher density of AMPA-type glutamate receptors (Andrasfalvy and Magee, 2001; Smith et al., 2003; Nicholson et al., 2006). However, both computer simulations and electron microscopy indicate that this principal of "synaptic scaling" to compensate for dendritic distance does not extend into the most distal apical dendrites, where the perforant-path fibers form synapses (Kali and Freund, 2005; Nicholson et al., 2006).

The perforant-path input to CA1 pyramidal neurons thus appears to be disadvantaged because EPSPs from this input attenuate so much on their way to the soma, and they apparently lack a conductance scaling mechanism to compensate. Exacerbating the problem is feedforward inhibition, which is so powerful, the excitatory nature of the perforant path inputs to CA1 was once in question (Buzsáki et al., 1995; Empson and Heinemann, 1995a,b; Soltesz, 1995; Andreasen and Lambert, 1998). It is now clear, however, that this input is excitatory (Doller and Weight, 1982; Yeckel and Berger, 1990,

1995) and that it is capable of discharging CA1 cells in vivo, even after lesions that reduce or eliminate input from Schaffer collaterals (McNaughton et al., 1989; Brun et al., 2002).

For perforant path synapses to have a significant impact on CA1 output, some mechanism must compensate for dendritic attenuation. One possibility is that distal synapses may result in significant somatic depolarization through amplification by voltage-gated channels in dendrites. Although this may occur in a graded fashion in the dendrites or the soma (Lipowsky et al., 1996; Cook and Johnston, 1997, 1999; Andreasen and Lambert, 1999), amplification may also occur through the generation of dendritic spikes (see Sections 5.2.11 through 5.5.13). Another possibility is that distal synapses normally do not exert a strong influence over action-potential initiation on their own but may interact effectively with more proximal synaptic activation to trigger action potentials (Remondes and Schuman, 2002). Such interactions may occur in two ways. First, the distal, perforant path EPSP may sum with more proximal, Schaffer collateral EPSPs to reach threshold for an action potential in the soma or the apical dendrite (Levy et al., 1995; Jarsky et al., 2005; Kali and Freund, 2005). Second, strong activation of perforant-path synapses can lead to dendritic spikes, which only propagate effectively to the soma when facilitated by coincident activation of the Schaffer collateral synapses (Jarsky et al., 2005).

5.2.10 Pyramidal Neuron Function: Passive Versus Active Dendrites

Even without much information about membrane properties, many neuroscientists predicted that synaptic potentials would attenuate severely as they propagate toward the soma if dendrites were truly passive. To counter the unlikely proposition that distal dendritic synapses are irrelevant, some investigators proposed that dendrites might contain voltage-gated conductances; others, however, took the view that voltage-gated channels were a unique property of the axon (reviewed in Llinás, 1988; Adams, 1992). Although the debate over passive versus active dendrites got started with studies of spinal motoneurons, the hippocampus soon took center stage, as its laminar structure and densely packed, uniformly oriented dendrites facilitated studies of dendritic function using extracellular electrodes. Field potential recordings in the CA1 region of the anesthetized rabbit indicated that spikes could be generated in the proximal dendrites of CA1 neurons and subsequently propagated actively away from this site (Cragg and Hamlyn, 1955; Andersen, 1960; Fujita and Sakata, 1962; Andersen and Lomo, 1966; Andersen et al., 1966). These conclusions were later confirmed and elaborated on by more detailed analyses using field potentials, both in vitro and in vivo (Turner et al., 1989, 1991; Herreras, 1990). Another important study was performed by Spencer and Kandel, who made intracellular recordings from CA1 neurons in the anesthetized cat (Spencer and Kandel, 1961). They observed fast, spike-like events that were smaller than action potentials and often preceded full-sized spikes. Based on the absence of such events following antidromic stimulation of the axon, Spencer and Kandel concluded that these "fast prepotentials" originated in dendrites. This view has received some support (Schwartzkroin, 1977; Wong and Stewart, 1992; Turner et al., 1993) but has remained controversial, as action potentials from CA1 neurons coupled by gap junctions have also been implicated (MacVicar and Dudek, 1981; Schmitz et al., 2001). Nevertheless, these studies collectively indicated that the dendrites of CA1 pyramidal neurons are capable of generating active responses owing to the presence of voltage-gated channels.

The view that CA1 dendrites are active received considerable support from studies using microelectrodes to record from CA1 dendrites in slices. These recordings indicated that action potentials could be observed in dendritic recordings, even when dendrites were physically or pharmacologically isolated from the soma (Wong et al., 1979; Benardo et al., 1982; Poolos and Kocsis, 1990; Turner et al., 1991, 1993; Wong and Stewart, 1992; Colling and Wheal, 1994; Andreasen and Lambert, 1995a). Calcium imaging studies also indicated that dendrites could generate active responses capable of activating voltage-gated Ca^{2+} channels and mediating significant Ca^{2+} entry into dendrites (Regehr et al., 1989; Jaffe et al., 1992; Regehr and Tank, 1992; Yuste and Denk, 1995; Yuste et al., 1999). By the late 1980s and early 1990s, such a wealth of data had been accumulated that it was undeniable that CA1 dendrites were active. Attention then shifted to answering more detailed questions about dendritic excitability, including what types of channels are present, what properties they possess, how they are distributed, and how they contribute to the integrative properties of CA1 neurons.

5.2.11 Dendritic Excitability and Voltage-Gated Channels in CA1 Neurons

Studies of dendritic excitability in the hippocampus and elsewhere have been greatly facilitated by the development of methods to routinely record from dendrites in brain slices using patch pipettes (Stuart et al., 1993). The ability to record simultaneously from the soma and the primary apical dendrite (up to about 400 μm from the soma) has been particularly useful. One of the first applications of this method was to address the question of where action potentials are initiated. The classic view was that action potentials are initiated in the axon, but several of the studies discussed above had led to the hypothesis that action potentials might actually be initiated in dendrites. Simultaneous somatic and dendritic recordings in CA1 neurons have indicated that fast, all-or-none action potentials begin near the soma (Spruston et al., 1995; Hoffman et al., 1997; Golding et al., 2001). Based on the sensitivity of the action potential threshold to local application to tetrodotoxin (TTX), the site of action potential initiation has been further narrowed to a region near the first node of Ranvier in the axon (Colbert et al., 1996). Similar results have been obtained in several other types of neurons, suggesting that the axon may have a low threshold for action potential initiation in most

neurons (Stuart et al., 1997). The reasons for this are not clear but are likely related to the density and/or properties of Na^+ channels in the axon (Colbert and Pan, 2002).

Following their initiation in the axon, action potentials invade the dendritic tree of CA1 neurons (Spruston et al., 1995; Golding et al., 2001) (Fig. 5–5A). Application of TTX to the dendrites dramatically reduces the amplitude of these back-propagating action potentials, indicating that Na^+ channels actively enhance action potential propagation in CA1 dendrites (Spruston et al., 1995; Magee and Johnston, 1997; Golding et al., 2002). In keeping with this, Na^+ channels have been recorded directly in cell-attached patches in CA1 dendrites (Magee and Johnston, 1995a,b; Colbert et al., 1997; Jung et al., 1997; Mickus et al., 1999). The amplitude of the back-propagating action potential, however, decreases with distance from the soma, indicating that back-propagation is not fully regenerative. At 300 μm, the back-propagating action potential amplitude is about half of its somatic amplitude (Golding et al., 2001). Attenuation of back-propagating action potentials in the distal half of the apical dendrites is variable. Within a given cell, back-propagation is controlled by the membrane potential and the availability of Na^+ and K^+ channels (Bernard and Johnston, 2003). Between cells, two populations of CA1 neurons have been identified (Golding et al., 2001). In about half of the CA1 neurons, attenuation of the backpropagating action potential from 300 to 400 μm continues at about the same rate as in more proximal dendrites. In the other half of the CA1 neurons, attenuation in this distal region is more pronounced. The relatively strong back-propagation may be promoted by somatic depolarization, as it is not observed with antidromic stimulation (Bernard and Johnston, 2003). The dichotomy of action potential back-propagation observed during somatic current injection suggests that there may be considerable cell-to-cell variability in the densities of ion channels that control action potential back-propagation (Golding et al., 2001).

Although patch-clamp recordings from the basal dendrites of CA1 neurons have not yet been obtained, models based on Na^+ and K^+ channel densities in the apical dendrites predict that action potential propagation into the shorter, basal dendrites is much more reliable (Golding et al., 2001). This finding is in keeping with imaging studies of the basal dendrites in neocortical pyramidal cells, which indicate reliable back-propagation in the basal dendrites (Schiller et al., 1995). Similarly, direct recordings from oblique branches of the apical dendrites have not been obtained, but Ca^{2+} imaging experiments suggest that action potentials actively invade these branches (Frick et al., 2003).

Attenuation of the back-propagating action potential amplitude is even more severe during repetitive spiking (Fig. 5–5A). Even at modest firing frequencies such as 20 Hz, the action potential amplitude, measured about 300 μm from the soma, attenuates to less than half of its amplitude at lower frequencies, equivalent to less than one-fourth of the somatic action potential amplitude (Andreasen and Lambert, 1995a; Callaway and Ross, 1995; Spruston et al., 1995; Golding et al.,

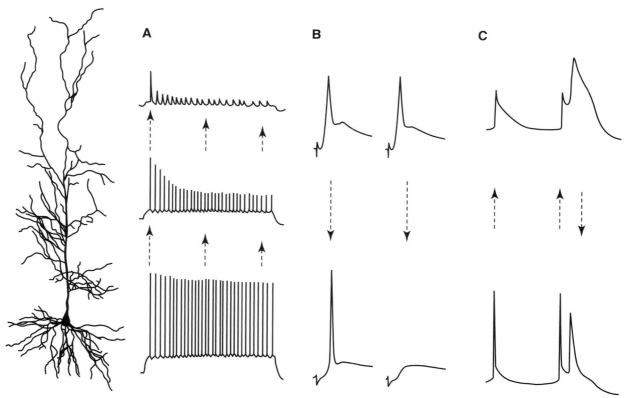

Figure 5–5. CA1 dendritic excitability. *Left.* Camera lucida drawing of a CA1 pyramidal neuron. Three types of dendritic excitability are indicated. (*Source*: Adapted from Golding et al., 1999.) *A.* Trains of back-propagating action potentials are initiated in the soma in response to step current injections and recorded in the dendrites with a second patch-clamp electrode. The somatic and mid-proximal recordings were obtained simultaneously from the same neuron. The more distal dendritic recording was obtained from a different cell. (*Source*: Adapted from Golding et al., 2001.) *B.* Dendritic Na$^+$ spikes were elicited by strong synaptic stimulation in the s.l.m. On one trial the dendritic spike is associated with a somatic action potential, whereas on the other trial only an EPSP is recorded at the soma (i.e., propagation failure). (*Source*: Adapted from Golding and Spruston, 1998.) *C.* Dendritic Ca^{2+} spikes were elicited by a step current injection via a dendritic patch-clamp electrode 160 μm from the soma. The second back-propagating action potential shown is followed by a large, broad dendritic Ca^{2+} spike. Simultaneous somatic recording shows that the dendritic Ca^{2+} spike caused an action potential burst in the soma. (*Source*: Adapted from Golding et al., 1999.)

2001). This activity-dependent back-propagation is mediated by a form of Na$^+$ channel inactivation that recovers very slowly (Colbert et al., 1997; Jung et al., 1997; Mickus et al., 1999). Patch-clamp recordings from CA1 somata and dendrites have revealed that repetitive depolarizations lead to cumulative Na$^+$ channel inactivation. Each brief depolarization forces a fraction of the available Na$^+$ channels into the prolonged inactivated state. Recovery from this state back to the closed (available) state has a time constant of about 1 second at the resting potential (Mickus et al., 1999). This kind of inactivation, which is especially pronounced in the dendrites, results in fewer and fewer dendritic Na$^+$ channels available to support action potential back-propagation during repetitive firing, resulting in progressive reduction in the amplitude of back-propagating action potentials.

Although simultaneous somatic and dendritic patch-clamp recordings indicated that the threshold for action potential initiation was lowest in the axon, these studies did not address the question of whether spikes could, under some conditions, be generated in the dendrites, as earlier studies had suggested (Spencer and Kandel, 1961; Schwartzkroin, 1977; Schwartzkroin and Slawsky 1977; Wong et al., 1979; Benardo et al., 1982; Masukawa and Prince, 1984; Andreasen and Lambert, 1995a). Direct evidence for dendritically generated spikes soon followed from simultaneous somatic and dendritic patch-clamp recordings. When the synaptic stimulus intensity was increased well above the threshold for action potential initiation in the axon, spikes were observed in apical dendritic recordings before the action potential was recorded in the soma (Golding and Spruston, 1998). With GABA$_A$ receptors blocked to increase the excitatory drive to dendrites, two kinds of dendritic spike could be elicited by synaptic stimulation: fast spikes mediated primarily by Na$^+$ channels and slower spikes mediated primarily by Ca^{2+} channels (Golding and Spruston, 1998; Golding et al., 1999) (Fig. 5–5B,C). Intriguingly, these two types of dendritic spike do not propagate reliably to the soma. Dendritic Na$^+$ spikes were often observed in dendritic recordings when no action potential reached the soma, suggesting that these events could be entirely restricted to the dendrites (Golding and Spruston, 1998). As is the case for back-propagation, forward propagation of dendritic Na$^+$ spikes is sensitive to both distance and membrane potential. Spikes initiated more distally are less likely to propagate to the soma successfully, and membrane depolarization enhances the forward propagation of distally generated spikes (Gasparini et al., 2004). Dendritic Ca^{2+} spikes often trigger multiple fast action potentials in the axon and soma but are also isolated to the dendrites in some circumstances (Golding et al., 1999; Wei et al., 2001; Golding et al., 2002). These findings indicate that dendritic Ca^{2+} spikes may function locally or may serve as a mechanism for producing bursts of action potentials in the soma and axon of CA1 neurons. Experiments combining imaging and electrophysiology suggest that spikes can also be generated locally in the basal dendrites of CA1 pyramidal neurons (Ariav et al., 2003).

An important question is whether the dendritic excitability observed in slice experiments also occurs under natural conditions in vivo. Only one study to date has addressed this question directly. Microelectrode recordings from the dendrites of CA1 neurons in anesthetized rats revealed a pattern of dendritic excitability similar to that seen in vitro. Three types of excitability were observed in the in vivo recordings that were putatively attributed to back-propagating action potentials, dendritically generated Na$^+$ spikes, and dendritically generated Ca^{2+} spikes (Kamondi et al., 1998). Putative back-propagating action potentials were identified by their rapid time course and decline in amplitude as a function of distance of the recording from the soma. These events also decayed in amplitude during repetitive firing in a manner similar to back-propagating action potentials in vitro (Kamondi et al., 1998; Golding et al., 2001). In addition to these events, which occurred both spontaneously and in response to current injection through the recording electrode, putative dendritically generated spikes were observed during hippocampal population discharges (sharp waves). These events were either small in amplitude and rapid in time course (putative dendritic Na$^+$ spikes) or large in amplitude and slow in time course (putative dendritic Ca^{2+} spikes).

The dendritic excitability of CA1 pyramidal neurons is not likely to be static but probably changes depending on the behavioral state of the animal. The best direct evidence for this is that dendritic spikes are primarily observed in vivo during sharp waves, which occur only during awake immobility, consummatory behaviors, and slow-wave sleep in rats (Kamondi et al., 1998) (see Chapter 11). Dendritic excitability may also be heterogeneous within CA1, as is seen for action potential invasion of the distal apical dendrites, which exhibits a dichotomy of strong and weak back-propagation (Golding et al., 2001). Several factors are likely to influence dendritic excitability in vivo: the balance and pattern of synaptic excitation and inhibition, previous experience-dependent synaptic and nonsynaptic plasticity, and the neuromodulatory state in the hippocampus.

Inhibition has been shown to influence dendritic excitability in two ways. First, in response to synaptic stimulation in the slice, dendritic spikes occur much more frequently when inhibition is blocked (Golding and Spruston, 1998; Golding et al., 1999). This is consistent with the notion that dendritic spikes are primarily observed during sharp waves, which occur because of strong, synchronous synaptic excitation (Kamondi et al., 1998). Second, inhibition has been shown to limit action potential back-propagation (Buzsáki, 1996; Tsubokawa and Ross, 1996). Both of these observations suggest that inhibition limits dendritic excitability, but it should be noted that it could, if appropriately timed prior to an excitatory input, enhance dendritic excitability by removing inactivation from dendritic Na$^+$ and Ca^{2+} channels.

Activation of neuromodulatory receptors and second messenger systems has also been shown to influence dendritic excitability in a variety of ways. Activation of mitogen-activated protein (MAP) kinase, protein kinase C (PKC), or protein kinase A (PKA) results in downregulation of A-type K$^+$ current in CA1 dendrites and, accordingly, produces an increase in the amplitude of back-propagating action potentials (Hoffman and Johnston, 1998; Yuan et al., 2002). Similar results are also produced by activation of β-adrenergic and muscarinic acetylcholine receptors, which activate the PKA and PKC systems, respectively. Activation of dopaminergic receptors produced a similar effect in a subset of CA1 neurons, suggesting heterogeneity in the responses of CA1 neurons to neuromodulators (Hoffman and Johnston, 1998). Arachidonic acid produces a complementary effect, enhancing the amplitude of back-propagating action potentials via a reduction in dendritic A-type K$^+$ current (Bittner and Müller, 1999; Colbert and Pan, 1999). Muscarinic receptor activation reduces the activity dependence of action potential back-propagation, presumably by reducing prolonged inactivation of Na$^+$ channels (Tsubokawa and Ross, 1997; Colbert and Johnston, 1998). A similar effect has also been observed following rises in intracellular Ca^{2+} evoked by repeated action potential firing (Tsubokawa et al., 2000).

Repeated synaptic activity can also modulate dendritic excitability. Frick and colleagues have shown that pairing of synaptic activity and action potential firing in a theta-burst pattern not only induces synaptic plasticity but also induces long-term enhancement of dendritic excitability (Frick et al., 2004). This enhancement is caused by a leftward shift in the voltage dependence of inactivation for A-type K$^+$ channels, which results in a reduction in the number of channels available to be activated from the resting potential and causes an increase in action potential back-propagation and dendritic Ca^{2+} entry (Frick et al., 2004).

5.2.12 Sources of Ca^{2+} Elevation in CA1 Pyramidal Neuron Dendrites

Calcium imaging experiments have provided considerable insight into the function of CA1 dendrites. These experiments have identified three sources of Ca^{2+} entry. First, dendritic depolarization can activate voltage-gated Ca^{2+} channels. Second, neurotransmitters can activate ligand-gated channels with significant Ca^{2+} permeability, such as the NMDA receptor. Third, Ca^{2+} can be released from intracellular stores in dendrites. Significant interactions have been identified among these mechanisms.

The large dendritic depolarizations produced by back-propagating action potentials and dendritic spikes result in activation of voltage-gated Ca^{2+} channels, which produces Ca^{2+} transients that are not uniform throughout the dendritic tree (Regehr et al., 1989; Jaffe et al., 1992; Yuste and Denk, 1995; Helmchen et al., 1996; Yuste et al., 1999; Golding et al., 2001; Frick et al., 2003). Spatial gradients in Ca^{2+} signals must be interpreted cautiously, as many factors may contribute. Larger Ca^{2+} transients may be produced by greater local depolarization, higher density of Ca^{2+} channels, larger surface-to-volume ratio (smaller dendrites), or weaker Ca^{2+} buffering and extrusion (Volfovsky et al., 1999; Majewska et al., 2000; Murthy et al., 2000). Careful interpretation of the available data suggests, however, that depolarization gradients contribute strongly to the gradients of Ca^{2+} entry observed. For example, back-propagating action potentials tend to produce smaller Ca^{2+} transients in distal dendrites than in proximal dendrites, largely due to the attenuation of the back-propagating action potential with distance from the soma (Jaffe et al., 1992; Christie et al., 1995; Golding et al., 2001). This gradient is enhanced during repetitive firing due to the activity dependence of back-propagation, which results in a steeper depolarization gradient along the dendrites (Golding et al., 2001). Neuromodulators coupled to G proteins reduce the dendritic calcium entry associated with back-propagating action potentials through membrane potential changes and a reduction in current through voltage-gated Ca^{2+} channels (Chen and Lambert, 1997; Sandler and Ross, 1999). Dendritically generated spikes produce a spatial gradient opposite to that produced by back-propagating action potentials, with the largest Ca^{2+} entry in more distal dendrites (Ariav et al., 2003).

Smaller depolarizations, such as those produced by EPSPs, tend to produce smaller Ca^{2+} transients that are even more spatially restricted (Regehr et al., 1989; Miyakawa et al., 1992; Regehr and Tank, 1992; Yuste and Denk, 1995; Yuste et al., 1999; Kovalchuk et al., 2000; Murthy et al., 2000). These Ca^{2+} transients may be produced by activation of NMDA receptors, but in some cases activation of voltage-gated Ca^{2+} channels also contributes. In fact, it can be difficult to dissect the relative contribution of these two mechanisms, as blocking either one reduces dendritic depolarization, which may reduce Ca^{2+} entry through either of these channel types.

Pairing EPSPs with back-propagating action potentials has been shown to produce Ca^{2+} entry that exceeds the sum of the two individual signals in dendritic shafts and spines (Yuste and Denk, 1995; Magee and Johnston, 1997; Yuste et al., 1999). This effect is likely to occur because EPSPs can increase the amplitude of back-propagating action potentials and because the additional depolarization provided by back-prop-

agating action potentials relieves the Mg^{2+} block of NMDA receptors.

Calcium release from intracellular stores has been observed in CA1 dendrites in response to elevation of Ca^{2+} via back-propagating action potentials and by activation of mGluRs coupled to inositol trisphosphate (IP_3) receptors (Bianchi et al., 1999; Nakamura et al., 1999, 2000; Sandler and Barbara, 1999). Again, these two means of activating Ca^{2+} release are not independent, as pairing of action potentials with EPSPs greatly enhances release (Nakamura et al., 1999, 2000). Although intracellular Ca^{2+} release has as yet been observed only in the proximal regions of the primary apical dendrite of CA1 neurons (Nakamura et al., 2000) and spine-restricted Ca^{2+} transients are primarily coupled to activation of NMDA receptors (Yuste and Denk, 1995; Kovalchuk et al., 2000), the presence of endoplasmic reticulum organelles in other regions of the dendrites, including spines (Spacek and Harris, 1997) is consistent with observations of spatially restricted Ca^{2+} release in dendritic spines under some conditions (Emptage et al., 1999).

5.2.13 Distribution of Voltage-Gated Channels in the Dendrites of CA1 Neurons

The subcellular distributions of various subtypes of voltage-gated ion channels have been investigated in CA1 neurons using physiological approaches, as well as antibody binding, in some cases combined with electron microscopy. Physiological studies fall into two categories: direct measurement of ion channel function using cell-attached or cell-excised patches from the soma, axon, and dendrites and indirect assessment of ion channel distribution using whole-cell recording or calcium imaging in combination with ion-channel pharmacology. Direct approaches offer a highly detailed picture of channel distribution and properties in various subcellular compartments, whereas indirect physiological observations have provided a broader perspective and are potentially informative about regions of the dendrites inaccessible to patch-clamp recording.

Early dendritic recordings strongly suggested the presence of voltage-gated Na^+ channels in CA1 apical dendrites, and the reduction of back-propagating action potentials by TTX confirmed this (see Section 5.2.11). Direct recordings of Na^+ channel activity in patches up to about 300 μm from the soma on the primary apical dendrite in CA1 neurons have revealed that Na^+ channels are distributed at an approximately constant density along this region of the dendrite (Magee and Johnston, 1995a) (Fig. 5–6A). Despite the relatively uniform channel density, the properties of the channels change with distance from the soma. Patches obtained at increasing distances from the soma exhibited a greater degree of prolonged inactivation, a feature of the Na^+ channel responsible for the activity dependence of action potential back-propagation (Colbert et al., 1997; Mickus et al., 1999). The reasons for this nonuniformity in channel function are not known but might be mediated by a unique subunit composition (α- and/or β-subunits), differential post-translational modification (e.g., phosphorylation), or protein-protein interactions (e.g., with the cytoskeleton). Little is known about the subcellular distribution of Na^+ channel α-subunits in the hippocampus, though the available data suggest that Nav1.2 is most abundant during the first few postnatal weeks, but that Nav1.6 is the dominant subunit in adults (Schaller and Caldwell, 2000).

Numerous Ca^{2+} imaging studies have demonstrated the presence of voltage-gated Ca^{2+} channels in CA1 dendrites. The presence of depolarization-induced Ca^{2+} transients in dendritic spines suggests that Ca^{2+} channels are also present in these postsynaptic specializations (Yuste and Denk, 1995; Sabatini et al., 2002). One imaging study used a pharmacological approach to determine that high-threshold Ca^{2+} channels are the major contributors to Ca^{2+} entry mediated by back-propagating action potentials in the soma and proximal dendrite, whereas low-threshold Ca^{2+} channels contribute more to the Ca^{2+} signal in the distal dendrites (Christie et al., 1995). The most direct information regarding Ca^{2+} channel distribution was provided by single-channel recordings along the length of the apical dendrite in CA1 neurons (Magee and Johnston, 1995a). This study revealed that the density of Ca^{2+} channels is approximately constant along the length of the apical dendrite, although there was a trend for more high-threshold channels to be encountered in the soma and proximal dendrites and more low-threshold channels to be encountered in more distal dendrites (Fig. 5–6B), which is consistent with the Ca^{2+} imaging results. Such a distribution is also consistent with an antibody-binding study for L-type (high-threshold) Ca^{2+} channels, which indicated the highest density of these channels is in the soma and proximal apical dendrites (Westenbroek et al., 1990). Unfortunately, more detailed information regarding the subcellular distribution of Ca^{2+} and Na^+ channels in hippocampal neurons is not available. The availability of a number of high-quality Ca^{2+} and Na^+ channel antibodies is required to provide this critical information in the future. Such studies will have to be performed using electron microscopy, as Ca^{2+} and Na^+ channels are abundant in both axons and dendrites, making it difficult to determine the presynaptic versus postsynaptic localization of these channels using light microscopy. Although no data are available regarding the subtypes of Ca^{2+} channels in CA1 axons, pharmacological studies of synaptic transmission and presynaptic Ca^{2+} entry indicate that N-, P-, Q-, and R-type Ca^{2+} channels are most abundant in other axon terminals of the hippocampus (Wu and Saggau, 1994; Gasparini et al., 2001; Qian and Noebels, 2001).

Information regarding K^+ channel distribution has also been obtained using both indirect and direct approaches. Cell-attached patch-clamp recordings have provided the most direct information regarding K^+ channel distribution in CA1 dendrites. Patches obtained at different distances from the soma revealed that the density of A-type K^+ channels increases approximately linearly along the primary apical dendrite, whereas the density of noninactivating (or slowly inactivating) K^+ channels is approximately constant (Hoffman et

al., 1997) (Fig. 5–6C). The farthest recordings, about 350 μm from the soma, indicate that the density of the A-type K^+ current is about five times its somatic level. This high density of dendritic A-type K^+ current contributes to a dramatic decline in amplitude of back-propagating action potentials (Hoffman et al., 1997) (see Section 5.2.11).

Ca^{2+} imaging experiments suggest that the density of A-type K^+ channels may be especially high in oblique apical dendrites (Frick et al.. 2003). Consistent with the high density of dendritic A-type K^+ channels, application of 4-AP to the bath or selectively to the apical dendrite results in an increased amplitude of back-propagating action potentials (Hoffman et al., 1997; Magee and Carruth, 1999). 4-AP application also increases the occurrence of dendritic Ca^{2+} spikes, an effect that is likely attributable to block of both A-type and D-type K^+ channels in the dendrites (Andreasen and Lambert, 1995a; Hoffman et al., 1997; Golding et al., 1999; Magee and Carruth, 1999; Cai et al., 2004). The most likely candidates for the α-subunits of the A-type K^+ channel in CA1 neurons are members of the Kv4 family (Sheng et al., 1992; Maletic-Savatic et al., 1995). Consistent with this, enhanced dendritic excitability has been observed in a mouse expressing a Kv4.2 dominant-negative construct (Cai et al., 2004). Pharmacological studies have also revealed that the AHP of back-propagating action potentials is much less sensitive to blockers of BK-type Ca^{2+}-activated K^+ channels than the AHP of somatic action potentials suggesting that there may be a higher density of these channels in the soma than in the apical dendrites (Andreasen and Lambert, 1995b; Poolos and Johnston, 1999). These channels are present in dendrites, however, and they have an important role in repolarizing dendritic Ca^{2+} spikes (Golding et al., 1999).

The hyperpolarization-activated, nonspecific cation current (I_h) is also distributed nonuniformly along the length of the CA1 apical dendrite. Cell-attached patch recordings reveal a linear increase in density along the apical dendrite, with currents at 350 μm approximately six times larger than in the soma (Magee, 1998) (Fig. 5–6D). In fact, I_h may reach an even higher density in more distal dendrites, as immunoreactivity for the channel is most intense in the distal dendrites (Santoro et al., 1997; Lorincz et al., 2002). This is also consistent with the dramatic increase in I_h observed in patch recordings from the distal dendrites of layer V pyramidal neurons (Williams and Stuart, 2000; Berger et al., 2001). In addition to the direct patch recordings, imaging studies reveal a large dendritic Na^+ entry activated by hyperpolarization in hippocampal neurons (Tsubokawa et al., 1999). Modeling the effects of blocking I_h on voltage attenuation in CA1 dendrites is also consistent with a high density of I_h in CA1 apical dendrites (Golding et al., 2005). Of the four I_h genes cloned so far, HCN 1, 2, and 4 are the most abundant in CA1 neurons (Moosmang et al., 1999; Santoro et al., 2000; Bender et al., 2001). The presence of a high density of I_h channels in CA1 dendrites has some interesting functional consequences, which are discussed below.

These examples highlight the point that many channels (e.g., A-type K^+ and I_h channels) are distributed nonuni-

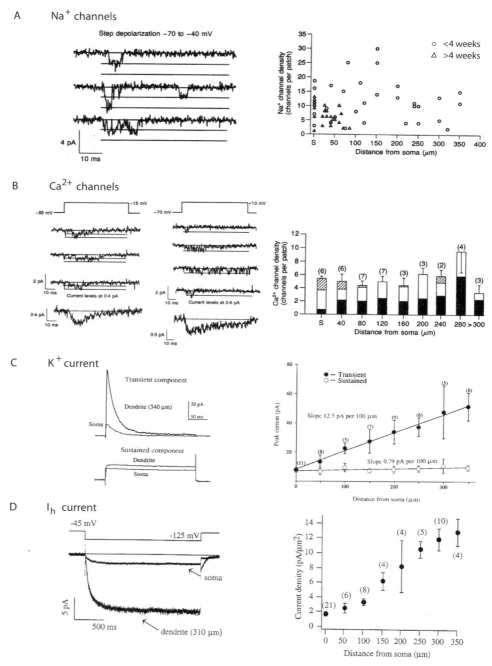

Figure 5–6. CA1 dendritic voltage-gated channels. *A*. Single-channel recordings of voltage-gated Na$^+$ channels in dendritic cell-attached patches (left) and a plot of Na$^+$ channel density as a function of distance from the soma (right). Circles and triangles are from rats younger and older than 4 weeks, respectively. (*Source:* Adapted from Magee and Johnston, 1995.) *B*. Single-channel recordings of voltage-gated Ca^{2+} channels in dendritic cell-attached patches [low-voltage activated (left) and high-voltage activated (middle); ensemble averages are also shown for each set of traces] and a plot of Ca^{2+} channel density as a function of distance from the soma (right). Black portions of the bars correspond to low-voltage activated channels; open bars correspond to high-voltage

activated, medium conductance channels; hatched bars correspond to high-voltage activated large conductance channels. (*Source:* Adapted from Magee and Johnston, 1995a.)*C*. Voltage-gated K$^+$ channels in cell-attached patches from dendrites and the soma, separated into sustained and transient components (left). The two components are plotted as a function of distance from the soma. The transient component is much larger in the dendrites. (*Source:* Adapted from Hofmann et al., 1997.) *D*. Hyperpolarization-activated current in cell-attached patches from dendrites and the soma (left). I$_h$ current density is plotted as a function of distance from the soma (right). I$_h$ is much larger in the dendrites. (*Source:* Adapted from Magee, 1998.)

formly along the somato-dendritic axis. Even when channel density is relatively uniform (e.g., Na^+ channels), the properties of the channels may differ between the soma and the dendrites. Although the mechanisms for establishing and maintaining these gradients are not known, more is known about the functional implications of ion channels and their nonuniform densities and properties in CA1 dendrites.

5.2.14 Functional Implications of Voltage-Gated Channels in CA1 Dendrites: Synaptic Integration and Plasticity

Knowing that the dendrites of CA1 neurons contain many voltage-gated channels, it is logical to ask: What for? Clearly, dendrites are able to generate a variety of active responses, including back-propagating action potentials and dendritic Na^+ and Ca^{2+} spikes. What is the purpose of these responses in excitable dendrites?

One obvious answer is that the occurrence of a dendritic spike generates output in the form of one or more axonal action potentials. This is correct for some dendritic spikes in CA1 neurons but not all. Large, broad Ca^{2+} spikes can trigger a burst of action potentials in the soma, indicating that these events produce a reliable axonal output (Golding et al., 1999), and under some conditions the forward propagation of dendritic spikes can be facilitated (Jarsky et al., 2005) (see Sections 5.2.10 and 5.2.11). Some dendritic Na^+ and Ca^{2+} spikes, however, do not propagate well to the soma, so their influence there can be quite small (Golding and Spruston, 1998; Golding et al., 2002). This observation hints at the possibility of local functions for dendritic spikes.

A likely function for back-propagating action potentials is to inform the dendrites and the synapses on them about the level of output in the axon. The most compelling evidence supporting such a role for dendritic spikes comes from the demonstration of their importance in the induction of long-term potentiation (LTP). At Schaffer collateral synapses (from CA3 axons), pairing of small EPSPs with somatic action potentials induces a form of LTP that disappears when action potentials are prevented from actively invading the dendrites (Magee and Johnston, 1997). Thus, back-propagating action potentials seem to have an important role in providing the postsynaptic depolarization necessary for the induction of some forms of Hebbian LTP (see Chapter 10). At more distal synapses on CA1 neurons, in particular the perforant path input from entorhinal cortex, LTP does not depend on back-propagating action potentials (Golding et al., 2002). Rather, dendritically generated Na^+ and Ca^{2+} spikes appear to provide an important component of the depolarization necessary to induce LTP at these synapses. A similar form of dendritic spike-induced LTP also occurs at the Schaffer collateral synapses if the stimulus intensity is increased to produce larger EPSPs during blockade of back-propagating action potentials (Golding et al., 2002). These findings indicate that both back-propagating action potentials and dendritically induced spikes can function to enhance the induction of LTP at synapses on the CA1 dendritic tree.

The function of dendritic Na^+ and Ca^{2+} channels at membrane potentials below threshold for the induction of regenerative dendritic events is less clear. In principle, each of these channel types (especially the low-threshold, T-type Ca^{2+} channels) could be activated during nonregenerative depolarizations (e.g., moderate EPSPs) and generate additional depolarization and Ca^{2+} entry. In fact, Na^+ channels have been shown to open during EPSPs, even when there are no obvious signs of regenerative activity (Magee and Johnston, 1995b). This finding is consistent with experiments showing that Na^+ and Ca^{2+} channel blockers can reduce postsynaptic EPSPs without affecting the presynaptic input (Lipowsky et al., 1996; Gillessen and Alzheimer, 1997). The ability of Na^+ and Ca^{2+} channels to amplify EPSPs effectively (without a dendritic spike), however, is compromised by coactivation of K^+ channels, which can cancel the effect of Na^+ and Ca^{2+} channel activation, resulting in linear summation of EPSPs (Cash and Yuste, 1998, 1999). It is likely, however, that neuromodulation, prior activity, and synaptic input pattern can alter the balance of Na^+, Ca^{2+}, and K^+ channel activation during synaptic integration, leading to nonlinearities in synaptic summation under some conditions.

The presence of a high density of hyperpolarization-activated, non-specific cation channels in CA1 dendrites has some interesting consequences for the temporal integration of EPSPs. Because some of I_h is active at the resting potential, it contributes a significant leak to the membrane. This has the effect of increasing attenuation of EPSPs as they propagate from the soma to the dendrite, as well as speeding the decay of EPSPs in the dendrite (Stuart and Spruston, 1998; Golding et al., 2005). This effect on the amplitude of EPSPs may be compensated in part by increased synaptic conductance at more distal synapses. Dendritic I_h has also been shown to normalize for the temporal filtering effects of dendrites (Magee, 1999). In passive dendrites, the filtering effects result in EPSPs generated at distal locations, producing slower EPSPs at the soma. As a result, distal dendritic EPSPs summate more at the soma than do size-matched EPSPs from more proximal locations. Dendritic I_h minimizes this spatial discrepancy of temporal summation by contributing a larger effective outward current (due to the turning off of inward I_h) for distal synapses, thus compensating for the additional temporal summation that would otherwise occur at the soma (Magee, 1999).

5.2.15 General Lessons Regarding Pyramidal Neuron Function

The CA1 pyramidal neuron is arguably the most extensively studied neuron with respect to resting membrane properties, dendritic function, and synaptic integration. These studies have produced a striking picture of the neuron in which the voltage attenuation in dendrites, is predicted to be enormous for the near-passive condition. CA1 dendrites impose powerful attenuation and filtering during both normal conditions and voltage clamp. The neuron appears to compensate for this by at least two key mechanisms: synapse conductance scaling and excitable dendrites containing myriad voltage-gated channels. On the other hand, such specialized properties are unlikely to exist exclusively to overcome the filtering properties of dendrites. Rather, the structure and ion channel expression are likely central to the specialized function of CA1 pyramidal neurons. For instance, one emergent property of the complexity of the CA1 dendritic tree appears to be coincidence detection for perforant-path and Schaffer-collateral synaptic inputs (Remondes and Schuman, 2002; Jarsky et al., 2005).

As becomes evident in the sections that follow, it would be inappropriate to generalize specific conclusions drawn from studies of one cell type and assume that other cells behave the same way. It is possible, however, to emphasize some conclusions based on studies of CA1 pyramidal neurons that are likely to direct studies of other neuronal cell types.

1. Morphology is stereotypical but variable. Although all CA1 cells have basal dendrites and a main apical dendrite that gives rise to oblique and tuft branches, dendritic morphology varies considerably from one CA1 neuron to the next. It is not known, but reasonable to postulate, that such morphological variability may have functional consequences.

2. Physiological properties are also variable. As with morphological variability, differences in physiological properties may be functionally relevant. Distinguishing inconsequential variability about a mean from significant functional variability is challenging but important. Physiological variability could arise as a result of genetic determinism, history-dependent development and plasticity, or both.

3. Channel and receptor distributions are often nonuniform. In CA1 neurons, as in layer V neocortical pyramidal neurons, distal dendrites contain a higher density of hyperpolarization-activated cation channels (Magee, 1998; Williams and Stuart, 2000; Berger et al., 2001; Lorincz et al., 2002) than the soma and more proximal dendritic regions. These two cell types differ, however, in that the high density of A-type K^+ channels in CA1 dendrites is not observed in layer V dendrites (Hoffman et al., 1997; Bekkers, 2000; Korngreen and Sakmann, 2000). Even though Na^+ and Ca^{2+} channel densities are uniform (on average) in CA1 dendrites, the properties of these channels vary systematically along the main apical dendrite. AMPA receptors have a higher density in mushroom-shaped spines and perforated synapses, whereas dopamine receptors have the highest density in distal apical dendrites of CA1 neurons. Additional inhomogeneities of channel and receptor density and function are likely to be revealed by future studies.

4. Population studies inform only about average behavior but cannot reveal functional variability across cells. For example, if some cells have increasing Na^+ channel density gradients from the soma into the dendrites, and others have decreasing gradients, they may have very different functional properties with respect to

dendritic excitability. A population approach to determining Na^+ channel distributions does not reveal such potentially important differences across cells.

5. Synaptic potentials attenuate dramatically between their site of origin in the dendrites and their final site of integration (with respect to action potential output) in the axon. Large synaptic depolarizations may serve local functions (e.g., release of retrograde messengers, initiation of dendritic spikes) independent of dendrosomatic attenuation. Because of the extensive filtering introduced by dendrites and the active responses that can be generated in dendrites, somatic voltage-clamp recordings must be interpreted with great caution.

6. Different excitatory and inhibitory inputs can target different subcellular domains. Excitatory inputs from different regions, such as the direct input from entorhinal cortex and the processed input from CA3 neurons in CA1, can contact distinct regions of the dendritic tree. Inhibitory interneurons, such as basket cells and oriens-alveus/lacunosum-moleculare (O-LM) neurons, can selectively innervate domains such as the soma or the distal apical dendrites. This differential targeting suggests important differences in postsynaptic actions, even among synapses using the same transmitter.

7. The threshold for action-potential initiation is lower in the axon than in the dendrites. This finding generalizes from CA1 neurons to many other neurons (Stuart et al., 1997). One possible exception has been noted: O-LM interneurons in the hippocampus have a low threshold for action potential initiation in the dendrites (Martina et al., 2000) (see section 5.9.7).

8. CA1 dendrites, like many other dendritic trees, contain voltage-gated channels that support action-potential back-propagation and dendritic spike initiation (Häusser et al., 2000). The presence of voltage-gated channels in dendrites is likely to have profound effects on synaptic integration.

These general conclusions share the common feature that they all imply a tremendous degree of complexity and specialization in neuronal function, even for a single cell type, such as the CA1 pyramidal neuron. As subsequent sections on the properties of other neurons in the hippocampus indicate, there are no shortcuts: The morphological and functional properties of each and every cell type must be explored in detail in the hippocampus as in the rest of the brain.

5.3 CA3 Pyramidal Neurons

Following the CA1 pyramidal layer back toward the dentate gyrus, one encounters the CA3 pyramidal layer. (Little is known about the physiology of neurons in the intervening CA2 region.) The CA3 pyramidal neurons have been studied extensively, in large part because of the unique functional specializations formed by the mossy fiber inputs from the dentate gyrus and because of the extensive axon collaterals between CA3 neurons, which create a highly interconnected and excitable network.

5.3.1 Dendritic Morphology

Pyramidal neurons in the CA3 region are structurally similar to CA1 neurons; they consist of pyramid-shaped somata that give rise to apical and basal dendritic trees (Fig. 5–7A). CA3 pyramidal neurons differ from their CA1 counterparts, however, in that the apical dendritic tree bifurcates closer to the soma. CA3 pyramidal neurons are typically somewhat larger than CA1 pyramidal cells, but their total dendritic length and organization is heterogeneous. The smallest CA3 pyramidal cells are located in the limbs of the dentate gyrus, and the largest cells are located in the distal portion of the CA3 subfield (Amaral et al., 1990).

Detailed morphometric analysis of dye-injected cells has allowed complete reconstruction of CA3 pyramidal neurons,

similar to that described above for CA1 pyramidal cells. CA3 pyramidal neurons, recovered from rat hippocampus in vitro slices from the mid-transverse hippocampal axis, possess extensive dendritic arborizations with four main features, (1) a basal arbor that extends throughout the stratum oriens, (2) a short apical trunk in the stratum lucidum that branches into two or more secondary trunks, (3) oblique apical dendrites in the stratum radiatum, and (4) an apical tuft that extends into the stratum lacunosum-moleculare. On average, the total dendritic length for the apical and basal dendritic arbors is similar to that of CA1, but with a larger range (9.3–15.8 mm) (Ishizuka et al., 1995; Henze et al., 1996). This variability of dendritic structure is attributable to systematic differences in the dendritic structure of pyramidal neurons in the various subregions of CA3 (Ishizuka et al., 1995) (see Section 5.3.3). Of particular interest, despite the greater total length and surface area of the apical arbor, the number of terminal branches and number of dendritic segments are similar for both the apical and basal arbors. This suggests that the distances between successive branch points are shorter for the basal dendrites (Henze et al., 1996). However, the basal dendrites

Figure 5–7. CA3 dendritic morphology, thorny excrescences, and synaptic inputs and outputs. *A.* Computer-generated plot showing dendritic morphology of a CA3 pyramidal neuron. Thorny excrescences are apparent on the proximal apical dendrites in the stratum pyramidale (s.p.) and stratum lucidum (s.l.). The major excitatory synaptic inputs to each layer are indicated, as are the major synaptic outputs. Bar = 50 μm. (*Source:* Adapted from Gonzales et al.,

2001.) *B.* Photomicrograph of dendrites in a filled CA3 pyramidal neuron providing clear examples of thorny excrescences. Particularly large spine clusters are indicated with arrows. Bar = 25 μm. (*Source:* Adapted from Gonzales et al., 2001.) *C.* Three-dimensional reconstruction of a large branched spine with 12 heads. The reconstructed thorn is light gray, and the PSDs are indicated in white. Bar = 1 μm. (*Source:* Adapted from Chicurel and Harris, 1992.)

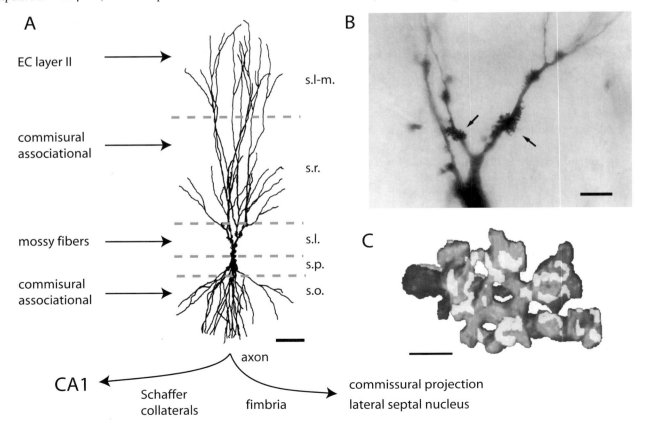

have approximately threefold fewer tips per primary dendrite (8.5 vs. 29.1). This, together with the lower maximum branch order for the basal dendrites (7.0 vs. 10.8), suggests that the individual basal dendritic trees are significantly less complex than the apical trees. Finally, in addition to being less complex, the mean distance to the basal dendritic tips is shorter than for the apical tree (212 vs. 425 μm) and suggests that synapses formed on the basal dendrites occupy a more restricted range of physical distances from the somata. The dendritic trees of CA3 pyramidal neurons also have a roughly symmetrical structure in their maximal transverse and septo-temporal extents (~ 300 and 270 μm, respectively).

5.3.2 Dendritic Spines and Synapses

Like their CA1 counterparts, CA3 pyramidal neuron dendrites are studded with thousands of spines. Even greater diversity of spine morphology is apparent in CA3. In addition to the spine shapes observed in CA1, the CA3 neurons also have another major spine class, the "thorny excrescences" (Fig. 5–7B,C). There are about 40 of these specialized spine clusters on each CA3 neuron (Blackstad and Kjaerheim, 1961; Chicurel and Harris, 1992; Amaral and Witter, 1995; Gonzales et al., 2001). In the proximal regions of CA3 (closest to the dentate gyrus) the thorny excrescences are distributed on apical and basal dendrites relatively close to the soma. In more distal CA3 neurons (closer to CA1), the excrescences are found primarily on the apical dendrite prior to the first branch point located at distances of 10 to 120 μm from the soma, where they form the postsynaptic targets of the mossy fiber synapses from granule cells of the dentate gyrus (Blackstad and Kjaerheim, 1961; Hamlyn, 1962; Chicurel and Harris, 1992; Gonzales et al., 2001). Three-dimensional reconstruction of thorny excrescences on CA3 pyramidal neurons have revealed many unusual features that are peculiar to the mossy fiber synapses and have not been described at other hippocampal synapses or indeed other brain areas. Typically, postsynaptic thorny excrescences at mossy fiber synapses comprise 1 to 16 branches that emerge from a single dendritic origin. These branched spines contain subcellular organelles typical of other spines (including ribosomes and multivesicular bodies), but they also contain organelles not found in other spines, such as mitochondria and microtubules. Multivesicular bodies occur most often in the spine heads, which also contain smooth endoplasmic reticulum; and ribosomes occur most often in spines that have spinules (nonsynaptic protruberances that emerge from the spine head). Branched spines are typically surrounded by a single mossy fiber bouton, which can establish synapses with multiple spine heads. The postsynaptic densities of these spines occupy ~ 10% to 15% of the spine head membrane. Individual mossy fiber boutons usually synapse with several branches belonging to more than one thorny spine excrescence but all originating from the same parent dendrite. Within a given branched spine, the dimension and volume of individual spine heads are comparable to those of the large mushroom spines found on CA1 pyramidal neurons, although the CA3 branches have more irregular

shapes (Blackstad and Kjaerheim, 1961; Chicurel and Harris, 1992).

The thorny excrescences (and hence the mossy fiber inputs) are concentrated in the first 100 μm or so of the apical dendritic tree of CA3 pyramidal neurons (stratum lucidum). Across the remaining portions of both the apical and basal dendrites, the shape and distribution of spines are somewhat similar to CA1 pyramidal neurons, described above. Various calculations put the number of simple spines close to 30,000, which is similar to estimates of total spine number on CA1 pyramidal neurons (Jonas et al., 1993;Trommald et al., 1995).

5.3.3 Excitatory and Inhibitory Synaptic Inputs

The CA3 pyramidal neurons receive three prominent forms of excitatory synaptic input. The aforementioned mossy fiber input from the dentate granule cells is the most extensively studied of these inputs. CA3 neurons also receive direct input from layer II of the entorhinal cortex via the perforant path. As in the CA1 region, this direct cortical input is limited to the distal regions of the apical dendrites, in the stratum lacunosum-moleculare. The third prominent input to CA3 neurons comes from the axons of other CA3 neurons. These "commissural/associational" (C/A) inputs are numerous and originate from CA3 neurons on both sides of the brain. This extensive network of recurrent collaterals has led to the postulate that the CA3 region may function as an autoassociative network involved in memory storage and recall (Bennett et al., 1994; Rolls, 1996) (see Chapter 14). A side effect of this extensive interconnectivity, however, is that the CA3 network is highly excitable and prone to seizure activity when inhibition is suppressed (Jung and Kornmuller, 1938; Ben-Ari, 1985) (see Section 5.3.5). CA3 neurons also receive cholinergic input from the medial septal nucleus and the nucleus of the diagonal band of Broca, which terminate mostly in the stratum oriens (Amaral and Witter, 1995).

The organization of the dendritic tree and its synaptic inputs are highly variable and strongly depend on the location of the cell body within CA3. Cells located in the limbs of the dentate gyrus have dendrites with a limited elaboration and do not extend dendrites into the stratum lacunosum-moleculare (Amaral et al., 1990). In contrast, cells toward the more distal portion of the CA3 subfield project their dendrites throughout the stratum radiatum and stratum lacunosum-moleculare. Of particular importance regarding this heterogeneous anatomical organization, CA3 pyramidal cells at the most proximal and distal ends of the CA3 subfield are under differential control by the various afferent pathways projecting into the CA3 hippocampus. Most notably, CA3 pyramidal neurons closest to the dentate gyrus receive the proportionally largest input from the dentate granule cells; these CA3 neurons receive mossy fiber axonal inputs onto both the apical and basal dendritic trees, whereas those located more distally in CA3 have mossy fiber inputs primarily onto the proximal portion of their apical dendritic tree (Blackstad et al., 1970). This limited mossy fiber projection to the basal CA3 pyramidal cell dendrites is referred to as the infrapyramidal projection and the granule cells in the infrapyramidal blade of the dentate gyrus are the primary source of this projection.

Although initial binding studies suggested that NMDA receptors were absent at mossy fiber synapses (Monaghan et al., 1983), subsequent physiological studies revealed that activation of NMDA receptors indeed occurs during activation of mossy fiber synapses (Jonas et al., 1993). Dendritic recordings from the apical dendrites of CA3 pyramidal cells in areas close to the mossy-fiber termination zone in stratum lucidum indicate that the properties of dendritic ionotropic glutamate receptors are remarkably similar to those expressed at the soma of CA3 pyramidal cells (Spruston et al., 1995). AMPA and NMDA-type glutamate receptors in CA3 neurons are also remarkably similar to these receptors in CA1 pyramidal neurons. One notable difference, however, is the deactivation kinetics of NMDA receptors, which were slower in CA1 than in CA3 pyramidal neurons. In addition, NMDA receptor-mediated Ca^{2+} entry is limited in CA3 spines (Reid et al., 2001; but see Pozzo-Miller et al., 1996). A comparison of the properties of mossy fiber synaptic transmission to AMPA receptor properties in CA3 dendrites suggests that a typical quantal event would consist of 35 AMPA receptors being activated by a single quantum of glutamate ($\times$10 pS single-channel conductance = 350 pS quantal conductance). About 70 receptors are estimated to be present at each release site, but only half of these receptors are open at the peak of the synaptic current (Jonas et al., 1993; Spruston et al., 1995). Immunocytochemical analysis suggests that about four times as many AMPA receptors are present at each mossy fiber synaptic specialization as at C/A synapses in CA3 or SC synapses in CA1 (Nusser et al., 1998). This high density of AMPA receptors and the large number of synaptic specializations on each thorny excrescence (Chicurel and Harris, 1992) accounts for the large size and variability of unitary mossy fiber synaptic currents, which have been estimated to comprise 2 to 16 quantal events (Jonas et al., 1993).

CA3 pyramidal neurons also receive substantial innervation from inhibitory interneurons. In addition to the somatic and axonal inhibition, which presumably limits action potential initiation, a number of interneurons target CA3 dendrites. This dendritic inhibition has been shown to limit the initiation and enhance termination of dendritic calcium spikes (Miles et al., 1996).

5.3.4 Axon Morphology and Synaptic Targets

Each CA3 pyramidal neuron gives rise to a single axon, which projects bilaterally to the CA3, CA2, and CA1 regions, as well as to the lateral septal nucleus (Ishizuka et al., 1990; Amaral and Witter, 1995). At the light microscopic level, individual axons are thin and myelinated with abundant en passant boutons or varicosities spaced, on average, 4.7 μm apart (Ishizuka et al., 1990; Shepherd and Harris, 1998; Shepherd et al., 2002). CA3 axons project primarily to the CA1 region but also collateralize extensively within CA3. The total length of the CA3 collaterals in the ipsilateral hippocampus has been estimated at 150 to 300 mm. These collaterals cover a large area in the longitudinal direction, extending more than one-third the length of the septo-temporal axis (Ishizuka et al., 1990; Sik et al., 1993; Li et al., 1994; Andersen et al., 2000). Pyramidal neurons in the CA3a subfield (closest to CA1) arborize primarily in the stratum oriens of CA1, whereas neurons in CA3c (closer to the hilus) collateralize more extensively in the stratum radiatum of CA1 (Ishizuka et al., 1990; Li et al., 1994). In one complete reconstruction, the highest density of boutons in CA1 clustered about 600 to 800 μm from the CA3 neuron in both the septal and temporal directions (Sik et al., 1993). These axons contribute to the Schaffer collateral inputs to CA1 pyramidal neurons. Another group of axon collaterals is localized in the stratum oriens and stratum radiatum of CA3, comprising the extensive associational connection common between CA3 pyramidal neurons. Boutons are located approximately every 4 μm along the CA3 axon, but boutons are distributed unevenly, with somewhat variable spacing (Shepherd et al., 2002). Estimates of the total number of synapses formed by a single axon in the ipsilateral hippocampus range from 15,000 to 60,000 (Sik et al., 1993; Li et al., 1994). A subset of the CA3 axon boutons contacts interneurons. Each axon contacts each interneuron at a single location, forming one synaptic release site. As in CA1, pyramidal cell-to-interneuron synapses are powerful enough that a single axon is capable of producing an action potential in postsynaptic interneurons (Miles, 1990; Gulyás et al., 1993a; Sik et al., 1993).

Three-dimensional reconstruction of CA3 pyramidal neuron axons in the CA1 region revealed that most of the varicosities or presynaptic boutons contained synaptic vesicles and were opposed to a postsynaptic specialization that comprised a single postsynaptic density (PSD). Approximately 20% of presynaptic varicosities were apposed to postsynaptic specializations comprising multiple PSDs (Shepherd and Harris, 1998). CA3 pyramidal neuron axonal varicosities are typically oblong in shape and demonstrate considerable variation in their length (~1 μm) and volume (~0.13 μm^3). The intervaricosity axonal shaft is narrow, tubular, and remarkably consistent in its diameter (~0.17 μm). The narrow axonal shafts resemble dendritic spine necks, an arrangement that raises the possibility of functional compartmentalization along individual axons. Importantly, serial electron microscopy has revealed that a small number of CA3 axons (~20%) may make multiple synapses on a single CA1 cell (Sorra and Harris, 1993).

5.3.5 Resting Potential and Action Potential Firing Properties

Like CA1 pyramidal cells, CA3 pyramidal cells possess a repertoire of conductances that allow them to respond to suprathreshold stimuli with either single action potentials or bursts. Although bursting also occurs in CA1 pyramidal neurons (see Section 5.2.5), bursting is more prominent in CA3, both in vivo and in the in vitro slice preparation (Kandel and Spencer, 1961; Spencer and Kandel, 1961; Wong and Prince, 1978) and is therefore considered a hallmark feature of CA3 pyramidal neurons. Bursts in CA3 neurons typically comprise several action potentials riding atop a depolarizing waveform, often accompanied by smaller calcium-dependent spikes late in the waveform. Each burst is an "all or nothing" event lasting approximately 30 to 50 ms, with the frequency of action potentials in the range of 100 to 300 Hz (Wong et al., 1979; Wong and Prince, 1981; Traub and Miles, 1991).

Bursts can be triggered in several ways in CA3 neurons, and the mechanism underlying bursting depends in large part on the way the burst is evoked. One mechanism for burst generation is entirely intrinsic to the neuron and does not require synaptic connectivity. A brief current injection via a somatic recording electrode can produce an all-or-none burst of action potentials in some CA3 neurons (Wong and Prince, 1981) (Fig. 5–8A), and in some cases these bursts occur spontaneously (Cohen and Miles, 2000). The burst is caused by an ADP that follows a single action potential, which is likely to be mediated by calcium current, as pharmacological blockade of calcium current converts burst firing to single spiking (Wong and Prince, 1981).

The CA3 neurons can also generate intrinsic bursts in response to brief synaptic activation or dendritic current injection (Wong et al., 1979; Masukawa et al., 1982; Masukawa and Prince, 1984). Under these conditions the ADP may contribute to the bursting, but dendritically generated calcium spikes are likely to be a more important mechanism driving the burst (Wong and Prince, 1978; Wong et al., 1979). Continuous current injection into the apical dendrites of CA3 pyramidal neurons evokes rhythmic bursts at frequencies of at least 8 Hz (Traub and Miles, 1991). The burst pattern in the dendrite differs markedly from that observed in the soma, with dendritic fast spikes (presumed Na$^+$) usually having a lower amplitude than slower spikes (presumed Ca^{2+}); this probably reflects a greater distance of the dendrite from the axon initial segment, a low density of Na$^+$ channels in the dendrite, or both (Traub et al., 1999).

The most robust bursts are generated in CA3 neurons when the entire network becomes synchronously active, usually in response to suppression of synaptic inhibition or reduction of K$^+$ currents (Prince and Connors, 1986). Under these conditions, the network produces a paroxysmal depolarization shift (PDS), which is a hallmark of seizure activity in cortical networks. The PDS is a synchronous network depolarization driven primarily by giant synaptic potentials (Johnston and Brown, 1981, 1984, 1986; Lebeda et al., 1982). Thus, intrinsic conductances can generate bursts that are likely to serve as important signals in a normally functional network, whereas massive, synchronous glutamate release contributes to synchronous bursting during hippocampal seizures (Fig. 5–8B,C). Because CA3 pyramidal neurons generate seizures, they have been extensively studied as the possible pacemakers of interictal epileptiform activity in a variety of animal models of electrographic seizures (see Schwartzkroin, 1993 for a number of relevant reviews).

Just as the mechanisms for generating normal and pathological bursts are different, the mechanisms for terminating them are different as well. During normal intrinsic burst-

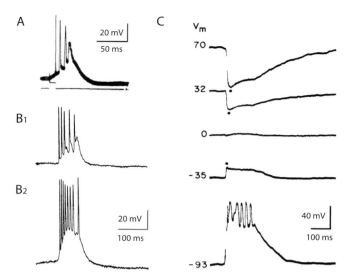

Figure 5–8. CA3 pyramidal neuron bursting and epilepsy. *A.* Intrinsic burst firing in response to a short current injection in a CA3 pyramidal neuron. (*Source*: Adapted from Wong and Prince, 1981.) *B.* Similar appearance of intrinsic and network-driven bursts in CA3 pyramidal neurons. B$_1$ shows an endogenous burst in a recording with the slice bathed in normal solution. B$_2$ shows a network-driven burst during a paroxysmal depolarization shift (PDS), a network discharge induced by bathing the slice in a solution containing penicillin. Recordings are from two different cells. (*Source*: Adapted from Johnston and Brown, 1984.) *C.* The synaptic nature of the PDS is shown by its reversal in polarity at a holding potential of around 0 mV. The PDS was induced by bathing the slice in a solution containing d-tubocurarine. (*Source*: Adapted from Lebeda et al., 1982.)

ing, each burst is terminated by a slow AHP (~1 second) mediated by a variety of voltage- and Ca^{2+}-activated K$^+$ conductances (Alger and Nicoll, 1980; Hotson and Prince, 1980; Schwartzkroin and Stafstrom, 1980; Lancaster and Adams, 1986; Lancaster and Nicoll, 1987; Storm, 1989). In contrast, there is good evidence that network bursts are terminated by depletion of glutamate-containing synaptic vesicles during the giant EPSPs that drive the PDS. Replenishment of these vesicle pools is an important factor determining the rate at which the PDS can recur during seizure activity (Staley et al., 1998).

Interestingly, not all CA3 pyramidal neurons respond to suprathreshold stimuli with intrinsic bursts. Intrinsic bursting is most typical of cells located at the distal portion of CA3, closest to CA2. In guinea pig slices, cells located closer to the dentate gyrus typically respond with only a series of single action potentials (Masukawa et al., 1982). Furthermore, CA3 pyramidal neurons with somata located close to the stratum pyramidale/oriens border are more predisposed to burst generation than those located closer to the stratum radiatum (Bilkey and Schwartzkroin, 1990). One notable morphological distinction between these two cell groups is the length of the initial portion of their apical dendrite; cells with somata closer to the stratum pyramidale/oriens border have a significantly longer initial apical dendrite. Consistent with the correlation between anatomy and burst behaviors, L-type voltage-gated Ca^{2+} channels are clustered with high density on the base of major dendrites of CA3 pyramidal neurons (Westenbroek et al., 1990). Such an arrangement would permit large Ca^{2+} fluxes in response to summed excitatory inputs and perhaps may account for the predisposition of certain "deep" CA3 pyramidal neurons to bursting activity.

5.3.6 Resting Membrane Properties

As discussed above for CA1 pyramidal neurons, accurate estimation of the resting membrane properties of central neurons has been problematic, so the conditions of any particular measurement must be carefully considered. At resting membrane potentials (−60 to −70 mV) and with I_h blocked, the input resistance of CA3 neurons is slightly higher than in CA1 neurons, at about 160 MΩ (Spruston and Johnston, 1992) (Fig. 5–9). Estimates of the membrane time constant of CA3 neurons in slices from adult guinea pig yield a mean value of 90 ms, which is considerably slower than for CA1 neurons under the same conditions (Spruston and Johnston, 1992). Similar estimates in slices from young rats at room temperature resulted in even slower membrane time constants (112 ms), also without block of I_h (Jonas et al., 1993). Assuming a C_m of 1 μF/cm² implies a membrane resistivity of 60,000 to 120,000 Ωcm² of CA3 neurons, which is more than twice as high as R_m in CA1 neurons. It is not known whether R_m is lower in dendrites of CA3 neurons than in the soma, as it is in CA1 neurons (Spruston and Johnston, 1992; Stuart and Spruston, 1998).

As with CA1 pyramidal neurons, estimates of τ_m and R_N are larger at more depolarized potentials, consistent with the notion that voltage-dependent conductances, active near the resting membrane potential, contribute to the resting membrane properties of CA3 neurons (Spruston and Johnston, 1992). Pharmacological elimination of I_h increases the magnitude of R_N and τ_m but did not alter their voltage dependence. This is in contrast to CA1 pyramidal cells, where blocking I_h reverses the voltage dependence of R_N and τ_m.

The high value of R_m for CA3 neurons implies that their dendrites may be electrically compact for the steady-state condition. As is the case for CA1 neurons, however, neuronal models indicate that attenuation of transient changes in membrane potential is substantial, and voltage control of synaptic and voltage-gated currents using a somatic electrode would be nearly impossible for conductances located in CA3 dendrites, even at rather modest distances from the soma (Spruston et al., 1993; Major et al., 1994).

5.3.7 Active Properties of CA3 Dendrites

Passive models of CA3 pyramidal neurons predict large attenuation of EPSPs between the dendrites and the soma (Carnevale et al., 1997; Jaffe and Carnevale, 1999). Although it is not known whether the conductance of distal synapses are larger to compensate for this attenuation (as shown in CA1) (Magee and Cook, 2000), dendritic attenuation is likely to be

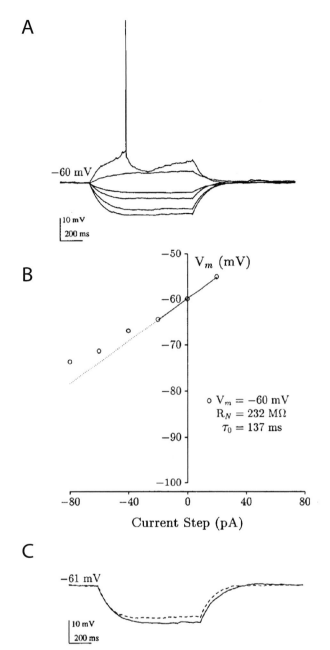

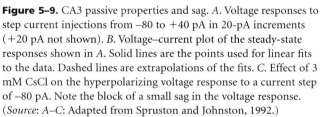

Figure 5–9. CA3 passive properties and sag. *A.* Voltage responses to step current injections from −80 to +40 pA in 20-pA increments (+20 pA not shown). *B.* Voltage–current plot of the steady-state responses shown in *A.* Solid lines are the points used for linear fits to the data. Dashed lines are extrapolations of the fits. *C.* Effect of 3 mM CsCl on the hyperpolarizing voltage response to a current step of −80 pA. Note the block of a small sag in the voltage response. (*Source*: A–C: Adapted from Spruston and Johnston, 1992.)

overcome, at least in part, by the presence of voltage-gated conductances in the dendrites. Although CA3 pyramidal neurons possess most if not all of the same intrinsic conductances described for the CA1 pyramidal cell, and in general these currents share many of the same properties and identities, the density of channels and/or the subcellular location often differ. For example, I_h is found in both CA1 and CA3 pyramidal neurons. However, the channels underlying the generation of this current in the two cell types appear to be different. Within the hippocampus two I_h subunit mRNA transcripts have been detected: HCN1 and HCN2. Labeling for HCN1 is heavy in the CA1 pyramidal cells, whereas only moderate expression is observed in the CA3 pyramidal cell layer. The opposite distribution pattern is true for HCN2. Functionally, despite the differing expression patterns of HCN1 and HCN2, there appears to be little overall difference between the biophysical properties of I_h in either cell type (Santoro et al., 2000; Fisahn et al., 2002). I_h measured at the CA3 pyramidal neuron soma is considerably smaller than those observed in CA1 pyramidal neurons (Santoro et al., 2000), however, suggesting a different I_h channel density in the two cell types. It is not known whether I_h is distributed at higher density in CA3 dendrites, as it is in CA1.

Because CA3 pyramidal cells lack a large primary apical dendrite such as that found in CA1, studies of dendritic excitability and ion channels in CA3 dendrites have lagged behind those in CA1. Consequently, little is known about the identities and properties of specific ion conductances in the dendrites of CA3 pyramidal neurons. A few studies have used sharp microelectrodes to record spikes from the dendrites of CA3 pyramidal neurons (Wong et al., 1979; Miles et al., 1996). Calcium imaging experiments also indicate that voltage-gated conductances are located in CA3 dendrites and spines (Pozzo-Miller et al., 1993; Jaffe and Brown, 1997). Although much of what we know about dendritic excitability in CA3 has been inferred from a relatively small number of dendritic recordings and calcium imaging, some interesting computer models have been developed for CA3 neurons. Roger Traub and colleagues used such computer models to demonstrate the importance of dendritic Ca^{2+} conductances in generating action potential bursts, as well as the importance of these bursts in the synaptic propagation of seizure activity through a model of the CA3 network (Traub and Miles, 1991; Traub et al., 1999). Another model of a CA3 pyramidal neuron demonstrated that bursting behavior does not require any special distribution of Ca^{2+}-dependent channels or mechanisms. Furthermore, a simple increase in the Ca^{2+}-independent K^+ conductances was sufficient to convert the firing mode of modeled CA3 pyramidal neurons from bursting to nonbursting (Migliore et al., 1995). Hopefully, these models will stimulate additional experimental studies of the excitable properties of CA3 dendrites.

5.4 Subicular Pyramidal Neurons

The subiculum lies on the opposite side of the CA1 region than CA3, directly adjacent to the distal extent of area CA1. It begins where the Schaffer collaterals end, a point distinguishable by the transition from the tightly packed CA1 pyramidal layer to the more diffuse pyramidal layer of subiculum. The subiculum plays an important role in the hippocampal formation, as it receives convergent input from numerous sources and constitutes the major output of the hippocampus (Naber et al., 2000) (see Chapter 3). Although neurons in this region have been studied much less than their neighbors in CA1 and CA3, the pronounced tendency of neurons in this region to fire bursts of action potentials has led to considerable interest in understanding the cell physiology of these neurons.

5.4.1 Dendritic Morphology

Almost all principal neurons in the subiculum have a typical pyramidal morphology, with apical dendrites extending into the molecular layer and in many cases reaching the hippocampal fissure (Harris et al., 2001) (Fig. 5–10). A quantitative comparison of dendritic branching in the subiculum and CA1 revealed that subicular pyramidal neurons have slightly fewer branches in both the basal and apical dendritic trees, with the largest difference in the proximal apical dendrites (Staff et al., 2000). No differences have been observed between the dendritic morphology of regular-spiking and bursting neurons in the subiculum (Mason, 1993; Taube, 1993; Greene and Totterdell, 1997; Staff et al., 2000; Harris et al., 2001).

5.4.2 Dendritic Spines and Synaptic Inputs

As in CA1, the dendrites of subicular pyramidal neurons are studded with spines. Virtually no quantitative data are available regarding spine density, however, and little is known about the distribution of the numerous cortical and subcortical inputs to the dendritic trees of subicular pyramidal neurons. Two of the most prominent inputs to subiculum include topographical projections from CA1 and the entorhinal cortex (see section 5.4.3 and Chapter 3 for details). The projection from the entorhinal cortex originates in both layer II (which also projects to the dentate gyrus and CA3) and layer III (which also projects to CA1) and forms synapses restricted to the distal portions of the apical dendrites (Witter and Amaral, 1991; Lingenhöhl and Finch, 1991; Tamamaki and Nojyo 1993; Amaral and Witter, 1995). These EC projections form functional excitatory synapses on subicular pyramidal neurons (van Groen and Lopes da Silva, 1986; Behr et al., 1998; Gigg et al., 2000). Axons from CA1 pyramidal neurons also form excitatory synapses on the dendrites of subicular pyramidal neurons (Finch and Babb, 1980, 1981; Tamamaki and Nojyo 1990; Amaral et al., 1991; Taube, 1993; Gigg et al., 2000).

Among the subcortical structures projecting to the subiculum are the thalamic nucleus reuniens and weak cholinergic projections from the septal nucleus and the nucleus of the diagonal band. Modulatory inputs from the brain stem also innervate the subiculum, including the locus coeruleus (noradrenergic), ventral tegmental area (dopaminergic), and raphe nuclei (serotonergic). In addition to a direct input from the entorhinal cortex, the subiculum receives inputs from many of the same cortical areas that project to the entorhinal cortex. Almost nothing is known about the inhibitory interneurons and their targeting of pyramidal neurons in the subiculum.

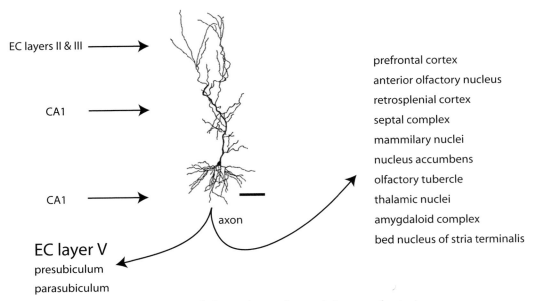

EC layers II & III

CA1

CA1

axon

EC layer V
presubiculum
parasubiculum

prefrontal cortex
anterior olfactory nucleus
retrosplenial cortex
septal complex
mammilary nuclei
nucleus accumbens
olfactory tubercle
thalamic nuclei
amygdaloid complex
bed nucleus of stria terminalis

Figure 5–10. Subiculum dendritic morphology, spines, and synaptic inputs and outputs. Camera lucida drawing shows the dendritic morphology of a subicular pyramidal neuron, with its major inputs and outputs indicated. Bar = 100 μm. (*Source*: Adapted from Staff et al., 2000.)

Synaptic stimulation in the CA1 region or entorhinal cortex results in apparently monosynaptic EPSPs that are blocked by AMPA-type glutamate receptor antagonists and are only modestly affected by NMDA receptor blockers (Stewart and Wong, 1993; Stewart, 1997; Stanford et al., 1998; Staff et al., 2000). When inhibition is not blocked, synaptic stimulation in CA1 also produces a strong inhibitory postsynaptic potential (IPSP), presumably mediated in part by feedforward inhibition resulting from activation of interneurons in the subiculum (Menendez de la Prida, 2003).

5.4.3 Axon Morphology and Synaptic Targets

The axons of subicular pyramidal neurons collateralize extensively in the subiculum as well as projecting out of the subiculum (Harris et al., 2001). The local collaterals are believed to form glutamatergic synapses contacts (Harris and Stewart, 2001). Pyramidal neurons with deeper cell bodies tend to form vertically oriented columns of local collaterals, whereas superficial pyramidal neurons exhibit a greater horizontal spread (toward CA1 and EC) in their local axon collaterals (Harris et al., 2001).

Projecting axon collaterals target a number of cortical and subcortical structures (Fig. 5–10). They do not project back to CA1 but do project to the entorhinal cortex and the pre- and parasubiculum (Amaral and Witter, 1995). The projection to the entorhinal cortex terminates primarily in layer V. These connections are organized such that subiculum projects back to the same regions of the entorhinal cortex from which it receives input. This reciprocal projection is organized in an arrangement similar to the CA1-subiculum projection, in that the proximal subiculum (closest to CA1) projects to the most distal regions of the entorhinal cortex (the lateral entorhinal area), and the distal subiculum projects to the proximal entorhinal cortex (the medial entorhinal area).

Among the other numerous targets of the subiculum are the medial prefrontal cortex, anterior olfactory nucleus, retrosplenial cortex, septal complex, mammilary nuclei, nucleus accumbens, olfactory tubercle, several thalamic nuclei (including reuniens), amygdaloid complex, and the bed nucleus of the stria terminalis (Amaral and Witter, 1995) (see Chapter 3 for more details). An interesting organizational feature of the axonal projections from the subiculum is that they are organized along the septo-temporal (dorsal-ventral) axis of the hippocampus as well as along the proximo-distal (CA1 to presubiculum) axis. Neurons from four regions defined by these axes (septal-proximal, septal-distal, ventral-proximal, ventral-distal) project to different targets, and most subicular neurons project to only a single cortical or subcortical target (Naber and Witter, 1998).

5.4.4 Resting and Active Properties

In awake, freely moving rats, subicular cells exhibit firing in "place fields," which are larger and noisier than those seen in CA1 (Sharp and Green, 1994; O'Mara et al., 2001) (see Chapter 11). A prominent feature of the firing patterns observed in vivo is action potential bursting. Indeed, bursting is much more prominent in the subiculum than in CA1. In both in vitro and in vivo studies, pyramidal cells in the subiculum have been shown to fall into two broad physiological categories: bursting cells and regular-spiking cells (Mason, 1993;

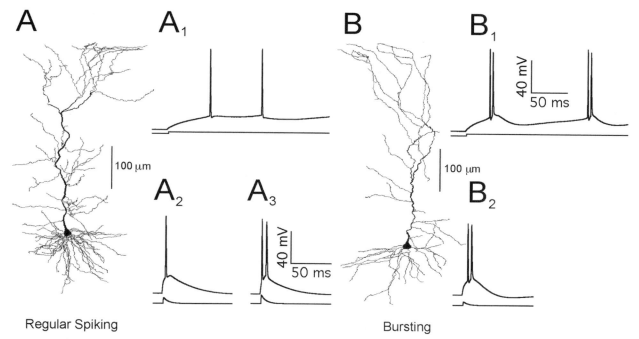

Regular Spiking   Bursting

Figure 5–11. Subiculum action potential bursting. *A.* Subicular pyramidal neuron classified as "regular spiking" because of its response to a threshold-level step current injection (A_1). A single spike occurs in response to a threshold-level current injection in the shape of an EPSC (A_2), but larger EPSC-like current injections produce bursting (A_3). *B.* Subicular pyramidal neuron classified as "bursting" because of its response to a threshold-level step current injection (B_1). A single two-spike burst occurs in response to a threshold-level current injection in the shape of an EPSC (B_2). (*Source*: *A, B*: Adapted from Cooper et al., 2003.)

Mattia et al., 1993; Stewart and Wong, 1993; Taube, 1993; Staff et al., 2000; Menendez de la Prida et al., 2003) (Fig. 5–11).

Given the large number of brain areas innervated by subicular neurons, it is tempting to speculate that strong bursting cells target different areas than weaker bursting or regular spiking cells. Some evidence supports this hypothesis, as it has been shown that bursting cells project preferentially to the presubiculum and parasubiculum, whereas regular-spiking cells project preferentially to the entorhinal cortex (Stewart, 1997; Funahashi et al., 1999). There is also some evidence for preferential localization of bursting and regular-spiking neurons in the subiculum, but the spatial gradients are weak. Two studies showed that regular spiking cells are more prevalent in superficial layers (Greene and Totterdell, 1997; Harris et al., 2001). Evidence for a proximo-distal gradient is less consistent. A microelectrode study in slices showed a preference for regular-spiking cells near the middle of the proximo-distal axis of the subiculum (Greene and Totterdell, 1997), whereas a patch-clamp study showed a slightly higher proportion of bursting cells in the distal subiculum (Staff et al., 2000). A variety of technical differences could account for these different conclusions, but the message emerging from these studies, taken together, is that proximo-distal gradients of bursting are weak, if they exist at all.

The resting and active properties of subicular pyramidal neurons have been examined in several studies. The measurements of resting potentials are remarkably consistent, ranging from −69 to −64 mV in microelectrode and patch-clamp recordings (Mason, 1993; Mattia et al., 1993, 1997a; Stewart and Wong, 1993; Greene and Totterdell, 1997; Staff et al., 2000). R_N ranged from 24 to 42 MΩ and τ_m from 7 to 20 ms. Most studies have revealed that these values are not significantly different between bursting and regular-spiking neurons in the subiculum (Taube, 1993; Staff et al., 2000). Compared to CA1 pyramidal neurons, however, a recent patch-clamp study showed that subicular neurons have significantly lower R_N and faster τ_m (Staff et al., 2000; but see Mason, 1993 and Taube, 1993). Like CA1 neurons, pyramidal neurons in the subiculum contain a substantial I_h current, which produces the characteristic sag toward the resting potential during hyperpolarizing or depolarizing current pulses (Stewart and Wong, 1993; Staff et al., 2000; Menendez de la Prida et al., 2003) (Fig. 5–12).

Action potentials were also found to be the same in bursting and regular spiking pyramidal neurons in the subiculum but were somewhat different from CA1 pyramidal neurons. Comparing single CA1 action potentials with subiculum action potentials (either the first in a burst or single action potentials in regular-spiking cells), the subicular action potentials were found to have slightly slower rise times and smaller amplitudes but shorter half widths (Staff et al., 2000). The dendritic morphology was also similar across all subicular neurons but distinct from that of CA1 cells (Staff et al., 2000). Taken together, these findings suggest that the dichotomy

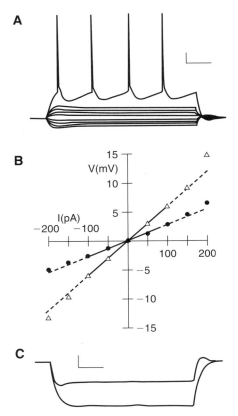

Figure 5–12. Subiculum passive properties and sag. *A.* Voltage responses to step current injections from –200 to +300 pA in 50-pA increments (+250 pA response not shown). Bar = 10 mV, 100 ms. *B.* Voltage–current plot of the steady-state responses shown in *A.* Solid lines are the points used for linear fits to the data. Dashed lines are extrapolations of the fits. *C.* Effect of 5 mM CsCl on the hyperpolarizing voltage response to a current step of –150 pA. Note the block of sag in the voltage response. Bar = 3 mV, 100 ms. (*Source*: Adapted from Staff et al., 2000.)

between bursting and regular-spiking neurons in the subiculum may be somewhat artificial. Another possibility is that subicular pyramidal neurons all have similar basic properties (yet distinct from those of CA1 cells), but that they vary along a continuum with respect to the strength of the burst-generating mechanism (Staff et al., 2000; Jung et al., 2001).

5.4.5 Mechanisms of Bursting

The mechanism responsible for bursting in the subiculum has been a matter of some controversy. Two early studies identified a calcium-dependent spike that could contribute to bursting, possibly as a result of dendritic spike initiation (Stewart and Wong, 1993; Taube, 1993). Another study, published about the same time, reported that bursting persisted in the presence of Ca^{2+} channel block but not Na^+ channel block and concluded that bursting is driven by Na^+ currents (Mattia et al., 1993; see also Mattia et al., 1997a). These seemingly contradictory findings were reconciled, to some extent, by a study showing that Ca^{2+} currents drive bursting, but they are acti-

vated by Na^+-dependent action potentials (Jung et al., 2001). Ca^{2+} channels are activated by each action potential, and current flows through these channels during spike repolarization as a result of an increased driving force and slow channel deactivation. The resulting Ca^{2+} tail current produces a spike afterdepolarization (ADP), which triggers additional spikes comprising the burst (Jung et al., 2001). This study also showed that block of Ca^{2+} channels can lead to an abnormal form of bursting in part due to indirect block of Ca^{2+}-activated K^+ channels. This finding reproduces and explains earlier demonstrations of the lack of effectiveness of some Ca^{2+} channel blockers to block bursting despite the fact that Ca^{2+} channels do play a pivotal role in producing the bursts under normal conditions. The results also explain the effectiveness of TTX as a blocker of bursting. Even at concentrations too low to eliminate the first spike, the threshold for the second spike was raised to a point that the ADP no longer triggers additional spikes (Jung et al., 2001).

5.4.6 Membrane Potential Oscillations

Another important feature of pyramidal neurons in the subiculum is their ability to generate subthreshold membrane potential oscillations in the theta frequency range of 4 to 9 Hz (Mattia et al., 1997b). These oscillations increase in amplitude as the membrane potential is depolarized above rest, reaching a peak amplitude of about 3 mV just below the action potential threshold. If the membrane is depolarized further, clusters of action potentials fire at a rate of about 1 to 2 Hz. Subthreshold theta oscillations in subicular pyramidal cells are abolished by the Na^+-channel blocker TTX but not by blockers of glutamate or GABA receptors or by Ca^{2+} channels, suggesting that oscillations are an intrinsic property that depends critically on voltage-gated Na^+ channels (Mattia et al., 1997b). Similar oscillations have also been observed in CA1 pyramidal neurons, where they have been shown to arise from interactions between voltage-gated Na^+ current, K^+ current (I_M), and I_h (Leung and Yu, 1998; Hu et al., 2002). Subicular pyramidal cells also participate in synaptically mediated oscillations in the gamma frequency range of 20 to 50 Hz. Bursting neurons in subiculum fire doublets of action potentials during these oscillations, which likely promote the spread of network activity in the gamma range (Stanford et al., 1998).

5.5 Dentate Granule Neurons

The main cell type of the dentate gyrus is the granule cell. These neurons have been studied extensively, in part because they were the first to be shown to exhibit LTP and in part because they receive spatially segregated synaptic inputs on different regions of their dendrites. Granule cells were also the first cell type in which it was shown that mRNA could be translated into proteins in dendrites, which has significant implications for plasticity and learning (Jiang and Schuman, 2002; Steward and Worley 2002).

5.5.1 Dendritic Morphology and Spines

The principal neurons of the dentate gyrus are distinctly different from all of the neurons discussed so far because they are not pyramidal in morphology. Rather, they comprise a small, ovoid cell body with a single, approximately conical (but somewhat elliptical) dendritic tree (Fig. 5–13). The granule cells lie in densely packed columnar stacks underneath the relatively cell-free molecular layer and the cell-rich polymorphic layer (also known as the hilus). Typically, granule cell somata are about 10 μm in diameter and about 18 μm in length, with their long axis oriented perpendicular to the granule cell layer. Interestingly, the packing density of dentate granule cells and CA3 pyramidal cells vary along the septo-temporal axis of the hippocampus but in opposite directions. Thus, the ratio of granule cells to CA3 cells ranges from about 12:1 at the septal pole to 2:3 at the temporal pole, implying substantial differences in connectivity along this axis (Amaral and Witter, 1995).

Granule cell dendrites all extend into the molecular layer and terminate near the hippocampal fissure. The number of dendritic branches is highly variable, with the calculated sum of the dendritic lengths ranging from 2.3 to 4.6 mm. These dendritic lengths are significantly shorter than those of the CA1 pyramidal neurons. Dendritic morphology also varies depending on the position in the dentate gyrus. Neurons located in the suprapyramidal blade (closest to CA1) are generally larger (greater total dendritic length, more dendritic segments, and a greater transverse spread) than those in the infrapyramidal blade (Desmond and Levy 1982, 1985; Claiborne et al., 1990).

Like pyramidal neurons, the dendrites of granule cells are heavily studded with spines. Estimates of spine density indicate that there are two to four spines per linear micrometer of dendrite. The number of spines increases (within this range) in progressively more distal dendrites, and there are slightly more spines in the suprapyramidal blade than in the infrapyramidal blade (Desmond and Levy 1982; Hama et al., 1989). The available data suggest that a granule cell located in the suprapyramidal layer would have close to 5600 spines, whereas a cell located in the infrapyramidal cell layer would have significantly fewer spines, at about 3600. These values are considerably lower than the spine densities and total spine numbers calculated for both CA1 and CA3 pyramidal neurons.

5.5.2 Excitatory and Inhibitory Synaptic Inputs

Dentate granule cells receive synaptic input from several sources. Granule cell dendrites are generally divided into thirds according to the differential inputs they receive. The proximal third (closest to the cell body) receives input from the commissural/associational fibers, which consist primarily of axons from the mossy cells (see Section 5.6). The middle

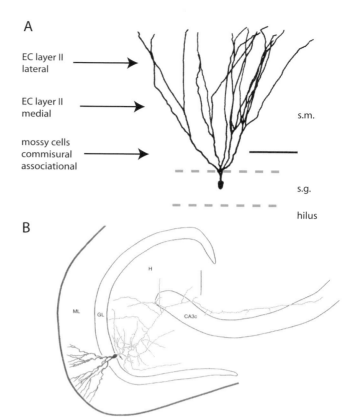

Figure 5–13. Dentate granule cell dendritic morphology, spines, and synaptic inputs and outputs. *A.* Computer-generated plot of a reconstructed granule cell from the suprapyramidal blade of the dentate gyrus showing the cell body in the stratum granulosum (s.g.) and the dendrites in the stratum moleculare (s.m.), with the major inputs indicated. (*Source*: Adapted from Claiborne et al. 1990, with permission.) *B.* Camera lucida drawing of the dendritic morphology and axonal arborization of a granule cell in the infrapyramidal blade of the dentate gyrus. The axons are in the molecular layer (ML, same as s.m.). The major targets of the mossy fiber axon (thin structure extending right of the granule layer, GL) are the mossy cells and CA3 pyramidal neurons, as well as interneurons in the hilus (H) and CA3 regions. (*Source*: Adapted from Lübke et al., 1998, with permission. A color version of this figure with the axon in red is available online.)

third receives input from relatively medial regions of the entorhinal cortex, and the distal third receives input from the lateral entorhinal cortex (Blackstad 1958; Amaral and Witter, 1995). Inputs to the dentate gyrus from layer II of the entorhinal cortex arrive via the perforant path. The spatial separation of lateral and medial perforant path inputs was elegantly exploited in early studies that described the cooperative and associative properties of LTP (McNaughton et al., 1978; Levy and Steward 1979) (see Chapter 10). Both inputs are primarily glutamatergic, although the medial perforant path inputs also contain cholecystokinin, and the lateral perforant path contains enkephalin (Amaral and Witter, 1995). Several differences between synaptic transmission at the medial and lateral perforant path have been reported, including differences in NMDA receptor activation as well as modulation by cholinergic, adrenergic, and metabotropic glutamate receptor activation (Abraham and McNaughton, 1984; Kahle and Cotman, 1989; Dahl et al., 1990; Pelletier et al., 1994; Macek et al., 1996).

The dentate gyrus receives several neuromodulatory inputs, including diffuse projections from the septal nuclei (acetylcholine), locus coeruleus (norepinephrine), and ventral tegmental area (dopamine). The supramammillary region of the hypothalamus (possibly containing substance P) projects to the proximal third of the molecular layer, and the raphe nuclei (serotonin) project primarily to the hilus (Amaral and Witter, 1995).

Granule cells also receive inputs from a variety of interneurons, mostly lying in the hilus. Basket cells and chandelier cells target primarily somata, whereas various interneurons target the dendrites. In addition, both the commissural/associational and perforant path inputs contain minor GABAergic components (Amaral and Witter, 1995). Of particular interest, almost all of the serotonergic input to the hilus terminates on GABAergic interneurons that project to the distal dendrites of granule cells (Halasy et al., 1992).

5.5.3 Axon Morphology and Synaptic Targets

The somata of granule cells taper at their base, where a single unmyelinated axon emerges and is directed toward the hilus. Ramon y Cajal termed the axons of granule cells "mossy fibers" for their anatomical similarity to the fibers in the cerebellum. The large varicosities and filopodial extensions are reminiscent of moss, thus providing the name for these pathways. Anatomically, as far as it is known these axons are unique among hippocampal and cortical neurons (and indeed throughout the mammalian CNS) in that they form anatomically specialized synapses depending on the nature of their postsynaptic targets.

Each granule cell gives rise to a single unmyelinated axonal fiber about 0.2 μm in diameter, with a total length (including collaterals) of more than 3 mm (Claiborne et al., 1986; Frotscher et al., 1991; Acsady et al., 1998). The axons form numerous collaterals throughout the hilus that innervate the numerous cell types present in the hilar subfield before projecting to the apical dendrites and in some cases basal dendrites of CA3 pyramidal neurons (Claiborne et al., 1986). The mossy-fiber projection to CA3 forms a tight bundle running parallel to the CA3 pyramidal cell body layer in a suprapyramidal region termed the stratum lucidum because of its appearance at the light microscopic level. This region corresponds to approximately the first 100 μm of the CA3 pyramidal neuron apical dendrite. After leaving the hilar region, the mossy fiber axon contains no further branch points.

Three basic types of mossy fiber terminal exist along the entire length of the main axon: large mossy terminals (4–10 μm), filopodial extensions that project from the large mossy boutons (0.5–2.0 μm), and small en passant varicosities (0.5–2.0 μm) (Amaral, 1979; Claiborne et al., 1986; Frotscher et al., 1991; Acsady et al., 1998). The latter two small terminals are somewhat larger than varicosities in axons of CA3 pyramidal neurons (Acsady et al., 1998). The total number of large

mossy terminals along a single axon is about 10 in the hilar region and about 12 (range 10–18) in the CA3 region, with the terminals being distributed more or less evenly along the mossy fiber axon. Mossy cells constitute the principal target of the large mossy terminals in the hilus (see Section 5.6), and the small filopodial and en passant terminals selectively innervate only inhibitory interneuron targets (Acsády et al., 1998). These terminals form only single, often perforated, asymmetrical synapses on the cell bodies, dendrites, and spines of GABAergic inhibitory interneurons. This anatomical arrangement stands in marked contrast to the large mossy fiber terminals, which contain numerous release sites housing thousands of both small, clear vesicles and large, dense-core vesicles. The mossy fibers are glutamatergic but also contain GABA (Sandler and Smith, 1991; Sloviter et al., 1996; Walker et al., 2001, 2002a) and the opiate peptide dynorphin (McGinty et al., 1983). Each mossy fiber bouton contains smooth endoplasmic reticulum and a large number of mitochondria (Chicurel and Harris, 1992). The main body of the large mossy bouton envelops the thorny excrescences of the CA3 pyramidal neuron, as described above.

Of particular interest, the filopodial extensions and small, en passant synapses outnumber the large mossy fiber terminals by about 10-fold, raising the intriguing idea that the primary targets of dentate gyrus granule cells are inhibitory interneurons (Acsády et al., 1998). This anatomical segregation of terminal types is unprecedented throughout the mammalian CNS and suggests that it may provide functional specialization of synaptic output.

Electrophysiological experiments have largely confirmed the hypothesis that the large and small synaptic specializations of the mossy fibers are functionally distinct. Individual mossy fiber release sites onto principal cells have a low initial release probability, which allows a high degree of short-term and frequency-dependent facilitation (Jonas et al., 1993; Salin et al., 1996; Toth et al., 2000; Lawrence et al., 2004). In contrast, mossy fiber synapses onto interneurons in the stratum lucidum demonstrate either mild facilitation or depression in response to brief stimulus trains (Toth et al., 2000). In addition, a form of NMDA receptor-independent LTP observed at mossy fiber synapses onto principal cells (which is thought to be expressed entirely in the presynaptic terminal) is absent at mossy fiber to interneuron synapses (Maccaferri et al., 1998) (see Chapter 10). Instead, paradigms that induce LTP at principal cell synapses induce two forms of long-term depression at interneuron synapses (Lei and McBain, 2002, 2004).

5.5.4 Resting Potential and Action Potential Firing Properties

The resting membrane potential of granule cells is typically more hyperpolarized than that of either CA1 or CA3 pyramidal neurons, being close to −84 mV, based on recordings made in vivo (Penttonen et al., 1997) and in vitro brain slices (Spruston and Johnston, 1992; Staley et al., 1992). Measurements of the action potential threshold have provided numbers similar to those observed for both CA1 and CA3 pyramidal cells: –45 mV. Given the relatively negative resting membrane potential of granule cells, larger depolarizations are required to bring single granule cells to threshold for action potential generation. These properties likely underlie the low spontaneous firing frequencies associated with granule cells in vivo (Penttonen et al., 1997). Surprisingly, little accurate information exists regarding granule cell firing patterns in vivo. This is due in part to the difficulty associated with unambiguously identifying granule cell activity during extracellular recordings. During behavioral tasks, granule cell firing frequencies are very low, except when the animal is in a place field (Jung and McNaughton, 1993; Skaggs et al., 1996) and during odor-guided tasks (Wiebe and Staubli, 1999) (see Chapter 11).

Upon reaching threshold for action potential initiation, in response to long depolarizing pulses granule cells typically fire trains of action potentials that demonstrate marked accommodation (Staley et al., 1992; Penttonen et al., 1997). As with pyramidal cells, spike accommodation is largely due to the activation of Ca^{2+}-dependent, voltage-gated K^+ conductances; addition of Ca^{2+} buffers to intracellular recording electrodes removes such accommodation (Staley et al., 1992).

5.5.5 Resting Membrane Properties

At the resting membrane potential granule cells have input resistances considerably higher than those of both CA1 and CA3 pyramidal cells, with estimates ranging from 230 to 450 $M\Omega$ (Spruston and Johnston, 1992; Staley et al., 1992) (Fig. 5–14) and a τ_m between 30 and 50 ms. These parameters are also developmentally regulated, a factor that is especially pertinent because granule cells continue to be born and develop in adults (Spigelman et al., 1992; Gould and Cameron, 1996; Liu et al., 1996). Lower values are obtained with sharp microelectrode recordings, but these values are likely to be affected by the microelectrode-induced leak (Spruston and Johnston, 1992; Staley et al., 1992). Leak-induced effects are likely to be larger in granule cells than in pyramidal cells because the smaller cell body and thinner dendrites mean that a leak constitutes a larger fraction of the total conductance.

As in pyramidal neurons, estimates of passive membrane properties are highly nonlinear across small deviations from the resting membrane potential (Spruston and Johnston, 1992), indicating that voltage-dependent conductances close to the resting membrane potential contribute to their passive membrane properties. Blockers of I_h have little effect on the passive membrane properties of granule cells (Spruston et al., 1992), thus implicating other conductances as influencing the resting membrane properties.

Granule cells have a relatively simple dendritic branching pattern. Their dendrites branch rather symmetrically, with each of the daughter branches being smaller in diameter than the parent dendrite. In fact, the branch points in granule cell dendrites come close to obeying the assumptions necessary to collapse the dendritic tree to an equivalent cylinder. In addition, each dendritic branch has similar geometry and terminates at approximately the same distance (the hippocampal

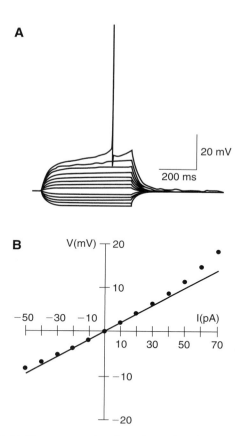

Figure 5–14. Dentate granule cell passive and active properties. *A.* Voltage responses to current injections of –50 to +80 pA in 10-pA increments. *B.* Voltage-current plot of the data in *A.* The line represents an extrapolated linear fit to the steady-state voltage responses to –20 to +20 pA current injections. (*Source:* Adapted from Lübke et al., 1998, with permission.)

fissure) as others in the same cell. Because of this dendritic geometry, it is reasonable to consider an equivalent cylinder model of granule cell dendrites (Durand et al., 1983; Turner and Schwartzkroin, 1983; Desmond and Levy, 1984; Turner, 1984). Unfortunately, the methods for determining electrotonic length (*L*) from the time course of somatic voltage transients (applied to granule cells and others by several investigators during the 1980s) are limited by the existence of a soma and further complicated by the presence of a microelectrode leak (Rall, 1969). Furthermore, anatomical data alone cannot be used to determine *L* because an important parameter, the intracellular resistivity (R_i) is not known for granule cells. The effects of a microelectrode leak on R_N and the apparent τ_m in granule cells, however, are strongly dependent on *L*. Using this approach, the electrotonic length of granule cells in the suprapyramidal blade of adult guinea pig slices has been estimated at 0.74 (Spruston and Johnston, 1992). In an equivalent cylinder of this length, a voltage imposed at the soma would be expected to attenuate only 22% by the end of the dendritic tree (Rall, 1959). Similar attenuation estimates were obtained independently using computer models (Carnevale et al., 1997).

Based on these analyses, one might be tempted to conclude that dentate granule cells are "electrotonically compact." However, steady-state voltage attenuation is much less than the attenuation of transient potentials, such as EPSPs. Furthermore, in the voltage-clamp condition, space-clamp errors are compounded because they are bidirectional (synapse to soma and back) and because escape of the dendritic potential from the command value introduces additional errors (Spruston et al., 1993). For these reasons, it may be argued that the descriptor "electrotonically compact" is at best misleading and at worst false for most neurons and experimental conditions. The term is best used as a comparator; indeed, computer models predict that granule cells are more electrotonically compact than most pyramidal neurons (Carnevale et al., 1997).

Despite the severity of EPSP attenuation, distal dendritic synapses on granule cells are likely to be more effective than synapses at similar distances on pyramidal cells. The reason is the absence of a large, main apical dendrite and the smaller soma in granule cells. A fixed current entering a synapse on a granule cell dendrite is not subject to as much attenuation as in pyramidal cell dendrites and can therefore generate a significant somatic EPSP even after its attenuation in the dendritic tree (Jaffe and Carnevale, 1999). In fact, because the diameter of granule-cell dendrites decreases with distance from the soma, the local depolarization from a fixed somatic current increases with distance from the soma in a way that largely cancels the effect of the increased voltage attenuation. Thus, synapses are at least partially normalized for their position on the dendritic tree. This effect has been called "passive normalization of synaptic integration" because the mechanism depends entirely on dendritic geometry and does not require any scaling of synaptic conductances with distance or interaction with voltage-gated conductances in the dendritic tree (Jaffe and Carnevale, 1999). Passive normalization has been shown to be plausible in other cell types that lack a large primary apical dendrite, including CA3 pyramidal neurons and interneurons. In CA1 neurons, passive normalization does not occur in the apical dendritic tree because of the long primary dendrite, but it could occur (at least partially) in the basal dendritic tree, which lacks a primary dendrite (Jaffe and Carnevale, 1999). These differences highlight the importance of dendritic architecture in synaptic integration and the functional relevance of variability of dendritic structure across the various regions of the hippocampus.

5.5.6 Active Properties of Granule Cells

Similar to pyramidal neurons, granule cells have a wide repertoire of voltage-gated currents. Granule cells express two forms of the voltage-gated, transient K+ current (Riazanski et al., 2001). One of these currents is indistinguishable from the transient currents expressed in most neurons, which have a low threshold for inactivation and block by 4-AP. The second current, however, activates at more depolarized potentials and is sensitive to low micromolar concentrations of TEA and the

anemone toxin BDS-I, properties consistent with it being carried by channels containing the Kv3.4 subunit. In granule cells this current has its highest density in nucleated patches excised from the basal end of the granule cell body, consistent with its immunohistochemical detection in the axons of granule cells.

In a technically superb series of experiments, Geiger and Jonas (2000) provided direct evidence for voltage-gated ion channels in the presynaptic mossy fiber terminals of granule cells (Fig. 5–15). In whole-cell recordings made directly from visually identified large mossy fiber boutons, action potential waveforms were observed to be remarkably brief (half duration 380 μs) compared to action potentials measured at the soma (half duration about 600 μs). Action potentials measured at the soma were typically followed by a prominent after-depolarization, whereas those at the mossy fiber terminal had a brief after-hyperpolarization followed by an after-depolarization. Action potentials at mossy fiber terminals were dynamically modulated during brief periods of high-frequency activity, with appreciable spike broadening occurring as a result of a decrease in the rate of repolarization. In contrast, only modest spike broadening was observed in similar experiments recorded at the granule cell soma, indicating differential expression of voltage-gated currents in the soma and the axon. Consistent with this hypothesis, voltage-gated K+ currents in axon terminals inactivated rapidly but recovered from inactivation very slowly, suggesting that cumulative channel inactivation mediated the activity-dependent spike broadening. Prolongation of the presynaptic spike waveform directly increased the amount of calcium that entered the presynaptic terminal during action potential activity, resulting in a significant increase in evoked synaptic currents. Pharmacological identification of the responsible conductance implicated channels formed by Kv1.1/Kv1.4 or Kv1.1/β-subunit combinations (Geiger and Jonas, 2000).

Propagation of action potentials into the granule cell dendritic structure has been much less studied than in pyramidal neurons. This is primarily due to the small diameter of granule-cell dendrites, which has made dendritic recording extremely difficult. Dendritic field potential recordings and current-source density analysis, however, have indicated that action potentials spread actively from an initiation zone near the soma into the dendrites (Jeffreys, 1979).

5.6 Mossy Cells in the Hilus

Numerous cell types are present in the polymorphic layer (hilus) between the dentate granule cells and the CA3 pyramidal neurons (Amaral, 1978). The most prominent and well studied principal neurons in this region are the mossy cells. These cells have been studied quite extensively because of the observation that they are among the first neurons to degenerate during epilepsy and ischemia (Sloviter, 1987, 1991; Hsu and Buzsáki, 1993; but see Ratzliff et al., 2002).

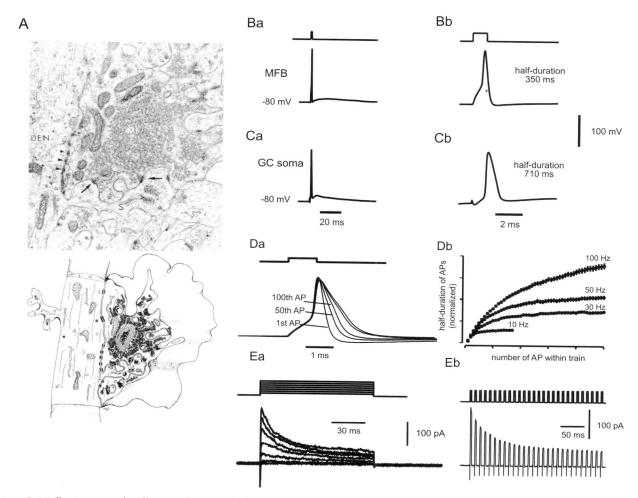

Figure 5–15. Dentate granule cell mossy fiber terminals. *A.* Ultrastructure of the mossy fiber synaptic complex. Upper panel: Electron micrograph through a mossy fiber synaptic complex. The postsynaptic CA3 pyramidal cell dendrite is indicated (DEN) to the left of the presynaptic mossy fiber terminal. The presynaptic terminal contains numerous small vesicles and mitochondria. The postsynaptic thorny excrescence is indicated (S) where it penetrates the terminal. Several symmetrical junctions between the dendritic shaft and the terminal are observed (arrowheads) and are representative of puncta adherentia. Note that these symmetrical junctions do not have any vesicles nearby. In contrast, asymmetrical junctions (arrows) onto the thorn show a significant clustering of vesicles. Lower panel: Representation of a mossy fiber synaptic complex depicting the various features observed at the electron microscopic level. (*Source*: Adapted from Amaral and Dent, 1981; from Henze et al., 2000.) *B, C.* Action potentials recorded from a presynaptic mossy fiber bouton (MFB, panel *B*) and in a granule cell soma (GC, panel *C*) evoked by a 1 ms current pulse and shown at different time bases. The properties of action potentials in the presynaptic mossy fiber bouton differ markedly from those in the granule cell somata, which had a significantly longer half duration and were followed by a more pronounced afterdepolarization. *D.* Action potentials in presynaptic mossy fiber boutons show marked activity-dependent broadening. Trains of action potentials were evoked at 50 Hz. *Da.* Every 50th action potential is shown superimposed with the first action potential in the train. *Db.* Plot of the action potential duration at half-maximal amplitude in whole cell recorded mossy fiber boutons against the number of action potentials in the train for the frequencies indicated. *E.* Frequency-dependent spike broadening is explained in part by the biophysical properties of voltage-gated outward potassium currents present in the presynaptic mossy fiber bouton. *Ea.* K$^+$ currents activated in a mossy fiber bouton outside-out patch by test pulses between –70 and +20mV. *Eb.* Cumulative inactivation of K$^+$ channels induced by repetitive activation. Traces are K$^+$ currents activated by a series of test pulses to +20 mV (3 ms duration, 7 ms interpulse interval). Such cumulative inactivation plays a significant role in shaping the action potential trajectory in response to high frequency stimulation. (*Source*: B–E: Geiger and Jonas, 2000.)

5.6.1 Dendritic Morphology and Spines

Mossy cells are located primarily in a C-shaped region of the hilus directly below the granule cell layer (zone 4 of Amaral, 1978). They consist of ovoid cell bodies that give rise to several primary dendrites (Fig. 5–16A,B). Each of these dendrites branches three or four times while remaining roughly parallel to the granule cell layer and with almost all branches remaining within the hilus (Amaral, 1978; Ribak et al., 1985; Buckmaster et al., 1992; but see Frotscher et al., 1991 and Scharfman, 1991).

The mossy cells are named for the mossy appearance created by the numerous thorny excrescences covering their proximal dendrites within 40 to 80 μm from the soma (Amaral, 1978; Ribak et al., 1985; Frotscher et al., 1991; Lübke et al., 1998) (Fig. 5–16B). These excrescences are similar, though not identical, to the thorny excrescences on CA3 pyramidal neurons. The major difference is a paucity of necks on the spines, with each excrescence formed by a cluster of spine heads (Amaral, 1978). The remaining portions of mossy cell dendrites are covered in more conventional spines.

5.6.2 Excitatory and Inhibitory Synaptic Inputs

Mossy cells receive direct excitatory input from the granule cell mossy fibers, which contact the thorny excrescences and at least some of the conventional spines on more distal dendrites (Frotscher et al., 1991; Buckmaster et al., 1992; Scharfman, 1994). An additional excitatory input arises from a subset of CA3 pyramidal neurons that send axon collaterals back into the hilus (Ishizuka et al., 1990; Scharfman, 1994). Intracellular recordings have revealed that mossy cells receive frequent, often large, spontaneous EPSPs (Scharfman and Schwartzkroin, 1988). Consistent with the large size of these spontaneous EPSPs, kinetic analysis has revealed that spontaneous EPSCs in mossy cells are slower than in aspiny hilar interneurons, a difference attributed to different glutamate receptor subtypes on these two classes of neurons (Livsey and Vicini, 1992; Livsey et al., 1993).

In addition to these powerful excitatory synaptic inputs, mossy cells receive substantial inhibitory inputs. After blocking glutamate receptors, a high frequency of spontaneous IPSCs are observed in all hilar neurons, including mossy cells (Scharfman, 1992; Soltesz and Mody, 1994; Acsady et al., 2000). It is likely that inhibitory synaptic input arrives from a variety of sources, including dentate basket cells, aspiny hilar interneurons (ipsilaterally and contralaterally), and GABAergic input from the medial septum.

5.6.3 Axon Morphology and Synaptic Targets

The mossy cell axon specifically targets the inner third of the molecular layer of the dentate gyrus (Ribak et al., 1985; Buckmaster et al., 1992). More than two-thirds of mossy cell axon collaterals ramify in this region, and the remainder

form synapses in the hilus and the granule cell layer (Buckmaster et al., 1996). The axon terminals in the inner molecular layer form asymmetrical synaptic contacts, primarily with granule cell dendrites. In the hilus, mossy cells form asymmetrical synapses on GABA-positive dendritic shafts and GABA-negative dendritic spines (Wenzel et al., 1997). Mossy cells stain positive for glutamate and negative for GABA, suggesting an excitatory function (Soriano and Frotscher, 1994; Wenzel et al., 1997), but may also contain peptide neurotransmitters (Fredens et al., 1987; Freund et al., 1997).

Two particularly important features of the mossy cell axon projection are that it is bilateral and it has an unusually extensive longitudinal component (Soltesz et al., 1993; Buckmaster et al., 1996) (Fig. 5–16C). In fact, each mossy cell forms synaptic contacts spanning more than half the length of the hippocampus, with most of the synaptic contacts formed by distal segments of the axon. These features imply that mossy cells allow granule cell activity to spread longitudinally and bilaterally in the dentate gyrus. Like the recurrent collaterals of the CA3 network, the positive feedback network formed by mossy cells has been suggested to contribute to the ability of the hippocampus to encode memories via an autoassociative network (Buckmaster and Schwartzkroin, 1994).

5.6.4 Resting and Active Properties

Mossy cells in vitro have resting potentials of –61 to –65 mV, R_N of 67 to 200 MΩ, and τ_m of 16 to 41 ms (Fig. 5–17). These ranges represent the mean values taken from sharp-microelectrode recordings and patch-clamp recordings, respectively (Scharfman and Schwartzkroin, 1988; Buckmaster et al., 1993; Lübke et al., 1998). Mossy cells can fire up to about 50 spikes during a 1-second current injection. Maximum spike rates can be higher, however, as mossy cells can exhibit both bursting and spike-frequency accommodation. These physiological features readily distinguish mossy cells from granule cells or basket cells of the dentate gyrus, but they are not easily distinguished from other neurons in the hilus (Scharfman, 1992; Lübke et al., 1998). Functionally, the most relevant functional features of mossy cells are likely to be their frequent and large EPSPs, which can trigger bursts of action potentials (Scharfman and Schwartzkroin, 1988). This unusual excitability of mossy cells has been proposed to be relevant during normal function and pathology (Sloviter, 1991; Buckmaster and Schwartzkroin, 1994; Ratzliff et al., 2002).

5.6.5 Other Spiny Neurons in the Hilus

A population of spiny neurons in the hilus that differs from mossy cells has also been identified. These neurons, fewer in number than mossy cells, are distinguishable by a lack of thorny excrescences and the presence of axon collaterals that extend to the outer molecular layer of the dentate gyrus

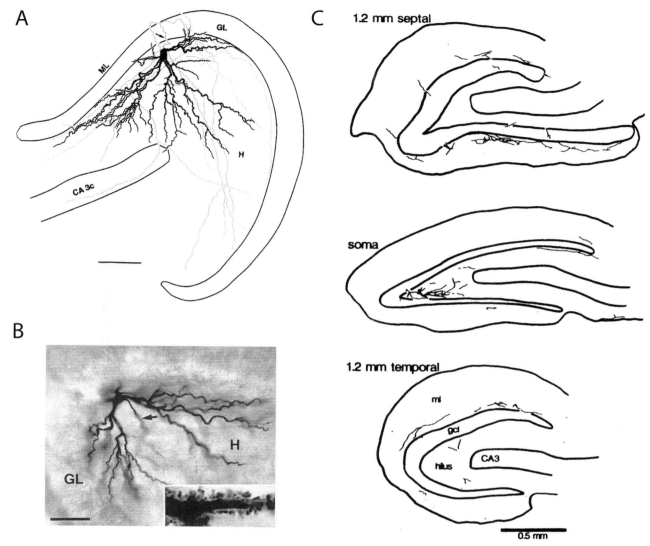

Figure 5–16. Mossy cell dendritic morphology, spines, and synaptic inputs and outputs. *A*. Camera lucida drawing of a mossy cell with the cell body in the hilus near the granule layer (GL) and dendrites extending farther into the hilus. (A color version of this figure with the axon in red is available online.) (*Source:* Adapted from Lübke et al. 1998, with permission.) *B*. Photomicrograph of a filled mossy cell showing the axon emerging from the cell body (arrow). The inset is a higher magnification view showing thorny excrescences covering a section of the dendrite. (*Source:* Adapted from Lübke et al., 1998, with permission.) *C*. Three sections showing axon collaterals from a single labeled mossy cell innervating nearly the full septotemporal extent of the hippocampus. Note that axon collaterals are restricted to the hilus and inner molecular layer (ml, near the granule cell layer, gcl). (*Source:* Adapted from Buckmaster et al., 1996, with permission.)

(Lübke et al., 1998). Although these neurons are spiny, it is not clear if they form excitatory or inhibitory synapses on their targets in the molecular layer. They have higher R_N than mossy cells (despite similar τ_m), presumably owing to more limited dendritic arborization. They can also fire at higher rates, on average, although the overlap in ranges of these values makes it difficult to distinguish them conclusively from mossy cells or aspiny hilar interneurons on the basis of physiological properties alone (Lübke et al., 1998).

5.7 Pyramidal and Nonpyramidal Neurons of Entorhinal Cortex

The entorhinal cortex is the major gateway between the hippocampal formation and the rest of the brain. It receives both intrinsic inputs from the hippocampus (primarily subiculum) and pre/parasubiculum as well as extrinsic inputs from numerous cortical areas. Various neurons in the entorhinal

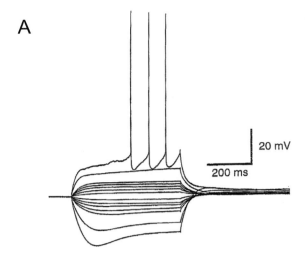

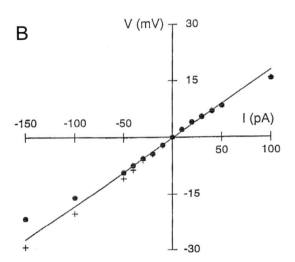

Figure 5–17. Mossy cell passive and active properties. *A.* Voltage responses of a mossy cell (same as Figure 5–16) to step current injections of −150 to +150 pA in 50-pA increments and −40 to +40 pA in 10-pA increments. Input resistance is 181 MΩ, and resting potential is −64 mV. *B.* Voltage-current relation of the steady-state (●) and peak (+) voltage responses shown in *A*. The line represents an extrapolated linear fit of the points between −50 and +50 pA. (*Source*: *A, B*: Adapted from Lübke et al., 1998, with permission.)

cortex provide the major input to the dentate gyrus and the hippocampus; they receive input back from the hippocampus and in turn project to other cortical areas, often the same areas that provide input to the entorhinal cortex.

The entorhinal cortex is a conventional six-layered structure comprising several excitatory cell types (Ramon y Cajal, 1904; Schwartz and Coleman, 1981; Carboni et al., 1990; Germroth et al., 1991; Belichenko, 1993; Mikkonen et al., 2000). Neurons in the superficial layers (II/III) receive most of their input from other cortical areas (largely olfactory in the rodent) as well as from presubiculum and parasubiculum. These layer II/III neurons then constitute the principal inputs to the dentate gyrus and hippocampus, and they provide feedback to other cortical areas. Neurons in the deep layers (IV-VI) receive extensive input from the hippocampus (subiculum) and presubiculum. In addition to projections back to other cortical areas, a projection from the deep layers back to the superficial layers of entorhinal cortex completes the closed-loop structure of the hippocampal formation (Chrobak and Buzsáki, 1994; Chrobak et al., 2000) (see Chapter 3 for more details). Here we consider three cell classes about which detailed physiological and morphological information is available: stellate cells in layer II, pyramidal cells in layers II/III, and pyramidal neurons in layers V/VI.

5.7.1 Stellate Cells of Layer II

Stellate cells are the most abundant cell type in layer II and are especially numerous in the medial entorhinal cortex. They derive their name from their star-like appearance, with numerous dendrites radiating out from the soma (Fig. 5–18A). In a typical stellate cell of rat medial entorhinal cortex, about five thick (5–6 μm diameter) primary dendrites emerge from the cell body (Klink and Alonso, 1997a). In most cases, one or two of the primary dendrites extend upward toward layer I, and a few primary dendrites extend downward toward layer III. Each of these two groups of dendrites branches extensively, giving rise to bitriangular dendritic arborization. On average, each primary dendrite gives rise to 15 terminal dendrites (Lingenhöhl and Finch, 1991). The upper dendritic tree (layer I) has a mediolateral expanse (up to 700 μm in the rat) that is greater than that of the lower dendritic tree (layer III) and exceeds that of most pyramidal neurons with apical dendrites in layer I (Klink and Alonso, 1997a). The dendrites of stellate cells are uniformly studded with spines, usually having a long, thin neck and a larger spine head. Dendritic branches often terminate in bouquets of about six dendritic spines (Klink and Alonso, 1997a). The dendritic spines presumably form the sites of contact for the synaptic inputs reaching layers I to III from other cortical areas as well as from the pre/parasubiculum.

The stellate cell axon usually emerges from a primary dendrite, close to the soma. The axon descends to the angular bundle, which eventually forms the perforant path. As described in Chapter 3, axons from stellate cells in the lateral entorhinal cortex terminate on the distal third of granule cell dendrites, whereas those from the medial entorhinal cortex terminate on the middle third of granule cell dendrites. Detailed reconstructions have revealed that the axonal arborization from a single layer II stellate cell is extensive, encompassing both the suprapyramidal and infrapyramidal blades of the dentate gyrus and encompassing more than two-thirds of the septo-temporal extent of the dentate gyrus (Tamamaki and Nojyo, 1993; Tamamaki, 1997; see also Paré and Llinás, 1994). The axons of layer II stellate cells also form synapses on CA3 pyramidal neurons. Importantly, many stellate cell axons do not cross the hippocampal fissure; rather, they project along one side of the fissure to CA3 and bend around the fissure toward the dentate gyrus. The presence of varicosities on axons in both CA3 and the dentate gyrus sug-

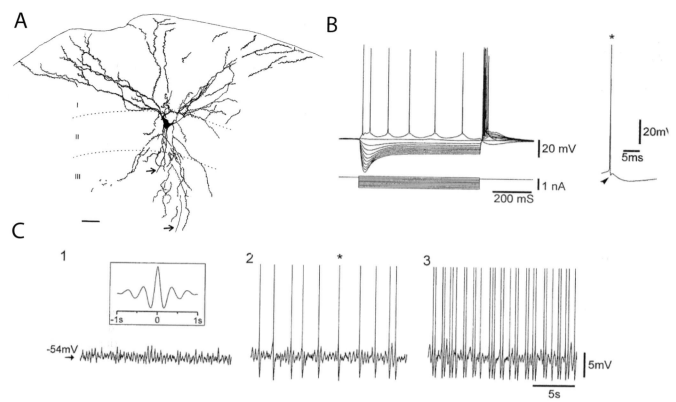

Figure 5–18. Stellate cells of layer II. *A.* Camera lucida drawing of a spiny stellate cell in layer II of entorhinal cortex showing its dendritic tree, which extends into layers I and III, and the axon emerging from the base of the soma (arrows). Bar = 40 μm. (*Source*: Adapted from Klink and Alonso, 1997a, with permission.) *B.* Voltage responses to step current injections as shown. Note the prominent sag in hyperpolarizing voltage responses and rebound firing at the offset of the current injection. The single action potential shown on an expanded time scale at the right (from C₂) shows a

fast AHP, an ADP, and a medium AHP. (*Source*: Adapted from Dickson et al., 2000a, with permission.) *C.* Membrane potential oscillations (1 and 2) and spike clustering (3) in a layer II stellate cell held at membrane potentials positive to –55 mV. Oscillations in 1–3 are at increasingly depolarized membrane potentials. The autocorrelation (inset in 1) demonstrates the rhythmicity of the subthreshold membrane potential oscillations. (*Source*: Adapted from Dickson et al., 2000a, with permission.)

gests that axons from individual stellate cells can project to both areas (Witter, 1989). Axon collaterals also branch and form synaptic connections within the entorhinal cortex (superficial and deep layers) and subiculum (Germroth et al., 1991; Lingenhöhl and Finch, 1991; Tamamaki and Nojyo, 1993; Klink and Alonso, 1997a).

In microelectrode recordings from layer II of rat medial entorhinal cortex, stellate cells have resting potentials of about –62 mV, R_N of about 36 MΩ, and τ_m of about 9 ms (Klink and Alonso, 1993; see also Jones, 1994). However, stellate cells also exhibit active nonlinearities near the resting potential, including TTX-sensitive amplification of subthreshold depolarizations and ZD-72688-sensitive sag of small hyperpolarizing and depolarizing responses (Fig. 5–18B). These two properties, mediated by voltage-gated Na⁺ channels and I_h channels, respectively, contribute to pronounced inward rectification (the voltage response to current injection is larger for depolarization than for hyperpolarization) in stellate cells (Klink and Alonso, 1993).

The action potential threshold is about –52 mV and the action potential duration about 1.2 ms in stellate cells. The

inward rectification properties of stellate cells contribute to a hump at the onset of depolarizing current pulses. Hence, action potential firing occurs near the beginning of long current injections above threshold. I_h and Na⁺ current also contribute to a depolarizing hump at the offset of hyperpolarizing current injections, which in some cases produce rebound spike firing (Fig. 5–18B). Action potentials in stellate cells are followed first by a fast AHP of about 10 mV, then a depolarizing after-potential of about 1 mV, and finally a medium AHP of about 11 mV. In response to long current injections stellate cells exhibit strong spike frequency accommodation; and a large, slow AHP occurs following the offset of the current injection (Klink and Alonso, 1993).

One of the most striking physiological features of layer II stellate cells in entorhinal cortex is the theta frequency oscillation that occurs during subthreshold depolarizations (Alonso and Llinás, 1989). These 5- to 15-Hz oscillations begin upon depolarization from rest and reach an amplitude of about 3 mV when V_m is around –55 mV (Fig. 5–18C). Further depolarization results in spike firing in a characteristic cluster pattern, with an interspike frequency of about 20 Hz and an intercluster frequency of 1 to 3 Hz (Alonso and Klink, 1993). Subthreshold theta oscillations in stellate cells are blocked by either TTX or ZD-72688, indicating that they result from interplay between voltage-gated Na^+ current and I_h (Klink and Alonso, 1993; Dickson et al., 2000a,b). The Na^+ dependence of the subthreshold oscillations in layer II stellate cells has prompted careful analysis of the voltage-gated Na^+ channels in these neurons. Na^+ currents in neurons dissociated from layer II have almost 10-fold larger Na^+ conductance than is seen in cells dissociated from layer III (Fan et al., 1994). Furthermore, compared to layer III neurons, Na^+ currents in layer II activate at lower voltages and inactivate at higher voltages, resulting in a substantial window current, a steady-state current in the voltage range where activation is significant but inactivation is incomplete (Fan et al., 1994). Biophysical analysis has revealed that a high-conductance, persistent Na^+ current is responsible for most of the window current, which is likely to produce subthreshold oscillations in layer II stellate cells (Magistretti et al., 1999a; Magistretti and Alonso, 1999). These currents are present in the dendrites as well as the soma of layer II neurons (Magistretti et al., 1999b). Although the subthreshold oscillations are blocked by high concentrations of TTX (Klink and Alonso, 1993), the Na^+ channels thought to mediate the oscillations have been termed "TTX resistant" because of the relatively high concentration of TTX required to block Na^+ currents in layer II neurons (White et al., 1993).

The membrane properties of layer II stellate cells are also subject to modulation by muscarinic receptor activation (Klink and Alonso, 1997b). Carbachol causes an increase in input resistance and membrane depolarization, which produces subthreshold voltage oscillations at a lower frequency (about 6 Hz) than the depolarization-induced theta oscillations that occur in the absence of the agonist. Because the effects of carbachol are potentiated by Ca^{2+} influx, it has been suggested that Ca^{2+}-activated, nonspecific-cation conductance may be activated by muscarinic receptor activation (Klink and Alonso, 1997c; Gloveli et al., 1999; Shalinsky et al., 2002).

5.7.2 Pyramidal Cells of Layer II

Most of the pyramidal neurons in layer II have their cell bodies in the deepest third of the layer. Their morphology is typical of pyramidal neurons, with a somewhat triangular soma, a thick apical dendrite extending into layer I, and thinner basal dendrites extending into layer III (Fig. 5–19A). Both apical and basal dendrites branch extensively and are studded with spines at even higher density than in layer II stellate cells (Klink and Alonso, 1997a).

The axon of layer II pyramidal neurons emerges from the base of the soma and extends through layers II and III toward the angular bundle. Extensive axon collaterals are also located within entorhinal cortex (Klink and Alonso, 1997a). The axons of layer II pyramidal cells, like those of the stellate cells in the same layer, form the perforant path, which projects to the dentate gyrus and CA3 (Schwartz and Coleman, 1981).

Many of the basic properties of layer II pyramidal neurons are similar to those of their stellate counterparts (V_{rest} −64 mV, R_N 40 MΩ, τ_m 12 ms, threshold −49 mV); both exhibit spike-frequency accommodation and a prominent TTX-resistant, persistent Na^+ current, which is also present in the dendrites (White et al., 1993; Magistretti et al., 1999) (Fig. 5–19C). However, several physiological properties clearly distinguish pyramidal cells from stellate cells in layer II (Alonso and Klink, 1993). First, the action potential duration is significantly longer in pyramidal cells than in stellate cells (1.8 vs. 1.2 ms at threshold). Second, pyramidal cells exhibit less sag than stellate cells, especially in the depolarizing direction. As a result, layer II pyramidal neurons do not exhibit rebound spike firing, even following large hyperpolarizations; and they exhibit longer latencies to spiking than do stellate cells (Fig. 5–19B). Third, pyramidal cells lack the outward rectification that is prominent in stellate cells in the presence of TTX. Fourth, spike repolarization in pyramidal cells is severely impaired in the absence of Ca^{2+} compared to the modest increase in spike duration observed under the same conditions in stellate cells (Alonso and Klink, 1993; Klink and Alonso, 1993). Finally, the membrane potential oscillations generated below threshold and the spike clusters occurring above threshold in stellate cells are absent in layer II pyramidal neurons (Alonso and Klink, 1993). Activation of muscarinic receptors, however, produces depolarization and low-frequency (0.2–0.5 Hz) oscillations of action potential bursting in layer II pyramidal neurons (Klink and Alonso, 1997b).

5.7.3 Pyramidal Cells of Layer III

Intracellular recordings followed by biocytin labeling have revealed two types of pyramidal neurons in layer III, each with distinct morphological and physiological properties (Gloveli et al., 1997a; but see Dickson et al., 1997). These two types of pyramidal neuron were distinguished primarily on the basis of dendritic spines, which are present on the dendrites of type 1 but not type 2 layer III pyramidal neurons (Gloveli et al., 1997a). Both types have pyramidal morphology (Fig. 5–20A), but the type 1 (spiny) cells cover broader expanses in both the apical and basal dendritic trees. The apical dendrites of both cell types extend toward the cortical surface, whereas basal dendrites remain largely restricted to layer III (Gloveli et al., 1997a; but see Dickson et al., 1997).

The axons of both types of layer III pyramidal neurons could be traced to the angular bundle, but only the axons of the type 1 (spiny) neurons could be followed to CA1 and the subiculum (Gloveli et al., 1997a). Thus, spiny pyramidal neurons give rise to the perforant-path projection to CA1 (or temporo-ammonic path), but the targets of type 2 (aspiny) neurons are less clear.

Layer III pyramidal neurons are easily distinguished from their layer II counterparts by the absence of sag (Dickson et al., 1997; Gloveli et al., 1997a; van der Linden and Lopes da Silva, 1998) (Fig. 5–20B). Type 1 (spiny) pyramidal neurons of layer III have relatively high R_N (70 MΩ) and long τ_m (20 ms),

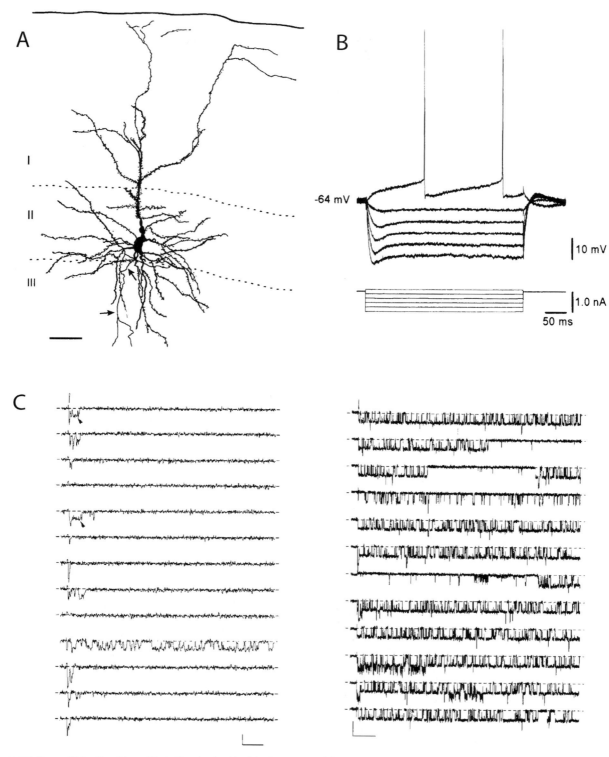

Figure 5–19. Pyramidal cells of layer II. *A.* Camera lucida drawing of a spiny pyramidal neuron in layer II of entorhinal cortex showing its dendritic morphology, which consists of an apical tree extending to the limit of layer I and a basal tree in layers II and III. The axon (arrows) emerges from the base of the soma. Bar = 40 μm. (*Source*: Adapted from Klink and Alonso, 1997a, with permission.) *B.* Voltage responses of a layer II pyramidal neuron to the current injections shown. (*Source*: Adapted from Alonso and Klink, 1993, with permission.) *C.* Voltage-gated Na$^+$ channels in the dendrites of layer II stellate cells showing transient (left) and persistent (right) gating. Channel activity was elicited by consecutive depolarizing voltage steps to –30 mV (beginning at arrow) in two cell-attached patches from the dendrites of isolated layer II pyramidal cells. Bars = 2 pA, 5 ms (left); 2 pA, 50 ms (right). (*Source*: Adapted from Magistretti et al. 1999b, with permission.)

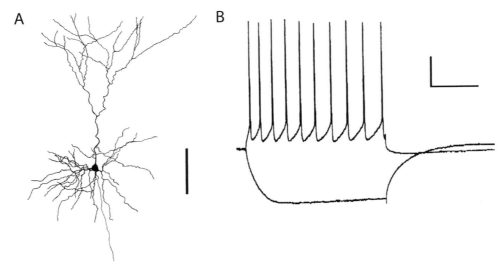

Figure 5–20. Pyramidal cells of layer III. *A.* Camera lucida drawing of a pyramidal neuron in layer III of medial entorhinal. Bar = 200 μm. *B.* Hyperpolarizing and depolarizing voltage responses to current injections of −300 and +300 pA. Bars = 20 mV, 100 ms. (*Source: A, B.* Adapted from van der Linden and Lopes da Silva, 1998, with permission.)

whereas type 2 (aspiny) pyramidal neurons have lower R_N (30 MΩ) and shorter τ_m (8 ms) (Gloveli et al., 1997a; see also Dickson et al., 1997). The resting potentials (about −70 mV) and action potential thresholds (about −55 mV) are similar in the two cell types, but type 2 (aspiny) pyramidal cells showed more spike-frequency accommodation than type 1 (spiny) cells (Gloveli et al., 1997a). An interesting difference between the pyramidal cells of layers II and III is that layer II neurons tend to be activated by synaptic activation at frequencies above 5 Hz, whereas layer III neurons respond best to frequencies below 10 Hz (Gloveli et al., 1997b).

5.7.4 Pyramidal Cells of Deep Layers

Layer III of the entorhinal cortex is separated from the next layer of cells by a cell-free zone called lamina dissecans. In Cajal's nomenclature, this acellular layer is synonymous with layer IV, in which case there are neurons in layers V and VI. In some other studies, however, the acellular layer is considered separately and the cellular layers are divided into layers IV to VI (see Chapter 3). At least two-thirds of the projecting neurons in the deep layers of entorhinal cortex are pyramidal neurons, and the rest are polymorphic or multipolar neurons (Lorente de No, 1933; Lingenhöhl and Finch, 1991; Hamam et al., 2000, 2002; Egorov et al., 2002a).

Although the pyramidal neurons and polymorphic neurons comprise heterogeneous groups of neurons, these groups are clearly distinguished by their dendritic architecture. Pyramidal neurons consist of a large apical dendrite extending to layer I or II and multiple basal dendrites with variable distributions, whereas polymorphic neurons consist of numerous dendrites radiating in all directions from the cell body. Pyramidal cells have been further subdivided into small and large pyramidal neurons. Small pyramidal cells have basal dendrites in layers V and VI, whereas large pyramidal cells have dendrites that extend horizontally within layer V and have therefore been alternately described as horizontal cells (Hamam et al., 2002) (Fig. 5–21A).

In layer V of the lateral entorhinal cortex, both small and large pyramidal neurons have an average of six to seven primary dendrites: one apical dendrite (average diameter 4.2 μm in small and 5.2 μm in large pyramidal cells) and three to eight primary basal dendrites (average diameter 1.7 μm in small and 3.3 μm in large pyramidal cells) for a total dendritic length of about 8 mm. Polymorphic cells also have an average of six to seven primary dendrites with an average diameter of 3.4 μm and a total dendritic length of about 10 mm (Hamam et al., 2002; see also Lingenhöhl and Finch, 1991; Hamam et al., 2000).

Spines are present on the dendrites of all deep-layer pyramidal neurons and polymorphic cells (Lingenhöhl and Finch, 1991; Hamam et al., 2000, 2002). The synaptic inputs to these principal neurons presumably originate from multiple sources, including other cortical areas, presubiculum, parasubiculum, and subiculum (Amaral and Witter, 1989; Lopes da Silva et al., 1990) (see Chapter 3).

The axons of deep-layer pyramidal and nonpyramidal projecting neurons of entorhinal cortex extend into the angular bundle, from which they project to other cortical areas, including many of the same regions that provide input to the superficial layers of entorhinal cortex (see Chapter 3). There is also considerable evidence, however, that deep-layer neurons project back to the dentate gyrus and hippocampus as part of the perforant path (Swanson and Cowan, 1977; Köhler, 1985; Deller et al., 1996b; Gloveli et al., 2001). In addition to entering the angular bundle, axons of both pyramidal and nonpyramidal neurons in the deep layers of the entorhinal cortex give off numerous branches, which are abundant in layers V and VI but in some cases also extend into the superficial layers (Gloveli et al. 2001; Hamam et al., 2000, 2002). Collaterals in layers V and VI form part of an associational system, which may contribute to the susceptibility of the entorhinal cortex to epileptic activity (Jones and Heinemann, 1988). Collaterals to the superficial layers complete a closed loop from layers II and III to the hippocampus, to layers V and VI, and back to layers II and III (Chrobak and Buzsáki, 1994; Chrobak et al., 2000).

Intracellular microelectrode recordings from deep-layer neurons in entorhinal cortex slices indicate that the basic electrophysiological properties of small pyramidal cells, large pyramidal cells (horizontal cells), and polymorphic cells are heterogeneous but not statistically different among the morphological groups (Hamam et al., 2000, 2002). Average resting potentials were -62 to -65 mV, R_N values were 50 to 80 MΩ, and τ_m values were 11 to 15 ms. Similar values have been reported in other studies (Jones and Heinemann, 1988; Egorov et al., 2002a). Voltage-current plots revealed inward rectification, in most cases consistent with a time-dependent

Figure 5–21. Pyramidal cells of layer V–VI. *A.* Reconstructions of three subtypes of neuron in layer V of lateral entorhinal cortex. Bar = 100 μm. (*Source*: Adapted from Hamam et al., 2002, with permission.) *B.* Responses of a layer V pyramidal neuron to successive current injections (300 pA, 4 seconds each) in the presence of the muscarinic AChR agonist carbachol (10 μM). Note the progressive increase in persistent action potential firing that continues after each current injection is terminated. Each depolarizing current step is 4 seconds in duration. (*Source*: Adapted from Egorov et al., 2002b, with permission.)

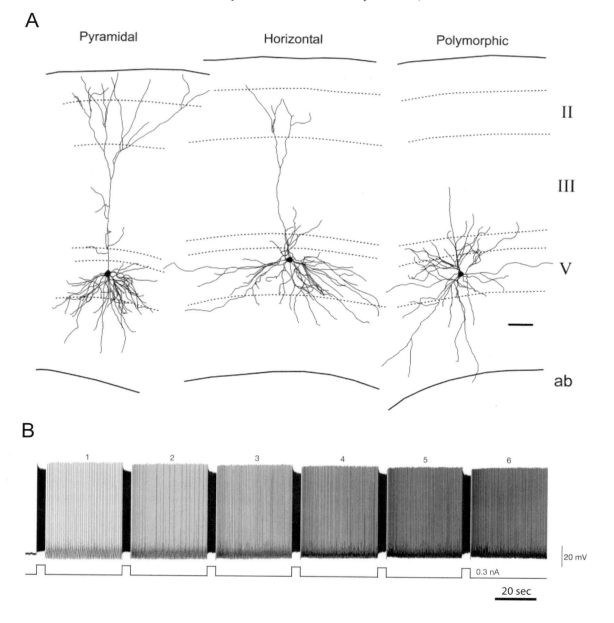

voltage sag, presumably due to activation of I_h (Hamam et al., 2000, 2002). In pyramidal neurons, sag was much smaller than reported for layer II stellate cells (Klink and Alonso, 1993), and one study reports that sag is absent from nonpyramidal neurons in the deep layers of the entorhinal cortex (Egorov et al., 2002a). Action potentials were about 65 mV in amplitude (threshold to peak) followed by an AHP of about 17 mV. Polymorphic neurons exhibit a voltage-dependent delay to spike firing, which is mediated by a D-type K^+ current (Egorov et al., 2002a). Repetitive firing was largely regular spiking with some spike-frequency accommodation, but burst firing was not observed (Hamam et al., 2000, 2002; Egorov et al., 2002a; but see Jones and Heinemann, 1988).

Another important characteristic of pyramidal neurons in the deep layers of the entorhinal cortex is that most exhibit membrane-potential oscillations in the theta range when held just below threshold for action potential firing (Dickson et al., 2000b). These oscillations have amplitudes of 2 to 7 mV and frequencies of 5 to 15 Hz (Dickson et al., 2000b; Hamam et al., 2000, 2002). Like the prominent oscillations in stellate cells of layer II, the oscillations in layer V neurons are TTX-sensitive and therefore require voltage-gated Na^+ current. An important difference, however, is that the oscillations in layer V do not seem to require I_h, as pyramidal cells lacking voltage sag still exhibit prominent theta oscillations (Dickson et al., 2000b). The relation between intracellular theta oscillations and the network theta, gamma, and ripple (sharp-wave) oscillations observed in the entorhinal cortex during various behavioral states remains unclear (Chrobak and Buzsáki, 1994, 1996; Buzsáki, 1996).

Perhaps the most intriguing property of layer V pyramidal cells in the entorhinal cortex is their ability to integrate neural activity over long periods of time. During activation of muscarinic acetylcholine receptors, stimuli lasting a few seconds can lead to sustained action potential firing for several minutes (Egorov et al., 2002b). Furthermore, repeated stimulation during cholinergic activation leads to sustained firing at higher frequencies (Fig. 5–21B). This unique form of neural integration, which is mediated by a calcium-activated, nonspecific cation current, has been proposed to contribute to the function of the entorhinal cortex in working and long-term memory (Egorov et al., 2002b).

5.8 Pyramidal and Nonpyramidal Neurons of Presubiculum and Parasubiculum

The presubiculum and parasubiculum are considered separately from the subiculum for two important reasons. First, these regions are distinct from the subiculum in that they are multilaminate (Fig. 5–22A). The parasubiculum has a conventional six-layered cortical structure. Presubiculum has also been described as a six-layered cortex, but the layers are not as well defined, so it may be more appropriately considered an anatomical transition zone between the three-layered hippocampus and the six-layered parasubiculum. The second reason for considering the pre- and parasubiculum separately from the subiculum is that these regions have distinctly different physiological properties (see below).

The major projection from the presubiculum is to layer III of the medial entorhinal cortex, whereas the major projection from the parasubiculum is to layer II of the medial and lateral entorhinal cortex. Both pre- and parasubiculum also project weakly back to the stratum lacunosum-moleculare of the hippocampus and to the superficial molecular layer of the dentate gyrus. Both regions also have numerous other cortical and subcortical inputs and outputs (see Chapter 3).

Microelectrode recordings have been used to study the electrophysiological properties of neurons in the pre- and parasubiculum (Funahashi and Stewart, 1997a). Despite the fact that pyramidal and nonpyramidal (stellate) neurons are present in all layers of the cortex, the basic resting and active properties of neurons in the pre- and parasubiculum are remarkably homogeneous, with resting potentials in the range of -60 to -68 mV, R_N of 42 to 84 MΩ, and τ_m of 8 to 12 ms. A modest degree of membrane sag was observed in superficial neurons, while sag was absent in deep-layer pyramidal and stellate neurons (Fig. 5–22B). In this respect, the properties of these neurons are functionally quite distinct from their neighbors in the subiculum and entorhinal cortex.

Another major difference between neurons in the pre- and parasubiculum and the subiculum is the absence of intrinsic burst firing. In response to depolarizing current injection, neurons in these regions were found to fire only regular trains of action potentials (Funahashi and Stewart, 1997a). Despite the absence of intrinsic burst firing, neurons in the deep layers of the pre- and parasubiculum exhibit synaptically driven burst discharges (Fig. 5–22C). In response to brief stimulation of either the subiculum or the deep medial entorhinal cortex, deep-layer neurons in the pre- and parasubiculum depolarize and fire for hundreds of milliseconds (Funahashi and Stewart, 1997b). These bursts are driven by giant, glutamatergic EPSPs and may be sustained by reciprocal connections with intrinsically bursting neurons in the subiculum (Funahashi et al., 1999). Neurons in the superficial layers of the pre- and parasubiculum respond to synaptic stimulation of the subiculum or entorhinal cortex with EPSPs and can produce synaptically driven bursts. The superficial neurons send axon collaterals to the deep layers of the pre- and parasubiculum, but reciprocal connections are absent (Funahashi and Stewart, 1997b).

5.9 Local Circuit Inhibitory Interneurons

Whereas most principal (i.e., glutamatergic) cell types of the hippocampus have their cell bodies organized into highly structured lamina (e.g., CA3/CA1 stratum pyramidale), the somata of local circuit GABAergic inhibitory interneurons

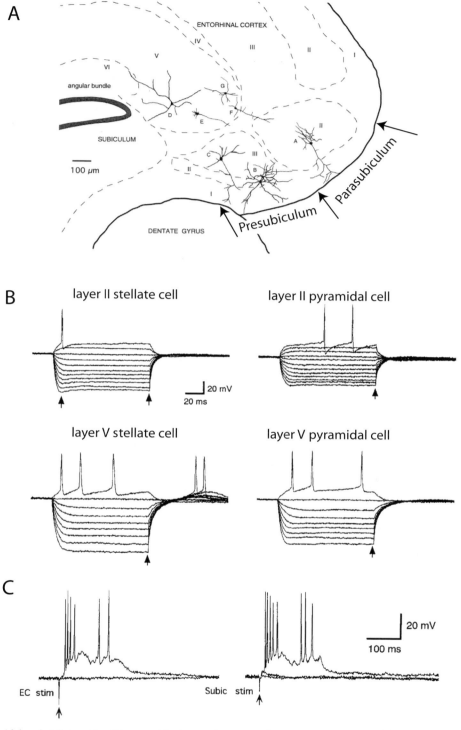

Figure 5–22. Pyramidal and stellate cells of the presubiculum and parasubiculum. *A*. Camera lucida drawings of several neurons in various layers of presubiculum and parasubiculum. A, pyramidal cell in layer II of parasubiculum; B, stellate cell in layer II of presubiculum; C, pyramidal cell in layer III of presubiculum; D, stellate cell in layer V of presubiculum; E, pyramidal cell in layer V of presubiculum; F, pyramidal cell in layer V parasubiculum; G, stellate cell in layer V of parasubiculum. *B*. Voltage responses of various neurons to current injections (approximately –1.5 to +0.5 nA). Note the similarity of response characteristics of different neurons within the same layers but differences in neurons between layers. *C*. Responses of a layer V neuron in the parasubiculum to synaptic stimulation of the entorhinal cortex or subiculum. Note also the burst-firing responses despite the absence of burst firing in response to current injections (*B*). (*Source*: *A–C*. Adapted from Funahashi and Stewart, 1997a, with permission.)

show no such apparent organization. In fact, the somata of this highly diverse population of neurons are scattered throughout almost all subfields and strata of the hippocampus (Fig. 5–23). Moreover, despite representing only ~10% of the total hippocampal neuronal population, inhibitory interneurons represent perhaps one of the most diverse cell populations, a claim based not only on their highly divergent anatomical properties but also on their functional properties.

The axons of this diverse cell population make mainly short-range projections and release the inhibitory neurotransmitter GABA onto their targets. Consequently, hippocampal inhibitory interneurons have traditionally been considered as little more than the regulators of principal neuron activity— the yin to the excitatory yang. Evidence suggests, however, that in addition to that role their network connectivity and properties of intrinsic voltage-gated currents are finely tuned to permit inhibitory interneurons to generate and control the rhythmic output of large populations of principal cells and other populations of inhibitory interneurons. The axons of these cells are often targeted to specific dendritic domains of pyramidal neurons as well as to other inhibitory interneuron types; this has led to the suggestion that specific interneuron

Figure 5–23. Inhibitory interneuron diversity. *A*. Composite drawing of characteristic hippocampal and dentate gyrus inhibitory interneuron types assembled from reconstructions of in vivo (5, 10–13) or in vitro (1–3, 6–9) intracellularly labeled or immunostained (4, 14, 15) neurons in the rat (1–5, 10–15) and guinea pig (6–9). Thick lines represent the dendritic trees; thin lines are the axons. *B*. Summary diagram shows the laminar distribution of dendritic and axonal arborizations of various types of calcium-binding protein- and neuropeptide-containing interneurons in the hippocampus. Filled circles mark the general cell body location of each interneuron type that gives rise to thick horizontal and/or vertical lines, indicating the predominant orientation and laminar distribution of the dendritic tree. Boxes represent the laminae, where the axon of each interneuron type typically arborizes. Shaded boxes indicate that other interneurons, rather than principal cells, are the primary targets. The transverse extent of the dendrites or axon is not indicated. (*Source*: Modified from Freund and Buzsáki, 1996; from McBain and Fisahn, 2001.)

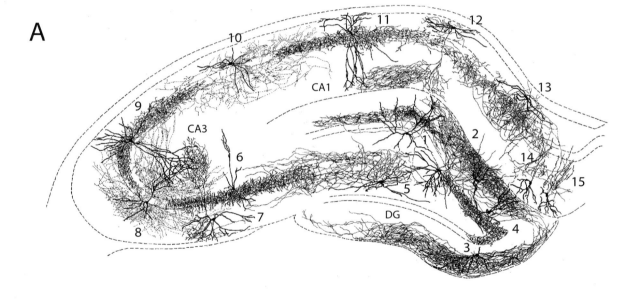

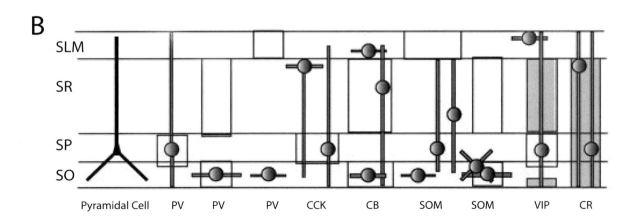

types are "tailor-made" to play fundamental roles in controlling the generation of Na^+- and Ca^+-mediated action potentials, the regulation of synaptic transmission and plasticity, and the generation and pacing of large-scale synchronous oscillatory activity.

5.9.1 Understanding Interneuron Diversity

By definition, all local circuit inhibitory interneurons synthesize and release GABA as their primary neurotransmitter. Anatomically, however, interneurons represent one of the most diverse populations in the mammalian CNS. To understand anything of inhibitory interneuron function one must first consider the diversity of the population and the efforts made by numerous anatomical and physiological investigators alike to break this population down into subpopulations based on anatomical, neurochemical, or functional properties. A major problem that has invariably plagued any study of interneuron function, however, has been the inability to classify interneurons neatly into functional or anatomical subpopulations. Even within a single region of the hippocampus, classifying interneurons is difficult and leads to different numbers of types depending on the classification scheme chosen. Because of this problem, we have chosen not to organize the discussion of hippocampal interneurons around an arbitrary classification scheme. Rather, this section is organized around a variety of commonly accepted features observed in interneurons. Such features can include anatomical, neurochemical, or functional commonalities that at the most elementary level allow identification of themes across neurons in different regions of the hippocampal formation. Ultimately, however, when such features are cross-referenced, such rigid classification schemes tend to break down and can often prove unhelpful, as is discussed below. Although we have chosen this approach, a detailed understanding of hippocampal function eventually requires that models be developed for several classes of interneurons, and different models may require different classification schemes. Thus, some discussion of the numerous attempts to classify these neurons into distinct subpopulations is warranted.

Historically, initial attempts to classify interneurons primarily used two approaches: classification based on anatomy or based on neurochemical markers (for review see Freund and Buzsáki, 1996). Classifications based solely on anatomy (Table 5–1) tell us little about interneuron function, but the recent mapping of axonal arbors to specific domains across the dendritic trees of their targets and the position of dendrites in specific hippocampal subfields have provided important clues to specific functional roles played by various interneuron subtypes (Fig. 5–23). For example, interneurons with axons that innervate either pyramidal cell somata or axon initial segments (basket cells, chandelier cells, axo-axonic cells) almost certainly regulate the local generation of Na^+-dependent action potentials. In contrast, inhibition arriving at dendritic locations likely has little direct influence over somatic action potential generation but may strongly influence local dendritic integra-

Table 5–1.
Morphological classification of hippocampal interneurons

Chandelier or Axo-axonic Cells

Basket Cells

Interneurons Innervating Principal Cell Dendrites

Dentate gyrus

Interneurons with hilar dendrites and ascending axons (HIPP cells)
Hilar border neurons with ascending axons and dendrites (HICAP cells)
Neurons with axons and dendrites in stratum moleculare (MOPP cells)
Hilar neurons with a projection to the hippocampus and subiculum
Hilar neurons with unknown projections

Hippocampus

Cells terminating in conjunction with entorhinal afferents (O-LM cells)
Interneurons innervating pyramidal cell dendrites in strata radiatum and oriens (bistratified and trilaminar cells)
Interneurons with axon collaterals and dendrites in stratum radiatum
Interneurons in stratum lacunosum-moleculare
Interneurons in stratum lucidum
Interneurons projecting across subfield boundaries

Interneurons Specialized to Innervate Other Interneurons
IS-1 neurons
IS-2 neurons
IS-3 neurons

Source: Adapted and extended from Freund and Buzsaki (1996).

tion, shunt excitatory inputs on their way to the soma, or regulate dendritic spike initiation and/or propagation. Each of these interneuron types exhibits both differences and similarities in their physiological properties. Even within a single layer of the hippocampus, interneurons with unique axon targeting and physiological properties can be identified (Fig. 5–24).

Perhaps one of the most useful characterizations of interneuron subtypes has been based on neurochemical content (Table 5–2). Although the precise physiological roles played by this wide repertoire of peptide transmitters and Ca^{2+}-binding proteins contained in specific inhibitory interneuron subpopulations is largely unclear, their role in aiding anatomical and functional characterization of interneurons cannot be overemphasized. Much of our current understanding of interneuron anatomy has its origins in studies utilizing antibodies raised against these markers. Neurochemically identical cells can, however, have surprisingly different functional properties, somewhat undermining this attempt to provide convenient interneuron subdivisions. For example, "fast-spiking" parvalbumin (PV)-containing interneurons were once considered to comprise only basket and axo-axonic cells types, but this interneuron class has

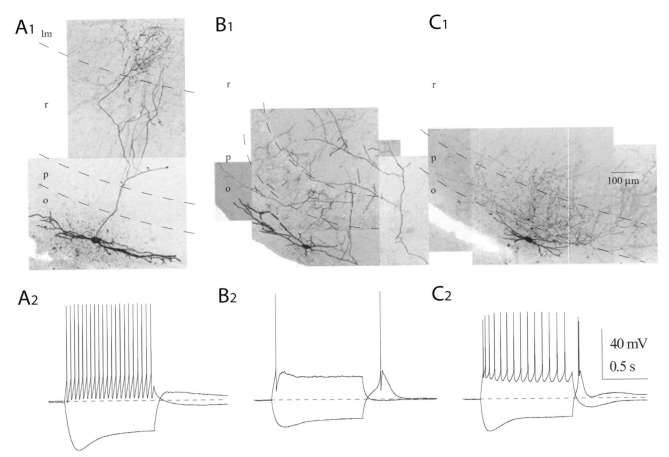

Figure 5–24. Differential axon targeting of various inhibitory interneurons. Three types of interneuron are shown, each with a cell body and dendrites in the stratum oriens of CA1 but having distinct axonal projection patterns and physiological properties. *A.* An O-LM cell targets the distal dendrites of CA1 pyramidal cells (A_1). Upon injection of a depolarizing current pulse, O-LM interneurons exhibit an accommodating train of action potentials followed by a slow AHP. A prominent sag indicative of I_h is present upon hyperpolarization (A_2). *B.* Interneuron type exhibiting a diffuse axonal arborization pattern suggestive of a septally projecting interneuron. These interneurons are typically somatostatin immunoreactive and target other interneurons (B_1) (Gulyás et al., 2003). In contrast to O-LM cells, this cell rapidly accommodated upon depolarization, firing only a single spike (B_2). Furthermore, upon repolarization, the cell fired a spike with a slow component suggestive of a T-type Ca^{2+} current. *C.* Stratum oriens interneuron type targeting the proximal dendritic trees of CA1 pyramidal cells (C_1). Also in contrast to O-LM interneurons, this cell exhibited a reduced fast AHP following each spike and a spike with a pronounced Ca^{2+} component upon repolarization (C_2). (*Source*: Lawrence and McBain, unpublished.)

recently seen new additions (Maccaferri et al., 2000). Interneurons with cell bodies in the stratum oriens and axons in the stratum lacunosum-moleculare (O-LM cells) or in both stratum radiatum and stratum oriens (bistratified cells) also contain PV. Given the dendritic location of their axonal targeting, it is highly unlikely that the latter cell types perform roles similar to those of the basket or axoaxonic cells. Similar additions to the somatostatin- and cholecystokinin (CCK)-containing families have also been described, further complicating classification systems based solely on neurochemical content (Oliva et al., 2000; Cope et al., 2002). Although these two methods of classification (morphology and neurochemistry) may be considered separately, substantial effort has been made to relate the two criteria. For example, neurons expressing distinct neurochemical markers have been found to also have different dendritic morphology (Gulyás et al., 1999) (Fig. 5–25).

Characterization based on function has proven even more problematic. The classic subdivisions were originally based solely on action potential firing patterns (e.g., fast-spiking versus regular spiking). However, action potential generation results from the combined activity of numerous voltage-gated channels, with each channel type potentially having a unique expression pattern throughout the interneuron subpopulations that imparts subtle characteristics to action potential firing. Therefore, although this classification has been historically useful, it has only limited value given the ever-expanding repertoire of voltage-gated channels being identi-

Table 5–2.
Neurochemical markers used to classify hippocampal interneurons

Classical Neurotransmitters of Hippocampal Neurons

GABAergic
Cholinergic?

Calcium-Binding Proteins

Parvalbumin
Calbindin D28k
Calretinin

Neuropeptides

Somatostatin
Neuropeptide Y
Cholecystokinin
Vasoactive intestinal polypeptide
Enkephalin
Neurokinin

Enzymes

Nitric oxide synthase

Neurotransmitter Receptors

Glutamate receptors
GABA receptors
Monoamine receptors
Acetylcholine receptors
Opiate receptors
Substance P receptor

Source: Adapted from Freund and Buzsáki (1996).

fied on inhibitory neurons. Subdivisions of interneurons based on responses to neuromodulators, properties of intrinsic currents and conductances, or expression of ligand-gated channels have all had limited success. Comparisons across these groups, however, have underscored problems with such classification systems and have threatened the very notion of homogeneous interneuron subpopulations. In fact, interneurons are excited or inhibited by a bewildering number of combinations of modulators; and when these properties are mapped onto their respective anatomical properties, a staggering number of subpopulations may exist (Parra et al., 1998).

Classifications based on the nature of excitatory synaptic transmission have become increasingly common. In hippocampal circuits, repetitive activation of glutamatergic afferents progressively increases (augmentation/facilitation) or decreases (depression) the amplitudes of excitatory synaptic events. The list of synapses that demonstrate facilitation or depression has become increasingly lengthy over the last few years primarily from studies involving connected pairs of neurons. One of the best examples of this characterization comes from studying CA1 pyramidal cell-mediated feedback excitation of interneurons in the stratum oriens (Pouille and

Scanziani, 2004). In this study, two groups of interneurons were identified: one whose probability of firing was highest at the onset of a series of presynaptic stimuli and then fell rapidly with subsequent stimuli ("onset transient interneurons") and a second where the probability of spike generation was lowest after the first stimuli but increased to a plateau in response to later events in the stimulus train ("late-persistent interneurons"). Of particular interest, the axons of onset transient interneurons were largely distributed around the somata of pyramidal cells (suggestive of basket, axo-axonic, or bistratified cells), whereas the axons of "late-persistent interneurons" largely innervated the stratum radiatum-lacunosum moleculare (indicative of dendrite-targeting O-LM interneurons). This anatomical and functional characterization suggests that two distinct inhibitory interneuron subclasses can be sequentially recruited to produce inhibition that first targets the soma of pyramidal cells followed by inhibition targeted to pyramidal cell dendrites.

This study, together with numerous others (Maccaferri et al., 1998; Markram et al., 1998; Scanziani et al., 1998), highlights an important feature of this type of classification scheme—that single axons may transmit information in a target-specific manner. This target specificity of transmission can be governed by both the transmitter release mechanisms of individual presynaptic boutons and the type of ionotropic or metabotropic receptors present at the postsynaptic face. In addition, this can be further complicated by the observation that whether a particular synapse demonstrates short-term depression or facilitation may be developmentally regulated (for further discussion see McBain and Fisahn, 2001; Maccaferri and Lacaille, 2003).

5.9.2 Dendritic Morphology

Despite representing only ~10% of the total hippocampal neuron population, inhibitory interneurons have highly variable morphologies even within distinct subpopulations (Figs. 5–23 to 5–25). For example, cells of a given neurochemical subclass can have dendrites that are organized in a widely heterogeneous orientation. Despite this marked heterogeneity, however, a few cell types are highly recognizable based on their cell morphology. A good example of this is the O-LM cell, which typically has its soma and dendrites oriented parallel to the pyramidal cell layer in the stratum oriens-alveus,. The O-LM cell typically projects its main axon across the stratum pyramidale to ramify predominantly in the stratum lacunosum-moleculare, with few collaterals projecting back to the stratum oriens-alveus. This cell belongs to the subpopulation of somatostatin-containing interneurons; but other than this neurochemical feature, it has little in common with other somatostatin-containing interneurons. As discussed above, this presents a problem when attempting to define the basic anatomical features of inhibitory interneurons. Consequently, we describe in detail only those interneuron subpopulations whose anatomical features have been subject to rigorous morphometric analysis.

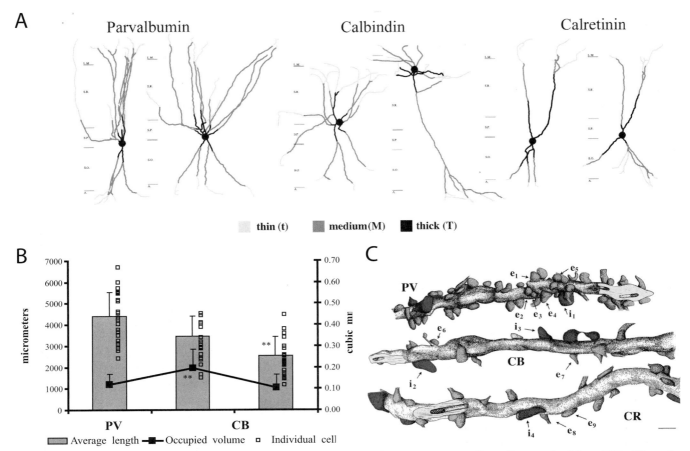

A Parvalbumin   Calbindin   Calretinin

thin (t)   medium (M)   thick (T)

B

C

PV

CB

CR

Average length — Occupied volume ▫ Individual cell

Figure 5–25. Inhibitory interneuron neurochemistry and dendritic morphology. *A*. Reconstructed dendritic trees of parvalbumin (PV)-, calbindin (CB)-, and calretinin (CR)-containing interneurons from the CA1 region of the rat hippocampus. Two examples of each cell type are shown, illustrating the characteristics of the branching patterns. The different types of dendritic segments separated on the basis of their diameter are indicated with different levels of gray. Note the variance in the total length of the dendrites of individual cells within a given group and the differential distribution of dendrites in distinct layers for the three cell populations. *B*. Parvalbumin cells have the largest dendritic tree and calretinin the smallest. The horizontal extent of the dendritic tree was widest for calbindin cells and is reflected in the largest occupied volume obtained for this class of cells. *C*. Distribution of excitatory and

inhibitory inputs on medium-diameter dendrites of PV-, CB-, and CR-containing interneurons in CA1 stratum radiatum. The dendrites and synapses were reconstructed from serial ultrathin sections immunostained for GABA. A large difference can be seen in the absolute and relative numbers of excitatory and inhibitory synapses terminating on the three types of dendrite. The surface of the PV-positive dendrite is densely covered by synapses, in contrast to the sparse innervation of CB- and CR-positive dendrites. On the other hand, the proportion of inhibitory terminals compared to all synaptic inputs is lowest on the PV and highest on the CB dendrites. Excitatory terminals are colored light gray (e.g., e1–e9), GABAergic boutons are dark (e.g., i1–i4). Note the large variance in the size of the axon terminals. (*Source*: Data are from Gulyás et al., 1999.)

Arguably the largest of all the inhibitory interneuron subpopulations, the PV-containing, fast-spiking basket cells are found throughout the hippocampal formation (Fig. 5–25). Their cell bodies in general are restricted to the stratum pyramidale, and its border with both the stratum oriens and stratum radiatum. Occasionally, however, PV-containing interneuron cell bodies are found in the stratum radiatum. Among interneurons, PV-containing cells have the most elaborate dendrites, which on average measure > 4 mm in their full extent (Gulyás et al., 1999). The surface area of PV-containing interneuron somata has been estimated at ~1000 μm^2. PV-containing interneurons have two to six (mean 5.5) primary dendrites that arise from the somata and run radially into the stratum oriens or through the stratum radiatum into the stratum lacunosum-moleculare making infrequent branches. Although PV-containing interneurons have the largest dendritic tree of all interneuron types, these cells demonstrate large variation in individual cell size, with a more than twofold variation in the range of dendritic length being reported (Gulyás et al., 1999). The distribution of dendrites among layers suggests that these cells are likely to collect most of their inputs in the strata radiatum and oriens and only a smaller portion in the strata lacunosum-moleculare and pyramidale (Gulyás et al., 1999).

The cross-sectional diameters of PV-containing interneuron dendrites are highly variable (0.3–2.7 μm) but are, in general, among the thickest of all interneuron classes studied to date. The thickest dendrites typically arise from the somata and then taper rapidly after the first branch point. Apical dendrites have about eight branch points, whereas basilar dendrites have about five. The number of terminal branches is also highly variable but is, on average, ten and seven for apical and basilar dendrites, respectively. Although PV-containing interneurons can be subclassified into several functionally distinct subgroups (i.e., basket and axo-axonic cells), there appears to be little anatomical difference between the measured somata and dendrites of these two subclasses.

Similar morphological estimates have been derived from physiologically characterized fast-spiking basket cells of the CA1 stratum pyramidale, which presumably represent either PV- or CCK-containing interneurons, although their neurochemical content was not determined (Thurbon et al., 1994). The mean total dendritic surface area of fast-spiking interneurons was estimated at ~5000 μm² and ~2000 μm² for apical and basilar dendrites, respectively. Thus, the total surface area of a CA1 fast-spiking basket cell is close to 7000 to 10,000 μm². By comparison the total surface area of CA1 pyramidal neurons has been estimated at around 24,400 μm² (Turner, 1984).

Calbindin (CB)-containing nonpyramidal neurons (some CA1 pyramidal neurons have high CB content) have the highest density within the stratum radiatum, with the greatest numbers of cells located at the border with the stratum lacunosum-moleculare. Smaller numbers of CB-containing interneurons are found in the strata oriens and pyramidale, with few cell bodies located in the stratum lacunosum-moleculare (Freund and Buzsáki, 1996). Two types of CB-containing interneuron can be distinguished based on morphology (Gulyás et al., 1999) (Fig. 5–25). The so-called type I cells are most numerous in the stratum radiatum, with lower numbers in the strata pyramidale and oriens. These cells have highly variable morphologies and are typically multipolar or bitufted with three to six primary dendrites (mean of four) running in all directions, often descending to the stratum oriens but only rarely entering the stratum lacunosum-moleculare. Their calculated somatic surface area is ~800 μm². The primary dendrites arising from the soma are thick and branch within 50 to 100 μm of the soma. The lengths of the dendrites of these cells are highly variable but, on average, they are in excess of 3000 μm (mean 3441 μm), with ~75% of the entire dendritic tree located in the stratum radiatum. Generally the dendritic diameter of CB-containing interneurons is small, ranging from 0.2 to 1.8 μm.

Type II CB-containing interneurons represent a special class of inhibitory interneurons; they are atypical because they project out of the hippocampus to the medial septum (i.e., axons are long-ranging and not "local circuit") (see Chapter 3). These cells, typically found in the stratum oriens, have large, fusiform cell bodies and several long horizontally oriented dendrites. Accurate morphometric analysis of this cell type has not been reported (Gulyás et al., 2003).

Similar to CB-containing interneurons, calretinin (CR)-containing interneurons can be subdivided into at least two classes based on morphology: a spiny type and a spine-free type (Fig. 5–25). In the CA1 subfield only spine-free CR-containing interneurons are found, whereas both classes are found in CA3, with spiny CR-containing interneurons being highly enriched in the stratum lucidum, suggesting they receive innervation primarily from mossy fiber axons of dentate gyrus granule cells (Gulyás et al., 1992). In the CA1 subfield, spine-free CR-containing interneurons are found throughout all layers, from the alveus to the hippocampal fissure. The cell bodies of this class of interneurons have surface areas about one-half that of PV-containing interneurons, with a mean surface area calculated at ~500 μm². The dendrites of CR-containing interneurons arise from highly diverse multipolar, bipolar, or fusiform cell bodies and primarily run radially, traversing several layers. Of particular interest, dendrites of CR-containing cells often form extensive dendrodendritic contacts with neighboring cells (Gulyás et al., 1999).

CR-containing interneurons have a comparatively small total dendritic length (mean ~2500 μm) and so are significantly smaller than both PV- and CB-containing interneurons. Unlike PV- and CB-containing interneurons, CR-containing interneurons have rather homogeneous features, with few primary dendrites (mean of three) that ascend or descend radially to invade all layers of the CA1 subfield. The diameters of CR-containing interneurons are approximately the same as those of CB-containing interneurons, with the surface of the thickest dendritic branches often being beaded.

Spiny CR-containing interneurons are present largely in the hilus of the dentate gyrus and the CA3 stratum lucidum (i.e., areas where mossy fiber axons of dentate gyrus granule cells are at their highest density). The dendrites of this cell class often bear numerous long protrusions that penetrate bundles of mossy fibers (Freund and Buzsáki, 1996). In the dentate gyrus, their dendrites are restricted to the hilus, never entering the granule cell layer. In CA3 stratum lucidum the dendrites run parallel with the pyramidal cell layer and typically do not penetrate the stratum pyramidale or stratum radiatum. Detailed morphometric analysis of this cell type has not been performed.

5.9.3 Dendritic Spines

The conspicuous absence of dendritic spines on most interneuron types undoubtedly has a major impact on their computational properties, in particular synapse specificity and intracellular calcium handling. Some well characterized interneurons are, however, covered densely by dendritic spines. These are the hippocampal O-LM and the dentate gyrus hilar perforant path-associated (HIPP) cells. Both cell types contain the neuropeptide somatostatin; and their dendrites, with prominent spines, can be visualized by immunostaining against mGluR1, substance P receptors, or in some cases calretinin (Freund and Buzsáki, 1996).

When present, spines on interneurons show profound differences from their counterparts on pyramidal neurons. For example, pyramidal cell spines have a spine apparatus, an organelle not detected in the spines of interneurons, despite examining many immunocytochemically visualized spines in serial sections (Gulyás et al., 1992; Acsady et al., 1998). Another important difference between interneuron and pyramidal cell spines is the number of synaptic boutons. The spines of interneurons are covered by numerous excitatory synaptic boutons (four to eight synapses per spine). By contrast, most pyramidal cell spines have only one bouton, occasionally two; typically, when a second synaptic bouton is encountered on a pyramidal cell spine, it forms a symmetrical, presumably GABAergic synapse (Gulyás et al., 1992; Acsady et al., 1998). The large number of excitatory synapses on interneuron spines raises the possibility that spines of interneurons serve to increase the synaptic surface area and do not function as a compartmentalization device as in pyramidal cells (McBain et al., 1999). Spines on pyramidal cells have traditionally been considered to be structures that provide functional microdomains or compartments essential for input-specific synaptic plasticity. Yuste and colleagues (Goldberg et al., 2003a) provided the first direct observation that functional microdomains restricted to less than 1 μm of dendritic space can exist on interneurons in the absence of spines. This compartmentalization was determined by the combination of rapid-kinetic, Ca^{2+}-permeable AMPA receptor-containing synapses located close to a fast extrusion mechanism governed by the Na^+/Ca^{2+} exchanger.

5.9.4 Excitatory and Inhibitory Synapses

Within the hippocampal circuit, interneurons receive afferent excitatory input from a number of intrinsic and extrinsic sources. The nature of the afferents innervating specific populations of interneurons depends of course on the location of their soma and the extent of their dendritic tree. For example, interneurons with somata and dendrites located in the CA1 stratum radiatum primarily receive excitatory input from the CA3 Schaffer collateral projections (i.e., are activated in a feedforward manner) (Gulyás et al., 1999; Pouille and Scanziani, 2001). In contrast, interneurons located in the stratum oriens/alveus receive little or no innervation from the Schaffer collateral input and are primarily excited by the axons of CA1 pyramidal neurons to provide feedback (recurrent) inhibition to CA1 pyramidal neurons (Blasco-Ibanez and Freund, 1995; Maccaferri and McBain, 1996). The myriad roles that interneurons play in neuronal networks are often crucially dependent on the rapid, temporally precise conversion of an excitatory synaptic input to an inhibitory synaptic output (Jonas et al., 2004). Consequently, glutamatergic inputs to interneurons are often very powerful; combined with the typically more depolarized resting membrane potentials and higher input resistances, these synapses tend to discharge the postsynaptic cell reliably and rapidly (within 1–2 ms) (Lawrence and McBain, 2003; Jonas et al., 2004).

In addition to their inhibitory inputs onto principal cells, interneurons provide inhibitory input to other interneurons. In contrast to our appreciation of inhibitory transmission onto principal cells, much less is known regarding the nature of inhibition between interneuron subpopulations. Although poorly appreciated, specificity appears to exist between the targets of identified populations of inhibitory interneurons. Both CCK- and PV-containing interneurons innervate the soma and proximal dendrites of other CCK- and PV-containing cells (as well as contacting other interneuron populations), respectively. Of particular interest, some subpopulations of interneurons [e.g., vasoactive inhibitory peptide (VIP)-containing, calretinin-containing] have axons that exclusively innervate only other interneurons. Moreover, the targets of these subpopulations of interneuron-selective interneurons are extremely specific; for example, the interneuron selective CR-positive cells innervate the CCK-containing cells but not the PV-containing cells (Gulyás et al., 1996). Like excitatory synaptic transmission onto interneurons, the time course of the GABA-mediated inhibitory postsynaptic currents (IPSCs) in cortical interneurons is markedly faster than the kinetics of IPSCs in principal neurons of the same circuit (Bartos et al., 2001; Jonas et al., 2004). Another distinction between inhibition on principal cells and inhibitory interneurons is that the inhibitory synaptic reversal potential in interneurons is often more depolarized and close to the resting membrane potential (Banke and McBain, 2005; Vida et al., 2006), such that inhibition in these cells is primarily shunting. In identified fast-spiking basket cells, this shunting inhibition improves the robustness of gamma oscillatory activity (Vida et al., 2006). In interneurons of the stratum lucidum, placing the inhibitory synaptic reversal potential close to the resting membrane potential allows rapid reversal of the polarity of synaptic inhibition during high-frequency transmission, such that $GABA_A$ receptor-mediated events depolarize other interneurons and recruit coordinated inhibitory input onto principal cell targets (Banke and McBain, 2005).

Precise estimates of synapse numbers and ratios of excitatory to inhibitory synapses have been performed for only a handful of interneuron subtypes, primarily the neurochemically defined PV-, CCK-, CB-, and CR-containing interneuron subtypes (Gulyás et al., 1999, Mátyás et al., 2004). Although the total number of synapses (excitatory plus inhibitory) is several-fold higher on PV-containing cells (~16,000) than on CCK- (~8200), CB- (~4000), or CR-containing (~2200) interneurons, the percentage of GABAergic inputs is higher in CB- (~30%), CCK- (~35%), and CR-containing interneurons (~20%) than in PV-containing interneurons (~6%). The pattern of excitatory innervation also varies among the three cell types. Whereas the dendritic and synaptic arrangements suggest that both PV- and CR-containing interneurons receive afferent input in all layers of the hippocampus, CB-containing cells receive input largely from Schaffer collateral afferents in the stratum radiatum (Gulyás et al., 1999). This high input specificity of CB-containing cells suggests that they are activated primarily in a feedforward manner, whereas PV- and CR-containing interneurons are activated in both a feedforward manner by CA3 (Schaffer collaterals), entorhinal cortex (perforant path), and thalamic (nucleus reuniens) afferents and a feedback manner by local CA1 recurrent collaterals.

Activation of inhibitory interneurons by feedforward or feedback afferent projections often permits individual interneurons to perform a dual role in the hippocampal circuit (Lei and McBain, 2002; Walker et al., 2002b). Indeed, glutamate receptors expressed at synapses formed between various afferent projections onto single interneurons are often comprised of AMPA and NMDA receptors of distinct molecular composition (Toth and McBain, 1998; Lei and McBain, 2002). AMPA receptors at synapses formed between the recurrent collaterals of CA3 pyramidal cells and interneurons of the stratum lucidum have a highly edited GluR2 content, making them essentially impermeable to calcium ions. In contrast, AMPA receptors at the synapses made by mossy fibers and the same interneuron lack, or have a low, GluR2 content, rendering these receptors highly permeable to calcium (Toth and McBain, 1998). It is particularly interesting that the time course of synaptic conductances associated with these two afferent projections are also markedly different despite the synapses having overlapping electrotonic locations (Walker et al., 2002b). Such an arrangement of synaptic receptors allows the output of the single interneurons to respond differentially to different afferent inputs, thus increasing the computational repertoire of the interneuron.

In addition to excitatory glutamatergic innervation, many interneurons also express muscarinic and nicotinic receptors and receive cholinergic input from the medial septum. There is also evidence for noradrenergic input from the locus coeruleus, serotonergic input from the raphe nucleus, and histaminergic input from the supramammillary nucleus, to name a few. Although the roles of many of these neuromodulatory systems are poorly understood, several studies have elucidated the roles of a few of these modulators in influencing interneuron activity. For example, histamine excitation of somatostatin- and PV-containing interneurons via H_2 receptors modulates the activity of voltage-gated potassium channels formed by Kv3.2 subunits (Atzori et al., 2000). Following H_2 receptor activation, PKA phosphorylates channels containing Kv3.2 to decrease their outward current, consequently reducing the upper firing frequency of these fast-spiking interneurons. This reduction in interneuron firing frequency has a major influence on high-frequency oscillatory activity in the CA3 hippocampus. Similarly, muscarinic receptor activation has a differential effect on interneuron function that depends on the subclass of interneuron being activated and suggests differential expression of muscarinic receptors (Hajos et al., 1998; McQuiston and Madison, 1999a,b). Activation of M1 and M3 muscarinic acetylcholine receptors on stratum oriens-lacunosum moleculare (O-LM) interneurons enhances their firing frequency and produces large, sustained after-depolarizations (Lawrence et al., 2006). The generation of after-depolarization results from the coordinated inhibition

of both an M current and a slow calcium-activated potassium current and activation of a calcium-dependent nonselective cationic current (I_{CAT}). In contrast, stratum oriens cell types with axon arborization patterns different from O-LM cells lacked this large muscarinic after-depolarization, suggesting that cholinergic specializations may be present in anatomically distinct subpopulations of hippocampal interneurons.

5.9.5 Axon Morphology and Synaptic Targets

The axonal arborization of local-circuit inhibitory interneurons constitutes another diverse feature of their anatomy. Each cell type or subclass of inhibitory neuron innervates distinct subcellular compartments of each of their targets. As described above, such an arrangement of axonal distribution predicts what role each interneuron plays in influencing activity of the postsynaptic cell. A detailed discussion of the axonal arborization of each type of interneuron is provided elsewhere (see Freund and Buzsáki, 1996). However, it is worthwhile discussing the axons of some of the most studied classes of inhibitory interneuron for comparison with the axons of CA1 and CA3 pyramidal neurons described earlier in the chapter.

Fast-spiking basket cells (presumably PV-containing) of the CA1 hippocampus (Halasy et al., 1996) typically have axons that emerge from either the soma or a proximal dendrite. The axon makes collaterals that extend into the stratum radiatum but primarily arborize throughout the pyramidal cell layer (Halasy et al., 1996). Basket cell axons have a mediolateral extent of > 700 μm. The initial part of the primary axon and secondary branches are typically myelinated, and axonal branches wrap around the somata and proximal dendrites of pyramidal cells establishing numerous synaptic contacts. In contrast, the axon initial segments and spines of pyramidal cells are rarely contacted by basket cell axons. A single basket cell can make up to 15 varicosities (presumably presynaptic specializations) on a single pyramidal neuron. In the case of one well filled basket cell, the total number of presumed synaptic boutons was in excess of 10,000 and was estimated to converge onto ~110 pyramidal neurons (Halasy et al., 1996).

Chandelier cells or axo-axonic cells of the dentate gyrus and hippocampus are so named because of the appearance of their axonal arborization. The cell type was first described by Szentagothai and Arbib (1974) in the neocortex and was subsequently found in the hippocampus (Kosaka, 1983; Somogyi et al., 1983a,b). The axons of the stratum pyramidale chandelier cells originate from the soma or primary dendrite and form rows of 2 to 30 boutons throughout the principal cell layers and in the stratum oriens. These rows of boutons are aligned parallel to the axon initial segments of principal cells (pyramidal cells in CA1 or CA3 and granule cells in the dentate gyrus) (Freund and Buzsáki, 1996) and drape the principal cell layer with a termination pattern reminiscent of a chandelier. The axonal arbor occupies an elliptical area of ~600 to 850 μm, elongated in the septo-temporal direction;

and a single chandelier cell is estimated to innervate ~1200 postsynaptic CA1 cells (Li et al., 1992). Interestingly, the number of cells targeted by a single chandelier cell in the CA3 subfield may be almost double that in CA1 (Gulyás et al., 1993b).

Although both fast spiking (PV- or CCK-containing interneurons) and axo-axonic interneurons predominantly innervate the somata, proximal dendrites, and axon initial segments of principal cells, respectively, other interneurons exclusively contact dendritic locations on principal cells. Two examples of dendritic projecting interneurons are the bistratified and the O-LM interneuron populations. These two cell types form an axonal plexus largely complementary to basket and axo-axonic cells. Bistratified cells (PV-positive, somatostatin-positive, CB-positive, neuropeptide Y-positive) have axons that innervate the dendrites of pyramidal cells in both the stratum radiatum and stratum oriens and largely spare the principal cell somata. In one confirmed CB-positive bistratified interneuron (Sik et al., 1995) the area occupied by the axon collaterals was 1860 μm (septotemporal) $\times$ 2090 μm (mediolateral). The total axon length was 78,800 μm, had 16,600 boutons, and innervated as many as 2500 pyramidal cells. O-LM cells (somatostatin-positive, mGluR1-positive, and to a lesser extent PV-positive) have horizontally oriented cell bodies residing deep within the stratum oriens and send out a largely nonbranching axon, often from a proximal dendrite, which crosses the strata pyramidale and radiatum to form an extensive axonal plexus in the stratum lacunosum moleculare, making synapses onto the distal dendrites of pyramidal cells. In one well-filled O-LM cell from an in vivo study (Sik et al., 1995) the axon had a rather limited septotemporal and mediolateral extent of its the termination field (840 μm by 500 μm). The total axon length of this cell was ~65,000 μm, and the calculated total number of presynaptic boutons was 16,874. Thus, even though the spatial extent of the terminal field was limited, the total number of putative synapses was typically higher than that of basket cells measured in the same study.

5.9.6 Resting Membrane Properties

Characterization of the passive membrane properties of inhibitory interneurons has been limited, with only a handful of studies providing reliable data. Given the numerous classes and subpopulations of inhibitory interneurons in the mammalian hippocampus, extrapolation of these numbers between subpopulations is to be avoided. Here, we discuss only those cells in which the anatomy is known and the passive membrane properties have been estimated using patch-clamp recording.

Where studied, inhibitory interneurons have resting membrane potentials that are slightly more depolarized than CA1 and CA3 pyramidal neurons. Estimates of interneuron resting membrane potentials have provided numbers spanning a wide range but typically lie 5 to 10 mV more depolarized than pyramidal neurons.

Inhibitory interneurons located in the CA1 pyramidal cell layer and morphologically identified as basket cells had highly variable input resistances, but on average the R_N was ~180 MΩ (Thurbon et al., 1994). Estimates of R_m in this cell population were also highly variable and ranged from 82,000 to 281,000 Ωcm^2 (mean 66,200 Ωcm^2). R_i was also highly variable and ranged from 60 to > 500 Ωcm (mean ~300 Ωcm). By combining the physical lengths of the apical and basal dendrites of these cells with their R_m and R_i, the electrotonic lengths (L) were calculated to be ~1.0 and 0.5 for the apical and basal dendrites, respectively. These values highlight an interesting aspect of interneuron physiology. Although the total surface area of the interneurons and the physical length of their dendrites are considerably shorter than for CA1 pyramidal neurons, their electrotonic profiles are often similar. This suggests that neurons with small physical profiles cannot simply be assumed to be more electrotonically compact than larger neurons.

The membrane time constants of both spiny and aspiny stratum lucidum interneurons (τ_m = ~40 and ~30 ms, respectively) are slower than that of CA1 pyramidal neurons but faster than that of CA3 pyramidal neurons, suggesting that these cells have R_m intermediate to both pyramidal neuron types (Spruston et al., 1997). Input resistances (R_N = ~350 and 290 MΩ, respectively), however, are typically higher than that of both CA1 and CA3 pyramidal neurons, presumably owing to the smaller somata and dendritic trees in these neurons.

Estimates of passive membrane parameters for a variety of interneuron types throughout all five laminar substrata in CA3 (stratum oriens through stratum lacunosum-moleculare) have also been determined (Chitwood et al., 1999). Although these numbers were not accompanied by a detailed analysis of the corresponding anatomy, the measured parameters provide worthwhile comparisons with other published data. Input resistances were significantly higher than those reported for basket cells but were similar to those obtained from identified stratum lucidum interneurons; on average they were ~440 MΩ. The membrane time constants of CA3 interneurons were also highly variable (27–69 ms) with a mean of ~60 ms. Interestingly, no significant differences in R_N, τ_m, R_m, or C_m were observed for interneurons located across the five substrata despite the marked heterogeneity in cell morphology across all subfields.

5.9.7 Voltage-Gated Channels in Inhibitory Interneurons

How an interneuron responds to afferent activity depends on many factors, in particular the synaptic conductance time course and the nature of the intrinsic channel proteins expressed on the cell surface. As was discussed in detail for CA1 pyramidal neurons, the properties, density, and distribution of these conductances determine how synaptic inputs are integrated and converted to unique patterns of action potential firing. Like most CNS neurons, interneurons differentially express a wide array of conductances with overlapping voltage dependence (e.g., activation by depolarization or hyperpolarization) and kinetics.

The first clue that interneurons might express voltage-gated ion channels distinct from their principal neuron counterparts came from inspection of action potential waveforms. Many interneurons fire brief action potentials with rapid repolarization, followed by only a simple fast after-hyperpolarization. Responses of interneurons to sustained depolarization are often quite distinct from both CA1 and CA3 pyramidal neurons, with many cell types showing high firing rates, brief interspike intervals, and little action potential accommodation. The most parsimonious explanation for these distinct properties was the presence of voltage-gated channel types unique to interneurons. The demonstration that low-threshold voltage-activated calcium channels conferred burst-firing properties on interneurons of the stratum lacunosum-moleculare provided the first direct evidence that interneurons expressed voltage-gated channels with properties distinct from principal cells (Fraser and MacVicar, 1991). Sodium channels with properties distinct from those of the principal cells have also been described (Martina and Jonas, 1997). Demonstration of the differential expression and func-

tional roles played by voltage-gated potassium channels has arguably provided the best insight into determinants of interneuron function (for review see McBain and Fisahn, 2001). Although attempts to correlate interneuron K$^+$ channel function with properties of recombinant K$^+$ channels has been problematic, major differences between principal cell and inhibitory interneuron voltage-gated potassium channels have emerged.

In recombinant systems, the K$^+$ channel subunits Kv3.1b and Kv3.2 confer currents that activate at highly depolarized potentials, show little inactivation during sustained depolarization, and deactivate rapidly upon repolarization (Rudy and McBain, 2001). Homo-tetramers formed by recombinant Kv3.1b and Kv3.2 have similar biophysical properties, with the notable difference that channels formed by Kv3.2 have a PKA-phosphorylation site that reduces currents through these channels when phosphorylated. In the hippocampus, Kv3.1b and Kv3.2 are expressed in all PV-containing interneurons, and Kv3.2 is also found in ~40% of somatostatin-containing interneurons; both are interneuron subpopulations with fast spiking phenotypes. Outward currents through Kv3 channels act to keep action potentials brief by activating at potentials close to the action potential peak, rapidly repolarizing the membrane potential, and limiting the duration of the after-

Figure 5–26. Inhibitory interneuron dendritic excitability. *A.* Camera lucida reconstruction of a biocytin-filled oriens-alveus interneuron. Soma and dendrites (thick lines) are typically restricted to the strata oriens and alveus. The axon (thin lines) projects across the pyramidal cell layer through the stratum radiatum to ramify extensively throughout the stratum lacunosum-moleculare.

B. Simultaneous current clamp (CC) recordings from a dendrite (gray) and soma (black). In response to long, threshold-level current injections, the action potential occurs first in the axon-bearing dendrite (top). With briefer, stronger-current injections, the action potential occurs first at the site of current injection (bottom). (*Source:* Data are from Martina et al., 2000.)

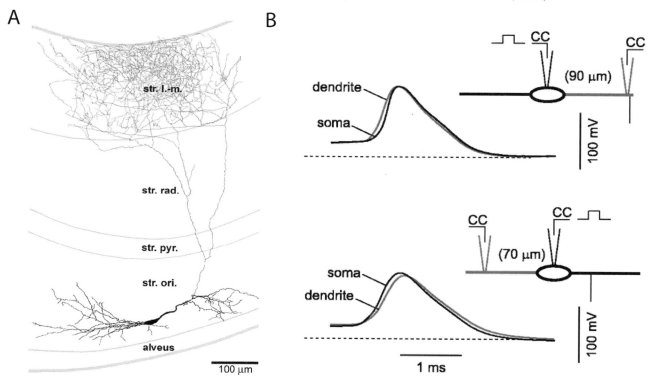

hyperpolarization by rapidly deactivating. High firing frequencies can be achieved by the ability of Kv3 channels to facilitate the recovery of both Na^+ channels and transient A-type potassium channels from inactivation. Of particular interest, PKA phosphorylation of Kv3.2 subunits is triggered by histamine via H_2 receptor activation, which reduces outward currents, broadens action potentials, and reduces the maximal firing frequency of dentate gyrus interneurons by altering Kv3.2 function.

Although the type of channels expressed by the cells are important determinants of interneuron function, the density and spatial distribution of those channels is also important. The density of both Na^+ and sustained K^+ currents are significantly higher and more uniform in dendrites of somatostatin-containing interneurons of the CA1 stratum oriens-alveus than those in the dendrites of neighboring principal cells (Martina et al., 2000). Consequently, action potentials in interneurons are initiated at sites across the dendritic tree and propagate rapidly to and from the soma with little decrement even during high-frequency firing (Fig. 5–26). Action potential initiation can switch between the soma and the axon-bearing dendrite, depending on the nature of the excitatory stimulus. Such organization of voltage-gated channels acts to ensure fast and reliable signaling in interneurons. This channel organization is in marked contrast to channel expression in principal cells, where dendritic action potentials are attenuated by a gradient of dendritic A-type K^+ channels (Hoffman et al., 1997; however, see Goldberg et al., 2003b) (see Section 5.2.11 for further discussion). Whether such organization of voltage-gated channels and dendritic initiation of action potentials exists in other interneurons remains to be seen, but it highlights another feature of interneuron design important for rapid signaling. Studies of the transcriptional regulation and selective targeting of both ligand- and voltage-gated channels will ultimately provide valuable insight into the molecular events regulating expression of these important membrane proteins.

ACKNOWLEDGMENTS

The authors thank members of their laboratories for helpful comments and discussion during the preparation of the chapter.

REFERENCES

Abraham WC, McNaughton N (1984) Differences in synaptic transmission between medial and lateral components of the perforant path. *Brain Res* 303:251–260.

Acsády L, Kamondi A, Sik A, Martinez-Guijarro FJ, Buzsáki G, Freund TF (1998) GABAergic cells are the major postsynaptic targets of mossy fibers in the rat hippocampus. *J Neurosci* 18:3386–3403.

Acsády L, Kamondi A, Sik A, Freund T, Buzsáki G (2000) Unusual target selectivity of perisomatic inhibitory cells in the hilar region of the rat hippocampus. *J Neurosci* 20:6907–6919.

Adams PR (1992) The platonic neuron gets the hots. *Curr Biol* 2:625–627.

Alger BE, Nicoll RA (1980) Epileptiform burst afterhyperpolarization: calcium-dependent potassium potential in hippocampal CA1 pyramidal cells. *Science* 210:1122–1124.

Ali AB, Deuchars J, Pawelzik H, Thomson AM (1998) CA1 pyramidal to basket and bistratified cell EPSPs: dual intracellular recordings in rat hippocampal slices. *J Physiol* (*Lond*) 507:201–217.

Alonso A, Klink R (1993) Differential electroresponsiveness of stellate and pyramidal-like cells of medial entorhinal cortex layer II. *J Neurophysiol* 70:128–143.

Alonso A, Llinás RR (1989) Subthreshold Na^+-dependent theta-like rhythmicity in stellate cells of entorhinal cortex layer II. *Nature* 342:175–177.

Amaral DG (1978) A Golgi study of cell types in the hilar region of the hippocampus in the rat. *J Comp Neurol* 182:851–914.

Amaral DG (1979) Synaptic extensions from the mossy fibers of the fascia dentata. *Anat Embryol* 155:241–251.

Amaral DG, Dent JA (1981) Development of the mossy fibers of the dentate gyrus. I. A light and electron microscopic study of the mossy fibers and their expansions. *J Comp Neurol* 195:51–86.

Amaral DG, Witter MP (1989) The three-dimensional organization of the hippocampal formation: a review of anatomical data. *Neuroscience* 31:571–591.

Amaral DG, Witter MP (1995) Hippocampal formation. In: *The rat nervous system* (Paxinos G, ed). San Diego: Academic Press.

Amaral DG, Ishizuka N, Claiborne B (1990) Neurons, numbers and the hippocampal network. *Prog Brain Res* 93:1–11.

Amaral DG, Dolorfo C, Alvarez-Royo P (1991) Organization of CA1 projections to the subiculum: a PHA-L analysis in the rat. *Hippocampus* 1:415–436.

Andersen P (1960) Interhippocampal impulses. II. Apical dendritic activation of CA1 neurons. *Acta Physiol Scand* 48:178–208.

Andersen P, Lømo T (1966) Mode of activation of hippocampal pyramidal cells by excitatory synapses on dendrites. *Exp Brain Res* 2:247–260.

Andersen P, Blackstad TW, Lomo T (1966a) Location and identification of excitatory synapses on hippocampal pyramidal cells. *Exp Brain Res* 1:236–248.

Andersen P, Holmqvist, Voorhoeve PE (1966b) Excitatory synapses on hippocampal apical dendrites activated by entorhinal stimulation *Acta Physiol Scand* 66:461–472.

Andersen P, Silfvenius H, Sundberg SH, Sveen O (1980) A comparison of distal and proximal dendritic synapses on CA1 pyramids in guinea-pig hippocampal slices in vitro. *J Physiol* 307:273–299.

Andersen P, Soleng AF, Raastad M (2000) The hippocampal lamella hypothesis revisited. *Brain Res* 886:165–171.

Andrade R, Nicoll RA (1987) Pharmacologically distinct actions of serotonin on single pyramidal neurones of the rat hippocampus recorded in vitro. *J Physiol* 394:99–124.

Andrasfalvy BK, Magee JC (2001) Distance-dependent increase in AMPA receptor number in the dendrites of adult hippocampal CA1 pyramidal neurons. *J Neurosci* 21:9151–9159.

Andreasen M, Lambert JD (1995a) Regenerative properties of pyramidal cell dendrites in area CA1 of the rat hippocampus. *J Physiol* 483:421–441.

Andreasen M, Lambert JD (1995b) The excitability of CA1 pyramidal cell dendrites is modulated by a local Ca^{2+}-dependent K^+-conductance. *Brain Res* 698:193–203.

Andreasen M, Lambert JD (1998) Factors determining the efficacy of distal excitatory synapses in rat hippocampal CA1 pyramidal neurones. *J Physiol* 507:441–462.

Andreasen M, Lambert JD (1999) Somatic amplification of distally generated subthreshold EPSPs in rat hippocampal pyramidal neurones. *J Physiol* 519:85–100.

Aniksztejn L, Demarque M, Morozov Y, Ben-Ari Y, Represa A (2001) Recurrent CA1 collateral axons in developing rat hippocampus. *Brain Res* 913:195–200.

Ariav G, Polsky A, Schiller J (2003) Submillisecond precision of the input-output transformation function mediated by fast sodium dendritic spikes in basal dendrites of CA1 pyramidal neurons. *J Neurosci* 23:7750–7758.

Atzori M, Lau D, Tansey EP, Chow A, Ozaita A, Rudy B, McBain CJ (2000) H_2 histamine receptor-phosphorylation of Kv3.2 modulates interneuron fast spiking. *Nat Neurosci* 3:791–798.

Azouz R, Alroy G, Yaari Y (1997) Modulation of endogenous firing patterns by osmolarity in rat hippocampal neurones. *J Physiol* 502:175–187.

Banke T, McBain CJ (2005) A frequency-dependent switch of synaptic inhibition polarity recruits a network of stratum lucidum interneurons [abstract 955.8]. Presented at the Annual Society for Neuroscience Meeting, San Diego.

Bannister NJ, Larkman AU (1995a) Dendritic morphology of CA1 pyramidal neurones from the rat hippocampus. I. Branching patterns. *J Comp Neurol* 360:150–160.

Bannister NJ, Larkman AU (1995b) Dendritic morphology of CA1 pyramidal neurones from the rat hippocampus. II. Spine distributions. *J Comp Neurol* 360:161–171.

Bartos M, Vida I, Frotscher M, Geiger JR, Jonas P (2001) Rapid signaling at inhibitory synapses in a dentate gyrus interneuron network. *J Neurosci* 21:2687–2698.

Behr J, Gloveli T, Heinemann U (1998) The perforant path projection from the medial entorhinal cortex layer III to the subiculum in the rat combined hippocampal-entorhinal cortex slice. *Eur J Neurosci* 10:1011–1018.

Bekkers JM (2000) Distribution and activation of voltage-gated potassium channels in cell-attached and outside-out patches from large layer 5 cortical pyramidal neurons of the rat. *J Physiol* 525:611–620.

Belichenko PV (1993) Neuronal cell types in entorhinal cortex and hippocampal formation of man and other mammalia: an interspecies comparison. *Hippocampus* 3:3–10.

Ben-Ari Y (1985) Limbic seizure and brain damage produced by kainic acid mechanisms and relevance to human temporal lobe epilepsy. *Neuroscience* 14:375–403.

Benardo LS, Prince DA (1982a) Ionic mechanisms of cholinergic excitation in mammalian hippocampal pyramidal cells. *Brain Res* 249:333–344.

Benardo LS, Prince DA (1982b) Cholinergic excitation of mammalian hippocampal pyramidal cells. *Brain Res* 249:315–331.

Benardo LS, Prince DA (1982c) Cholinergic pharmacology of mammalian hippocampal pyramidal cells. *Neuroscience* 7:1703–1712.

Benardo LS, Prince DA (1982d) Dopamine modulates a Ca^{2+}-activated potassium conductance in mammalian hippocampal pyramidal cells. *Nature* 297:76–79.

Benardo LS, Prince DA (1982e) Dopamine action on hippocampal pyramidal cells. *J Neurosci* 2:415–423.

Benardo LS, Masukawa LM, Prince DA (1982) Electrophysiology of isolated hippocampal pyramidal dendrites. *J Neurosci* 2:1614–1622.

Bender RA, Brewster A, Santoro B, Ludwig A, Hofmann F, Biel M, Baram TZ (2001) Differential and age-dependent expression of hyperpolarization-activated, cyclic nucleotide-gated cation channel isoforms 1–4 suggests evolving roles in the developing rat hippocampus. *Neuroscience* 106:689–698.

Benson DM, Blitzer RD, Landau EM (1988) An analysis of the depolarization produced in guinea-pig hippocampus by cholinergic receptor stimulation. *J Physiol* 404:479–496.

Bernard C, Johnston D (2003) Distance-dependent modifiable threshold for action potential back-propagation in hippocampal dendrites. *J Neurophysiol* 90:1807–1816.

Bennett MR, Gibson WG, Robinson J (1994) Dynamics of the CA3 pyramidal neuron autoassociative memory network in the hippocampus. *Philos Trans R Soc Lond B Biol Sci* 343:167–187.

Berger T, Larkum ME, Luscher HR (2001) High I_h channel density in the distal apical dendrite of layer V pyramidal cells increases bidirectional attenuation of EPSPs. *J Neurophysiol* 85:855–868.

Bianchi R, Young SR, Wong RK (1999) Group I mGluR activation causes voltage-dependent and -independent Ca^{2+} rises in hippocampal pyramidal cells. *J Neurophysiol* 81:2903–2913.

Bilkey DK, Schwartzkroin PA (1990) Variation in electrophysiology and morphology of hippocampal CA3 pyramidal cells. *Brain Res* 514:77–83.

Bittner K, Muller W (1999) Oxidative downmodulation of the transient K-current IA by intracellular arachidonic acid in rat hippocampal neurons. *J Neurophysiol* 82:508–511.

Blackstad TW (1956) Commissural connections of the hippocampal region in the rat, with special reference to their mode of termination. *J Comp Neurol* 105:417–537.

Blackstad TW (1958) On the termination of some afferents to the hippocampus and fascia dentata; an experimental study in the rat. *Acta Anat (Basel)* 35:202–214.

Blackstad TW, Kjaerheim A (1961) Special axo-dendritic synapses in the hippocampal cortex: electron and light microscopic studies on the layer of mossy fibers. *J Comp Neurol* 117:133–159.

Blackstad TW, Brink K, Hem J, Jeune B (1970) Distribution of hippocampal mossy fibers in the rat: an experimental study with silver impregnation methods. *J Comp Neurol* 138:433–450.

Blasco-Ibanez JM, Freund TF (1995) Synaptic input of horizontal interneurons in stratum oriens of the hippocampal CA1 subfield: structural basis of feed-back activation. *Eur J Neurosci* 7:2170–2180.

Bonhoeffer T, Yuste R (2002) Spine motility: phenomenology, mechanisms, and function. *Neuron* 35:1019–1027.

Bowden SHE, Fletcher S, Loane DJ, Marrion NV (2001) Somatic colocalization of rat SK1 and D class ($Ca_v1.2$) L-type calcium channels in rat CA1 hippocampal neurons. *J Neurosci* 21:RC175 (1–6).

Brown TH, Fricke RA, Perkel DH (1981) Passive electrical constants in three classes of hippocampal neurons. *J Neurophysiol* 46:812–827.

Brun VH, Otnass MK, Molden S, Steffenach HA, Witter MP, Moser MB, Moser EI (2002) Place cells and place recognition maintained by direct entorhinal-hippocampal circuitry. *Science* 296:2243–2246.

Buckmaster PS, Schwartzkroin PA (1994) Hippocampal mossy cell function: a speculative view. *Hippocampus* 4:393–402.

Buckmaster PS, Strowbridge BW, Kunkel DD, Schmiege DL, Schwartzkroin PA (1992) Mossy cell axonal projections to the dentate gyrus molecular layer in the rat hippocampal slice. *Hippocampus* 2:349–362.

Buckmaster PS, Strowbridge BW, Schwartzkroin PA (1993) A comparison of rat hippocampal mossy cells and CA3c pyramidal cells. *J Neurophysiol* 70:1281–1299.

Buckmaster PS, Wenzel HJ, Kunkel DD, Schwartzkroin PA (1996) Axon arbors and synaptic connections of hippocampal mossy cells in the rat in vivo. *J Comp Neurol* 366:270–292.

Burnashev N, Monyer H, Seeburg PH, Sakmann B (1992) Divalent ion permeability of AMPA receptor channels is dominated by the edited form of a single subunit. *Neuron* 8:189–198.

Buzsáki G (1996) The hippocampo-neocortical dialogue. *Cereb Cortex* 6:81–92.

Buzsáki G, Penttonen M, Bragin A, Nadasdy Z, Chrobak JJ (1995) Possible physiological role of the perforant path-CA1 projection. *Hippocampus* 5:141–146.

Cai X, Liang CW, Muralidharan S, Kao JP, Tang CM, Thompson SM (2004) Unique roles of SK and Kv4.2 potassium channels in dendritic integration. *Neuron* 44:351–364.

Cajal SR (1911) *Histology of the nervous system of man and vertebrates* (Swanson N, Swanson L, translators). Oxford: Oxford University Press, 1995.

Callaway JC, Ross WN (1995) Frequency-dependent propagation of sodium action potentials in dendrites of hippocampal CA1 pyramidal neurons. *J Neurophysiol* 74:1395–1403.

Carboni AA, Lavelle WG, Barnes CL, Cipolloni PB (1990) Neurons of the lateral entorhinal cortex of the rhesus monkey: a Golgi, histochemical, and immunochemical characterization. *J Comp Neurol* 291:583–608.

Carnevale NT, Tsai KY, Claiborne BJ, Brown TH (1997) Comparative electronic analysis of three classes of rat hippocampal neurons. *J Neurophysiol* 78:703–720.

Cash S, Yuste R (1998) Input summation by cultured pyramidal neurons is linear and position-independent. *J Neurosci* 18:10–15.

Cash S, Yuste R (1999) Linear summation of excitatory inputs by CA1 pyramidal neurons. *Neuron* 22:383–394.

Chen H, Lambert NA (1997) Inhibition of dendritic calcium influx by activation of G-protein-coupled receptors in the hippocampus. *J Neurophysiol* 78:3484–3488.

Chicurel ME, Harris KM (1992) Three-dimensional analysis of the structure and composition of CA3 branched dendritic spines and their synaptic relationships with mossy fiber boutons in the rat hippocampus. *J Comp Neurol* 325:169–182

Chitwood RA, Hubbard A, Jaffe DB (1999) Passive electrotonic properties of rat hippocampal CA3 interneurons. *J Physiol* (*Lond*) 515:743–756.

Christie BR, Eliot LS, Ito K, Miyakawa H, Johnston D (1995) Different Ca^{2+} channels in soma and dendrites of hippocampal pyramidal neurons mediate spike-induced Ca^{2+} influx. *J Neurophysiol* 73:2553–2557.

Chrobak JJ, Buzsáki G (1994) Selective activation of deep layer (V–VI) retrohippocampal cortical neurons during hippocampal sharp waves in the behaving rat. *J Neurosci* 14:6160–6170.

Chrobak JJ, Buzsáki G (1996) High-frequency oscillations in the output networks of the hippocampal-entorhinal axis of the freely behaving rat. *J Neurosci* 16:3056–3066.

Chrobak JJ, Lörincz A, Buzsáki G (2000) Physiological patterns in the hippocampal-entorhinal cortex system. *Hippocampus* 10:457–465.

Claiborne BJ, Amaral DG, Cowan WM (1986) A light and electron microscopic analysis of the mossy fibers of the rat dentate gyrus. *J Comp Neurol* 246:435–458.

Claiborne BJ, Amaral DG, Cowan WM (1990) Quantitative, three-dimensional analysis of granule cell dendrites in the rat dentate gyrus. *J Comp Neurol* 302:206–219.

Cohen I, Miles M (2000) Contributions of intrinsic and synaptic activities to the generation of neuronal discharges in in vitro hippocampus. *J Physiol* 524:485–502.

Colbert CM, Johnston D (1996) Axonal action-potential initiation and Na$^+$ channel densities in the soma and axon initial segment of subicular pyramidal neurons. *J Neurosci* 16:6676–6686.

Colbert CM, Johnston D (1998) Protein kinase C activation decreases activity-dependent attenuation of dendritic Na$^+$ current in hippocampal CA1 pyramidal neurons. J Neurophysiol 79:491–495.

Colbert CM, Pan E (1999) Arachidonic acid reciprocally alters the availability of transient and sustained dendritic K$^+$ channels in hippocampal CA1 pyramidal neurons. *J Neurosci* 19:8163–8171.

Colbert CM, Pan E (2002) Ion channel properties underlying axonal action potential initiation in pyramidal neurons. *Nat Neurosci* 5:533–538.

Colbert CM, Magee JC, Hoffman DA, Johnston D (1997) Slow recovery from inactivation of Na$^+$ channels underlies the activity-dependent attenuation of dendritic action potentials in hippocampal CA1 pyramidal neurons. *J Neurosci* 17:6512–6521.

Colling SB, Wheal HV (1994) Fast sodium action potentials are generated in the distal apical dendrites of rat hippocampal CA1 pyramidal cells. *Neurosci Lett* 172:73–96.

Cook EP, Johnston D (1997) Active dendrites reduce location-dependent variability of synaptic input trains. *J Neurophysiol* 78:2116–2128.

Cook EP, Johnston D (1999) Voltage-dependent properties of dendrites that eliminate location-dependent variability of synaptic input. *J Neurophysiol* 81:535–543.

Cooney JR, Hurlburt JL, Selig DK, Harris KM, Fiala JC (2002) Endosomal compartments serve multiple hippocampal dendritic spines from a widespread rather than a local store of recycling membrane. *J Neurosci* 22:2215–2224.

Cooper DC, Moore SJ, Staff NP, Spruston N (2003) Psychostimulant-induced plasticity of intrinsic neuronal excitability in ventral subiculum. *J Neurosci* 23:9937–9946.

Cope DW, Maccaferri G, Marton LF, Roberts JD, Cobden PM, Somogyi P (2002) Cholecystokinin-immunopositive basket and Schaffer collateral-associated interneurones target different domains of pyramidal cells in the CA1 area of the rat hippocampus. *Neuroscience* 109:63–80.

Cragg BG, Hamlyn LH (1955) Action potentials of the pyramidal neurones in the hippocampus of the rabbit. *J Physiol* 129:608–627.

Csicsvari J, Hirase H, Czurko A, Buzsáki G (1998) Reliability and state dependence of pyramidal cell–interneuron synapses in the hippocampus: an ensemble approach in the behaving rat. *Neuron* 21:179–189.

Dahl D, Burgard EC, Sarvey JM (1990) NMDA receptor antagonists reduce medial, but not lateral, perforant path-evoked EPSPs in dentate gyrus of rat hippocampal slice. *Exp Brain Res* 83:172–177.

Dailey ME, Smith SJ (1996) The dynamics of dendritic structure in developing hippocampal slices. *J Neurosci* 16:2983–2994.

Deller T, Adelmann G, Nitsch R, Frotscher M (1996a) The alvear pathway of the rat hippocampus. *Cell Tissue Res* 286:293–303.

Deller T, Martinez A, Nitsch R, Frotscher M (1996b) A novel entorhinal projection to the rat dentate gyrus: direct innervation of proximal dendrites and cell bodies of granule cells and GABAergic neurons. *J Neurosci* 16:3322–3333.

Desmond NL, Levy WB (1982) A quantitative anatomical study of the granule cell dendritic fields of the rat dentate gyrus using a novel probabilistic method. *J Comp Neurol* 212:131–145.

Desmond NL, Levy WB (1984) Dendritic caliber and the 3/2 power relationship of dentate granule cells. *J Comp Neurol* 227: 589–596.

Desmond NL, Levy WB (1985) Granule cell dendritic spine density in the rat hippocampus varies with spine shape and location. *Neurosci Lett* 54:219–224.

Destexhe A, Paré D (1999) Impact of network activity on the integrative properties of neocortical pyramidal neurons in vivo. *J Neurophysiol* 81:1531–1547.

Deuchars J, Thomson AM (1996) CA1 pyramid-pyramid connections in rat hippocampus in vitro: dual intracellular recordings with biocytin filling. *Neuroscience* 74:1009–1018.

Dickson CT, Mena AR, Alonso A (1997) Electroresponsiveness of medial entorhinal cortex layer III neurons in vitro. *Neuroscience* 81:937–950.

Dickson CT, Magistretti J, Shalinsky MH, Fransén E, Hasselmo ME, Alonso A (2000a) Properties and role of I_h in the pacing of subthreshold oscillations in entorhinal cortex layer II neurons. *J Neurophysiol* 83:2562–2579.

Dickson CT, Magistretti J, Shalinsky M, Hamam B, Alonso A (2000b) Oscillatory activity in entorhinal neurons and circuits. *Ann NY Acad Sci* 911:127–150.

Dolleman-Van der Weel MJ, Witter MP (1996) Projections from the nucleus reuniens thalami to the entorhinal cortex, hippocampal field CA1, and the subiculum in the rat arise from different populations of neurons. *J Comp Neurol* 364:637–650.

Dolleman-Van der Weel MJ, Lopes da Silva FH, Witter MP (1997) Nucleus reuniens thalami modulates activity in hippocampal field CA1 through excitatory and inhibitory mechanisms. *J Neurosci* 17:5640–5650.

Doller HJ, Weight FF (1982) Perforant pathway activation of hippocampal CA1 stratum pyramidale neurons: electrophysiological evidence for a direct pathway. *Brain Res* 237:1–13.

Durand D, Carlen PL, Gurevich N, Ho A, Kunov H (1983) Electrotonic parameters of rat dentate granule cells measured using short current pulses and HRP staining. *J Neurophysiol* 50:1080–1097.

Egorov AV, Heinemann U, Müller W (2002a) Differential excitability and voltage-dependent Ca^{2+} signaling in two types of medial entorhinal cortex layer V neurons. *Eur J Neurosci* 16:1305–1312.

Egorov AV, Hamam BN, Fransen E, Hasselmo ME, Alonso AA (2002b) Graded persistent activity in entorhinal cortex neurons. *Nature* 420:173–178.

Empson RM, Heinemann U (1995a) The perforant path projection to hippocampal area CA1 in the rat hippocampal-entorhinal cortex combined slice. *J Physiol* 484:707–720.

Empson RM, Heinemann U (1995b) Perforant path connections to area CA1 are predominantly inhibitory in the rat hippocampal-entorhinal cortex combined slice preparation. *Hippocampus* 5:104–107.

Emptage N, Bliss TV, Fine A (1999) Single synaptic events evoke NMDA receptor-mediated release of calcium from internal stores in hippocampal dendritic spines. *Neuron* 22:115–124.

Engert F, Bonhoeffer T (1999) Dendritic spine changes associated with hippocampal long-term synaptic plasticity. *Nature* 399:66–70.

Fan S, Stewart M, Wong RKS (1994) Differences in voltage-dependent sodium currents exhibited by superficial and deep layer neu-

rons of guinea pig entorhinal cortex. *J Neurophysiol* 71:1986–1991.

Fiala JC, Feinberg M, Popov V, Harris KM (1998) Synaptogenesis via dendritic filopodia in developing hippocampal area CA1. *J Neurosci* 18:8900–8911.

Fiala JC, Kirov SA, Feinberg MD, Petrak LJ, George P, Goddard CA, Harris KM (2003) Timing of neuronal and glial ultrastructure disruption during brain slice preparation and recovery in vitro. *J Comp Neurol* 465:90–103.

Finch DM, Babb TL (1980) Neurophysiology of the caudally directed hippocampal efferent system in the rat: projections to the subicular complex. *Brain Res* 197:11–12.

Finch DM, Babb TL (1981) Demonstration of caudally directed hippocampal efferents in the rat by intracellular injection of horseradish peroxidase. *Brain Res* 214:405–410.

Fisahn A, Yamada M, Duttaroy A, Gan J-W, Deng C-X, McBain CJ, Wess J (2002) Muscarinic induction of hippocampal gamma oscillations requires coupling of the M1 receptor to two mixed cation currents. *Neuron* 33:615–624.

Fox S, Ranck JB (1975) Localization and anatomical identification of theta and complex spike cells in dorsal hippocampal formation of rats. *Exp Neurol* 49:299–313.

Frank LM, Brown EN, Wilson MA (2001) A comparison of the firing properties of putative excitatory and inhibitory neurons from CA1 and the entorhinal cortex. *J Neurophysiol* 86: 2029–2040.

Fraser DD, MacVicar BA (1991) Low-threshold transient calcium current in rat hippocampal lacunosum-moleculare interneurons: kinetics and modulation by neurotransmitters. *J Neurosci* 11:2812–2820.

Fraser DD, MacVicar BA (1996) Cholinergic-dependent plateau potential in hippocampal CA1 pyramidal neurons. *J Neurosci* 16:4113–4128.

Fredens K, Stengaard-Pedersen K, Wallace MN (1987) Localization of cholecystokinin in the dentate commissural-associational system of the mouse and rat. *Brain Res* 401:68–78.

Freund TF, Buzsáki G (1996) Interneurons of the hippocampus. *Hippocampus* 6:347–470.

Freund TF, Hajos N, Acsady L, Gorcs TJ, Katona I (1997) Mossy cells of the rat dentate gyrus are immunoreactive for calcitonin gene-related peptide (CGRP). *Eur J Neurosci* 9:1815–1830.

Frick A, Magee J, Koester HJ, Migliore M, Johnston D (2003) Normalization of Ca^{2+} signals by small oblique dendrites of CA1 pyramidal neurons. *J Neurosci* 23:3243–3250.

Frick A, Magee J, Johnston D (2004) LTP is accompanied by an enhanced local excitability of pyramidal neuron dendrites. *Nat Neurosci* 7:126–135.

Fricker D, Verheugen JAH, Miles R (1999) Cell-attached measurements of the firing threshold of rat hippocampal neurons. *J Physiol (Lond)* 517:791–804.

Frotscher M, Seress L, Schwerdtfeger WK, Buhl E (1991) The mossy cells of the fascia dentata: a comparative stuy of their fine structure and synaptic connections in rodents and primates. *J Comp Neurol* 312:145–163.

Fujita Y, Sakata H (1962) Electrophysiological properties of CA1 and CA2 apical dendrites of rabbit hippocampus. *J Neurophysiol* 25:209–222.

Funahashi M, Stewart M (1997a) Presubicular and parasubicular cortical neurons of the rat: electrophysiological and morphological properties. *Hippocampus* 7:117–129.

Funahashi M, Stewart M (1997b) Presubicular and parasubicular cortical neurons of the rat: functional separation of deep and superficial neurons in vitro. *J Physiol (Lond)* 501:387–403.

Funahashi M, Harris E, Stewart M (1999) Re-entrant activity in pre-subiculum-subiculum circuit generates epileptiform activity in vitro. *Brain Res* 849:139–146.

Ganeshina O, Berry RW, Petralia RS, Nicholson DA, Geinisman Y (2004a) Differences in the expression of AMPA and NMDA receptors between axospinous perforated and nonperforated synapses are related to the configuration and size of postsynaptic densities. *J Comp Neurol* 468:86–95.

Ganeshina O, Berry RW, Petralia RS, Nicholson DA, Geinisman Y (2004b) Synapses with a segmented, completely partitioned postsynaptic density express more AMPA receptors than other axospinous synaptic junctions. *Neuroscience* 125:615–623.

Gasparini S, Kasyanov AM, Pietrobon D, Voronin LL, Cherubini E (2001) Presynaptic R-type calcium channels contribute to fast excitatory synaptic transmission in the rat hippocampus. *J Neurosci* 21:8715–8721.

Gasparini S, Migliore M, Magee JC (2004) On the initiation and propagation of dendritic spikes in CA1 pyramidal neurons. *J Neurosci* 24:11046–11056.

Gentet LJ, Stuart GJ, Clements JD (2000) Direct measurement of specific membrane capacitance in neurons. *Biophys J* 79:314–320.

Geiger JRP, Jonas P (2000) Dynamic control of presynaptic Ca^{2+} inflow by fast inactivating K^+ channels in hippocampal mossy fiber boutons. *Neuron* 28:927–939.

Geinisman Y (2000) Structural synaptic modifications associated with hippocampal LTP and behavioral learning. *Cereb Cortex* 10:952–962.

Germroth P, Schwerdtfeger WK, Buhl EH (1991) Ultrastructure and aspects of functional organization of pyramidal and nonpyramidal entorhinal projection neurons contributing to the perforant path. *J Comp Neurol* 305:215–231.

Gigg J, Finch DM, O'Mara SM (2000) Responses of rat subicular neurons to convergent stimulation of lateral entorhinal cortex and CA1 in vivo. *Brain Res* 884:35–50.

Gillessen T, Alzheimer C (1997) Amplification of EPSPs by low Ni^{2+}- and amiloride-sensitive Ca^{2+} channels in apical dendrites of rat CA1 pyramidal neurons. *J Neurophysiol* 77:1639–1643.

Gloveli T, Schmitz D, Empson RM, Dugladze T, Heinemann U (1997a) Morphological and electrophysiological characterization of layer III cells of the medial entorhinal cortex of the rat. *Neuroscience* 77:629–648.

Gloveli T, Schmitz D, Empson RM, Heinemann U (1997b) Frequency-dependent information flow from the entorhinal cortex to the hippocampus. *J Neurophysiol* 78:3444–3449.

Gloveli T, Egorov AV, Schmitz D, Heinemann U, Müller W (1999) Carbachol-induced changes in excitability and $[Ca^{2+}]_i$ signaling in projection cells of medial entorhinal cortex layers II and III. *Eur J Neurosci* 11:3626–3636.

Gloveli T, Dugladze T, Schmitz D, Heinemann U (2001) Properties of entorhinal cortex deep layer neurons projecting to the rat dentate gyrus. *Eur J Neurosci* 13:413–420.

Goldberg JH, Tamas G, Aronov D, Yuste R (2003a) Calcium microdomains in aspiny dendrites. *Neuron* 40:807–821.

Goldberg JH, Tamas G, Yuste R (2003b) Ca^{2+} imaging of mouse neocortical interneurone dendrites: Ia-type K^+ channels control action potential backpropagation. *J Physiol* 551:49–65.

Golding NL, Spruston N (1998) Dendritic spikes are variable triggers of axonal action potentials in hippocampal CA1 pyramidal neurons. *Neuron* 21:1189–1200.

Golding NL, Kath WL, Spruston N (2001) Dichotomy of action potential backpropagation in CA1 pyramidal neurons. *J Neurophysiol* 86:2998–3010.

Golding NL, Jung H, Mickus TJ, Spruston N (1999) Dendritic calcium spike initiation and repolarization are controlled by distinct potassium channel subtypes in CA1 pyramidal neurons. *J Neurosci* 19:8789–8798.

Golding N, Staff NP, Spruston N (2002) Dendritic spikes as a mechanism for cooperative long-term potentiation. *Nature* 418:326–331.

Golding N, Mickus T, Katz Y, Kath WL, Spruston N (2005) Factors mediating powerful voltage attenuation along CA1 dendrites. *J Physiol* 568:69–82.

Goldsmith SK, Joyce JN (1994) Dopamine D2 receptor expression in hippocampus and parahippocampal cortex of rat, cat, and human in relation to tyrosine hydroxylase-immunoreactive fibers. *Hippocampus* 4:354–373.

Gonzales RB, DeLeon Galvan CJ, Rangel YM, Claiborne BJ (2001) Distribution of thorny excrescences on CA3 pyramidal neurons in the rat hippocampus. *J Comp Neurol* 430:357–368.

Gould E, Cameron HA (1996) Regulation of neuronal birth, migration and death in the rat dentate gyrus. *Dev Neurosci* 18:22–35.

Gray EG (1959) Electron microscopy of synaptic contacts on dendrite spines of the cerebral cortex. *Nature* 183:1592–1593.

Greene JRT, Totterdell S (1997) Morphology and distribution of electrophysiologically defined classes of pyramidal and nonpyramidal neurons in rat ventral subiculum in vitro. *J Comp Neurol* 380:395–408.

Grutzendler J, Kasthuri N, Gan WB (2002) Long-term dendritic spine stability in the adult cortex. *Nature* 420:812–816.

Gulyás AI, Miettinen R, Jacobowitz DM, Freund TF (1992) Calretinin is present in non-pyramidal cells of the rat hippocampus. I. A new type of neuron specifically associated with the mossy fibre system. *Neuroscience* 48:1–27.

Gulyas AI, Miles R, Sik A, Toth K, Tamamaki N, Freund T (1993a) Hippocampal pyramidal cells excite inhibitory neurons through a single release site. *Nature* 366:683–687.

Gulyas AI, Miles R, Hajos N, Freund TF (1993b) Precision and variability in postsynaptic target selection of inhibitory cells in the hippocampal CA3 region. *Eur J Neurosci* 5:1729–1751.

Gulyás AI, Hajos N, Freund TF (1996) Interneurons containing calretinin are specialized to control other interneurons in the rat hippocampus. *J Neurosci* 16:3397–3411.

Gulyás AI, Toth K, McBain CJ, Freund TF (1998) Stratum radiatum giant cells: a type of principal cell in the rat hippocampus. *Eur J Neurosci* 10:3813–3822.

Gulyás A, Megias M, Emri Z, Freund TF (1999) Total number and ratio of excitatory and inhibitory synapses converging onto single interneurons of different types in the CA1 area of the rat hippocampus. *J Neurosci* 19:10082–10097.

Gulyás AI, Hajos N, Katona I, Freund TF (2003) Interneurons are the local targets of hippocampal inhibitory cells which project to the medial septum. *Eur J Neurosci* 17:1861–1872.

Hajos N, Papp EC, Acsady L, Levey AI, Freund TF (1998) Distinct interneuron types express m2 muscarinic receptor immunoreactivity on their dendrites or axon terminals in the hippocampus. *Neuroscience* 82:355–376.

Halasy K, Miettinen R, Szabat E, Freund TF (1992) GABAergic interneurons are the major postsynaptic targets of median raphe afferents in the rat dentate gyrus. *Eur J Neurosci* 4:144–153.

Halasy K, Buhl EH, Lorinczi Z, Tamas G, Somogyi P (1996) Synaptic target selectivity and input of GABAergic basket and bistratified interneurons in the area CA1 of the rat hippocampus. *Hippocampus* 6:306–329.

Halliwell JV, Adams PR (1982) Voltage-clamp analysis of muscarinic excitation in hippocampal neurons. *Brain Res* 250:71–92.

Hama K, Arii T, Kosaka T (1989) Three-dimensional morphometrical study of dendritic spines of the granule cell in the rat dentate gyrus with HVEM stereo images. *J Electron Microsc Tech* 12:80–87.

Hamam BN, Kennedy TE, Alonso A, Amaral DG (2000) Morphological and electrophysiological characteristics of layer V neurons of the rat medial entorhinal cortex. *J Comp Neurol* 418:457–472.

Hamam BN, Amaral DG, Alonso A (2002) Morphological and electrophysiological characteristics of layer V neurons of the rat lateral entorhinal cortex. *J Comp Neurol* 451:45–61.

Hamlyn LH (1962) The fine structure of the mossy fiber endings in the hippocampus of the rabbit. *J Anat* 96:112–120.

Harris E, Stewart M (2001) Intrinsic connectivity of the rat subiculum. II. Properties of synchronous spontaneous activity and a demonstration of multiple generator rhythms. *J Comp Neurol* 436:506–518.

Harris E, Witter MP, Weinstein G, Stewart M (2001) Intrinsic connectivity of the rat subiculum. I. Dendritic morphology and patterns of axonal arborization by pyramidal neurons. *J Comp Neurol* 436:490–505.

Harris KM, Kater SB (1994) Dendritic spines: cellular specializations imparting both stability and flexibility to synaptic function. *Annu Rev Neurosci* 17:341–371.

Harris KM, Stevens JK (1989) Dendritic spines of CA1 pyramidal cells in the rat hippocampus: serial electron microscopy with reference to their biophysical characteristics. *J Neurosci* 9:2982–2997.

Harris KM, Jensen FE, Tsao B (1992) Three-dimensional structure of dendritic spines and synapses in rat hippocampus (CA1) at postnatal day 15 and adult ages: implications for the maturation of synaptic physiology and long-term potentiation. *J Neurosci* 12:2685–2705.

Hausser M, Spruston N, Stuart GJ (2000) Diversity and dynamics of dendritic signaling. *Science* 290:739–744.

Helmchen F, Imoto K, Sakmann B (1996) Ca^{2+} buffering and action potential-evoked Ca^{2+} signaling in dendrites of pyramidal neurons. *Biophys J* 70:1069–1081.

Henze DA, Buzsáki G (2001) Action potential threshold of hippocampal pyramidal cells in vivo is increased by recent spiking activity. *Neuroscience* 105:121–130.

Henze DA, Cameron WE, Barrionuevo GJ (1996) Dendritic morphology and its effects on the amplitude and rise-time of synaptic signals in hippocampal CA3 pyramidal cells. *J Comp Neurol* 369:331–344.

Henze DA, Urban NN, Barrionuevo G (2000) The multifarious hippocampal mossy fiber pathway: a review. *Neuroscience* 98:407–427.

Hering H, Sheng M (2001) Dendritic spines: structure, dynamics and regulation. *Nat Rev Neurosci* 2:880–888.

Herreras O (1990) Propagating dendritic action potential mediates synaptic transmission in CA1 pyramidal cells in situ. *J Neurophysiol* 64:1429–1441.

Hjorth-Simonsen A (1973) Some intrinsic connections of the hippocampus in the rat: an experimental analysis. *J Comp Neurol* 147:145–161.

Hoffman DA, Johnston D (1998) Downregulation of transient K^+ channels in dendrites of hippocampal CA1 pyramidal neurons by activation of PKA and PKC. *J Neurosci* 18:3521–3528.

Hoffman DA, Magee JC, Colbert CM, Johnston D (1997) K^+ channel regulation of signal propagation in dendrites of hippocampal pyramidal neurons. *Nature* 387:869–875.

Hosokawa T, Rusakov DA, Bliss TV, Fine A (1995) Repeated confocal imaging of individual dendritic spines in the living hippocampal slice: evidence for changes in length and orientation associated with chemically induced LTP. *J Neurosci* 15:5560–5573.

Hotson JR, Prince DA (1980) A calcium-activated hyperpolarization follows repetitive firing in hippocampal neurons. *J Neurophysiol* 43:409–419.

Hotson JR, Prince DA, Schwartzkroin PA (1979) Anomalous inward rectification in hippocampal neurons. *J Neurophysiol* 42:889–895.

Hsu M, Buzsáki G (1993) Vulnerability of mossy fiber targets in the rat hippocampus to forebrain ischemia. *J Neurosci* 13:3964–3979.

Hu H, Vervaeke K, Storm JF (2002) Two forms of electrical resonance at theta frequencies, generated by M-current, h-current and persistent Na^+ current in rat hippocampal pyramidal cells. *J Physiol* 545:783–805.

Ishizuka N, Weber J, Amaral DG (1990) Organization of intrahippocampal projections originating from CA3 pyramidal cells in the rat. *J Comp Neurol* 295:580–623.

Ishizuka N, Cowan WM, Amaral DG (1995) A quantitative analysis of the dendritic organization of pyramidal cells in the rat hippocampus. *J Comp Neurol* 362:17–45.

Isaac JT (2003) Postsynaptic silent synapses: evidence and mechanisms. *Neuropharmacology* 45:450–460.

Isaac JT, Nicoll RA, Malenka RC (1995) Evidence for silent synapses: implications for the expression of LTP. *Neuron* 15:427–434.

Jaffe DB, Brown TH (1997) Calcium dynamics in thorny excrescences of CA3 pyramidal neurons. *J Neurophysiol* 78:10–18.

Jaffe DB, Carnevale NT (1999) Passive normalization of synaptic integration influenced by dendritic architecture. *J Neurophysiol* 82:3268–3285.

Jaffe DB, Johnston D, Lasser-Ross N, Lisman JE, Miyakawa H, Ross WN (1992) The spread of Na^+ spikes determines the pattern of dendritic Ca^{2+} entry into hippocampal neurons. *Nature* 357:244–246.

Jarsky T, Roxin A, Kath WL, Spruston N (2005) Conditional dendritic spike propagation following distal synaptic activation of hippocampal CA1 pyramidal neurons. *Nat Neurosci* 8:1667–1676.

Jay TM, Glowinski J, Thierry AM (1989) Selectivity of the hippocampal projection to the prelimbic area of the prefrontal cortex in the rat. *Brain Res* 505:337–340.

Jefferys JGR (1979) Initiation and spread of action potentials in granule cells maintained in vitro in slices of guinea-pig hippocampus. *J Physiol (Lond)* 289:375–388.

Jensen MS, Azouz R, Yaari Y (1994) Variant firing patterns in rat hippocampal pyramidal cells modulated by extracellular potassium. *J Neurophysiol* 71:831–839.

Jiang C, Schuman EM (2002) Regulation and function of local protein synthesis in neuronal dendrites. *Trends Biochem Sci* 27:506–513.

Johnston D (1981) Passive cable properties of hippocampal CA3 pyramidal neurons. *Cell Mol Neurobiol* 1:41–45.

Johnston D, Brown TH (1981) Giant synaptic potential hypothesis for epileptiform activity. *Science* 211:294–297.

Johnston D, Brown TH (1984) The synaptic nature of the paroxysmal depolarizing shift in hippocampal neurons. *Ann Neurol* 16(Suppl):S65–S71.

Johnston D, Brown TH (1986) Control theory applied to neural networks illuminates synaptic basis of interictal epileptiform activity. *Adv Neurol* 44:263–274.

Jonas P, Major G, Sakmann B (1993) Quantal components of unitary EPSCs at the mossy fibre synapse on CA3 pyramidal cells of rat hippocampus. *J Physiol (Lond)* 472:615–663.

Jonas P, Bischofberger J, Fricker D, Miles R (2004) Interneuron diversity series: fast in, fast out–temporal and spatial signal processing in hippocampal interneurons. *Trends Neurosci* 27:30–40.

Jones R (1994) Synaptic and intrinsic properties of neurons of origin of the perforant path in layer II of the rat entorhinal cortex in vitro. *Hippocampus* 4:335–353.

Jones RSG, Heinemann U (1988) Synaptic and intrinsic responses of medial entorhinal cortical cells in normal and magnesium-free medium in vitro. *J Neurophysiol* 59:1476–1496.

Jung H, Mickus T, Spruston N (1997) Prolonged sodium channel inactivation contributes to dendritic action potential attenuation in hippocampal pyramidal neurons. *J Neurosci* 17:6639–6646.

Jung H, Staff NP, Spruston N (2001) Action potential bursting in subicular pyramidal neurons is driven by a calcium tail current. *J Neurosci* 21:3312–3321.

Jung MW, McNaughton BL (1993) Spatial selectivity of unit activity in the hippocampal granular layer. *Hippocampus* 3:165–182.

Jung R, Kornmueller AE (1938) Eine Metodik der Ableitung lokalisierter Potentialschwankungen aus subcorticalen Hirngebieten. *Arch Psychiatr Nervenkr* 109:1–30.

Kahle JS, Cotman CW (1989) Carbachol depresses synaptic responses in the medial but not the lateral perforant path. *Brain Res* 482:159–163.

Kali S, Freund TF (2005) Distinct properties of two major excitatory inputs to hippocampal pyramidal cells: a computational study. *Eur J Neurosci* 22:2027–2048.

Kamondi A, Acsady L, Buzsaki G (1998) Dendritic spikes are enhanced by cooperative network activity in the intact hippocampus. *J Neurosci* 18:3919–3928.

Kandel ER, Spencer WA (1961) Electrophysiology of hippocampal neurons. II. Afterpotentials and repetitive firing. *J Neurophysiol* 24:243–259.

Kemppainen S, Jolkkonen E, Pitkanen A (2002) Projections from the posterior cortical nucleus of the amygdala to the hippocampal formation and parahippocampal region in rat. *Hippocampus* 12:735–755.

Klink R, Alonso A (1993) Ionic mechanisms for the subthreshold oscillations and differential electroresponsiveness of medial entorhinal cortex layer II neurons. *J Neurophysiol* 70:144–157.

Klink R, Alonso A (1997a) Morphological characteristics of layer II projection neurons in the rat medial entorhinal cortex. *Hippocampus* 7:571–583.

Klink R, Alonso A (1997b) Muscarinic modulation of the oscillatory and repetitive firing properties of entorhinal cortex layer II neurons. *J Neurophysiol* 77:1813–1828.

Klink R, Alonso A (1997c) Ionic mechanisms of muscarinic depolarization in entorhinal cortex layer II neurons. *J Neurophysiol* 77:1829–1843.

Knowles WD, Schwartzkroin PA (1981) Axonal ramifications of hippocampal Ca1 pyramidal cells. *J Neurosci* 1:1236–1241.

Koch C, Zador A (1993) The function of dendritic spines: devices subserving biochemical rather than electrical compartmentalization. *J Neurosci* 13:413–422.

Köhler C (1985) A projection from the deep layers of the entorhinal area to the hippocampal formation in the rat brain. *Neurosci Lett* 56:13–19.

Korngreen A, Sakmann B (2000) Voltage-gated K$^+$ channels in layer 5 neocortical pyramidal neurones from young rats: subtypes and gradients. *J Physiol* 525:621–639.

Kosaka T (1983) Axon initial segments of the granule cell in the rat dentate gyrus: synaptic contacts on bundles of axon initial segments. *Brain Res* 274:129–134.

Kovalchuk Y, Eilers J, Lisman J, Konnerth A (2000) NMDA receptor-mediated subthreshold Ca^{2+} signals in spines of hippocampal neurons. *J Neurosci* 20:1791–1799.

Krettek JE, Price JL (1977) The cortical projections of the mediodorsal nucleus and adjacent thalamic nuclei in the rat. *J Comp Neurol* 171:157–191.

Laatsch RH, Cowan WM (1966) Electron microscopic studies of the dentate gyrus of the rat. I. Normal structure with special reference to synaptic organization. *J Comp Neurol* 128:359–395.

Lancaster B, Adams PR (1986) Calcium-dependent current generating the afterhyperpolarization of hippocampal neurons. *J Neurophysiol* 55:1268–1282.

Lancaster B, Nicoll RA (1987) Properties of two calcium-activated hyperpolarizations in rat hippocampal neurones. *J Physiol* 389:187–203.

Lawrence JJ, McBain CJ (2003) Interneuron diversity series: containing the detonation–feedforward inhibition in the CA3 hippocampus. *Trends Neurosci* 26:631–640.

Lawrence JJ, Grinspan ZM, McBain CJ (2004) Quantal transmission at mossy fibre targets in the CA3 region of the rat hippocampus. *J Physiol* 554:175–193.

Lawrence JJ, Statland JM, Grinspan ZM, McBain CJ (2006) Cell type-specific dependence of muscarinic signaling in mouse hippocampal stratum oriens interneurons. *J Physiol* 570:595–610.

Lebeda FJ, Hablitz JJ, Johnston D (1982) Antagonism of GABA-mediated responses by d-tubocurarine in hippocampal neurons. *J Neurophysiol* 48:622–632.

Lei S, McBain CJ (2002) Distinct NMDA receptors provide differential modes of transmission at mossy fiber-interneuron synapses. *Neuron* 33:921–933.

Lei S, McBain CJ (2004) Two loci of expression for long-term depression at hippocampal mossy fiber-interneuron synapses. *J Neurosci* 24:2112–2121.

Leung LS, Yu HW (1998) Theta-frequency resonance in hippocampal CA1 neurons in vitro demonstrated by sinusoidal current injection. *J Neurophysiol* 79:1592–1596.

Levy WB, Steward O (1979) Synapses as associative memory elements in the hippocampal formation. *Brain Res* 175:233–245.

Levy WB, Colbert CM, Desmond NL (1995) Another network model bites the dust: entorhinal inputs are no more than weakly excitatory in the hippocampal CA1 region. *Hippocampus* 5:137–140.

Li XG, Somogyi P, Tepper JM, Buzsaki G (1992) Axonal and dendritic arborization of an intracellularly labeled chandelier cell in the CA1 region of rat hippocampus. *Exp Brain Res* 90:519–525.

Li XG, Somogyi P, Ylinen A, Buzsaki G (1994) The hippocampal CA3 network: an in vivo intracellular labeling study. *J Comp Neurol* 339:181–208.

Liao D, Hessler NA, Malinow R (1995) Activation of postsynaptically silent synapses during pairing-induced LTP in CA1 region of hippocampal slice. *Nature* 375:400–404.

Lingenhöhl K, Finch DM (1991) Morphological characterization of rat entorhinal neurons in vivo: soma-dendritic structure and axonal domains. *Exp Brain Res* 84:57–74.

Lipowsky R, Gillessen T, Alzheimer C (1996) Dendritic Na$^+$ channels amplify EPSPs in hippocampal CA1 pyramidal cells. *J Neurophysiol* 76:2181–2191.

Liu YB, Lio PA, Pasternak JF, Trommer BL (1996) Developmental changes in membrane properties and postsynaptic currents of granule cells in rat dentate gyrus. *J Neurophysiol* 76:1074–1088.

Livsey CT, Vicini S (1992) Slower spontaneous excitatory postsynaptic currents in spiny versus aspiny hilar neurons. *Neuron* 8:745–755.

Livsey CT, Costa E, Vicini S (1993) Glutamate-activated currents in outside-out patches from spiny versus aspiny hilar neurons of rat hippocampal slices. *J Neurosci* 13:5324–5333.

Llinas RR (1988) The intrinsic electrophysiological properties of mammalian neurons: insights into central nervous system function. *Science* 242:1654–1664.

Lopes da Silva FH, Witter MP, Boeijinga PH, Lohman AH (1990) Anatomic organization and physiology of the limbic cortex. *Physiol Rev* 76:453–511.

Lorente de No R (1933) Studies on the structure of the cerebral cortex. I. The area entorhinalis. *J Psychol Neurol* 45:381–438.

Lorente de No R (1934) Studies on the structure of the cerebral cortex. II. Continuation of the study of ammonic system. *J Psychol Neurol* 46:113–177.

Lorincz A, Notomi T, Tamas G, Shigemoto R, Nusser Z (2002) Polarized and compartment-dependent distribution of HCN1 in pyramidal cell dendrites. *Nat Neurosci* 5:1185–1193.

Lübke J, Frotscher M, Spruston N (1998) Specialized electrophysiological properties of anatomically identified neurons in the hilar region of the rat fascia dentata. *J Neurophysiol* 79:1518–1534.

Lujan R, Nusser Z, Roberts JD, Shigemoto R, Somogyi P (1996) Perisynaptic location of metabotropic glutamate receptors mGluR1 and mGluR5 on dendrites and dendritic spines in the rat hippocampus. *Eur J Neurosci* 8:1488–1500.

Maccaferri G, McBain CJ (1996) Long-term potentiation in distinct subtypes of hippocampal nonpyramidal neurons. *J Neurosci* 16:5334–5343.

Maccaferri G, Lacaille JC (2003) Interneuron diversity series: hippocampal interneuron classifications—making things as simple as possible, not simpler. *Trends Neurosci* 26:564–571.

Maccaferri G, Toth K, McBain CJ (1998) Target-specific expression of presynaptic mossy fiber plasticity. *Science* 279:1368–1370.

Maccaferri G, Roberts JD, Szucs P, Cottingham CA, Somogyi P (2000) Cell surface domain specific postsynaptic currents evoked by identified GABAergic neurones in rat hippocampus in vitro. *J Physiol* 524:91–116.

Macek TA, Winder DG, Gereau RW 4th, Ladd CO, Conn PJ (1996) Differential involvement of group II and group III mGluRs as autoreceptors at lateral and medial perforant path synapses. *J Neurophysiol* 76:3798–3806.

MacVicar BA, Dudek FE (1981) Electrotonic coupling between pyramidal cells: a direct demonstration in rat hippocampal slices. *Science* 213:782–785.

Madison DV, Nicoll RA (1982) Noradrenaline blocks accommodation of pyramidal cell discharge in the hippocampus. *Nature* 299:636–638.

Madison D, Nicoll RA (1984) Control of the repetitive discharge of rat CA1 pyramidal neurons in vitro. *J Physiol* 354:319–331.

Madison DV, Lancaster B, Nicoll RA (1987) Voltage clamp analysis of cholinergic action in the hippocampus. *J Neurosci* 7:733–741.

Magee JC (1998) Dendritic hyperpolarization-activated currents modify the integrative properties of hippocampal CA1 pyramidal neurons. *J Neurosci* 18:7613–7624.

Magee JC (1999) Dendritic I_h normalizes temporal summation in hippocampal CA1 neurons. *Nat Neurosci* 2:508–514.

Magee JC, Carruth M (1999) Dendritic voltage-gated ion channels regulate the action potential firing mode of hippocampal CA1 pyramidal neurons. *J Neurophysiol* 82:1895–1901.

Magee JC, Cook EP (2000) Somatic EPSP amplitude is independent of synapse location in hippocampal pyramidal neurons. *Nat Neurosci* 3:895–903.

Magee JC, Johnston D (1995a) Characterization of single voltage-gated Na$^+$ and Ca^{2+} channels in apical dendrites of rat CA1 pyramidal neurons. *J Physiol* 487:67–90.

Magee JC, Johnston D (1995b) Synaptic activation of voltage-gated channels in the dendrites of hippocampal pyramidal neurons. *Science* 68:301–304.

Magee JC, Johnston D (1997) A synaptically controlled, associative signal for Hebbian plasticity in hippocampal neurons. *Science* 275:209–213.

Magistretti J, Alonso A (1999) Biophysical properties and slow voltage-dependent inactivation of a sustained sodium current in entorhinal cortex layer-II principal neurons: a whole-cell and single-channel study. *J Gen Physiol* 115:491–509.

Magistretti J, Ragsdale DS, Alonso A (1999a) High conductance sustained single-channel activity responsible for the low-threshold persistent Na$^+$ current in entorhinal cortex neurons. *J Neurosci* 19:7334–7341.

Magistretti J, Ragsdale DS, Alonso A (1999b) Direct demonstration of persistent Na$^+$ channel activity in dendritic processes of mammalian cortical neurones. *J Physiol* 521:629–636.

Mainen ZF, Carnevale NT, Zador AM, Claiborne BJ, Brown TH (1996) Electrotonic architecture of hippocampal CA1 pyramidal neurons based on three-dimensional reconstructions. *J Neurophysiol* 76:1904–1923.

Majewska A, Brown E, Ross J, Yuste R (2000) Mechanisms of calcium decay kinetics in hippocampal spines: role of spine calcium pumps and calcium diffusion through the spine neck in biochemical compartmentalization. *J Neurosci* 20:1722–1734.

Major G, Larkman AU, Jonas P, Sakmann B, Jack JJ (1994) Detailed passive cable models of whole-cell recorded CA3 pyramidal neurons in rat hippocampal slices. *J Neurosci* 14:4613–4638.

Maletic-Savatic M, Lenn NJ, Trimmer JS (1995) Differential spatiotemporal expression of K$^+$ channel polypeptides in rat hippocampal neurons developing in situ and in vitro. *J Neurosci* 15:3840–3851.

Maletic-Savatic M, Malinow R, Svoboda K (1999) Rapid dendritic morphogenesis in CA1 hippocampal dendrites induced by synaptic activity. *Science* 283:1923–1927.

Markram H, Wang Y, Tsodyks M (1998) Differential signaling via the same axon of neocortical pyramidal neurons. *Proc Natl Acad Sci USA* 95:5323–5328.

Marrion NV, Tavalin SJ (1998) Selective activation of Ca^{2+}-activated K$^+$ channels by co-localized Ca^{2+} channels in hippocampal neurons. *Nature* 395:900–905.

Marshall L, Henze DA, Hirase H, Leinekugel X, Dragoi G, Buzsaki G

(2002) Hippocampal pyramidal cell-interneuron spike transmission is frequency dependent and responsible for place modulation of interneuron discharge. *J Neurosci* 22:RC197(1–5).

Martina M, Jonas P (1997) Functional differences in Na$^+$ channel gating between fast-spiking interneurones and principal neurones of rat hippocampus. *J Physiol* 505:593–603.

Martina M, Vida I, Jonas P (2000) Distal initiation and active propagation of action potentials in interneuron dendrites. *Science* 287:295–300.

Mason A (1993) Electrophysiology and burst-firing of rat subicular pyramidal neurons in vitro: a comparison with area CA1. *Brain Res* 600:174–178.

Masukawa LM, Prince DA (1984) Synaptic control of excitability in isolated dendrites of hippocampal neurons. *J Neurosci* 4:217–227.

Masukawa LM, Benardo LS, Prince DA (1982) Variations in electrophysiological properties of hippocampal neurons in different subfields. *Brain Res* 242:341–344.

Matsuzaki M, Ellis-Davies GC, Nemoto T, Miyashita Y, Iino M, Kasai H (2001) Dendritic spine geometry is critical for AMPA receptor expression in hippocampal CA1 pyramidal neurons. *Nat Neurosci* 4:1086–1092.

Matsuzaki M, Honkura N, Ellis-Davies GC, Kasai H (2004) Structural basis of long-term potentiation in single dendritic spines. *Nature* 429:761–766.

Mattia D, Hwa GGC, Avoli M (1993) Membrane properties of rat subicular neurons in vitro. *J Neurophysiol* 70:1244–1248.

Mattia D, Kawasaki H, Avoli M (1997a) In vitro electrophysiology of rat subicular bursting neurons. *Hippocampus* 7:48–57.

Mattia D, Kawasaki H, Avoli M (1997b) Repetitive firing and oscillatory activity of pyramidal-like bursitng neurons in the rat subiculum. *Exp Brain Res* 114:507–517.

Mátyás F., Freund TF, Gulyás AI (2004) Convergence of excitatory and inhibitory inputs onto CCK-containing basket cells in the CA1 area of the rat hippocampus. *Eur J Neurosci* 19:12–43.

McBain CJ, Fisahn A (2001) Interneurons unbound. *Nat Rev Neurosci* 2:11–23.

McBain CJ, Freund T, Mody I (1999) Glutamatergic synapses onto hippocampal interneurons: precision timing without lasting plasticity. *Trends Neurosci* 22:228–235.

McGinty JF, Henriksen SJ, Goldstein A, Terenius L, Bloom FE (1983) Dynorphin is contained within hippocampal mossy fibers: immunochemical alterations after kainic acid administration and colchicine-induced neurotoxicity. *Proc Natl Acad Sci USA* 80:589–593.

McNaughton BL, Douglas RM, Goddard GV (1978) Synaptic enhancement in fascia dentata: cooperativity among coactive afferents. *Brain Res* 157:277–293.

McNaughton BL, Barnes CA, Meltzer J, Sutherland RJ (1989) Hippocampal granule cells are necessary for normal spatial learning but not for spatially-selective pyramidal cell discharge. *Exp Brain Res* 76:485–496.

McQuiston AR, Madison DV (1999a) Muscarinic receptor activity induces an afterdepolarization in a subpopulation of hippocampal CA1 interneurons. *J Neurosci* 19:5703–5710.

McQuiston AR, Madison DV (1999b) Muscarinic receptor activity has multiple effects on the resting membrane potentials of CA1 hippocampal interneurons. *J Neurosci* 19:5693–5702.

Megias M, Emri Z, Freund TF, Gulyas AI (2001) Total number and distribution of inhibitory and excitatory synapses on hippocampal CA1 pyramidal cells. *Neuroscience* 102:527–540.

Menendez de la Prida L (2003) Control of bursting by local inhibition in the rat subiculum in vitro. *J Physiol* 549:219–230.

Menendez de la Prida L, Suarez F, Pozo MA (2003) Electrophysiological and morphological diversity of neurons from the rat subicular complex in vitro. *Hippocampus* 13:728–744.

Metz A, Jarsky T, Martina M, Spruston N (2005) R-type calcium channels produce an afterdepolarization and bursting in hippocampal CA1 pyramidal neurons. *J Neurosci* 25:5763–5773.

Mickus T, Jung H, Spruston N (1999) Properties of slow, cumulative sodium channel inactivation in rat hippocampal CA1 pyramidal cells. *Biophys J* 76:846–860.

Migliore M, Cook EP, Jaffe DB, Turner DA, Johnston D (1995) Computer simulations of morphologically reconstructed CA3 hippocampal neurons. *J Neurophysiol* 73:1157–1168.

Mikkonen M, Pitkänen A, Soininen H, Alafuzoff I, Miettinen R (2000) Morphology of spiny neurons in the human entorhinal cortex: intracellular filling with lucifer yellow. *Neuroscience* 96:515–522.

Miles R (1990) Variation in strength of inhibitory synapses in the CA3 region of guinea-pig hippocampus in vitro. *J Physiol (Lond)* 431:659–676.

Miles R, Toth K, Gulyas AI, Hajos N, Freund TF (1996) Differences between somatic and dendritic inhibition in the hippocampus. *Neuron* 16:815–823.

Miyakawa H, Ross WN, Jaffe D, Callaway JC, Lasser-Ross N, Lisman JE, Johnston D (1992) Synaptically activated increases in Ca^{2+} concentration in hippocampal CA1 pyramidal cells are primarily due to voltage-gated Ca^{2+} channels. *Neuron* 9:1163–1173.

Monaghan DT, Holets VR, Toy DW, Cotman CW (1983) Anatomical distributions of four pharmacologically distinct ^{3}H-L-glutamate binding sites. *Nature* 306:176–179.

Moosmang S, Biel M, Hofmann F, Ludwig A (1999) Differential distribution of four hyperpolarization-activated cation channels in mouse brain. *Biol Chem* 380:975–980.

Murthy VN, Sejnowski TJ, Stevens CF (2000) Dynamics of dendritic calcium transients evoked by quantal release at excitatory hippocampal synapses. *Proc Natl Acad Sci USA* 97:901–906.

Naber PA, Witter MP (1998) Subicular efferents are organized mostly as parallel projections: a double labeling, retrograde-tracing study in the rat. *J Comp Neurol* 393:284–297.

Naber PA, Witter MP, Lopes da Silva FH (2000) Networks of hippocampal memory system of the rat. *Ann NY Acad Sci* 911:392–403.

Nafstad PHJ, Blackstad TW (1966) Distribution of mitochondria in pyramidal cells and boutons in hippocampal cortex. *Z Zellforsch Mikrosk Anat* 3:234–245.

Nakamura T, Barbara JG, Nakamura K, Ross WN (1999) Synergistic release of Ca^{2+} from IP3–sensitive stores evoked by synaptic activation of mGluRs paired with backpropagating action potentials. *Neuron* 24:727–737.

Nakamura T, Nakamura K, Lasser-Ross N, Barbara JG, Sandler VM, Ross WN (2000) Inositol 1,4,5–trisphosphate (IP3)-mediated Ca^{2+} release evoked by metabotropic agonists and backpropagating action potentials in hippocampal CA1 pyramidal neurons. *J Neurosci* 20:8365–8376.

Nicholson D, Katz Y, Trana R, Kath WL, Spruston N, Geinisman Y (2006) Distance-dependent differences in synapse number and

AMPA receptor expression in hippocampal CA1 pyramidal neurons. *Neuron* 50:431–442.

Nikonenko I, Jourdain P, Alberi S, Toni N, Muller D (2002) Activity-induced changes of spine morphology. *Hippocampus* 12:585–591.

Nimchinsky EA, Sabatini BL, Svoboda K (2002) Structure and function of dendritic spines. *Annu Rev Physiol* 64:313–353.

Nimchinsky EA, Yasuda R, Oertner TG, Svoboda K (2004) The number of glutamate receptors opened by synaptic stimulation in single hippocampal spines. *J Neurosci* 24:2054–2064.

Nusser Z, Lujan R, Laube G, Roberts JD, Molnar E, Somogyi P (1998) Cell type and pathway dependence of synaptic AMPA receptor number and variability in the hippocampus. *Neuron* 21:545–559.

Oertner TG, Sabatini BL, Nimchinsky EA, Svoboda K (2002) Facilitation at single synapses probed with optical quantal analysis. *Nat Neurosci* 5:657–664.

Oliva AA Jr, Jiang M, Lam T, Smith KL, Swann JW (2000). Novel hippocampal interneuronal subtypes identified using transgenic mice that express green fluorescent protein in GABAergic interneurons. *J Neurosci* 20:3354–3368.

O'Mara SM, Commins S, Anderson M, Gigg J (2001) The subiculum: a review of form, physiology and function. *Prog Neurobiol* 64:129–155.

Otmakhova NA, Lisman JE (1999) Dopamine selectively inhibits the direct cortical pathway to the CA1 hippocampal region. *J Neurosci* 19:1437–1445.

Otmakhova NA, Lisman JE (2000) Dopamine, serotonin, and noradrenaline strongly inhibit the direct perforant path-CA1 synaptic input, but have little effect on the Schaffer collateral input. *Ann NY Acad Sci* 911:462–464.

Paré D, Llinás R (1994) Non-lamellar propagation of entorhinal influences in the hippocampal formation: multiple electrode recordings in the isolated guinea pig brain in vitro. *Hippocampus* 4:403–409.

Parnass Z, Tashiro A, Yuste R (2000) Analysis of spine morphological plasticity in developing hippocampal neurons. *Hippocampus* 10:561–568.

Parra P, Gulyas AI, Miles R (1998) How many subtypes of inhibitory cells in the hippocampus? *Neuron* 20:983–993.

Pasquier DA, Reinoso-Suarez F (1978) The topographic organization of hypothalamic and brain stem projections to the hippocampus. *Brain Res Bull* 3:373–389.

Pearce RA (1993) Physiological evidence for two distinct GABAA responses in rat hippocampus. *Neuron* 10:189–200.

Pedarzani P, Storm JF (1996) Evidence that Ca/calmodulin-dependent protein kinase mediates the modulation of the Ca^{2+}-dependent K^{+} current, IAHP, by acetylcholine, but not by glutamate, in hippocampal neurons. *Pflugers Arch* 431:723–728.

Pelletier MR, Kirkby RD, Jones SJ, Corcoran ME (1994) Pathway specificity of noradrenergic plasticity in the dentate gyrus. *Hippocampus* 4:181–188.

Penttonen M, Kamondi A, Sik A, Acsady L, Buzsaki G (1997) Feed-forward and feed-back activation of the dentate gyrus in vivo during dentate spikes and sharp wave bursts. *Hippocampus* 7:437–450.

Peters A, Kaiserman-Abramof IR (1970) The small pyramidal neuron of the rat cerebral cortex: the perikaryon, dendrites and spines. *Am J Anat* 127:321–355.

Poolos NP, Kocsis JD (1990) Dendritic action potentials activated by NMDA receptor-mediated EPSPs in CA1 hippocampal pyramidal cells. *Brain Res* 524:342–346.

Poolos NP, Johnston D (1999) Calcium-activated potassium conductances contribute to action potential repolarization at the soma but not the dendrites of hippocampal CA1 pyramidal neurons. *J Neurosci* 19:5205–5212.

Popov VI, Davies HA, Rogachevsky VV, Patrushev IV, Errington ML, Gabbott PL, Bliss TV, Stewart MG (2004) Remodelling of synaptic morphology but unchanged synaptic density during late phase long-term potentiation (LTP): a serial section electron micrograph study in the dentate gyrus in the anaesthetised rat. *Neuroscience* 128:251–262.

Pouille F, Scanziani M (2001) Enforcement of temporal fidelity in pyramidal cells by somatic feed-forward inhibition. *Science* 293:1159–1163.

Pouille F, Scanziani M (2004) Routing of spike series by dynamic circuits in the hippocampus. *Nature* 429:717–723.

Pozzo-Miller LD, Petrozzino JJ, Mahanty NK, Connor JA (1993) Optical imaging of cytosolic calcium, electrophysiology, and ultrastructure in pyramidal neurons of organotypic slice cultures from rat hippocampus. *Neuroimage* 1:109–120.

Pozzo-Miller LD, Petrozzino JJ, Golarai G, Connor JA (1996) Ca^{2+} release from intracellular stores induced by afferent stimulation of CA3 pyramidal neurons in hippocampal slices. *J Neurophysiol* 76:554–562.

Prince DA, Connors BW (1986) Mechansims of interictal epileptogenesis. *Adv Neurol* 44:275–299.

Pyapali GK, Sik A, Penttonen M, Buzsaki G, Turner DA (1998) Dendritic properties of hippocampal CA1 pyramidal neurons in the rat: intracellular staining in vivo and in vitro. *J Comp Neurol* 391:335–352.

Qian J, Noebels JL (2001) Presynaptic Ca^{2+} channels and neurotransmitter release at the terminal of a mouse cortical neuron. *J Neurosci* 21:3721–3728.

Racca C, Stephenson FA, Streit P, Roberts JD, Somogyi P (2000) NMDA receptor content of synapses in stratum radiatum of the hippocampal CA1 area. *J Neurosci* 20:2512–222.

Rall W (1959) Branching dendritic trees and motoneuron membrane resistivity. *Exp Neurol* 1:491–527.

Rall W (1964) Theoretical significance of dendritic trees for neuronal input-output relations. In: *Neural theory and modeling* (Reiss RF, ed). Palo Alto: Stanford University Press.

Rall W (1969) Time constants and electrotonic length of membrane cylinders and neurons. *Biophys J* 9:1483–1508.

Ramon y Cajal S (1904, 1995) *Histology of the nervous system*, vol 2 (Swanson N, Swanson L, translators). New York: Oxford University Press.

Ranck JB (1973) Studies on single neurons in dorsal hippocampal formation and septum in unrestrained rats. Part I. Behavioral correlates and firing repertoires. *Exp Neurol* 41:461–531.

Ratzliff AdH, Santhakumar V, Howard A, Soltesz I (2002) Mossy cells in epilepsy: rigor mortis or vigor mortis? *Trends Neurosci* 25:140–144.

Regehr WG, Tank DW (1992) Calcium concentration dynamics produced by synaptic activation of CA1 hippocampal pyramidal cells. *J Neurosci* 12:4202–4223.

Regehr WG, Connor JA, Tank DW (1989) Optical imaging of calcium accumulation in hippocampal pyramidal cells during synaptic activation. *Nature* 341:533–536.

Reid CA, Fabian-Fine R, Fine A (2001) Postsynaptic calcium transients evoked by activation of individual hippocampal mossy fiber synapses. *J Neurosci* 21:2206–2214.

Remondes M, Schuman EM (2002) Direct cortical input modulates plasticity and spiking in CA1 pyramidal neurons. *Nature* 416:736–740.

Riazanski V, Becker A, Chen J, Sochivko D, Lie A, Wiestler OD, Elger CE, Beck H (2001) Functional and molecular analysis of transient voltage-dependent K$^+$ currents in rat hippocampal granule cells *J Physiol* 537:391–406.

Ribak CE, Seress L, Amaral DG (1985) The development, ultrastructure and synaptic connections of the mossy cells of the dentate gyrus. *J Neurocytol* 14:835–857.

Rolls ET (1996) A theory of hippocampal function in memory. Hippocampus 6:601–620.

Ropert N (1988) Inhibitory action of serotonin in CA1 hippocampal neurons in vitro. *Neuroscience* 26:69–81.

Rudy B, McBain CJ (2001) Kv3 channels: voltage-gated K$^+$ channels designed for high-frequency repetitive firing. *Trends Neurosci* 24:517–526.

Sabatini BL, Oertner TG, Svoboda K (2002) The life cycle of Ca^{2+} ions in dendritic spines. *Neuron* 33:439–452.

Salin PA, Scanziani M, Malenka RC, Nicoll RA (1996) Distinct short-term plasticity at two excitatory synapses in the hippocampus. *Proc Natl Acad Sci USA* 93:13304–13309.

Sandler R, Smith AD (1991) Coexistence of GABA and glutamate in mossy fiber terminals of the primate hippocampus: an ultrastructural study. *J Comp Neurol* 303:177–192.

Sandler VM, Barbara JG (1999) Calcium-induced calcium release contributes to action potential-evoked calcium transients in hippocampal CA1 pyramidal neurons. *J Neurosci* 19:4325–4336.

Sandler VM, Ross WN (1999) Serotonin modulates spike backpropagation and associated [Ca^{2+}]$_i$ changes in the apical dendrites of hippocampal CA1 pyramidal neurons. *J Neurophysiol* 81:216–224.

Santoro B, Grant SG, Bartsch D, Kandel ER (1997) Interactive cloning with the SH3 domain of N-src identifies a new brain specific ion channel protein, with homology to eag and cyclic nucleotide-gated channels. *Proc Natl Acad Sci USA* 94:14815–14820.

Santoro B, Chen S, Luthi A, Pavlidis P, Shumyatsky GP, Tibbs GR, Siegelbaum SA (2000) Molecular and functional heterogeneity of hyperpolarization-activated pacemaker channels in the mouse CNS. *J Neurosci* 20:5264–5275.

Scanziani M, Gahwiler BH, Charpak S (1998) Target cell-specific modulation of transmitter release at terminals from a single axon. *Proc Natl Acad Sci USA* 95:12004–12009.

Schaffer K (1892) Beitrag zur Histologie der Ammons Horn-formation. *Arch Mikrosc Anat* 39:611–632.

Schaller KL, Caldwell JH (2000) Developmental and regional expression of sodium channel isoform NaCh6 in the rat central nervous system. *J Comp Neurol* 420:84–97.

Scharfman HE (1991) Dentate hilar cells with dendrites in the molecular layer have lower thresholds for synaptic activation by perforant path than granule cells. *J Neurosci* 11:1660–1673.

Scharfman HE (1992) Differentiation of rat dentate neurons by morphology and electrophysiology in hippocampal slices: granule cells, spiny hilar cells and aspiny 'fast-spiking' cells. *Epilepsy Res Suppl* 7:93–109.

Scharfman HE (1994) Evidence from simultaneous intracellular recordings in rat hippocampal slices that area CA3 pyramidal cells innervate dentate hilar mossy cells. *J Neurophysiol* 72:2167–2180.

Scharfman HE, Schwartzkroin PA (1988) Electrophysiology of morphologically identified mossy cells of the dentate hilus recorded in guinea pig hippocampal slices. *J Neurosci* 8:3812–3821.

Schiller J, Helmchen F, Sakmann B (1995) Spatial profile of dendritic calcium transients evoked by action potentials in rat neocortical pyramidal neurones. *J Physiol* 487:583–600.

Schmitz D, Schuchmann S, Fisahn A, Draguhn A, Buhl EH, Petrasch-Parwez E, Dermietzel R, Heinemann U, Traub RD (2001) Axo-axonal coupling: a novel mechanism for ultrafast neuronal communication. *Neuron* 31:831–840.

Schwartz SP, Coleman PD (1981) Neurons of origin of the perforant path. *Exp Neurol* 74:305–312.

Schwartzkroin PA (1977) Further characteristics of hippocampal CA1 cells in vitro. *Brain Res* 128:53–68.

Schwartzkroin PA (1993) *Epilepsy; models, mechanisms and concepts.* Cambridge: Cambridge University Press.

Schwartzkroin PA, Slawsky M (1977) Probable calcium spikes in hippocampal neurons. *Brain Res* 135:157–161.

Schwartzkroin PA, Stafstrom CE (1980) Effects of EGTA on the calcium-activated afterhyperpolarization in hippocampal CA3 cells. *Science* 210:1125–1126.

Segev I, Rinzel J, Shepherd GM (1995) *The theoretical foundation of dendritic function: selected papers of Wilfrid Rall with commentaries.* Cambridge, MA: MIT Press.

Shalinsky MH, Magistretti J, Ma L, Alonso A (2002) Muscarinic activation of a cation current and associated current noise in entorhinal-cortex layer-II neurons. *J Neurophysiol* 88:1197–1211.

Sharp PE, Green C (1994) Spatial correlates of firing patterns of single cells in the subiculum of the freely moving rat. *J Neurosci* 14:2339–2356.

Sheng M (2001) Molecular organization of the postsynaptic specialization. *Proc Natl Acad Sci USA* 98:7058–7061.

Sheng M, Tsaur M-L, Jan YN, Jan LY (1992) Subcellular segregation of two A-type K$^+$ channel proteins in rat central neurons. *Neuron* 9:271–284.

Shepherd GMG, Harris KM (1998) Three dimensional structure and composition of CA3-CA1 axons in rat hippocampal slices: implications for presynaptic connectivity and compartmentalization. *J Neurosci* 18:8300–8310.

Shepherd GMG, Raastad M, Andersen P (2002) General and variable features of varicosity spacing along unmyelinated axons in the hippocampus and cerebellum. *Proc Natl Acad Sci USA* 99:6340–6345.

Sik A, Tamamaki N, Freund TF (1993) Complete axon arborization of a single CA3 pyramidal cell in the rat hippocampus, and its relationship with postsynaptic parvalbumin-containing interneurons. *Eur J Neurosci* 5:1719–1728.

Sik A, Penttonen M, Ylinen A, Buzsaki G (1995) Hippocampal CA1 interneurons: an in vivo intracellular labeling study. *J Neurosci* 15:6651–6665.

Skaggs WE, McNaughton BL, Wilson MA, Barnes CA (1996) Theta phase precession in hippocampal neuronal populations and the compression of temporal sequences. *Hippocampus* 6:149–172.

Sloviter RS (1987) Decreased hippocampal inhibition and a selective loss of interneurons in experimental epilepsy. *Science* 235:73–76.

Sloviter RS Somogyi P (1991) Permanently altered hippocampal structure, excitability, and inhibition after experimental status epilepticus in the rat: the "dormant basket cell" hypothesis and its possible relevance to temporal lobe epilepsy. *Hippocampus* 1:41–66.

Sloviter RS, Dichter MA, Rachinsky TL, Dean E, Goodman JH, Sollas AL, Martin DL (1996) Basal expression and induction of glutamate decarboxylase and GABA in excitatory granule cells of the rat and monkey hippocampal dentate gyrus. J Comp Neurol 373:593–618.

Smith MA, Ellis-Davies GC, Magee JC (2003) Mechanism of the distance-dependent scaling of Schaffer collateral synapses in rat CA1 pyramidal neurons. J Physiol 548:245–258.

Soltesz I (1995) Brief history of cortico-hippocampal time with a special reference to the direct entorhinal input to CA1. Hippocampus 5:120–124.

Soltesz I, Mody I (1994) Patch-clamp recordings reveal powerful GABAergic inhibition in dentate hilar neurons. J Neurosci 14:2365–2376.

Soltesz I, Bourassa J, Deschenes M (1993) The behavior of mossy cells of the rat dentate gyrus during theta oscillations in vivo. Neuroscience 57:555–564.

Somogyi P, Nunzi MG, Gorio A, Smith AD (1983a) A new type of specific interneuron in the monkey hippocampus forming synapses exclusively with the axon initial segments of pyramidal cells. Brain Res 259:137–142.

Somogyi P, Smith AD, Nunzi MG, Gorio A, Takagi H, Wu JY (1983b) Glutamate decarboxylase immunoreactivity in the hippocampus of the cat: distribution of immunoreactive synaptic terminals with special reference to the axon initial segment of pyramidal neurons. J Neurosci 3:1450–1468.

Soriano E, Frotscher M (1993) Spiny nonpyramidal neurons in the CA3 region of the rat hippocampus are gluatmate-like immunoreactive and receive convergent mossy fiber input. J Comp Neurol 332:435–448.

Soriano E, Frotscher M (1994) Mossy cells of the rat fascia dentata are glutamate-immunoreactive. Hippocampus 4:65–69.

Sorra KE, Harris KM (1993) Occurrence and three-dimensional structure of multiple synapses between individual radiatum axons and their target pyramidal cells in hippocampal area CA1. J Neurosci 13:3736–3748.

Sorra KE, Harris KM (2000) Overview on the structure, composition, function, development, and plasticity of hippocampal dendritic spines. Hippocampus 10:501–511.

Spacek J, Harris KM (1997) Three-dimensional organization of smooth endoplasmic reticulum in hippocampal CA1 dendrites and dendritic spines of the immature and mature rat. J Neurosci 17:190–203.

Spencer WA, Kandel ER (1961) Electrophysiology of hippocampal neurons IV. Fast prepotentials. J Neurophysiol 24:272–285.

Spigelman I, Zhang L, Carlen PL (1992) Patch-clamp study of postnatal development of CA1 neurons in rat hippocampal slices: membrane excitability and K$^+$ currents. J Neurophysiol 68:55–69.

Spruston N, Johnston D (1992) Perforated patch-clamp analysis of the passive membrane properties of three classes of hippocampal neurons. J Neurophysiol 67:508–529.

Spruston N, Jaffe DB, Williams SH, Johnston D (1993) Voltage- and space-clamp errors associated with the measurement of electrotonically remote synaptic events. J Neurophysiol 70:781–802.

Spruston N, Jaffe DB, Williams SH, Johnston D (1994) Dendritic attenuation of synaptic potentials and currents: the role of passive membrane properties. Trends Neurosci 17:161–166.

Spruston N, Jonas P, Sakmann B (1995) Dendritic glutamate receptor channels in rat hippocampal CA3 and CA1 pyramidal neurons. J Physiol (Lond) 482:325–352.

Spruston N, Lübke J, Frotscher M (1997) Interneurons in the stratum lucidum of the rat hippocampus: an anatomical and electrophysiological characterization. J Comp Neurol 385: 427–440.

Staff NP, Jung H, Thiagarajan T, Yao M, Spruston N (2000) Resting and active properties of pyramidal neurons in subiculum and CA1 of rat hippocampus. J Neurophysiol 84:2398–2408.

Staley KJ, Otis TS, Mody I (1992) Membrane properties of dentate gyrus granule cells: comparison of sharp microelectrode and whole cell recordings. J Neurophysiol 67:1346–1358.

Staley KJ, Longacher M, Bains JS, Yee A (1998) Presynaptic modulation of CA3 network activity. Nat Neurosci 1:201–209.

Stanford IM, Traub RD, Jefferys JGR (1998) Limbic gamma rhythms. II. Synaptic and intrinsic mechanisms underlying spike doublets in oscillating subicular neurons. J Neurophysiol 80:162–171.

Stanzione P, Calabresi P, Mercuri N, Bernardi G (1984) Dopamine modulates CA1 hippocampal neurons by elevating the threshold for spike generation: an in vitro study. Neuroscience 13:1105–1116.

Steward O, Worley P (2002) Local synthesis of proteins at synaptic sites on dendrites: role in synaptic plasticity and memory consolidation? Neurobiol Learn Mem 78:508–527.

Steward O, Falk PM, Torre ER (1996) Ultrastructural basis for gene expression at the synapse: synapse-associated polyribosome complexes. J Neurocytol 25:717–734.

Stewart M (1997) Antidromic and orthodromic responses by subicular neurons in rat brain slices. Brain Res 769:71–85.

Stewart M, Wong RKS (1993) Intrinsic properties and evoked responses of guinea pig subicular neurons in vitro. J Neurophysiol 70:232–245.

Storm JF (1987) Action potential repolarization and a fast afterhyperpolarization in rat hippocampal pyramidal cells. J Physiol 385:733–759.

Storm JF (1989) An afterhyperpolarization of medium duration in rat hippocampal pyramidal cells. J Neurophysiol 409:171–190.

Storm JF (1990) Potassium currents in hippocampal pyramidal cells. Prog Brain Res 83:161–187.

Storm-Mathisen J (1977) Localization of transmitter candidates in the brain: the hippocampal formation as a model. Prog Neurobiol 8:119–181.

Storm-Mathisen J, Fonnum F (1972) Localization of transmitter candidates in the hippocampal region. Prog Brain Res 36:41–58.

Stuart G, Spruston N (1998) Determinants of voltage attenuation in neocortical pyramidal neuron dendrites. J Neurosci 18:3501–3510.

Stuart GJ, Dodt HU, Sakmann B (1993) Patch-clamp recordings from the soma and dendrites of neurons in brain slices using infrared video microscopy. Pflugers Arch 423:511–518.

Stuart G, Spruston N, Sakmann B, Häusser M (1997) Action potential initiation and backpropagation in neurons of the mammalian central nervous system. Trends Neurosci 20:125–131.

Su H, Alroy G, Kirson ED, Yaari Y (2001) Extracellular calcium modulates persistent sodium current-dependent burst-firing in hippocampal pyramidal neurons. J Neurosci 21:4173–4182.

Suzuki SS, Smith GK (1985) Burst characteristics of hippocampal complex spike cells in the awake rat. Exp Neurol 89:90–95.

Swanson LW, Cowan WM (1977) An autoradiographic study of the organization of the efferent connections of the hippocampal formation in the rat. J Comp Neurol 172:49–84.

Swanson LW, Köhler C, Björklund A (1987) The limbic region. I. The septo-hippocampal system. In: Integrated systems of the CNS (Björklund A, Hökfelt T, Swanson L, eds), pp. 125–269. New York: Elsevier.

Szentagothai J, Arbib MA (1974) Conceptual models of neural organization. *Neurosci Res Prog Bull* 12:307–510.

Takumi Y, Rami'rez-Leo'n V, Laake P, Rinvik E, Ottersen OP (1999) Different modes of expression of AMPA and NMDA receptors in hippocampal synapse. *Nat Neurosci* 2:618–624.

Tamamaki N (1997) Organization of the entorhinal projection to the rat dentate gyrus revealed by DiI anterograde labeling. *Exp Brain Res* 116:250–258.

Tamamaki N, Nojyo Y (1990) Disposition of slab-like modules formed by axon branches originating from single CA1 pyramidal neurons in the rat hippocampus. *J Comp Neurol* 291:509–519.

Tamamaki N, Nojyo Y (1993) Projection of the entorhinal layer II neurons in the rat as revealed by intracellular pressure-injection of neurobiotin. *Hippocampus* 3:471–480.

Tamamaki N, Abe K, Nojyo Y (1987) Columnar organization in the subiculum formed by axon branches originating from single CA1 pyramidal neurons in the rat hippocampus. *Brain Res* 412:156–160.

Taube JS (1993) Electrophysiological properties of neurons in the rat subiculum. *Exp Brain Res* 96:304–318.

Thurbon D, Field A, Redman S (1994) Electronic profiles of interneurons in stratum pyramidale of the CA1 region in the rat hippocampus. *J Neurophysiol* 71:1948–1958.

Toth K, McBain CJ (1998) Afferent-specific innervation of two distinct AMPA receptor subtypes on single hippocampal interneurons. *Nat Neurosci* 1:572–578.

Toth K, Suares G, Lawrence JJ, Philips-Tansey E, McBain CJ (2000) Differential mechanisms of transmission at three types of mossy fiber synapse. *J Neurosci* 20:8279–8289.

Trachtenberg JT, Chen BE, Knott GW, Feng G, Sanes JR, Welker E, Svoboda K (2002) Long-term in vivo imaging of experience-dependent synaptic plasticity in adult cortex. *Nature* 420:788–794.

Traub RD, Miles R (1991) *Neuronal networks of the hippocampus.* Cambridge, UK: Cambridge University Press.

Traub RD, Jefferys JGR, Whittington MA (1999) *Fast oscillations in cortical circuits.* Cambridge, MA: MIT Press.

Trommald M, Hulleberg G (1997) Dimensions and density of dendritic spines from rat dentate granule cells based on reconstructions from serial electron micrographs. *J Comp Neurol* 377:15–28.

Trommald M, Jensen V, Andersen P (1995) Analysis of dendritic spines in rat CA1 pyramidal cells intracellularly filled with a fluorescent dye. *J Comp Neurol* 353:260–274.

Tsubokawa H, Ross WN (1996) IPSPs modulate spike backpropagation and associated $[Ca^{2+}]_i$ changes in the dendrites of hippocampal CA1 pyramidal neurons. *J Neurophysiol* 76:2896–2906.

Tsubokawa H, Ross WN (1997) Muscarinic modulation of spike backpropagation in the apical dendrites of hippocampal CA1 pyramidal neurons. *J Neurosci* 17:5782–5791.

Tsubokawa H, Miura M, Kano M (1999) Elevation of intracellular Na^+ induced by hyperpolarization at the dendrites of pyramidal neurones of mouse hippocampus. *J Physiol* 517:135–142.

Tsubokawa H, Offermanns S, Simon M, Kano M (2000) Calcium-dependent persistent facilitation of spike backpropagation in the CA1 pyramidal neurons. *J Neurosci* 20:4878–4884.

Turner DA (1984) Segmental cable evaluation of somatic transients in hippocampal neurons (CA1, CA3 and dentate) *Biophys J* 46:73–84.

Turner DA, Schwartzkroin PA (1983) Electrical characteristics of dendrites and dendritic spines in intracellularly stained CA3 and dentate hippocampal neurons. *J Neurosci* 3:2381–2394.

Turner RW, Meyers DE, Barker JL (1989) Localization of tetrodotoxin-sensitive field potentials of CA1 pyramidal cells in the rat hippocampus. *J Neurophysiol* 62:1375–1387.

Turner RW, Meyers DE, Richardson TL, Barker JL (1991) The site for initiation of action potential discharge over the somatodendritic axis of rat hippocampal CA1 pyramidal neurons. *J Neurosci* 11:2270–2280.

Turner RW, Meyers DE, Barker JL (1993) Fast pre-potential generation in rat hippocampal CA1 pyramidal neurons. *Neuroscience* 53:949–959.

Van der Linden S, Lopes da Silva FH (1998) Comparison of the electrophysiology and morphology of layers III and II neurons of the rat medial entorhinal cortex in vitro. *Eur J Neurosci* 10:1479–1489.

Van Groen T, Wyss JM (1990) Extrinsic projections from area CA1 of the rat hippocampus: olfactory, cortical, subcortical, and bilateral hippocampal formation projections. *J Comp Neurol* 302:515–528.

Van Groen T, Lopes da Silva FH (1986) Organization of the reciprocal connections between the subiculum and the entorhinal cortex in the cat. II. An electrophysiological study. *J Comp Neurol* 251:111–120.

Verdoorn TA, Burnashev N, Monyer H, Seeburg PH, Sakmann B (1991) Structural determinants of ion flow through recombinant glutamate receptor channels. *Science* 252:1715–1718.

Vida I, Bartos M, Jonas P (2006) Shunting inhibition improves robustness of gamma oscillations in hippocampal interneuron networks by homogenizing firing rates. *Neuron* 49:107–117.

Vissavajjhala P, Janssen WG, Hu Y, Gazzaley AH, Moran T, Hof PR, Morrison JH (1996) Synaptic distribution of the AMPA-GluR2 subunit and its colocalization with calcium-binding proteins in rat cerebral cortex: an immunohistochemical study using a GluR2-specific monoclonal antibody. *Exp Neurol* 142:296–312.

Volfovsky N, Parnas H, Segal M, Korkotian E (1999) Geometry of dendritic spines affects calcium dynamics in hippocampal neurons: theory and experiments. *J Neurophysiol* 82:450–462.

Walker MC, Ruiz A, Kullmann DM (2001) Monosynaptic GABAergic signaling from dentate to CA3 with a pharmacological and physiological profile typical of mossy fiber synapses. *Neuron* 29:703–715.

Walker MC, Ruiz A, Kullmann DM (2002a) Do mossy fibers release GABA? *Epilepsia* 43:196–202.

Walker HC, Lawrence JJ, McBain CJ (2002b) Activation of kinetically distinct synaptic conductances on inhibitory interneurons by electrotonically overlapping afferents. *Neuron* 35:161–171.

Wei DS, Mei YA, Bagal A, Kao JP, Thompson SM, Tang CM (2001) Compartmentalized and binary behavior of terminal dendrites in hippocampal pyramidal neurons. *Science* 293:2272–2275.

Wenthold RJ, Petralia RS, Blahos J II, Niedzielski AS (1996) Evidence for multiple AMPA receptor complexes in hippocampal CA1/CA2 neurons. *J Neurosci* 16:1982–1989.

Wenzel HJ, Buckmaster PS, Anderson NL, Wenzel ME, Schwartzkroin

PA (1997) Ultrastructural localization of neurotransmitter immunoreactivity in mossy cell axons and their synaptic targets in the rat dentate gyrus. *Hippocampus* 7:559–570.

Westenbroek RE, Ahlijanian MK, Catterall WA (1990) Clustering of L-type Ca^{2+} channels at the base of major dendrites in hippocampal pyramidal neurons. *Nature* 347:281–284.

White JA, Alonso A, Kay AR (1993) A heart-like Na^+ current in the medial entorhinal cortex. *Neuron* 11:1037–1047.

Wickens J (1988) Electrically coupled but chemically isolated synapses: dendritic spines and calcium in a rule for synaptic modification. *Prog Neurobiol* 31:507–528.

Wiebe SP, Staubli UV (1999) Dynamic filtering of recognition memory codes in the hippocampus. *J Neurosci* 19:10562–10574.

Williams SR, Stuart GJ (2000) Site independence of EPSP time course is mediated by dendritic I(h) in neocortical pyramidal neurons. *J Neurophysiol* 83:3177–3182.

Witter MP (1989) Connectivity of the rat hippocampus. In: *The hippocampus: new vistas*, pp 53–69. New York: Alan R. Liss.

Witter MP, Amaral DG (1991) Entorhinal cortex of the monkey. V. Projections to the dentate gyrus, hippocampus, and subicular complex. *J Comp Neurol* 307:437–459.

Wong RKS, Prince DA (1978) Participation of calcium spikes during intrinsic burst firing in hippocampal neurons. *Brain Res* 159:385–390.

Wong RKS, Prince DA, Basbaum AI (1979) Intradendritic recordings from hippocampal neurons. *Proc Natl Acad Sci USA* 76:986–990.

Wong RKS, Prince DA (1981) Afterpotential generation in hippocampal pyramidal cells. *J Neurophysiol* 45:86–97.

Wong RKS, Stewart M (1992) Different firing patterns generated in dendrites and somata of CA1 pyramidal neurones in guinea-pig hippocampus. *J Physiol* 457:675–687.

Wong RKS, Traub RD, Miles R (1986) Cellular basis of neuronal synchrony in epilepsy. *Adv Neurol* 44:583–592.

Wouterlood FG, Saldana E, Witter MP (1990) Projection from the nucleus reuniens thalami to the hippocampal region: light and electron microscopic tracing study in the rat with the anterograde tracer Phaseolus vulgaris-leucoagglutinin. *J Comp Neurol* 296:179–203.

Wu LG, Saggau P (1994) Pharmacological identification of two types of presynaptic voltage-dependent calcium channels at CA3-CA1 synapses of hippocampus. *J Neurosci* 14:5613–5622.

Xiao B, Tu JC, Worley PF (2000) Homer: a link between neural activity and glutamate receptor function. *Curr Opin Neurobiol* 10:370–374.

Yasuda R, Sabatini BL, Svoboda K (2003) Plasticity of calcium channels in dendritic spines. *Nat Neurosci* 6:948–955.

Yeckel MF, Berger TW (1990) Feedforward excitation of the hippocampus by afferents from the entorhinal cortex: redefinition of the role of the trisynaptic pathway. *Proc Natl Acad Sci USA* 87:5832–6583.

Yeckel MF, Berger TW (1995) Monosynaptic excitation of hippocampal CA1 pyramidal cells by afferents from the entorhinal cortex. *Hippocampus* 5:108–114.

Yuan LL, Adams JP, Swank M, Sweatt JD, Johnston D (2002) Protein kinase modulation of dendritic K^+ channels in hippocampus involves a mitogen-activated protein kinase pathway. *J Neurosci* 22:4860–4868.

Yue C, Remy S, Su H, Beck H, Yaari Y (2005) Proximal persistent Na^+ channels drive spike afterdepolarizations and associated bursting in adult CA1 pyramidal cells. *J Neurosci* 25:9704–9720.

Yuste R, Denk W (1995) Dendritic spines as basic functional units of neuronal integration. *Nature* 375:682–684.

Yuste R, Majewska A, Cash SS, Denk W (1999) Mechanisms of calcium influx into hippocampal spines: heterogeneity among spines, coincidence detection by NMDA receptors, and optical quantal analysis. *J Neurosci* 19:1976–1987.

6

Dimitri Kullmann

Synaptic Function

6.1 Overview

Ever since Sherrington coined the term "synapse" (from the Greek "hold together"), this organelle has attracted intense interest for several reasons. First, the information passing through the synapses supplied by an individual neuron reflects the outcome of its integrative functions. Second, with some notable exceptions it acts as a one-way "valve," transmitting information from the pre- to the postsynaptic neuron. Third, plasticity of synaptic transmission is the leading candidate for the cellular substrate of memory formation and storage. This chapter addresses some of the ways that individual synapses in the hippocampus are specialized to transmit signals and encode a history of their recent activity. It also provides the physiological context to Chapter 7, which examines the function of many of the molecules underlying synaptic transmission. The mechanisms of induction and expression of long-term changes in synaptic strength are addressed in Chapter 10.

Although the hippocampus has provided extensive information on the mechanisms by which neurons communicate with one another, many important principles underlying synaptic transmission were originally elucidated at the mammalian or arthropod neuromuscular junction. Indeed, many of the mechanisms underlying the trafficking of presynaptic vesicles are shared with other intracellular membrane-bound compartments and are even present in prokaryotes. We therefore start by summarizing some general features of interneuronal communication that are shared with other systems without going into detail into the experimental basis for these generally agreed upon principles. A detailed treatment of this subject is given in *Synapses* (Cowan et al., 2003). We then examine the various types of hippocampal synapse (classified anatomically) to see how their functional properties differ and how these distinct characteristics shed light on their roles.

For the purpose of this chapter a synapse is taken to represent the specialized structural and functional unit that is composed of one or more contiguous synaptic specializations occurring at the interface between two neurons (the presynaptic and postsynaptic partners). Thus, a single synapse can contain more than one presynaptic active zone (where neurotransmitter molecules are released) and postsynaptic specialization (where receptors detect them). However, a pair of pre- and postsynaptic neurons can also be connected via more than one synapse. Although this definition of a synapse is morphological, it should be borne in mind that major insights into synaptic function have relied principally on electrophysiological, pharmacological, and biochemical methods, often in the absence of histological reconstruction of the underlying elements.

Not all communication between neurons is via synapses: Some neurotransmitters are released from axonal varicosities in the absence of postsynaptic specialization. The fact that receptors are sometimes relatively remote from the site of release of their endogenous ligands (e.g., monoamines, peptides, acetylcholine) has been taken as evidence that two distinct forms of signaling exist: (1) "point-to-point" or "wiring" transmission at synapses and (2) a more diffuse "spillover," "extrasynaptic," or "volume" transmission mediated by diffusion of neuroactive substances through the extracellular space (Agnati et al., 1995). As is argued below, the distinction between these concepts is blurred by the existence of numerous types of receptor at variable distances from the release sites of their endogenous agonists. Neurons can also exert effects on their neighbors via mechanisms that do not involve neurotransmitters at all, for instance via field effects (Jefferys, 1995) or gap junctions (Galarreta and Hestrin, 1999; Gibson et al., 1999). These act as relatively low-impedance pathways that permit the passive flow of electrical signals among connected neurons. They can also permit ions to flow down their electrochemical gradients, thereby dissipating their local accumulation and depletion. Preliminary data also imply that axons of neighboring pyramidal neurons may be coupled through electrical contacts (Schmitz et al., 2001b). Moreover, not all hippocampal synapses are formed between neurons: Morphological and electrophysiological evidence supports the existence of excitatory synapses between hippocampal neurons and a subset of oligodendrocyte precursors (Bergles et al., 2000).

6.2 General Features of Synaptic Transmission: Structure

Synaptic transmission can be broken down into neurotransmitter release from a presynaptic specialization, diffusion of the neurotransmitter across the synaptic cleft, and activation of postsynaptic receptors. These phenomena must be understood in the context of the detailed ultrastructure of the synapse.

The electron micrograph shown in Figure 6–1, see color insert illustrates some features of hippocampal synapses. The pre- and postsynaptic elements are separated by a synaptic cleft. This cleft is often narrower than the gap separating non-synaptic membranes and appears relatively dense, reflecting the presence of a "basal substance" containing intercellular adhesion molecules. These molecules, some of which are

described in detail in Chapter 7, are thought to contribute to the formation, stabilization, and plasticity of synapses (see also Chapter 10).

The presynaptic element is readily identified by the presence of vesicles containing neurotransmitter molecules. These vesicles are generally of relatively uniform size and are aggregated near a membrane specialization that is often identified ultrastructurally as a thickening. This is thought to represent the "active zone," which is the site of exocytosis; and the thickening reflects the presence of membrane proteins necessary for exocytosis. Among them are proteins that interact with vesicular partners (SNARE proteins, see below), as well as voltage-dependent channels that mediate the influx of Ca^{2+}, which triggers exocytosis upon action potential invasion. It is almost universally agreed that vesicles are the morphological counterpart of the "quanta," that make up synaptic signals (see below). In addition, mitochondria are frequently present, reflecting the energetic demands of transmitter release (principally represented by the work required for transmitter synthesis, vesicular packaging, exocytosis, and reuptake) (Shepherd and Harris, 1998).

On the postsynaptic side, there is also an increased density of the membrane. Synapses with obvious postsynaptic thickening are known as asymmetrical, or type I, synapses (Gray, 1959) and were shown to be excitatory by Andersen and colleagues (1966), who examined the ultrastructural consequences of lesioning monosynaptic excitatory pathways. The

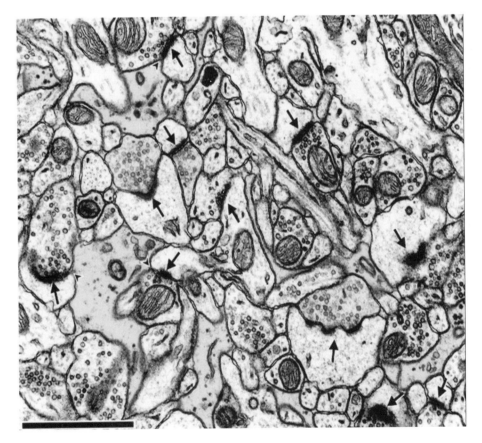

Figure 6–1. Fine structure of the hippocampal neuropil. Arrows point to individual asymmetrical (glutamatergic) synapses in a section taken from the stratum radiatum of CA1 in the rat. The presynaptic boutons contain numerous vesicles, which are frequently clustered close to membrane specializations (the active zone). A proportion of "docked" vesicles are in contact with the presynaptic membrane and are thought to be ready for exocytosis. The electron-dense area is the postsynaptic density, which distinguishes these synapses from numerically less abundant symmetrical (inhibitory) synapses (see Fig. 6–9). Astrocyte profiles, colored in blue, lacking vesicles and postsynaptic densities, contact the synaptic perimeter in some cases (arrowheads). Bar = 1 μm. (*Source:* Ventura and Harris, 1999, with permission.)

"postsynaptic density" (PSD) is a relatively detergent-resistant structure containing glutamate receptors and associated macromolecules (Kennedy, 1997) (discussed in Chapter 7). Some synapses lack this specialization and are therefore known as "symmetrical," or type II, synapses (Gray, 1959). They are thought to be principally GABAergic inhibitory synapses (see Chapter 8). Although they represent a small number of synapses in the hippocampus as a whole, they play numerous important roles, including setting the overall excitability of the structure and its rhythms. GABAergic synapses are concentrated around the soma and axonal initial segment of many neurons but are also found on dendrites.

In addition to the pre- and postsynaptic elements that make up a synapse, astrocyte processes commonly occur in close proximity to the synaptic cleft. As is shown below, they play a critical role in clearing neurotransmitter from the extracellular space. They also play an important role in buffering extracellular ion transients and in providing for the energetic demands of synaptic transmission. Although astrocyte processes are often thought of as an obligatory partner, making up the third element of a "tripartite" synapse, their presence at excitatory and inhibitory synapses is much more haphazard in the hippocampus than in other regions of the brain, such as the cerebellar cortex (Spacek, 1985; Lehre et al., 1995; Ventura and Harris, 1999). Indeed, many synapses in the hippocampus are not contacted by an obvious astrocytic process at all (Ventura and Harris, 1999).

6.2.1 Transmitter Release and Diffusion

Anatomical, biochemical, and electrophysiological methods have converged on the following general account of transmitter release (Zucker et al., 1998; Chen and Scheller, 2001; Sudhof, 2004) (Fig. 6–2).

On the presynaptic side, neurotransmitter molecules are translocated from the cytoplasm into vesicles by specific transporters, which exploit a proton gradient formed by vesicular ATPases. The two principal vesicular amino acid neurotransmitters differ slightly in their uptake mechanisms. The glutamate anion is driven into vesicles by the vesicle potential gradient formed by the high intraluminal H^+ concentration. A family of proteins that mediate glutamate uptake (VGLUT1-3) has recently been identified (Bellocchio et al., 2000; Takamori et al., 2000). In the case of GABA (γ-aminobutyric acid), in addition to uptake driven by the potential gradient, another mechanism exists: Cl^- is driven in by the potential gradient, and then exchanged for the GABA anion (Fykse and Fonnum, 1996). The vesicular transporter VGAT appears to be responsible for GABA uptake (McIntire et al., 1997).

Vesicles are reversibly tethered by synapsin molecules to a presynaptic actin scaffold. A subset of vesicles are especially closely apposed to the presynaptic active zone and have been described as beging "docked," presumably ready for exocytosis (Harris and Sultan, 1995). These vesicles may correspond to a population of quanta that are available for release on a relatively rapid time scale (defined physiologically as the "readily releasable pool") (Stevens and Tsujimoto, 1995; Rosenmund and Stevens, 1996). Evidence obtained in isolated preparations suggests that vesicle docking may be reversible (Steyer et al., 1997; Murthy and Stevens, 1999), and there may be a further stage of preparation for exocytosis that is not resolved ultrastructurally (named "priming").

Considerable effort has gone into identifying the molecular identity of the proteins that mediate and detect the influx of Ca^{2+} and trigger the fusion of the vesicle membrane with the presynaptic neuronal membrane (Augustine, 2001).

Voltage-dependent Ca^{2+} channels clearly play a critical role, and it is important to understand their properties to explain use-dependent plasticity and pharmacological modulation of transmitter release. Of the various pharmacologically and biophysically defined classes, P/Q− and N-type channels (also known as $Ca_V 2.1$ and $Ca_V 2.2$, respectively) account for most of the Ca^{2+} influx that triggers exocytosis (Dunlap et al., 1995). A third class of Ca^{2+} channels, R type ($Ca_V 2.3$), play a relatively small role at most synapses. Because of their high depolarization threshold, all three types are normally kept shut at resting potentials. They open rapidly upon depolarization; but because their closure lags slightly behind action

Figure 6–2. Stages of the vesicle cycle. 1, Vesicle filling. 2, Trafficking to the release site. 3, Docking/priming. 4, Fusion/release. 5, Membrane flattening. 6, Clathrin coating. 7, Endocytosis. 8, Clathrin uncoating. 9, Merging with endosome. 10, Recycling. Some evidence suggests that docking/priming and fusion/release may be reversible (indicated by broken line arrows).

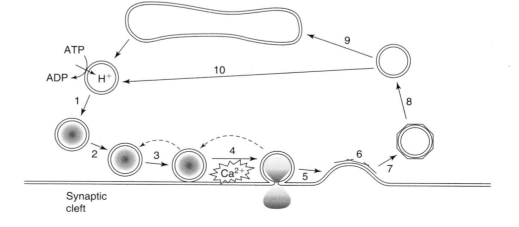

potential repolarization, they are still able to carry Ca^{2+} flux when the presynaptic membrane potential has returned close to the resting value. The bulk of the Ca^{2+} influx triggering exocytosis therefore probably occurs during repolarization, because the inward driving force for Ca^{2+} ions is maximal at this time point. Interestingly, whereas both N- and P/Q-type channels contribute to triggering glutamate release at individual synapses, many GABAergic terminals appear to fall into two classes: those that rely mainly on N-type channels and those that predominantly use P/Q-type channels (Poncer et al., 1997). It is not known if the Ca^{2+} channel identity is somehow tailored to the firing patterns of the presynaptic neurons.

Measurement of the intraterminal spatiotemporal Ca^{2+} concentration profile that occurs following action potential invasion is technically difficult in relatively small hippocampal synapses. Nevertheless, it has been estimated that the average concentration of free Ca^{2+} in a presynaptic varicosity rises to about 500 nM (Koester and Sakmann, 2000). This underestimates the peak concentration seen by the Ca^{2+} sensors responsible for triggering exocytosis. Based on studies at other synapses, the concentration at the site of exocytosis is thought to rise transiently approximately 100-fold, to approach 10 μM (Bollmann et al., 2000; Schneggenburger and Neher, 2000). Estimates of the size of the Ca^{2+} ion flux through an individual Ca^{2+} channel and the distance separating them from docked vesicles are consistent with the view that relatively few voltage-sensitive Ca^{2+} channels (possibly fewer than 100) must open to trigger exocytosis of a single vesicle (Borst and Sakmann, 1996).

Transmitter release shows a steep dependence on the extracellular Ca^{2+} concentration. A fourth-power relation has been observed at some synapses (Dodge and Rahamimoff, 1967), although this saturates at supraphysiological concentrations so the curve relating transmitter release to Ca^{2+} concentration is actually sigmoid. Several possible explanations exist for the steep Ca^{2+} dependence, including summation of Ca^{2+} influx via multiple channels, saturation of buffers, and cooperativity of Ca^{2+} sensors, in particular the vesicle-associated protein synaptotagmin I (Fernandez-Chacon et al., 2001). Synaptotagmin I contains two Ca^{2+}-binding domains, and genetic deletion of this protein severely disrupts fast Ca^{2+}-dependent exocytosis, making it a strong candidate for the Ca^{2+} sensor responsible for triggering transmitter release (Geppert et al., 1994). Ca^{2+} binding is thought to trigger a conformational change in a macromolecular complex consisting of three groups of proteins: vesicular, target membrane-associated, and soluble proteins (Chen and Scheller, 2001). The membrane-associated proteins are known as the SNAREs, from "SNAP-receptors" (SNAP: synaptosomal-associated proteins). The vesicular SNAREs (v-SNAREs) include VAMP (vesicle-associated membrane protein, also known as synaptobrevin); and the target membrane SNAREs (t-SNAREs) include SNAP-25 and syntaxin. These key proteins form a complex consisting of four helices (one α helix contributed by each of VAMP/synaptobrevin and syntaxin, and two α helices contributed by SNAP-25). Each of these proteins can be

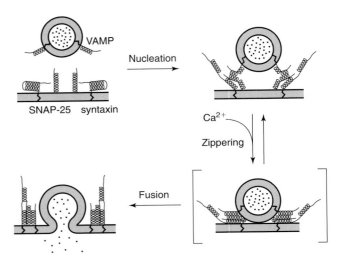

Figure 6–3. Proposed mechanism of SNARE-mediated exocytosis. Assembly of the core complex (VAMP/synaptobrevin, syntaxin, SNAP-25) is seen as a "nucleation" event necessary to prepare the vesicle for exocytosis. Ca^{2+} influx induces a conformational change of the core complex ("zippering"), which brings the vesicle and plasma membranes into contact, followed by transmitter release. (*Source*: Lin and Scheller, 2000, with permission.)

cleaved by at least one clostridial toxin (botulinum toxins A–G and tetanus toxin), which results in blockade of neurotransmitter release.

A compelling suggestion for the role of the core complex formed by VAMP/synaptobrevin, syntaxin, and SNAP-25 is that it forces together the vesicular and target membranes in preparation for their fusion. Nevertheless, the precise sequence of events that leads up to the conformational change underlying exocytosis is incompletely understood. In particular, it remains unclear precisely how synaptotagmin interacts with the SNARE complex and how the cascade overcomes the steep energy barrier to fusion of the vesicular and target membrane bilayers. Ultimately, the transmitter is released into the synaptic cleft. An outline of this cascade is summarized in Figure 6–3.

Before considering the consequence of transmitter release into the synaptic cleft, it is worth examining the fate of Ca^{2+} ions. Powerful presynaptic Ca^{2+} buffers exist in the form of proteins and mitochondria (Klingauf and Neher, 1997; Tang and Zucker, 1997). These, together with Ca^{2+} extrusion mechanisms, contribute to terminating the Ca^{2+} transient in such a way that the system is returned to the resting state. Nevertheless, it may take several minutes for this to be achieved, during which time successive action potentials may become increasingly effective in triggering transmitter release (Kamiya and Zucker, 1994; Zucker and Regehr, 2002). Genetic manipulation of Ca^{2+}-buffering proteins can alter the dependence of synaptic strength on the recent history of activity, underlining the importance of this phenomenon (Caillard et al., 2000). However, this is only one of several mechanisms that contribute to short-term use-dependent plasticity of synaptic transmission (see below).

It remains unclear whether exocytosis always involves complete fusion of the vesicle, flattening and merging with the presynaptic membrane, or can occur through the reversible opening of a "fusion pore," allowing the escape of all or part of the vesicle contents. Early reports of incomplete exocytosis came from ultrastructural studies at the neuromuscular junction and from two types of electrophysiological measurement that offer very good temporal resolution: voltammetric recordings of monoamine release (Chow et al., 1992; Bruns and Jahn, 1995) and capacitance measurements of the release of secretory granules (Breckenridge and Almers, 1987). None of these measurements was obtained at hippocampal synapses, so their relevance to this structure remains indirect. However, recent optical measurements of dyes taken up by presynaptic vesicles in hippocampal neurons in culture have suggested that individual vesicles can retain their identity through the cycle of release and reuptake (Murthy and Stevens, 1998), consistent with the proposal that they discharge their contents without completely fusing with the presynaptic membrane. This behavior raises the possibility that a vesicle may release less than its entire contents (so-called kiss-and-run release) before separating from the presynaptic membrane and mixing with a pool of vesicles in the terminal. Electrophysiological evidence has also been reported from hippocampal neurons in culture suggesting that glutamate can be released through two interchangeable modes, corresponding to full exocytosis or escape through a fusion pore (Renger et al., 2001).

Once fusion has occurred, the SNARE proteins must be dissociated and made available for another round of exocytosis. This step involves the soluble ATPase NSF (*N*-ethylmaleimide-sensitive factor) and α-SNAP (soluble NSF attachment protein). The requirement for ATP hydrolysis probably reflects the energetically unfavorable reversal of the formation of the core complex (Chen and Scheller, 2001; Jahn et al., 2003). The vesicle membrane, together with the membrane-associated proteins (including the vesicular ATPase and transporters, v-SNAREs, and synaptotagmin) must also be endocytosed if full fusion has occurred. This retrieval proceeds by formation of a lattice of clathrin molecules on the cytoplasmic face of the vesicle membrane. This lattice imposes a concavity on the membrane that is eventually pinched off by the action of dynamin, following which the recycled vesicle reenters the presynaptic pool (Cremona and De Camilli, 1997). Whether the vesicle merges immediately with the pool available to be released or is targeted specifically to an intermediate endosomal compartment is unclear.

Numerous mechanisms regulate the availability of vesicles for release. Among them is ATP-dependent mobilization of vesicles tethered to presynaptic microfilaments by synapsins (Rosahl et al., 1995). Rab3A is a GTP-binding protein that reversibly associates with vesicles as they go through the exocytosis–endocytosis cycle. Genetic deletion of Rab3A interferes with the expression of long-term potentiation at mossy fibers (see below) (Castillo et al., 1997a), suggesting a regulatory role; but its precise function in the vesicle cycle is unclear.

It is known to interact with two other proteins, rabphilin and RIM (Rab-interacting molecule), that contain putative Ca^{2+}-binding domains. There may also be a mechanism that regulates vesicle trafficking as a function of the neurotransmitter contents: Interfering with vesicular ATPase has been reported not to reduce the quantal amplitude but only to reduce the number of quanta available for release (Zhou et al., 2000). This observation suggests that a form of quality control exists to prevent underfilled vesicles from docking and/or releasing.

Following release, neurotransmitter molecules diffuse across the cleft to activate postsynaptic receptors. Because the synaptic cleft spans only approximately 20 nm, the time taken by neurotransmitter molecules to reach the nearest possible postsynaptic receptors is negligible: Assuming that neurotransmitter molecules diffuse readily in the extracellular space, they should reach most of the receptors in the synaptic cleft within 100 μs. However, although many receptors occur in the postsynaptic membrane opposite the active zone, others are farther away. Several classes of receptors (considered in detail below) show distinct patterns of localization: in the presynaptic membrane within the synaptic cleft or in a perisynaptic halo around the synapse, either pre- or postsynaptically (Takumi et al., 1998). Some receptors are even found in the axonal membrane relatively far from the synaptic cleft (Yokoi et al., 1996). To assess the functional role of these types of receptor, it is important to understand how the endogenous ligands reach them following release from presynaptic varicosities. The factors that determine the activation of these receptors are as follows.

- Amount of neurotransmitter released
- Temporal profile of release
- Distance from release site to receptors
- Diffusion coefficient (or diffusivity) of the neurotransmitter in the cleft and in the extracellular medium
- Diffusional obstacles
- Neurotransmitter transporters, their affinity and kinetics, and other binding sites
- Kinetics of the receptors

Astrocytes play an important role in determining receptor activation because they frequently extend processes that contact the perimeter of the synaptic cleft and because they express transporters and receptors on their surface, which buffer and/or sequester the neurotransmitter molecules. A further role played by astrocytes in the case of glutamate, is to convert it enzymatically to glutamine (see below).

6.2.2 Receptors and Receptor Activation

Receptors fall into two distinct classes. Ionotropic receptors, also known as ligand-gated ion channels, contain binding sites for neurotransmitters. Binding of the transmitter molecules causes the channel to open, allowing charged ions to travel down their chemical and electrical gradients. The biophysical principles and molecular mechanisms underlying ion selectivity and permeation are described in detail in *Ion Channels of Excitable Membranes* (Hille, 2001). With the other type, known as metabotropic receptors, ligand binding triggers an intracellular biochemical cascade beginning with dissociation of GTP-binding proteins (G proteins).

Ionotropic receptors generally occur postsynaptically, although they can also occur presynaptically in some areas of the brain (MacDermott et al., 1999), and mediate depolarizing or hyperpolarizing synaptic signals that activate within milliseconds. Depolarizing signals mediated by glutamate receptors take the form principally of an influx of Na^+ ions, accompanied by variable amounts of Ca^{2+} influx. Other excitatory ionotropic receptors (purinergic P2x receptors, nicotinic acetylcholine receptors, and serotonergic $5HT_3$ receptors) are present in far smaller numbers. The ion flux constitutes the excitatory postsynaptic current (EPSC), whose size is determined by the membrane potential, the reversal potential for each ion species, its permeability through the receptor, and the mean number of receptor channels opening. The EPSC depolarizes the postsynaptic membrane, and gives rise to an excitatory postsynaptic potential (EPSP), which if it is sufficiently large and/or sums with other EPSPs can activate regenerative currents. Such currents can reach threshold to trigger an action potential in the axon initial segment, although under some conditions an action potential can also arise in the parent dendrite (see Chapter 5). Box 6–1 summarizes some principles underlying voltage-clamp recording techniques, which have shed much light on the mechanisms underlying the generation of synaptic signals.

Conversely, inhibitory ionotropic signals are mediated principally by $GABA_A$ receptors. Although glycine receptors also contribute to inhibition in spinal and brain stem neurons, they are not known to play an important role in the hippocampus. Inhibitory postsynaptic currents (IPSCs) are carried by Cl^- and HCO_3^- ions flowing down their electrochemical gradients. Because the permeability of $GABA_A$ receptors for Cl^- is greater than that for HCO_3^- and the equilibrium potential for Cl^- is relatively negative, the IPSC generally hyperpolarizes the neuron, giving rise to an inhibitory postsynaptic potential (IPSP). Synaptic inhibition has two effects on neuronal excitability. First, it drives the membrane potential farther away from the threshold for activating regenerative depolarizing currents; and, second, by lowering the membrane resistivity it shunts EPSCs that would normally depolarize the neuron.

Although IPSPs and EPSPs contribute to the excitability of the neuron, they do not sum linearly because of several factors addressed in Chapter 5. Briefly, voltage- and time-dependent electrical properties of dendrites cause synaptic currents to dissipate or amplify as they propagate, the results of which depend strongly on the initial spatial profile of the membrane voltage, on the geometric distribution of active synapses, and on the density and kinetics of a set of voltage-gated ion channels.

Metabotropic receptors occur both pre- and postsynaptically, although different types, which have distinct pharmaco-

---

Box 6–1
Voltage-Clamp Techniques

Early studies of ion channels in neurons relied on measuring the effects of drugs and stimuli on the membrane potential. However, an ion flux through a population of channels can itself alter the membrane potential. This has two consequences: It alters the driving force for further ion flux and can cause voltage-sensitive channels to open or close, thereby potentially setting off regenerative currents. Thus, it is difficult to characterize the properties of different types of receptors on the basis of voltage recordings alone. The voltage-clamp method circumvents this problem by keeping the membrane potential at a fixed value and estimating the current flowing through the membrane. The method relies on a feedback circuit that pumps enough current back into the neuron to clamp its voltage at the desired level. The amplitude and time course of this current in relation to various stimuli (for instance, synaptic release or exogenous application of neurotransmitters or changes in the command voltage itself) then give an indication of the properties of the ion channels. As originally developed to study muscle fibers and axons, the method required separate electrodes to detect the membrane potential and to pass the current. This was not feasible in any but the largest cells. The patch-clamp method overcomes this difficulty by using the same low-resistance electrode to detect the membrane potential *and* pass the current. It relies on the finding that a glass pipette applied to the surface of a neuron can make a very high resistance seal with the plasmalemma. The method can work in various configurations.

1. Currents passing through individual ion channels under the membrane can be recorded in the "cell attached" mode.
2. The membrane under the pipette can be ruptured to allow the entire neuron to be voltage-clamped ("whole cell" mode—the most versatile method for recording synaptic currents).
3. Another way to access the entire cell electrically while minimizing the perturbation of its biochemical milieu is to add an ionophore to the pipette solution while remaining in the cell attached mode. This is the "perforated patch" technique.
4. In the whole cell configuration, slowly withdrawing the pipette causes a patch of membrane to seal over the pipette mouth ("outside-out configuration"). This allows the effects of brief pulses of agonists on small numbers of receptors to be studied in great detail.
5. It is also possible to rupture a vesicle of membrane in such a way that the cytoplasmic face is exposed to the bath ("inside-out configuration"). This is useful for studying the regulation of ion channels by second messengers.

---

logical profiles, have specific patterns of distribution. Most such receptors exert their actions over a slower time scale, lasting up to seconds. As a general principle, presynaptic metabotropic receptors depress transmitter release (Pin and Duvoisin, 1995; Schoepp, 2002). This effect is mediated partly through G protein regulation of presynaptic Ca^{2+} channels.

N-type Ca^{2+} channels in particular are directly modulated by the G protein subunit $G_{\beta\gamma}$ (Zhang et al., 1996; Dolphin, 1998); but in addition, some metabotropic receptors affect transmitter release indirectly via inactivation of adenylate cyclase (Tzounopoulos et al., 1998). Some metabotropic receptors may decrease transmitter release separately from an effect on Ca^{2+} influx (Scanziani et al., 1995; Blackmer et al., 2001).

On the postsynaptic side, metabotropic receptors have more diverse actions, although again most of these effects involve G proteins. The effector mechanisms include opening of K^+ channels, giving rise to a slow hyperpolarization (Pin and Duvoisin, 1995; Luscher et al., 1997). Some metabotropic glutamate receptors in contrast trigger the closure of specific K^+ channel subtypes, leading to depolarization or a change in the temporal profile of repetitive action potentials. Activation of yet other metabotropic receptors can lead to a depolarizing current by opening a cation channel with high permeability to Na^+ (Heuss et al., 1999). Other effects of metabotropic receptor activation include activation of phospholipase C, generating inositol trisphosphate (IP3) and diacylglycerol (DAG). IP3 is intimately involved in regulating the release of Ca^{2+} from internal stores, which may lead to triggering regenerative Ca^{2+} release and more remote effects such as modulation of gene transcription.

Receptor activation must eventually terminate. The most important mechanism that underlies this is rapid dissipation of the neurotransmitter pulse by diffusion into the large extracellular space, which can drop the concentration 100-fold within a few milliseconds. This phenomenon, on its own, thus causes a rapid decrease in ligand concentration to levels that may fall below those required to activate receptors. Nevertheless, some receptors remain bound for several hundred milliseconds because they have very high affinity (Lester et al., 1990). Uptake also plays a major role in the clearance of neurotransmitter through both the rapid quenching of neurotransmitter molecules binding to unoccupied transporters and their translocation into the cytoplasm. A third mechanism that can underlie the termination of receptor activation is desensitization: In the continued presence of agonist molecules, ionotropic receptors generally enter a state that is no longer able to open. (Much less is known about the desensitization mechanisms of metabotropic receptors.) The relative importance of diffusion, uptake, and desensitization in terminating activation may vary among receptors and even among synapses. However, even if uptake plays little role in the rapid termination of receptor activation, the neurotransmitters must eventually be cleared from the extracellular space by active transport because, apart from acetylcholine, ATP, and some neuroactive peptides, there are no extracellular mechanisms to break them down.

6.2.3 Quantal Transmission

The conventional view of synaptic function—originating from studies by Katz and coworkers at the neuromuscular junction—is that transmission is quantized; that is, repeated presynaptic action potentials give rise to postsynaptic signals that fluctuate from trial to trial among discrete levels (Katz, 1969; Zucker et al., 1998). These discrete levels occur at integral multiples (0, 1, 2, ...) of an underlying unit, the "quantum." This model of transmission has received only partial support from studies in the central nervous system (CNS). As already hinted above, if exocytosis is incomplete or the neurotransmitter is discharged slowly, a single vesicle may give a graded postsynaptic effect, even if it originally contained a fixed amount of neurotransmitter. Moreover, nonuniformities in the distribution of receptors available to detect transmitter released at different synapses or in the degree of distortion that the postsynaptic signals undergo as they propagate to the cell body are likely to conceal any quantal "structure" in the amplitude fluctuations of postsynaptic signal recorded at the soma. Finally, unlike the neuromuscular junction, where a single presynaptic end-plate has a large number of relatively uniform, well separated release sites, most hippocampal synapses probably contain only one or a few release sites (Schikorski and Stevens, 1997), which probably interact nonlinearly. Nevertheless, recordings of synaptic signals have reported large trial-to-trial fluctuations in the size of the postsynaptic response to activation of a single or a small number of presynaptic axons. In some cases, it has even been possible to discern clustering of postsynaptic response amplitudes at integral multiples of the unit value, perhaps reflecting the fortuitous case where underlying release events gave similar responses, and where they summed relatively linearly across the various active synapses or release sites (e.g., Kullmann and Nicoll, 1992). These cases probably represent only a small number of recordings but have helped shed light on the parameters that underlie transmission. Box 6–2 summarizes the principles of "quantal analysis" (Zucker et al., 1998).

The more general finding is that although transmission is stochastic and can even fail on occasion EPSCs, EPSPs, IPSCs, and IPSPs tend not to cluster systematically at preferred amplitudes (Raastad, 1995). It has nevertheless been possible to extract some information on the mechanisms of modulation of synaptic strength from examining the trial-to-trial variability of such signals. This application of quantal analysis relies on making a few assumptions, but some of them have been found to be reasonably robust. For instance, if it is assumed that failures of transmission reflect cases where the presynaptic action potential did not trigger exocytosis, it may be possible to use the frequency of such failures as an indirect witness of the state of the presynaptic terminal. That is, if a physiological or pharmacological event decreases the rate at which presynaptic action potentials elicit postsynaptic responses, it may be inferred that the presynaptic release probability has decreased. Other approaches rely on estimating the coefficient of variation of the postsynaptic signal (see Box 6–2). These approaches, however, must be used with caution. They have been at the center of a controversy surrounding the mechanisms of expression of long-term potentiation (see Chapter 10), and some of the disagreements

Box 6–2
Quantal Analysis

Chemical synaptic transmission occurs via the presynaptic release of packages of neurotransmitter, which diffuse to and act upon postsynaptic receptors. This phenomenon was originally elucidated at the neuromuscular junction on the basis of electrophysiological recordings from the postsynaptic muscle cells. Under certain conditions, the size of the postsynaptic response to presynaptic stimulation fluctuates from stimulus to stimulus among discrete levels, reflecting 0, 1, 2… quanta released. These levels correspond to integral multiples of an underlying unit, which coincide with the size of a spontaneous event arising from the spontaneous release of a single package of neurotransmitter. From a wealth of other data, it has been established that the quantum corresponds to the postsynaptic response to the neurotransmitter packaged in an individual vesicle. The quantal description of neurotransmission not only gives a powerful insight into the biophysics of transmitter release and receptor activation, it provides a shortcut for investigating the mechanisms of synaptic signaling modulation. Thus, factors that reduce or increase the presynaptic release of transmitter almost universally affect the average number of quanta released across a population of release sites (the quantal content m, which is the product of the number of available quanta n, and their average release probability p). Factors that modulate the state of the postsynaptic receptors alter the size of the response to an individual package of neurotransmitter (the quantal amplitude Q).

Extrapolation of the quantal model to the central nervous system (CNS) has uncovered some subtle but important differences. Unlike the neuromuscular junction—which is often a long ribbon-like structure with numerous vesicles available to be released—active zones in the CNS tend to be small structures with only a few vesicles in close apposition to the presynaptic membrane ("docked" vesicles). Correspondingly, postsynaptic signals often fluctuate between failures and an amplitude that may reflect the release of only one vesicle (0 or 1 quantum). Moreover, because the peak occupancy of postsynaptic receptors in response to release of a single vesicle may be high ($> 50\%$), release of two vesicles may not yield a signal whose amplitude is twice as large. Nevertheless, some synapses (such as mossy fiber synapses on CA3 pyramidal neurons) have numerous active zones and postsynaptic densities; and at these synapses, multiquantal release can be detected. Another difference between quantal transmission in the CNS and neuromuscular juction is that different synapses are probably not electrically equivalent: Differences in the number of receptors and degrees of electrotonic attenuation at distinct synapses may conceal any clear quantal increments in the distribution of amplitudes of the postsynaptic signal obtained by repeatedly sampling the connections between pre- and postsynaptic neurons.

Despite the differences in quantal neurotransmission between the CNS and neuromuscular junction, measuring the trial-to-trial fluctuations in the amplitudes of postsynaptic currents or potentials yields a powerful insight into the loci of alterations in synaptic strength. In particular, a change in the fraction of presynaptic stimuli evoking failure of transmission implies an alteration in p or n. A more indirect method relies on measuring the trial-to-trial variability of the signal, as estimated by the coefficient of variation (CV: standard deviation/mean). Although the evidence is more circumstantial, changes in CV are again generally associated with alterations in p or n. Conversely, if the average size of the postsynaptic response is not associated with a change in either the failure rate or the CV, the simplest inference is that it is mediated by a change in Q. An important application of quantal analysis is for understanding the mechanisms of the expression of synaptic plasticity, and some of the results and pitfalls of this approach are discussed in Chapter 10.

can be attributed to unjustified assumptions about the underlying mechanisms.

6.2.4 Short-term Plasticity

Implicit in the outline of quantal transmission given above is the assumption that action potentials repeatedly invading a presynaptic terminal trigger neurotransmitter release with a constant probability. In fact, synapses show numerous forms of memory of their activation history. Some of the most interesting forms of synaptic plasticity (long-term potentiation and depression, LTP and LTD, respectively) persist for hours if not longer and are considered in detail in Chapter 10. There are, however, other forms of use-dependent plasticity that last up to a few minutes and that may play an equally important role in the second-to-second traffic of information through synapses. Phenomenologically, they are divided into increases and decreases in transmission: facilitation, augmentation, and potentiation on the one hand and depression on the other (Zucker and Regehr, 2002). There is some redundancy in these terms. Facilitation describes the enhancement of transmission frequently seen following a preceding action potential. If the synapse is stimulated twice in rapid succession and the second response is larger than the first, the phenomenon is often referred to as "paired pulse facilitation." Augmentation refers to a gradual increase in synaptic strength with repeated stimulation. Potentiation (often referred to as post-tetanic potentiation to distinguish it from long-term potentiation) requires a high-frequency train of stimuli for its induction and persists for up to a few minutes after the end of the train. Many synapses do not show these phenomena and, instead, depress when repeatedly stimulated. At some hippocampal synapses early facilitation gives way to later depression with prolonged trains of stimulation.

These distinct patterns of short-term plasticity result from a large number of processes occurring principally in the presynaptic terminals (Thomson, 2000; Zucker and Regehr, 2002). The following is an incomplete list of events that contribute to short-term plasticity.

1. Facilitation/augmentation/potentiation
   - If the presynaptic free Ca^{2+} concentration has not returned to baseline levels or if the occupancy of Ca^{2+} buffers is high, successive action potentials may give rise to larger increments of Ca^{2+}, thereby enhancing exocytosis.
   - High-affinity Ca^{2+} sensors detect a slow build-up of Ca^{2+} in the presynaptic varicosity and contribute to triggering exocytosis.
   - Some presynaptic protein kinases activated with repeated Ca^{2+} influx may phosphorylate proteins involved in making vesicles available for exocytosis or in triggering exocytosis itself.
2. Depression
   - The readily releasable pool of quanta (possibly equivalent to docked vesicles) may become depleted.
   - Repeated depolarizing pulses inactivate presynaptic voltage-dependent Ca^{2+} channels, reducing the amount of Ca^{2+} entry following successive action potentials.
   - Depletion of extracellular Ca^{2+} from the restricted synaptic cleft may reduce its availability for the presynaptic terminal.
   - Presynaptic autoreceptors activated by released neurotransmitters decrease further transmitter release during subsequent action potentials.

The above list focuses on presynaptic mechanisms that contribute to short-term plasticity. However, postsynaptic mechanisms also contribute. In particular, depolarizing synaptic potentials can summate, leading to activation of regenerative currents in the postsynaptic dendrite. Interactions with dendritic action potentials further complicate the relation between voltage signals measured at the soma and presynaptic transmitter release: Orthodromically or antidromically propagating action potentials can either amplify or shunt synaptic potentials, depending on many

variables, such as their temporal relation and the distribution of voltage-gated channels (Johnston et al., 1996; Larkum et al., 1999; Hausser et al., 2001; Stuart and Hausser, 2001). Nonlinearities in the secondary message cascade may also amplify metabotropic receptor-mediated signals. Another postsynaptic mechanism contributing to the facilitation of some glutamatergic signals is relief from voltage-dependent block of the ion channel by polyamines (Rozov and Burnashev, 1999). Conversely, at some synapses desensitization of receptors can contribute to use-dependent depression of neurotransmission (Brenowitz and Trussell, 2001).

Because principal neurons frequently discharge in bursts of action potentials, the degree of postsynaptic facilitation or depression during such bursts may contain much of the information transmitted through the network. Indeed, it has been argued that lasting changes in short-term plasticity are of greater importance for information encoding than synaptic strength per se (defined as the size of an EPSP or IPSP evoked after an interval sufficiently long for short-term plasticity phenomena to have dissipated) (Markram and Tsodyks, 1996). However, because short-term plasticity is mediated predominantly through use-dependent alteration in release probability, the information contained in a facilitating or depressing burst is inevitably corrupted by the stochastic nature of transmitter release. That is, the degree of facilitation or depression at a synapse can be reliably detected by the network only by averaging out the response to a stereotyped sequence of action potentials repeatedly delivered to the presynaptic neuron. This has led to an almost diametrically opposite view of the importance of bursts: Because high-probability synapses often depress and low-probability synapses often facilitate, the function of bursts is to cancel out the effects of the initial release probability and minimize the sampling error arising from stochastic release. Thus, it is argued that the most important modifiable parameter relevant to information transmission is the quantal amplitude (Lisman, 1997). Against this background, there has recently been considerable interest in the long-term consequences of particular timing patterns of pre- and postsynaptic action potentials. Notably, it has been reported at several cortical synapses that if presynaptic glutamate release occurs shortly before a postsynaptic action potential it can lead to persistent enhancement of transmission. If, on the other hand, the presynaptic stimulus lags behind the postsynaptic action potential, it can be followed by depression of transmission (Bi and Poo, 2001). The mechanisms underlying these phenomena and their relevance to learning are further considered in Chapter 10.

6.3 Glutamatergic Synaptic Transmission

The main excitatory transmitter in the hippocampus, as elsewhere in the mammalian CNS, is glutamate. Although the earliest evidence for this was principally obtained in the spinal cord, many important insights have come from work on rodent hippocampal tissue: Glutamate depolarizes hippocampal neurons (Biscoe and Straughan, 1966), and tritiated glutamate is avidly taken up by areas enriched in synapses (Storm-Mathisen and Iversen, 1979). Moreover, electrical stimulation evokes glutamate release (Dolphin et al., 1982; Walker et al., 1995), and antibodies raised against glutamate stain presynaptic terminals at asymmetrical synapses (Ottersen et al., 1990). Importantly, glutamate activates the three principal types of receptors that mediate ionotropic excitatory transmission: α-amino-3-hydroxy-5-methyl-isoxazole-propionic acid (AMPA), kainate, and N-methyl-D-aspartate (NMDA). Finally, a vesicular glutamate transporter has recently been identified (Bellocchio et al., 2000; Takamori et al., 2000).

Although there is abundant evidence that glutamate mediates fast excitatory transmission at "glutamatergic" synapses, there are persistent reports that aspartate also can be released from hippocampal slices in an activity-dependent manner (Szerb, 1988; Nadler et al., 1990). Aspartate immunoreactivity has also been found in certain presynaptic glutamate-releasing terminals, and the abundance of this signal decreases following intense synaptic activity (Gundersen et al., 1998). Because aspartate is a weak agonist at NMDA receptors (although inactive at AMPA or kainate receptors), these observations raise the possibility that it may be co-released with glutamate. However, aspartate is not taken up effectively by isolated vesi-

cles, so it is unclear how it could be packaged appropriately to fulfill a role as a fast neurotransmitter.

Following release, glutamate is taken up into neurons and glia, although this process takes place at a much slower rate than passive diffusion away from the release site (see below). Of the cloned glutamate transporters, the most abundant in the rodent hippocampus is GLT (also known as EAAT2), followed by GLAST (EAAT1) and EAAC1 (EAAT3) (Danbolt, 2001). In the hippocampus, GLT and GLAST are almost exclusively expressed in astrocytes. EAAC1 is principally expressed in neurons although at a relatively low level, so it probably contributes relatively little to clearing glutamate following exocytosis. However, it has been proposed to supply glutamate for GABA synthesis in inhibitory boutons (Sepkuty et al., 2002; Mathews and Diamond, 2003).

Glutamate taken up into astrocytes is decarboxylated by glutamine synthetase (Fig. 6–4). The intracellular concentration of glutamate in astrocytes is thereby kept low, which is necessary to make continued uptake of glutamate energetically favorable. The energy required for uptake of glutamate comes from the co-transport of three Na^+ ions down their electrochemical gradient. In addition, flux measurements have shown that one H^+ ion accompanies glutamate, and one K^+ ion is countertransported (Zerangue and Kavanaugh, 1996). Because the net movement of glutamate is dictated by the electrochemical gradients for these other species, it is pos-

Figure 6–4. Glutamate–glutamine cycle. The excitatory neurotransmitter glutamate is synthesized from α-ketoglutarate, which is produced by the Krebs cycle, and recycled from glutamine. Following release, glutamate is taken up by glial cells, where it is rapidly decarboxylated to form glutamine. Glutamine can diffuse across the extracellular space back to presynaptic varicosities. The diagram also shows the arrangement of several types of glutamate receptors: AMPA and NMDA receptors tend to be located opposite release sites, and group I metabotropic receptors [mGluR (I)] tend to be located in a perisynaptic distribution. Group II and III metabotropic receptors tend to be located presynaptically.

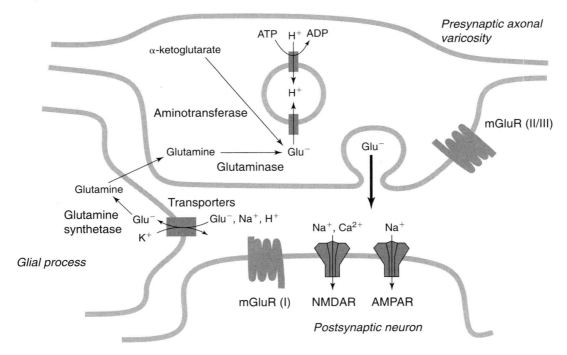

sible to reverse uptake; moreover, evidence exists that such reversed uptake can take place during ischemia, when extracellular K^+ builds up and cells become depolarized because of ATP depletion (Rossi et al., 2000). Because the extracellular accumulation of glutamate can exacerbate depolarization of neurons by acting at glutamate receptors, there is the possibility of triggering a positive feedback loop. This cascade may underlie part of the "excitotoxic" role of glutamate in stroke.

Astrocytic glutamine, formed from decarboxylation of glutamate, can enter metabolic pathways in astrocytes; but it can also diffuse passively down its concentration gradient into the extracellular space, a phenomenon facilitated by several transporters. From here it is taken up into presynaptic terminals, where it can be converted back to glutamate and repackaged into vesicles.

The three major classes of ionotropic glutamate receptors (Table 6–1) take their names from agonists that activate them in a relatively selective fashion (Watkins and Evans, 1981; Nakanishi et al., 1998; Ozawa et al., 1998). These agonists do not normally exist in the brain. At most excitatory hippocampal synapses, EPSCs are mediated by AMPA and NMDA receptors, which have strikingly different biophysical and pharmacological properties. Kainate receptors play a relatively poorly understood role in synaptic transmission. All three receptor types are heteromultimeric structures probably made up of four pore-forming subunits. These subunits are coded for by several genes that show considerable homology and exist in several splice variants, which contribute to defining their kinetic properties. The importance of the molecular variability of the subunits making up each class of receptors is considered further in Chapter 7. Here, we concentrate on the major pharmacological and biophysical differences that exist among the various receptors. Much of the information summarized here has been obtained by studying the behavior of small numbers of receptors present in membrane patches exposed to brief pulses of glutamate and studied with voltage-clamp methods. These patches are taken from the somata of neurons in acute hippocampal slices or in cultures (reflecting the properties of native, although not necessarily synaptic, receptors) or from cells expressing recombinant receptors.

6.3.1 AMPA Receptors

AMPA receptors are composed of different combinations of four subunits (GluR1-4, also known as GluRA-B) (Hollmann et al., 1989; Keinanen et al., 1990; Hollmann and Heinemann, 1994; Nakanishi et al., 1998; Ozawa et al., 1998). They occur at almost all excitatory synapses in the hippocampus and gate a cation-selective channel. At resting membrane potentials, Na^+ influx accounts for most of the current, but the channel is also permeant to other small monovalent cations, so K^+ efflux can also occur at depolarized potentials. Most AMPA receptors in pyramidal neurons of the adult hippocampus (at least in rodents) are thought to be GluR1-2 or GluR2-3 tetramers (Wenthold et al., 1996).

AMPA receptors require a rapid pulse of glutamate in excess of approximately 100 μM to open. When a membrane patch taken from the soma or proximal dendrite of a hippocampal neuron is exposed to a pulse of 1 mM glutamate (roughly corresponding to the synaptic glutamate transient; see below) a current is generated with a rapid rise time (100–600 μs at physiological temperature). This reflects both very fast binding kinetics and a high opening probability: the peak probability that a bound receptor is in the open state has been estimated at approximately 0.6 (Jonas et al., 1993).

Native AMPA receptors deactivate rapidly following clearance of synaptic glutamate (with a time constant of 2.3–3.0 ms) (Colquhoun et al., 1992). Deactivation is probably sufficient to explain the termination of AMPA receptor-mediated EPSCs on the grounds that glutamate is cleared from the synaptic cleft faster than this. If glutamate is not cleared, however, AMPA receptors close rapidly and enter a desensitized state from which they recover relatively slowly. The time course of desensitization depends on the subunit composition of the receptors and is affected by alternative splicing of the subunit mRNA (so-called flip and flop variants; see

Table 6–1.
Ionotropic Glutamate Receptors

Receptor type	Agonists	Subunits	Permeant ions	Examples of antagonists
AMPA (α-amino-3-hydroxy-5-methyl-4-isoxazolepropionic acid)	Glutamate (endogenous), AMPA, kainate	GluR1-4 (GluRA-D)	Na^+, K^+ (Ca^{2+})	Kynurenic acid 6-Cyano-7-nitroquinoxaline-2,3-dione (CNQX) GYKI53655
Kainate	Glutamate (endogenous), kainate	Glur5-7, KA1,2	Na^+, K^+ (Ca^{2+})	Kynurenic acid CNQX LY382884 (GluR5-specific)
NMDA (N-methyl-D-aspartic acid)	Glutamate, glycine, D-serine (endogenous co-agonists), NMDA	NR1, NR2A-D	Na^+, K^+, Ca^{2+}	Kynurenic acid D-Aminophosphonovalerate (D-AP5) 3-[(RS)-2-carboxypiperazine-4-yl]-propyl-1-phosphonate (CPP)

Chapter 7), but it usually proceeds with a decay time constant of the order of 5–10 ms) (Mosbacher et al., 1994). AMPA receptors can even desensitize in the presence of glutamate concentrations that are insufficient to open them or if the glutamate concentration rises sufficiently slowly. This form of desensitization may be an adaptation that prevents excessive receptor activation under pathological conditions where extracellular glutamate accumulates. Desensitization may also occur with extremely brief (millisecond) exposure to the agonist, so if a second pulse is applied a smaller response is obtained. However, this phenomenon does not contribute appreciably to frequency-dependent plasticity of transmission in the hippocampus (Hjelmstad et al., 1999).

Depending on their subunit composition, AMPA receptors can also show significant permeability to Ca^{2+} ions. This permeability is determined by the presence or absence of a critical amino acid (arginine, R) in a pore-lining segment of the GluR2 subunit. This subunit undergoes post-transcriptional RNA editing resulting in a change of the amino acid at this position from glutamine (Q), encoded by the genomic sequence, to arginine (Sommer et al., 1991). The presence of the edited form of GluR2 ensures that the receptor is impermeable to Ca^{2+}, which is the case for most of the glutamate receptors in principal cells. If the GluR2 subunit is absent, the receptor has significant Ca^{2+} permeability. Such receptors are present in some hippocampal interneurons (Geiger et al., 1995). In addition, some fetal GluR2 subunits are not edited.

"Q/R editing" has several other consequences for AMPA receptor function (Swanson et al., 1997). If the edited (R)

form of GluR2 is present in the receptor, its conductance is relatively small and is independent of the transmembrane voltage. If the edited GluR2 is absent from the receptor, the current–voltage relation becomes highly nonlinear (Fig. 6–5). That is, the receptor functions as a rectifier, with a conductance that increases with the transmembrane potential difference. This transition between low- and high-conductance states is due to blockade of the receptor by polyamine molecules, which enter the ion channel but can be expelled in a voltage-dependent manner (Bowie and Mayer, 1995; Donevan and Rogawski, 1995; Kamboj et al., 1995; Koh et al., 1995).

The single-channel conductance of native receptors varies broadly from < 1 pS to approximately 30 pS, depending not only the presence of GluR2 but also on the identity of other subunits (Swanson et al., 1997). Bound receptors do not remain open continuously. In common with other ligand-gated ion channels, they flicker between open and closed states; and even in their open state they fluctuate among distinct preferred conductance levels. Although most kinetic schemes assume that two glutamate molecules must bind for the receptor to open (Jonas et al., 1993; Diamond and Jahr, 1997), there is little direct experimental data to support this assumption. Indeed, it has been proposed that four binding steps to a tetrameric receptor take place, and that the conductance level of an individual channel increases with the number of glutamate molecules bound (Rosenmund et al., 1998). Both the opening probability and the conductance of the channel can be modulated by phosphorylation (Derkach et al., 1999; Banke et al., 2000), phenomena that may play an important role in synaptic plasticity (see Chapter 10).

Figure 6–5. Rectification of unedited GluR2-containing AMPA receptors. *A*, Current (I)–voltage (V) relationships of glutamate-evoked currents obtained in a cell expressing Ca^{2+}-permeable unedited GluR2 (GluRB) subunits. The open circles show a nonlinear, rectifying, I–V relation 1 minute after beginning whole-cell recording. This is explained by a blockade of the ion pore by endogenous polyamines, which is relieved by increasing the voltage gradient across the membrane. Fifteen minutes after beginning the

recording with an intracellular solution devoid of polyamines (filled symbols) the I–V relation becomes more linear, explained by washout of endogenous polyamines from the cytoplasm. *B*, I–V relation measured with a pipette solution containing 25 µM spermine, an endogenous polyamine. The rectification is more marked and persists despite prolonged recording. (*Source*: Rozov et al., 1998, with permission.)

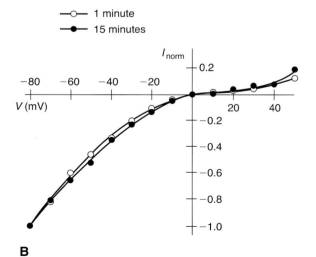

A   **B**

6.3.2 Kainate Receptors

Kainate receptors share many features with AMPA receptors (Lerma et al., 1997, 2001; Bleakman, 1999; Chittajallu et al., 1999; Ben-Ari and Cossart, 2000; Frerking and Nicoll, 2000; Kullmann, 2001). They too are heteromultimeric, made up of different combinations of five subunits: GluR5-7 and KA1-2. However, not all of these subunits have the same status because receptors made up of KA1 or KA2 alone are nonfunctional. GluR5-6 undergo Q/R editing with similar consequences as for GluR2, although the proportion of edited subunits falls considerably below 100%. This means that the Ca^{2+} permeability, single-channel conductance, and rectification of the receptor cannot be inferred easily from the subunit composition.

The biophysical properties of recombinant kainate receptors are similar to those of AMPA receptors. That is, they open and desensitize rapidly, and they have single-channel conductances, rectification properties, and Ca^{2+} permeabilities that depend on Q/R editing (Bowie and Mayer, 1995; Kamboj et al., 1995). However, there are some unexplained discrepancies between the relatively low affinity and rapid kinetics of kainate receptors studied in isolated cells and the finding that synaptic kainate receptor-mediated signals exhibit very slow kinetics (Castillo et al., 1997b; Lerma et al., 1997, 2001; Vignes and Collingridge, 1997; Cossart et al., 1998; Frerking et al., 1998). Some kainate receptor-mediated EPSCs can last more than 100 ms, at which time they would have been expected to have deactivated following clearance of glutamate or desensitized if glutamate persisted. Several explanations have been proposed for this discrepancy, including the possibility that synaptic kainate receptors differ from nonsynaptic receptors in their subunit composition because of the actions of accessory proteins or because of site-specific phosphorylation (Garcia et al., 1998). Among other possible explanations for the slow kinetics of kainate receptor-mediated EPSCs is that glutamate needs to diffuse a long distance to reach the receptors, perhaps because they are relatively remote from the site of exocytosis. Finally, synaptic co-release of a modulatory substance might alter the response of kainate receptors to glutamate. Another puzzle is that, although kainate receptors are abundant in the hippocampus, synaptic responses mediated by them are very small and generally require trains of high-frequency stimuli to be detected. Recently, however, relatively fast, apparently monoquantal kainate receptor-mediated EPSCs have been described in interneurons and CA3 pyramidal neurons (Cossart et al., 2002). Why such currents have been overlooked previously is unclear.

Evidence has emerged for a major role of presynaptic kainate receptors in modulating transmitter release (Chittajallu et al., 1996; Rodriguez-Moreno et al., 1997; Vignes et al., 1998; Kamiya and Ozawa, 2000; Cossart et al., 2001; Jiang et al., 2001; Schmitz et al., 2001a), axon excitability (Semyanov and Kullmann, 2001), and synaptic plasticity (Contractor et al., 2001; Lauri et al., 2001). Surprisingly, kainate receptors at various synapses, activated by different concentrations of agonists, either enhance or depress transmitter release. The mechanisms underlying these phenomena are incompletely understood (Kullmann, 2001) and may include depolarization, Ca^{2+} influx via permeable receptors, and coupling to a metabotropic cascade (Rodriguez-Moreno and Lerma, 1998). Controversy also surrounds the subunit composition of the kainate receptors mediating postsynaptic and presynaptic kainate receptor-mediated signaling. Some pharmacological data suggest a major role for GluR5-containing receptors at mossy fibers (Bortolotto et al., 1999; Lauri et al., 2001). However, the results of genetic deletion experiments are more consistent with a role for GluR6-containing receptors at mossy fibers and GluR5-containing receptors on interneurons (Contractor et al., 2000, 2001; Mulle et al., 2000). Although presynaptic kainate receptors exert a powerful influence on synaptic function, the adaptive significance of the enhancement and depression of transmitter release remains a subject of speculation.

6.3.3 NMDA Receptors

NMDA receptors consist of subunits belonging to two relatively distinct subtypes (McBain and Mayer, 1994); they exist as heteromultimers of NR1 and NR2A-D subunits. (A recently described NR3 subunit does not appear to play an important role in the hippocampus.) The NR1 subunit is encoded by one gene but exists in several alternatively spliced isoforms. It does not bind glutamate but, instead, contains an important binding site for another amino acid, glycine or D-serine, which acts as a co-agonist (see below). The NR2A-D subunits, on the other hand, contain the glutamate-binding site (Laube et al., 1997). They are encoded by four genes and are variably expressed in different regions of the brain and at different stages of development (see Chapter 7).

NMDA receptors show many striking properties that mark them out as quite different from AMPA and kainate receptors. Notably, they have very slow kinetics and can continue to mediate an ion flux for several hundreds of milliseconds after the glutamate pulse has terminated (activation time constant is approximately 7 ms; deactivation time constants are approximately 200 ms and 1–3 s). The slow kinetics are explained by an extremely slow receptor unbinding rate (Lester et al., 1990). That is, once glutamate molecules have become bound to NMDA receptors, they remain bound for a long time, during which time the ionophore can undergo repeated opening. The maximal probability that a bound receptor is in the open state has been estimated at between 0.05 and 0.3, which is lower than the corresponding probability for AMPA receptors (Jahr, 1992; Rosenmund et al., 1995). The range of estimates reflects alterations in NMDA receptor kinetics as a function of intracellular factors, including Ca^{2+} ions. Reflecting the very slow dissociation rate, the apparent affinity of NMDA receptors under steady-state conditions is much higher than that of AMPA receptors (the EC_{50} is in the range of 1–10 μM, instead of 100–500 μM) (Patneau and Mayer, 1990). This distinction may explain several striking properties of glutamatergic EPSCs (discussed further below). In addition to their slow kinetics, NMDA receptors have three other important features.

First, a second agonist-binding site (the "strychnine-insensitive glycine site") must be occupied before glutamate is able to activate them (Johnson and Ascher, 1987; Kleckner and Dingledine, 1988). However, some estimates of the tonic extracellular glycine concentration in the brain suggest that the glycine-binding site is normally occupied. Alternatively, D-serine can substitute for glycine, and it has been proposed that this amino acid plays a physiological role in regulating NMDA receptor function (Schell et al., 1995; Baranano et al., 2001).

Second, they are highly permeable to Ca^{2+} ions and monovalent cations (Ascher and Nowak, 1988). Ca^{2+} influx via NMDA receptors plays a central role in several forms of long-term synaptic plasticity (see Chapter 10). Ca^{2+} ions are actually ubiquitous secondary messengers, and NMDA receptor activation has been shown to trigger further release of Ca^{2+} from intracellular stores (Emptage et al., 1999). Accompanying the high Ca^{2+} permeability of NMDA receptors is a relatively high single-channel conductance (40–50 pS), which is greater than that of most AMPA receptors (Jahr and Stevens, 1987; Gibb and Colquhoun, 1992).

Third, Mg^{2+} ions block the ionophore in a voltage-dependent manner (Mayer et al., 1984; Nowak et al., 1984). Thus, at resting membrane potentials (more negative than approximately −50 mV), NMDA receptors are unable to mediate an EPSC even if glutamate and glycine (or D-serine) are present. They mediate an ion flux only when the membrane is depolarized.

The Ca^{2+} permeability and Mg^{2+} blockade of NMDA receptors explain their role as synaptic coincidence detectors: Ca^{2+} influx occurs only if there is a conjunction of presynaptic glutamate release and postsynaptic depolarization, a situation that arises when pre- and postsynaptic activity occur together (Wigstrom and Gustafsson, 1986). The significance of this phenomenon for long-term modification of synaptic strength is addressed in Chapter 10.

6.3.4 Co-localization of Glutamate Receptors

Both AMPA and NMDA receptors are present at a roughly 100-fold higher density at synapses than in extrasynaptic membranes (Bekkers and Stevens, 1989; Nusser et al., 1998; Bolton et al., 2000). However, some synapses may be devoid of AMPA receptors, especially early in postnatal development (Nusser et al., 1998; Takumi et al., 1998; Petralia et al., 1999). Less is known about the subcellular location of kainate receptors because adequate antibodies have not been developed.

Reflecting the co-localization of AMPA and NMDA (and possibly kainate) receptors, EPSCs generally show several pharmacologically, electrophysiologically, and kinetically distinct components (Forsythe and Westbrook, 1988; Hestrin et al., 1990). At most hippocampal synapses, at negative membrane potentials, the EPSC has fast kinetics and is blocked by the AMPA/kainate receptor blocker 6-cyano-7-nitroquinoxaline-2,3-dione (CNQX). Subsequent studies, taking advantage of more selective AMPA receptor antagonists (in particular the 2,3-benzodiazepine GYKI53655), have established that AMPA receptors account for the fast EPSC at negative potentials. This EPSC is analogous to the fast synaptic current carried by acetylcholine receptors at the neuromuscular junction, which "short-circuits" the transmembrane potential difference. At depolarized membrane potentials, a slower component of the EPSC emerges that is blocked by the NMDA receptor antagonist D-amino-5-phosphonovalerate (APV). This NMDA receptor-mediated current accounts for most of the charge transfer because of the very slow receptor kinetics. Both AMPA and NMDA receptor-mediated components disappear near 0 mV because this represents the reversal potential for the mixture of monovalent cations that account for the bulk of the current. However, a small Ca^{2+} influx still occurs at this membrane potential because the reversal potential for Ca^{2+} is positive. If the neuron is held at a positive membrane potential, the dual-component EPSC appears again, although it is now an outward current (Fig. 6–6).

Kainate receptors generally do not contribute appreciably to the fast EPSC recorded in principal neurons. However, a low-amplitude kainate receptor-mediated current can be detected in some neurons in response to high-frequency trains of action potentials (especially in CA3 pyramidal neurons in response to mossy fiber stimulation and in some interneurons) (Castillo et al., 1997a; Vignes and Collingridge, 1997; Cossart et al., 1998, 2002). Because it has very slow kinetics, it may account for a sizable fraction of the total charge injected. Although kainate receptor-mediated EPSCs have been described as "synaptic," it remains to be determined whether they arise from the activation of kainate receptors in synapses rather than by spillover of glutamate onto more remote extrasynaptic receptors.

6.3.5 Metabotropic Glutamate Receptors

Metabotropic receptors contain seven transmembrane segments and are coupled to nucleotide-binding G proteins, which mediate most of their actions. They assemble as dimers, which are thought to be in a dynamic equilibrium between two conformations: Binding of a glutamate molecule stabilizes them in the active state (Kunishima et al., 2000). Metabotropic glutamate receptors fall into three classes, although eight genes have been identified (Pin and Duvoisin, 1995; Ozawa et al., 1998; Schoepp, 2002) (Table 6–2).

Group I receptors (mGluR1 and 5) are generally localized to postsynaptic membranes and tend to occur in a halo around the synaptic cleft (Baude et al., 1993). They are coupled via G proteins to phospholipase C, and their activation leads to an increase in both inositol trisphosphate and diacylglycerol (Fagni et al., 2000). Activation of these receptors at mossy fiber synapses can elicit a slow EPSP mediated by cation-selective conductance and can trigger Ca^{2+} release from intracellular stores (Heuss et al., 1999; Yeckel et al.,

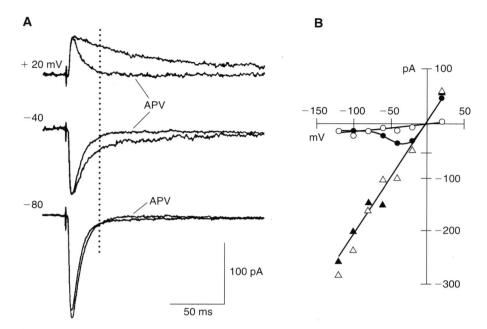

Figure 6–6. Dual-component glutamatergic transmission at hippocampal synapses. *A*, EPSCs recorded in a pyramidal neuron at various voltages. As the postsynaptic cell is depolarized, a slow component appears. This slow current is abolished by the NMDA receptor blocker traces marked APV. *B*, Current-voltage (I–V) relation is plotted for the peak of the EPSCs (triangles) and for a later time point indicated by the vertical dotted line in *A*. Filled symbols, control conditions; open symbols, in the presence of APV. The I–V rela-tion of the APV-sensitive component (circles, measured at a time shown by the dotted line in *A*) shows a region of negative slope (that is, increasing conductance as the cell is depolarized) characteristic of voltage-dependent relief of blockade of NMDA receptors by Mg^{2+} ions. In contrast, the peak of the EPSC (triangles) has an approximately linear I–V relation because the AMPA receptors in pyramidal neurons mainly contain edited GluR2 subunits. (*Source*: Hestrin et al., 1990 with permission).

1999). Some responses appear not to involve G proteins, implying that group I receptors may be coupled to other second messenger cascades (Heuss et al., 1999).

Group II (mGluR 2, 3) and group III (mGluR4, 6, 7, 8) receptors tend to be located in presynaptic membranes. At mossy fibers, mGluR2 receptors are located relatively far from glutamate release sites—in axonal membranes—implying that they detect only glutamate molecules that have escaped from the synaptic cleft (Yokoi et al., 1996).

Several group III receptors, on the other hand, tend to be located in synapses, that is, very close to or even within active zones (Shigemoto et al., 1996, 1997). Both types are negatively coupled to adenylate cyclase via G proteins. The distinction between group II and group III receptors is pharmacological: L-AP4 is a selective agonist at group III, but not group II, receptors. However, the EC_{50} for L-AP4 differs markedly between the individual receptors in group III, so this classification is somewhat arbitrary (Wu et al., 1998).

The physiological roles of metabotropic receptors are not fully understood. The perisynaptic postsynaptic group I receptors may preferentially respond to trains of action potentials that result in the prolonged presence of glutamate in their vicinity. Indeed, such stimulus patterns have been used to evoke postsynaptic currents and Ca^{2+} signals mediated by

Table 6–2.
Metabotropic Glutamate Receptors

Group	Subtypes	Transduction mechanisms	Agonists	Examples of antagonists
I	mGluR1,5	Phospholipase C ↑	Glutamate, (S)-3,5-dihydroxyphenylglycine (DHPG) 1S,3R-1-aminocyclopentane-1, 3-dicarboxylic acid (1S,3R-ACPD)	3,5-Methyl-4-carboxyphenylglycine (MCPG)
II	mGluR2,3	Adenylyl cyclase ↓	Glutamate 1S,3R-ACPD (2S,2′R,3′R)-2-(2′,3′-dicarboxycyclopropyl) glycine (DCG-IV)	MCPG LY341495
III	mGluR4,6-8	Adenylyl cyclase ↓	Glutamate L-Amino-phosphonobutyrate (L-AP4)	Methylserine-O-phosphate (MSOP)

group I receptors (Heuss et al., 1999; Yeckel et al., 1999). As for group II receptors, their predominantly extrasynaptic presynaptic location implies that they detect the extracellular build-up of glutamate and that they therefore act as autoreceptors that regulate neurotransmitter release as a function of the volume-averaged excitatory traffic (Scanziani et al., 1997). The intrasynaptic presynaptic location of some group III receptors prompts the speculation that they act as autoreceptors on a smaller spatial scale. However, they are also present at some GABAergic terminals (Shigemoto et al., 1997), which are not known to release glutamate. There is evidence that they detect glutamate released from neighboring synapses (Semyanov and Kullmann, 2000), so their role may be akin to that of group II receptors.

6.3.6 Receptor Targeting and Anchoring

A major challenge is to understand how receptors are targeted and anchored to postsynaptic densities and how they are trafficked to and from the synapse. These issues are considered from a molecular perspective in Chapter 7. AMPA receptor insertion plays a major role in synapse maturation and long-term potentiation (further considered in Chapter 10). Briefly, considerable evidence is emerging for two types of interaction between AMPA receptor subunits and intracellular proteins involved in trafficking (Shi et al., 2001). One process is mediated by an interaction between the cytoplasmic C-termini of GluR1 (and possibly GluR4) subunits with protein(s) containing a consensus motif known as a PDZ domain (see Chapter 7). This process is triggered by activation of Ca^{2+}-calmodulin-dependent protein kinase II (CaMKII) and contributes to long-term potentiation. Another process involves an interaction between the C-terminus of GluR2 subunits and both NSF (the ATPase involved in dissociating the SNARE core complex; see above) and PDZ proteins.

NMDA receptors are anchored to a large number of scaffolding, signaling, and transduction proteins (Husi et al., 2000; Sheng and Sala, 2001). This anchoring is mediated via an interaction between the C-termini of NR2 subunits and several PDZ domain proteins, in particular PSD-95 and SAP97. Some group I metabotropic glutamate receptors are also anchored via a PDZ domain protein, Homer (Brakeman et al., 1997). Relatively less is known of the mechanisms that target and/or anchor other metabotropic receptors: One splice variant of mGluR7 interacts with another intracellular protein, PICK1 (Perroy et al., 2002), but how other receptors are localized to presynaptic terminals is unclear.

6.4 GABAergic Synaptic Transmission

The major inhibitory transmitter GABA is synthesized by decarboxylation of glutamate. Two isoforms of glutamic acid decarboxylase exist. GAD67 is widespread in the cytoplasm, whereas GAD65 is more closely associated with presynaptic

terminals of GABAergic neurons. Its expression varies in response to changes in neuronal activity, implying that it may play a regulatory role in GABAergic transmission (Soghomonian and Martin, 1998). Uptake into vesicles is facilitated by the vesicular GABA transporter VGAT, which can also mediate vesicular glycine transport, although this enzyme may not be essential for vesicular GABA accumulation because it is absent from a subset of GABAergic terminals (Chaudhry et al., 1998). Following exocytosis, GABA diffuses out of the synaptic cleft and is taken up by a family of four transporters: GAT1-4 (Schousboe, 2000) (Fig. 6–7). These transporters are located not only in astrocytes but also in interneurons and principal cells. GABA uptake is electrogenic; that is, the amino acid is transported together with two Na^+ ions (and possibly one Cl^- ion) (Kavanaugh et al., 1992; Cammack et al., 1994). This stoichiometry normally ensures that GABA is taken up into cells because the driving force provided by the Na^+ electrochemical gradient is sufficient to overcome the gradient for GABA. However, because the transport stoichiometry is less electrogenic than for glutamate, it has been suggested that GABA uptake can be reversed when cells are depolarized (Richerson and Wu, 2003). The various GABA transporters show some differences in localization and substrate specificity: For instance, GAT1 is relatively abundant in neurons and is relatively insensitive to β-alanine compared to the other major transporter GAT3. Although GABA transport shows many similarities with glutamate uptake, there are suggestions that it may be less efficient, either because individual transporters function more slowly or because they are present in a lower concentration. In particular, synaptically released GABA appears to exert actions at high-affinity, remotely located receptors; and GABA escaping from the synaptic cleft can even be detected by recording from a membrane patch containing $GABA_A$ receptors positioned on the surface of a slice (Isaacson et al., 1993). In contrast, although glutamate also exerts extrasynaptic actions, they are spatially much more restricted (see below).

GABA receptors are divided into ionotropic ($GABA_A$) and metabotropic ($GABA_B$) receptors (Table 6-3). $GABA_C$ receptors are ionotropic receptors with an unusual pharmacological profile and are made up of ρ subunits. They are arguably a variant of $GABA_A$ receptors (Barnard et al., 1998; Bormann, 2000). Because they are not known to play a major role in the hippocampus, they are not considered here.

6.4.1 GABA_A Receptors

$GABA_A$ receptors are heteropentameric, and consist of subunits drawn from at least 7 different families: α_{1-6}, β_{1-3}, γ_{1-3}, δ, ϵ, π, and θ (Mehta and Ticku, 1999). Of these, α_6, ϵ, π, and θ appear to be excluded from the rodent hippocampus or to occur at very low levels. The remaining subunits show differential distributions at a macroscopic level. Thus, α_1, α_2, α_4, β_3, γ_2, and δ are present in the dentate gyrus. In the hippocampus proper, the principal subunits are α_1, α_2, α_5, β_3, and γ_2, with relatively lower levels of α_4, β_1, $\beta2$, γ_3, and δ; α_3 and γ_1 are

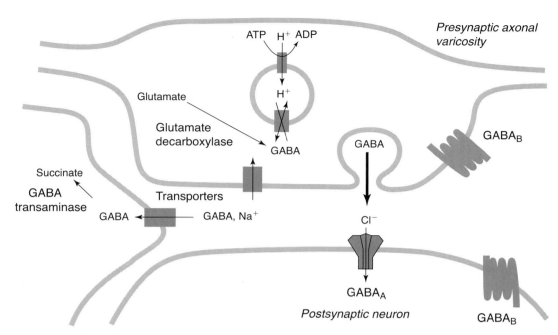

Figure 6–7. GABA cycle. The inhibitory neurotransmitter GABA is synthesized from glutamate via the action of two enzymes, GAD-65 and GAD-67. Following release, GABA is taken up by both neurons and glial cells. GABA can be converted back to glutamate or to succinate by the mitochondrial enzyme GABA transaminase. The diagram also shows the arrangement of $GABA_A$ and $GABA_B$ receptors. Ionotropic $GABA_A$ receptors tend to be located opposite release sites, although extrasynaptic receptors also occur in dentate granule cells. $GABA_B$ receptors occur both pre- and postsynaptically.

present only at very low levels (Sperk et al., 1997). Most hippocampal $GABA_A$ receptors probably contain two α subunits and two β subunits, together with either a γ subunit or the δ subunit but not both (Chang et al., 1996; Farrar et al., 1999; Whiting et al., 1999). The α subunits in particular play important roles in determining the affinity for GABA and the sensitivity to numerous modulatory agents such as Zn^{2+} ions, steroids, ethanol, and exogenous pharmacological agents such as benzodiazepines, barbiturates, and general anesthetics (Barnard et al., 1998). The γ subunits also affect several of these parameters and, in addition, mediate anchoring of $GABA_A$ receptors to synapses via an indirect interaction with gephyrin, a scaffolding protein that plays an important role in the formation and stabilization of both GABAergic and glycinergic synapses (Essrich et al., 1998). The δ-containing receptors tend not to be confined to synapses but have a high affinity for GABA and are relatively insensitive to benzodiazepines. These δ-containing receptors are strong candidates for mediating a $GABA_A$ receptor-dependent tonic inhibition in dentate granule cells (Overstreet and Westbrook, 2001; Nusser and Mody, 2002). The $\alpha_4\beta_2\delta$ receptors have recently been shown to be strongly potentiated by ethanol at low concentrations, making them a candidate for some of the psychotropic properties of this drug (Sundstrom-Poromaa et al., 2002).

$GABA_A$ receptor-mediated IPSCs have a fast onset, although their decay is generally slower than that of AMPA receptor-mediated EPSCs. Their single-channel conductance is highly variable, ranging from < 1 to > 30 pS, depending on their subunit composition.

Table 6–3.
GABA receptors

Receptor type	Subunits	Ions	Agonists	Antagonists	Modulators
$GABA_A$	$\alpha_{1-6}, \beta_{1-3}, \gamma_{1-3}, \delta, \epsilon, \pi, \theta$	Cl^-, HCO_3^- (ion channel)	GABA Muscimol	Picrotoxin Bicuculline SR 95531	Benzodiazepines, barbiturates, Zn^{2+}, ethanol, neurosteroids
$GABA_B$	GBR1 GBR2	G protein-gated inward rectifying K^+ (GIRK) channels $\uparrow$ Ca^{2+} channels $\downarrow$	GABA Baclofen	Saclofen CGP35348	

Depending on the subunit composition, benzodiazepines enhance the affinity of $GABA_A$ receptors for the agonist. This causes prolongation of the IPSC and also usually increases the peak amplitude, implying that the occupancy of the receptors is normally incomplete (Perrais and Ropert, 1999; Hajos et al., 2000). However, because benzodiazepines can, in addition, increase single-channel conductance (Eghbali et al., 1997), estimating the occupancy of receptors from their effects on IPSC amplitude is problematic. Barbiturates, on the other hand, enhance and prolong the IPSC by increasing the proportion of the time that GABA-liganded channels remain open (Study and Barker, 1981). Both these classes of drugs have the effect of potentiating GABAergic transmission, possibly accounting for their usefulness as sedative, anxiolytic, and antiepileptic agents. Combined genetic and pharmacological manipulation of the receptors has suggested that α_1-containing receptors preferentially mediate the sedative, but not the anxiolytic, effects of systemic benzodiazepines (Rudolph et al., 1999), although whether and how the hippocampal formation contributes to these phenomena remains to be determined.

$GABA_A$ receptors are permeable only to anions. The current is carried overwhelmingly by Cl^- ions, but receptors are also permeable to HCO_3^- ions (Kaila, 1994). Because neurons are normally depolarized relative to the Cl^- reversal potential, $GABA_A$ receptor-mediated IPSCs are generally hyperpolarizing. The situation is different in neurons at early stages of development (Ben-Ari et al., 1989). The intracellular Cl^- concentration is relatively high because the principal extrusion mechanism (the K^+/Cl^- co-transporter KCC2) is not expressed abundantly (Rivera et al., 1999). The electrochemical gradient then dictates that Cl^- ions flow out of the cell, making the current depolarizing. Somewhat confusingly, this is sometimes referred to as a "depolarizing IPSC." Such depolarizing GABAergic signals can bring neurons to firing threshold and trigger Ca^{2+} influx, and they may play an important role in the early stages of neural circuit formation (Ben-Ari et al., 1997). An analogous depolarizing response to GABA has also been observed in response to exogenous agonist application to the dendrites of pyramidal neurons in acute slices taken from adult brains (Andersen et al., 1980a). A major mechanism underlying this phenomenon is that prolonged and intense activation of $GABA_A$ receptors results in accumulation of intracellular Cl^-, which eventually alters the reversal potential for the receptors (Staley et al., 1995). In addition, because $GABA_A$ receptors have a significant permeability to HCO_3^-, alterations in the electrochemical gradient for this anion can contribute to the phenomenon. Extracellular K^+ also accumulates through the action of KCC2, further contributing to neuronal depolarization (Kaila et al., 1997). Although depolarizing responses can be achieved by iontophoretic application of GABA and possibly during seizures (Bracci et al., 2001), it is not clear that they occur with synaptic activity under physiological conditions in adult animals, which generally activates only a small proportion of the receptors on a neuron and for a short time.

6.4.2 $GABA_B$ Receptors

Metabotropic $GABA_B$ receptors occur as heterodimers composed of GBR_1 and GBR_2 (Jones et al., 1998), both of which can undergo alternative splicing (Kuner et al., 1999). $GABA_B$ receptors are widespread at both pre- and postsynaptic elements of synapses and also in extrasynaptic membranes (Fritschy et al., 1999). The $GABA_B$ receptor agonist baclofen powerfully depresses the synaptic release of both glutamate and GABA, so the presynaptic targeting of $GABA_B$ receptors and/or their linkage to effector mechanisms is presumably not confined to GABAergic terminals. Conversely, some GABAergic terminals appear to be insensitive to baclofen (Lambert and Wilson, 1993). Among possible explanations for this finding are the absence of receptors at some terminals and heterogeneity in the identity of the presynaptic Ca^{2+} channels (see above).

$GABA_B$ receptors in the presynaptic membrane are negatively coupled to N- and P/Q- type Ca^{2+} channels via a G-protein cascade (Anwyl, 1991; Mintz and Bean, 1993), although this may not account entirely for their effect on transmitter release (Capogna et al., 1996). On the postsynaptic side, the $GABA_B$-triggered cascade leads to the opening of G protein-gated inward-rectifying K^+ (GIRK) channels (Andrade et al., 1986; Misgeld et al., 1995). Activation of these channels causes a slow IPSP, lasting several hundred milliseconds. This is easily distinguished from the $GABA_A$ receptor-mediated IPSP, not only because of its slow kinetics but also because it is independent of the Cl^- reversal potential.

In contrast to $GABA_A$ receptor-mediated IPSCs, it has proved difficult to elicit $GABA_B$ receptor-mediated synaptic responses by activating individual presynaptic neurons. This observation is difficult to reconcile with data that $GABA_B$ receptors generally have a higher affinity for GABA than do $GABA_A$ receptors. A possible resolution of the paradox is that the receptors are principally extrasynaptic, and that GABA released from multiple presynaptic terminals must accumulate to activate them (Destexhe and Sejnowski, 1995; Scanziani, 2000). This argument suggests that uptake mechanisms are insufficient to isolate GABAergic terminals functionally from one another, at least as far as high affinity $GABA_B$ receptors are concerned.

6.5 Other Neurotransmitters

In comparison with glutamate and GABA, other neurotransmitters are present at far fewer synapses. Some of them appear to carry a diffuse signal in the extracellular space and may therefore play extensive roles in determining the overall state of the hippocampal circuitry. Relatively little is known about the mechanisms underlying their release and postsynaptic actions.

ATP is thought to be co-released with other neurotransmitters, and activates ionotropic P_{2X} receptors linked to a cation-selective channel. In the presence of broad-spectrum antagonists of amino acid receptors, a fast depolarizing purinergic postsynaptic current has been reported in hippocampal neurons (Pankratov et al., 1998; Mori et al., 2001). However, to detect such a current it is often necessary to stimulate many presynaptic fibers synchronously, implying that the receptors are present in very low density or that little ATP is released. The physiological or pathological role of this class of receptors is not known. ATP undergoes extracellular enzymatic degradation, which eventually results in the formation of adenosine. Adenosine is probably also released by neurons directly, and extracellular adenosine accumulation occurs under conditions of metabolic stress. Presynaptic adenosine receptors (mainly A_1 in the hippocampus) are widespread on excitatory terminals, where they depress glutamate release via a G protein-dependent mechanism (Wu and Saggau, 1994). This phenomenon contributes to the potent depressant effect of hypoxia on excitatory synaptic transmission. GABA release is relatively less sensitive to adenosine (Yoon and Rothman, 1991; Lambert and Wilson, 1993).

Among other small molecules that act as neurotransmitters are the monoamines noradrenaline (norepinephrine), dopamine (DA), serotonin (5-HT), and histamine (Nicoll et al., 1990) Norepinephrine acts at metabotropic β-adrenergic receptors, serotonin activates both ionotropic depolarizing 5-HT_3 receptors and a large number of metabotropic receptors, and histamine acts at metabotropic H_{1-3} receptors. The monoamines tend to be released from varicosities of extrinsic afferent fibers, mainly originating in hindbrain structures. Norepinephrine, acting via β receptors, increases the action potential frequency and reduces spike frequency adaptation during continued depolarizing current injection (Madison and Nicoll, 1982, 1984). This effect is mediated by a relatively selective inhibition of Ca^{2+}-gated K^+ channels responsible for the slow after-hyperpolarization following an action potential (Haas and Konnerth, 1983) and requires a signaling cascade involving protein kinase A (Pedarzani and Storm, 1993). Serotonin and histamine have effects similar to those of norepinephrine but, in addition, exert other actions. Serotonin, in particular, activates GIRK channels (Andrade et al., 1986). The role of the ionotropic 5-HT_3 receptors is poorly understood. Histamine has been reported to enhance NMDA receptor-mediated currents (Bekkers, 1993).

The hippocampus receives dopaminergic projections from both the substantia nigra pars compacta and the ventral tegmental area. Dopamine acts at two groups of metabotropic receptors (Sealfon and Olanow, 2000). D1-like receptors (D1 and D5) are positively coupled to adenylate cyclase, which activates protein kinase A and leads to phosphorylation of the protein phosphatase inhibitor DARPP-32, whereas D2-like receptors (D2, D3, D4) are negatively coupled to this cascade. Transcripts for all of these receptors can be detected in the hippocampus. Relatively little is known about the synaptic function of this transmitter. Exogenous dopamine hyperpolarizes a proportion of pyramidal neurons, an action that is principally mediated by D1 receptors (Berretta et al., 1990).

However, whether this is relevant to the role of endogenous dopamine depends on how and where it is released, which remains to be determined. An alternative possibility is that the main role of dopamine is to modulate synaptic transmission. Such a possibility is prompted by analogy with the effects of dopamine in the striatum, which receives a much stronger projection from the substantia nigra. In this system, dopaminergic projections terminate on the necks of dendritic spines that receive glutamatergic terminals (Kotter, 1994). Activation of such dopamine receptors results in inhibition of EPSCs (Calabresi et al., 1997), an action that has also been reported at some hippocampal synapses (Otmakhova and Lisman, 1999).

Acetylcholine is also released from extrinsic afferents, although in this case their cell bodies lie in diencephalic structures, in particular the medial septal nuclei and the nucleus of the diagonal band (see Chapter 3). Acetylcholine acts on both ionotropic (nicotinic) and metabotropic (muscarinic) receptors.

Nicotinic receptors are pentameric, and two main types occur in the hippocampus: homomeric $α_7$ and heteromeric $α_4β_2$. These receptors can be distinguished by their affinity for acetylcholine, by the desensitization kinetics, and by selective agonists and antagonists. Homopentameric $α_7$ receptors have a lower affinity for the endogenous agonist than do $α_4β_2$ receptors, desensitize fast, and are inhibited by methyllaconitine (MLA) and α-bungarotoxin. Activation of these receptors by exogenous agonist application has been reported to enhance evoked glutamate and GABA release (McGehee et al., 1995; Albuquerque et al., 1997; Dani, 2001). This observation implies that they are located presynaptically (MacDermott et al., 1999), a conclusion that has recently been supported by immunohistochemical evidence for abundant α-bungarotoxin staining co-localized with both glutamatergic and GABAergic terminals in the hippocampus (Fabian-Fine et al., 2001). However, postsynaptic staining was also seen in this study. Heteromeric $α_4β_2$ receptors have a relatively higher affinity for acetylcholine and nicotine, desensitize slowly, and are antagonized by dihydro-β-erythroidine and mecamylamine. Activation of these receptors has been reported to depolarize a subset of neocortical interneurons (Porter et al., 1999). A major limitation of these studies is that they have mainly relied on application of exogenous agonists. Thus, although they shed light on possible mechanisms of action of nicotine, it is not known under what conditions endogenously released acetylcholine is able to activate these receptors.

Four muscarinic receptors (M_{1-4}) are found in the hippocampus. Activation of muscarinic receptors has several effects. The so-called M current is active at resting potentials (Brown and Adams, 1980) and is inhibited by muscarinic receptor agonists, thereby facilitating burst-firing of neurons. It is mediated at least in part by heteromultimeric K^+ channels containing KCNQ2 and KCNQ3 subunits (Wang et al., 1998; Selyanko et al., 1999; Shapiro et al., 2000). Muscarinic receptors have recently been reported to influence the M current by activation of phospholipase C, which leads to the breakdown of phosphatidylinositol-4,5-bisphosphate (Suh and Hille, 2002). The depolarizing actions of muscarinic agonists are especially prominent in some interneurons (Pitler and Alger, 1992; Behrends and ten Bruggencate, 1993). This phenomenon may also play an important role in generating the hippocampal θ rhythm (Fischer et al., 1999), although the precise synaptic and nonsynaptic mechanisms underlying this rhythm in vivo are far from clear (see Chapter 8). Other consequences of muscarinic receptor activation include prolongation of action potential duration (Figenschou et al., 1996) and activation of GIRK channels (Seeger and Alzheimer, 2001). The inhibition of Ca^{2+}-sensitive K^+ channels by muscarinic receptors is reminiscent of the effect of β receptor activation by norepinephrine (see above). However, this action of muscarinic receptors is mediated not by protein kinase A but by Ca^{2+}/calmodulin-dependent protein kinase II (Pedarzani and Storm, 1996). Muscarinic receptors also exist presynaptically, where they depress transmitter release (Behrends and ten Bruggencate, 1993). This action is likely to be mediated by G protein-mediated inhibition of Ca^{2+} channels. Again, the physiological role of this effect is unknown.

In contrast to the amino acids glutamate and GABA, several of the transmitters considered in this section tend not to subserve conventional point-to-point (or "wiring") transmission. Instead, they probably act principally by diffusing a relatively long distance from the axonal varicosities where they are released. Indeed, many such varicosities exist in the absence of identifiable postsynaptic structures. Although this principle would argue against an important role in the fast transmission of information through the hippocampal formation, these transmitters actually play crucial roles in regulating the excitability of the circuitry. The involvement of the cholinergic projection to the hippocampus in setting the theta rhythm is an important example of such a phenomenon (see Chapters 8 and 11).

A large number of peptides have also been shown to exist in axonal varicosities and to bind to specific receptors in the hippocampus (Hökfelt et al., 1980). They include the opioid peptides, somatostatin, neuropeptide Y, galanin, and cholecystokinin. Of these, the opioid peptides (enkephalins, endorphins, dynorphin, endomorphins) have been studied most extensively. They act at receptors that fall into three classes with distinct pharmacological profiles (κ, δ, μ), although there is evidence that these receptors can heterodimerize (Jordan and Devi, 1999).

Peptides are thought to be contained in dense-core vesicles, which occur in GABAergic synapses and at mossy fiber synapses. Many peptides probably act principally via spillover to modulate either pre- or postsynaptic metabotropic receptors in the vicinity of the site where they are released (Weisskopf et al., 1993; Simmons and Chavkin, 1996).

Recently, brain-derived neurotrophic factor (BDNF) applied to hippocampal neurons was shown to evoke fast depolarizing currents mediated by an interaction between the TrkB receptor and $Na_V1.9$ Na^+ channels (Blum et al., 2002). This finding is unexpected, not least because peptides gener-

ally exert only indirect control over membrane potentials via G proteins. Before BDNF is elevated to the rank of neurotransmitters, it is important to determine whether endogenous BDNF can evoke the same effect.

Some molecules have an uncertain status as neurotransmitters in the hippocampus. Glycine receptors occur in the hippocampus, where they open Cl^- conductance. However, glycinergic synaptic transmission has not been demonstrated (in contrast to the spinal cord). The amino acids taurine and β-alanine have recently been proposed to act as endogenous agonists at glycine receptors, although it is unclear whether they can be released in an activity-dependent manner (Mori et al., 2002).

The Zn^{2+} ion is associated with synaptic vesicles of glutamatergic synapses throughout the hippocampus but is especially prominent in mossy fibers. Zn^{2+} inhibits $GABA_A$ and NMDA receptors, as well as glutamate uptake, although it is unclear whether this occurs during synaptic transmission under physiological conditions (Draguhn et al., 1990; Smart et al., 1994; Spiridon et al., 1998; Frederickson et al., 2000; Vogt et al., 2000). The dipeptide N-acetylaspartate may also be released from presynaptic terminals and acts as an agonist at metabotropic glutamate receptors (Wroblewska et al., 1993).

Nitric oxide (NO) and carbon monoxide (CO) deserve mention, although they do not appear to function as synaptic neurotransmitters in the conventional sense. NO is synthesized in neurons expressing nitric oxide synthase (principally a subset of interneurons) in a Ca^{2+}-dependent manner and diffuses through membranes to its targets, which include soluble guanylyl cyclase (Baranano et al., 2001). This agent potentially acts as a retrograde messenger, but evidence to support this—let alone to indicate a physiological role for the phenomenon—is scanty.

Products of lipid metabolism may also play a role in intercellular communication. Notable among these products are arachidonic acid (AA) (Piomelli, 1994), and the endocannabinoids anandamide and 2-arachidonylglycerol (Davies et al., 2002). Both AA and endocannabinoids are synthesized in a Ca^{2+}-dependent manner and are potential retrograde messengers. The role of endocannabinoid signaling in modulation of inhibition is considered further below.

6.6 Special Features of Individual Hippocampal Synapses

In contrast to the neuromuscular junction, hippocampal synapses usually occur at axonal varicosities (the widely used term "terminal" is thus misleading). These varicosities occur at regular intervals along many axons. Their spacing is approximately 4 μm for Schaffer collaterals and associational-commissural fibers and approximately 5 μm for mossy fibers (Shepherd et al., 2002) (see Chapter 3). They often contain mitochondria, reflecting the energetic demands of transmitter synthesis, vesicular packaging, release, and re-endocytosis (Shepherd and Harris, 1998).

Only one type of axo-axonic synapse is known in the hippocampus: the GABAergic synapse made by chandelier cells on axon initial segments (see Chapters 3 and 8). In contrast to the spinal cord, presynaptic specializations have not been reported in contact with distal axons or axonal varicosities. It can thus be inferred that heterosynaptic modulation of transmitter release by activation of metabotropic receptors occurs via spillover transmission (see below).

6.6.1 Small Excitatory Spine Synapses

The most abundant type of synapse in the hippocampus is the small glutamatergic synapse made on dendritic spines. This subserves transmission from the perforant path to dentate granule cells, as well as associational/commissural projections to CA3 pyramidal neurons and Schaffer collateral/commissural transmission to CA1 pyramidal neurons. The monosynaptic projection from the perforant path to the distal dendrites of CA1 and CA3 pyramidal neurons has received less attention but probably has broadly similar biophysical properties (Berzhanskaya et al., 1998; Otmakhova et al., 2002). Similar synapses relay excitatory signals from CA1 pyramidal neurons to subicular pyramidal cells and from the latter to the entorhinal cortex. Just over half of the presynaptic varicosities in CA1 appear to contain mitochondria (Shepherd and Harris, 1998). The postsynaptic densities range widely in area: from less than 0.07 μm^2 at synapses on thin spines to at least 0.42 μm^2 (Harris and Sultan, 1995). Dendritic spines in the dentate gyrus measure up to 0.8 μm in diameter and approximately 1 μm in length (Trommald and Hulleberg, 1997), and generally receive only one presynaptic bouton. However, the presynaptic varicosity is sometimes in synaptic contact with more than one spine (Westrum and Blackstad, 1962; Sorra and Harris, 1993). Spines are thought to represent principally biochemical compartments rather than electrical barriers or amplifiers for the propagation of synaptic currents to the dendrite (Yuste et al., 2000).

The synaptic cleft is often closely apposed by an astrocytic process, although this is highly variable: In one study as few as 57% of glutamatergic synapses in CA1 were contacted, and of these only approximately 43% of the perimeter of the synaptic cleft was found to be bounded by an astrocytic process (Ventura and Harris, 1999). Because astrocytes express abundant glutamate transporters, this implies that there may be considerable variability in the spatiotemporal profile of glutamate in the vicinity of the synapse following exocytosis.

A combination of immunohistochemical and ultrastructural techniques has shown that both AMPA and NMDA receptors are localized to the postsynaptic density (Nusser et al., 1998; Takumi et al., 1998, 1999; Racca et al., 2000). Whether kainate receptors are also present is not known. However, glutamatergic EPSCs at Schaffer collateral–CA1 synapses are entirely blocked by antagonists of AMPA and NMDA receptors, leaving little room for the involvement of postsynaptic kainate receptors (Castillo et al., 1997b; Vignes and Collingridge, 1997). The AMPA receptors at small spine synapses on principal neurons have a low permeability to Ca^{2+} and are nonrectifying, reflecting the presence of edited GluR2 subunits in almost all receptors (Jonas et al., 1994). Most AMPA receptors are thought to be GluR1/2 and GluR2/3 heteromers (Wenthold et al., 1996). Ca^{2+} influx, however, occurs as an indirect consequence of AMPA receptor activation because the consequent depolarization allows Ca^{2+}-permeable NMDA receptors to open (Yuste et al., 1999). In addition, the depolarization allows voltage-gated Ca^{2+} channels in the dendritic spine and nearby region of the dendrite to open. A final source of Ca^{2+} is from intracellular stores, triggered by second messengers including inositol trisphosphate and Ca^{2+} itself (Emptage et al., 1999). However, the latter is controversial as some studies have not found a substantial role for Ca^{2+} release from stores at these synapses (Kovalchuk et al., 2000). Some of the disagreement about the relative importance of the various sources of Ca^{2+} probably reflects differences in recording methods: Although whole-cell recordings allow voltage control of the dendrite, they may interfere with intracellular Ca^{2+} homeostasis. Intracellular microelectrode recordings, though minimizing this source of error, sacrifice voltage control.

Although AMPA and NMDA receptors both contribute to EPSCs evoked by simultaneous stimulation of numerous presynaptic fibers, EPSCs evoked by action potentials in single presynaptic axons sometimes lack an AMPA receptor-mediated component (Kullmann, 1994; Isaac et al., 1995; Liao et al., 1995). Such EPSCs are evoked only under conditions where the postsynaptic neuron is depolarized or Mg^{2+} ions are omitted from the extracellular solution to reveal the NMDA receptor-mediated component. This observation has led to the hypothesis that AMPA receptors are absent or nonfunctional at a proportion of synapses, which are consequently often referred to as "silent synapses." Immunohistochemical studies provide some indirect support for this hypothesis: Some small and/or immature synapses appear not to stain for AMPA receptors (Nusser et al., 1998; Petralia et al., 1999; Takumi et al., 1999). However, given the finite sensitivity of the antibodies, inferring that the receptors are genuinely absent relies on extrapolation. In contrast, NMDA receptor density appears to be more uniform across synapses of different size (Racca et al., 2000). Taken together with the observation that the proportion of silent synapses diminishes with age, it is tempting to conclude that synaptic maturation develops by an initial expression of NMDA receptors, followed later by insertion of AMPA receptors (Durand et al., 1996). This phenomenon may share mechanisms in common with long-term potentiation.

Alternative explanations for silent synapses exist: Because NMDA receptors have a much higher steady-state affinity for glutamate than AMPA receptors (Patneau and Mayer, 1990), they might respond to a relatively low and prolonged pulse of glutamate that is insufficient to activate AMPA receptors. Such a glutamate profile could arise by diffusion from neighboring synapses ("spillover") (Asztely et al., 1997; Kullmann and Asztely, 1998). Thus, the NMDA receptors of the recorded cell might be acting as bystanders, eavesdropping on the excitatory traffic through many synapses formed on neighboring cells. In favor of this model is the observation that raising the recording temperature from room temperature (thereby enhancing glutamate uptake) reduces the discrepancy between the number of quanta detected by NMDA and AMPA receptors. Conversely, blocking glutamate uptake pharmacologically increases the ratio of NMDA to AMPA receptor-mediated signaling, consistent with an exacerbation of cross-talk among synapses. Further evidence in favor of glutamate spillover comes from examining the effects of manipulations of release probabilities and competitive glutamate antagonists on the time course of NMDA receptor-mediated EPSCs (Lozovaya et al., 1999; Diamond, 2001; Arnth-Jensen et al., 2002).

Another possible explanation for selective activation of NMDA receptors is that the glutamate released from the presynaptic terminal to activate AMPA receptors is insufficient. This could occur if release took place via a "fusion pore." That is, glutamate could slowly escape from a vesicle via a small, possibly flickering, opening to the synaptic cleft. Evidence for this phenomenon comes in part from the observation that enhancing the affinity of AMPA receptors for glutamate with pharmacological tools can unsilence such a "whispering" synapse (Choi et al., 2000; Renger et al., 2001). Moreover, manipulation of the presynaptic release probability can differentially affect AMPA and NMDA receptor-mediated components of EPSCs (Gasparini et al., 2000).

The various explanations for silent synapses (absence of functional AMPA receptors, spillover, fusion pore release) are not mutually exclusive. Their relative importance is also unresolved. Indeed, a silent synapse could be "deaf" (that is, devoid of functional AMPA receptors) early in its development but be "mute" (presynaptically silent but potentially susceptible to spillover of glutamate from a neighbor) at a later stage.

Because these issues have profound implications for the interpretation of changes in quantal parameters following long-term potentiation or depression, they will no doubt continue to attract considerable attention (Kullmann, 2003) (see Chapter 10). One critical question that bears on the interpretation of silent synapses is the degree of occupancy of AMPA and NMDA receptors following presynaptic glutamate release. Despite much effort, there is still considerable uncertainty over the extent to which AMPA and NMDA receptors are bound by glutamate released from the presynaptic terminal. It is also unclear whether presynaptic terminals are able to release more than one vesicle of glutamate. Three approaches have been used to estimate the occupancy of receptors following a presynaptic action potential.

- First, by assuming that a single vesicle contains between 2000 and 5000 molecules of glutamate, and that all of them are released through a rapidly expanding pore, one can simulate diffusion of the glutamate molecules

and their interaction with receptors and transporters around the synapse (Wahl et al., 1996; Rusakov and Kullmann, 1998; Barbour, 2001). There are considerable uncertainties in several critical parameters, including the diffusion coefficient of glutamate in the extracellular space and the fraction of the local volume accounted for by the extracellular space. Nevertheless, some studies applying this approach have arrived at the conclusion that the glutamate concentration in the synaptic cleft reaches a peak of approximately 1 to 3 mM almost instantaneously and then drops rapidly with a multiexponential time course. Taking into account the kinetic properties of NMDA receptors, this glutamate profile implies that the NMDA receptors opposite a release site should be almost saturated by a single vesicle. The occupancy of AMPA receptors is generally found to be slightly lower than that of NMDA receptors, reflecting their lower affinity. Another result from numerical simulations is that glutamate spreads outside the synaptic cleft, although the extent of this extrasynaptic glutamate escape is sharply curtailed by transporters. Some studies have suggested that a significant proportion of NMDA receptors within a radius of approximately 500 nm are activated by such glutamate spillover (Rusakov and Kullmann, 1998). This roughly corresponds to the typical distance separating one synapse in the CA1 neuropil from its nearest neighbor, taking into account the fact that synapses are not arranged as a regular lattice (Rusakov et al., 1998; Kirov et al., 1999). One report arrived at lower estimates for the glutamate concentrations in both the synaptic cleft and the perisynaptic space (Barbour, 2001); however, the discrepancy is mainly explained by assuming a larger extracellular space fraction, which gives rise to a greater degree of dilution of neurotransmitter following release.

- The second approach to estimate receptor occupancy is to compare the effects of receptor antagonists with different properties on the amplitude of the postsynaptic response (Clements et al., 1992). Low-affinity antagonists should be more easily displaced from the receptors by a pulse of glutamate than high-affinity antagonists. By titrating the concentration of the antagonists and establishing the kinetic properties of the receptors in patches of membranes exposed to known concentrations of agonists and antagonists, this approach can yield information about the glutamate concentration profile in the synapse. This method relies on the assumption that receptors in somatic membrane patches are representative of synaptic receptors. Nevertheless, it leads to the conclusion that glutamate reaches a concentration in excess of 1 mM for 100 μs, subsequently decaying with an exponential time constant of approximately 1 to 2 ms. These results have again argued for a relatively high occupancy of NMDA receptors (> 95% bound). Extending this method to AMPA receptors has been difficult because of the lack of suitable antagonists; but driving kinetic models of AMPA receptors with a similar concentration profile leads to the prediction that they should be only approximately 60% bound at the peak of the response.

- The third approach has given a different picture of receptor occupancy. High-resolution optical methods have shown Ca^{2+} transients in single dendritic spines, which reflects NMDA receptor opening in response to presynaptic glutamate release and which can be distinguished from transmission failure (Mainen et al., 1999). When two presynaptic stimuli were given in rapid succession (with an interval too short to allow appreciable NMDA receptor unbinding), the Ca^{2+} transient was frequently larger than when only one stimulus was given. This implies that the receptors were not saturated by the first transient. This approach again depends on a number of assumptions, not least that voltage-sensitive Ca^{2+} channels and postsynaptic Ca^{2+} stores do not contribute to the signals and that the visualized synapses are representative of the overall population. Notwithstanding these caveats, it implies that NMDA receptors are less than 60% bound following a single release event. Again, it is difficult to extend this approach to AMPA receptors because normally they are not sufficiently permeable to Ca^{2+} for a postsynaptic signal to be detected directly. Nevertheless, the conclusion that NMDA receptor occupancy is less than 60% does not automatically imply that AMPA receptor occupancy should be less than this: The 100-fold difference in affinities of the two receptors applies to steady-state agonist application. With a very brief pulse of transmitter, the occupancy is determined principally by the binding rate, not by the balance of binding and unbinding rates (Kullmann, 1999). Because the binding rates of the two receptor types are similar, it is not impossible that both are equally and incompletely occupied by glutamate following a single release event.

Overall, the average release probability at Schaffer collateral-CA1 pyramidal neuron synapses is probably less than 50% (Raastad, 1995), although it is highly variable from synapse to synapse (Hessler et al., 1993; Rosenmund et al., 1993). In fact, it is difficult to estimate the mean probability because there may be a large number of release sites with a release probability close to 0. Moreover, the release probability at neocortical synapses has been reported to increase with the temperature of the preparation (Hardingham and Larkman, 1998), so estimates obtained at room temperature may be biased. Recent electrophysiological and optical approaches have suggested that more than one vesicle can be simultaneously released at small glutamatergic synapses (Bolshakov et al., 1997; Oertner et al., 2002). Spontaneous "miniature" EPSCs (mEPSCs), recorded in the presence of tetrodotoxin to block Na^+-dependent action potentials, have conventionally been taken to reflect the postsynaptic effect of individual quanta, corresponding to single vesicles released from presy-

naptic terminals. Equating mEPSCs with vesicles, however, relies on two assumptions: first, that exocytosis proceeds in the same way in the presence and absence of presynaptic action potentials; and second, that spontaneous presynaptic Ca^{2+} fluctuations do not trigger the simultaneous release of multiple vesicles. Nevertheless, mEPSCs recorded in individual pyramidal neurons show a broad, skewed distribution, ranging from detection threshold ($<$ 5 pA) up to approximately 50 pA (Manabe et al., 1992). Part of this variability may be due to different degrees of cable filtering of EPSCs originating in different parts of the dendritic tree. Nevertheless, the median amplitude probably corresponds to about 100 AMPA receptor-gated channels opening.

It has been suggested that quantal parameters are positively correlated across different synapses (Schikorski and Stevens, 1997). Thus, synapses with large presynaptic elements tend to have many docked vesicles (as well as more vesicles in total), large active zones and PSDs, and large postsynaptic spines (Harris and Sultan, 1995). Thus, if multivesicular release occurs, it should do so preferentially at such synapses and give rise to large postsynaptic signals. Conversely, small synapses, some of which are possibly devoid of AMPA receptors, may not contribute appreciably to the excitatory traffic impinging on the postsynaptic neuron.

Even though a pyramidal neuron has 10,000 to 30,000 spine synapses (see Chapters 3 and 5), it has been estimated that only 16 to 26 need to fire synchronously to bring it to action potential threshold (Otmakhov et al., 1993). Clearly, fewer large quanta are required than small ones, and physiological patterns of discharges further complicate this equation. Because the dendrites of CA1 pyramidal neurons can extend up to 500 μm from the soma, an important question is whether distal synapses are as effective as proximal ones (Andersen et al., 1980b). If the dendrites acted as passive cables, and the same synaptic current was injected irrespective of position, distal synapses would give rise to a somatic EPSP whose peak amplitude was considerably smaller than that generated by proximal synapses. However, if the total charge transfer is estimated, the difference between proximal and distal synapses decreases. It has recently been reported that EPSCs generated at different positions on the dendritic tree show a location-related scaling that further compensates for the effect of cable attenuation (Magee and Cook, 2000). This finding remains to be confirmed independently, and the biophysical mechanisms underlying such a scaling have yet to be resolved. Finally, voltage-dependent conductances may modulate the anterograde and retrograde propagation of electrical signals in the dendrites. These issues are considered further in Chapter 5.

Dentate granule cells are much smaller and have fewer total spines than pyramidal neurons, although they have the same spine density per unit length of dendrite (Trommald and Hulleberg, 1997). The two extrinsic excitatory projections to granule cells show a striking difference in their short-term plasticity when two presynaptic stimuli are delivered in rapid succession. Lateral perforant path synapses exhibit marked facilitation of the second EPSC compared to the first EPSC ("paired pulse facilitation"). This behavior is essentially the same as at Schaffer collateral synapses on CA1 pyramidal neurons. In contrast, medial perforant path synapses show less pronounced paired-pulse facilitation or even depression (McNaughton, 1980). This phenomenon is seen under conditions where inhibitory transmission is blocked, and it appears to reflect intrinsic differences between the glutamatergic synapses in the two pathways. Indeed, medial perforant path synapses appear to have a higher initial release probability than lateral perforant path synapses (Min et al., 1998).

Medial and lateral perforant path synapses also show several differences in sensitivity to neurotransmitters acting on presynaptic receptors. Notably, metabotropic glutamate receptor agonists depress transmission in the two pathways via distinct receptors (Macek et al., 1996), in approximate agreement with the distribution of subtypes resolved with immunohistochemical methods (Shigemoto et al., 1997). Muscarinic receptor agonists depress the medial perforant path input relatively selectively (Kahle and Cotman, 1989), and norepinephrine has also been reported to have pathway-specific actions (Dahl and Sarvey, 1989). It remains to be determined whether these differences have functional consequences.

Another difference between the two pathways is that LPP but not MPP synapses exhibit the silent synapse phenomenon seen at Schaffer collateral synapses (Min et al., 1998a). The pharmacological and/or morphological differences that underlie this difference are unknown.

6.6.2 Mossy Fiber Synapses

Mossy fibers are the thin, unmyelinated axons of dentate granule cells. They form several distinct types of synapse (Henze et al., 2000). Those formed on CA3 pyramidal neurons are in many ways unique (Fig. 6–8). First, they are much larger than any other synapses in the hippocampus, with a diameter up to 10 μm. Second, the large presynaptic element (volume approximately 50 μm^3) contains numerous dense-core vesicles in addition to the small clear vesicles that predominate in other glutamatergic terminals. These dense-core vesicles are thought to contain dynorphin, Zn^{2+}, and other molecules, many of which are released in an activity-dependent manner. Although mossy fibers are excitatory, they contain abundant GABA (Sandler and Smith, 1991; Sloviter et al., 1996), raising the possibility that they may also package this neurotransmitter in some vesicles and release it following action potential invasion. Indeed, this possibility has been given indirect

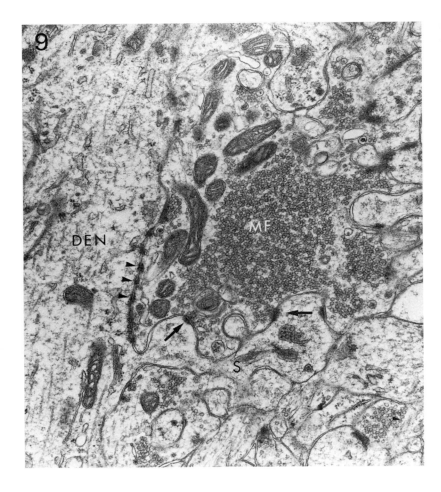

Figure 6–8. Mossy fiber structure. The mossy fiber terminal (MF) contains numerous small (approximately 40 nm diameter) vesicles as well as mitochondria and larger vesicles, some of which are dense-cored. Some vesicles are found close to membrane specializations (arrows) that represent release sites in contact with a postsynaptic complex spine (S) belonging to a CA3 pyramidal neuron. DEN, dendrite. Arrowheads point to puncta adhaerentia, symmetrical membrane specializations often seen at synapses. (*Source*: Amaral and Dent, 1981, with permission.)

experimental support (Gutierrez, 2000; Walker et al., 2001). Third, the postsynaptic element is a highly branched structure ("thorny excrescence") akin to a large, complex spine, occurring in the proximal part of the apical dendrite of the CA3 pyramidal neuron. These structures are also found in relatively small numbers in the proximal basal dendrites, although their incidence increases following intense excitatory traffic such as occurs during a prolonged seizure (see Chapter 15). The postsynaptic excrescence invaginates the presynaptic terminal. Mossy fiber synapses on CA3 pyramidal neurons can contain between 3 and 80 active zones, each of which is apposed to a PSD (Henze et al., 2000)

Mirroring their anatomical complexity, mossy fiber–CA3 synapses show many physiological and pharmacological peculiarities. EPSCs contain a kainate receptor-mediated component in addition to the AMPA receptor-mediated component (Castillo et al., 1997b; Vignes and Collingridge, 1997), whereas the NMDA component is relatively small (Jonas et al., 1993). These pharmacological features are in agreement with the relatively high kainate and low NMDA binding densities observed in the stratum lucidum (Monaghan et al., 1983; Benke et al., 1993). The kainate component is generally thought to be carried by GluR6-containing receptors (Mulle et al., 1998), although it remains unclear why this component of the EPSC is slow compared to the kinetics of recombinant GluR6-containing receptors. High-frequency stimuli also evoke a postsynaptic metabotropic glutamate receptor-mediated depolarizing current (Heuss et al., 1999; Yeckel et al., 1999).

Mossy fiber EPSCs exhibit pronounced facilitation with very modest increases in discharge frequency, and part of this facilitation is mediated by presynaptic kainate autoreceptors (Schmitz et al., 2001c). Following a high-frequency burst of action potentials in the presynaptic axons, transmission at mossy fibers can remain elevated for hours (Henze et al., 2000). This form of long-term potentiation is distinct from that seen at other spine synapses in the hippocampus in that it is not dependent on NMDA receptors. Its underlying mechanisms are considered further in Chapter 10.

Transmission at mossy fiber synapses can be profoundly depressed by activation of several classes of presynaptic receptors, including group II (and in some species group III) metabotropic glutamate receptors (Yamamoto et al., 1983; Lanthorn et al., 1984; Kamiya et al., 1996), $GABA_B$ receptors (Min et al., 1998b; Vogt and Nicoll, 1999) and opioid receptors (Weisskopf et al., 1993). Presynaptic kainate receptors have a paradoxical function: With low concentrations of agonists, probably corresponding to that achieved with synaptic glutamate release, they facilitate transmission (Schmitz et al., 2001c), whereas with higher concentrations transmission is depressed (Chittajallu et al., 1996; Vignes et al., 1998; Kamiya and Ozawa, 2000; Kullmann, 2001; Schmitz et al., 2001c). The degree to which presynaptic receptors on mossy fibers are activated by neurotransmitters released from their own terminals, in contrast to neighboring axons (whether mossy fiber or

other afferent fibers) remains unclear. The functional role of presynaptic modulation of mossy fiber transmission is also unclear: It may act as a brake on further transmitter release or subserve a form of center-surround inhibition to sharpen the projection from the dentate gyrus. Such a role has been proposed for the release of dynorphin, which acts at κ receptors (Weisskopf et al., 1993; Simmons and Chavkin, 1996).

Although mossy fiber synapses on CA3 pyramidal neurons are large and complex, this projection is sparse: Each mossy fiber makes only about 14 synapses in CA3 (see Chapter 3). Moreover, at low frequencies unitary mossy fiber EPSCs evoked in individual CA3 pyramidal neurons have a peak amplitude corresponding to a synaptic conductance of approximately 1 nS and consist of approximately 5 quanta (Jonas et al., 1993). This conductance is only approximately fivefold larger than at the far more abundant glutamatergic input to CA3 pyramidal neurons, the associational-commisural fibers. However, because mossy fiber EPCS can increase up to 10-fold with high-frequency activity (Regehr et al., 1994), the projection sometimes becomes powerful for depolarizing CA3 neurons. A brief train of action potentials in a single mossy fiber can bring a CA3 pyramidal neuron to firing threshold in vivo (Henze et al., 2002). The sparse connectivity of granule cells to CA3 pyramidal neurons has impeded detailed biophysical study of this pathway.

A second type of mossy fiber synapse is formed on glutamatergic mossy cells of the dentate hilus. The presynaptic varicosities are also large and contain pleomorphic vesicles. Numerically far more important are small synapses on other hilar interneurons (Acsady et al., 1998). They have a very different shape in that the presynaptic element is a filopodial extension off the shaft of the mossy fiber itself, which makes a single contact with the target interneuron. These synapses are much smaller than the synapses on CA3 pyramidal neurons and probably contain only a single release site. Several physiological studies of mossy fiber–interneuron transmission have not systematically identified the postsynaptic neurons (Maccaferri et al., 1998; Toth et al., 2000; Lei and McBain, 2002). However, because small filopodial synapses far outnumber large synapses on mossy cells, they probably principally reflect the properties of the former. Although they are highly susceptible to presynaptic modulation via metabotropic glutamate receptors, many mossy fiber synapses on interneurons appear not to exhibit marked frequency-dependent facilitation or NMDA receptor-independent LTP (Maccaferri et al., 1998). However, this conclusion may not apply universally to the interneuronal targets of mossy fibers: Short- and long-term potentiation have recently been reported in identified basket cells in response to high-frequency trains of stimuli delivered to single presynaptic granule cells (Alle et al., 2001) (see Chapter 10).

Another peculiarity of mossy fiber transmission to some interneurons is that Ca^{2+}-permeable AMPA receptors have been reported to mediate transmission (Toth et al., 2000). This property is shared with other excitatory synapses on interneurons and probably depends on whether the interneuron expresses GluR2 receptors (see below). However, there may be a further level of refinement because it has been proposed that a given interneuron targets Ca^{2+}-permeable and Ca^{2+}-impermeable receptors to different synapses (Toth and McBain, 1998).

The fourth type of synapse formed by mossy fibers is on the proximal dendrites of other granule cells. Although this projection is normally sparse, it increases following intense seizure activity, in common with the infrapyramidal projection to CA3 ("mossy fiber sprouting") (see Chapter 16).

6.6.3 Other Glutamatergic Synapses on Interneurons

Excitatory synapses on interneurons made by pyramidal neurons are generally small and are made directly on the soma and dendrites (Box 6–3). From limited ultrastructural and electrophysiological data obtained in parallel, they contain a single release site (Gulyas et al., 1993). Two important pharmacological features distinguish them from small spine synapses on principal neurons. First, at a subset of synapses the AMPA receptors are permeable to Ca^{2+} (Jonas et al., 1994), which can be explained by the absence of the GluR2 subunit that confers Ca^{2+} impermeability at other receptors. Interestingly, many of the same interneurons express neuronal nitric oxide synthase (NOS) (Catania et al., 1995). It is tempting to speculate that Ca^{2+} influx via AMPA synaptic receptors may trigger the release of NO from these neurons, which could act as a diffuse messenger, affecting several target neurons within a small distance. This property is, however, not ubiquitous among interneurons; and many appear neither to express NOS nor to have Ca^{2+}-permeable AMPA receptors. Another highly variable property of glutamatergic synapses at interneurons is that some have a kainate receptor-mediated component (Cossart et al., 1998; Frerking et al., 1998), although it does not occur ubiquitously (Semyanov and Kullmann, 2001). In contrast to mossy fiber–CA3 synapses, interneurons are enriched in GluR5. It is not known whether the presence or absence of a kainate receptor-mediated component to EPSCs in interneurons correlates with the postsynaptic interneuron's morphological or immunocytochemical identity (see Chapter 7).

The kinetics of AMPA receptor-mediated EPSCs vary extensively among the various excitatory synapses in the hippocampus. In general, the rise times and decay time constants are slow in pyramidal neurons, intermediate in granule cells, and fast in interneurons (Geiger et al., 1997). Although this matches the passive membrane time constants of the various neurons, the difference persists once the cable properties of the neurons have been taken into account. That is, the different kinetics appear to be an intrinsic property of the neurons and/or synapses (Colquhoun et al., 1992) and, indeed, appear to reflect the subunit composition and splice variants of AMPA receptors expressed in each neuron (Lambolez et al., 1996).

Box 6–3
Methods Used to Study Transmission at Excitatory Hippocampal Synapses

The hippocampus has yielded many of the most important insights into synaptic transmission in the CNS. This is because of two principal factors. First, the hippocampal formation has a remarkable laminar organization: Many of the fibers making excitatory synapses run parallel to one another, and target neurons and their projections are tightly packed (see Chapter 3). Second, development of the slice preparation allowed neurons and their connections to be studied in vitro, where the chemical and physical environment of the synapses could be manipulated experimentally. An important consequence of the laminar structure of the hippocampus is that the currents evoked by synchronous activity in many synapses can be detected via extracellular electrodes. Because synapses represent a current sink (current moves from the extracellular medium into neurons), field EPSPs (fEPSPs) are detected as negative voltage deflections in the dendritic regions where most excitatory synapses occur (the stratum radiatum or stratum oriens of the hippocampus proper or the stratum moleculare of the dentate gyrus). In the cell body layer, there is a corresponding positive wave (representing current flowing out of the principal neurons) that completes the local circuit. With stimuli of sufficient amplitude, however, a sharp negative deflection is superimposed on the positive fEPSP in the cell body layer. This "population spike" reflects the synchronous discharge of principal cells that are brought to firing threshold by the EPSP propagating to the cell body (Andersen et al., 1971).

Intracellular records from hippocampal neurons in vivo have lent direct support for the identification of population spikes with somatic action potentials (Kandel and Spencer, 1961). With the development of the hippocampal slice, Schwartzkroin (1975) showed that the dendritic negative fEPSP was indeed due to activation of synaptic potentials generated at the dendritic level, recorded as an intracellular depolarizing EPSP in the soma. More recently, patch-clamp recordings have been widely used, either from somata or from dendrites close to the excitatory synapses. They have shown even more directly that EPSCs result from the local activation of afferent fibers (Hestrin et al., 1990).

Another difference between the synapses is the expression of presynaptic group III metabotropic glutamate receptors. As already mentioned, these receptors are present at mossy fiber synapses in some species (for instance in guinea pigs) but not at Schaffer collateral synapses in CA1 pyramidal neurons. However, excitatory transmission to interneurons is highly sensitive to agonists of group III metabotropic receptors (Scanziani et al., 1998). Small synapses on pyramidal neurons, in contrast, are insensitive. This differential sensitivity to group III agonists parallels the distribution of some subtypes of group III receptors imaged with high-resolution immunohistochemical methods. For instance, mGluR7 appears to be expressed in presynaptic active zones apposed to interneurons and not at active zones apposed to pyramidal neurons (Shigemoto et al., 1996, 1997). This target cell dependence in the distribution of presynaptic receptors implies that a retrograde signal instructs the presynaptic membrane whether to anchor these receptors.

Many glutamatergic synapses on interneurons show similar patterns of short-term use-dependent plasticity as Schaffer collateral synapses on CA1 pyramidal neurons. That is, they show frequency-dependent facilitation with brief trains of action potentials. However, a subset of basket and bistratified cells receive glutamatergic synapses that depress prominently (Thomson, 2000). The molecular basis of this distinction has not been elucidated in the hippocampus but may again imply a retrograde signal from the target neuron that specifies some of the properties of the presynaptic terminal. Such a principle is supported by the finding that different synapses supplied by the same neocortical neurons can show either depression or facilitation with repeated stimulation, depending on the identity of the postsynaptic neurons (Reyes et al., 1998).

Finally, glutamatergic synapses to interneurons frequently appear not to express NMDA receptor-dependent LTP, although a form of LTD has been described (McMahon and Kauer, 1997). One report implicates a coincidence of Ca^{2+} influx via Ca^{2+}-permeable AMPA receptors and activation of presynaptic metabotropic receptors in the induction of this phenomenon (Laezza et al., 1999). This depression of inhibition potentially leads to a disynaptic disinhibition of principal cells (Lu et al., 2000).

6.6.4 Inhibitory Synapses

GABAergic inhibition of principal neurons plays an essential role in regulating the transmission of information through the hippocampal formation (see Box 6–4). The wide range of interneuron morphologies is summarized in Chapter 3, and their connectivities are considered in Chapter 8. Not all interneurons are GABAergic: Mossy cells in the dentate hilus and giant spiny interneurons in the stratum radiatum are glutamatergic and more akin to pyramidal neurons. Because relatively little is known about synapses made by glutamatergic interneurons, this section restricts its attention to GABAergic signaling (Fig. 6–9). Complementing the variability of interneuron morphology, GABAergic synapses fall into various types depending on their location on the target neuron. Three main types are recognized: axo-axonic, axo-somatic, and axo-dendritic. This distinction appears to be valid whether the postsynaptic target is a pyramidal neuron or another interneuron.

Axo-axonic synapses are made by chandelier cells and occur 50 to 70 μm from the soma of the target neuron. In pyramidal neurons, postsynaptic α_2 $GABA_A$ subunits are restricted principally to these synapses (Nusser et al., 1996). They are also distinguished from other GABAergic synapses by the presence of a postsynaptic Ca^{2+}-sequestering organelle (Benedeczky et al., 1994). Situated at the strategic point for impulse initiation, these synapses probably exert extremely powerful control over the discharge of target cells. From the small number of published paired recordings of pre- and

Box 6–4

Early Insights into Inhibitory Synaptic Signaling in the Hippocampus

Early intracellular recordings from principal neurons in the hippocampus showed that following a strong afferent stimulus the initial discharge was often followed by a pause in spontaneous activity (Albe-Fessard and Buser, 1955). fEPSP recordings also showed that intense activation was followed by a temporarily reduced ability to excite CA1 pyramidal cells and dentate granule cells synaptically. These observations led to the hypothesis that inhibitory processes are entrained by the stimulus. The synaptic basis for this inhibition was not immediately established because intracellular recordings revealed long-lasting depolarizing waves. However, it was subsequently discovered that they were IPSPs whose polarity was artificially reversed by the leakage of Cl^- ions into the neurons from the recording microelectrodes (Spencer and Kandel, 1961). This inhibition was shown to be generated across the soma membrane (Andersen et al., 1964), as would be expected if it was mediated by the perisomatic terminals of basket cells. Extracellular stimuli not only recruited basket cells via axon collaterals of principal neurons (disynaptic "feedback inhibition") but could also directly activate inhibitory interneurons, yielding a monosynaptic IPSP ("feedforward inhibition"). Both types of inhibition play an important role in regulating the excitability of the circuitry and in synchronizing the activity of populations of neurons (see Chapter 8). A potential role for feedforward inhibition in sharpening the temporal resolution of pattern discrimination has recently been proposed (Pouille and Scanziani, 2001).

postsynaptic neurons, these synapses appear to yield large-amplitude IPSCs with relatively fast kinetics and activity-dependent depression (Pawelzik et al., 1999; Maccaferri et al., 2000).

Axo-somatic synapses are made by basket cells, whose axon collaterals form clusters of boutons surrounding the soma of the target neurons (see Chapter 3). Basket cells mediate powerful inhibition of principal neurons by synchronous release of GABA from the multiple synapses. These synapses also tend to depress with repeated activation (Hefft et al., 2002). Interestingly, two subtypes of basket cells appear to signal via different postsynaptic $GABA_A$ receptors: Cholecystokinin-positive cells make synapses with a high α_2 content, and parvalbumin-containing basket cells signal preferentially via synapses containing α_1 subunits (Klausberger et al., 2002). How this complementary distribution of receptors fits with the physiological roles of these two subsets of interneurons is unknown.

Axo-dendritic synapses on pyramidal cells are made by a variety of interneurons whose cell bodies are found in the strata oriens, radiatum, and lacunosum-moleculare. Synapses formed on the distal dendrites are thought to control the excitability of the postsynaptic neuron relatively indirectly. They are unlikely to hyperpolarize the cell body effectively because they are electrically remote, but they may be highly

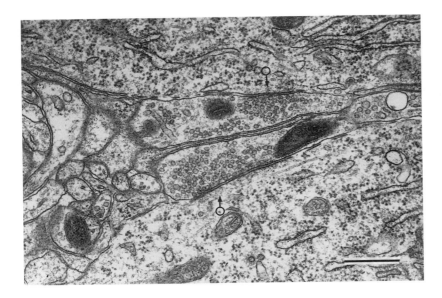

Figure 6–9. Inhibitory synapse structure. The arrows point to two symmetrical synapses on neighboring CA1 pyramidal cell bodies. Bar = 0.5 μm. (*Source*: Harris and Landis, 1986, with permission).

effective in shunting locally evoked EPSCs (Staley and Mody, 1992).

Possibly reflecting the different sites at which GABAergic synapses contact postsynaptic neurons, GABAergic IPSCs in pyramidal neurons have bimodal kinetics. So-called GABA$_{A-Fast}$ IPSCs have a faster rise-time (< 2 ms) and a correspondingly faster decay time constant (< 20 ms) than GABA$_{A-Slow}$ IPSCs (Pearce, 1993). This distinction is greater than can be explained entirely by cable filtering by the dendritic tree and suggests, instead, that different GABA$_A$ receptor subunits with differing kinetics are segregated to different synapses. Indeed, GABA$_{A-Fast}$ IPSCs are sensitive to furosemide (Pearce, 1993), which is consistent with presence of the α_4 subunit (Wafford et al., 1996). Circumstantial evidence suggests that they originate from basket cells and may be primarily responsible for generating relatively high-frequency (gamma range, approximately 40 Hz) oscillations in the hippocampus (Banks et al., 2000). In contrast, GABA$_{A-Slow}$ IPSCs are insensitive to furosemide, are more likely to arise from dendritic synapses equipped with α_1-containing receptors, and may play a more important role in generating theta-rhythm (approximately 8 Hz) oscillations.

Although GABA is the principal transmitter released at all of the synapses considered above, some are also thought to release peptides from dense-core vesicles. Basket cells contain either cholecystokinin (CCK) or parvalbumin but not both. Although little is known about differences in the physiology of the synapses supplied by these two cell types, only cholecystokinin-positive neurons appear to express CB1 cannabinoid receptors (Marsicano and Lutz, 1999; Tsou et al., 1999). The evidence for a synaptic role for cholecystokinin and other neuro-active peptides such as somatostatin, CCK, and substance P is scanty.

In contrast to most glutamatergic synapses, most GABAergic synapses show marked depression with repetitive activity at moderate frequencies (Thomson, 2000). This may reflect a high baseline release probability, but the presence of Ca^{2+}-buffering proteins also attenuates the accumulation of

free Ca^{2+} with repeated action potential invasion (Caillard et al., 2000). Another phenomenon that may underlie differences in use-dependent plasticity is that some GABAergic synapses rely exclusively on either N- or P/Q-type Ca^{2+} channels to trigger transmitter release (Poncer et al., 1997; Wilson et al., 2001) in contrast to glutamatergic synapses, which tend to use a mixture of both types. Because N-type channels tend to inactivate more rapidly and are a more sensitive to G protein-mediated inhibition (Zhang et al., 1996), it is tempting to speculate that synapses relying on this Ca^{2+} channel subtype depress more readily.

Although GABAergic IPSCs evoked by a single basket cell are generally multiquantal (Edwards et al., 1990), this probably reflects the numerous synapses made by a single neuron (Kraushaar and Jonas, 2000). The number of vesicles released at a single synapse is not known with certainty. Evidence exists for multivesicular release at some cerebellar GABAergic synapses (Auger et al., 1998), but whether this also holds for hippocampal synapses is not known. Because the occupancy of postsynaptic GABA$_A$ receptors following release of a single vesicle may be greater than 50% (Perrais and Ropert, 1999), it cannot be inferred that release of two vesicles gives rise to a response twice as large.

GABAergic synapses in the hippocampus show a different profile of modulation by presynaptic receptors than most glutamatergic synapses. Thus, μ opioid receptors depress GABA release relatively selectively (Simmons and Chavkin, 1996). Cannabinoid receptors have a similar effect at some basket cell synapses (Katona et al., 1999; Hoffman and Lupica, 2000) and mediate an unusual form of short-term depression triggered by Ca^{2+} transients in postsynaptic pyramidal neurons (Ohno-Shosaku et al., 2001; Wilson and Nicoll, 2001). Because the CB1 cannabinoid receptors mediating this phenomenon are apparently restricted to CCK-positive basket cells, this form of retrograde signaling could exert a powerful disinhibitory effect. Moreover, it could relatively selectively interfere with rhythmogenesis, possibly contributing to the cognitive and hallucinatory effects of exogenous cannabinoid agonists.

In contrast to glutamatergic synapses, GABA release is relatively resistant to adenosine (Yoon and Rothman, 1991; Lambert and Wilson, 1993). Surprisingly, GABAergic synapses on interneurons are as sensitive to group III metabotropic glutamate agonists as glutamatergic synapses (Semyanov and Kullmann, 2000) even though only the latter actually release the endogenous agonist. GABAergic transmission to pyramidal neurons, however, is relatively insensitive to group III agonists, mirroring the lack of sensitivity of Schaffer collateral synapses on pyramidal neurons. Thus, the expression of presynaptic group III receptors appears to be determined in large part by the target cell identity. The presence of these receptors on GABA-releasing synapses is difficult to explain unless they have evolved to detect glutamate released from neighboring synapses. Evidence that glutamate spillover modulates inhibition via these receptors has been reported (Semyanov and Kullmann, 2000).

There is relatively little evidence for long-term use-dependent plasticity at GABAergic synapses akin to long-term potentiation (see Chapter 10). However, some manipulations in neuronal cultures can enhance the surface expression of $GABA_A$ receptors (Wan et al., 1997), underlining the importance of this phenomenon for the development of synapses, if not their regulation in adults.

$GABA_A$ receptors in cerebellar granule cells can mediate a continuous current, a phenomenon known as "tonic" inhibition (to distinguish it from "phasic" inhibition represented by the occurrence of IPSCs) (Brickley et al., 1996; Wall and Usowicz, 1997). Tonic $GABA_A$ receptor-mediated inhibition also occurs in hippocampal granule cells (Overstreet and Westbrook, 2001; Stell and Mody, 2002). In the hippocampus proper, interneurons appear to express tonic inhibition relatively selectively, possibly reflecting a homeostatic role in regulating circuit excitability (Semyanov et al., 2003).

Inhibitory synapses are also made among interneurons. These synapses appear to show use-dependent depression similar to that seen at most GABAergic synapses on principal cells, although the kinetics of the IPSCs are generally faster (Bartos et al., 2001). Some parvalbumin-positive basket cells are also coupled by gap junctions (Fukuda and Kosaka, 2000). Genetic deletion of connexion 36 perturbs γ frequency oscillations, possibly because of impaired electrical coupling among these interneurons (Hormuzdi et al., 2001).

6.7 Unresolved Issues

There are numerous unresolved issues surrounding synaptic function that cannot be listed completely here. Many are fundamental questions concerning transmitter release, such as the mechanisms by which synaptotagmin transduces the Ca^{2+} surge to trigger exocytosis, how the degree of filling of a vesicle affects its readiness for release, and whether and under what conditions exocytosis can take place via a fusion pore. Other important questions concern postsynaptic mechanisms. Some of these questions, such as the targeting and clustering of glutamate receptors at synapses, have attracted intense interest because of their potential role in the development and plasticity of excitatory transmission. They are taken up in greater detail in Chapter 7. Other areas, such as the detailed postsynaptic signaling cascades, leading to effects as remote as nuclear transcription, are discussed, in the context of LTP, in Chapter 10.

As in so many areas of neuroscience, insights at a molecular level are outpacing progress at a more macroscopic level. It is some of these areas that ultimately may require major breakthroughs to relate the mechanisms of synaptic function to the function of the network as a whole. For instance, although the involvement of cholinergic mechanisms in theta rhythms is on a relatively secure footing, this understanding remains at a qualitative level. Many critical parameters remain far from established: What is the temporal profile of acetylcholine release? Where are the target receptors in relation to the sites of release? How many individual terminals cooperate to activate muscarinic and nicotinic receptors? Which of the numerous actions of these receptors actually take place in vivo?

Similar questions occur for each of the other neurotransmitters described here. Most of this chapter has concentrated on the fast ionotropic signaling by glutamate and GABA; this is because, to a great extent, electrophysiological methods are so powerful in detecting and quantifying EPSP/Cs and IPSP/Cs. More diffuse types of signaling mediated by metabotropic receptors or even by extrasynaptic actions at ionotropic receptors may be of similar or even greater importance for understanding the roles of these transmitters in intercellular signaling. As for the monoamines and peptides, they are considered less important only on the grounds that the releasing axons are relatively sparse. However, not until their actions have been put on a sound quantitative footing similar to that of the amino acid neurotransmitters will it be possible to know if this ranking is correct.

ACKNOWLEDGMENTS

My thanks to the editors, in particular Per Andersen, for helpful input to this chapter.

REFERENCES

Acsady L, Kamondi A, Sik A, Freund T, Buzsaki G (1998) GABAergic cells are the major postsynaptic targets of mossy fibers in the rat hippocampus. *J Neurosci* 18:3386–3403.

Agnati LF, Zoli M, Stromberg I, Fuxe K (1995) Intercellular communication in the brain: wiring versus volume transmission. *Neuroscience* 69:711–726.

Albe-Fessard D, Buser P (1955) Intracellular activities collected in the sigmoid cortex of the cat; participation of the pyramidal neurons in the somesthetic evoked potential. *J Physiol (Paris)* 47:67–69.

Albuquerque EX, Alkondon M, Pereira EF, Castro NG, Schrattenholz A, Barbosa CT, Bonfante-Cabarcas R, Aracava Y, Eisenberg HM, Maelicke A (1997) Properties of neuronal nicotinic acetylcholine receptors: pharmacological characterization and modulation of synaptic function. *J Pharmacol Exp Ther* 280:1117–1136.

Alle H, Jonas P, Geiger JR (2001) PTP and LTP at a hippocampal mossy fiber–interneuron synapse. *Proc Natl Acad Sci USA* 98:14708–14713.

Amaral DG, Dent JA (1981) Development of the mossy fibers of the dentate gyrus. I. A light and electron microscopic study of the mossy fibers and their expansions. *J Comp Neurol* 195:51–86.

Andersen P, Eccles JC, Loyning Y (1964) Pathway of postsynaptic inhibition in the hippocampus. *J Neurophysiol* 27:608–619.

Andersen P, Blackstad TW, Lomo T (1966) Location and identification of excitatory synapses on hippocampal pyramidal cells. *Exp Brain Res* 1:236–248.

Andersen P, Bliss TV, Skrede KK (1971) Unit analysis of hippocampal polulation spikes. *Exp Brain Res* 13:208–221.

Andersen P, Dingledine R, Gjerstad L, Langmoen IA, Laursen AM (1980a) Two different responses of hippocampal pyramidal cells to application of gamma-amino butyric acid. *J Physiol* 305:279–296.

Andersen P, Silfvenius H, Sundberg SH, Sveen O (1980b) A comparison of distal and proximal dendritic synapses on CA1 pyramids in guinea-pig hippocampal slices in vitro. *J Physiol* 307:273–299.

Andrade R, Malenka RC, Nicoll RA (1986) A G protein couples serotonin and $GABA_B$ receptors to the same channels in hippocampus. *Science* 234:1261–1265.

Anwyl R (1991) Modulation of vertebrate neuronal calcium channels by transmitters. *Brain Res Rev* 16:265–281.

Arnth-Jensen N, Jabaudon D, Scanziani M (2002) Cooperation between independent hippocampal synapses is controlled by glutamate uptake. *Nat Neurosci* 5:325–331.

Ascher P, Nowak L (1988) The role of divalent cations in the N-methyl-D-aspartate responses of mouse central neurones in culture. *J Physiol* 399:247–266.

Asztely F, Erdemli G, Kullmann DM (1997) Extrasynaptic glutamate spillover in the hippocampus: dependence on temperature and the role of active glutamate uptake. *Neuron* 18:281–293.

Auger C, Kondo S, Marty A (1998) Multivesicular release at single functional synaptic sites in cerebellar stellate and basket cells. *J Neurosci* 18:4532–4547.

Augustine GJ (2001) How does calcium trigger neurotransmitter release? *Curr Opin Neurobiol* 11:320–326.

Banke TG, Bowie D, Lee H, Huganir RL, Schousboe A, Traynelis SF (2000) Control of GluR1 AMPA receptor function by cAMP-dependent protein kinase. *J Neurosci* 20:89–102.

Banks MI, White JA, Pearce RA (2000) Interactions between distinct GABA(A) circuits in hippocampus. *Neuron* 25:449–457.

Baranano DE, Ferris CD, Snyder SH (2001) Atypical neural messengers. *Trends Neurosci* 24:99–106.

Barbour B (2001) An evaluation of synapse independence. *J Neurosci* 21:7969–7984.

Barnard EA, Skolnick P, Olsen RW, Mohler H, Sieghart W, Biggio G, Braestrup C, Bateson AN, Langer SZ (1998) International Union of Pharmacology. XV. Subtypes of gamma-aminobutyric acid A receptors: classification on the basis of subunit structure and receptor function. *Pharmacol Rev* 50:291–313.

Bartos M, Vida I, Frotscher M, Geiger JR, Jonas P (2001) Rapid signaling at inhibitory synapses in a dentate gyrus interneuron network. *J Neurosci* 21:2687–2698.

Baude A, Nusser Z, Roberts JD, Mulvihill E, McIlhinney RA, Somogyi P (1993) The metabotropic glutamate receptor (mGluR1 alpha) is concentrated at perisynaptic membrane of neuronal subpopulations as detected by immunogold reaction. *Neuron* 11:771–787.

Behrends JC, ten Bruggencate G (1993) Cholinergic modulation of synaptic inhibition in the guinea pig hippocampus in vitro: excitation of GABAergic interneurons and inhibition of GABA-release. *J Neurophysiol* 69:626–629.

Bekkers JM (1993) Enhancement by histamine of NMDA-mediated synaptic transmission in the hippocampus. *Science* 261:104–106.

Bekkers JM, Stevens CF (1989) NMDA and non-NMDA receptors are co-localized at individual excitatory synapses in cultured rat hippocampus. *Nature* 341:230–233.

Bellocchio EE, Reimer RJ, Fremeau RT Jr, Edwards RH (2000) Uptake of glutamate into synaptic vesicles by an inorganic phosphate transporter. *Science* 289:957–960.

Ben-Ari Y, Cossart R (2000) Kainate, a double agent that generates seizures: two decades of progress. *Trends Neurosci* 23:580–587.

Ben-Ari Y, Cherubini E, Corradetti R, Gaiarsa JL (1989) Giant synaptic potentials in immature rat CA3 hippocampal neurones. *J Physiol* 416:303–325.

Ben-Ari Y, Khazipov R, Leinekugel X, Caillard O, Gaiarsa JL (1997) $GABA_A$, NMDA and AMPA receptors: a developmentally regulated "menage a trois." *Trends Neurosci* 20:523–529.

Benedeczky I, Molnar E, Somogyi P (1994) The cisternal organelle as a Ca(2+)-storing compartment associated with GABAergic synapses in the axon initial segment of hippocampal pyramidal neurones. *Exp Brain Res* 101:216–230.

Benke TA, Jones OT, Collingridge GL, Angelides KJ (1993) N-Methyl-D-aspartate receptors are clustered and immobilized on dendrites of living cortical neurons. *Proc Natl Acad Sci USA* 90:7819–7823.

Bergles DE, Roberts JD, Somogyi P, Jahr CE (2000) Glutamatergic synapses on oligodendrocyte precursor cells in the hippocampus. *Nature* 405:187–191.

Berretta N, Berton F, Bianchi R, Capogna M, Francesconi W, Brunelli M (1990) Effects of dopamine, D-1 and D-2 dopaminergic agonists on the excitability of hippocampal CA1 pyramidal cells in guinea pig. *Exp Brain Res* 83:124–130.

Berzhanskaya J, Urban NN, Barrionuevo G (1998) Electrophysiological and pharmacological characterization of the direct perforant path input to hippocampal area CA3. *J Neurophysiol* 79:2111–2118.

Bi G, Poo M (2001) Synaptic modification by correlated activity: Hebb's postulate revisited. *Annu Rev Neurosci* 24:139–166.

Biscoe TJ, Straughan DW (1966) Micro-electrophoretic studies of neurones in the cat hippocampus. *J Physiol* 183:341–359.

Blackmer T, Larsen EC, Takahashi M, Martin TF, Alford S, Hamm HE (2001) G protein betagamma subunit-mediated presynaptic inhibition: regulation of eocytotic fusion downstream of Ca^{2+} entry. *Science* 292:293–297.

Bleakman D (1999) Kainate receptor pharmacology and physiology. *Cell Mol Life Sci* 56:558–566.

Blum R, Kafitz KW, Konnerth A (2002) Neurotrophin-evoked depolarization requires the sodium channel Na(V)1.9. *Nature* 419:687–693.

Bollmann JH, Sakmann B, Borst JG (2000) Calcium sensitivity of glutamate release in a calyx-type terminal. *Science* 289:953–957.

Bolshakov VY, Golan H, Kandel ER, Siegelbaum SA (1997)

Recruitment of new sites of synaptic transmission during the cAMP- dependent late phase of LTP at CA3-CA1 synapses in the hippocampus. *Neuron* 19:635–651.

Bolton MM, Blanpied TA, Ehlers MD (2000) Localization and stabilization of ionotropic glutamate receptors at synapses. *Cell Mol Life Sci* 57:1517–1525.

Bormann J (2000) The 'ABC' of GABA receptors. *Trends Pharmacol Sci* 21:16–19.

Borst JG, Sakmann B (1996) Calcium influx and transmitter release in a fast CNS synapse. *Nature* 383:431–434.

Bortolotto ZA, Clarke VR, Delany CM, Parry MC, Smolders I, Vignes M, Ho KH, Miu P, Brinton BT, Fantaske R, Ogden A, Gates M, Ornstein PL, Lodge D, Bleakman D, Collingridge GL (1999) Kainate receptors are involved in synaptic plasticity. *Nature* 402:297–301.

Bowie D, Mayer ML (1995) Inward rectification of both AMPA and kainate subtype glutamate receptors generated by polyamine-mediated ion channel block. *Neuron* 15:453–462.

Bracci E, Vreugdenhil M, Hack SP, Jefferys JG (2001) Dynamic modulation of excitation and inhibition during stimulation at gamma and beta frequencies in the CA1 hippocampal region. *J Neurophysiol* 85:2412–2422.

Brakeman PR, Lanahan AA, O'Brien R, Roche K, Barnes CA, Huganir RL, Worley PF (1997) Homer: a protein that selectively binds metabotropic glutamate receptors. *Nature* 386:284–288.

Breckenridge LJ, Almers W (1987) Final steps in exocytosis observed in a cell with giant secretory granules. *Proc Natl Acad Sci USA* 84:1945–1949.

Brenowitz S, Trussell LO (2001) Minimizing synaptic depression by control of release probability. *J Neurosci* 21:1857–1867.

Brickley SG, Cull-Candy SG, Farrant M (1996) Development of a tonic form of synaptic inhibition in rat cerebellar granule cells resulting from persistent activation of GABA_A receptors. *J Physiol (Lond)* 497:753–759.

Brown DA, Adams PR (1980) Muscarinic suppression of a novel voltage-sensitive K$^+$ current in a vertebrate neurone. *Nature* 283:673–676.

Bruns D, Jahn R (1995) Real-time measurement of transmitter release from single synaptic vesicles. *Nature* 377:62–65.

Caillard O, Moreno H, Schwaller B, Llano I, Celio MR, Marty A (2000) Role of the calcium-binding protein parvalbumin in short-term synaptic plasticity. *Proc Natl Acad Sci USA* 97:13372–13377.

Calabresi P, Pisani A, Centonze D, Bernardi G (1997) Synaptic plasticity and physiological interactions between dopamine and glutamate in the striatum. *Neurosci Biobehav Rev* 21:519–523.

Cammack JN, Rakhilin SV, Schwartz EA (1994) A GABA transporter operates asymmetrically and with variable stoichiometry. *Neuron* 13:949–960.

Capogna M, Gahwiler BH, Thompson SM (1996) Presynaptic inhibition of calcium-dependent and -independent release elicited with ionomycin, gadolinium, and alpha-latrotoxin in the hippocampus. *J Neurophysiol* 75:2017–2028.

Castillo PE, Janz R, Sudhof TC, Tzounopoulos T, Malenka RC, Nicoll RA (1997a) Rab3A is essential for mossy fibre long-term potentiation in the hippocampus. *Nature* 388:590–593.

Castillo PE, Malenka RC, Nicoll RA (1997b) Kainate receptors mediate a slow postsynaptic current in hippocampal CA3 neurons. *Nature* 388:182–186.

Catania MV, Tolle TR, Monyer H (1995) Differential expression of AMPA receptor subunits in NOS-positive neurons of cortex, striatum, and hippocampus. *J Neurosci* 15:7046–7061.

Chang Y, Wang R, Barot S, Weiss DS (1996) Stoichiometry of a recombinant GABA_A receptor. *J Neurosci* 16:5415–5424.

Chaudhry FA, Reimer RJ, Bellocchio EE, Danbolt NC, Osen KK, Edwards RH, Storm-Mathisen J (1998) The vesicular GABA transporter, VGAT, localizes to synaptic vesicles in sets of glycinergic as well as GABAergic neurons. *J Neurosci* 18: 9733–9750.

Chen YA, Scheller RH (2001) SNARE-mediated membrane fusion. *Nat Rev Mol Cell Biol* 2:98–106.

Chittajallu R, Vignes M, Dev KK, Barnes JM, Collingridge GL, Henley JM (1996) Regulation of glutamate release by presynaptic kainate receptors in the hippocampus. *Nature* 379:78–81.

Chittajallu R, Braithwaite SP, Clarke VR, Henley JM (1999) Kainate receptors: subunits, synaptic localization and function. *Trends Pharmacol Sci* 20:26–35.

Choi S, Klingauf J, Tsien RW (2000) Postfusional regulation of cleft glutamate concentration during LTP at 'silent synapses.' *Nat Neurosci* 3:330–336.

Chow RH, von Ruden L, Neher E (1992) Delay in vesicle fusion revealed by electrochemical monitoring of single secretory events in adrenal chromaffin cells. *Nature* 356:60–63.

Clements JD, Lester RA, Tong G, Jahr CE, Westbrook GL (1992) The time course of glutamate in the synaptic cleft. *Science* 258:1498–1501.

Colquhoun D, Jonas P, Sakmann B (1992) Action of brief pulses of glutamate on AMPA/kainate receptors in patches from different neurones of rat hippocampal slices. *J Physiol (Lond)* 458:261–287.

Contractor A, Swanson GT, Sailer A, O'Gorman S, Heinemann SF (2000) Identification of the kainate receptor subunits underlying modulation of excitatory synaptic transmission in the CA3 region of the hippocampus. *J Neurosci* 20:8269–8278.

Contractor A, Swanson G, Heinemann SF (2001) Kainate receptors are involved in short- and long-term plasticity at mossy fiber synapses in the hippocampus. *Neuron* 29:209–216.

Cossart R, Esclapez M, Hirsch JC, Bernard C, Ben-Ari Y (1998) GluR5 kainate receptor activation in interneurons increases tonic inhibition of pyramidal cells. *Nat Neurosci* 1:470–478.

Cossart R, Tyzio R, Dinocourt C, Esclapez M, Hirsch JC, Ben-Ari Y, Bernard C (2001) Presynaptic kainate receptors that enhance the release of GABA on CA1 hippocampal interneurons. *Neuron* 29:497–508.

Cossart R, Epsztein J, Tyzio R, Becq H, Hirsch J, Ben-Ari Y, Crepel V (2002) Quantal release of glutamate generates pure kainate and mixed AMPA/kainate EPSCs in hippocampal neurons. *Neuron* 35:147–159.

Cowan WM, Südhof TC, Stevens CF (eds) (2003) *Synapses.* Baltimore: Johns Hopkins University Press.

Cremona O, De Camilli P (1997) Synaptic vesicle endocytosis. *Curr Opin Neurobiol* 7:323–330.

Dahl D, Sarvey JM (1989) Norepinephrine induces pathway-specific long-lasting potentiation and depression in the hippocampal dentate gyrus. *Proc Natl Acad Sci USA* 86:4776–4780.

Danbolt NC (2001) Glutamate uptake. *Prog Neurobiol* 65:1–105.

Dani JA (2001) Overview of nicotinic receptors and their roles in the central nervous system. Biol Psychiatry 49:166–174.

Davies SN, Pertwee RG, Riedel G (2002) Functions of cannabinoid receptors in the hippocampus. *Neuropharmacology* 42:993–1007.

Derkach V, Barria A, Soderling TR (1999) Ca^{2+}/calmodulin-kinase II enhances channel conductance of alpha-amino-3- hydroxy-5-methyl-4-isoxazolepropionate type glutamate receptors. *Proc Natl Acad Sci USA* 96:3269–3274.

Destexhe A, Sejnowski TJ (1995) G protein activation kinetics and spillover of gamma-aminobutyric acid may account for differences between inhibitory responses in the hippocampus and thalamus. *Proc Natl Acad Sci USA* 92:9515–9519.

Diamond JS (2001) Neuronal glutamate transporters limit activation of NMDA receptors by neurotransmitter spillover on CA1 pyramidal cells. *J Neurosci* 21:8328–8338.

Diamond JS, Jahr CE (1997) Transporters buffer synaptically released glutamate on a submillisecond time scale. *J Neurosci* 17:4672–4687.

Dodge FA Jr, Rahamimoff R (1967) Co-operative action a calcium ions in transmitter release at the neuromuscular junction. *J Physiol* 193:419–432.

Dolphin AC (1998) Mechanisms of modulation of voltage-dependent calcium channels by G proteins. *J Physiol* 506:3–11.

Dolphin AC, Errington ML, Bliss TV (1982) Long-term potentiation of the perforant path in vivo is associated with increased glutamate release. *Nature* 297:496–498.

Donevan SD, Rogawski MA (1995) Intracellular polyamines mediate inward rectification of Ca(2+)- permeable alpha-amino-3-hydroxy-5-methyl-4-isoxazolepropionic acid receptors. *Proc Natl Acad Sci USA* 92:9298–9302.

Draguhn A, Verdorn TA, Ewert M, Seeburg PH, Sakmann B (1990) Functional and molecular distinction between recombinant rat GABAA receptor subtypes by Zn^{2+}. *Neuron* 5:781–788.

Dunlap K, Luebke JI, Turner TJ (1995) Exocytotic Ca^{2+} channels in mammalian central neurons. *Trends Neurosci* 18:89–98.

Durand GM, Kovalchuk Y, Konnerth A (1996) Long-term potentiation and functional synapse induction in developing hippocampus. *Nature* 381:71–75.

Edwards FA, Konnerth A, Sakmann B (1990) Quantal analysis of inhibitory synaptic transmission in the dentate gyrus of rat hippocampal slices: a patch-clamp study. *J Physiol* 430:213–249.

Eghbali M, Curmi JP, Birnir B, Gage PW (1997) Hippocampal GABA(A) channel conductance increased by diazepam. Nature 388:71–75.

Emptage N, Bliss TV, Fine A (1999) Single synaptic events evoke NMDA receptor-mediated release of calcium from internal stores in hippocampal dendritic spines. *Neuron* 22:115–124.

Essrich C, Lorez M, Benson JA, Fritschy JM, Luscher B (1998) Postsynaptic clustering of major GABAA receptor subtypes requires the gamma 2 subunit and gephyrin. *Nat Neurosci* 1:563–571.

Fabian-Fine R, Skehel P, Errington ML, Davies HA, Sher E, Stewart MG, Fine A (2001) Ultrastructural distribution of the alpha7 nicotinic acetylcholine receptor subunit in rat hippocampus. *J Neurosci* 21:7993–8003.

Fagni L, Chavis P, Ango F, Bockaert J (2000) Complex interactions between mGluRs, intracellular Ca^{2+} stores and ion channels in neurons. *Trends Neurosci* 23:80–88.

Farrar SJ, Whiting PJ, Bonnert TP, McKernan RM (1999) Stoichiometry of a ligand-gated ion channel determined by fluorescence energy transfer. *J Biol Chem* 274:10100–10104.

Fernandez-Chacon R, Konigstorfer A, Gerber SH, Garcia J, Matos MF, Stevens CF, Brose N, Rizo J, Rosenmund C, Sudhof TC (2001) Synaptotagmin I functions as a calcium regulator of release probability. *Nature* 410:41–49.

Figenschou A, Hu GY, Storm JF (1996) Cholinergic modulation of the action potential in rat hippocampal neurons. *Eur J Neurosci* 8:211–219.

Fischer Y, Gahwiler BH, Thompson SM (1999) Activation of intrinsic hippocampal theta oscillations by acetylcholine in rat septo-hippocampal cocultures. *J Physiol* 519(Pt 2):405–413.

Forsythe ID, Westbrook GL (1988) Slow excitatory postsynaptic currents mediated by *N*-methyl-D-aspartate receptors on cultured mouse central neurones. *J Physiol (Lond)* 396:515–533.

Frederickson CJ, Suh SW, Silva D, Thompson RB (2000) Importance of zinc in the central nervous system: the zinc-containing neuron. *J Nutr* 130:1471S(1483S.

Frerking M, Nicoll RA (2000) Synaptic kainate receptors. *Curr Opin Neurobiol* 10:342–351.

Frerking M, Malenka RC, Nicoll RA (1998) Synaptic activation of kainate receptors on hippocampal interneurons. *Nat Neurosci* 1:479–486.

Fritschy JM, Meskenaite V, Weinmann O, Honer M, Benke D, Mohler H (1999) GABA$_B$-receptor splice variants GB1a and GB1b in rat brain: developmental regulation, cellular distribution and extrasynaptic localization. *Eur J Neurosci* 11:761–768.

Fukuda T, Kosaka T (2000) Gap junctions linking the dendritic network of GABAergic interneurons in the hippocampus. *J Neurosci* 20:1519–1528.

Fykse EM, Fonnum F (1996) Amino acid neurotransmission: dynamics of vesicular uptake. *Neurochem Res* 21:1053–1060.

Galarreta M, Hestrin S (1999) A network of fast-spiking cells in the neocortex connected by electrical synapses. *Nature* 402:72–75.

Garcia EP, Mehta S, Blair LA, Wells DG, Shang J, Fukushima T, Fallon JR, Garner CC, Marshall J (1998) SAP90 binds and clusters kainate receptors causing incomplete desensitization. *Neuron* 21:727–739.

Gasparini S, Saviane C, Voronin LL, Cherubini E (2000) Silent synapses in the developing hippocampus: lack of functional AMPA receptors or low probability of glutamate release? *Proc Natl Acad Sci USA* 97:9741–9746.

Geiger JR, Melcher T, Koh DS, Sakmann B, Seeburg PH, Jonas P, Monyer H (1995) Relative abundance of subunit mRNAs determines gating and Ca^{2+} permeability of AMPA receptors in principal neurons and interneurons in rat CNS. *Neuron* 15:193–204.

Geiger JR, Lubke J, Roth A, Frotscher M, Jonas P (1997) Submillisecond AMPA receptor-mediated signaling at a principal neuron–interneuron synapse. *Neuron* 18:1009–1023.

Geppert M, Goda Y, Hammer RE, Li C, Rosahl TW, Stevens CF, Sudhof TC (1994) Synaptotagmin I: a major Ca^{2+} sensor for transmitter release at a central synapse. *Cell* 79:717–727.

Gibb AJ, Colquhoun D (1992) Activation of *N*-methyl-D-aspartate receptors by L-glutamate in cells dissociated from adult rat hippocampus. *J Physiol (Lond)* 456:143–179.

Gibson JR, Beierlein M, Connors BW (1999) Two networks of electrically coupled inhibitory neurons in neocortex. *Nature* 402:75–79.

Gray EG (1959) Electron microscopy of synaptic contacts on dendrite spines of the cerebral cortex. *Nature* 183:1592–1593.

Gulyas AI, Miles R, Sik A, Toth K, Tamamaki N, Freund TF (1993) Hippocampal pyramidal cells excite inhibitory neurons through a single release site. *Nature* 366:683–687.

Gundersen V, Chaudhry FA, Bjaalie JG, Fonnum F, Ottersen OP, Storm-Mathisen J (1998) Synaptic vesicular localization and exocytosis of L-aspartate in excitatory nerve terminals: a quantitative immunogold analysis in rat hippocampus. *J Neurosci* 18:6059–6070.

Gutierrez R (2000) Seizures induce simultaneous GABAergic and glutamatergic transmission in the dentate gyrus–CA3 system. *J Neurophysiol* 84:3088–3090.

Haas HL, Konnerth A (1983) Histamine and noradrenaline decrease calcium-activated potassium conductance in hippocampal pyramidal cells. *Nature* 302:432–434.

Hajos N, Nusser Z, Rancz EA, Freund TF, Mody I (2000) Cell type- and synapse-specific variability in synaptic GABAA receptor occupancy. *Eur J Neurosci* 12:810–818.

Hardingham NR, Larkman AU (1998) Rapid report: the reliability of excitatory synaptic transmission in slices of rat visual cortex in vitro is temperature dependent. *J Physiol* 507:249–256.

Harris KM, Landis DM (1986) Membrane structure at synaptic junctions in area CA1 of the rat hippocampus. *Neuroscience* 19:857–872.

Harris KM, Sultan P (1995) Variation in the number, location and size of synaptic vesicles provides an anatomical basis for the nonuniform probability of release at hippocampal CA1 synapses. *Neuropharmacology* 34:1387–1395.

Hausser M, Major G, Stuart GJ (2001) Differential shunting of EPSPs by action potentials. *Science* 291:138–141.

Hefft S, Kraushaar U, Geiger JR, Jonas P (2002) Presynaptic short-term depression is maintained during regulation of transmitter release at a GABAergic synapse in rat hippocampus. *J Physiol* 539:201–208.

Henze DA, Urban NN, Barrionuevo G (2000) The multifarious hippocampal mossy fiber pathway: a review. *Neuroscience* 98:407–427.

Henze DA, Wittner L, Buzsaki G (2002) Single granule cells reliably discharge targets in the hippocampal CA3 network in vivo. *Nat Neurosci* 5:790–795.

Hessler NA, Shirke AM, Malinow R (1993) The probability of transmitter release at a mammalian central synapse. *Nature* 366:569–572.

Hestrin S, Nicoll RA, Perkel DJ, Sah P (1990) Analysis of excitatory synaptic action in pyramidal cells using whole-cell recording from rat hippocampal slices. *J Physiol (Lond)* 422:203–225.

Heuss C, Scanziani M, Gahwiler BH, Gerber U (1999) G-protein-independent signaling mediated by metabotropic glutamate receptors. *Nat Neurosci* 2:1070–1077.

Hille B (2001) *Ion channels of excitable membranes,* 3rd ed. Sunderland, MA: Sinauer.

Hjelmstad GO, Isaac JT, Nicoll RA, Malenka RC (1999) Lack of AMPA receptor desensitization during basal synaptic transmission in the hippocampal slice. *J Neurophysiol* 81:3096–3099.

Hoffman AF, Lupica CR (2000) Mechanisms of cannabinoid inhibition of GABA(A) synaptic transmission in the hippocampus. *J Neurosci* 20:2470–2479.

Hökfelt T, Johansson O, Ljungdahl A, Lundberg JM, Schultzberg M (1980) Peptidergic neurones. *Nature* 284:515–521.

Hollmann M, Heinemann S (1994) Cloned glutamate receptors. *Annu Rev Neurosci* 17:31–108.

Hollmann M, O'Shea-Greenfield A, Rogers SW, Heinemann S (1989) Cloning by functional expression of a member of the glutamate receptor family. *Nature* 342:643–648.

Hormuzdi SG, Pais I, LeBeau FE, Towers SK, Rozov A, Buhl EH, Whittington MA, Monyer H (2001) Impaired electrical signaling disrupts gamma frequency oscillations in connexin 36-deficient mice. *Neuron* 31:487–495.

Husi H, Ward MA, Choudhary JS, Blackstock WP, Grant SG (2000) Proteomic analysis of NMDA receptor(adhesion protein signaling complexes. *Nat Neurosci* 3:661–669.

Isaac JT, Nicoll RA, Malenka RC (1995) Evidence for silent synapses: implications for the expression of LTP. *Neuron* 15:427–434.

Isaacson JS, Solis JM, Nicoll RA (1993) Local and diffuse synaptic actions of GABA in the hippocampus. *Neuron* 10:165–175.

Jahn R, Lang T, Sudhof TC (2003) Membrane fusion. *Cell* 112:519–533.

Jahr CE (1992) High probability opening of NMDA receptor channels by L-glutamate. *Science* 255:470–472.

Jahr CE, Stevens CF (1987) Glutamate activates multiple single channel conductances in hippocampal neurons. *Nature* 325:522–525.

Jefferys JG (1995) Nonsynaptic modulation of neuronal activity in the brain: electric currents and extracellular ions. *Physiol Rev* 75:689–723.

Jiang L, Xu J, Nedergaard M, Kang J (2001) A kainate receptor increases the efficacy of GABAergic synapses. *Neuron* 30:503–513.

Johnson JW, Ascher P (1987) Glycine potentiates the NMDA response in cultured mouse brain neurons. *Nature* 325:529–531.

Johnston D, Magee JC, Colbert CM, Cristie BR (1996) Active properties of neuronal dendrites. *Annu Rev Neurosci* 19:165–186.

Jonas P, Major G, Sakmann B (1993) Quantal components of unitary EPSCs at the mossy fibre synapse on CA3 pyramidal cells of rat hippocampus. *J Physiol (Lond)* 472:615–663.

Jonas P, Racca C, Sakmann B, Seeburg PH, Monyer H (1994) Differences in Ca^{2+} permeability of AMPA-type glutamate receptor channels in neocortical neurons caused by differential GluR-B subunit expression. *Neuron* 12:1281–1289.

Jones KA, Borowsky B, Tamm JA, Craig DA, Durkin MM, Dai M, Yao WJ, Johnson M, Gunwaldsen C, Huang LY, Tang C, Shen Q, Salon JA, Morse K, Laz T, Smith KE, Nagarathnam D, Noble SA, Branchek TA, Gerald C (1998) GABA(B) receptors function as a heteromeric assembly of the subunits GABA(B)R1 and GABA(B)R2. *Nature* 396:674–679.

Jordan BA, Devi LA (1999) G-protein-coupled receptor heterodimerization modulates receptor function. *Nature* 399:697–700.

Kahle JS, Cotman CW (1989) Carbachol depresses synaptic responses in the medial but not the lateral perforant path. *Brain Res* 482:159–163.

Kaila K (1994) Ionic basis of GABA$_A$ receptor channel function in the nervous system. *Prog Neurobiol* 42:489–537.

Kaila K, Lamsa K, Smirnov S, Taira T, Voipio J (1997) Long-lasting GABA-mediated depolarization evoked by high-frequency stimulation in pyramidal neurons of rat hippocampal slice is attributable to a network-driven, bicarbonate-dependent K^+ transient. *J Neurosci* 17:7662–7672.

Kamboj SK, Swanson GT, Cull-Candy SG (1995) Intracellular spermine confers rectification on rat calcium-permeable AMPA and kainate receptors. *J Physiol* 486:297–303.

Kamiya H, Ozawa S (2000) Kainate receptor-mediated presynaptic inhibition at the mouse hippocampal mossy fibre synapse. *J Physiol (Lond)* 523(Pt 3):653–665.

Kamiya H, Zucker RS (1994) Residual Ca^{2+} and short-term synaptic plasticity. *Nature* 371:603–606.

Kamiya H, Shinozaki H, Yamamoto C (1996) Activation of metabotropic glutamate receptor type 2/3 suppresses transmission at rat hippocampal mossy fibre synapses. *J Physiol (Lond)* 493:447–455.

Kandel ER, Spencer WA (1961) Electrophysiology of hippocampal neurons. II. Afterpotentials and repetitive firing. *J Neurophysiol* 24:305–322.

Katona I, Sperlagh B, Sik A, Kafalvi A, Vizi ES, Mackie K, Freund TF (1999) Presynaptically located CB1 cannabinoid receptors regulate GABA release from axon terminals of specific hippocampal interneurons. *J Neurosci* 19:4544–4558.

Katz B (1969) *The release of neural transmitter substances.* Livepool, UK: Liverpool University Press.

Kavanaugh MP, Arriza JL, North RA, Amara SG (1992) Electrogenic uptake of gamma-aminobutyric acid by a cloned transporter expressed in *Xenopus* oocytes. *J Biol Chem* 267:22007–22009.

Keinanen K, Wisden W, Sommer B, Werner P, Herb A, Verdoorn TA, Sakmann B, Seeburg PH (1990) A family of AMPA-selective glutamate receptors. *Science* 249:556–560.

Kennedy MB (1997) The postsynaptic density at glutamatergic synapses. *Trends Neurosci* 20:264–268.

Kirov SA, Sorra KE, Harris KM (1999) Slices have more synapses than perfusion-fixed hippocampus from both young and mature rats. *J Neurosci* 19:2876–2886.

Klausberger T, Roberts JD, Somogyi P (2002) Cell type- and input-specific differences in the number and subtypes of synaptic GABA(A) receptors in the hippocampus. *J Neurosci* 22: 2513–2521.

Kleckner NW, Dingledine R (1988) Requirement for glycine in activation of NMDA-receptors expressed in *Xenopus* oocytes. *Science* 241:835–837.

Klingauf J, Neher E (1997) Modeling buffered Ca^{2+} diffusion near the membrane: implications for secretion in neuroendocrine cells. *Biophys J* 72:674–690.

Koester HJ, Sakmann B (2000) Calcium dynamics associated with action potentials in single nerve terminals of pyramidal cells in layer 2/3 of the young rat neocortex. *J Physiol* 529(Pt 3): 625–646.

Koh DS, Burnashev N, Jonas P (1995) Block of native $Ca(2+)$-permeable AMPA receptors in rat brain by intracellular polyamines generates double rectification. *J Physiol* 486:305–312.

Kotter R (1994) Postsynaptic integration of glutamatergic and dopaminergic signals in the striatum. *Prog Neurobiol* 44:163–196.

Kovalchuk Y, Eilers J, Lisman J, Konnerth A (2000) NMDA receptor-mediated subthreshold $Ca(2+)$ signals in spines of hippocampal neurons. *J Neurosci* 20:1791–1799.

Kraushaar U, Jonas P (2000) Efficacy and stability of quantal GABA release at a hippocampal interneuron–principal neuron synapse. *J Neurosci* 20:5594–5607.

Kullmann DM (1994) Amplitude fluctuations of dual-component EPSCs in hippocampal pyramidal cells: implications for long-term potentiation. *Neuron* 12:1111–1120.

Kullmann DM (1999) Excitatory synapses: neither too loud nor too quiet. *Nature* 399:111–112.

Kullmann DM (2001) Presynaptic kainate receptors in the hippocampus: slowly emerging from obscurity. *Neuron* 32: 561–564.

Kullmann DM (2003) Silent synapses: what are they telling us about long-term potentiation? *Philos Trans R Soc Lond B Biol Sci* 358:727–733.

Kullmann DM, Asztely F (1998) Extrasynaptic glutamate spillover in the hippocampus: evidence and implications. *Trends Neurosci* 21:8–14.

Kullmann DM, Nicoll RA (1992) Long-term potentiation is associated with increases in quantal content and quantal amplitude. *Nature* 357:240–244.

Kuner R, Kohr G, Grunewald S, Eisenhardt G, Bach A, Kornau HC (1999) Role of heteromer formation in $GABA_B$ receptor function. *Science* 283:74–77.

Kunishima N, Shimada Y, Tsuji Y, Sato T, Yamamoto M, Kumasaka T, Nakanishi S, Jingami H, Morikawa K (2000) Structural basis of glutamate recognition by a dimeric metabotropic glutamate receptor. *Nature* 407:971–977.

Laezza F, Doherty JJ, Dingledine R (1999) Long-term depression in hippocampal interneurons: joint requirement for pre- and postsynaptic events. *Science* 285:1411–1414.

Lambert NA, Wilson WA (1993) Heterogeneity in presynaptic regulation of GABA release from hippocampal inhibitory neurons. *Neuron* 11:1057–1067.

Lambolez B, Ropert N, Perrais D, Rossier J, Hestrin S (1996) Correlation between kinetics and RNA splicing of alpha-amino-3-hydroxy- 5-methylisoxazole-4-propionic acid receptors in neocortical neurons. *Proc Natl Acad Sci USA* 93:1797–1802.

Lanthorn TH, Ganong AH, Cotman CW (1984) 2-Amino-4-phosphonobutyrate selectively blocks mossy fiber-CA3 responses in guinea pig but not rat hippocampus. *Brain Res* 290:174–178.

Larkum ME, Zhu JJ, Sakmann B (1999) A new cellular mechanism for coupling inputs arriving at different cortical layers. *Nature* 398:338–341.

Laube B, Hirai H, Sturgess M, Betz H, Kuhse J (1997) Molecular determinants of agonist discrimination by NMDA receptor subunits: analysis of the glutamate binding site on the NR2B subunit. *Neuron* 18:493–503.

Lauri SE, Bortolotto ZA, Bleakman D, Ornstein PL, Lodge D, Isaac JT, Collingridge GL (2001) A critical role of a facilitatory presynaptic kainate receptor in mossy fiber LTP. *Neuron* 32:697–709.

Lehre KP, Levy LM, Ottersen OP, Storm-Mathisen J, Danbolt NC (1995) Differential expression of two glial glutamate transporters in the rat brain: quantitative and immunocytochemical observations. *J Neurosci* 15:1835–1853.

Lei S, McBain CJ (2002) Distinct NMDA receptors provide differential modes of transmission at mossy fiber–interneuron synapses. *Neuron* 33:921–933.

Lerma J, Morales M, Vicente MA, Herreras O (1997) Glutamate receptors of the kainate type and synaptic transmission. *Trends Neurosci* 20:9–12.

Lerma J, Paternain AV, Rodriguez-Moreno A, Lopez-Garcia JC (2001) Molecular physiology of kainate receptors. *Physiol Rev* 81:971–998.

Lester RA, Clements JD, Westbrook GL, Jahr CE (1990) Channel kinetics determine the time course of NMDA receptor-mediated synaptic currents. *Nature* 346:565–567.

Liao D, Hessler NA, Malinow R (1995) Activation of postsynaptically silent synapses during pairing-induced LTP in CA1 region of hippocampal slice. *Nature* 375:400–404.

Lin RC, Scheller RH (2000) Mechanisms of synaptic vesicle exocytosis. *Annu Rev Cell Dev Biol* 16:19–49.

Lisman JE (1997) Bursts as a unit of neural information: making unreliable synapses reliable. *Trends Neurosci* 20:38–43.

Lozovaya NA, Kopanitsa MV, Boychuk YA, Krishtal OA (1999)

Enhancement of glutamate release uncovers spillover-mediated transmission by *N*-methyl-D-aspartate receptors in the rat hippocampus. *Neuroscience* 91:1321–1330.

Lu YM, Mansuy IM, Kandel ER, Roder J (2000) Calcineurin-mediated LTD of GABAergic inhibition underlies the increased excitability of CA1 neurons associated with LTP. *Neuron* 26:197–205.

Luscher C, Jan LY, Stoffel M, Malenka RC, Nicoll RA (1997) G protein-coupled inwardly rectifying K⁺ channels (GIRKs) mediate postsynaptic but not presynaptic transmitter actions in hippocampal neurons. *Neuron* 19:687–695. Erratum: *Neuron* 1997;19;following 945.

Maccaferri G, Toth K, McBain CJ (1998) Target-specific expression of presynaptic mossy fiber plasticity. *Science* 279:1368–1370.

Maccaferri G, Roberts JD, Szucs P, Cottingham CA, Somogyi P (2000) Cell surface domain specific postsynaptic currents evoked by identified GABAergic neurones in rat hippocampus in vitro. *J Physiol* 524(Pt 1):91–116.

MacDermott AB, Role LW, Siegelbaum SA (1999) Presynaptic ionotropic receptors and the control of transmitter release. *Annu Rev Neurosci* 22:443–485.

Macek TA, Winder DG, Gereau RWt, Ladd CO, Conn PJ (1996) Differential involvement of group II and group III mGluRs as autoreceptors at lateral and medial perforant path synapses. *J Neurophysiol* 76:3798–3806.

Madison DV, Nicoll RA (1982) Noradrenaline blocks accommodation of pyramidal cell discharge in the hippocampus. *Nature* 299:636–638.

Madison DV, Nicoll RA (1984) Control of the repetitive discharge of rat CA 1 pyramidal neurones in vitro. *J Physiol* 354:319–331.

Magee JC, Cook EP (2000) Somatic EPSP amplitude is independent of synapse location in hippocampal pyramidal neurons. *Nat Neurosci* 3:895–903.

Mainen ZF, Malinow R, Svoboda K (1999) Synaptic calcium transients in single spines indicate that NMDA receptors are not saturated. *Nature* 399:151–155.

Manabe T, Renner P, Nicoll RA (1992) Postsynaptic contribution to long-term potentiation revealed by the analysis of miniature synaptic currents. *Nature* 355:50–55.

Markram H, Tsodyks M (1996) Redistribution of synaptic efficacy between neocortical pyramidal neurons. *Nature* 382:807–810.

Marsicano G, Lutz B (1999) Expression of the cannabinoid receptor CB1 in distinct neuronal subpopulations in the adult mouse forebrain. *Eur J Neurosci* 11:4213–4225.

Mathews GC, Diamond JS (2003) Neuronal glutamate uptake contributes to GABA synthesis and inhibitory synaptic strength. *J Neurosci* 23:2040–2048.

Mayer ML, Westbrook GL, Guthrie PB (1984) Voltage-dependent block by Mg²⁺ of NMDA responses in spinal cord neurones. *Nature* 309:261–263.

McBain CJ, Mayer ML (1994) *N*-Methyl-D-aspartic acid receptor structure and function. *Physiol Rev* 74:723–760.

McGehee DS, Heath MJ, Gelber S, Devay P, Role LW (1995) Nicotine enhancement of fast excitatory synaptic transmission in CNS by presynaptic receptors. *Science* 269:1692–1696.

McIntire SL, Reimer RJ, Schuske K, Edwards RH, Jorgensen EM (1997) Identification and characterization of the vesicular GABA transporter. *Nature* 389:870–876.

McMahon LL, Kauer JA (1997) Hippocampal interneurons express a novel form of synaptic plasticity. *Neuron* 18:295–305.

McNaughton BL (1980) Evidence for two physiologically distinct perforant pathways to the fascia dentata. *Brain Res* 199:1–19.

Mehta AK, Ticku MK (1999) An update on GABA_A receptors. *Brain Res Brain Res Rev* 29:196–217.

Min MY, Asztely F, Kokaia M, Kullmann DM (1998a) Long-term potentiation and dual-component quantal signaling in the dentate gyrus. *Proc Natl Acad Sci USA* 95:4702–4707.

Min MY, Rusakov DA, Kullmann DM (1998b) Activation of AMPA, kainate, and metabotropic receptors at hippocampal mossy fiber synapses: role of glutamate diffusion. *Neuron* 21:561–570.

Mintz IM, Bean BP (1993) GABAB receptor inhibition of P-type Ca²⁺ channels in central neurons. *Neuron* 10:889–898.

Misgeld U, Bijak M, Jarolimek W (1995) A physiological role for GABA_B receptors and the effects of baclofen in the mammalian central nervous system. *Prog Neurobiol* 46:423–462.

Monaghan DT, Holets VR, Toy DW, Cotman CW (1983) Anatomical distributions of four pharmacologically distinct ³H-L- glutamate binding sites. *Nature* 306:176–179.

Mori M, Heuss C, Gahwiler BH, Gerber U (2001) Fast synaptic transmission mediated by P2X receptors in CA3 pyramidal cells of rat hippocampal slice cultures. *J Physiol* 535:115–123.

Mori M, Gahwiler BH, Gerber U (2002) Beta-alanine and taurine as endogenous agonists at glycine receptors in rat hippocampus in vitro. *J Physiol* 539:191–200.

Mosbacher J, Schoepfer R, Monyer H, Burnashev N, Seeburg PH, Ruppersberg JP (1994) A molecular determinant for submillisecond desensitization in glutamate receptors. *Science* 266:1059–1062.

Mulle C, Sailer A, Perez-Otano I, Dickinson-Anson H, Castillo PE, Bureau I, Maron C, Gage FH, Mann JR, Bettler B, Heinemann SF (1998) Altered synaptic physiology and reduced susceptibility to kainate- induced seizures in GluR6-deficient mice. *Nature* 392:601–605.

Mulle C, Sailer A, Swanson GT, Brana C, O'Gorman S, Bettler B, Heinemann SF (2000) Subunit composition of kainate receptors in hippocampal interneurons. *Neuron* 28:475–484.

Murthy VN, Stevens CF (1998) Synaptic vesicles retain their identity through the endocytic cycle. *Nature* 392:497–501.

Murthy VN, Stevens CF (1999) Reversal of synaptic vesicle docking at central synapses. *Nat Neurosci* 2:503–507.

Nadler JV, Martin D, Bustos GA, Burke SP, Bowe MA (1990) Regulation of glutamate and aspartate release from the Schaffer collaterals and other projections of CA3 hippocampal pyramidal cells. *Prog Brain Res* 83:115–130.

Nakanishi S, Nakajima Y, Masu M, Ueda Y, Nakahara K, Watanabe D, Yamaguchi S, Kawabata S, Okada M (1998) Glutamate receptors: brain function and signal transduction. *Brain Res Brain Res Rev* 26:230–235.

Nicoll RA, Malenka RC, Kauer JA (1990) Functional comparison of neurotransmitter receptor subtypes in mammalian central nervous system. *Physiol Rev* 70:513–565.

Nowak L, Bregestovski P, Ascher P, Herbet A, Prochiantz A (1984) Magnesium gates glutamate-activated channels in mouse central neurones. *Nature* 307:462–465.

Nusser Z, Mody I (2002) Selective modulation of tonic and phasic inhibitions in dentate gyrus granule cells. *J Neurophysiol* 87:2624–2628.

Nusser Z, Sieghart W, Benke D, Fritschy JM, Somogyi P (1996) Differential synaptic localization of two major gamma-aminobutyric acid type A receptor alpha subunits on hippocampal pyramidal cells. *Proc Natl Acad Sci USA* 93: 11939–11944.

Nusser Z, Lujan R, Laube G, Roberts JD, Molnar E, Somogyi P (1998) Cell type and pathway dependence of synaptic AMPA receptor number and variability in the hippocampus. *Neuron* 21:545–559.

Oertner TG, Sabatini BL, Nimchinsky EA, Svoboda K (2002) Facilitation at single synapses probed with optical quantal analysis. *Nat Neurosci* 5:657–664.

Ohno-Shosaku T, Maejima T, Kano M (2001) Endogenous cannabinoids mediate retrograde signals from depolarized postsynaptic neurons to presynaptic terminals. *Neuron* 29:729–738.

Otmakhova NA, Lisman JE (1999) Dopamine selectively inhibits the direct cortical pathway to the CA1 hippocampal region. *J Neurosci* 19:1437–1445.

Otmakhov N, Shirke AM, Malinow R (1993) Measuring the impact of probabilistic transmission on neuronal output. *Neuron* 10:1101–1111.

Otmakhova NA, Otmakhov N, Lisman JE (2002) Pathway-specific properties of AMPA and NMDA-mediated transmission in CA1 hippocampal pyramidal cells. *J Neurosci* 22:1199–1207.

Ottersen OP, Storm-Mathisen J, Bramham C, Torp R, Laake J, Gundersen V (1990) A quantitative electron microscopic immunocytochemical study of the distribution and synaptic handling of glutamate in rat hippocampus. *Prog Brain Res* 83:99–114.

Overstreet LS, Westbrook GL (2001) Paradoxical reduction of synaptic inhibition by vigabatrin. *J Neurophysiol* 86:596–603.

Ozawa S, Kamiya H, Tsuzuki K (1998) Glutamate receptors in the mammalian central nervous system. *Prog Neurobiol* 54:581–618.

Pankratov Y, Castro E, Miras-Portugal MT, Krishtal O (1998) A purinergic component of the excitatory postsynaptic current mediated by P2X receptors in the CA1 neurons of the rat hippocampus. *Eur J Neurosci* 10:3898–3902.

Patneau DK, Mayer ML (1990) Structure-activity relationships for amino acid transmitter candidates acting at N-methyl-D-aspartate and quisqualate receptors. *J Neurosci* 10:2385–2399.

Pawelzik H, Bannister AP, Deuchars J, Ilia M, Thomson AM (1999) Modulation of bistratified cell IPSPs and basket cell IPSPs by pentobarbitone sodium, diazepam and Zn^{2+}: dual recordings in slices of adult rat hippocampus. *Eur J Neurosci* 11:3552–3564.

Pearce RA (1993) Physiological evidence for two distinct $GABA_A$ responses in rat hippocampus. *Neuron* 10:189–200.

Pedarzani P, Storm JF (1993) PKA mediates the effects of monoamine transmitters on the K^+ current underlying the slow spike frequency adaptation in hippocampal neurons. *Neuron* 11:1023–1035.

Pedarzani P, Storm JF (1996) Evidence that Ca/calmodulin-dependent protein kinase mediates the modulation of the Ca^{2+}-dependent K^+ current, IAHP, by acetylcholine, but not by glutamate, in hippocampal neurons. *Pflugers Arch* 431:723–728.

Perrais D, Ropert N (1999) Effect of zolpidem on miniature IPSCs and occupancy of postsynaptic $GABA_A$ receptors in central synapses. *J Neurosci* 19:578–588.

Perroy J, El Far O, Bertaso F, Pin JP, Betz H, Bockaert J, Fagni L (2002) PICK1 is required for the control of synaptic transmission by the metabotropic glutamate receptor 7. *EMBO J* 21:2990–2999.

Petralia RS, Esteban JA, Wang YX, Partridge JG, Zhao HM, Wenthold RJ, Malinow R (1999) Selective acquisition of AMPA receptors over postnatal development suggests a molecular basis for silent synapses. *Nat Neurosci* 2:31–36.

Pin JP, Duvoisin R (1995) The metabotropic glutamate receptors: structure and functions. *Neuropharmacology* 34:1–26.

Piomelli D (1994) Eicosanoids in synaptic transmission. *Crit Rev Neurobiol* 8:65–83.

Pitler TA, Alger BE (1992) Cholinergic excitation of GABAergic interneurons in the rat hippocampal slice. *J Physiol* 450:127–142.

Poncer JC, McKinney RA, Gahwiler BH, Thompson SM (1997) Either N- or P-type calcium channels mediate GABA release at distinct hippocampal inhibitory synapses. *Neuron* 18:463–472.

Porter JT, Cauli B, Tsuzuki K, Lambolez B, Rossier J, Audinat E (1999) Selective excitation of subtypes of neocortical interneurons by nicotinic receptors. *J Neurosci* 19:5228–5235.

Pouille F, Scanziani M (2001) Enforcement of temporal fidelity in pyramidal cells by somatic feed-forward inhibition. *Science* 293:1159–1163.

Raastad M (1995) Extracellular activation of unitary excitatory synapses between hippocampal CA3 and CA1 pyramidal cells. *Eur J Neurosci* 7:1882–1888.

Racca C, Stephenson FA, Streit P, Roberts JD, Somogyi P (2000) NMDA receptor content of synapses in stratum radiatum of the hippocampal CA1 area. *J Neurosci* 20:2512–2522.

Regehr WG, Delaney KR, Tank DW (1994) The role of presynaptic calcium in short-term enhancement at the hippocampal mossy fiber synapse. *J Neurosci* 14:523–537.

Renger JJ, Egles C, Liu G (2001) A developmental switch in neurotransmitter flux enhances synaptic efficacy by affecting AMPA receptor activation. *Neuron* 29:469–484.

Reyes A, Lujan R, Rozov A, Burnashev N, Somogyi P, Sakmann B (1998) Target-cell-specific facilitation and depression in neocortical circuits. *Nat Neurosci* 1:279–285.

Richerson GB, Wu Y (2003) Dynamic equilibrium of neurotransmitter transporters: not just for reuptake anymore. *J Neurophysiol* 90:1363–1374.

Rivera C, Voipio J, Payne JA, Ruusuvuori E, Lahtinen H, Lamsa K, Pirvola U, Saarma M, Kaila K (1999) The K^+/Cl^- co-transporter KCC2 renders GABA hyperpolarizing during neuronal maturation. *Nature* 397:251–255.

Rodriguez-Moreno A, Lerma J (1998) Kainate receptor modulation of GABA release involves a metabotropic function. *Neuron* 20:1211–1218.

Rodriguez-Moreno A, Herreras O, Lerma J (1997) Kainate receptors presynaptically downregulate GABAergic inhibition in the rat hippocampus. *Neuron* 19:893–901.

Rosahl TW, Spillane D, Missler M, Herz J, Selig DK, Wolff JR, Hammer RE, Malenka RC, Sudhof TC (1995) Essential functions of synapsins I and II in synaptic vesicle regulation. *Nature* 375:488–493.

Rosenmund C, Stevens CF (1996) Definition of the readily releasable pool of vesicles at hippocampal synapses. *Neuron* 16:1197–1207.

Rosenmund C, Clements JD, Westbrook GL (1993) Nonuniform probability of glutamate release at a hippocampal synapse. *Science* 262:754–757.

Rosenmund C, Feltz A, Westbrook GL (1995) Synaptic NMDA receptor channels have a low open probability. *J Neurosci* 15:2788–2795.

Rosenmund C, Stern-Bach Y, Stevens CF (1998) The tetrameric structure of a glutamate receptor channel. *Science* 280:1596–1599.

Rossi DJ, Oshima T, Attwell D (2000) Glutamate release in severe brain ischaemia is mainly by reversed uptake. *Nature* 403:316–321.

Rozov A, Burnashev N (1999) Polyamine-dependent facilitation of postsynaptic AMPA receptors counteracts paired-pulse depression. *Nature* 401:594–598.

Rozov A, Zilberter Y, Wollmuth LP, Burnashev N (1998) Facilitation of currents through rat Ca^{2+}-permeable AMPA receptor channels by activity-dependent relief from polyamine block. *J Physiol* 511:361–377.

Rudolph U, Crestani F, Benke D, Brunig I, Benson JA, Fritschy JM, Martin JR, Bluethmann H, Mohler H (1999) Benzodiazepine actions mediated by specific gamma-aminobutyric acid(A) receptor subtypes. *Nature* 401:796–800.

Rusakov DA, Kullmann DM (1998) Extrasynaptic glutamate diffusion in the hippocampus: ultrastructural constraints, uptake, and receptor activation. *J Neurosci* 18:3158–3170.

Rusakov DA, Harrison E, Stewart MG (1998) Synapses in hippocampus occupy only 1–2% of cell membranes and are spaced less than half-micron apart: a quantitative ultrastructural analysis with discussion of physiological implications. *Neuropharmacology* 37:513–521.

Sandler R, Smith AD (1991) Coexistence of GABA and glutamate in mossy fiber terminals of the primate hippocampus: an ultrastructural study. *J Comp Neurol* 303:177–192.

Scanziani M (2000) GABA spillover activates postsynaptic GABA(B) receptors to control rhythmic hippocampal activity. *Neuron* 25:673–681.

Scanziani M, Gahwiler BH, Thompson SM (1995) Presynaptic inhibition of excitatory synaptic transmission by muscarinic and metabotropic glutamate receptor activation in the hippocampus: are Ca^{2+} channels involved? *Neuropharmacology* 34:1549–1557.

Scanziani M, Salin PA, Vogt KE, Malenka RC, Nicoll RA (1997) Use-dependent increases in glutamate concentration activate presynaptic metabotropic glutamate receptors. *Nature* 385:630–634.

Scanziani M, Gahwiler BH, Charpak S (1998) Target cell-specific modulation of transmitter release at terminals from a single axon. *Proc Natl Acad Sci USA* 95:12004–12009.

Schell MJ, Molliver ME, Snyder SH (1995) D-Serine, an endogenous synaptic modulator: localization to astrocytes and glutamate-stimulated release. *Proc Natl Acad Sci USA* 92:3948–3952.

Schikorski T, Stevens CF (1997) Quantitative ultrastructural analysis of hippocampal excitatory synapses. *J Neurosci* 17:5858–5867.

Schmitz D, Mellor J, Nicoll RA (2001c) Presynaptic kainate receptor mediation of frequency facilitation at hippocampal mossy fiber synapses. *Science* 291:1972–1976.

Schmitz D, Mellor J, Frerking M, Nicoll RA (2001a) Presynaptic kainate receptors at hippocampal mossy fiber synapses. *Proc Natl Acad Sci USA* 98:11003–11008.

Schmitz D, Schuchmann S, Fisahn A, Draguhn A, Buhl EH, Petrasch-Parwez E, Dermietzel R, Heinemann U, Traub RD (2001b) Axo-axonal coupling. a novel mechanism for ultrafast neuronal communication. *Neuron* 31:831–840.

Schneggenburger R, Neher E (2000) Intracellular calcium dependence of transmitter release rates at a fast central synapse. *Nature* 406:889–893.

Schoepp DD (2002) Metabotropic glutamate receptors. *Pharmacol Biochem Behav* 73:285–286.

Schousboe A (2000) Pharmacological and functional characterization of astrocytic GABA transport: a short review. *Neurochem Res* 25:1241–1244.

Schwartzkroin PA (1975) Characteristics of CA1 neurons recorded intracellularly in the hippocampal in vitro slice preparation. *Brain Res* 85:423–436.

Sealfon SC, Olanow CW (2000) Dopamine receptors: from structure to behavior. *Trends Neurosci* 23:S34–S40.

Seeger T, Alzheimer C (2001) Muscarinic activation of inwardly rectifying K(+) conductance reduces EPSPs in rat hippocampal CA1 pyramidal cells. *J Physiol* 535:383–396.

Selyanko AA, Hadley JK, Wood IC, Abogadie FC, Delmas P, Buckley NJ, London B, Brown DA (1999) Two types of K(+) channel subunit, Erg1 and KCNQ2/3, contribute to the M-like current in a mammalian neuronal cell. *J Neurosci* 19:7742–7756.

Semyanov A, Kullmann DM (2000) Modulation of GABAergic signaling among interneurons by metabotropic glutamate receptors. *Neuron* 25:663–672.

Semyanov A, Kullmann DM (2001) Kainate receptor-dependent axonal depolarization and action potential initiation in interneurons. *Nat Neurosci* 4:718–723.

Semyanov A, Walker MC, Kullmann DM (2003) GABA uptake regulates cortical excitability via cell type-specific tonic inhibition. *Nat Neurosci* 6:484–490.

Sepkuty JP, Cohen AS, Eccles C, Rafiq A, Behar K, Ganel R, Coulter DA, Rothstein JD (2002) A neuronal glutamate transporter contributes to neurotransmitter GABA synthesis and epilepsy. *J Neurosci* 22:6372–6379.

Shapiro MS, Roche JP, Kaftan EJ, Cruzblanca H, Mackie K, Hille B (2000) Reconstitution of muscarinic modulation of the KCNQ2/KCNQ3 K(+) channels that underlie the neuronal M current. *J Neurosci* 20:1710–1721.

Sheng M, Sala C (2001) PDZ domains and the organization of supramolecular complexes. *Annu Rev Neurosci* 24:1–29.

Shepherd GM, Harris KM (1998) Three-dimensional structure and composition of CA3→CA1 axons in rat hippocampal slices: implications for presynaptic connectivity and compartmentalization. *J Neurosci* 18:8300–8310.

Shepherd GM, Raastad M, Andersen P (2002) General and variable features of varicosity spacing along unmyelinated axons in the hippocampus and cerebellum. *Proc Natl Acad Sci USA* 99:6340–6345.

Shi S, Hayashi Y, Esteban JA, Malinow R (2001) Subunit-specific rules governing AMPA receptor trafficking to synapses in hippocampal pyramidal neurons. *Cell* 105:331–343.

Shigemoto R, Kulik A, Roberts JD, Ohishi H, Nusser Z, Kaneko T, Somogyi P (1996) Target-cell-specific concentration of a metabotropic glutamate receptor in the presynaptic active zone. *Nature* 381:523–525.

Shigemoto R, Kinoshita A, Wada E, Nomura S, Ohishi H, Takada M, Flor PJ, Neki A, Abe T, Nakanishi S, Mizuno N (1997) Differential presynaptic localization of metabotropic glutamate receptor subtypes in the rat hippocampus. *J Neurosci* 17:7503–7522.

Simmons ML, Chavkin C (1996) Endogenous opioid regulation of hippocampal function. *Int Rev Neurobiol* 39:145–196.

Sloviter RS, Dichter MA, Rachinsky TL, Dean E, Goodman JH, Sollas AL, Martin DL (1996) Basal expression and induction of glutamate decarboxylase and GABA in excitatory granule cells of the rat and monkey hippocampal dentate gyrus. *J Comp Neurol* 373:593–618.

Smart TG, Xie X, Krishek BJ (1994) Modulation of inhibitory and excitatory amino acid receptor ion channels by zinc. *Prog Neurobiol* 42:393–341.

Soghomonian JJ, Martin DL (1998) Two isoforms of glutamate decarboxylase: why? *Trends Pharmacol Sci* 19:500–505.

Sommer B, Kohler M, Sprengel R, Seeburg PH (1991) RNA editing in brain controls a determinant of ion flow in glutamate-gated channels. *Cell* 67:11–19.

Sorra KE, Harris KM (1993) Occurrence and three-dimensional structure of multiple synapses between individual radiatum axons and their target pyramidal cells in hippocampal area CA1. *J Neurosci* 13:3736–3748.

Spacek J (1985) Three-dimensional analysis of dendritic spines. III. Glial sheath. *Anat Embryol* 171:245–252.

Spencer WA, Kandel ER (1961) Electrophysiology of hippocampal neurons. IV. Fast pre-potentials. *J Neurophysiol* 24:272–285.

Sperk G, Schwarzer C, Tsunashima K, Fuchs K, Sieghart W (1997) GABA(A) receptor subunits in the rat hippocampus. I. Immunocytochemical distribution of 13 subunits. *Neuroscience* 80:987–1000.

Spiridon M, Kamm D, Billups B, Mobbs P, Attwell D (1998) Modulation by zinc of the glutamate transporters in glial cells and cones isolated from the tiger salamander retina. *J Physiol* 506:363–376.

Staley KJ, Mody I (1992) Shunting of excitatory input to dentate gyrus granule cells by a depolarizing GABA$_A$ receptor-mediated postsynaptic conductance. *J Neurophysiol* 68:197–212.

Staley KJ, Soldo BL, Proctor WR (1995) Ionic mechanisms of neuronal excitation by inhibitory GABA$_A$ receptors. *Science* 269:977–981.

Stell BM, Mody I (2002) Receptors with different affinities mediate phasic and tonic GABA(A) conductances in hippocampal neurons. *J Neurosci* 22:RC223.

Stevens CF, Tsujimoto T (1995) Estimates for the pool size of releasable quanta at a single central synapse and for the time required to refill the pool. *Proc Natl Acad Sci USA* 92:846–849.

Steyer JA, Horstmann H, Almers W (1997) Transport, docking and exocytosis of single secretory granules in live chromaffin cells. *Nature* 388:474–478.

Storm-Mathisen J, Iversen LL (1979) Uptake of [^{3}H]glutamic acid in excitatory nerve endings: light and electron microscopic observations in the hippocampal formation of the rat. *Neuroscience* 4:1237–1253.

Stuart GJ, Hausser M (2001) Dendritic coincidence detection of EPSPs and action potentials. *Nat Neurosci* 4:63–71.

Study RE, Barker JL (1981) Diazepam and (−)-pentobarbital: fluctuation analysis reveals different mechanisms for potentiation of gamma-aminobutyric acid responses in cultured central neurons. *Proc Natl Acad Sci USA* 78:7180–7184.

Sudhof TC (2004) The synaptic vesicle cycle. *Annu Rev Neurosci* 27:509–547.

Suh B, Hille B (2002) Recovery from muscarinic modulation of m current channels requires phosphatidylinositol 4,5-bisphosphate synthesis. *Neuron* 35:507.

Sundstrom-Poromaa I, Smith DH, Gong QH, Sabado TN, Li X, Light A, Wiedmann M, Williams K, Smith SS (2002) Hormonally regulated alpha(4)beta(2)delta GABA(A) receptors are a target for alcohol. *Nat Neurosci* 5:721–722.

Swanson GT, Kamboj SK, Cull-Candy SG (1997) Single-channel properties of recombinant AMPA receptors depend on RNA editing, splice variation, and subunit composition. *J Neurosci* 17:58–69.

Szerb JC (1988) Changes in the relative amounts of aspartate and glutamate released and retained in hippocampal slices during stimulation. *J Neurochem* 50:219–224.

Takamori S, Rhee JS, Rosenmund C, Jahn R (2000) Identification of a vesicular glutamate transporter that defines a glutamatergic phenotype in neurons. *Nature* 407:189–194.

Takumi Y, Bergersen L, Landsend AS, Rinvik E, Ottersen OP (1998) Synaptic arrangement of glutamate receptors. *Prog Brain Res* 116:105–121.

Takumi Y, Ramirez-Leon V, Laake P, Rinvik E, Ottersen OP (1999) Different modes of expression of AMPA and NMDA receptors in hippocampal synapses. *Nat Neurosci* 2:618–624.

Tang Y, Zucker RS (1997) Mitochondrial involvement in post-tetanic potentiation of synaptic transmission. *Neuron* 18:483–491.

Thomson AM (2000) Facilitation, augmentation and potentiation at central synapses. *Trends Neurosci* 23:305–312.

Toth K, McBain CJ (1998) Afferent-specific innervation of two distinct AMPA receptor subtypes on single hippocampal interneurons. *Nat Neurosci* 1:572–578.

Toth K, Suares G, Lawrence JJ, Philips-Tansey E, McBain CJ (2000) Differential mechanisms of transmission at three types of mossy fiber synapse. *J Neurosci* 20:8279–8289.

Trommald M, Hulleberg G (1997) Dimensions and density of dendritic spines from rat dentate granule cells based on reconstructions from serial electron micrographs. *J Comp Neurol* 377:15–28.

Tsou K, Mackie K, Sanudo-Pena MC, Walker JM (1999) Cannabinoid CB1 receptors are localized primarily on cholecystokinin-containing GABAergic interneurons in the rat hippocampal formation. *Neuroscience* 93:969–975.

Tzounopoulos T, Janz R, Sudhof TC, Nicoll RA, Malenka RC (1998) A role for cAMP in long-term depression at hippocampal mossy fiber synapses. *Neuron* 21:837–845.

Ventura R, Harris KM (1999) Three-dimensional relationships between hippocampal synapses and astrocytes. *J Neurosci* 19:6897–6906.

Vignes M, Collingridge GL (1997) The synaptic activation of kainate receptors. *Nature* 388:179–182.

Vignes M, Clarke VR, Parry MJ, Bleakman D, Lodge D, Ornstein PL, Collingridge GL (1998) The GluR5 subtype of kainate receptor regulates excitatory synaptic transmission in areas CA1 and CA3 of the rat hippocampus. *Neuropharmacology* 37:1269–1277.

Vogt KE, Nicoll RA (1999) Glutamate and gamma-aminobutyric acid mediate a heterosynaptic depression at mossy fiber synapses in the hippocampus. *Proc Natl Acad Sci USA* 96:1118–1122.

Vogt K, Mellor J, Tong G, Nicoll R (2000) The actions of synaptically released zinc at hippocampal mossy fiber synapses. *Neuron* 26:187–196.

Wafford KA, Thompson SA, Thomas D, Sikela J, Wilcox AS, Whiting PJ (1996) Functional characterization of human gamma-aminobutyric acid A receptors containing the alpha 4 subunit. *Mol Pharmacol* 50:670–678.

Wahl LM, Pouzat C, Stratford KJ (1996) Monte Carlo simulation of fast excitatory synaptic transmission at a hippocampal synapse. *J Neurophysiol* 75:597–608.

Walker MC, Galley PT, Errington ML, Shorvon SD, Jefferys JG (1995) Ascorbate and glutamate release in the rat hippocampus after perforant path stimulation: a "dialysis electrode" study. *J Neurochem* 65:725–731.

Walker MC, Ruiz A, Kullmann DM (2001) Monosynaptic GABAergic signaling from dentate to CA3 with a pharmacological and physiological profile typical of mossy fiber synapses. *Neuron* 29:703–715.

Wall MJ, Usowicz MM (1997) Development of action potential-dependent and independent spontaneous GABA$_A$ receptor-mediated currents in granule cells of postnatal rat cerebellum. *Eur J Neurosci* 9:533–548.

Wan Q, Xiong ZG, Man HY, Ackerley CA, Braunton J, Lu WY, Becker LE, MacDonald JF, Wang YT (1997) Recruitment of functional GABA(A) receptors to postsynaptic domains by insulin. *Nature* 388:686–690.

Wang HS, Pan Z, Shi W, Brown BS, Wymore RS, Cohen IS, Dixon JE, McKinnon D (1998) KCNQ2 and KCNQ3 potassium channel subunits: molecular correlates of the M-channel. *Science* 282: 1890–1893.

Watkins JC, Evans RH (1981) Excitatory amino acid transmitters. *Annu Rev Pharmacol Toxicol* 21:165–204.

Weisskopf MG, Zalutsky RA, Nicoll RA (1993) The opioid peptide dynorphin mediates heterosynaptic depression of hippocampal mossy fibre synapses and modulates long-term potentiation. *Nature* 362:423–427.

Wenthold RJ, Petralia RS, Blahos J, II, Niedzielski AS (1996) Evidence for multiple AMPA receptor complexes in hippocampal CA1/CA2 neurons. *J Neurosci* 16:1982–1989.

Westrum LE, Blackstad TW (1962) An electron microscopic study of the stratum radiatum of the rat hippocampus (regio superior CA1) with particular emphasis on synaptology. *J Comp Neurol* 119:281–309.

Whiting PJ, Bonnert TP, McKernan RM, Farrar S, Le Bourdelles B, Heavens RP, Smith DW, Hewson L, Rigby MR, Sirinathsinghji DJ, Thompson SA, Wafford KA (1999) Molecular and functional diversity of the expanding GABA-A receptor gene family. *Ann NY Acad Sci* 868:645–653.

Wigstrom H, Gustafsson B (1986) Postsynaptic control of hippocampal long-term potentiation. *J Physiol* 81:228–236.

Wilson RI, Nicoll RA (2001) Endogenous cannabinoids mediate retrograde signalling at hippocampal synapses. *Nature* 410: 588–592.

Wilson RI, Kunos G, Nicoll RA (2001) Presynaptic specificity of endocannabinoid signaling in the hippocampus. *Neuron* 31:453–462.

Wroblewska B, Wroblewski JT, Saab OH, Neale JH (1993) *N*-Acetylaspartylglutamate inhibits forskolin-stimulated cyclic AMP levels via a metabotropic glutamate receptor in cultured cerebellar granule cells. *J Neurochem* 61:943–948.

Wu LG, Saggau P (1994) Adenosine inhibits evoked synaptic transmission primarily by reducing presynaptic calcium influx in area CA1 of hippocampus. *Neuron* 12:1139–1148.

Wu S, Wright RA, Rockey PK, Burgett SG, Arnold JS, Rosteck PR, Jr., Johnson BG, Schoepp DD, Belagaje RM (1998) Group III human metabotropic glutamate receptors 4, 7 and 8: molecular cloning, functional expression, and comparison of pharmacological properties in RGT cells. *Brain Res Mol Brain Res* 53:88–97.

Yamamoto C, Sawada S, Takada S (1983) Suppressing action of 2-amino-4-phosphonobutyric acid on mossy fiber-induced excitation in the guinea pig hippocampus. *Exp Brain Res* 51:128–134.

Yeckel MF, Kapur A, Johnston D (1999) Multiple forms of LTP in hippocampal CA3 neurons use a common postsynaptic mechanism. *Nat Neurosci* 2:625–633.

Yokoi M, Kobayashi K, Manabe T, Takahashi T, Sakaguchi I, Katsuura G, Shigemoto R, Ohishi H, Nomura S, Nakamura K, Nakao K, Katsuki M, Nakanishi S (1996) Impairment of hippocampal mossy fiber LTD in mice lacking mGluR2. *Science* 273: 645–647.

Yoon KW, Rothman SM (1991) Adenosine inhibits excitatory but not inhibitory synaptic transmission in the hippocampus. *J Neurosci* 11:1375–1380.

Yuste R, Majewska A, Cash SS, Denk W (1999) Mechanisms of calcium influx into hippocampal spines: heterogeneity among spines, coincidence detection by NMDA receptors, and optical quantal analysis. *J Neurosci* 19:1976–1987.

Yuste R, Majewska A, Holthoff K (2000) From form to function: calcium compartmentalization in dendritic spines. *Nat Neurosci* 3:653–659.

Zerangue N, Kavanaugh MP (1996) Flux coupling in a neuronal glutamate transporter. *Nature* 383:634–637.

Zhang JF, Ellinor PT, Aldrich RW, Tsien RW (1996) Multiple structural elements in voltage-dependent Ca^{2+} channels support their inhibition by G proteins. *Neuron* 17:991–1003.

Zhou Q, Petersen CC, Nicoll RA (2000) Effects of reduced vesicular filling on synaptic transmission in rat hippocampal neurones. *J Physiol* 525(Pt 1):195–206.

Zucker RS, Regehr WG (2002) Short-term synaptic plasticity. *Annu Rev Physiol* 64:355–405.

Zucker RS, Kullmann DM, Bennett M (1998) Release of neurotransmitters. In: *Fundamental neuroscience* (Zigmond MJ, Bloom FE, Landis SC, Roberts JL, Squire LR, eds), pp 155–192. San Diego: Academic Press.

7 ▦ Pavel Osten, William Wisden, and Rolf Sprengel

Molecular Mechanisms of Synaptic Function in the Hippocampus: Neurotransmitter Exocytosis and Glutamatergic, GABAergic, and Cholinergic Transmission

7.1 Overview

In the hippocampus, excitatory (also termed principal or pyramidal) neurons, the basic working units of the mammalian central nervous system (CNS), form a highly organized three-layer circuit. Excitatory input from the entorhinal cortex enters the hippocampus largely via dentate gyrus granular cells, which in turn connect through the mossy fiber synapses to the CA3 pyramidal neurons. CA3 pyramids process the input via a dense network of recurrent connections and send their output through the Schaffer collaterals synapsing onto the CA1 pyramidal cells. Finally, CA1 pyramids send the hippocampus-processed information via the subiculum back to the cortex. Within this circuit, fast excitatory synaptic transmission is mediated by inward excitatory postsynaptic currents (EPSCs) flowing through the ionotropic α-amino-3-hydroxy-5-methyl-4-isoxazolepropionate (AMPA) and, to a lesser extent, kainate types of glutamate receptors. Slower hippocampal EPSCs are the result of activation of N-methyl-D-aspartate (NMDA) receptors and certain subtypes of metabotropic glutamate receptors.

The activity of hippocampal principal neurons is tightly controlled and synchronized by an inhibitory system comprised of γ-aminobutyric acid (GABA)ergic interneurons interspersed throughout the hippocampus. Fast inhibitory postsynaptic currents (IPSCs) are the result of ionotropic $GABA_A$ receptor activation, and slow IPSCs are due to the activation of metabotropic $GABA_B$ receptors. In addition, activation of some metabotropic glutamate receptors may also have inhibitory rather than excitatory effects. Cholinergic projections in the hippocampus comprise a prominent modulatory system, where acetylcholine binds to muscarinic and nicotinic receptors and produces either excitatory or inhibitory effects depending on the receptor type, the cell type that expresses the receptor, and the synaptic location of the receptors in a given cell. Finally, a set of neuropeptide receptors [e.g., receptors for somatostatin, neuropeptide Y (NPY)] and receptors that bind

modulators such as serotonin, steroids, and endocannabinoids play important roles in the hippocampus, as does electrical transmission through gap junctions.

In this chapter, we primarily restrict ourselves to a description of the molecular biology of excitatory and inhibitory transmission. We start by describing the basis of all signal transmission processes, the release of the signaling transmitter from the presynaptic terminal. Next we give details of the key glutamate and GABA receptors responsible for the "nuts and bolts" of hippocampal chemical transmission. We end by discussing—as an example of modulatory transmission—how acetylcholine muscarinic and nicotinic receptors influence information flow in the hippocampal cell types. To fully integrate our chapter into the overall theme of the book, we focus in detail on hippocampal-specific features of synaptic transmission, such as the hippocampal distribution of the individual receptor types. In addition, we discuss the growing number of mouse models aimed at genetic analysis of presynaptic or postsynaptic functions, which are typically assayed for behavioral phenotype in a battery of hippocampus-dependent tasks. As these mouse models are becoming increasingly more refined, particularly with improved spatiotemporal control over the onset of the genetic manipulation, this line of work is beginning to uncover previously unsuspected differences in the molecular and cellular mechanisms of various hippocampus-based functions, such as the differences in synaptic transmission and plasticity underlying hippocampal working and spatial memory.

7.2 Neurotransmitter Exocytosis

7.2.1 Introduction: Proteins Involved in Synaptic Release

Neurotransmitter release occurs at specialized sites of the presynaptic axon terminals, termed the active zones, and is tightly linked to intraterminal influx of extracellular Ca^{2+}. The event itself is a culmination of numerous trafficking steps of the synaptic vesicle cycle that was introduced in general terms in Chapter 6. The temporal and spatial complexity of these processes is accomplished by the highly synchronized "collaboration" of a large number of presynaptic proteins. On the basis of their function during the synaptic vesicle cycle, they can be grouped as proteins regulating (1) the reserve pool of vesicles, (2) mobilization of vesicles toward the active zone, (3) docking and priming of vesicles at the active zone, (4) Ca^{2+}-triggered neurotransmitter release, and (5) vesicle endocytosis, recycling, and refilling.

7.2.2 Reserve Pool of Synaptic Vesicles

Synaptic vesicles are kept in two spatially and functionally distinct pools: the reserve pool and the readily releasable pool. The reserve pool, approximately 200 to 500 nm away from the active zone plasma membrane, provides a supply of vesicles after depletion of the readily releasable pool. The equilibrium between the reserve and the releasable pool is maintained largely by abundant synaptic vesicle proteins termed synapsins, which tether the vesicles to the presynaptic cytoskeletal network made up of filamentous actin (F-actin), microtubules and brain spectrin (for review see Hilfiker et al., 1999; Doussau and Augustine, 2000). Synapsins comprise a family of three phosphoproteins, termed synapsin I, II, and III, each of which undergoes alternative splicing in the variable C-terminal part of the molecule, generating isoforms termed "a" and "b." Whereas the distribution of synapsin I and II is highly overlapping throughout the CNS (Südhof et al., 1989), differences in function between the two isoforms in the hippocampus were recently revealed in synapsin I and II knockout mice (see below). In contrast, synapsin III is largely restricted to mossy fiber terminals of the granule cells in the adult hippocampus (Pieribone et al., 2002).

The function of synapsins is tightly regulated by protein kinases: During repetitive synaptic release, activated protein kinases phosphorylate synapsins on several residues, inducing their unbinding from synaptic vesicles and subsequent mobilization of the vesicles toward the active zone. Two kinases implicated in the phosphorylation of synapsin I are Ca^{2+}/calmodulin-dependent protein kinase (CaM kinase) and mitogen-activated protein kinase (MAPK). Interestingly, the two kinases regulate synapsin I function in response to different rates of activity: A lower rate of presynaptic stimulation activates phosphorylation of synapsin I by CaM kinase, whereas a higher rate is more selective for MAPK phosphorylation (Chi et al., 2003). Even though the functional significance of the two kinase pathways is presently not clear, these observations suggest that synapsins may be fine-tuned to different firing frequencies in vivo and may participate in regulating the mobilization of synaptic vesicles during different patterns of activity.

Direct experimental support for the above proposed role of synapsins comes from mice lacking synapsin I and/or II, which indeed have a decreased number of reserve vesicles at hippocampal synapses (Rosahl et al., 1993, 1995; Li et al., 1995; Takei et al., 1995). In addition, the mice show interesting phenotypes with respect to synapsin I and II functions in the hippocampus. First, synapsin I, II, or I/II knockout mice all have normal long-term synaptic plasticity as assessed by measurements of long-term potentiation (LTP) at either mossy fiber to CA3 or CA3 to CA1 synapses. Thus maintaining a reserve pool of synaptic vesicles is not necessary for LTP in the hippocampus. However, the mice show changes in short-term plasticity. Synapsin I knockout mice show an increase in paired pulse facilitation (PPF) but no change in posttetanic potentiation (PTP) at CA3 to CA1 synapses, whereas mice lacking synapsin II and I/II show a loss of PTP but no change of PPF. Even more interestingly, synapsin II and I/II but not synapsin I knockout mice show impaired hippocampus-dependent contextual learning (Silva et al., 1996). This suggests that a deficit in short-term plasticity (i.e., in PTP) in the presence of normal LTP can cause an impairment of hippocampus-dependent learning; this finding, although perhaps surprising, is supported by a similar result from animals lacking the presynaptic protein RIM1α (see Section 7.2.5).

7.2.3 Synaptic Vesicle Docking and Priming at the Active Zone: Role of the SNARE Complex, Munc18, and Munc13

Synaptic vesicles, after their mobilization toward the active zone, undergo a number of trafficking steps before achieving a state at which they are ready to fuse with the presynaptic plasma membrane, the so called readily releasable state. Although the functions of numerous proteins involved in these processes are now understood in some detail, a complete "unified" model that would explain how synaptic vesicles dock and become primed at the active zone is yet to be established. Perhaps the least-understood step during the vesicle mobilization concerns the initial docking (tethering) of synaptic vesicles at the active zone membrane. It seems likely, based on data from membrane fusion in many secretory pathways, that vesicle tethering is mediated by small guanosine triphosphate (GTP)-binding proteins of the Rab family: A vesicle-associated, GTP-bound Rab links the vesicle to a Rab effector protein (tether) that is present selectively at the target membrane. Several Rab proteins are associated with synaptic vesicles, the most abundant of which is Rab3A (other Rab3 isoforms are Rab3B, -C, and -D). Analysis of knockout mice, however, revealed that Rab3A functions during neurotransmitter release, after docking and priming (Geppert et al., 1994a, 1997). (See Section 7.2.5 on the role of Rab3A in the later stages of the synaptic vesicle cycle.) Furthermore, quadruple Rab3A/B/C/D knockout mice have normal gross brain and synaptic morphology (the mice die at birth owing to respiratory failure), and cultured hippocampal neurons prepared from these mice have normal spontaneous and only partially reduced evoked release (Schlüter et al., 2004). Thus, other proteins, perhaps yet another Rab isoform or a protein with a different function altogether, are sufficient for docking of synaptic vesicles at hippocampal synapses in the absence of Rab3.

Past the initial docking step, proteins principally involved in the regulation of priming of synaptic vesicles at the active zone include the SNARE (SNAp REceptor) complex, Sec1/Munc18 homologues (SM proteins), Munc13-1, and complexins (reviewed in Rizo and Südhof, 2002). The role of synaptotagmin 1 is discussed in the section relating directly to Ca^{2+}-triggered release (see Section 7.2.4). The SNARE complex is a critical component of most if not all intracellular membrane fusion events. Assembly of the SNARE complex from proteins of the vesicular and target membranes (v- and t-SNAREs) is believed to bring the two membranes into close contact; this primed state is a prerequisite for initiation of membrane fusion (Fig. 7–1) (see Chapter 6). At the presynaptic terminals, the SNAREs involved in neurotransmitter release are a v-SNARE termed synaptobrevin (also VAMP) and two t-SNAREs present at the active zone termed SNAP25 and syntaxin1; synaptobrevin and syntaxin are single transmembrane proteins, and SNAP25 is a membrane-attached protein. The critical importance of the SNAREs for synaptic functions was first demonstrated in experiments with clostridial neurotoxins, which cause site-specific cleavage of the individual SNARE proteins: A loss of SNARE function abolished neurotransmitter release (reviewed in Rizo and Südhof, 2002). These experiments also showed that in the absence of the SNARE assembly synaptic vesicles can accumulate at the active zone in a similar way as at wild-type synapses, indicating that SNAREs are not involved in synaptic vesicle docking.

The molecule key to understanding the function of the SNARE complex during synaptic release is the t-SNARE syntaxin1, a neuronal isoform of the syntaxin protein family.

Syntaxin1 comprises a large cytoplasmic domain, one transmembrane domain, and a short extracellular C-terminus. Functionally, Syntaxin1 exists in three conformational states (Fig. 7–1) (reviewed in Brose et al., 2000; Rizo and Südhof, 2002). In the "closed" state, syntaxin1 binds to Munc18-1 (also known as nSec1, a neuronal isoform of the sec1/Munc18 protein family). Because the binding of syntaxin1 to Munc18-1 and to SNAP25 is mutually exclusive, it is postulated that Munc18-1 controls the pool of free syntaxin1 and inhibits formation of the SNARE complex. However, surprisingly, genetic deletion of Munc18-1 in mice caused complete loss of neurotransmitter release despite an apparently normal number of docked vesicles at the presynaptic membrane (Verhage et al., 2000). This indicates that in addition to its restrictive function in binding to syntaxin1 Munc18-1 plays a more positive and yet to be identified role during late steps of the synaptic vesicle cycle prior to synaptic release. Strikingly, these mice are born with essentially normal gross brain anatomy and morphologically defined synapses, demonstrating that SNARE-dependent neurotransmitter release is not required for brain assembly or formation of synaptic contacts; the mice, however, die immediately after birth owing to complete paralysis and exhibit widespread apoptosis in the brain.

In the next step, before formation of the SNARE complex, syntaxin1 undergoes conformational transition, from a "closed" to an "open" state, which disinhibits the binding of Munc18-1. Based on the following evidence, the main candidate for initiating this transition is Munc13 (reviewed in Brose et al., 2000; Rizo and Südhof, 2002). First, the carboxy-terminal region of Munc13-1 binds to syntaxin1 and displaces the binding of Munc18-1 in vitro. Second, double knockout mice lacking two Munc13 isoforms (Munc13-1 and Munc13-2) exhibit complete loss of neurotransmitter release at hippocampal synapses but no change in the total or docked number of vesicles at synapses; this demonstrates that

Figure 7–1. Three conformations of syntaxin during assembly of the ternary SNARE complex. *A.* Syntaxin in a "close" conformation is bound with Munc18 via its N-terminal H_{abc} (also termed $H_A H_B H_C$) domain (checkered region of the syntaxin molecule) and a part of its juxtamembrane H3 domain (dashed region). *B.* During a switch from a "closed" to an "open" state, Munc18 is displaced

from syntaxin by Munc13. In the "open" state, syntaxin can interact with SNAP25 and synaptobrevin from a docked vesicle. *C.* The resulting "assembled" state corresponds to syntaxin binding within the ternary SNARE complex. The vesicle is now primed for synaptic release triggered by Ca^{2+} entry into the terminal (see Fig. 7–2). (*Source*: Brose et al., 2000, with permission.)

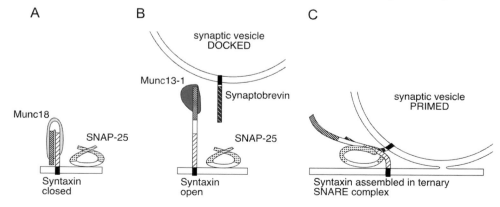

Munc13-1 and 13-2 function after synaptic vesicle docking, during priming, and prior to synaptic release (Varoqueaux et al., 2002). Importantly, a constitutively "open" mutant of syntaxin1, which does not bind Munc18-1, rescues the loss of Unc-13 (homologue of Munc13) in *Caenorhabditis elegans* (Richmond et al., 2001); these data provide further evidence that the Munc-13/Unc-13 proteins function during a conformational switch of syntaxin1 into the "open" state (see Section 7.2.5 for another role of Munc13-1 in binding with RIM1 and Rab3A). Other potential mechanisms that may modulate syntaxin1 transition to the open state include syntaxin1 binding to tomosyn, which also displaces Munc18-1, and/or a direct modulation of Munc18-1 by phosphorylation or by an interaction with other presynaptic proteins (reviewed in Rizo and Südhof, 2002).

The third conformational state of syntaxin corresponds to its binding in the SNARE complex, initially forming a binary complex with SNAP25, which is followed by assembly of the ternary SNARE complex with SNAP25 and synaptobrevin (Fig. 7–1). The complete "zipped" SNARE complex is formed by a tight four-helix bundle formed among coil-coil domains of all three SNAREs (one coil domain of syntaxin and synaptobrevin, and two of SNAP25). The orientation of the coil-coil domains in the complex is in parallel, which brings the docked vesicle in close contact with the active zone membrane, resulting in a primed readily releasable state. The unstable nature of the primed vesicles is reflected by occasional spontaneous miniature release events, electrophysiologically measured as miniature excitatory and inhibitory postsynaptic currents: mEPSCs and mIPSCs, respectively; these events can thus be seen as failures of the mechanism(s) that normally prevent Ca^{2+}-independent release at the synaptic terminals (see Section 7.1.5 for the role of synaptotagmin in the initiation of Ca^{2+}-triggered synaptic exocytosis).

Mice engineered to lack either synaptobrevin or SNAP-25 were generated to explore the SNARE complex function in vivo (Schoch et al., 2001; Washbourne et al., 2002). Both genotypes were born with normal brain anatomy but died immediately after birth, likely owing to respiratory failure. Strikingly, although they showed drastically reduced (in the case of synaptobrevin knockout mice) or completely abolished (SNAP-25 knockout) action potential-evoked neurotransmitter release in hippocampal cultured neurons, spontaneous synaptic release was either only 10-fold decreased (synaptobrevin knockout) or occurred at wild-type frequency and amplitude (SNAP-25 knockout). These mice thus confirm that the SNARE complex is not required for synaptic vesicle docking, as previously indicated by the experiments with clostridial neurotoxins (see above). In addition, the persistence of spontaneous release indicates that the SNARE complex is not essential for fusion of docked vesicles at the active zone membrane. It remains to be determined if the release in the absence of synaptobrevin or SNAP-25 is due to compensation by other cellular SNAREs or is mediated via a truly SNARE-independent mechanism.

During or closely following formation of the SNARE complex, low-molecular-weight proteins termed complexins bind to the core complex at 1:1 stoichiometry in a groove between the synaptobrevin and syntaxin coil-coil domains. It has been proposed that complexins stabilize the SNARE complex prior to evoked neurotransmitter release. Mice lacking both complexin 1 and 2 isoforms show normal brain anatomy but die a few hours after birth (Reim et al., 2001). Analysis of synaptic functions in hippocampal cultured neurons revealed normal spontaneous release but dramatically reduced probability of evoked synaptic release. Complexins thus appear to fine-tune the competence of the docked vesicles to respond to a cytoplasmic influx of Ca^{2+}.

7.2.4 Ca^{2+}-triggered Synaptic Release: Role of Synaptotagmin

The first step in the sequence of events underlying Ca^{2+}-triggered exocytosis is the activation of voltage-gated Ca^{2+} channels of the N and P/Q types by action potential-driven depolarization of the nerve terminal membrane (for review see Meir et al., 1999). For transmitter release to occur, the intracellular Ca^{2+} concentration must reach a threshold, which is set by the sensitivity of a Ca^{2+} sensor responsible for triggering the release. The bulk Ca^{2+} concentration in the presynaptic terminal reaches about 500 nM following an action potential. However, the Ca^{2+} concentration required for synaptic release is estimated to be as high as 10 μM (from measurements made at the large calyx of the Held synapse) (Bollmann et al., 2000; Schneggenburger and Neher, 2000). Because such a high Ca^{2+} concentration is likely to be reached only in close proximity to the openings of the Ca^{2+} channels, it is important to maintain a close link between the channels and proteins of the presynaptic release machinery. This is mediated, at least in part, by direct protein–protein coupling of Ca^{2+} channels to the SNARE complex as well as to synaptotagmin 1 and 2, vesicular proteins proposed to function as presynaptic Ca^{2+} sensors (fora review on Ca^{2+} channel interactions with the active zone proteins, see Seagar et al., 1999). In addition, because neurotransmitter release at the CNS synapses is comprised of two kinetically distinct components—a major fast component followed by a smaller slower component—it is likely that at least two distinct Ca^{2+} sensors are employed to regulate the event.

Synaptotagmins constitute an 11-gene family of Ca^{2+}-binding proteins, the most abundant of which in the brain is synaptotagmin 1. The molecular structure of synaptotagmin consists of a small intravesicular domain, a single transmembrane domain, and a large cytoplasmic C-terminal domain, which contains two Ca^{2+}-binding C_2-domains (C_2A and C_2B). The Ca^{2+} affinity of the C_2 domains of synaptotagmin is highly increased by binding to phospholipid membranes. In the primed state, synaptotagmin C_2 domains bind to the SNARE complex and to phospholipids of the active zone plasma membrane; upon Ca^{2+} entry, the C_2 domains insert

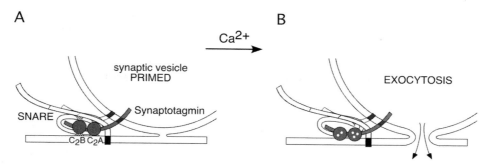

Figure 7–2. Synaptotagmin role as a Ca^{2+} sensor for synaptic release. *A.* In the primed state, synaptotagmin C_2 domains (C_2A and C_2B) bind with phospholipids of the active zone plasma membrane and the SNARE complex (the SNARE components are shown as in Fig. 7–1). *B.* Upon Ca^{2+} entry, synaptotagmin binds Ca^{2+} ions (marked as white dots; three per C_2A and two per C_2B), which may further insert the C_2 domains into the plasma membrane phospholipids. Such conformational change was proposed to act as the final trigger for synaptic exocytosis (*Source*: Südhof, 2004, with permission.)

themselves farther into the plasma membrane, a step that may act as a final trigger for fusion between the synaptic vesicle and active zone membranes during synaptic exocytosis (reviewed in Südhof, 2004) (Fig. 7–2).

Perhaps the best evidence for the role of synaptotagmin in Ca^{2+}-induced synaptic release comes from synaptotagmin 1 knockout mice, which exhibit a severely depressed fast phase and a normal slow (asynchronous) phase of Ca^{2+}-dependent synaptic release in cultured hippocampal neurons. Note that the mice die after birth, indicating that the fast Ca^{2+}-dependent release is essential for life (Geppert et al., 1994b). As expected, presynaptic vesicle docking appears normal in these mice, with the readily releasable pool of synaptic vesicles, frequency of mEPSCs, and Ca^{2+}-independent neurotransmitter release all comparable to that in wild-type terminals. In addition, Fernandez-Chacon et al. (2001) used a sophisticated knock-in approach to introduce a single point mutation in the synaptotagmin 1 C_2A domain, which decreased its Ca^{2+} affinity by 50%. This genetic manipulation resulted in a proportional decrease of Ca^{2+} sensitivity of neurotransmitter release in cultured hippocampal neurons prepared from the mutant mice (Fernandez-Chacon et al., 2001). (See Section 7.2.5 for a discussion of behavioral phenotype of synaptotagmin mutant mice.) Taken together, these findings strongly indicate that synaptotagmin 1 functions after docking and priming, during the fast phase of Ca^{2+}-triggered release.

7.2.5 Ca^{2+}-triggered Synaptic Release: Role of Rab3A and RIM1

The abundant synaptic vesicle-associated protein Rab3A, a member of the Rab family of low-molecular-weight GTP-binding proteins, cycles between two functional states: a synaptic vesicle-associated GTP-bound form and a cytoplasmic GDP-bound form. Rab3A GTP hydrolysis, which occurs during or after neurotransmitter exocytosis, releases Rab3A from its association with the vesicular membrane. Cytoplasmic Rab3A-GDP is then recognized by the Rab3-GDP/GTP exchange factor, and Rab3A-GTP rebinds with synaptic vesicles.

Rab3A interacts, in a GTP-dependent manner, with two proteins proposed to function as its effectors, rabphilin and RIM1 (reviewed in Südhof, 2004). Both proteins have an N-terminal zinc finger domain (which mediates the binding with Rab3A) and two C-terminal Ca^{2+}-binding C_2 domains. Rabphilin, a cytoplasmic protein, is recruited to synaptic vesicles by its interaction with Rab3A-GTP. RIM1, which is stably associated with the active zone membrane, binds via its zinc finger to Rab3A and Munc13-1, via its C_2B domain to synaptotagmin 1 and 2, and to liprins.

Rab3A does not play an essential role in docking or priming of synaptic vesicles as initially believed, as Rab3A knockout mice have a normal gross brain as well as synaptic morphology and normal spontaneous transmitter release (Geppert et al., 1994a). Rather, the function of Rab3A seems to be to modulate synaptic release, with distinct roles at various hippocampal synapses. At the CA3 to CA1 synapses, loss of Rab3A results in altered short-term plasticity with enhanced paired-pulse facilitation (Geppert et al., 1994a, 1997). In contrast, the mossy fiber to CA3 synapse shows normal short-term plasticity, but mossy fiber LTP (mfLTP) is abolished (Castillo et al., 1997a). Somewhat surprisingly, knockout of rabphilin showed no phenotype, indicating that rabphilin is not an essential Rab3A effector in the synaptic vesicle cycle (Schlüter et al., 1999). However, knockout of the major brain RIM isoform, RIM1α, showed a broader phenotype than that of Rab3A, indicating additional roles for RIM1α in synaptic release. First, mfLTP is abolished, as in the Rab3A knockout mice, suggesting that RIM1α is the main effector of Rab3A at the mossy fiber to CA3 synapse (Castillo et al., 2002). Second, both the probability of evoked synaptic release and short-term plasticity are altered, but LTP can still be induced at CA3 to CA1 synapses (Schoch et al., 2002; Calakos et al., 2004).

Although the exact molecular mechanisms underlying the RIM1α-based deficits remain to be explained, recent behavioral experiments showed that the synaptic functions that are disturbed in the RIM1α knockout mice are crucial for hippocampus-based behavior. The mice showed normal coordination and anxiety-like behavior but were deficient in two forms of hippocampus-dependent associative learning and memory: context-dependent fear conditioning and spatial learning in the Morris watermaze (Powell et al., 2004). In parallel experiments, the same authors found that mice lacking Rab3A, which are selectively deficient in mfLTP (see above), showed normal behavior. Thus, mfLTP is not essential for these hippocampus-dependent forms of learning. In addition, mice with a synaptotagmin C_2A point mutation, which exhibit a decrease in the probability of release at hippocampal excitatory synapses similar to that seen in RIM1α knockout mice (see Section 7.2.4), also showed normal behavior. The RIM1α knockout behavioral phenotype thus cannot be simply correlated with the decreased release probability at excitatory synapses. The observed behavioral deficits in the RIM1α knockout may result from the combined alterations in mossy fiber to CA3 transmission and CA3 to CA1 transmission. Alternatively, short-term plasticity, even in the presence of normal LTP, may play an important role in learning, as was already suggested with experiments using the synapsin II and I/II knockout mice (Silva et al., 1996) (see Section 7.2.2).

7.2.6 NSF-mediated Disassembly of the SNARE Complex

The SNARE complex, assembled by the α-helical domains of t- and v-SNAREs during the steps of docking and priming, is thermodynamically stable. To initiate recycling of SNARE proteins for the next round of synaptic vesicle cycle after synaptic exocytosis, the SNARE complex must be first disassembled by a chaperon protein, the hexameric ATPase *N*-ethylmaleimide-sensitive fusion protein (NSF) (for review see May et al., 2001). The NSF molecule consists of three domains: an N-terminal domain responsible for binding with the α-SNAP–SNARE complex (below) and two C-terminal ATP-binding domains, termed D1 and D2. The D1 domain is essential for NSF ATPase activity, and the D2 domain is required for NSF hexameric assembly. The association between NSF and the SNARE complex is not direct but mediated by an adaptor protein termed α-SNAP (soluble NSF-attachment protein). NSF binds to the α-SNAP–SNARE complex only in the presence of ATP, forming the so-called 20 S particle. The quick-freeze/deep-etch electron microscopic image of the 20 S particle shows α-SNAP and NSF wrapping as a "sleeve" along the rod-like α-helical domains of the SNARE complex (Hanson et al., 1997). Binding of NSF to the α-SNAP–SNARE complex stimulates NSF ATPase activity, resulting in subsequent disassembly of the SNARE complex driven by NSF-mediated ATP hydrolysis. The monomeric SNARE proteins syntaxin1, synaptobrevinm and SNAP25 are then sorted for the next round of vesicular cycling during endocytotic uptake of the components of the vesicular membrane (see below).

7.2.7 Synaptic Vesicle Endocytosis, Recycling, and Refilling

Currently, the model of recycling of the synaptic vesicular membrane and its integral proteins at the CNS synapses includes two pathways: "kiss-and-run" and clathrin-mediated endocytosis.

The kiss-and-run hypothesis proposes that the lumen of the synaptic vesicle briefly opens and closes again, without the vesicle membrane collapsing to the active zone plasma membrane; in the next step, the vesicle is recaptured mostly intact. Compelling evidence for kiss-and-run recycling comes from fluorescence imaging of single-vesicle release in hippocampal primary cultures, documenting partial loss of the vesicular content and recovery of the same vesicle afterward (Aravanis et al., 2003; Gandhi and Stevens, 2003). However, many questions about the molecular mechanisms that may regulate this form of release remain unanswered; for example, it is not known what prevents full collapse of the vesicle into the presynaptic membrane or how the vesicle is pinched off before it can "run" again.

The mechanisms of clathrin-mediated endocytosis of synaptic vesicles, in contrast, are understood in much more detail (reviewed in Slepnev and De Camilli, 2000). The general outline of the distinct molecular steps include formation of clathrin-coated invaginations (pits) followed by fission of the coated pits to generate free clathrin-coated vesicles, rapid loss of the clathrin coat, and reentry into the synaptic vesicle cycle. The formation of the clathrin-coated pits is initiated by binding of adaptor proteins AP-2 and AP-180 to synaptic vesicle proteins, such as synaptotagmin, that are undergoing sorting at the plasma membrane after neurotransmitter release and to phospholipids. The adapters then recruit the three-legged clathrin triskelia and synergistically induce clathrin polymerization, resulting in membrane invagination.

In addition to adaptor proteins, a number of accessory proteins are involved in the mechanisms of invagination of the clathrin-coated pit and formation of a uniform-size vesicle. Amphiphysin 1 and 2 are multifunctional adapters that bind to clathrin, AP-2, and synaptojanin and dynamin, which are involved in uncoating and fission of the vesicles (see below). In addition to their adaptor role, amphiphysins may also participate in the formation of membrane curvature during endocytosis via its N-terminal Bin/Amphiphysin/Rvs (BAR) domain; amphiphysins directly bind the membrane lipid bilayer and force membrane curving via BAR domains dimerized into a banana-like shape. As with many other synaptic proteins, the role of amphiphysins in the CNS has been examined by mouse genetics. Amphiphysin 1 knockout mice showed drastically diminished levels of amphiphysin 2, indicating that the proteins exist as functional heterodimers; and in vitro assays using lysates and cultured hippocampal cells from the knockout animals revealed defects in the assembly of the synaptic endocytotic protein machinery as well as decreased rates of activity-dependent endocytosis and recycling of the vesicles (Di Paolo et al., 2002). Interestingly, the mice have morphologically normal presynaptic terminals and unaffected evoked glutamate release, but they are prone to seizures and show cognitive deficits in hippocampus-based spatial learning (Di Paolo et al., 2002). Thus the exact role of amphiphysins in clathrin-mediated endocytosis remains to be established.

Another gene family of clathrin accessory proteins comprises the endophilins (endophilin 1, 2, and 3, of which endophilin 1 is the major isoform in the brain). Endophilins share the BAR and SH3-domain structure with amphiphysins and, in addition, exhibit enzymatic lysophosphatidic acid acyl transferase (LPAAT) activity. Endophilin 1 is proposed to promote negative membrane curvature directly during endocytosis by LPAAT activity-induced change in the composition of the plasma membrane and to act as an adaptor in recruiting synaptojanin and dynamin.

The key molecule during the fission of clathrin-coated vesicles is the GTPase dynamin (for review see Schmid et al., 1998). GTP-bound dynamin, which is recruited to the clathrin-coated membrane by its interaction with SH3 domains of amphiphysin, endophilin, and other accessory proteins, forms rings around the stalk of the clathrin pit. It has been proposed that dynamin-driven GTP hydrolysis induces conformational change in the dynamin ring and pinches off the coated vesicle by either restricting or elongating the stalk membrane.

It has been proposed that clathrin uncoating, a final step in clathrin-dependent endocytosis, is mediated by synaptojanins (synaptojanin 1 and 2—synaptojanin 1 is the main isoform in the brain). Synaptojanins have polyphosphoinositide phosphatase activity and degrade phoshatidylinositol-4,5-biphosphate, $PI(4,5)P_2$, to phosphatidylinositol (for review see Slepnev and De Camilli, 2000). because $PI(4,5)P_2$ is a positive regulator of clathrin assembly, its degradation is believed to be the mechanism for vesicle uncoating after dynamin-mediated fission. Mice lacking synaptojanin 1 die shortly after birth (indicating a crucial role of the gene for life) and show increased levels of $PI(4,5)P_2$ in cortical neurons, accumulation of clathrin-coated vesicles in nerve terminals, and depression of hippocampal Schaffer collateral CA1 transmission, rather than LTP, after high-frequency stimulation (Cremona et al., 1999).

Finally, before the vesicles are re-sorted back to the active zone membrane or to the reserve pool, they must be refilled with a corresponding neurotransmitter. The energy necessary for uptake of a specific neurotransmitter is provided by an electrochemical gradient with positively charged, acidic vesicle lumen; this gradient is generated by an ATP-driven proton pump termed "vacuolar H^+-ATPase" (V-ATPase) (reviewed in Nishi and Forgac, 2002). The uptake is mediated by vesicular neurotransmitter transporters (VNTs), which pump neurotransmitter in exchange for protons. There are three types of VNT in the brain: vesicular amine transporters, vesicular inhibitory amino acid transporters, and vesicular excitatory amino acid transporters (reviewed in Eiden, 2000; Torres et al., 2003; Fremeau et al., 2004). The type of VNT expressed in a specific cell type determines the neurotransmitter that is loaded into vesicles and subsequently released at axon terminals.

The vesicular monoamine transporter 2 (VMAT2) is responsible for synaptic vesicle uptake of catecholamines, serotonin, and histamine; and the vesicular acetylcholine transporter (VAChT) mediates uptake of acetylcholine. The two transporters are closely related, with the same protein topology consisting of 12 transmembrane domains and cytoplasmic N- and C-terminal domains. The vesicular GABA transporter (VGAT), also termed the vesicular inhibitory amino acid transporter (VIAAT), is responsible for loading of neurotransmitters GABA and glycine. VGAT has a topology of 10 predicted transmembrane domains. Finally, vesicular uptake of glutamate is mediated by a protein family of the vesicular glutamate transporters (VGLUT1-3). Interestingly, the first identified vesicular transporter for glutamate (termed "VGLUT1") was originally cloned as a gene upregulated in cerebellar granule cells after treatment with NMDA; the gene was termed "Brain, Na^+-dependent P_i transporter1" (BNP1) because of its 32% amino acid identity with the Na^+-dependent P_i transporter from the kidney. However, 5 years later, BNP1 was localized selectively to glutamatergic synaptic vesicles and was shown to mediate vesicular glutamate uptake. The fact that VGLUT1 expression can be regulated by activation of NMDA-type glutamate receptors suggests that the levels of VGLUT1 may have a functional relevance for regulation of synaptic transmission. At the molecular level, VGLUT1 is a protein with predicted six to eight transmembrane domains. VGLUT1 and VGLUT2 show largely complementary expression in the CNS, with hippocampal glutamatergic neurons expressing mainly the VGLUT1 transporter (Fremeau et al., 2004).

7.3 Glutamate Receptors: Structure, Function, and Hippocampal Distribution

7.3.1 Introduction: Ionotropic and Metabotropic Receptors

Glutamatergic synaptic transmission and, in particular, synaptic plasticity play a central role in hippocampus-dependent learning and memory. Activation of the ionotropic glutamate receptors provides an essential mechanism required for the induction of at least some forms of Hebbian synaptic plasticity; the metabotropic receptors play more modulatory roles in these processes. After a brief introduction to the nomenclature of the receptors (see Fig. 7–3 for an overview of ligand-gated receptor types), we discuss the molecular principles that enable the receptors to mediate their functions, the distribution of receptors in hippocampal neurons, and the mechanisms of the transport of receptors to excitatory synapses, with a particular focus on how glutamate receptor trafficking may regulate synaptic plasticity. Finally, we con-

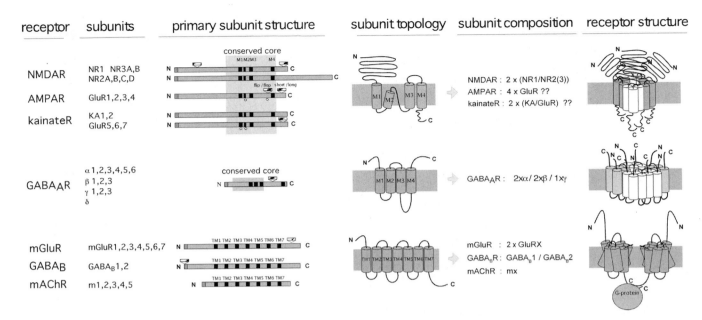

Figure 7–3. Molecular organization of neurotransmitter receptors. From top to down: Receptors are grouped into NMDA, AMPA, and kainate receptor ion channels (iGluRs), GABA$_A$ receptor ion channels (GABA$_A$Rs), and GABA$_B$, mGlu, and mACh receptors (GABA$_B$Rs, mGluRs, mAChRs). From left to right: (1) Receptor nomenclature. (2) Individual subunit nomenclature. (3) Primary structure of the subunits with indicated amino-termini (N) and carboxy-termini (C). The N-terminal signal peptides and the positions of membrane domains are indicated in dark gray and black boxes, respectively; the positions of alternative spliced exons are indicated in striped boxes and RNA-edited sites in open circles; con-served regions between subunits of a receptor family have a gray background. (4) Membrane topology of the receptor subunits. Membrane spanning alpha helixes are numbered and depicted as barrels; the cell membrane areas are in gray. (5) The subunit composition of the receptors is given as a formula. For example, NMDAR = 2 × [NR1/NR2(3)] – NMDA receptors are tetramers consisting of two NR1 and two NR2 or NR3 subunits. (6) The oligomeric receptor structure shows the formation of the receptors from the individual subunits; in the cell membrane they are given as gray background.

sider how genetically modified mice can be models of gluta-mate receptor function in vivo.

Ionotropic glutamate receptors (iGluRs) are ligand-gated ion channels that mediate most of the excitatory neurotransmission in the hippocampus (and elsewhere in the brain). Traditionally, iGluRs are classified into NMDA and non-NMDA (AMPA and kainate) receptors. The receptors are heteromeric assemblies of four subunits, with each distinct subunit encoded by its own gene. The molecular structure–function complexity is further extended by alternative splicing of the primary transcripts and by recoding through posttranscriptional RNA editing. The receptor subunits are glycosylated membrane-spanning polypeptides with an average length of 900 amino acids. According to our current understanding, the subunit segments M1, M3, and M4 are membrane-spanning; the M2 segment, which does not traverse the membrane bilayer, forms a pore-loop region, which determines the ion selectivity of the channel. The complete channel pore is built by amino acid residues of M1 and M3 together with the M2 loop; it is permeable to monovalent and, in some instances, divalent cations. The extracellular ligand-binding site is formed by the S1 region of the N-terminal domain and the S2 region of the extracellular loop between M3 and M4. The carboxy-terminal domain of each subunit is intracellular and carries binding sites for several proteins regulating trafficking and signaling of the receptors at synapses.

The expression of most iGluR subunits in the hippocampus increases with development and reaches peak levels approximately 2 weeks after birth (Fig. 7–4). This developmental profile closely resembles that of the α subunit of CaMKII, a kinase that critically contributes to the conversion of glutamatergic synaptic transmission into intracellular signaling during synaptic plasticity and learning. The iGluRs and α-CaMKII can be viewed as the molecular core of hippocampal synaptic plasticity and learning.

In addition to the direct feedforward excitatory role mediated by activation of the iGluRs, glutamate plays modulatory roles in regulating its own release as well as GABA release and neuronal excitability in the hippocampus. This is achieved by activation of the kainate and metabotropic glutamate receptors (mGluRs). mGluRs are G protein-coupled receptors, which exhibit excitatory or inhibitory effects depending on the receptor subtype and the cell context: EPSPs are often reduced by presynaptic mGluR activation and enhanced by activation of postsynaptic mGluRs. Localization of mGluRs is often outside of pre- and postsynaptic sites, which suggests that optimal activation of mGluRs takes place during intense synaptic activity resulting in neurotransmitter spillover.

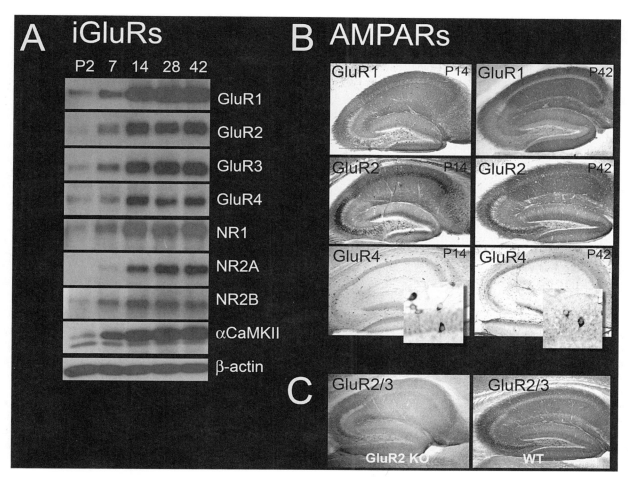

Figure 7–4. AMPA receptor subunit expression in mouse hippocampus. *A.* Immunoblots of mouse hippocampal extracts at postnatal day 2 (P2), P7, P14, P28, and P42 probed with antibodies against ionotropic glutamate receptor subunits and the α-subunit of CaMKII (indicated on the right side of the panel). Anti-β-actin staining was used for normalization of the amount of protein loaded (bottom lane). *B.* Expression of the GluR1, 2, and 4 subunits in the mouse hippocampus at P14 and P42 visualized by immunohistochemistry with subunit-specific antibodies. For GluR4 expression, higher magnification inserts demonstrate strong expression in interneurons in the pyramidal cell layer. (*Source*: Modified from Jensen et al., 2003b, with permission). *C.* GluR3 expression was visualized by an anti-GluR2/3 antibody in the hippocampus of adult GluR2 knockout mice (GluR2 KO, left panel); the right panel shows staining with the same antibody in wt hippocampus; the GluR2/3 signal represents mainly the GluR2 subunit (compare to GluR2-specific staining in the GluR2 panel, second from the top).

7.3.2 AMPA Receptors

The non-NMDA ionotropic receptors consist of two subgroups: AMPA and kainate receptors. In the hippocampus, AMPA receptors are responsible for "general purpose" transmission at all excitatory synapses. The properties of AMPA receptors allow high temporal precision and short latency of action potential initiation.

Posttranscriptional Modifications of AMPA Receptor Subunits

AMPA receptors are heterotetramers of GluR1 to GluR4 (or GluR-A to -D) subunits, all of which are expressed in the hippocampus. Of the four subunits, GluR2 plays the most critical role in determining ion channel properties: GluR2-containing channels have low Ca^{2+} permeability and a linear I/V function relating evoked current to membrane potential. This electrophysiological profile is determined by a single amino acid residue of the GluR2 M2 pore-loop segment. Whereas GluR1, 3, and 4 subunits contain glutamine (Q) in this position, the GluR2 primary transcript undergoes selective RNA editing that changes the glutamine into an arginine (R)—so-called Q/R site editing (for review see Seeburg et al., 1998). In the hippocampus, the mature GluR2 transcript is 100% edited, and the Q-to-R coding change is essential for normal brain function (see Section 7.4.3 for consequences of disrupted Q/R editing in mice). In addition, GluR2, 3, and 4 transcripts are edited at an R/G site (the glycine codon replacing genomically encoded arginine), which is located just before the flip/flop exons (see below). R/G editing is somewhat less efficient, resulting in the editing of approximately 80% to 90% of

GluR2, 3, and 4, except for GluR4 flip, which is only 50% edited. Editing at the R/G site was shown to reduce the amplitude of and accelerate recovery from desensitization for recombinant GluR3 and GluR4; the physiological role for this AMPA receptor modification, however, is still unclear.

In addition to RNA editing, a second type of posttranscriptional modification—alternative splicing—modulates the properties of AMPA receptor channels in the hippocampus at distinct synapses (for review, see Dingledine et al., 1999) (see below for hippocampal distribution of different subunit splice forms). All AMPA receptor primary transcripts undergo alternative splicing of two exons encoding a 38-amino-acid segment of the extracellular loop between M3 and M4, just before the start of the M4 domain. Each subunit thus exists as either a "flip" or a "flop" variant, depending on which exon is retained. The flip/flop domain influences receptor desensitization: Flip forms desensitize with slower kinetics compared to flop forms. The GluR2 and GluR4 primary transcripts undergo, in addition to flip/flop splicing, alternative splicing of their C-terminal domain-coding sequences. The AMPA receptor subunit C-terminal domains are grouped into "long" (~70 to 80 amino acids; e.g., 81 aa in the rat GluR1 sequence) and "short" (~50 amino acids; e.g., 50 aa in rat

GluR3). The prevalent splice of the GluR2 transcript codes for a short C-terminal tail (50 amino acids); the 68 amino acid long splice form, termed GluR2$_{long}$, is expressed at significantly lower levels but may be functionally important in the young postnatal hippocampus, where it mediates a juvenile GluR1-independent form of LTP (see Section 7.3.1). The GluR4 subunit is expressed in the hippocampus only in its long form, with a 68-amino-acid residue C-terminal domain. The role of the AMPA receptor subunit C-terminal peptides in mediating subunit-specific interactions with proteins regulating intracellular trafficking of the receptors is discussed further in Section 7.4.

Hippocampal Distribution of AMPA Receptor Subunits

AMPA receptor subunit distribution varies significantly among hippocampal cell types (Fig. 7–4), resulting in different receptor properties between, for example, excitatory and inhibitory neurons. Hippocampal principal cells express mainly GluR1 and GluR2, whereas GluR3 is present at lower levels and GluR4 only in embryonic and early postnatal principal cells (see mRNA in situ detection in Keinanen et al.,

Figure 7–5. Expression of AMPA receptor-subunit splice variants in rodent hippocampus. *A.* In situ hybridization with specific oligonucleotides detects the mRNAs of the "flip" and "flop" versions of each AMPA receptor subunit in rat hippocampus at P15. (*Source*: Modified from Monyer et al., 1991, with permission). *B.* Developmentally regulated expression of the GluR2$_{long}$ subunit

in the mouse hippocampus, visualized by in situ hybridization with GluR2$_{long}$-specific oligonucleotides at P7, P15, and mice older than P42 (P>42). For an approximate comparison of mRNA expression of both GluR2 isoforms, GluR2$_{short}$ (marked as GluR2) in situ is shown on the right.

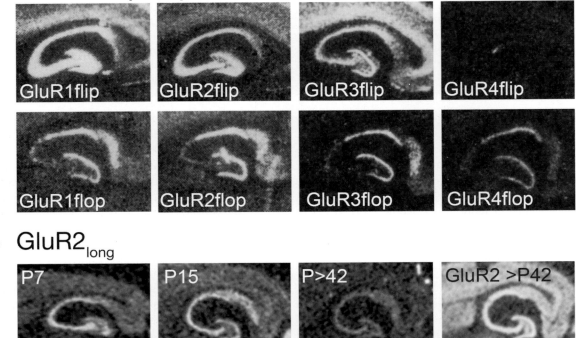

A AMPAR flip/flop isoforms

GluR1flip GluR2flip GluR3flip GluR4flip

GluR1flop GluR2flop GluR3flop GluR4flop

B GluR2$_{long}$

P7 P15 P>42 GluR2 >P42

1990; protein detection in Petralia and Wenthold, 1992). The receptor assemblies are predominantly GluR1/2 channels, with some GluR2/3 and GluR1 homomeric channels. The fact that most AMPA receptor assemblies in the principal cells contain the edited GluR2 subunit guarantees that they conduct AMPA currents with low Ca^{2+} permeability. (Note that GluR1 does not appear to form channel assemblies with GluR3 in the principal cells, even though the GluR1/GluR3 channels are efficiently formed from recombinant subunits in heterologous expression systems; the mechanism of this selective AMPA receptor assembly is not understood.)

Both flip and flop splice versions of GluR1, 2, and 3 are expressed in CA1 pyramidal cells (Fig. 7–5). In contrast, CA3 pyramidal neurons synthesize only the flip versions of GluR1, 2, and 3. Dentate granule cells express GluR1, 2, and 3 flip and flop forms, with flop > flip forms (Sommer et al., 1990; Monyer et al., 1991) (Fig. 7–5). In addition, the flip and flop splice variants are also differently regulated during the development. The flop versions are expressed at low levels prior to postnatal day 8 (P8), and their characteristic high expression in CA1 pyramidal cells becomes apparent only during the second postnatal week, in parallel with synaptic maturation. In contrast, flip mRNA levels are already substantial in pyramidal cells at birth (Monyer et al., 1991). Hippocampal pyramidal cells also express both C-terminal splice forms GluR2 and GluR2$_{long}$. GluR2$_{long}$ is expressed as early as the embryonic stage and reaches peak expression between P7 and P15. However, GluR2$_{long}$ is considerably less abundant than GluR2 (at the protein level, the GluR2$_{long}$/GluR2 ratio is 1:5 in young hippocampus and 1:20 in adult hippocampus) (Kolleker et al., 2003).

Hippocampal interneurons express mainly GluR1 and GluR4 subunits. The fact that interneurons lack significant levels of GluR2 means that their synaptic AMPA currents show voltage dependence with high permeability to Ca^{2+} ions (Geiger et al., 1995). Both GluR1 and GluR4 are expressed mainly as the flop splice form in hippocampal interneurons (Monyer et al., 1991).

In addition to the cell type-specific expression patterns, there is now evidence that receptors with different subunit compositions are selectively targeted to distinct subcellular locations in individual neurons; this could potentially allow selective tuning of postsynaptic responses to glutamate release at different anatomical inputs projecting onto a particular cell. In the hippocampus, stratum lucidum interneurons express both Ca^{2+}-permeable (GluR2-lacking) and Ca^{2+}-impermeable (GluR2-containing) AMPA receptors at synapses receiving mossy fiber input, whereas synapses receiving input from CA3 pyramidal neurons express selectively Ca^{2+}-impermeable AMPA receptors (Toth and McBain, 1998). Functionally, whereas induction of synaptic plasticity (LTD) requires an elevation of postsynaptic Ca^{2+} at both synapse types, the requirement for NMDA receptor activation is restricted to the Ca^{2+}-impermeable synapses (Laezza et al., 1999; Lei and McBain, 2002).

In addition to synapse-specific targeting, AMPA receptors are selectively distributed in the proximal versus the distal dendritic segments of hippocampal CA1 pyramidal neurons, with an increasing density toward more distal localization (Magee and Cook, 2000). This distance-dependent scaling of AMPA receptor distribution provides a mechanism that may help normalize the amplitudes of distal versus proximal synaptic inputs onto the same cell.

7.3.3 NMDA Receptors

NMDA receptors differ from AMPA receptors in several important properties, including voltage-dependent Mg^{2+} block of the channel pore, high permeability to Ca^{2+} ions, slower activation kinetics, longer open time, and higher affinity for glutamate (reviewed in Dingledine et al., 1999). At resting and slightly depolarized membrane potentials, the ion channel is blocked by the binding of extracellular Mg^{2+} in the ion pore. However, this Mg^{2+} block is released when the postsynaptic membrane is sufficiently depolarized (for example, due to strong activation of AMPA receptors). This unique feature gives NMDA receptors the ability to act as coincidence detectors for presynaptic activity (glutamate release) and postsynaptic activity (sufficient depolarization of the postsynaptic membrane). The subsequent postsynaptic influx of Ca^{2+} transduces the activation of NMDA receptors into Ca^{2+}-dependent intracellular signaling. These integrative and ion channel properties of NMDA receptor function underlie the induction of NMDA receptor-dependent synaptic plasticity, a process involved in many types of learning and memory formation (see Section 7.5.2 for genetic dissection of NMDA receptor-dependent plasticity in hippocampal learning in mice and Chapter 10 for a full account of synaptic plasticity in the hippocampus).

Seven genes encode the family of NMDA receptor subunits termed NR1; NR2A, 2B, 2C, 2D; and NR3A and 3B. The NR1 and NR3 subunits contain a binding site for glycine; and NR2 subunits bind glutamate. As demonstrated in mice with genetic deletion of the NR1 gene, NR1 is the essential subunit of all NMDA receptor channels; and in its absence, no functional NMDA receptors are formed in the brain (Forrest et al., 1994). Native tetrameric NMDA receptor assemblies are probably built of two NR1 and two NR2 or NR3 subunits. Depending on the presence of the NR2 and NR3 subunits, the NMDA receptors can be subdivided into the NR2A subtype (tetramer of two NR1 plus two NR2A), NR2B subtype (two NR1 plus two NR2B), and so on. The NR2 subunits determine the electrophysiological and pharmacological profile of the channels, affecting its open time, conductance, and Mg^{2+} sensitivity. The NR2B receptors stay open longer, providing a larger time window for coincidence detection than the NR2A receptor type. Compared to the NR2A or NR2B subtypes, the NR2D-type receptors show slow activation and deactivation kinetics (in the range of seconds rather than hundreds of milliseconds) as well as lower sensitivity to voltage-dependent Mg^{2+} block. Similarly, NR3 subunits determine that NR1/NR3 assemblies function as glycine-gated ion channels (Chatterton et al., 2002). With the exception of the NR3B subtype, all NMDA receptor subtypes are expressed in the hippocampus; the NR2A and NR2B subtypes are the major hippocampal forms.

Hippocampal Distribution of NR1 and NR1 Splice Variants

The NR1 subunit is expressed in dentate granule cells, in all pyramidal neurons, and in many interneurons (Laurie and Seeburg, 1994; Monyer et al., 1994). Alternative splicing generates eight splice forms of the NR1 subunit. First, there are NR1 splice forms that either lack (NR1a) or contain (NR1b) exon 5 of the NR1 gene, which encodes the so-called N1 cassette; this cassette influences gating kinetics and is a part of the extracellular N-terminal domain of the receptor. A second group of NR1 forms is generated by alternative splicing of the last two carboxyl-terminal exons, 21 and 22. Exon 21 encodes the C-terminal domain C1 and exon 22 the C-terminal domains C2 and C2′. In the first set of splice forms, exon 21 is excluded and C2 or C2′ are used for coding the NR1 C-terminal domain (NR1-2 and NR1-4). In the second set, exon 21 is present, which leads to C1-C2 and C1-C2′ carboxy-termini (NR1-1 and NR1-3). The eight NR1 isoforms are then termed NR1a-1, NR1a-2, NR1a-3, NR1a-4, NR1b-1, NR1b-2, NR1b-3, and NR1b-4.

The NR1 splice forms are differentially expressed in the hippocampus (Laurie and Seeburg, 1994) (Fig. 7–6). The NR1a, NR1-1, and NR1-2 splice forms are prominently expressed in all pyramidal cell layers of the hippocampus throughout development. In general, NR1-4 and NR1b are less expressed but show more prominent levels in CA3 pyramidal cells. NR1-3 expression is not detectable in the embryonic hippocampus and remains low in adult rats. The proposed roles of the various NR1 C-terminal splice forms in NMDA receptor trafficking and function, through mediating splice form-specific protein–protein interactions, are discussed in Section 7.4.2.

Hippocampal Distribution of NR2 Subunits

Functionally, NR2A and NR2B receptor subtypes differ in their channel kinetics. As already discussed, NR2B receptors stay open longer, providing a larger time window for coincidence detection compared to the NR2A receptor type. Both NR2A and NR2B are prominently expressed in all cell layers of the hippocampus (Fig. 7–6). The NR2A/NR2B expression ratio increases strongly during postnatal development, indicating that the NR2B-type NMDA receptors are more important at the early postnatal stage, whereas the NR2A receptors play a major role at mature hippocampal synapses (Monyer et al., 1994). In addition to the developmental differences, NR2A and NR2B receptors are also selectively targeted to different synapses in the CA1 and CA3 principal cells. In CA3 cells, the NR2A receptors are preferentially located at commissural/associational synapses and the NR2B receptors

at the fimbrial–CA3 synapses (Ito et al., 1997). The NR2B-type receptors are also reported to be selectively targeted to the apical versus the basal dendrites of CA1 neurons of the mouse hippocampus at synapses receiving either ipsilateral or contralateral CA3 inputs (Kawakami et al., 2003). Finally, the NR2A- and NR2B-type receptors are distinctly localized in the same synapse, with the NR2B type placed more extrasynaptically and the NR2A type restricted to the center of glutamatergic synapses in hippocampal principal neurons (Tovar and Westbrook, 1999). The distinct expression profiles of the two subunits thus provide a mechanism for expression of different types of NMDA receptor-dependent synaptic plasticity at different synapses and developmental stages in the hippocampus (see Section 7.5.2 for NR2 mutant mice).

The NR2C receptor type is not significantly expressed in the hippocampus. NR2D expression is restricted to hippocampal GAD67-, parvalbumin-, and somatostatin-positive interneurons in the stratum radiatum of the CA1 and CA3 regions (Standaert et al., 1996). Functionally, as noted above, the NR1/NR2D receptors show slower activation and deactivation kinetics (in the range of seconds rather than hundreds of milliseconds) and lower sensitivity to voltage-dependent Mg^{2+} block than do the NR1/NR2A or NR1/NR2B receptors (Monyer et al., 1994). Cells expressing the NR1/NR2D receptors would thus be expected to conduct NMDA currents without the need for strong coincident depolarization. However, hippocampal interneurons do not show the expected NR2D-type channel characteristics, possibly because NR2B has dominance over channel properties in NR1/NR2B/NR2D assemblies (cf. the NMDA receptor responses of NR1-, NR2B-, and NR2D-expressing cholinergic interneurons in the caudate-putamen) (Götz et al., 1997).

As with NR2D, the NR3A subunit is expressed in the hippocampus during embryogenesis and early postnatally, mainly in area CA1 and the subiculum (Ciabarra et al., 1995; Sucher et al., 1995). In the adult hippocampus, NR3A mRNA remains expressed in CA1 pyramidal cells, possibly forming NR1/NR3A glycine-gated excitatory cation channels. NR3B subtype receptors are not expressed in the hippocampus.

7.3.4 Kainate Receptors

Kainate receptors are tetrameric assemblies composed of GluR5, -6, -7 and KA1 and KA2 subunits, depending on which genes are expressed in a given cell type (Wisden et al., 2000). Recombinant GluR5, -6, and -7 subunits form functional homomeric as well as heteromeric channels; but most native receptors probably coassemble from both GluR and KA subunits.

Characterization of native kainate currents in the hippocampus has been made possible by using an antagonist (GYKI 53655), which selectively inhibits AMPA but not kainate receptors. With this pharmacological approach, kainate receptor-mediated currents were identified in the hippocampus at the mossy fiber synapses onto CA3 principal cells and the Schaffer collateral projections onto CA1

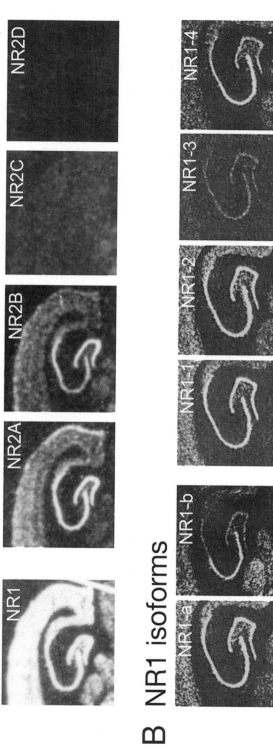
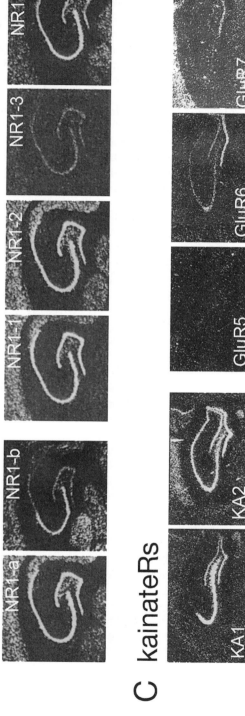

Figure 7–6. Expression of NMDA receptor subunits in rat hippocampus. *A.* In situ hybridization with specific oligonucleotides detects the mRNAs of NR1 and NR2A-D subunits. *B.* Expression of NR1 splice variant mRNAs visualized by in situ hybridization with splice form-specific oligonucleotides. *C.* Expression of kainate receptor subunit mRNAs in the adult rat hippocampus. (*Sources: A:* Modified from Monyer et al., 1994; *B:* modified from Laurie and Seeburg, 1994; *C:* modified from Wisden and Seeburg, 1993, all with permission.)

interneurons (Castillo et al., 1997b; Vignes and Collingridge, 1997; Cossart et al., 1998; Frerking et al., 1998). Further characterization of kainate receptor function was made possible by the development of knockout mice for the receptor subunit genes. At the mossy fiber–CA3 pyramidal cell synapse, kainate receptors participate in multiple aspects of transmission both pre- and postsynaptically. GluR6/KA2 receptors provide the postsynaptic response; GluR6/KA2/KA1 receptors contribute to presynaptic modulation (Contractor et al., 2003) (see more below). For the presynaptic component, applying low concentrations of kainate facilitates glutamate release; high concentrations depress release because of a depolarizing block of axonal conduction.

Kainate receptor currents constitute only about 10% of the total peak current generated by AMPA receptors on hippocampal pyramidal cells. However, the slow deactivation kinetics of kainate receptor currents means that during a mossy fiber composite EPSC a significant proportion of the total charge transfers through kainate receptors. Kainate receptors thus contribute to glutamate transmission by enhancing as well as extending the postsynaptic membrane depolarization. In addition, repetitive stimulation of the mossy fibers markedly increases kainate receptor currents; there is evidence that kainate receptors on mossy fiber terminals positively modulate synaptic release at higher firing frequencies of dentate granule cells (reviewed in Lerma, 2003).

Posttranscriptional Modifications of Kainate Receptor Subunits

As with AMPA receptors, the structural/functional complexity of kainate receptors is increased by posttranscriptional modifications (reviewed in Dingledine et al., 1999). The subunits GluR6 and GluR7 each come in two splice forms, with different C-terminal sequences (GluR6-1, 2; GluR7a, b). The GluR5 subunit displays four alternatively splice C-tails; additionally, an exon encoding 15 amino acids in the N-terminal domain occurs in some transcripts. Functionally, recombinant homomeric GluR7a channels have 5- to 10-fold larger currents in HEK 293 cells compared to GluR7b, suggesting that the C-tail splicing may regulate kainate receptor function. In addition, the various C-terminal domains are likely to play distinct roles in receptor trafficking by binding with splice form-specific regulatory proteins.

The GluR5 and GluR6 subunits are also regulated by site-selective RNA editing. Like the AMPA receptor GluR2 subunit (see Section 7.2.2), RNA editing at the Q/R site (a glutamine to arginine coding change) in the M2 domain of the GluR5 and GluR6 subunits reduces the single-channel conductance and Ca^{2+} permeability and changes the I–V relation. In contrast to GluR2, however, the glutamine residue is edited only in some GluR5 and GluR6 transcripts, with a gradual increase in the expression of the edited forms of both subunits during postnatal development. In the adult, approximately 50% of GluR5 and 80% of GluR6 are edited at the Q/R site. In addition, GluR6 undergoes editing at the I/V and Y/C sites in the M1 segment. Editing efficiency at these site is variable, giving a rise to a high number of functional variants (reviewed in Seeburg et al., 1998).

Hippocampal Distribution of Kainate Receptor Subunits

In hippocampal principal cells, the KA1 gene is mainly expressed in CA3 cells and dentate granule cells, with markedly weaker expression in CA1 pyramidal cells (Werner et al., 1991; Wisden and Seeburg, 1993) (Fig. 7–6). At the electron microscopic level, KA1 immunoreactivity was found on presynaptic mossy fiber boutons and, to a lesser degree, in postsynaptic spines (Darstein et al., 2003). KA2 mRNA is abundant in both CA1 and CA3 pyramidal cells and in the dentate granule cells (Bahn et al., 1994). The GluR6 subunit is moderately expressed in all CA pyramidal cells and in the dentate granule cells, with expression in CA3 higher than in CA1 (Egebjerg et al., 1991; Wisden and Seeburg, 1993). Using a GluR7 knockout mouse and a GluR6/7-selective antibody, GluR6 immunoreactivity was strong in the stratum lucidum (suggesting mossy fibers) and the CA3 pyramidal cell layer (Darstein et al., 2003). GluR7 mRNA is present in dentate granule cells but absent from CA pyramidal cells (Bettler et al., 1992). Using a GluR6 knockout mouse and the GluR6/7-selective antibody showed that GluR7 immunoreactivity was confined to the somatodendritic regions of dentate gyrus granule cells (Darstein et al., 2003); thus, GluR7 may not contribute to the KA1/KA2/GluR6 receptors on the mossy fiber terminals (alternatively, GluR7 axonal transport may require subunit coassembly with GluR6). Taken together, based on the subunit distributions, immunoprecipitation assays, and electrophysiological analyses from knockout mice, kainate receptors in hippocampal principal cells are assemblies of KA2/GluR6 in CA1 pyramidal cells; KA2/GluR6 and KA1/GluR6 or KA1/KA2/GluR6 in CA3 pyramidal cells; and KA1-, KA2-, GluR6-, and GluR7-derived receptors in dentate granule cells. A significant expression of KA1/KA2/GluR6 receptors is presynaptically assembled on mossy fiber terminals. Note that KA1 and KA2 subunits selectively assemble with GluR6 but not GluR7 subunits in the mouse hippocampus (Darstein et al., 2003).

In hippocampal interneurons, the most prominent kainate receptor subunit is GluR5 (Bettler et al., 1990; Wisden and Seeburg, 1993; Bahn et al., 1994); approximately half of the interneurons in the stratum oriens of adult CA1 express GluR5 (Paternain et al., 2000). Some of these GluR5-positive cells are probably oriens/alveus/lacunosum-moleculare (OLM) interneurons. In addition, there are a few GluR5-positive cells in the stratum radiatum (approximately 14% of all GABAergic cells), and in the pyramidal cell layer itself (approximately 30% of all GABAergic cells located in the pyramidal cell layer). However, disruption of the GluR5 gene does not cause a loss or reduction of functional kainate receptors in CA1 stratum radiatum interneurons, indicating that other kainate receptor subunits are also expressed in hippocampal interneurons (Mulle et al., 2000). Indeed, most of the GABAergic cells in the pyramidal cell layer also express GluR6 (Paternain et al., 2000), and combined deletion of GluR5 and GluR6 abolishes their kainate receptor-mediated currents. In addition, presynaptic GluR6- but not GluR5-containing receptors modulate synaptic transmission between inhibitory interneurons, indicating synapse-specific distribution of kainate receptor subunits in interneurons (Mulle et al., 2000).

Considering the GluR-6 expressing interneurons in more detail, there are a few GluR6-positive cells in theCA1 stratum oriens (6% of total GABAergic cells) and the stratum radiatum (approximately 3%); however, there are many GluR6-positive cells in the CA3 stratum lucidum; 85% of these GluR6-expressing stratum lucidum cells are also GAD65-positive. There are a few GluR6 mRNA-positive cells in the mouse stratum oriens and radiatum layers of both CA1 and CA3 (Bureau et al., 1999). Kainate receptor-mediated modulation of synaptic transmission between inhibitory interneurons in the stratum radiatum is impaired in GluR6 knockout mice (Mulle et al., 1998). However, excitation of the interneurons by activation of kainate receptors was still possible, suggesting the existence of two populations of kainate receptors in hippocampal interneurons (Mulle et al., 2000). GluR7 is expressed in occasional cells in the pyramidal cell layer; it is unknown if they are pyramidal cells or interneurons. There are a few GluR7 mRNA-positive cells in the mouse stratum oriens and stratum radiatum (Bureau et al., 1999).

7.3.5 Metabotropic Glutamate Receptors

Metabotropic glutamate receptors (mGluRs) are G protein-coupled and modulate glutamate release, GABA release, and neuronal excitability (for a review, see De Blasi et al., 2001). Metabotropic glutamate receptor activation inhibits or excites, depending on the receptor subtype and cell context. EPSPs are often reduced by presynaptic mGluR activation and enhanced by activation of postsynaptic mGluRs. An interesting aspect of the function of mGluRs in synaptic transmission comes from their subcellular localization: The mGluRs are typically outside of the pre- and postsynaptic membranes, indicating that they are selectively activated during intense synaptic activity, such as repetitive high-frequency firing, leading to a spillover of neurotransmitter into the perisynaptic space (Baude et al., 1993; Lujan et al., 1996; Shigemoto et al., 1997).

The eight mGluR receptor subtypes, each consisting of a large extracellular N-terminal domain with a binding site for glutamate, seven transmembrane domains, and an intracellular C-terminal peptide, are closely related to the family of GABA$_B$ receptors but have low sequence identity with "classic" G protein-coupled receptors such as the muscarinic receptors

(considered later in the chapter). Unlike the heteromeric GABA$_B$ receptors (see Section 7.5.3), all mGluR receptors are homodimers. The mGluR family subdivides into three groups based on their pharmacological and functional properties: group I (mGluR1, mGluR5), II (mGluR2, mGluR3), and III (mGluR4, mGluR6, mGluR7, mGluR8) (Shigemoto et al., 1997). Group I mGluRs are selectively activated by 3,5-dihydroxyphenylglycine (DHPG) and positively couple via Gq to phospholipase C, thus stimulating protein kinase C activation and inositol triphosate (IP3) production. Group I mGluRs have a somatodendritic distribution (see below); and their activation leads to enhanced excitability of hippocampal neurons via modulation of Ca^{2+}, K$^+$, and nonselective cation channels and to an increase in postsynaptic intracellular Ca^{2+} via IP3-mediated release from internal Ca^{2+} stores. Group II and III mGluRs are selectively activated by 2-(2,3-dicarboxycyclopropyl)glycine (DCG-IV) and 2-amino-4-phosphonobutyrate (L-AP4), respectively, and negatively couple via Gi to adenylate cyclase, thus inhibiting cAMP production. The mGluRs 2, 3, 4, 7, and 8 are located in axons near and within presynaptic terminals (see below). They suppress neurotransmitter release by inhibiting voltage-dependent Ca^{2+} channels and/or by interfering directly with the release machinery. In the hippocampus, group III mGluRs mediate inhibition of excitatory transmission in the Schaffer collateral(CA1 cell synapses, whereas both group II and group III mGluRs contribute to presynaptic inhibition in the perforant path–granule cell synapses.

mGluR Distribution in the Hippocampus

All mGluR genes, except mGluR6, are expressed in the hippocampus and show a diverse cellular distribution (Fig. 7–7). Their expression has been studied in detail by in situ hybridization and with subtype-specific antibodies.

From group I mGluRs, mGluR1 mRNA is in all principal cells, with the order of expression level DG $\gg$ CA3 $\gg$ CA1 (Shigemoto et al., 1992). Many interneurons in the CA1 stratum oriens and the stratum oriens and radiatum in CA3 are strong mGluR1 expressors (Shigemoto et al., 1992). Within the detection limits of the method, double-labeling in situ hybridization shows that mGluR1 mRNA is in somatostatin-positive but not parvalbumin-positive interneurons (Kerner et al., 1997). mGluR-5 mRNA is abundant in the hippocampus, expressed strongly in CA pyramidal cells, dentate granule cells, and many types of GABAergic interneurons (Fotuhi et al., 1994). mGluR-5 mRNA was also detected by double-labeling in situ hybridization in somatostatin-positive and parvalbumin-positive interneurons (Kerner et al., 1997). Group I mGluRs have a selective somatodendritic perisynaptic distribution in principal neurons and are typically located at the outer edge of postsynaptic densities of dendritic spines (Lujan et al., 1996; Shigemoto et al., 1997).

From group II and III mGluRs, mGluR3 mRNA is abundant in dentate granule cells but absent from pyramidal cells;

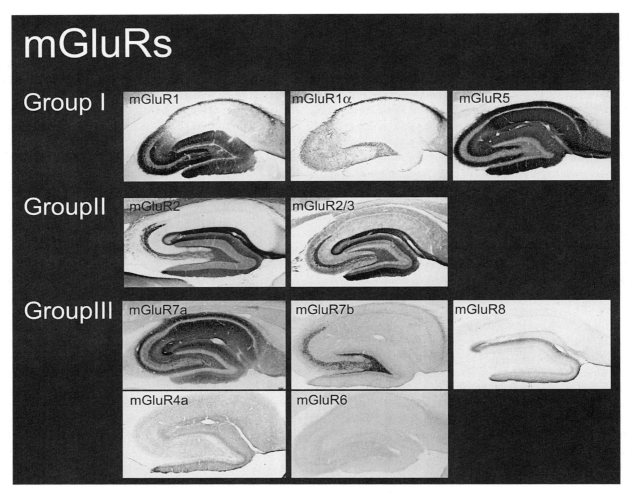

Figure 7–7. Expression of mGluRs in the rat hippocampus. Immunohistochemistry with subunit-specific antibodies was used to visualize expression patterns of individual mGluRs in adult hippocampus. (*Source*: Modified from Shigemoto et al., 1997, with permission.)

mGluR3 is also expressed in hippocampal white matter tracts, the fimbria, and the fornix (Ohishi et al., 1993). In contrast to the largely presynaptic localization of most group II and III mGluRs, mGluR3 protein is expressed perisynaptically in dendrites of the dentate granule cells in a pattern reminiscent of mGluR1 and mGluR5 expression (Tamaru et al., 2001). mGluR4 and mGluR7 mRNAs are both expressed in CA1 and CA3 pyramidal cells, dentate granule cells, and scattered interneurons (Ohishi et al., 1995). mGluR4 is more marked in CA2 pyramidal cells. The mGluR2 and mGluR7a proteins are on axons and terminals of the medial perforant path, whereas the lateral perforant path is prominently immunoreactive for mGluR8 in the dentate gyrus and the CA3 area. Mossy fibers contain mGluR2, mGluR7a, and mGluR7b, whereas Schaffer collateral axons display only mGluR7a. Group II (mGluR2) and group III (mGluR4, 7, and 8) mGluRs are in different parts of the presynaptic elements: Group III receptors predominate in presynaptic active zones of both asymmetrical (glutamatergic) and symmetrical (GABAergic) synapses, whereas group II receptors are found in the preterminal portions of axons (Shigemoto et al., 1997).

7.4 Trafficking of Glutamate Receptors and Hippocampal Synaptic Plasticity

In mammalian neurons, subcellular compartments, often located in near proximity to each other, comprise distinct protein complexes. For example, in principal neurons, excitatory synapses are positioned on dendritic spines, which contain glutamatergic receptors and cytoskeletal and signaling proteins relevant to their functions—all components of the so-called postsynaptic density (PSD). GABA receptors and their specialized cytoskeletal proteins, on the other hand, are positioned at GABAergic synapses scattered between the dendritic spines; whereas dendritic voltage-gated ion channels, regulating integration of the excitatory and inhibitory inputs along the dendritic branches, are mostly excluded from the synaptic sites and show either uniform or gradient-like distributions in the dendrites. To maintain such function-specific subcellular distribution of proteins, neurons have a variety of trafficking proteins that mediate intracellular targeting, retention, and removal of particular receptors, channels, kinases, phosphatases, and other molecules at their corresponding destination sites.

The most prevalent type of protein–protein interaction underlying intracellular trafficking is between a short amino acid motif typically present at the C-terminal end of the trafficked protein and a PDZ domain of its cytoskeletal interactor. The PDZ abbreviation is derived from three proteins originally identified to contain this approximately 90-amino-acid structural motif: PSD-95 (postsynaptic density protein of 95 kD molecular weight), DlgA (*Drosophila* discs-large protein; present in septate junctions) and ZO-1 (protein of epithelial tight junctions). There are three PDZ domains that bind different amino acid sequences. The class 1 PDZ domain recognizes the X-S/T-X-V/L motif (where X is any amino acid), class 2 the X-f-X-f motif (f = hydrophobic aa), and class 3 the X-D-X-V motif (reviewed in Sheng and Sala, 2001). Next to the carboxyl sequence, PDZ domains can also bind to an internal motif that forms a β-hairpin structure, although this form of PDZ interaction is much less frequent.

7.4.1 Synaptic Transport of AMPA Receptors in LTP and LTD

Intracellular trafficking of ionotropic glutamate receptors includes selective somatodendritic transport to the postsynaptic membrane of glutamatergic synapses and anchoring of the receptors by cytoskeletal proteins. In addition, AMPA receptors undergo activity-dependent cycling between two pools: the functional pool of AMPA receptors inserted at the synaptic surface and the reserve pool of AMPA receptors present either intracellularly (in which case the movement is regulated by local endo- and exocytosis) or at the extrasynaptic surface membrane (in which case the receptors are transported by lateral diffusion). Such activity-dependent local synaptic recycling of AMPA receptors is believed to be one mechanism by which hippocampal pyramidal neurons—particularly in the CA1 region—can regulate the strength of their synaptic transmission.

GluR1-dependent Trafficking and GluR1-binding Proteins: Relevance to Hippocampal LTP

Trafficking mechanisms mediated by the GluR1 C-terminal domain were proposed to regulate synaptic insertion of GluR1-containing AMPA receptors at the Schaffer collateral to CA1 synapses. The initial evidence for this came from a series of electrophysiological experiments studying synaptic delivery of recombinant receptors in organotypic slice cultures (reviewed in Malinow and Malenka, 2002). In this work, synaptic insertion of recombinant GFP-tagged GluR1 recep-

tors, either homomeric GluR1 or heteromeric GluR1/2 channels, was shown to be triggered during the induction of LTP and to depend on the activation of NMDA receptors as well as α-CaMKII. Direct evidence of the role of GluR1 in LTP and in specific forms of learning came from mice that either lack the GluR1 gene altogether or contain the gene with knock-in mutations in its C-terminal phosphorylation sites (Zamanillo et al., 1999; Reisel et al., 2002; Lee et al., 2003) (these mouse models are discussed in detail in Section 7.5.3).

The search for trafficking proteins binding specifically to the GluR1 C-terminal domain has yet to yield a clear candidate for mediating synaptic delivery of GluR1-containing AMPA receptors. To date, the list of GluR1 C-tail interactors includes 4.1N protein, which binds at juxtamembrane C-tail region; PDZ domain-containing protein SAP-97, which binds at the class I PDZ binding motif at the C-tail carboxyl end; and PDZ and LIM domain-containing protein RIL (reverse-induced LIM domain protein), which binds at the last 10 amino residues of GluR1 C-tail via its LIM domain (reviewed in Malinow and Malenka, 2002; Song and Huganir, 2002). Note that the PDZ domain-binding motif of the GluR1 C-tail is not required for synaptic delivery/accumulation of the receptors or for synaptic plasticity in the CA1 hippocampus (Lee et al., 2003). Functionally, 4.1N protein was proposed to anchor GluR1-containing AMPA receptors at the synaptic surface by a linkage to spectrin/actin cytoskeleton; SAP-97 may regulate the transport of newly synthesized receptors through Golgi and ER compartments; and RIL was proposed to link the intracellular transport of the receptors in the dendritic spine compartment to the actin/α-actinin cytoskeleton (Song and Huganir, 2002; Schulz et al., 2004).

GluR2-dependent Trafficking and GluR2-binding Proteins: Relevance to Hippocampal LTD

It has been proposed that the prevalent C-terminal splice form of GluR2, with its 50-amino-acid residue "short" C-terminal tail, regulates activity-independent (constitutive) synaptic delivery of GluR2/3 receptors in the CA1 pyramidal neurons (this model of transport is again primarily based on electrophysiology experiments with recombinant channels) (reviewed in Malinow and Malenka, 2002). Interestingly, the GluR2/3 receptor insertion does not change the overall strength of synaptic transmission but, rather, replaces the GluR1/2-containing receptors. The GluR2-containing receptors, however, undergo activity-dependent endocytosis from the synaptic surface during protocols resulting in the induction of LTD. Based on these experiments, it was suggested that the synaptic transport of AMPA receptors is regulated by subunit-specific interactions where the GluR1 subunit plays a critical role in upregulating the strength of AMPA receptor-mediated transmission during LTP, and the GluR2 subunit mediates downregulation of the glutamatergic transmission seen in LTD.

Trafficking proteins that bind to the GluR2 C-terminal domain include N-ethylmaleimide-sensitive fusion protein

(NSF), glutamate receptor interacting protein (GRIP) and a closely related AMPA receptor-binding protein (ABP, also termed GRIP2), protein interacting with C-kinase (PICK1), and clathrin adaptor protein complex AP2 (reviewed in Song and Huganir, 2002). In general, the function of individual GluR2 interactors is not clearly resolved; the overall conclusions, however, tend to agree with the proposed role of GluR2-interacting proteins in endocytosis and recycling of the receptors and support the electrophysiology findings that GluR2-dependent transport plays a role in LTD. NSF is an ATPase that is essential for SNARE-dependent intracellular membrane fusion (see Section 7.2.6 for the role of NSF in neurotransmitter release). It was proposed that NSF binding to the GluR2 C-tail regulates the recycling of GluR2-containing AMPA receptors after their endocytosis from synaptic sites toward new synaptic insertion. One model of NSF function suggests that the ATPase regulates disassembly of the internalized receptors from their binding with PICK1 (Hanley et al., 2002). The binding by GRIP/ABP (proteins containing 6/7 PDZ domains) and PICK1 (single PDZ domain protein) at the same class II PDZ-binding motif of the GluR2 C-tail is regulated by phosphorylation: PICK1, but not GRIP/ABP, binds to the phosphorylated TEV motif. Functionally, GRIP/ABP binding was proposed to mediate anchoring of the GluR2-containing receptors at the hippocampal CA1 synapses (Osten et al., 2000), and PICK1 binding may regulate internalization of GluR2-containing receptors during LTD (Kim et al., 2001). Interestingly, PICK1-based GluR2 trafficking may also enhance the proportion of synaptic Ca^{2+}-permeable (GluR2-lacking) AMPA receptors, suggesting a further, more complex role for PICK1 in hippocampal synaptic functions (Terashima et al., 2004). The role of the AP2 adaptor, in agreement with its well established role in clathrin-dependent endocytosis (see also Section 7.1.7), appears to be necessary for activity-dependent internalization of the GluR2-containing receptors during LTD (Lee et al., 2002).

Glutamatergic "Silent Synapses": GluR2$_{long}$-dependent and GluR4-dependent Trafficking

Mature glutamatergic synapses contain both AMPA- and NMDA-type receptors. In contrast, electrophysiological recordings of synaptic currents in hippocampal slices prepared from rats less than 2-weeks old demonstrated that a large portion of young synapses contain only NMDA receptors and lack functional AMPA receptors. Because NMDA receptors are inhibited by their voltage-dependent Mg^{2+} block at a resting membrane potential (see Section 7.3.3), glutamate release at these sites fails to evoke postsynaptic currents; and hence such synapses were named "silent synapses" (reviewed in Malinow and Malenka, 2002). In addition to the electrophysiological demonstration of silent synapses, anatomical support for their existence was provided by an electron microscopy-based analysis of AMPA and NMDA receptor distribution, which confirmed the predicted large portion of AMPA receptor-lacking synapses in the young hippocampus (Nusser et al., 1998b; Petralia et al., 1999).

The initial delivery of AMPA receptors to silent synapses—the conversion of silent to functional AMPA receptor-expressing synapses—has been proposed to be mediated primarily by two subunits, GluR4 and GluR2$_{long}$, with closely related C-terminal domains (Zhu et al., 2000; Kolleker et al., 2003); GluR2$_{long}$ is a C-terminal splice form of GluR2 (see section 7.2.2). Both subunits are synaptically inserted during the induction of LTP as well as by synchronized spontaneous synaptic activity resembling the giant depolarizing potentials (GDPs) that frequently occur in the juvenile hippocampus. Interacting proteins specific for the GluR4 and/or GluR2$_{long}$ subunits, which could potentially regulate the trafficking of AMPA receptors to the silent synapses, are yet to be identified.

AMPA Receptor Pan-subunit-interacting Proteins: Narp and Stargazin

Two proteins, neuronal activity-regulated pentraxin (Narp) and stargazin (also termed γ2), were shown to bind to AMPA receptors without selectivity for individual subunits (reviewed in Bredt and Nicoll, 2003). Narp is a secreted immediate early gene product that binds to the extracellular portions of the GluR1/2/3 subunits. Narp was shown to induce AMPA receptor clustering and may function during glutamatergic synaptogenesis (O'Brien et al., 1999).

The stargazin gene was originally identified because of its spontaneous loss-of-function mutation in a mouse line with head-tossing movements (hence the name stargazer for the mouse and stargazin for the gene), ataxic gait, impaired eyeblink conditioning, and spike-wave seizures characteristic of absence epilepsy (reviewed in Letts, 2005). Stargazin is a four-transmembrane protein, with three closely related brain-specific isoforms: γ3, γ4, and γ8. The trafficking function of stargazin with respect to AMPA receptors was revealed first in stargazer cerebellar granule cells, which show a striking failure of AMPA receptor synaptic delivery (Chen et al., 2000). Note that these cells appear to express only stargazin, whereas most other CNS neurons express multiple stargazin isoforms (Tomita et al., 2003). Thus, the cerebellar granule cells can be considered a cellular model of a complete γ2, γ3, γ4, and γ8 knockout. In the hippocampus, γ8 is the most prominent isoform but γ2, γ3, and γ4 are also expressed; cellularly, stargazin and its isoforms are expressed in pyramidal neurons and interneurons (Tomita et al., 2003). In agreement with the overlapping expression in the hippocampus, genetic deletion of γ8 did not cause complete breakdown of AMPA receptor trafficking: Synaptic AMPA receptor-mediated currents in the CA1 pyramidal neurons were only modestly decreased in the γ8 knockout; however, the total protein levels of GluR1 and GluR2/3 receptors were strongly reduced, a portion of the remaining receptors appeared retained somatically, and extrasynaptic receptor pools were depleted; furthermore, LTP in the CA1 neurons was also impaired (Rouach et al., 2005).

How does this phenotype, which strikingly resembles genetic deletion of GluR1 in the hippocampus (see Section 7.4.3), compare to what is known about stargazin functions? Stargazin appears to be stably associated (as an auxiliary subunit) with a large portion of native AMPA receptors (Nakagawa et al., 2005; Vandenberghe et al., 2005) and was proposed to chaperone the transport of the receptors through early endoplasmatic reticulum and Golgi compartments (Vandenberghe et al., 2005). In the hippocampal CA1 pyramidal neurons, most mature AMPA receptor complexes thus appear to require the presence of GluR1 (see Section 7.4.3) and γ8. In addition, stargazin and its γ isoforms are also likely to play direct roles in synaptic functions of AMPA receptors in the hippocampus: first, by anchoring the receptors to the postsynaptic cytoskeletal protein PSD-95 (Chen et al., 2000) (see Section 7.3.2 for PSD-95 role in synaptic function of NMDA receptors) and, second, by reducing the receptor desensitization in response to synaptic glutamate (Priel et al., 2005; Tomita et al., 2005; Turetsky et al., 2005). These functions may be sufficiently compensated by γ2, γ3, and/or γ4 in the γ8-knockout hippocampus.

7.4.2 NMDA Receptor-associated Cytoskeletal and Signaling Proteins

Until recently, NMDA receptors were believed to be less synaptically "mobile" than AMPA receptors, and the trafficking of NMDA receptors was originally proposed to be largely limited to their synaptic delivery and subsequently transport for degradation. However, it is becoming evident that NMDA receptors undergo activity-dependent trafficking, which may be quite similar (for example, with regard to the subunit-specific transport mechanisms) to that of AMPA receptors, though perhaps happening on a slower time scale. At the same time, synaptic functions of NMDA receptors appear to depend critically on interactions with cytoskeletal and signaling proteins of the postsynaptic density, which directly or indirectly bind to the C-terminal domains of the receptor subunits. As described in Section 7.2.3, the major NMDA receptor types in the hippocampus are the NR1/NR2A, NR1/NR2B, and to a lesser extent NR1/NR2A/NR2B subunit assemblies. The NMDA receptor C-terminal domains are quite large, varying from approximately 100 amino acid residues for the longer NR1 splice forms to more than 600 amino acid residues for the NR2A/2B subunits. These receptor domains are thus well suited to accommodate a large number of interacting proteins and their associated protein complexes.

Regulation of NMDA Receptor Function via PSD-95 and Its Interacting Proteins

The identification of PSD-95 as an NMDA receptor-binding protein (which incidentally was also the first identification of a protein–protein interaction at a C-terminal tail of a glutamate receptor subunit) came from a yeast two-hybrid screen with the entire 627-amino-acid residue NR2A C-terminal domain (Kornau et al., 1995). The yeast two-hybrid method is used to identify protein interactions by screening a cDNA library, such as a brain or hippocampal library, with a transcription-reporter system in yeast; it has been used for isolation of most of the glutamate receptor-interacting proteins described to date. NR2A, as well as the other NR2 subunits, binds to the second and third PDZ domains of PSD-95 via a conserved class I PDZ-binding motif; in addition, NR1 splice forms containing the C2′ segment, NR1-3, and NR-4, may also bind to PSD-95 via a different PDZ-binding sequence (reviewed in Sheng and Sala, 2001).

PSD-95 is an abundant postsynaptic protein that contains three PDZ domains, an SH3 domain, and a nonfunctional guanylate kinase (GK) domain. The PSD-95 protein family consists of three additional closely related proteins: SAP102, SAP97, and PSD-93 (note that SAP97 binds to GluR1) (see Section 7.3.1). Functionally, PSD-95 acts as a scaffold linking a number of other postsynaptic proteins to the NMDA receptor complex (reviewed in Sheng and Pak, 2000). For example, PSD-95 binds, via its GK domain, to a protein termed GKAP. GKAP binds to Shank, and Shank in turn binds to Homers and cortactin. Dimers of Homer may link the NMDA receptors to internal Ca^{2+} stores or to the metabotropic receptors, as Homer also binds to the IP3 and/or ryanodine receptors of the Ca^{2+} stores and to the C-terminal domains of mGluR1a/mGluR5 (see more on Homer in Section 7.3.3). Cortactin, on the other hand, links the NMDA receptors to the actin cytoskeleton. Other proteins are associated with PSD-95 via binding to one of its three PDZ domains; these proteins include the neuronal nitric oxide synthase (nNOS); neuronal cell adhesion proteins neuroligins, microtubule-binding protein CRIPT; synaptic GTPase-activating protein for Ras termed SynGAP; Rho effector citron; nonreceptor tyrosine kinase Fyn; and possibly Src. Taken together, the scaffold function of PSD-95 is twofold: First, PSD-95 anchors the receptors to postsynaptic cytoskeletal proteins; and second, it links signaling molecules to the near proximity of the receptors. In addition, PSD-95 directly clusters NMDA receptors at the postsynaptic membrane, a function that depends on its ability to multimerize and to associate with membrane lipids via palmitoylation of cysteine residues in the N-terminal portion of the PSD-95 molecule (reviewed in el-Husseini Ael and Bredt, 2002).

The importance of PSD-95 for NMDA receptor function was directly tested in mice engineered to lack the PSD-95 gene (Migaud et al., 1998). Somewhat surprisingly, the subcellular distribution of the receptors in hippocampal CA1 neurons was normal, indicating that PSD-95 is not essential for NMDA receptor targeting to and accumulation at excitatory synapses. In contrast, synaptic plasticity at the Schaffer collateral to CA1 synapses was altered: The frequency threshold for the induction of NMDA receptor-dependent LTD and LTP was shifted in favor of LTP, resulting in strikingly enhanced LTP at stimulation frequencies ranging from 1 to 100 Hz. In agreement with the belief that LTP and LTD are both required for normal learning and memory, the PSD-95 knockout mice showed a profound deficit in hippocampus-based spatial learning in the Morris watermaze (Migaud et al., 1998). One possible explanation of the PSD-95 null phenotype is that other members of the PSD-95 family are able to compensate for the trafficking and clustering functions but are not sufficient to bind one or more of the signaling molecules that are normally linked by PSD-95 in the proximity of NMDA receptors (see above). Presently, it is not clear which PSD-95-dependent signaling molecules/cascades may be impaired in the knockout mice. The cellular and behavioral phenotypes do, however, provide evidence regarding the importance of the NMDA receptor subunit C-terminal domains for normal NMDA receptor function. This conclusion was even more dramatically established in mice engineered to lack the complete C-terminal peptides of the NRA, NR2B, or NR2C (Sprengel et al., 1998) (see Section 7.5.2).

NMDA Receptor-interacting Proteins (Other than PSD-95)

In addition to PSD-95, a number of other postsynaptic proteins bind directly to the NMDA receptor complex—primarily to the NR1 C-terminal domain (see above for NR1 C-terminal splice forms). The juxtamembrane region of the NR1 C-terminal peptide, termed C0, serves as a binding site for α-actinin, an actin-binding protein. This interaction may contribute to anchoring of the receptors at the postsynapse, as actin is the major cytoskeleton of dendritic spines. (Note that there are at least three other possible ways for linking NMDA receptors to actin cytoskeleton: via NR2B binding to α-actinin, via NR1/2A/2B binding to spectrin, and via the PSD-95-GKAP-Shank-spectrin complex—as reviewed by Sheng and Pak, 2000.) Other interactions give rise to functional changes. Calmodulin binds to the C0 and C1 segment of NR1; this interaction is Ca^{2+}-dependent and causes an approximately fourfold reduction of open NMDA channel probability. It has been proposed that competitive binding between α-actinin and Ca^{2+}/calmodulin at the C0 segment mediates activity/Ca^{2+}-dependent inactivation of NMDA receptors (Zhang et al., 1998; Krupp et al., 1999). In addition to calmodulin, two other proteins bind to the NR1 C1 segment: yotiao and neurofilament L. Yotiao may serve to link the type I protein phosphatase (PP1) and the adenosine 3',5'-monophosphate (cAMP)-dependent protein kinase (PKA) to the proximity of the receptor (Sheng and Pak, 2000). This close physical association of kinases and phosphatases with the NMDA receptors is an elegant mechanism that enhances the coupling of the Ca^{2+} influx to downstream signaling molecules. Perhaps the best example of such "symbiosis" is the binding of the most abundant postsynaptic kinase, CaMKII, to the NR2A/NR2B subunits.

CaMKII plays a critical role in plasticity at Schaffer collateral to CA1 synapses, where it has been shown to be both necessary and sufficient for the induction of LTP (see Section 7.5.1 on deficits in LTP and learning in mice lacking the α-isoform of the kinase). The current model of CaMKII in LTP suggests that the kinase, after its activation by postsynaptic Ca^{2+} influx through the NMDA receptors, undergoes a molecular switch by autophosphorylation of a single residue in the regulatory domain (Thr286 in α-CaMKII), which allows the dodecameric holoenzyme to become persistently active even in the absence of Ca^{2+}/calmodulin; as a next step, the kinase translocates to the NMDA receptor complex and binds to the C-tails of NR2A/B and/or NR1 (reviewed in Lisman et al., 2002). The switch back to a normal state requires dephosphorylation of the kinase; similar dephosphorylation by PP1 may occur during LTD (note that PP1 is also localized to the NMDA receptor complex by its interactions with yotiao, see above). In addition, binding of activated CaMKII selectively to the NR2B C-tail locks the kinase in an autoactive state that does not require autophosphorylation (Bayer et al., 2001). Once at the PSD site, CaMKII can phosphorylate the GluR1 C-terminal Ser831, which directly increases the channel conductance of GluR1-containing AMPA receptors; furthermore, CaMKII-mediated phosphorylation of a yet to be identified protein(s) was proposed to regulate the synaptic insertion of AMPA receptors during the induction of LTP (see Section 7.4.1) (reviewed in Malinow and Malenka, 2002).

Synaptic Trafficking of NMDA Receptors: Relevance to Homeostatic Plasticity and LTP

Intracellular transport of NMDA receptors appears to be tightly regulated at several levels, from the assembly and trafficking in the endoplasmatic reticulum to agonist induced internalization at synapses. As discussed in Section 7.3.3, the NR2B receptors are more prevalent at young and NR2A at mature hippocampal synapses; in the adult, NR2B receptors are expressed at lower levels and perhaps mainly extrasynaptically. Some of the first evidence for regulated synaptic trafficking of NMDA receptors came from studies showing that long-term changes in overall synaptic activity regulate the synaptic expression of both AMPA and NMDA receptors, a phenomenon termed "homeostatic plasticity." Chronic (several hours or even days) suppression of excitatory network activity upregulates AMPA and NMDA receptor-mediated responses, whereas chronic elevation of excitatory network activity has the opposite effect (reviewed in Turrigiano and Nelson, 2004). This form of plasticity was proposed to protect excitatory circuits from both runaway excitation and too little excitation (in other words, to maintain an overall balance between synaptic input and spiking output in excitatory networks).

Synaptic delivery of the NR2A and NR2B receptors at hippocampal synapses is also differently regulated by activity: NR2B insertion at synapses occurs constitutively, whereas the exchange of NR2B for NR2A receptors is driven by synaptic activity (Barria and Malinow, 2002). This transport mechanism may guarantee that NR2B receptors are freely inserted during development and prior to and/or during the formation of synaptic contacts, whereas the NR2A receptors are delivered only to preexisting synapses. Recently, synaptic recruitment of NMDA receptors was also observed during LTP, analogous to the delivery of AMPA receptors but with a delay of approximately 2 hours (Watt et al., 2004); this finding provides a mechanism for maintaining a constant ratio of AMPA to NMDA receptors at synapses, as observed on a longer time scale during the homeostatic form of plasticity.

7.4.3 Proteins Regulating Transport and Function of mGluRs

As with ionotropic glutamate receptors, the subcellular trafficking and function of mGluRs are also regulated via proteins binding at their intracellular C-terminal domains. However, fewer mGluR-binding partners have been identified so far (see below). In view of the numerous mGluR C-terminal splice variants, further mGluR trafficking proteins may be expected to be found in the coming years (mGluR C-terminal variations due to alternative RNA splicing include four versions of mGluR1, termed mGluR1a to d; and two versions each of mGluR4, 7, and 8, termed mGluR4a and b, mGluR5a and b, mGluR7a and b, and mGluR8a and b).

Both members of the mGluR I group (mGluR1 and mGluR5) bind to proteins of the Homer gene family, which, in turn, interact with the NMDA receptor–PSD-95 complex (see above). Homers exist in two forms: constitutively expressed Homers (Homer 1b and c, 2, and 3), which contain an N-terminal EVH domain and a C-terminal dimerizing coil-coil domain; and an immediate early gene (IEG) homer (Homer 1a), which lacks the coil-coil domain (reviewed in Xiao et al., 2000; Fagni et al., 2002). Due to the lack of the coil-coil domain, Homer1a cannot dimerize; it can, however, act as a competitive decoy and disrupt the interactions between full-length Homer dimers and their associated proteins. Homers bind via their EVH domain to the Pro–Pro–X–X–Phe motif present in the distal part of the mGluR1a/5 C-terminal domains. The mGluR–Homer interaction may serve several functions. First, Homer proteins may direct the targeting of mGluR1a/5 to dendrites rather than axons, and anchor mGluR1a/5 within intracellular membrane compartments. In this scenario, the induction of the IEG Homer1a would act to release the intracellular anchor and lead to the delivery of the receptors at the perisynaptic membrane. Second, as with NMDA receptors, the Homer dimer complex may link group I mGluRs to the cytoskeleton of dendritic spines via a mGluR1a/5-Homer-Homer-Shank complex. However, because NMDARs and mGluR1a/5 are differentially localized in spines (the former in the postsynaptic density, the latter perisynaptically), it seems likely that protein(s) other than Homers mediate the precise localization of mGluR1a/5 at the cellular membrane. Third, Homers may couple mGluR1a/5 directly to intracellular Ca^{2+} stores via the mGluR1a/5-Homer-Homer-IP3/ryanodine receptor complex. Fourth, and finally, Homers may directly regulate the function of mGluR1a/5, as full-length Homer forms have been shown to

inhibit the constitutive activity of this mGluR species. Under this last scenario, the induction of Homer1a would not only increase the surface expression of mGluR1a/5, as described above, but also enhance mGluR activation even in the absence of glutamate.

Axonal transport of the presynaptic mGluR7 in hippocampal neurons is directed by a sequence in the mid-region of its C-terminal peptide (Stowell and Craig, 1999). The distal region of the mGluR7 C-terminal tail interacts with the PDZ domain-containing protein PICK1 (Boudin et al., 2000), a protein that also binds to the C-terminal domains of the AMPA receptor subunits GluR2 and GluR3. The mGluR7–PICK1 interaction may mediate the clustering of metabotropic receptors at the presynaptic terminal membrane.

7.5 Glutamate Receptor Mutant Mice: Genetic Analysis of Hippocampal Function

7.5.1 Introduction: Building of Hippocampus-specific Genetic Models

As discussed in detail in Chapter 10, modulation of excitatory synaptic transmission between principal neurons, typically via Hebbian synaptic plasticity, is believed to constitute the principal neural mechanism of hippocampus-dependent learning and memory. Mouse models engineered to lack a specific gene related to functions underlying synaptic plasticity or to express a modified version of such a gene with an altered function, are becoming increasingly powerful in addressing molecular and cellular mechanisms underlying the various types of hippocampal learning and memory that are studied in rodents (see Chapter 10 for hippocampus-based learning in rats and mice). A pioneering work in this direction was the generation of mice lacking the a subunit of the Ca^{2+}/calmodulin-dependent protein kinase (CaMKII), an enzyme postulated to be a critically important player in the process of memory formation in the hippocampus (see Section 7.4.2 and Chapter 10 for activation of CaMKII in LTP). The α-CaMKII knockout mice showed impairment of LTP at CA3 to CA1 synapses, as well as deficits in hippocampus-dependent learning (Silva et al., 1992a,b). This was a critical piece of evidence highlighting the importance of α-CaMKII in LTP; even more importantly, together with the contemporaneous study of the fyn mutant (Grant et al., 1992), it provided the first genetic evidence that LTP is involved in hippocampal memory formation.

In many other genetic studies, however, the correlation between the introduced manipulation and hippocampus-based memory formation is not as easily interpretable. Typically, this is due to lack of a spatiotemporal regulation over the onset of the manipulation, resulting in alteration of a specific gene function that is present in many different brain regions and throughout development. The straightforward explanation of the results of Silva et al. was possible because of the prominent expression of α-CaMKII in the hippocampus as well as the fact that the onset of α-CaMKII expression is limited to a later stage of postnatal development. For other genes one wishes to study with respect to their hippocampal functions, this problem has been overcome, at least to some extent, by the development of genetic techniques that are spatially restricted to the frontal cortex including the hippocampus or to hippocampal pyramidal cell types (e.g., CA1 neurons or dentate gyrus granule cells) (see Box 7–1). So far, such hippocampus-specific mutations have been mainly used to examine the functions of AMPA and NMDA receptors. As described below, these studies not only support the conclusions of Silva et al. and Grant et al. and those of the earlier pharmacological studies (Morris et al., 1986) regarding the role of LTP in learning, they also threw light on the importance of glutamate receptors for both the induction and expression of synaptic plasticity. The experiments showed that different mechanisms are used to establish and maintain different forms of LTP used in different forms of learning (for example, spatial working versus reference memory).

7.5.2 NMDA Receptor Mutant Mice

The first mouse model aimed at studying NMDA receptor function was a knockout of the NR1 subunit (Forrest et al., 1994); these mice showed that NR1 is essential for formation of functional NMDA receptor channels (the mice died 8–15 hours after birth). Mice with reduced expression of the NR1 gene were generated by insertion of the "neo gene cassette" in an intronic region of the NR1 gene, which resulted in silencing NR1 gene expression and subsequent reduction of NR1 protein expression down to 5% of the wild-type level (Mohn et al., 1999). Note that the neo gene cassette serves as a selection marker during preparation of knockout targeting constructs (see Box 7–1); the presence of the cassette sometimes interferes with normal mRNA processing of the transcribed gene product, causing indirect silencing of gene expression. The NR1 "neo" mice survived to adulthood, showed normal AMPA and kainate receptor functions, but displayed deficits in social and sexual interactions, increased motor activity, and stereotypical behavior that was similar to the behavior observed in pharmacologically induced animal models of schizophrenia.

Hippocampal Region-specific NR1 Knockout Mice

Hippocampal CA1-specific NR1 knockout mice were generated using the Cre/lox-recombination system, with the Cre recombinase expressed under the control of the α-CaMKII promoter (see Box 7–1) (Tsien et al., 1996a,b). Although this promoter is typically active in most postnatal excitatory forebrain neurons, a transgenic line with Cre expression restricted almost exclusively to the CA1 region (due to a chromosomal integration effect) was selected. The CA1 cell-specific NR1 gene deletion had no apparent effect on mRNA levels of

(text continued on page 265)

Box 7–1
Tools to Generate Conditional Mouse Mutants

Conditional mouse mutants are used for temporally and spatially regulated transgene expression, gene deletion, or gene activation. The two most commonly used systems are the tTA system and the *Cre system*. In both systems, two genetic modules are introduced separately into the mouse genome: the *activator gene*, which regulates expression of the second module, and the *responsive target gene*, the function of which one wishes to study. After first obtaining independent, "activator" and "responder" mouse lines, the two are bred together to create the "conditional mouse" line (see Box Table 7–1).

Activator mice function in two ways (see Box Fig. 7–1). First, the expression of the activator gene is controlled spatially and, to some extent, temporally by the selection of a specific promoter. The promoters that have been used to drive activator genes include the following: the *α-CaMKII promoter*, which restricts expression of the activator to pyramidal neurons in postnatal brain (spatially ranging from most pyramidal cells of the forebrain to only selective hippocampal CAI expression, depending on the integration of the transgenic construct, and the *kainate receptor subunit KA-I promoter*, which restricts the expression to CA1 and CA3 pyramidal neurons. Second, the activator itself can be controlled pharmacologically, typically by systemic drug application (for example, in drinking water). The transactivators tTA and rtTA are regulated by tetracycline (or its analogue doxycycline); tTA is inactivated, which means that it does not bind to the *tet operators* in the promoter of the target gene in the presence of doxycycline (often referred to as a "let off" protocol); rtTA is regulated in the opposite way ("tet on"). Fusion protein of Cre recombinase and the hormone-binding portion of the estrogen receptor, named CreERt2, was developed for temporal activation of the Cre recombinase: In the cell, CreERt2 is present in the cytoplasm, thus restricting the nuclear localization of Cre; but it translocates into the nucleus in the presence of drugs such as tamoxifen. Finally, expression of Cre recombinase alone from various cell-specific promoters, such as the α-CaMKII promoter, has been used for conditional knockout of target genes in selected neuronal populations.

Box Table 7–1.
Activator, Responder, and Conditional Mice

Activator Mice	Responder Mice
Activator genes tTA or rtTA Cre or CreERt2	*Responder Genes* Any transgene (wt or mutant) under the control of a promoter with tet operon regulation Floxed genes for conditional gene knockout, floxed hypomorphic alleles for gene activation
Activator genes determine *where* and *when* genetic manuipulation occurs	Responder genes determine the type of the genetic manipulation in the responder gene
No phenotype	No phenotype

Conditional Mice (obtained by breeding activator and responder mice)

Type of Genetic Manipulation	Responder Involved	Activator Involved
Knockout rescue	wt "flagged" transgene	tTA or rtTA in knockout mice
Expression of mutant genes	Mutant "flagged" transgenes	tTA or rtTA
Conditional gene knockout	Floxed gene	Cre or CreERt2
Conditional gene activation	Floxed hypomorphic alleles	Cre or CreERt2

Conditional phenotype is mediated by activation of the genetic manipulation of the responder gene in brain regions where activator gene is expressed.

There are two types of responder mice (see Box Fig. 7–1), depending on the activator used. Mice regulated by tTA or rtTA expression are typically generated by transgenic insertion of the responder gene under control of a pol II transcription initiation site containing several upstream tet operators. After binding of tTA/rtTA at the tet operators, transcription of the target gene is initiated by the tTA/rtTa VP16 activation domain. In contrast, the target genes in mice regulated by the expression of Cre recombinase are endogenous genes with genetically introduced Cre-recognition (lox P) sites in two intronic regions flanking one or several functionally important exons. The Cre recombinase binds to the loxP elements and eliminates the in-between genomic sequence by DNA recombination, creating a knockout form of the target gene. As an alternative use of the Cre-based approach, a loxP-flanked neo gene is sometimes inserted into a small intron of a target gene, which in most cases inhibits the target gene expression by disturbing its transcription or RNA processing (such target genes are called hypomorphic). Expression of the hypomorphic target allele can be activated by Cre-mediated removal of the floxed neo gene. Because this activation can be performed in mice heterozygous or homozygous for the hypomorphic alleles, it can be also used for studying gene-dose effects.

tTA = tetracycline-regulated transactivator; rtTA-reverse tetracycline-regulated transactivator; Floxed = exon(s) of a gene flanked by loxP site; flagged = proteins tagged by GFP or a short epitope recognized by selective antibody, such as Myc or Flag -epitopes.

Conditional mutagenesis: an approach to disease models. In: *Handbook of Experimental Pharmacology* (Starke K, Editor-in-chief Feil R, Series editors Metzger). D, Heidelberg: Springer Verlag.

(Continued)

Box 7-1
Tools to Generate Conditional Mouse Mutants *(Continued)*

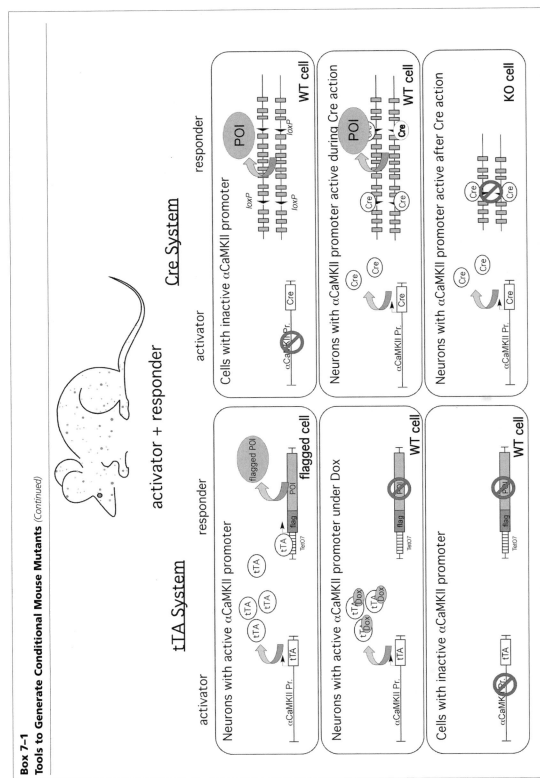

Box Figure 7-1. Principles of conditional expression systems. *Left.* tTA System. Upper box: α-CaMKII promoter regulates the expression of tTA, which can bind to the tet operator region (TetO7) in front of a transcription unit for a protein of interest (POI) labeled with a flag (GEF) or epitopes; flagged POI). In neurons with active a-CaMKII promoter, the binding of tTA at TetO7 initiates transcription of flagged POI. Middle box: In the presence of doxycycline (DOX), the binding affinity of tTA to its operators is drastically reduced, and POI is not expressed. Lower box: In cells where α-CaMKII is not active, neither tTA nor POI are expressed. *Right,* Cre system. Upper box: α-CaMKII promoter regulates the expression of Cre recombinase, which can bind to loxP elements inserted by gene targeting into a mouse gene. In cells where α-CaMKII promoter is not active, Cre is not expressed, which leaves expression of the floxed gene (POI) intact. Middle box: In cells with active α-CaMKII promoter, Cre is expressed and binds to the loxP elements in both alleles of a gene. Lower box: In Cre-expressing cells, the floxed gene segment is removed in both alleles, and the POI is "knocked-out."

NR2A or NR2B but caused severe reduction of NR2A and NR2B protein; in addition, both subunits were retained and aggregated in the somata of CA1 cells, indicating that the NR1 subunit is necessary for the release of NR2 subunits from the endoplasmic reticulum in hippocampal pyramidal cells, and that in the absence of NR1 no functional NMDA receptor channels can be formed in CA1 cells (Fukaya et al., 2003).

The loss of NMDA receptor-mediated synaptic currents in CA1-specific knockout mice resulted in impaired LTP at Schaffer collateral to CA1 synapses. Confirming the specificity of the genetic manipulation, no changes in synaptic transmission or plasticity were found at other synaptic connections in the hippocampus. Behaviorally, the mice showed regular development and normal nonspatial learning in the water-maze. However, adult mice had impaired learning during the acquisition phase of the hidden version of the Morris water-maze and in the postacquisition probe (Tsien et al., 1996b). These mice thus provided the first direct genetic evidence that NMDA receptor-mediated synaptic plasticity at the CA1 synapses is involved in the formation of spatial memory in mice. In addition, further analysis showed a number of other cellular and behavioral deficits. The mice failed to learn an association between a conditional and an unconditional stimulus (separated by 30 seconds) in trace fear conditioning, indicating that in addition to spatial information temporal information is processed in an NMDA receptor-dependent manner in the mouse hippocampus (Huerta et al., 2000). Mice also had impaired nonspatial memory formation, including object recognition, olfactory discrimination, and contextual fear memory; interestingly, the last three deficits were rescued by keeping the mice in an enriched environment (Rampon et al., 2000). The same study showed that the enriched environment led to an increase in synapse density in the CA1 region in the knockouts (as well as in the control littermates), suggesting that NMDA receptor activity is not essential for experience-induced synaptic structural changes, and that such structural plasticity may compensate for normal synaptic plasticity at least to some extent. Further deficits were found in place cell properties in area CA1: McHugh and colleagues found a striking deficit in the coordinated firing of pairs of neurons tuned to similar spatial locations. However CA1 cells retained place-related activity, indicating that the formation of place cells as such is not NMDA receptor-dependent (McHugh et al., 1996).

CA1-specific NR1 knockout mice were also used to study the consolidation phase of learning. Shimizu et al. described a mouse model termed iCA1-KO in which gene expression in CA1 neurons could be temporally controlled (Shimizu et al., 2000). As with the previous model for NMDA receptor depletion, the α-CaMKII promoter-driven Cre transgene is used to excise the floxed NR1 gene, but now it leads to simultaneous induction of a doxycycline-sensitive transcriptional activator (tTA) in the affected CA1 cells (see Box 7–1). In the absence of doxycycline, tTA is active and induces expression of the tTA-controlled transgene, which in the case of the iCA1-KO of NR1 was the GFP-tagged wild-type NR1 subunit (NR1-GFP). However, when the mice are fed doxycycline, tTA is inacti-

vated and NR1-GFP expression is switched off. Using this "on–off" mouse model, the study showed that when NR1-GFP expression was switched off in CA1 at day 1 to 6 after learning a spatial memory task retention of the acquired memory was significantly impaired compared to control mice or mice with the NR1-GFP expression switched off at post-training day 9 to 14 (Shimizu et al., 2000). Contextual fear memory was affected in a similar way. These experiments showed that memory retrieval relies on NMDA receptor-mediated synaptic transmission/plasticity for the first 6 days after learning; thereafter, retrieval becomes NR1-independent. In a follow-up study, α-CaMKII promoter-Cre transgenic line with Cre expression in forebrain principal neurons was used to switch off NR1-GFP expression during memory storage, 6 months after the initial training, and at least 2 months prior to memory retrieval. The retention of 9-month contextual and cued fear memories was severely disrupted by a long (30-day) but not short (7-day) doxycycline treatment suppressing NR1-GFP expression, indicating an unexpected role for NMDA receptors in long-term memory storage (Cui et al., 2004). The proposed role of NMDA receptors in memory consolidation and storage, however, contradicts earlier pharmacological experiments (reviewed in Riedel et al., 2003). Further experiments are necessary to settle the question of NMDA receptor function in memory consolidation, storage, and retrieval.

Hippocampal CA3-specific NR1 knockout mice were generated by Cre recombinase driven from a promoter of the kainate receptor subunit KA-1 (Nakazawa et al., 2002). In this case, electrophysiological analysis of the mice revealed impaired LTP in the recurrent commissural/associational pathway but not in mossy fiber synapses of CA3 cells. The mice showed regular performance in the Morris watermaze but had clear deficits when some of the spatial guiding cues were removed or when rapid memory formation was tested in a delayed matching-to-place version of the watermaze. This led to a model proposing a critical role for the CA3 region in "filling in the blanks" (pattern completion) after partial cue removal. Similarly, CA1 pyramidal cells in these mice displayed normal place-related activity in a full-cue environment but reduced activity upon partial cue removal and increased field size in a novel environment (Nakazawa et al., 2002, 2003).

In summary, the NR1 cell-type specific knockouts unequivocally demonstrated the critical role of NMDA receptors in synaptic plasticity and learning in both CA3 and CA1 regions of the hippocampus. This work initiated a novel strategy to determine the role of specific synapses in a complex memory system.

Mice with Point Mutations in the NR1 Subunit

Two knock-in mouse models were designed to study the role of glycine modulation in NMDA receptor function: NR1 K483Q mutation causes severe reduction of glycine affinity of the NMDA receptors, whereas NR1 D481N mutation has a milder effect (Kew et al., 2000). Mice homozygous for the

K483Q mutation do not feed and die early after birth, essentially exhibiting a phenotype similar to that of the complete NR1 knockout. This indicates that the high-affinity glycine binding site is crucial for normal NMDA receptor function. The mild reduction of glycine affinity in NR1 D481N mice was not lethal, and the mutants exhibited reduced theta burst-induced LTP and slightly impaired acquisition in the Morris watermaze.

The postulated function of the NMDA receptor with respect to synaptic plasticity in the hippocampus, and elsewhere in the brain, is to act as a Hebbian-type coincidence detection mechanism for post- and presynaptic activity owing to its dual ligand and voltage-dependent ion channel activation (see Section 7.2.3); once the receptors open, Ca^{2+} influx initiates postsynaptic signaling cascades leading to changes in synaptic efficacy. To test this model of NMDA receptor function directly, mice with altered NMDA receptor ion permeability were generated. A single asparagine residue N598 in the M2 segment of the NR1 subunit, which determines Ca^{2+} permeability, was changed to glutamine (Q) or arginine (R) (Single et al., 2000). Like NR1 knockout mice, mice exclusively expressing the mutated NR1 alleles—NR1(Q/Q) and NR1 (-/R) mice—died perinatally. Electrophysiological recordings from nucleated patches of CA1 cells in slices from NR1 (Q/Q) mice revealed the expected reduction of Ca^{2+} permeability and voltage-dependent Mg^{2+} block. Furthermore, even heterozygous NR1(+/Q) mice exhibited reduced life expectancy, and NR1(+/R) mice displayed signs of underdevelopment and died before weaning. This shows that Ca^{2+} influx via NMDA receptors remains critically important throughout life.

To address the importance of NMDA receptor-controlled Ca^{2+} influx for adult hippocampal functions, the N598R mutation was expressed conditionally in the forebrain using the Cre/lox system (see Box 7–1). First, expression of the dominant negative NR1(R) allele was inhibited by a floxed neo gene cassette in an intron of the NR1(R) allele. In these mice, the intronic neo gene can be deleted by Cre recombinase expressed, for example, from the α-CaMKII promoter, resulting in activation of the NR1(R) allele. Analysis of the NR1(R) forebrain-specific mice revealed a role for NMDA receptor-mediated Ca^{2+} influx in hippocampal homeostatic and Hebbian synaptic plasticity. The developmental synaptic scaling was lacking in CA1 cells, and LTP was induced by high-frequency but not low-frequency stimulation (Pawlak et al., 2005a,b). The mortality of these mutants, unfortunately, was still elevated; to assess the role of NMDA receptor Ca^{2+} signaling for learning and memory, it is thus necessary to develop more restricted NR1(R) expression, limited, for example, to expression only in CA1 or CA3 pyramidal neurons.

NR2 Mutant Mice

In agreement with the high expression of NR2A in mature compared to juvenile hippocampus, adult NR2A knockout mice showed a significant reduction of NMDA receptor-mediated synaptic currents in CA1 neurons. Nonetheless, LTP at the hippocampal Schaffer collateral to CA1 synapses and spatial learning were only slightly impaired. This indicates that in the absence of the NR2A subunit the NR1/NR2B heteromeric receptors are generally sufficient for adult hippocampal LTP and spatial learning (Sakimura et al., 1995; Kiyama et al., 1998). The same phenotype was also observed when only the NR2A C-terminal domain was genetically deleted (Sprengel et al., 1998). The truncated NMDA receptor subunits NR2AΔC participated in synaptic hippocampal NMDA receptor functions, as indicated by immunoisolation of synaptic NR2AΔC-containing receptor complexes, NR2AΔC immunogold labeling at hippocampal synapses, and the existence of spinous Ca^{2+} transients in the presence of NR2B blockers. LTP induced by a single tetanic stimulation in CA1 neurons was strongly reduced but could be restored to wild-type levels by repeated tetanic stimulation; this paradigm thus may preferentially activate NMDA receptors containing the NR2B subtype. Because the NR2AΔC-containing receptors allowed synaptically evoked Ca^{2+} influx in dendritic spines, these results indicate that NR2A C-terminal domain-based function (e.g., a scaffold role for various cytoskeletal and signaling proteins) is critical for normal LTP induction. In juvenile (P14) mice, when NR2B-mediated LTP induction pathway was more pronounced, the NR2AΔC mice showed no deficits in synaptic plasticity (Köhr et al., 2003). Notably, NR2A-dependent LTP as well as hippocampus-dependent spatial and associative learning are impaired in mice with forebrain-specific knockout of the transcription factor c-fos, indicating that NR2A-dependent plasticity involves activation of the c-fos pathways (note that NR2B-dependent LTP induced by repetitive tetanic stimulation was normal) (Fleischmann et al., 2003). The results from genetic mouse models, however, remain to be reconciled with pharmacological studies indicating a selective role of NR2A in LTP and NR2B in LTD (Liu et al., 2004; but see also Berberich et al., 2005). Thus, it seems most likely that the two NMDA receptor subunits play distinct roles in different synaptic plasticity paradigms by activating selective signaling pathways; however, further experimental work is necessary to determine the exact mechanisms and pathways.

NR2B knockout mice die shortly after birth owing to lack of a suckling response. In mice kept alive for several days by hand-feeding, synaptic NMDA receptor currents and LTD were abolished at CA1 synapses; this confirms that the NR2B subunit is critical for NMDA receptor function during early postnatal development (Kutsuwada et al., 1996).

Selective truncation of the NR2B C-terminal domain in mice caused the same phenotype as complete deletion of the subunit (Mori et al., 1998; Sprengel et al., 1998); homozygous NR2BΔC mice died a few days after birth, NMDA receptor-mediated EPSCs were reduced, with an accompanying reduction in synaptic NR2B immunosignal in the dendritic regions of the hippocampus. This suggests that the NR2B C-terminal domain is important for efficient synaptic transport of the NR2B-type receptors.

A striking finding regarding the function of the NR2B subunit and of NMDA receptors in general came from mice with forebrain-specific overexpression of the NR2B gene, driven from the α-CaMKII promoter; these mice showed not only increased LTP at the CA3 to CA1 synapses but also enhanced associative learning and memory (Tang et al., 1999). The authors proposed that the enhanced synaptic and behavioral performance was primarily the result of the increased opening time of the NR2B receptors, leading to overall enhanced coincidence detection by NMDA receptors.

The phenotype of NR2C knockout mice relates to the prominent expression of the NR2C subunit in cerebellar granule cells: The mice show deficits in fine-tuning motor coordination. The same impairment was also observed in mice with the C-terminally truncated NR2C subunit, providing a third confirmation of the importance of the C-terminal intracellular domain for normal synaptic function of each NR subunit (Ebralidze et al., 1996; Kadotani et al., 1996; Sprengel et al., 1998). No deficits were observed in hippocampus-based functions.

The NR2D subunit shows its highest expression in the embryonic brain and declines by P2. NR2D knockout mice are viable, indicating that the subunit function is not essential for development; in addition, no synaptic or memory deficiencies have been described in NR2D knockouts (Ikeda et al., 1995).

In contrast to the NR2B-overexpressing mice, α-CaMKII promoter-driven forebrain-specific overexpression of NR2D did not improve CA3 to CA1 LTP or memory performance in mice (Okabe et al., 1998). In NR2D-overexpressing mice, NMDA receptor-mediated currents in CA1 pyramidal cells had smaller amplitudes and slower kinetics, with selective impairment of LTD at juvenile and of LTP at mature Schaffer collateral to CA1 synapses. Thus, expression of NMDA receptors with NR2D-specific channel characteristics—leading to high affinity for glutamate and glycine, slow gating, and low sensitivity to Mg^{2+}—significantly altered NMDA receptor-dependent plasticity; surprisingly, these changes did not affect learning in the Morris watermaze task (Ikeda et al., 1995).

7.5.3 AMPA Receptor Mutant Mice

As discussed in the section about AMPA receptor trafficking (see Section 7.4.1), the two major subunits GluR1 and GluR2 appear to have distinct functions in hippocampal synaptic plasticity. Using mouse genetics, the GluR1 subunit was unequivocally identified as a key molecule in LTP at the hippocampal CA3 to CA1 connections (Zamanillo et al., 1999). The importance of the GluR2 subunit at the behavioral level is at the moment less clear, and the GluR3 subunit appears not to play a critical role in hippocampal functions.

GluR1 Mutant Mice

Genetic depletion of the GluR1 subunit has major effects on hippocampal functions (Fig. 7–8). CA1 pyramidal neurons showed a dramatic loss of AMPA receptor-mediated extrasynaptic currents in both the soma and the dendrites; synaptic

currents were only slightly reduced but showed a loss of a density scaling toward the apical dendrites (Zamanillo et al., 1999; Andrasfalvy et al., 2003). These findings demonstrated that GluR1 is necessary to establish and/or maintain an extrasynaptic AMPA receptor pool as well as distance-dependent synaptic scaling. The GluR2 subunit, in the absence of GluR1, showed a strong reduction in overall dendritic distribution and increased somatic accumulation in CA1 principal neurons when examined by immunostaining at the light microscopy level. However, consistent with the preservation of synaptic currents, synaptic GluR2 expression, as detected by immunogold labeling, was comparable to that in wild-type cells. Taken together, these data indicate that in wild-type animals a large proportion of AMPA receptors is maintained as a reserve pool at extrasynaptic sites, not immediately participating in synaptic signal transduction.

The function of the extrasynaptic pool of AMPA receptors became evident from analysis of synaptic plasticity in GluR1 knockout mice; the NMDA receptor-dependent LTP at adult Schaffer collateral to CA1 synapses was largely abolished (Zamanillo et al., 1999). Interestingly, whereas the loss of LTP in CA1 was observed after various stimulation protocols—e.g., tetanic stimulation (1×100 Hz or 4×100 Hz "field" LTP) or 3-minute pairing of postsynaptic depolarization and low-frequency Schaffer collateral stimulation ("cellular" LTP)—a protocol using theta-burst frequency of pairing pre- and postsynaptic activity induced a slow-onset LTP that reached normal levels within ~20 minutes after induction. This was the first evidence that two forms of LTP coexist at the Schaffer collateral to CA1 synapses: one dependent on and the other independent of the extracellular pool of GluR1-containing AMPA receptors (Hoffman et al., 2002). Similarly, at the perforant path to dentate gyrus granular cell synapses, GluR1-independent LTP was detected in adult GluR1 knockout mice (Zamanillo et al., 1999); this indicates that in wild-type animals LTP at these synapses is at least partly GluR1-independent.

Molecular mechanisms underlying synaptic plasticity in the hippocampus also change during development. In contrast to adult GluR1-deficient mice, juvenile (2-week-old) knockout mice have normal field and cellular LTP in CA1 (Jensen et al., 2003b). This "juvenile" LTP may rely on expression of other AMPA receptor subunits, such as $GluR2_{long}$, a GluR2 form with an alternatively spliced C-terminal domain (Kolleker et al., 2003) (see Section 7.3.2). The notion that GluR1-dependent function is not critical in juvenile mice is consistent with the observation that hippocampal LTP in adult GluR1 knockout mice can be rescued by transgenic forebrain-specific expression of GFP-tagged GluR1 with an onset from the second to the third postnatal week (Mack et al., 2001). This indicates that a GluR1-independent form(s) of synaptic plasticity is (are) sufficient for development of normal hippocampal synaptic circuits. Later in development, as the extrasynaptic AMPA receptor pool increases, GluR1-dependent plasticity becomes the dominant form of LTP (Jensen et al., 2003b).

Does hippocampal CA3 to CA1 LTP in the adult rely on

A Functional depletion of GluR1 in the mouse

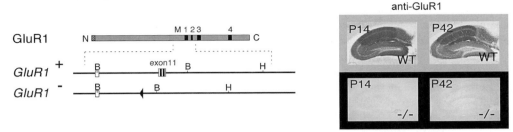

B LTP in junvenile and adult WT and GluR1 deficient mice

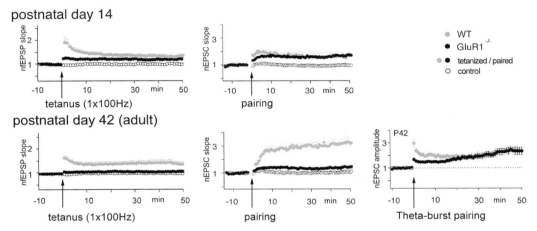

C GluR1 deficient mice are impaired in spatial working memory

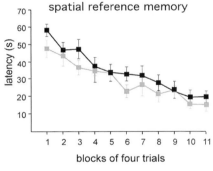
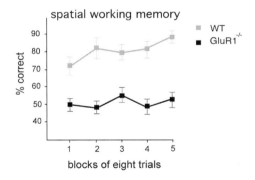

Figure 7–8. Various forms of LTP at CA3-to-CA1 synapses revealed by analysis of GluR1-deficient mice. *A*. GluR1 knockout was generated by gene targeting of the M1- and M2-encoding exon 11 (Zamanillo et al., 1999). Right panel: GluR1 immunoreactivity was detected in the hippocampi of wild-type (WT) but not GluR1-deficient mice (-/-) at P14 and P42. *B*. Residual CA3-to-CA1 LTP is present in the GluR1-deficient mice at P14, as revealed by tetanic stimulation and pairing LTP protocols (Jensen et al., 2003b). These two forms of LTP are absent at P42 in the GluR1-deficient mice. However, theta-burst pairing can still induce LTP at P42 in these mice (Hoffman et al., 2002). *C*. GluR1-deficient mice show regular learning in the hidden platform task of the Morris water-maze (left) but cannot learn the rewarded alternation in the T-maze task (Reisel et al., 2002).

any extracellular reserve pool of AMPA receptors, or does it specifically require a GluR1-containing reserve pool? A specific role for the GluR1 subunit was suggested from studies examining the function of GluR1 C-terminal phosphorylation. First, experiments in hippocampal slice cultures suggested that PKA phosphorylation of GluR1 C-tail serine 845 is necessary for synaptic insertion of GluR1-containing AMPA

receptors after LTP induction (Esteban et al., 2003); and second, gene-targeted mice carrying a mutation of GluR1 serine 845 showed reduced LTP despite normal levels of extrasynaptic AMPA receptors (Lee et al., 2003). These results provide evidence for a specific role of the GluR1 subunit in LTP at CA1 synapses.

Behavioral analysis of the GluR1-deficient mice revealed

two striking findings. First, it came as a surprise that these mice showed normal spatial reference memory in the Morris watermaze task, the paddling-pool escape task, and the appetitive elevated plus-maze and Y-maze tasks (Zamanillo et al., 1999; Reisel et al., 2002; Bannerman et al., 2003; Schmitt et al., 2004b). Importantly, the spatial learning in the watermaze and Y-maze was still dependent on hippocampal function, as bilateral hippocampal lesions in the GluR1-deficient mice profoundly impaired their performance in both tasks. These findings thus established that GluR1-dependent LTP in the CA1 region of the hippocampus is not necessary for the formation of spatial reference memory. Second, the GluR1-deficient mice did show a drastic reduction in spatial working memory during tests of nonmatching to place in a Y-maze and elevated T-maze. This impairment was partially rescued by transgenic expression of GFP-GluR1 that was largely restricted to the dorsal hippocampus of GluR1 knockout mice (Schmitt et al., 2005). These experiments thus provide a close link between hippocampal CA1 LTP and a specific form of memory formation, as a genetic LTP rescue in adult mice was paralleled by a gain of function in the behavior of the mice.

GluR1-dependent synaptic plasticity appears to be critical for a form of learning that involves processing rapid interactions between spatial cues and response requirements (Schmitt et al., 2004b). When mice were allowed to navigate through a T-maze by using textural conditional cues (all floor areas were covered with either white Perspex or wire mesh, depending on the position of the food reward) the knockout mice learned as well as wild-type mice; this is consistent with their having normal spatial reference memory. When the floor cues were present only in the start arm (not in the goal arms) of the maze, the GluR1-deficient mice again failed to learn the task. This shows that the absence of the conditional cue at the time when the place/reward association was processed critically determines whether the mice can learn. Hippocampal GluR1-dependent synaptic plasticity at the CA1 region thus contributes to a memory system that in rodents encodes both the spatial and temporal contexts associated with a particular event, a paradigm that may be analogous to human episodic memory (Schmitt et al., 2004a).

The lack of GluR1 in the brain, despite the prominent, widespread expression of the subunit, does not have major effects on general sensorimotor behavior. The GluR1 knockout mice are slightly more hyperactive, anxious, and aggressive, with only a subtle lack of motor coordination (Bannerman et al., 2004; Vekovischeva et al., 2004).

GluR2 and GluR2/3 Mutant Mice

According to the model for NMDA receptor-dependent LTP at Schaffer collateral to CA1 synapses, it is important that AMPA receptors have low permeability for Ca^{2+}, which is determined by the presence of the Q to R edited GluR2 subunit (see Section 7.3.2); NMDA receptor-mediated Ca^{2+} influx then acts as a selective trigger for Hebbian coincidence detection of pre- and postsynaptic activity. To test this

hypothesis directly and to examine the overall role of GluR2 in synaptic transmission, mice were generated that either completely lack GluR2 or contain targeted mutations eliminating the editing of the Q codon in the M2 membrane segment.

In contrast to the GluR1-deficient mice, GluR2 knockout mice are compromised in development and overall behavior. Juvenile GluR2-deficient mice are about half the size of their wild-type littermates, and some succumb to preweaning mortality. Even though the surviving mice "catch up" in weight by 8 weeks of age, they remain impaired in several aspects of their behavior, ranging from reduced sensory stimulus processing to reduced motivation and learning; deficits are associated with hippocampus-dependent behaviors as well as behaviors associated with other brain regions, including the neocortex and cerebellum. The overall lower activity of the GluR2-deficient mice and the reduction in synaptic AMPA receptor-mediated currents (Jia et al., 1996; Meng et al., 2003) suggest that GluR2 is necessary for maintaining a steady-state level of AMPA receptor-mediated transmission, in contrast to GluR1, which is more critical for activity-dependent synaptic plasticity (see also discussion of subunit-specific AMPA receptor trafficking in Section 7.4.1).

At the cellular level, GluR1 distribution in the absence of GluR2 was unchanged in the hippocampus, indicating that GluR2 is not necessary for the extracellular AMPA receptor pool in dendrites; the aberrant receptor assemblies of GluR1/GluR3 and GluR1 or GluR3 homomeric channels are less efficiently expressed at synapses, again supporting the idea that GluR2 is necessary for synaptic stabilization of AMPA receptors (Sans et al., 2003). However, the GluR1/3-based receptors, which are permeable to Ca^{2+}, are sufficient even at their low synaptic levels to mediate CA3 to CA1 LTP; furthermore, this LTP is partially independent of NMDA receptor activation—about twofold enhanced compared to that of their wild-type littermates and nonsaturating (Jia et al., 1996). Thus, it appears that activity-dependent GluR1-based synaptic delivery of AMPA receptors is still operative, but now changes in synaptic transmission can be achieved in an atypical manner, without relying on NMDA receptor-based coincidence detection. It is unfortunate that the overall low behavioral performance of the mice makes it difficult to analyze learning under these altered synaptic conditions. One approach to getting around this problem was to analyze hippocampal place cell firing, as there is a strong correlation between Hebbian NMDA receptor-dependent LTP, place-cell function, and learning and memory. In the GluR2 knockout mice, CA1 place cells were impaired, with only 25% (down from 46%) of CA1 neurons showing detectable place fields; moreover, the remaining place cells were less precise and unstable (Yan et al., 2002). This suggests that CA1 depletion of GluR2 leads to impaired hippocampal learning and memory functions.

Mice lacking GluR2 selectively in postnatal forebrain were generated to directly circumvent the global behavioral impairments in the complete knockout animals (a floxed GluR2 gene was again excised by CRE recombinase under control of the α-CaMKII promoter (Shimshek et al., 2005, 2006). The mice showed less overall behavioral deficits but had impaired spatial reference and working memory; interestingly, LTP at the CA3 to CA1 synapses was induced to a wild-type level of potentiation and was entirely dependent on activation of NMDA receptors.. Detailed analysis of hippocampal functions in these mice revealed the following morphological and synaptic changes: loss of CA3 pyramidal cells and parvalbumin-positive interneurons in the dentate gyrus; diminished neurogenesis in the subgranular zone; reduced presynaptic fiber excitability at CA3 to CA1 synapses and reduced threshold for evoking population spikes at the CA3 to CA1 synapses.

At least some of the changes observed in the forebrain-specific GluR2 knockout mice are likely due to aberrant Ca^{2+} influx through the remaining GluR1/3 receptors; this is also supported by observations in mice with Ca^{2+}-permeable (but GluR2-containing) AMPA receptors due to genetically induced deficiency in the GluR2 Q to R editing (Brusa et al., 1995; Feldmeyer et al., 1999; Krestel et al., 2004; Shimshek et al., 2005). In these mice, AMPA receptors are stabilized by GluR2 at excitatory synapses, and the overall Ca^{2+} load during neurotransmission is larger. When the unedited GluR2 is expressed in the whole brain, the mice develop severe seizures and typically die by 3 weeks of age (Brusa et al., 1995). The severity of the phenotype correlates with the level of GluR2(Q586) expression, as mice with GluR2(Q586) expressed in the brain at only the 5% level of the endogenous GluR2 survive substantially longer and show a low tendency to epileptic attacks (Feldmeyer et al., 1999). In young mice, the deficiency of GluR2 Q to R editing induces an NMDA receptor-independent LTP at Schaffer collateral to CA1 synapses, the magnitude of which correlates with the expression level of the GluR2(Q586) subunit (Feldmeyer et al., 1999).

Interestingly, lethality and seizures do not occur in mice with GluR2(Q586) expression conditionally restricted to postnatal hippocampus, suggesting that additional expression of GluR2(Q586) in forebrain, striatum, and/or amygdala is necessary for global epileptic attacks (Krestel et al., 2004). In mice with forebrain-restricted GluR2(Q586) expression, the presynaptic fiber excitability at CA3 to CA1 synapses is unchanged, but excitatory postsynaptic responses are smaller, suggesting compensatory downscaling of the AMPA receptor-mediated Ca^{2+}-permeable currents; nonetheless, CA1 neurons are more excitable, as revealed by a lower threshold for an evoked population spike and epileptic activity in these mice; increased gliosis and mossy fiber sprouting are clear signs of recurrent seizures. Thus, in both postnatally induced forebrain-specific GluR2 knockout and editing-deficient animals, an AMPA receptor-mediated increase of a postsynaptic Ca^{2+} load induces long-term changes in hippocampal circuits affecting normal hippocampal functions and spatial learning.

GluR3 is not as highly expressed as GluR1 and GluR2 in the hippocampus. GluR3 knockout mice showed normal basal synaptic transmission in CA1; LTP at CA3 to CA1 synapses

was increased but was still fully dependent on activation of NMDA receptors (Meng et al., 2003). In addition, GluR2/GluR3 double knockout mice showed a phenotype similar to that of the GluR2-deficient mice, with general retardation of postnatal development and increased mortality, without detectable abnormalities in the gross anatomy of the central nervous system, including the hippocampus (Meng et al., 2003). Although synaptic transmission at CA1 synapses was reduced several-fold, the GluR2/3-deficient mice were competent in establishing LTD and LTP as well as depotentiation and dedepression at the Schaffer collateral to CA1 synapses. This indicates that GluR1 receptors are sufficient, in the absence of GluR2/3, to mediate the major types of synaptic plasticity in CA1 principal neurons. The overall behavioral retardation of the animals, however, prevented tests of learning and memory in the double knockout mice.

7.5.4 Kainate Receptor Mutant Mice

At present, there are no reports on mice lacking the KA1 subunit; however, the other kainate receptor subunit mutants have been extremely useful in mapping kainate receptor function in different hippocampal cell types and at distinct subcellular localizations (see also Section 7.3.4).

KA2, GluR5, and GluR6 Knockout Mice

Genetic depletion of KA2 identified this subunit as an important functional component of both pre- and postsynaptic kainate receptors at the mossy fiber to CA3 synapses (Contractor et al., 2003). First, whereas the function of the presynaptic facilitatory kainate receptor, which is responsible for the marked frequency facilitation at the mossy fiber terminals, was normal, heterosynaptic facilitation resulting from a spillover of glutamate from CA3 collateral synapses was absent. This finding agrees with the idea that KA2 plays a role as a high-affinity glutamate-binding subunit, specifically required for sensing low concentrations of glutamate. Second, postsynaptic kainate receptor-mediated EPSCs in CA3 pyramidal cells showed faster decay. Mossy fiber LTP in these mice, however, was normal (Contractor et al., 2003).

Whereas the GluR5 subunit is prominently expressed in hippocampal interneurons, disruption of the GluR5 gene did not cause a loss or reduction of functional kainate receptors in these cells; this suggests that other kainate receptor subunits can compensate for the lack of GluR5 in hippocampal interneurons (Mulle et al., 2000). In contrast, kainate receptor-mediated enhancement of the amplitude of synaptic currents at the perforant path to CA3 synapses was abolished in the GluR5 and the GluR6 knockout animals (Contractor et al., 2000).

Gene-targeted mice lacking GluR6 revealed that the subunit plays a critical role at the mossy fiber to CA3 synapses, where postsynaptic kainate receptors mediate a small EPSC component that is completely abolished in the GluR6-deficient mice (Mulle et al., 1998). Importantly, synaptic plasticity of mossy fiber connections is also affected; mossy fiber LTP—the expression of which is known to depend on presynaptic mechanisms—is reduced, and short-term synaptic facilitation is impaired in the absence GluR6. This suggests that kainate receptors act as presynaptic autoreceptors that mediate frequency-dependent synaptic facilitation at the mossy fiber terminals, a form of short-term plasticity in which the strength of transmission increases with repetitive stimulation (Contractor et al., 2001). In addition, several other roles for GluR6 in the hippocampus were revealed during analysis of the GluR6 knockout mice. Kainate receptor-mediated modulation of synaptic transmission between inhibitory interneurons in the stratum radiatum was impaired; however, a loss of postsynaptic kainate currents was observed only in double GluR5/GluR6 knockouts, suggesting the existence of two populations of kainate receptors in hippocampal interneurons (Mulle et al., 1998, 2000). GluR6-deficient mice also provided evidence of a functional role of GluR6-containing kainate receptors in CA1 cells, which showed reduced kainate- and domoate-induced CA1 inward currents in the mutant mice.

GluR5(Q636R) and GluR6(Q636R) Mutant Mice

The Ca^{2+} permeability of GluR5- and GluR6-containing receptors is controlled by site-selective RNA editing in the coding region for the channel pore-forming segment M2 (see Section 7.3.4). Mice with deficient editing of the GluR6 Q/R site show several phenotypic changes at the levels of synaptic transmission and behavior. First, LTP at medial perforant path to dentate gyrus synapses had an NMDA receptor-independent component, suggesting that, at this synapse too, kainate receptor-mediated Ca^{2+}-signaling can lead to an atypical NMDAR coincidence-deficient form of synaptic plasticity (Vissel et al., 2001). The GluR6(Q) mice were also more vulnerable to kainate-induced seizures than were their wild-type littermates. Together with the seizure-prone phenotypes of the GluR2(Q856) mice, these results provide further support for the hypothesis that increased postsynaptic Ca^{2+} influx and NMDAR coincidence-deficient synaptic plasticity lead to changes in hippocampal neuronal circuits, resulting in epileptic activity. In addition, the GluR6(Q) mice showed that GluR6-containing receptors are located on dendrites of dentate gyrus granule cells as well as on mossy fiber boutons. No phenotypic changes as yet have been found in the GluR5(Q) mice carrying the same mutation as the GluR6(Q) mice (Sailer et al., 1999).

7.5.5 mGluR Mutant Mice

The role of group I metabotropic receptors in synaptic plasticity is well documented at both mossy fiber to CA3 and Schaffer collateral to CA1 synapses (see Chapter 10). Accordingly, mice lacking the mGluR1 subtype show reduced LTP at the Schaffer collateral CA1 synapse (Aiba et al., 1994) and possibly also at the mossy fiber to CA3 synapse (Conquet et al., 1994; but see also Hsia et al., 1995). Behaviorally, the

mGluR1 null mice showed impaired context-specific associative learning (Aiba et al., 1994; Conquet et al., 1994); note that the mice showed much stronger deficits in cerebellar plasticity and related behavior. Mice deficient in the mGluR5 subunit had a phenotype similar to that of the mGluR1 null mice, with reduced LTP in CA1 neurons, intact LTP at the mossy fiber to CA3 neurons, and somewhat impaired spatial learning and contextual fear conditioning. Thus, these animal models reveal that group I mGluRs play at least modulatory roles in hippocampal learning and memory.

Mice with targeted deletions of the group II/III mGluRs were also generated in a number of laboratories during the late 1990s. Among them, mice lacking the mGluR2 subtype, in agreement with its prominent expression in mossy fibers, show a loss of mossy fiber LTD (Yokoi et al., 1996). Interestingly, in the same study, no deficits were found in mossy fiber LTP or in watermaze tasks, suggesting that neither mGluR2 nor mossy fiber LTD are required for hippocampal spatial learning. Mice deficient in mGluR7 were found to be more prone to developing seizures, with a concomitant increase in population excitability of principal neurons in hippocampal slices (Sansig et al., 2001). Thus, mGluR7 may play an important role in presynaptic control of hippocampal excitability.

7.5.6 Synopsis of the Section

Studies on genetic mouse mutants with altered excitatory neurotransmission in the hippocampus have greatly enhanced our understanding of the principles of glutamatergic synaptic transmission and synaptic plasticity, as well as of complex hippocampus-dependent behavior, learning, and memory. First, work with NMDA receptor mutant mice has provided important evidence for a causal link between NMDA receptor-mediated LTP at CA3 to CA1 synapses and spatial memory formation, as well as between this form of LTP and the formation of stable hippocampal place fields. In addition, NMDA receptor mutant mice have also revealed that different NMDA receptor subtypes contribute to different signaling pathways for LTP induction, such as the NR2A- and NR2B-specific pathways. During juvenile development the NR2B pathway is dominant, whereas in adult mice the NR2A pathway is more prominent.

The importance of hippocampal LTP in learning and memory, as well as the existence of subunit-specific forms of LTP in CA1 neurons were further substantiated by experiments using mice with altered AMPA receptors. Adult GluR1-deficient mice showed complete loss of field CA1 LTP, which correlated with spatial working memory impairment. The fact that spatial reference memory in these mice is intact suggests that different forms of NMDA receptor-dependent plasticity may underlie different forms of hippocampal memory. In juvenile mice, GluR1 is not essential for normal synaptic plasticity; juvenile LTP may be mediated by other AMPA receptor subunits (e.g., GluR4 and/or GluR2$_{long}$). Genetic conversion of AMPA receptors to Ca^{2+}-permeable ion channels in pyramidal neurons by depletion of GluR2 or by the inhibition of GluR2 Q/R site editing leads to long-term changes in hippocampal activity with increased excitability of CA1 cells and subsequent epileptic activity. This points to the critical importance of the edited GluR2 subunit, which determines the monovalent ion selectivity of the AMPA receptors in establishing and/or maintaining normal hippocampal functions and the survival of the animal. Finally, genetically modified mice showed unequivocally that kainate receptors act as important modulators of synaptic transmission in the hippocampus; their function is critical for maintaining normal synaptic transmission, especially for the dentate gyrus and CA3 neurons.

In summary, it seems clear that mouse genetics will continue to be an important source for unraveling complex molecular processes that underlie hippocampal functions. Currently, the global gene knockout strategy is being replaced by an approach aimed at generating mice deficient for receptor subtypes at specific hippocampal connections and at defined developmental stages. This will enable geneticists to study the role of glutamate receptors at distinct hippocampal connections without the interference of developmental disturbances. These new generations of mouse mutants promise to enhance our understanding of the relations between various forms of hippocampal synaptic plasticity and hippocampus-dependent learning and memory.

7.6 GABAergic Receptors: Structure, Function, and Hippocampal Distribution

7.6.1 Introduction: Synaptic and Extrasynaptic GABAergic Receptors Mediate Tonic and Phasic Inhibition in the Hippocampus

The flow of excitation through the hippocampus (dentate granule cells to CA3 pyramidal cells to CA1 pyramidal cells) is paced by GABA pulses from interneurons. A typical synaptic pulse of GABA (1 mM, 1 ms) initiates fast (milliseconds) point-to-point inhibition via ionotropic type A ($GABA_A$) receptors forming Cl^--permeable channels. This fast $GABA_A$ receptor activation controls action potential frequency and inhibits dendritic Ca^{2+} spikes. Slower responses (e.g., late inhibitory postsynaptic potentials caused by opening of K^+ channels), lasting 500 to 2000 ms, originate from metabotropic $GABA_B$ receptors and extrasynaptic or perisynaptic $GABA_A$ receptors. Both receptor types can be pre- or postsynaptic, as well as extrasynaptic or perisynaptic (reviewed in Kullmann et al., 2005). Indeed, there is likely to be substantial extrasynaptic activation of both $GABA_A$ and $GABA_B$ receptors via GABA spillover. Extrasynaptic GABA does not provide a clean time-dependent signal, unlike the phasic GABA pulses at the synapse. Hence extrasynaptic inhibition is termed "tonic inhibition." Repetitive stimulation acti-

vates $GABA_B$ receptors more effectively than single stimuli: Enough GABA has to build up and diffuse away from the cleft. $GABA_B$ receptors are perhaps optimally activated by short bursts of inhibitory afferent activation coming from groups of interneurons. However, even the GABA released by a single interneuron—provided it fires at least three action potentials at high frequency—is sufficient to activate postsynaptic $GABA_B$ receptors. On the other hand, extrasynaptic activation of $GABA_A$ receptors is likely to be continually present, constituting background conductance.

The functions of background inhibitory conductances in neuronal circuits are unknown. Small, persistent tonic chloride conductances alter input resistance and membrane time constants; these in turn influence synaptic efficacy and integration. Manipulating background inhibitory currents, for example, may influence epileptic thresholds. Additionally, allosteric modulators active on $GABA_A$ receptors, such as benzodiazepines, steroids, and general anesthetics, may be more potent on extrasynaptic than synaptic receptors because of the much lower GABA concentration outside the synapse (allosteric modulators produce effects at the receptor only at submaximal GABA concentrations).

GABA transporter activity helps set the extracellular GABA level and so governs the extent of extrasynaptic tonic and perisynaptic $GABA_A$ receptor activation and presynaptic $GABA_B$ activation. For example, in the hippocampus of GABA transporter-1 (GAT-1)-deficient mice, complex layers of feedback emerge: A large increase in tonic postsynaptic $GABA_A$ conductance occurs in these mice, but the frequency of spontaneous quantal GABA release is one-third of normal (Jensen et al., 2003a).

In summary, the GABAergic system in the hippocampus has various modes. First, there is point-to-point $GABA_A$ receptor-mediated synaptic transmission and a continually present background of extrasynaptic tonic $GABA_A$-mediated inhibition. In this case, interneurons act as individual units to release GABA. This mode does not provide enough GABA to activate $GABA_B$ receptors (because of their low affinity/efficacy). Second, during oscillatory activity, with synaptic activity from many inhibitory neurons, substantially more GABA is released, allowing the concentration of GABA to build up extrasynaptically. When this diffuse mode comes into play, a new population of receptors, extrasynaptic $GABA_B$ receptors, is recruited as well as more extrasynaptic $GABA_A$ receptors. Specific behavioral states might use different levels of diffuse inhibitory transmission.

7.6.2 $GABA_A$ Receptors

$GABA_A$ receptors are anion-permeable channels, with an HCO_3^-/Cl^- permeability ratio of approximately 0.2 to 0.4. In adult cells, Cl^- ions usually move into the cell to produce strong inhibitory hyperpolarization, as the reversal potential for Cl^- is 15 to 20 mV more negative than the resting membrane potential. The Cl^- gradient is maintained by K/Cl co-transporters. HCO_3^- ions move out of the cells through the $GABA_A$ receptor channel; the HCO_3^- efflux is mildly depolarizing (HCO_3^- has a reversal potential of -12 mV), but this is normally offset by the Cl^- hyperpolarization. The HCO_3^- efflux is encouraged by the actions of extracellular carbonic anhydrase; in fact, these enzymes are essential for maintaining the HCO_3^- gradient. With an increased HCO_3^-/Cl^- permeability ratio, the outward HCO_3^- flux would depolarize the membrane at the resting membrane potential. Depending on the local internal Cl^- concentration, Cl^- ions can also move out after $GABA_A$ receptor activation and depolarize the cell; this happens especially during embryonic and postnatal hippocampal development. Even in the adult hippocampus, when interneurons are strongly stimulated in the presence of ionotropic glutamate receptor antagonists, a biphasic postsynaptic GABAergic response is produced in pyramidal cells. An initial hyperpolarizing IPSP is followed by slow depolarization of the pyramidal cell. The slow depolarization causes action potential firing, and so is excitatory—it is termed a GABA-mediated *d*epolarizing *p*ostsynaptic *p*otential (GDSP) (Kaila et al., 1997).

$GABA_A$ receptors form as pentameric assemblies of subunits (reviewed in Ernst et al., 2003). A gene family encodes the subunits ($\alpha1$–$\alpha6$, $\beta1$–$\beta3$, $\gamma1$–$\gamma3$, δ, ϵ, θ, π, and $\rho1$-$\rho3$). The $GABA_A$ receptor subunits belong to the acetylcholine receptor subunit gene superfamily; consequently, our working models of the $GABA_A$ receptor structures are based on the extracellular domain of the nicotinic acetylcholine receptor structure. As for other brain regions, the $GABA_A$ receptor subunit genes are differentially transcribed in the hippocampus (Fig. 7–9) (Persohn et al., 1992; Wisden et al., 1992; Sperk et al., 1997). Genes expressed at significant levels in the hippocampus are: $\alpha1$ $\alpha2$ $\alpha4$ $\alpha5$, $\beta1$-$\beta3$, $\gamma2$ and δ. The subunits assemble into different combinations, depending on the cell-type. The large family of subunit genes produces considerable receptor diversity. These $GABA_A$ receptors differ in their affinity for neurotransmitter and allosteric modulators, activation rate, desensitization rate, channel conductance and location on the cell (reviewed in Korpi et al., 2002).

Principal $GABA_A$ receptor subtypes relevant for hippocampal function contain: $\alpha1\beta\gamma2$, $\alpha2\beta\gamma2$, $\alpha3\beta\gamma2$, $\alpha4\beta\gamma2$, $\alpha5\beta\gamma2$, and $\alpha\beta\delta$ (mainly $\alpha4\beta\delta$). Most hippocampal $GABA_A$ receptors are probably $\alpha\beta\gamma2$ combinations, and a small number are $\alpha\beta\delta$: The subunit ratio in the receptor pentamer is probably $2\alpha/2\beta/1\gamma$ or $2\alpha2\beta1\delta$ (Ernst et al., 2003). Note that some receptors may contain a mixture of α and β subunits (e.g., $\alpha1\alpha2\beta2\gamma2$, and perhaps $\alpha x\alpha4\beta\delta$ where x is 1, 2, 3, or 5). The single channel conductance of $\alpha\beta\gamma2$ or $\alpha\beta\delta$ receptors is 25 to 30 pS. As discussed in detail below, receptors with the $\gamma2$ subunit can be both synaptic and extrasynaptic; receptors with the δ subunit are probably principally perisynaptic, localized around the edge of synapses (Wei et al., 2003).

The question of the function(s) of $GABA_A$ receptor diversity has been partially addressed by pharmacological and genetic studies (reviewed in Rudolph and Mohler, 2004).

Some receptors specialize as extra or perisynaptic sensors of GABA; others enrich in particular synaptic locations. For some types of extrasynaptic or perisynaptic receptors that contain the δ subunit, the key properties are high affinity for neurotransmitter and limited desensitization, enabling them to contribute to tonic background conductance. Another important consequence of differences in subunit expression between cells or on different parts of the same cell is that $GABA_A$ receptor kinetics differ at different synapses (from, for example, distinct interneurons synapsing onto the pyramidal cell). This may influence the oscillation frequency of principal cells, as different interneuronal subtypes innervate different domains of pyramidal or dentate granule cells or each other (Bartos et al., 2002). In recombinant $\alpha n\beta\gamma2$ combinations, the α subunits determine receptor kinetics (Goldstein et al., 2002). The decay time constants of $\alpha1\beta2$ subunits are fast, whereas those of $\alpha2$- and $\alpha3$-containing receptors are slower; for example, currents from recombinant $\alpha3\beta2\gamma2$ receptors decay more slowly than $\alpha1\beta2\gamma2$ receptors in response to a synaptic pulse of GABA. The $\alpha1$ subunit knockout mice provide direct support for this. Synaptic $GABA_A$ receptor-mediated currents in hippocampal neurons (pyramidal and interneurons) from wild-type mice decay more rapidly than those in $\alpha1$ knockout mice; loss of the $\alpha1$ subunit in synaptically localized receptors leads to a population of synaptic receptors, probably containing the $\alpha2$ subunit, with slower deactivation kinetics (Goldstein et al., 2002). Differences in $GABA_A$ receptor subunit expression between hippocampal cells and synapses likely directly influence circuit properties. Parvalbumin interneurons, for example, express mainly $\alpha1\beta\gamma2$-containing $GABA_A$ receptors (Klausberger et al., 2002). The fast $GABA_A$-conveyed inhibition between these cell types helps pace the oscillation frequency in the pyramidal cell network (Bartos et al., 2002). Similarly, the mean decay time constant of the IPSC at the basket cell to basket cell synapse in the dentate gyrus is twofold faster than at the basket cell to granule cell synapse (Bartos et al., 2001). Again, this almost certainly reflects differences in receptor subunit expression.

Distribution of $GABA_A$ Receptor Subunits in Hippocampal Dentate Granule Cells

Inhibitory terminals originate from several types of interneuron. Of the total number of inhibitory GABAergic terminals synapsing onto hippocampal granule cells, 25% occur on the cell body or axon initial segments, with the remaining 75% synapsing onto dendrites in the molecular layer (Halasy and Somogyi, 1993). At $GABA_A$ receptors on the somatic synapses of rat dentate granule cells, there is a high probability of receptor opening ($P_o = 0.8$), and all receptors are occupied by the released transmitter (reviewed in Nusser, 1999); these synapses have, on average, 26 $GABA_A$ receptors, with an average conductance of 21 pS. Rat dentate granule cells have been shown to express an extensive set of subunit mRNAs: $\alpha1$–$\alpha5$,

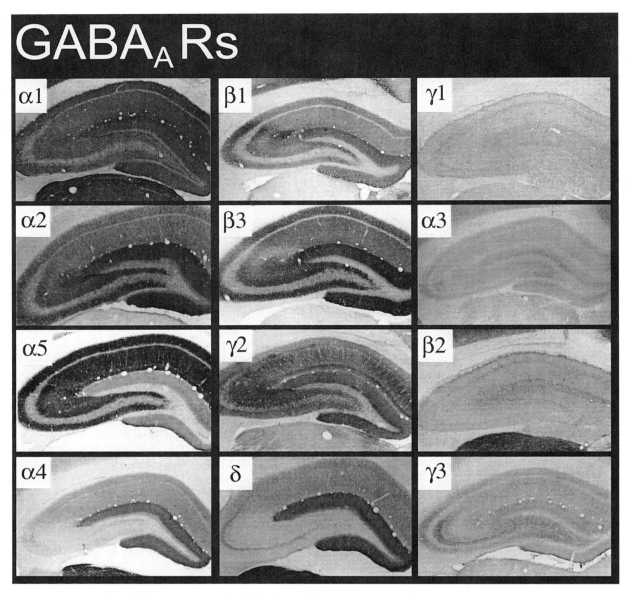

Figure 7–9. Expression of GABA$_A$ receptor subunits in the rat hippocampus. Expression pattern of the 12 GABA$_A$ subunits in the adult dorsal rat hippocampus was visualized by immunohistochemistry with subunit-specific antibodies. Note: the β2 subunit staining is artificially reduced because of the low antibody concentration used. (*Source*: Modified from Sperk et al., 1997, with permission.)

β1–β3, and γ1–γ3, although the α3, γ1, and γ3 mRNAs are rare (Persohn et al., 1992; Wisden et al., 1992; Brooks-Kayal et al., 2001). The α2 and α4 subunit mRNAs are strongly expressed; the α1 and α5 mRNAs are at moderate levels. Of the βs, the β3 gene has the highest expression level, but β1 and β2 are also significantly expressed.

Immunocytochemical results generally agree with the in situ hybridization data. The α2, α4, α5, β1, β3, and δ protein staining is high in the dentate molecular layer, indicating a dendritic location on granule cells (Pirker et al., 2000; Peng et al., 2002). There is weaker staining of the granule cell soma. Many of the α subunits co-localize in the same synapses on dentate granule cells: Double labeling immunocytochemistry shows that most of the α2-positive synapses also contains α1. Autoradiography with an α5-selective ligand, [^{3}H]L-655,708, highlights the molecular layer of the dentate gyrus, confirming α5 protein enrichment on granule cell dendrites (Sur et al., 1999). The α4 and/or α1 and δ subunits probably assemble as perisynaptic α4βδ, α1βδ-, or α1α4βδ-type receptors localized around the edge of the synapse (Peng et al., 2002; Wei et al., 2003). These receptors, based on analysis of their cloned counterparts, are predicted to be high-affinity and nondesensitizing, designed for their role in sensing extrasynaptic GABA and contributing to tonic inhibition.

Kullmann's group has identified presynaptic $GABA_A$ receptors on mossy fibers of dentate granule cells that inhibit axonal excitability; these receptors are tonically active in the absence of evoked GABA release or exogenous agonist application (Ruiz et al., 2003). In the presence of glutamate receptor blockers, stimulation of mossy fibers provokes monosynaptic GABA-mediated responses in their target cells; this mossy fiber-released GABA may also contribute to negative feedback via the presynaptic $GABA_A$ receptors. Alternatively, or in addition, these receptors may sense ambient GABA released from interneurons, allowing axons from granule cells to rapidly integrate the activity of surrounding neurons.

What is the identity of this presynaptic receptor? It is activated by muscimol, is antagonized by SR 95531, and has GABA responses potentiated by zolpidem (0.2 μM) (Ruiz et al., 2003), a selective agonist for $\alpha1\beta2\gamma2$ receptors if used at the appropriate concentration, although at higher concentrations zolpidem also potentiates GABA's actions at $\alpha2\beta2$ and $\alpha3\beta2$ receptors. The zolpidem sensitivity of these presynaptic receptors suggests an $\alpha1\beta\gamma2$ or $\alpha2\beta\gamma2$ combination. Ruiz et al. found punctate $\alpha2$ subunit immunoreactivity in rat stratum lucidum, the termination zone of mossy fibers (Ruiz et al., 2003); however, immunoreactivity for the $\alpha3$ subunit was also reported at the rat mossy fibers (Pirker et al., 2000).

Several modulators of hippocampal $GABA_A$ receptors were shown to have special relevance to dentate granule cells. Neuroactive steroids modulate $GABA_A$ receptor function in the hippocampus and other brain regions. Naturally occurring steroid metabolites form locally in the brain, independently of their peripheral concentrations. 5α-Reductase transforms progesterone to 5α-DPH, which in turn is reduced by 3α-hydroxysteroid oxidoreductase to allopregnanolone. Allopregnanolone potently activates $GABA_A$ receptors. No absolute specificity of neurosteroids for particular $GABA_A$ receptor subunit combinations has been found. Many $GABA_A$ receptors are sensitive to the steroid tetrahydrodeoxycorticosterone (THDOC), but receptors with the δ subunit are particularly sensitive: 30 nM THDOC enhances the peak currents of $\alpha1\beta3\delta$ $GABA_A$ receptors (with 1 μM GABA) by up to 800%; currents of other receptor isoforms (e.g., $\alpha1\beta3\gamma2$) are enhanced by less (15–50%) (Mihalek et al., 1999; Wohlfarth et al., 2002; Stell et al., 2003). Thus, endogenous allopregnanolone may act on perisynaptic $\alpha\beta\delta$ $GABA_A$ receptor isoforms on dentate granule cells to increase basal levels of inhibition. Mice without functional δ subunits have decreased sensitivity to the sedative/hypnotic, anxiolytic, and pro-absence effects of neuroactive steroids (Mihalek et al., 1999).

Zinc inhibits $GABA_A$ receptors. Glutamatergic neurons provide most of the extracellular zinc in the hippocampus. Zinc is stored in synaptic vesicles, notably in mossy fiber terminals; strong stimulation of mossy fibers induces co-release of glutamate and zinc into the synaptic cleft. In hippocampal neurons, zinc can reduce the amplitude, slow the rise time, and accelerate the decay of mIPSCs (e.g., Wei et al., 2003). On recombinant $GABA_A$ receptors, zinc has an inhibitory potency

3400 times higher on $\alpha\beta$ receptors than on $\alpha\beta\gamma2$ receptors (reviewed in Hosie et al., 2003). Thus the $\gamma2$ subunit lowers the sensitivity of the $GABA_A$ receptor complex to zinc. Hosie et al. suggested that the concentrations of extracellular zinc occurring in the hippocampus inhibit $\alpha\beta\delta$ receptors but do not affect $\alpha\beta\gamma2$ receptors (presumably $\alpha1$-, $\alpha2$-, $\alpha3$-containing), so zinc would be a specific modulator of tonic inhibition. They hypothesized that in addition to its role in promoting synaptic targeting and single channel conductance the $\gamma2$ subunit evolved to retain the fidelity of GABAergic inhibition in the presence of zinc. Nevertheless, zinc's potency is also α subunit- and δ subunit-dependent. The IC_{50} for zinc inhibition of $\alpha4\beta3\delta$ and $\alpha4\beta3\gamma2$ receptors is, in fact, similar (2 μM).

Blood alcohol levels of 1 to 3 mM can result from drinking half a glass of wine or less. Ethanol influences various channels, including the NMDA glutamate receptor; but among $GABA_A$ receptor subunit combinations, low concentrations of ethanol (about 3 mM, a concentration six times lower than the legal blood alcohol limit for driving in many states in the United States) specifically potentiate GABA responses of cloned $\alpha4\beta2\delta$ receptors expressed in *Xenopus* oocytes; this effect is β subunit-dependent, as $\beta3$ subunits are needed for maximal sensitivity to ethanol (Sundstrom-Poromaa et al., 2002; Wallner et al., 2003).

Distribution of $GABA_A$ Receptors in Hippocampal Pyramidal Cells

A pyramidal cell is covered with GABAergic terminals; a typical rat CA1 pyramidal cell receives around 1700 GABAergic synapses, with the highest density on the perisomatic region (Megias et al., 2001). Inhibition on the various domains affects different aspects of pyramidal cell function. $GABA_A$ receptor-mediated IPSCs can be generated along the whole somatodendritic domain and on the axon initial segment of CA1 pyramidal cells (Maccaferri et al., 2000). The apical dendritic trunk has a high density of GABAergic terminals relative to the rest of the dendrite (Papp et al., 2001); strong GABAergic stimulation on this apical trunk region isolates the dendritic compartment from the cell body. Inhibition on the more distal dendrites controls Ca^{2+} spike propagation. Inhibiting the axon initial segment powerfully clamps down the pyramidal cell's activity, as this is where action potentials initiate: A typical rat CA1 pyramidal cell has more than 25 GABAergic terminals per 50 μm of the axon initial segment (AIS). Thus, $GABA_A$ receptors in the AIS deliver inhibition that controls the overall level of output activity of pyramidal cells.

Hippocampal pyramidal cells assemble many $GABA_A$ receptor subtypes (Fritschy and Brunig, 2003). By in situ hybridization and immunocytochemistry, rat pyramidal cells are seen to express the $\alpha1$, $\alpha2$, $\alpha4$, $\beta5$, $\beta1$, $\beta2$, $\beta3$, $\gamma1$, and $\gamma2$ genes; expression of $\alpha3$ and $\gamma1$ genes is present but weak (Wisden et al., 1992). For the α subunits, $\alpha2$ mRNA is the most abundant; of the β genes, $\beta1$ and $\beta3$ are more abundant than $\beta2$; $\gamma2$ mRNA is at about the same level as $\alpha1$ and $\beta2$

(Wisden et al., 1992). The in situ hybridization and immunocytochemical data are in agreement. β1 immunoreactivity is enriched at the CA2 pyramidal cell boundary (Pirker et al., 2000), as is β1 mRNA (Wisden et al., 1992).

As seen by immunocytochemistry with the light microscope, α1, α2, α5, β1, β2, β3, and γ2 proteins distribute evenly on pyramidal cell dendrites and are sparser on the cell body (Sperk et al., 1997). Autoradiography with the α5-selective ligand [^{3}H]L-655708 highlights the stratum radiatum, confirming α5 protein enrichment on pyramidal cell dendrites (Sur et al., 1999). Subcellularly, the α5 subunit appears predominantly extrasynaptic, with about 25% synaptic component (Brunig et al., 2002; Crestani et al., 2002). Note that the reduction in spontaneous IPSC amplitude on CA1 pyramidal cells in hippocampal slices of α5 knockout mice supports the conclusion that at least some α5 subunits are synaptically located (Collinson et al., 2002).

As already mentioned, the cell bodies of pyramidal cells do not heavily stain with GABA$_A$ receptor subunit-specific antibodies. However, gold-labeled antibodies combined with immunocytochemistry at the electron microscopic level have revealed GABA$_A$ subunits at synapses on the cell body; these somatic GABAergic synapses do not all have the same GABA$_A$ receptor subunit composition (Nusser et al., 1996; Somogyi et al., 1996; Nyiri et al., 2001) (see below).

GABA$_A$ receptors are also differentially sorted to specific pyramidal cell synapses. This is indicated by three levels of evidence: kinetically distinct IPSPs depending on subcellular location; GABA$_A$ receptors with different pharmacology at different synaptic inputs; and direct visualization of different receptor subunits at different synapses and extrasynaptic sites.

Different synaptic locations on pyramidal neurons have kinetically distinct IPSCs (Banks et al., 1998). At least two different IPSCs are found on CA1 pyramidal cells. A fast component (decay time constant of 9 ms) on the soma is mediated by basket cells and other interneurons; the slow component is dendritic, with a decay time constant of 50 ms, and is activated by interneurons in the stratum lacunosum-moleculare. These two decay types may be due to different receptors, although there are no subunits on the dendrite that are not on the cell body (Banks et al., 1998). In fact, a better explanation for location-dependent IPSCs is electrotonic filtering and/or the lack of voltage-clamp at the more distal recording locations (Maccaferri et al., 2000).

GABA$_A$ receptors at different GABAergic inputs onto pyramidal cells have differing sensitivities to zinc and benzodiazepines, suggestive of different subunit compositions. Zolpidem sensitivity (a selective agonist for α1β2/3γ2 receptors if used at the appropriate concentration) was used to probe the subunit composition of synapses on the pyramidal cell body (Thomson et al., 2000). IPSPs in pyramidal cells elicited by fast-spiking basket cells (possibly corresponding to the parvalbumin-positive basket cells) were enhanced more by zolpidem than IPSCs elicited by regular spiking basket cells. Both types of synapse have IPSCs equally enhanced by diazepam. Thus, by pharmacological inference, α1β2/3γ2 receptors dominate postsynaptic responses in synapses formed on pyramidal cells from fast-spiking cells, whereas the α2 (and α3) subunits also contribute to receptors, together with α1, in the regular spiking basket cell to pyramidal cell synapses. This is directly supported by anatomical work (see below).

Indirect evidence for α4β3γ2-type GABA$_A$ receptors participating in synaptic transmission on the soma of CA1 pyramidal cells comes from studies on "chronic intermittent ethanol" (CIE)-treated rats. In this model, rats are exposed to intermittent episodes of ethanol and then ethanol withdrawal, producing a kindled-like state of excitability; this is accompanied by changes in GABA$_A$ receptor expression in, among other areas, the hippocampus (Cagetti et al., 2003). In CA1 pyramidal cells of CIE-treated rats, mIPSCs become insensitive to diazepam but can still be modulated by the benzodiazepine bretazenil (diazepam is active on α1βγ2 receptors, but not α4βγ2 receptors, whereas bretazenil is active on both). In CA1 pyramidal cells of control rats, mIPSCs are enhanced only slightly by the benzodiazepine "partial inverse agonist" Ro 15-4513 but are substantially enhanced by this drug in CIE-treated rats.

GABA$_A$ receptors also show differential subunit distribution at different synapses of the same pyramidal cell. On hippocampal pyramidal cells, the α2 subunit is enriched in the axon initial segment but is present at only a small number of cell body synapses and synapses on dendrites (Nusser et al., 1996; Fritschy et al., 1998). The axon initial segment synapse also contains the α1 subunit and possibly the α4 and α5 subunits. GABA$_A$ receptors at the axon initial segment are positioned to exert strong inhibitory influence over action potential generation.

Synapses formed by two types of basket cell on CA1 pyramidal cells contain distinct GABA$_A$ receptor subtypes: Only those synapses coming from parvalbumin-negative/CCK and VIP-positive basket cell interneurons contain the α2 subunit; synapses from parvalbumin-positive basket cells are often α2-immunonegative (Nyiri et al., 2001). This is preferential targeting or enrichment of the α2 in a particular type of synapse, not absolute selectivity. Both synapse types contain the same level of immunoreactivity for the β2/3 subunits; both types of synapse made by basket cells onto pyramidal cell somata also contain the α1 and the γ2 subunits (Somogyi et al., 1996). However, the α1 subunit is less abundant in the parvalbumin-negative pyramidal cell synapses than in the parvalbumin-positive ones. This work fits well with the pharmacological experiments (zolpidem sensitivity) described above. Thus, (fast-spiking) PV-basket cells probably act through α1β2/3γ2, α2β2/3γ2, and/or α1α2β2/3γ2 subunit-containing receptors. The subcellular location of other α subunits (α4 and α5) on pyramidal cells has not yet been established by electron microscopy. Despite these differences in GABA$_A$ receptor subunit composition among synapses, paired intracellular recordings between pyramidal cells and basket cells did not reveal significant differences in the kinetic parameters of postsynaptic responses evoked by PV- or CCK-containing basket cells (Maccaferri et al., 2000; Pawelzik et al., 2002). Different $GABA_A$ receptor subunit compositions at the synapse do not necessarily produce different kinetics.

$GABA_A$ receptors are also expressed at the dentate granule cell mossy fiber to CA3 pyramidal cell synapse, a synapse traditionally considered glutamatergic (Walker et al., 2001). Dentate granule cells can induce a partial GABAergic phenotype after seizure by expressing glutamic acid decarboxylase (reviewed in Gutierrez, 2003). The $\alpha 1$ and $\beta 2/3$ subunits were found by immunogold cytochemistry in some rat mossy fiber to CA3 synapses and co-localized with GluR2/3 AMPA receptor subunits (95% of AMPA receptor-positive mossy fiber to CA3 synapses were also $GABA_A$ receptor-positive) (Bergersen et al., 2003). What is the function of GABA release and $GABA_A$ receptor activation in mossy fiber synapses? It may be a brake on the AMPA system, although the GABAergic signal is small compared with the AMPA receptor EPSP. Note also that mossy fibers have a particularly high concentration of zinc, which when released may inhibit extrasynaptic δ subunit-containing receptors; on the other hand, the $\gamma 2$ subunit may serve to reduce zinc sensitivity of the synaptic $GABA_A$ receptor complex (Hosie et al., 2003).

Distribution of $GABA_A$ Receptors in Hippocampal Interneurons

GABAergic interneuronsand innervating principal cells also innervate each other and thus reciprocally inhibit each other. The amount of GABAergic input onto hippocampal interneurons varies with cell type, as seen from a detailed study of three types of CA1 interneuron: The ratio of GABAergic to glutamatergic inputs was about 30% for calbindin-expressing D_{28K} cells, 20% for calretinin-expressing cells, and only 6% for parvalbumin-expressing cells (Gulyas et al., 1999). Regardless of the exact interneuronal type, GABAergic terminals onto interneurons are concentrated in the perisomatic region and on proximal dendrites; GABAergic synapses are also on distal dendrites, although at reduced density. Because of the high diversity of the interneuronal GABAergic population in the hippocampus, the available information on $GABA_A$ subunit expression in hippocampal interneurons is patchy. Based on immunocytochemistry and zolpidem sensitivity, many rat hippocampal interneurons probably use the $\alpha 1\beta 2\gamma 2$ receptor subunit combination. The $\alpha 1$ immunoreactivity is found in all parvalbumin-positive interneurons and about half of calretinin-positive cells but in no calbindin-containing cells (Gao and Fritschy, 1994; Klausberger et al., 2002); much of the $\alpha 1$ immunoreactivity on parvalbumin-positive cells is attributable to extrasynaptic receptors. The $\alpha 1$ immunoreactivity is found in most NPY- and some somatostatin-containing cells, but not in CCK- or VIP-positive cells (Gao and Fritschy, 1994). However, at least 40% of hippocampal interneurons do not express the $\alpha 1$ subunit and so probably use other types of

$GABA_A$ receptor. For example, as seen by the single-cell reverse transcription-polymerase chain reaction (RT-PCR), the most prominently expressed $GABA_A$ receptor subunit genes in rat dentate basket-like cells are $\alpha 2$, $\beta 3$, and $\gamma 2$ (Berger et al., 1998), although by immunocytochemistry there is only weak (Fritschy and Mohler, 1995) or no (Sperk et al., 1997) $\alpha 2$ subunit immunoreactivity detectable in this cell type. Some other interneurons (unidentified) in the polymorph cell layer of the dentate gyrus may assemble multiple $GABA_A$ receptor types: Such cells are immunoreactive for the $\alpha 3$, $\beta 1$, and the δ subunits as well as for the $\alpha 1$, $\alpha 2$, and $\gamma 2$ subunits (Fritschy and Mohler, 1995; Pirker et al., 2000). The $\alpha 3$-positive cells in the hilus may be mossy cells. Some $\alpha 3$-positive cells (small cells, three to five parallel dendrites) are present in the stratum oriens of the CA1 region (Brunig et al., 2002). Peng et al (2002) and Wei et al (2003) reported δ subunit immunoreactivity in scattered, unidentified interneurons throughout the hippocampus. Double-labeling studies are needed to confirm subunit co-expression and interneuron type.

$GABA_A$ Receptor Subtypes and Network Oscillation Frequency in the Hippocampus

Modeling predicts that IPSC kinetics between basket cell–basket cell groupings and between basket cells and principal cells strongly influence network oscillations in the gamma frequency range, although models differ in their assumption of the actual values of IPSC parameters (reviewed in Bartos et al., 2002). Empirically, synapses in the hippocampus differ with respect to their IPSC kinetics; the kinetics of interneuron–interneuron IPSCs are always faster than interneuron–principal cell IPSCs (Bartos et al., 2002). For example, the time course of the GABAergic postsynaptic conductance change at basket cell to basket cell synapses in the dentate gyrus is fast (decay time constant 1.8 ms), whereas basket cell to granule cell synapses are slower (decay time constant 5.2 ms). The differing subunit combinations between cell types can explain the differing IPSC kinetics; the predominant receptor subtype on many hippocampal interneurons is $\alpha 1\beta\gamma 2$, and this receptor subtype has faster decay kinetics than those of the $\alpha 2\beta\gamma 2$ receptors enriched at some synapses on pyramidal and dentate cell bodies. Whether these IPSC kinetic differences are really due to the distinct $GABA_A$ receptor subunit compositions at specific synapses or have some other explanation remains to be tested. Indeed, the decay time constants between basket cell–basket cell pairs vary among hippocampal regions (DG faster than CA3, in turn faster than CA1), although they are always faster than the corresponding interneuron–principal cell IPSCs. Factors in addition to subunit composition that might affect IPSC kinetics include the phosphorylation status of the $GABA_A$ receptors; synaptic geometry (differing distances of receptors from transmitter release sites); and differences in GABA reuptake kinetics via transporters. These factors could be synapse- and cell type-dependent.

7.6.3 GABA_B Receptors

The GABA_B receptors consist of seven transmembrane-domain proteins, GABA_BR1, and GABA_BR2 (reviewed in Bettler et al., 2004). Most GABA_B receptors are heterodimers of GABA_BR1 and GABA_BR2. Inactivation of the GABA_BR1 gene in mice removes all biochemical and electrophysiological GABA_B responses, demonstrating that GABA_BR1 is an essential component of all GABA_B receptors. The lack of the GABA_B response causes generalized epilepsy (Prosser et al., 2001; Schuler et al., 2001). There are two R1 versions, GABA_BR1a and GABA_BR1b, produced by different promoters of the GABA_BR1 gene; the proteins differ in their N-termini, the first 147 amino acids in GABA_BR1a being replaced by an equivalent region in GABA_BR1b differing in 18 amino acids. In many neurons, such as pyramidal cells and dentate granule cells, GABA_B receptors are formed as heteromers of GABA_BR1 and GABA_BR2 in a stoichiometric 1:1 ratio. Most GABA_B receptors are likely to be GABA_BR1a/GABA_BR2 or GABA_BR1b/GABA_BR2 heteromers. In the GABA_BR complex, the GABA_BR1 subunit binds GABA and all competitive GABA_B ligands, whereas the GABA_BR2 subunit is essential for the translocation of GABA_BR1 subunits to the cell surface and for targeting of the receptor to distal dendrites (Pagano et al., 2001; Gassmann et al., 2004); the GABA_BR2 subunit contributes to activating the G protein but is not absolutely essential, as GABA_BR2 knockout mice still have (atypical) electrophysiological GABA_B responses (Gassmann et al., 2004).

GABA_B receptors act through G proteins to, for example, open K^+ channels (GIRK type), inhibit high-voltage-activated Ca^{2+} channels (P/Q- and N-type) and inhibit/stimulate adenyl cyclase; the opposite effects on cAMP production might be due to different G proteins (Bettler et al., 2004). GABA_B receptor effects on K^+ channels are mainly postsynaptic and cause long-lasting membrane hyperpolarization, which can take up to 200 ms to peak and 450 to 2000 msec to decay. In contrast, Ca^{2+} effects are mainly presynaptic. GABA_B receptors can act as inhibitory autoreceptors to block GABA release from interneurons (Poncer et al., 2000); the resulting disinhibition plays an important role in the induction of LTP (see Chapter 10). In CA1 pyramidal cells of mice lacking the GABA_BR2 subunit, GABA_B receptors inhibit rather than activate K^+ channels, but whether this is physiologically relevant is unclear—it may be a side effect of GABA_BR1 having no proper partner (Gassmann et al., 2004).

In keeping with the long-term effects produced by GABA_B receptor activation, various signaling proteins, including transcription factors, may link to the GABA_B receptor complex, forming a signaling scaffold. Examples include the direct interactions between the C-terminal tails of GABA_BR1 and GABA_BR2 with two related transcription factors, CREB2 (ATF4) and ATFx (Nehring et al., 2000; White et al., 2000); both these transcription factors activate target genes with CRE sites in their regulatory regions. On cultured hippocampal neurons, immunocytochemistry shows that GABA_B receptors and ATF4 co-cluster in the soma and at the dendritic membrane surface. This suggests a model in which activation of the receptor releases the transcription factors, which then translocate to the nucleus to activate/repress target gene expression. NGF and BDNF genes are candidate target genes (White et al., 2000).

Distribution of GABA_B Receptors in Hippocampal Principal Cells

Both GABA_BR1 and GABA_BR2 are expressed in hippocampal pyramidal cells and dentate granule cells, as shown by in situ hybridization and immunocytochemistry (Fig. 7–10A) (Kulik et al., 2003). Most GABA_B receptors are on dendrites. There is a differential subcellular distribution of GABA_B receptors on hippocampal pyramidal cells: GABA_BR1b immunoreactivity is enriched on distal dendrites (stratum lacunosum-moleculare) of rat pyramidal cells, whereas the GABA_BR1a form is found predominantly on the cell body. The somatic receptors are probably not functional; electron microscopy with gold particle-tagged antibodies shows that the strong somatic labeling results from GABA_B receptor immunoreactivity in the endoplasmic reticulum (Kulik et al., 2003). On dentate granule cells, GABA_B receptor immunoreactivity is enriched in the molecular layer, suggesting a dendritic location. Throughout the hippocampus, GABA_BR2 immunoreactivity corresponds to the sum of the R1a and R1b patterns. The subunits co-localize in the same intracellular compartments. The targeting of GABA_B receptors to distal dendrites requires the GABA_BR2 subunit; in mouse hippocampal neurons lacking GABA_BR2 the soma of pyramidal cells and dentate granule cells become prominently labeled by a GABA_BR1 antibody, whereas in wild-type animals cell bodies have only weak, diffuse staining, and GABA_BR1 immunoreactivity is distributed throughout the neuropil (Gassmann et al., 2004).

Distribution of GABA_B Receptors in Hippocampal Interneurons

GABA_B receptor responses are detected on some interneurons and are similar to those of principal cells (Mott et al., 1999). Both GABA_BR1a- and GABA_BR1b-like immunoreactivity is found on subsets of hippocampal GABAergic interneurons (Kulik et al., 2003; Gassmann et al., 2004); however, these interneurons do not stain with an antibody recognizing the GABA_A receptor β2/β3 subunits. This implies that GABA_A and GABA_B receptors may be on distinct interneuronal cell populations, or that these GABA_B-expressing interneurons use GABA_A receptors with the β1 subunit (Fritschy et al., 1999). Not all hippocampal interneurons seem to have GABA_B receptors; there are some in the dentate hilus border region in which GABA_B-activated K^+ currents are not produced (Mott et al., 1999). By double labeling for glutamic acid decarboxy-

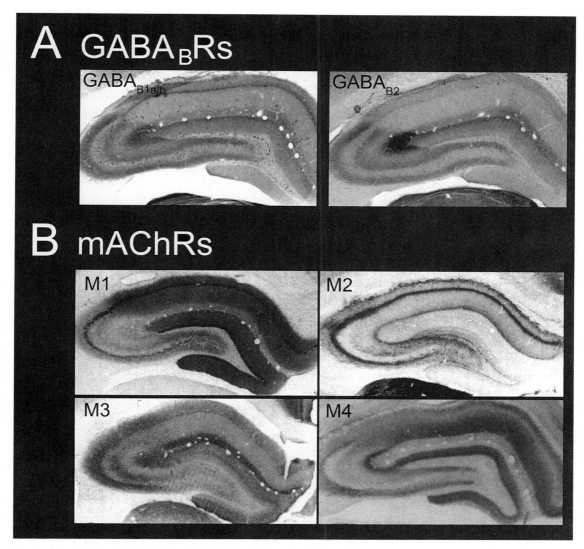

Figure 7–10. Expression of GABA$_B$ and mAChR receptors in the hippocampus. *A*. Immunohistochemistry with subunit-specific antibodies was used to visualize the expression pattern of GABA$_B$ receptor subunits. (*Source*: Modified from Kulik et al., 2003, with permission.) *B*. Immunohistochemistry with mAChR type-specific antibodies in the adult rat hippocampus. (*Source*: Modified from Levey et al., 1995, with permission.)

lase 67 (GAD67) mRNA, Kulik et al, estimated that only 50% of GABAergic interneurons contain GABA$_B$ receptor immunoreactivity (Kulik et al., 2003).

Subcellular Localization of GABA$_B$ Receptors in Hippocampal Neurons

Presynaptic GABA$_B$ receptor subunits are localized to GABAergic and putative glutamatergic axon terminals. Functional GABA$_B$ receptors can be found, for example, on mossy fiber terminals, where they provide heterosynaptic depression (Vogt and Nicoll, 1999). The subunits are found at the extrasynaptic membrane but also at the presynaptic membrane specialization. GABA$_B$ receptors on inhibitory synaptic terminals autoinhibit GABA release. Presynaptic GABA$_B$ receptors on glutamatergic terminals likely function as heteroreceptors regulating glutamate receptor release (Kulik et al., 2003).

Postsynaptically, the most intense labeling for GABA$_B$ receptor subunits was found in CA1 and CA3 pyramidal cell spines associated with glutamatergic terminals (Kulik et al., 2003). The functional relevance of this is unclear. In dendritic shafts, the GABA$_B$ receptor subunits localize to the extrasynaptic membrane, with no association with inhibitory synapses. Thus, activation of these receptors requires GABA spillover. Activation of GABA$_B$ receptors depends on transients in the ambient GABA concentration and may serve to detect enhanced and/or simultaneous activity of GABAergic interneurons, as occurs in population oscillations when many interneurons fire simultaneously.

7.7 Trafficking of GABA Receptors and Hippocampal Synaptic Function

How $GABA_A$ receptor subunits/subtypes target GABAergic synapses, and differentially target between synapses on the same hippocampal cell (e.g., the $\alpha2$ subunit enriched in the axon initial segment of pyramidal cells) is not well understood. In vivo most $GABA_A$ receptors on hippocampal neurons are located opposite GABAergic terminals, not opposite glutamatergic terminals. How does this selective targeting occur? There is evidence that targeting of $GABA_A$ receptors to specific domains of hippocampal neurons is partially cell-intrinsic. In cultured hippocampal neurons, 40% of pyramidal axon initial segments have enrichment of the $\alpha2$ subunit, as seen by co-staining with the axon-specific type II voltage-gated Na channel (Brunig et al., 2002), and a similar proportion is seen in vivo (Nusser et al., 1996). Thus, specific innervation patterns on the hippocampal pyramidal cells (e.g., from the axo-axonic interneurons in vivo) are not required to establish $\alpha2$ enrichment at the axon initial segment during development.

7.7.1 Role of Gephyrin in $GABA_A$ Receptor Localization

Placing $GABA_A$ receptors at synapses requires specific proteins that interact directly or indirectly with the $\gamma2$ subunit. For example, targeting some $GABA_A$ receptor subtypes to GABAergic terminals involves the microtubule-binding protein gephyrin. In hippocampal neurons in vitro and in vivo, gephyrin either helps convey some $GABA_A$ receptor subtypes to the synapse or anchors them there; this requires the $\gamma2$ subunit (Kneussel et al., 1999; Brunig et al., 2002). Without the $\gamma2$ subunit, no $GABA_A$ receptors are found in synapses in the developing or adult hippocampus (Gunther et al., 1995; Essrich et al., 1998; Schweizer et al., 2003); and without gephyrin, much reduced numbers of some synaptic $GABA_A$ receptor subtypes, especially $\alpha2$-containing, are found. Some receptor clusters, especially those containing the $\alpha1$ subunit, persist in hippocampal gephyrin knockout neurons (Levi et al., 2004). Gephyrin, however, does not bind the $\gamma2$ $GABA_A$ receptor subunit intracellular loop directly, as it does for the glycine β receptor subunit. The identity of the missing link(s) between gephyrin and $GABA_A$ receptor subunits is unknown.

As mentioned above, the targeting of $\gamma2$-containing receptors to hippocampal synapses must depend on both the α subunit and the $\gamma2$ subunit. According to some investigators $\alpha5\beta\gamma2$ receptors seem largely extrasynaptic and not co-localized with gephyrin (Crestani et al., 2002), and when $\alpha6\beta\gamma2$ receptors (normally found only in cerebellar granule cells) are

ectopically expressed in hippocampal pyramidal cells, these receptors remain extrasynaptic (Wisden et al., 1992). The determinants of synaptic/extrasynaptic $GABA_A$ receptor location may be cell type-specific and subunit-specific. In hippocampal "fireball" interneurons, the $\alpha3$ subunit is extrasynaptic (not co-localized with gephyrin); whereas in interneurons described as "small multipolar," $\alpha3$ immunoreactivity clusters with that of gephyrin (Brunig et al., 2002). Thus, in addition to gephyrin, other clustering proteins must contribute to the synaptic localization of selected $GABA_A$ receptor subtypes.

7.7.2 Role of Dystrophin-associated Protein Complex in $GABA_A$ Receptor Function

The dystrophin-associated protein complex (DAPC) connects the cytoskeleton to the extracellular matrix via a transmembrane link. The DAPC's integrative role has been best studied in muscle and Duchenne muscular dystrophy. However, DAPC components are also expressed in both neurons and glia, and some that are not found at excitatory synapses seem to be specialized for GABAergic synaptic function (Kneussel et al., 1999; Brunig et al., 2002; Levi et al., 2002; Fritschy and Brunig, 2003). Because the DAPC binds intracellular and extracellular components, it could function as an organizer of GABAergic synaptic structure in the hippocampus. The DAPC comprises dystroglycan (extracellular α subunits and transmembrane β subunits derived from a common precursor protein by cleavage). The α-dystroglycan binds laminin and agrin and the transmembrane β-dystroglycan. The β-dystroglycan binds the intracellularly located dystrophin and/or related utrophin. Dystrophin (Dp) is a cytoskeletal protein of the α-actinin/β-spectrin family. The main brain isoform of dystrophin is Dp71. Dp71 binds to α-dystrobrevin. Dystrophin and α-dystrobrevin each bind up to two syntrophins (pleckstrin homology domain and PDZ-containing proteins). The PDZ domain of the syntrophins serves as an adaptor to bind membrane channels, receptors, kinases, and other signaling proteins. Dystrophin and dystroglycan selectively associate with subsets of GABAergic synapses in the hippocampus (Kneussel et al., 1999; Levi et al., 2002). Dystrophin immunoreactivity is present in the CA1 and CA3 regions but not in the dentate gyrus; extensive co-localization between the $\alpha2$, $\gamma2$, and dystrophin immunoreactivities was observed in the soma and dendrites of hippocampal pyramidal cells; but the axon initial segment, which was prominently stained for $GABA_A$ receptor subunits, was negative for dystrophin staining (Kneussel et al., 1999). Similarly, β-dystroglycan is present at only a subset of GABAergic synapses in cultured hippocampal neurons, including synapses positive for $\alpha1$, $\alpha2$, $\gamma2$, and $\beta2/3$ subunits (Levi et al., 2002). However, many clusters of glutamic acid decarboxylase, gephyrin, and $\gamma2$ subunits were not co-localized with β-dystroglycan, which, like dystrophin, is present only in a subset of GABAergic synapses. There is no interaction between the gephyrin and DAPC systems. The number and size of gephyrin-immunoreactive clusters were unaffected by the absence of dystrophin in *mdx* mice; hippocampal neurons from gephyrin knockout mice have normal dystroglycan and dystrophin immunoreactive clusters.

7.7.3 Plasticity of GABA$_A$ Receptor Expression at Hippocampal Synapses

It is important to keep in mind that, as for ionotropic glutamate receptors, GABA$_A$ receptor expression on the surface of hippocampal cells is dynamic; receptors rapidly recycle and leave from or insert into the synapse (reviewed in Kittler and Moss, 2003). For some inhibitory hippocampal synapses, a direct relation exists between the number of synaptic GABA$_A$ receptors and the strength of the synapse (reviewed in Nusser, 1999). As for glutamate receptors at excitatory synapses, neurons probably recycle GABA$_A$ receptors as an important strategy for setting their degree of excitability. GABA$_A$ receptors constitutively internalize by clathrin-dependent endocytosis; this requires interactions between the β and γ2 subunits and the AP2 adaptin complex. Again, as for glutamatergic synapses, the properties of inhibitory GABAergic synapses alter with activity through changes in GABA$_A$ receptor properties or receptor number.

Plasticity in GABA Receptor Expression in Dentate Granule Cells

Dentate granule cells exhibit pronounced plasticity in their patterns of gene expression; although their phenotype is predominantly glutamatergic, after prolonged seizure activity granule cells can display a partial GABAergic phenotype by expressing glutamic acid decarboxylase (reviewed in Gutierrez, 2003). Moreover, seizure activity in the hippocampus—for example, pilocarpine-induced epilepsy or kindling—causes changes in GABA$_A$ receptor subunit expression in dentate granule cells (Brooks-Kayal et al., 1998). There are also long-term changes in receptor number. After kindling, the amplitudes of elementary synaptic GABA$_A$ currents on dentate granule cells increased 66% owing to a corresponding 75% increase in GABA$_A$ receptor number in GABAergic synapses on granule cell somata and axon initial segments, as assessed with immunogold labeling with an antibody to the β2 and β3 subunits (Nusser et al., 1998a); immunostaining of granule cells with α1, α2, and γ2 subunit antibodies was also increased. This demonstrates directly that under these conditions the efficacy of GABAergic synapses is enhanced by the insertion of extra GABA$_A$ receptors postsynaptically. Using single-cell mRNA amplification, Brooks-Kayal et al. (1998) studied the relative changes in GABA$_A$ receptor subunit expression in isolated dentate granule cells from normal rats and chronically epileptic rats in which temporal lobe epilepsy was produced by pilocarpine injection. The largest changes found were a marked decease in α1 and a strong increase in α4

subunit mRNA levels, as well as increases in β and δ subunit transcript levels (Brooks-Kayal et al., 1998).

Other forms of stimulation eliciting GABA$_A$ receptor plasticity in dentate granule cells include ethanol, steroids, and prenatal handling. Expression of the α4 subunit gene seems particularly plastic with regard to ethanol and steroid treatments. Chronic in vivo administration and withdrawal of progesterone, which mimics hormonal changes of the menstrual cycle, increases the expression of hippocampal α4βδ receptors (Smith et al., 1998a,b); long-term treatment and withdrawal from ethanol (in CIE-treated rats) elevates hippocampal α4 mRNA and protein in CA1 pyramidal cells (Mahmoudi et al., 1997). Brief traumatic stress during infancy can permanently alter expression of GABA$_A$ receptors in dentate granule cells of the adult hippocampus (Hsu et al., 2003). In adult rats that have experienced two episodes of separation from their mothers and human handling, dentate granule cells recorded in vitro significantly reduced responses to zolpidem application; by single-cell RNA amplification, α1 subunit mRNA levels decrease in handled individuals, whereas those of the α2 subunit increase.

7.8 Genetic Analysis of GABA Receptor Function in the Hippocampus

7.8.1 GABA$_A$ Receptor Mutant Mice

The widespread expression of most GABA$_A$ receptor subunit genes makes it difficult to attribute behavioral changes in knockout animals specifically to changes in the hippocampus (reviewed in Rudolph and Mohler, 2004). Nevertheless, various studies on genetically engineered mice have provided insight into the role of GABA$_A$ receptors in hippocampal function.

Expression of the α5 gene is highly enriched in pyramidal cells of the hippocampus compared with other brain regions, making the knockout phenotype relatively easy to interpret as "hippocampal" (Collinson et al., 2002). Homozygous α5 subunit knockout mice show no overt phenotypic abnormalities, breed normally, and have no spontaneous seizures. However, in a "matching-to-place" watermaze task, in which the hidden platform is moved between trials, α5 knockout mice had enhanced performance compared with their wild-type littermates, whereas performance in non-hippocampal-dependent learning and anxiety tasks was unaltered. In the CA1 region of hippocampal slices from α5 knockout mice, the IPSC amplitude was decreased and paired-pulse facilitation of field EPSP amplitudes was enhanced. In complementary data, mice engineered to express α5 subunits with a histidine to arginine mutation at position 105 of α5 have a fortuitous CA1-specific knockdown of the α5 subunit expression (Crestani et al., 2002). In these α5 CA1 knockdown mice, trace fear conditioning (a hippocampal-dependent process) is selectively enhanced. These combined data suggest that α5-containing GABA$_A$ receptors contribute to cognitive processes by controlling a component of synaptic transmission in CA1 (Collinson et al., 2002).

In terms of network properties, γ oscillations (20–80 Hz) are modified in α5 knockout hippocampal slices (Towers et al., 2004). The peak power of oscillations evoked by kainic acid was significantly greater in α5 knockout than in wild-type slices; however, the frequency change of γ oscillations that normally occurs with increasing network drive was absent in α5 knockout slices. The enriched expression of the α5 subunit in the hippocampus has therapeutic potential. The drugs L-655,708 (partial inverse agonist at the BZ site) and "43" (a thiophene analogue and a full inverse agonist at the BZ site) are α5βγ2-selective modulatory ligands (Chambers et al., 2003); "43" can increase, relatively selectively, neuronal activity in the hippocampus; "43" enhances cognitive performance in rats in the delayed matching-to-place Morris watermaze. In principle, it and similar α5 subunit-selective drugs are potential "cognition enhancers" in humans.

Further useful information on hippocampal signaling has also been gleaned from some of the other GABA$_A$ receptor subunit knockouts. The δ subunit knockout mice were instrumental in showing the selective contribution of the α4δ-containing GABA$_A$ receptors to extrasynaptic tonic inhibition on dentate granule cells (Stell et al., 2003). In the hippocampus of α1 subunit knockout mice, synaptic GABA$_A$ receptor-mediated currents (pyramidal and interneuronal) decay more slowly than those from wild-type mice (Goldstein et al., 2002). Loss of the α1 subunit in synaptically localized receptors leads to a population of synaptic receptors with slower deactivation kinetics, in which the α1 subunit is probably replaced by an α2 or α3 subunit, thus confirming the role of α subunits in determining GABA$_A$ receptor kinetics.

7.8.2 GABA$_B$ Receptor Mutant Mice

Two independent GABA$_B$R1 knockout lines were established (Prosser et al., 2001; Schuler et al., 2001). Although both lines show a loss of GABA$_B$ responses in hippocampal pyramidal cells, demonstrating the absolute requirement for the GABA$_B$R1 subunit in forming GABA$_B$ receptors, the genetic background of the two lines dramatically affects their mortality. The responsible strain-dependent modifier genes have not been identified.

Balb/c GABA$_B$R1 knockout mice (BALB/c (BALB/c, F1) generated from BALB/c embryonic stem cells have spontaneous epileptiform activity but are otherwise viable. In addition, the mice are hyperalgesic, show hyperlocomotor activity, and are severely impaired in passive avoidance learning (Schuler et al., 2001). The second line—genetic background 129SVJ × C57Bl6/J,—GABA$_B$R1 knockout mice have spontaneous generalized seizures and die after several seizure events; an increased ictal discharge pattern of epileptiform activity

was observed in hippocampal slices from mice that had repetitive seizures (Prosser et al., 2001).

A knockout mouse line has also been made for the other GABA$_B$ receptor subunit gene, GABA$_B$R2 (Gassmann et al., 2004). Adult GABA$_B$R2 knockout mice (BALB/c) display several episodes of spontaneous seizures per day. The recorded seizures are exclusively clonic. This is in contrast to GABA$_B$R1 knockout mice (BALB/c), in which additionally absence-type and spontaneous tonic-clonic seizures occur with low frequency. GABA$_B$R2 knockout mice exhibit impaired passive avoidance learning, similar to GABA$_B$R1 knockout mice. Thus, the GABA$_B$R2 subunit is needed for functional GABA$_B$ receptors in vivo.

7.9 Cholinergic Receptors

7.9.1 Introduction: Muscarinic and Nicotinic Receptors

Cholinergic neurotransmission modulates glutamatergic and GABAergic transmission in the hippocampus, and cholinergic projections into the hippocampus regulate the hippocampal theta rhythm in vivo (reviewed in Kimura, 2000). The neurotransmitter acetylcholine activates both metabotropic G protein-coupled muscarinic receptors and neuronal nicotinic receptors constituting ligand-gated cation channels. Acetylcholine is delivered to the hippocampus primarily by cholinergic neurons projecting from the medial septum/diagonal band complex; in addition, infrequent choline acetyl transferase (ChAT)-positive interneurons in the hippocampus produce local acetylcholine (ACh).

Activation of muscarinic receptors on both principal cells and interneurons causes a variety of cellular effects, including inhibition of K$^+$ currents, membrane depolarization, and IP3 production (reviewed in Wess, 2004). A prominent effect of muscarinic agonists on pyramidal cells is the potentiation of NMDA-induced currents (Marino et al., 1998). Muscarinic effects on hippocampal function can be modulated by activation of autoreceptors on cholinergic terminals of the afferents from the septo-hippocampal pathway, with a resultant reduction in hippocampal ACh release.

Nicotinic receptors are used for fast transmission at the nerve–muscle synapse and at autonomic nervous system ganglia; however, in the brain, nicotinic receptors play modulatory roles—an interesting case of a fast-ligand-gated neurotransmitter receptor working as a modulator. The timing of nicotinic receptor activation depends on activity in the medial septum–diagonal band complex (Ji et al., 2001). Presynaptic nicotinic acetylcholine receptors (nAChRs) can increase the probability of neurotransmitter release, increasing the fidelity of synaptic transmission. Postsynaptic nAChRs can increase the depolarization and Ca^{2+} signal associated with successful transmission, helping initiate intracellular cascades. On the other hand, nicotinic activity can strongly excite GABAergic interneurons, thus regulating the excitability of circuits. To quote Ji et al., "the location of nAChR activity and the moment-by-moment change in that activity can tip the balance in favor or against the induction of synaptic plasticity" (Ji et al., 2001).

Nicotinic acetylcholine receptors in the hippocampus are important for learning and memory. In addition to findings from mice lacking distinct nicotinic acetylcholine receptor genes (see Section 7.8.3), evidence for this role comes also from behavioral pharmacology showing that infusion of the nicotinic receptor antagonist mecamylamine into the ventral hippocampus impairs memory performance in rats; conversely, injection of nicotine and nicotinic receptor agonists improves memory performance (reviewed in Levin et al., 2002). In the ventral hippocampus, cholinergic transmission thus boosts memory-related functions. In contrast, the cholinergic tone in the dorsal hippocampus is associated with anxiolysis (reviewed in File et al., 2000).

7.9.2 Hippocampal Muscarinic Receptors

Five subtypes (M1–M5) of muscarinic receptors exist: M1, M3, and M5 couple to Gq/G11 G proteins; M2 and M4 prefer Gi/Go (reviewed in Wess, 2004). Muscarinic receptors are "classic" G protein-coupled receptors that are distantly related, if at all, to metabotropic glutamate and $GABA_B$ receptors. As seen by in situ hybridization and immunocytochemistry, M1 is the most prominent muscarinic receptor in the hippocampus. The M1 gene is abundantly expressed in CA1 and CA3 pyramidal cells, dentate granule cells, and scattered interneurons; M1 protein is on somata and dendrites (Buckley et al., 1988; Levey et al., 1995). In CA1 pyramidal cells, M1 and the NR1a NMDA receptor subunits co-localize and may directly interact via an intracellular signaling scaffold (Marino et al., 1998). This may explain how muscarinic agonists potentiate NMDA-induced currents (see above). Mice lacking the M1 gene show various cellular and behavioral phenotypes related to hippocampal functions (see below), confirming the importance of M1 in the hippocampus.

M2 and M4 couple to the Gi family and share similar ligand-binding properties, making it difficult to distinguish pharmacologically between the two subtypes. However, studies with M2 and M4 knockouts revealed that various physiological functions are mediated by a mixture of M2 and M4 activation (Wess, 2004) (see below). M2 is expressed mostly in interneurons in the oriens/alveus border; the M2 protein is on the GABAergic terminals of the interneurons and might account for the observation that presynaptic muscarinic receptors depress inhibitory responses in the hippocampus (Levey et al., 1995). M2 is not found in pyramidal cells or dentate granule cells. In contrast, M4 mRNA and protein are mainly in CA pyramidal cells; they have lower expression in the dentate granule cells, with CA3 pyramidal cells containing slightly more M4 than CA1 cells.

In the hippocampus, M3 mRNA and protein have distributions similar to those of M4 mRNA (see above) (Buckley et al., 1988; Levey et al., 1995). M5 mRNA is restricted to CA1 pyramidal cells, but the expression is weak (Vilaro et al., 1990); M5 protein has not been detected in the hippocampus.

Muscarinic Receptor Mutant Mice

M1 knockout mice exhibit a mild reduction in hippocampal LTP (Schaffer-CA1 synapse) in response to theta burst stimulation (Anagnostaras et al., 2003). M1 knockouts have normal or enhanced memory for tasks involving contextual fear conditioning and the Morris watermaze, but they are impaired in non-matching-to-sample working memory and consolidation (win-shift radial arm and social discrimination learning). The conclusion drawn from these mice was that M1 receptors are not essential for memory formation or initial stability of memory in the hippocampus but are more likely to contribute to processes requiring interactions between the neocortex and hippocampus. A possible substrate for binding distant populations of cells is γ oscillations. Muscarine-induced γ oscillations are absent in hippocampal slices (CA3 area) from M1 knockout mice but are still present in the M2 to M5 knockouts (Fisahn et al., 2002). These muscarine-induced γ oscillations depend on M1-mediated depolarization of CA3 pyramidal cells by activation of the mixed Na^+/K^+ current (I_h) and the Ca^{2+}-dependent nonspecific cation current (I_{cat}).

M2 knockout mice have significant performance deficits in passive avoidance tests. The increase in hippocampal ACh induced by local administration of scopolamine was markedly reduced in M2 knockout mice and completely abolished in M2/M4 double knockouts (as measured by in vivo microdialysis), probably due to a lack of M2 and M4 autoreceptors on septal-hippocampal afferents (Tzavara et al., 2003). In M2 and M4 knockouts, and to a much greater extent in M2/M4 double knockouts, the increase in hippocampal ACh triggered by exposure to a novel environment was more pronounced than in wild types (both amplitude and duration).

7.9.3 Hippocampal Nicotinic Receptors

Nicotinic acetylcholine receptors are ligand-gated cation channels of the superfamily that also includes the $GABA_A$ receptors; and like the $GABA_A$ receptors, they are pentameric assemblies of subunits. Neuronal nicotinic receptor subunit genes comprise $\alpha2$ to $\alpha10$ and $\beta2$ to $\beta4$ subtypes. In the hippocampus, prominent neuronal nicotinic receptors are $(\alpha4)_2(\beta2)_3$, $(\alpha3)_2(\beta4)_3$, and $(\alpha7)_5$ (Zoli et al., 1998; Fabian-Fine et al., 2001). The $\alpha7$ receptors are fast-inactivating nonselective cation channels with high Ca^{2+} permeability. The $(\alpha4)_2(\beta2)_3$ receptors are mainly permeable to Na^+ and K^+ and are the main targets for nicotine. Both the $\alpha7$ and $(\alpha4)_2(\beta2)_3$ receptors can be pre- and postsynaptic. Although the $(\alpha4)_2(\beta2)_3$ and $(\alpha3)_2(\beta4)_3$ receptors are expressed on pyramidal cells, their function is not clear.

The α7 gene is expressed in many hippocampal cell types, including interneurons, dentate granule cells, and pyramidal cells (Fabian-Fine et al., 2001). Many GABAergic and glutamatergic synapses in the hippocampus contain α7 receptors; postsynaptically, α7 receptors are on dendritic spines in a perisynaptic annulus. The large Ca^{2+} entry through α7 nicotinic receptors may play a key role in synaptic plasticity, evoking transmitter release (e.g., from mossy fiber terminals) and/or triggering Ca^{2+}-induced Ca^{2+} release from internal stores (Khiroug et al., 2003). In hippocampal principal neurons, nicotinic α7 receptors mediate activation of Ca^{2+}/calmodulin-dependent protein kinase and the ERK/MAPK cascade, resulting in sustained phosphorylation of the transcription factor CREB. Presynaptic α7 receptors enhance the probability of hippocampal LTP, presumably via Ca^{2+} entry through these receptors (Dajas-Bailador and Wonnacott, 2004). Interestingly, β-amyloid peptide ($A\beta_{1-42}$) antagonizes α7 receptors on hippocampal neurons (Liu et al., 2001), suggesting that in patients with early Alzheimer's disease this antagonist effect could be an additional factor that contributes to cognitive defects. This also provides indirect support for the role of the α7 subunit in cognition under normal conditions. In hippocampal interneurons, α7 receptors constitute 38 pS, inwardly rectifying channels that produce strong excitatory effects, including generation of action potentials.

Nicotinic Receptor Mutant Mice

Strong pharmacological evidence suggests that nicotinic transmission is essential for healthy cognition and learning; but as is often the case with knockouts of modulatory systems, studies on nicotinic receptor subunit knockout mice have failed to provide convincing support for this conclusion (see the informed commentary by Champtiaux and Changeux, 2002, for possible reasons). Thus, despite the proposed roles of α7 receptors in hippocampal function alluded to above, mice lacking the α7 subunit have no deficits in hippocampal learning tasks (Paylor et al., 1998). Thus, either there is compensation (always a possibility), or the α7 receptors regulate behavioral effects too subtle to pick up with current techniques. Similarly, young adult β2 knockout animals performed normally in spatial learning (Morris watermaze) and Pavlovian fear conditioning (reviewed in Champtiaux and Changeux, 2002). However, the performance of aged β2 knockout mice was significantly impaired in the watermaze compared with age-matched wild-type mice. These deficits were mainly attributed to increased neurodegeneration in hippocampal and neocortical areas of β2 knockout brains.

Instead of studying loss of function, dominant-negative mutations can sometimes provide more insight into receptor function. Non-α7 nAVh responses (e.g., from α4β2 receptors) are more difficult to characterize on central neurons, so knock-in mice with hypersensitive α4 subunit-containing receptors have been used to amplify the effect of these receptors (Fonck et al., 2003). In these mice, the α4 subunits have a leucine to serine mutation in the channel pore-lining region of TM2, a 9′ position that renders α4 receptors hypersensitive to agonists. Homozygous animals die soon after birth (the same lethal phenotype was also observed for knock-in mice with an L250T mutation in the α7 subunit gene that increases the α7 currents) (Orr-Urtreger et al., 2000). However, mice heterozygous for the α4 TM2 mutation survive but show increased anxiety. In these mice, the hippocampus is hypersensitive to nicotine; much lower doses of nicotine are needed to elicit increases in the amplitude of the electroencephalography trace; and compared with wild-type mice, a large (threefold) nicotine-induced increase in power density at ϑ frequencies (7 Hz) occurs (Fonck et al., 2003). Thus α4-containing nicotinic receptors could contribute to oscillatory network behavior in the wild-type hippocampus.

ACKNOWLEDGMENTS

We thank Peter H. Seeburg for long-term support. We also gratefully acknowledge our collaborators Per Andersen, David Bannerman, Øvind Hvalby, Vidar Jensen, Nick Rawlins, and Bert Sakmann. W.W. thanks Hannah Monyer for long-term support. The work in P.O.'s laboratory was funded in part by Deutsche Forschungsgemeinschaft, the German Israeli Foundation, and the Human Frontier Science Program. The work in W.W.'s laboratory was funded by the Volkswagen Stiftung, the Fonds der Chemischen Industrie, the Deutsche Forschungsgemeinschaft, and the Schilling Foundation (grant to Prof. H. Monyer). The work in R.S.'s laboratory was funded in part by the Deutsche Forschungsgemeinschaft and Volkswagen Stiftung.

REFERENCES

Aiba A, Chen C, Herrup K, Rosenmund C, Stevens CF, Tonegawa S (1994) Reduced hippocampal long-term potentiation and context-specific deficit in associative learning in mGluR1 mutant mice. *Cell* 79:365–375.

Anagnostaras SG, Murphy GG, Hamilton SE, Mitchell SL, Rahnama NP, Nathanson NM, Silva AJ (2003) Selective cognitive dysfunction in acetylcholine M1 muscarinic receptor mutant mice. *Nat Neurosci* 6:51–58.

Andrasfalvy BK, Smith MA, Borchardt T, Sprengel R, Magee JC (2003) Impaired regulation of synaptic strength in hippocampal neurons from GluR1-deficient mice. *J Physiol* 552:35–45.

Aravanis AM, Pyle JL, Tsien RW (2003) Single synaptic vesicles fusing transiently and successively without loss of identity. *Nature* 423:643–647.

Bahn S, Volk B, Wisden W (1994) Kainate receptor gene expression in the developing rat brain. *J Neurosci* 14:5525–5547.

Banks MI, Li TB, Pearce RA (1998) The synaptic basis of GABA(A,slow). *J Neurosci* 18:1305–1317.

Bannerman DM, Deacon RM, Seeburg PH, Rawlins JN (2003) GluR-A-deficient mice display normal acquisition of a hippocampus-dependent spatial reference memory task but are impaired during spatial reversal. *Behav Neurosci* 117:866–870.

Bannerman DM, Deacon RM, Brady S, Bruce A, Sprengel R, Seeburg PH, Rawlins JN (2004) A comparison of GluR-A-deficient and wild-type mice on a test battery assessing sensorimotor, affective, and cognitive behaviors. *Behav Neurosci* 118:643647.

Barria A, Malinow R (2002) Subunit-specific NMDA receptor trafficking to synapses. *Neuron* 35:345–353.

Bartos M, Vida I, Frotscher M, Geiger JR, Jonas P (2001) Rapid signaling at inhibitory synapses in a dentate gyrus interneuron network. *J Neurosci* 21:2687–2698.

Bartos M, Vida I, Frotscher M, Meyer A, Monyer H, Geiger JR, Jonas P (2002) Fast synaptic inhibition promotes synchronized gamma oscillations in hippocampal interneuron networks. *Proc Natl Acad Sci USA* 99:13222–13227.

Baude A, Nusser Z, Roberts JD, Mulvihill E, McIlhinney RA, Somogyi P (1993) The metabotropic glutamate receptor (mGluR1 alpha) is concentrated at perisynaptic membrane of neuronal subpopulations as detected by immunogold reaction. *Neuron* 11:771–787.

Bayer KU, De Koninck P, Leonard AS, Hell JW, Schulman H (2001) Interaction with the NMDA receptor locks CaMKII in an active conformation. *Nature* 411:801–805.

Berberich S, Punnakkal P, Jensen V, Pawlak V, Seeburg PH, Hvalby O, Köhr G (2005) Lack of NMDAR subtype selectivity for hippocampal LTP. *J Neurosci* 25:6907–6910.

Berger T, Schwarz C, Kraushaar U, Monyer H (1998) Dentate gyrus basket cell GABAA receptors are blocked by Zn^{2+} via changes of their desensitization kinetics: an in situ patch-clamp and single-cell PCR study. *J Neurosci* 18:2437–2448.

Bergersen L, Ruiz A, Bjaalie JG, Kullmann DM, Gundersen V (2003) GABA and GABA$_A$ receptors at hippocampal mossy fibre synapses. *Eur J Neurosci* 18:931–941.

Bettler B, Boulter J, Hermans-Borgmeyer I, O'Shea-Greenfield A, Deneris ES, Moll C, Borgmeyer U, Hollmann M, Heinemann S (1990) Cloning of a novel glutamate receptor subunit, GluR5: expression in the nervous system during development. *Neuron* 5:583–595.

Bettler B, Egebjerg J, Sharma G, Pecht G, Hermans-Borgmeyer I, Moll C, Stevens CF, Heinemann S (1992) Cloning of a putative glutamate receptor: a low affinity kainate-binding subunit. *Neuron* 8:257–265.

Bettler B, Kaupmann K, Mosbacher J, Gassmann M (2004) Molecular structure and physiological functions of GABA$_B$ receptors. *Physiol Rev* 84:835–867.

Bollmann JH, Sakmann B, Borst JG (2000) Calcium sensitivity of glutamate release in a calyx-type terminal. *Science* 289:953–957.

Boudin H, Doan A, Xia J, Shigemoto R, Huganir RL, Worley P, Craig AM (2000) Presynaptic clustering of mGluR7a requires the PICK1 PDZ domain binding site. *Neuron* 28:485–497.

Bredt DS, Nicoll RA (2003) AMPA receptor trafficking at excitatory synapses. *Neuron* 40:361–379.

Brooks-Kayal AR, Shumate MD, Jin H, Rikhter TY, Coulter DA (1998) Selective changes in single cell GABA(A) receptor subunit expression and function in temporal lobe epilepsy. *Nat Med* 4:1166–1172.

Brooks-Kayal AR, Shumate MD, Jin H, Rikhter TY, Kelly ME, Coulter DA (2001) Gamma-aminobutyric acid(A) receptor subunit expression predicts functional changes in hippocampal dentate granule cells during postnatal development. *J Neurochem* 77:1266–1278.

Brose N, Rosenmund C, Rettig J (2000) Regulation of transmitter release by Unc-13 and its homologues. *Curr Opin Neurobiol* 10:303–311.

Brunig I, Scotti E, Sidler C, Fritschy JM (2002) Intact sorting, targeting, and clustering of gamma-aminobutyric acid A receptor subtypes in hippocampal neurons in vitro. *J Comp Neurol* 443:43–55.

Brusa R, Zimmermann F, Koh D-S, Feldmeyer D, Gass P, Seeburg PH, Sprengel R (1995) Early-onset epilepsy and postnatal lethality associated with an editing-deficient GluR-B allele in mice. *Science* 270:1677–1680.

Buckley NJ, Bonner TI, Brann MR (1988) Localization of a family of muscarinic receptor mRNAs in rat brain. *J Neurosci* 8:4646–4652.

Bureau I, Bischoff S, Heinemann SF, Mulle C (1999) Kainate receptor-mediated responses in the CA1 field of wild-type and GluR6-deficient mice. *J Neurosci* 19:653–663.

Cagetti E, Liang J, Spigelman I, Olsen RW (2003) Withdrawal from chronic intermittent ethanol treatment changes subunit composition, reduces synaptic function, and decreases behavioral responses to positive allosteric modulators of GABA$_A$ receptors. *Mol Pharmacol* 63:53–64.

Calakos N, Schoch S, Südhof TC, Malenka RC (2004) Multiple roles for the active zone protein RIM1alpha in late stages of neurotransmitter release. *Neuron* 42:889–896.

Castillo PE, Janz R, Südhof TC, Tzounopoulos T, Malenka RC, Nicoll RA (1997b) Rab3A is essential for mossy fibre long-term potentiation in the hippocampus. *Nature* 388:590–593.

Castillo PE, Malenka RC, Nicoll RA (1997a) Kainate receptors mediate a slow postsynaptic current in hippocampal CA3 neurons. *Nature* 388:182–186.

Castillo PE, Schoch S, Schmitz F, Südhof TC, Malenka RC (2002) RIM1alpha is required for presynaptic long-term potentiation. *Nature* 415:327–330.

Chambers MS, Atack JR, Broughton HB, Collinson N, Cook S, Dawson GR, Hobbs SC, Marshall G, Maubach KA, Pillai GV, Reeve AJ, MacLeod AM (2003) Identification of a novel, selective GABA(A) alpha5 receptor inverse agonist which enhances cognition. *J Med Chem* 46:2227–2240.

Champtiaux N, Changeux JP (2002) Knock-out and knock-in mice to investigate the role of nicotinic receptors in the central nervous system. *Curr Drug Targets CNS Neurol Disord* 1:319–330.

Chatterton JE, Awobuluyi M, Premkumar LS, Takahashi H, Talantova M, Shin Y, Cui J, Tu S, Sevarino KA, Nakanishi N, Tong G, Lipton SA, Zhang D (2002) Excitatory glycine receptors containing the NR3 family of NMDA receptor subunits. *Nature* 415:793–798.

Chen L, Chetkovich DM, Petralia RS, Sweeney NT, Kawasaki Y, Wenthold RJ, Bredt DS, Nicoll RA (2000) Stargazin regulates synaptic targeting of AMPA receptors by two distinct mechanisms. *Nature* 408:936–943.

Chi P, Greengard P, Ryan TA (2003) Synaptic vesicle mobilization is regulated by distinct synapsin I phosphorylation pathways at different frequencies. *Neuron* 38:69–78.

Ciabarra AM, Sullivan JM, Gahn LG, Pecht G, Heinemann S, Sevarino KA (1995) Cloning and characterization of chi-1: a developmentally regulated member of a novel class of the ionotropic glutamate receptor family. *J Neurosci* 15:6498–6508.

Collinson N, Kuenzi FM, Jarolimek W, Maubach KA, Cothliff R, Sur C, Smith A, Otu FM, Howell O, Atack JR, McKernan RM,

Seabrook GR, Dawson GR, Whiting PJ, Rosahl TW (2002) Enhanced learning and memory and altered GABAergic synaptic transmission in mice lacking the alpha 5 subunit of the GABA$_A$ receptor. *J Neurosci* 22:5572–5580.

Conquet F, Bashir ZI, Davies CH, Daniel H, Ferraguti F, Bordi F, Franz-Bacon K, Reggiani A, Matarese V, Conde F, et al. (1994) Motor deficit and impairment of synaptic plasticity in mice lacking mGluR1. *Nature* 372:237–243.

Contractor A, Swanson GT, Sailer A, O'Gorman S, Heinemann SF (2000) Identification of the kainate receptor subunits underlying modulation of excitatory synaptic transmission in the CA3 region of the hippocampus. *J Neurosci* 20:8269–8278.

Contractor A, Swanson G, Heinemann SF (2001) Kainate receptors are involved in short- and long-term plasticity at mossy fiber synapses in the hippocampus. *Neuron* 29:209–216.

Contractor A, Sailer AW, Darstein M, Maron C, Xu J, Swanson GT, Heinemann SF (2003) Loss of kainate receptor-mediated heterosynaptic facilitation of mossy-fiber synapses in KA2-/- mice. *J Neurosci* 23:422–429.

Cossart R, Esclapez M, Hirsch JC, Bernard C, Ben-Ari Y (1998) GluR5 kainate receptor activation in interneurons increases tonic inhibition of pyramidal cells. *Nat Neurosci* 1:470–478.

Cremona O, Di Paolo G, Wenk MR, Luthi A, Kim WT, Takei K, Daniell L, Nemoto Y, Shears SB, Flavell RA, McCormick DA, De Camilli P (1999) Essential role of phosphoinositide metabolism in synaptic vesicle recycling. *Cell* 99:179–188.

Crestani F, Keist R, Fritschy JM, Benke D, Vogt K, Prut L, Bluthmann H, Mohler H, Rudolph U (2002) Trace fear conditioning involves hippocampal alpha5 GABA(A) receptors. *Proc Natl Acad Sci USA* 99:8980–8985.

Cui Z, Wang H, Tan Y, Zaia KA, Zhang S, Tsien JZ (2004) Inducible and reversible NR1 knockout reveals crucial role of the NMDA receptor in preserving remote memories in the brain. *Neuron* 41:781–793.

Dajas-Bailador F, Wonnacott S (2004) Nicotinic acetylcholine receptors and the regulation of neuronal signalling. *Trends Pharmacol Sci* 25:317–324.

Darstein M, Petralia RS, Swanson GT, Wenthold RJ, Heinemann SF (2003) Distribution of kainate receptor subunits at hippocampal mossy fiber synapses. *J Neurosci* 23:8013–8019.

De Blasi A, Conn PJ, Pin J, Nicoletti F (2001) Molecular determinants of metabotropic glutamate receptor signaling. *Trends Pharmacol Sci* 22:114–120.

Dingledine R, Borges K, Bowie D, Traynelis SF (1999) The glutamate receptor ion channels. *Pharmacol Rev* 51:7–61.

Di Paolo G, Sankaranarayanan S, Wenk MR, Daniell L, Perucco E, Caldarone BJ, Flavell R, Picciotto MR, Ryan TA, Cremona O, De Camilli P (2002) Decreased synaptic vesicle recycling efficiency and cognitive deficits in amphiphysin 1 knockout mice. *Neuron* 33:789–804.

Doussau F, Augustine GJ (2000) The actin cytoskeleton and neurotransmitter release: an overview. *Biochimie* 82:353–363.

Ebralidze AK, Rossi DJ, Tonegawa S, Slater NT (1996) Modification of NMDA receptor channels and synaptic transmission by targeted disruption of the NR2C gene. *J Neurosci* 16:5014–5025.

Egebjerg J, Bettler B, Hermans-Borgmeyer I, Heinemann S (1991) Cloning of a cDNA for a glutamate receptor subunit activated by kainate but not AMPA. *Nature* 351:745–748.

Eiden LE (2000) The vesicular neurotransmitter transporters: current perspectives and future prospects. *FASEB J* 14:2396–2400.

El-Husseini Ael D, Bredt DS (2002) Protein palmitoylation: a regulator of neuronal development and function. *Nat Rev Neurosci* 3:791–802.

Ernst M, Brauchart D, Boresch S, Sieghart W (2003) Comparative modeling of GABA(A) receptors: limits, insights, future developments. *Neuroscience* 119:933–943.

Essrich C, Lorez M, Benson JA, Fritschy JM, Luscher B (1998) Postsynaptic clustering of major GABA$_A$ receptor subtypes requires the gamma 2 subunit and gephyrin. *Nat Neurosci* 1:563–571.

Esteban JA, Shi SH, Wilson C, Nuriya M, Huganir RL, Malinow R (2003) PKA phosphorylation of AMPA receptor subunits controls synaptic trafficking underlying plasticity. *Nat Neurosci* 6:136–143.

Fabian-Fine R, Skehel P, Errington ML, Davies HA, Sher E, Stewart MG, Fine A (2001) Ultrastructural distribution of the alpha7 nicotinic acetylcholine receptor subunit in rat hippocampus. *J Neurosci* 21:7993–8003.

Fagni L, Worley PF, Ango F (2002) Homer as both a scaffold and transduction molecule. *Sci STKE* 2002:RE8.

Feldmeyer D, Kask K, Brusa R, Kornau HC, Kolhekar R, Rozov A, Burnashev N, Jensen V, Hvalby O, Sprengel R, Seeburg PH (1999) Neurological dysfunctions in mice expressing different levels of the Q/R site-unedited AMPAR subunit GluR-B. *Nat Neurosci* 2:57–64.

Fernandez-Chacon R, Konigstorfer A, Gerber SH, Garcia J, Matos MF, Stevens CF, Brose N, Rizo J, Rosenmund C, Südhof TC (2001) Synaptotagmin I functions as a calcium regulator of release probability. *Nature* 410:41–49.

File SE, Kenny PJ, Cheeta S (2000) The role of the dorsal hippocampal serotonergic and cholinergic systems in the modulation of anxiety. *Pharmacol Biochem Behav* 66:65–72.

Fisahn A, Yamada M, Duttaroy A, Gan JW, Deng CX, McBain CJ, Wess J (2002) Muscarinic induction of hippocampal gamma oscillations requires coupling of the M1 receptor to two mixed cation currents. *Neuron* 33:615–624.

Fleischmann A, Hvalby O, Jensen V, Strekalova T, Zacher C, Layer LE, Kvello A, Reschke M, Spanagel R, Sprengel R, Wagner EF, Gass P (2003) Impaired long-term memory and NR2A-type NMDA receptor-dependent synaptic plasticity in mice lacking c-Fos in the CNS. *J Neurosci* 23:9116–9122.

Fonck C, Nashmi R, Deshpande P, Damaj MI, Marks MJ, Riedel A, Schwarz J, Collins AC, Labarca C, Lester HA (2003) Increased sensitivity to agonist-induced seizures, straub tail, and hippocampal theta rhythm in knock-in mice carrying hypersensitive alpha 4 nicotinic receptors. *J Neurosci* 23:2582–2590.

Forrest D, Yuzaki M, Soares HD, Ng L, Luk DC, Sheng M, Stewart CL, Morgan JI, Connor JA, Curran T (1994) Targeted disruption of NMDA receptor 1 gene abolishes NMDA response and results in neonatal death. *Neuron* 13:325–338.

Fotuhi M, Standaert DG, Testa CM, Penney JB Jr, Young AB (1994) Differential expression of metabotropic glutamate receptors in the hippocampus and entorhinal cortex of the rat. *Brain Res Mol Brain Res* 21:283–292.

Fremeau RT Jr, Voglmaier S, Seal RP, Edwards RH (2004) VGLUTs define subsets of excitatory neurons and suggest novel roles for glutamate. *Trends Neurosci* 27:98–103.

Frerking M, Malenka RC, Nicoll RA (1998) Synaptic activation of kainate receptors on hippocampal interneurons. *Nat Neurosci* 1:479–486.

Fritschy JM, Brunig I (2003) Formation and plasticity of GABAergic synapses: physiological mechanisms and pathophysiological implications. *Pharmacol Ther* 98:299–323.

Fritschy JM, Mohler H (1995) GABA_A-receptor heterogeneity in the adult rat brain: differential regional and cellular distribution of seven major subunits. *J Comp Neurol* 359:154–194.

Fritschy JM, Weinmann O, Wenzel A, Benke D (1998) Synapse-specific localization of NMDA and GABA(A) receptor subunits revealed by antigen-retrieval immunohistochemistry. *J Comp Neurol* 390:194–210.

Fritschy JM, Meskenaite V, Weinmann O, Honer M, Benke D, Mohler H (1999) GABA_B-receptor splice variants GB1a and GB1b in rat brain: developmental regulation, cellular distribution and extrasynaptic localization. *Eur J Neurosci* 11:761–768.

Fukaya M, Kato A, Lovett C, Tonegawa S, Watanabe M (2003) Retention of NMDA receptor NR2 subunits in the lumen of endoplasmic reticulum in targeted NR1 knockout mice. *Proc Natl Acad Sci USA* 100:4855–4860.

Gandhi SP, Stevens CF (2003) Three modes of synaptic vesicular recycling revealed by single-vesicle imaging. *Nature* 423:607–613.

Gao B, Fritschy JM (1994) Selective allocation of GABA_A receptors containing the alpha 1 subunit to neurochemically distinct sub-populations of rat hippocampal interneurons. *Eur J Neurosci* 6:837–853.

Gassmann M, Shaban H, Vigot R, Sansig G, Haller C, Barbieri S, Humeau Y, Schuler V, Muller M, Kinzel B, Klebs K, Schmutz M, Froestl W, Heid J, Kelly PH, Gentry C, Jaton AL, Van der Putten H, Mombereau C, Lecourtier L, Mosbacher J, Cryan JF, Fritschy JM, Luthi A, Kaupmann K, Bettler B (2004) Redistribution of GABA_B(1) protein and atypical GABA_B responses in GABA_B(2)-deficient mice. *J Neurosci* 24:6086–6097.

Geiger JR, Melcher T, Koh DS, Sakmann B, Seeburg PH, Jonas P, Monyer H (1995) Relative abundance of subunit mRNAs determines gating and Ca^{2+} permeability of AMPA receptors in principal neurons and interneurons in rat CNS. *Neuron* 15:193–204.

Geppert M, Bolshakov VY, Siegelbaum SA, Takei K, De Camilli P, Hammer RE, Südhof TC (1994a) The role of Rab3A in neurotransmitter release. *Nature* 369:493–497.

Geppert M, Goda Y, Hammer RE, Li C, Rosahl TW, Stevens CF, Südhof TC (1994b) Synaptotagmin I: a major Ca^{2+} sensor for transmitter release at a central synapse. *Cell* 79:717–727.

Geppert M, Goda Y, Stevens CF, Südhof TC (1997) The small GTP-binding protein Rab3A regulates a late step in synaptic vesicle fusion. *Nature* 387:810–814.

Goldstein PA, Elsen FP, Ying SW, Ferguson C, Homanics GE, Harrison NL (2002) Prolongation of hippocampal miniature inhibitory postsynaptic currents in mice lacking the GABA(A) receptor alpha1 subunit. *J Neurophysiol* 88:3208–3217.

Götz T, Kraushaar U, Geiger J, Lubke J, Berger T, Jonas P (1997) Functional properties of AMPA and NMDA receptors expressed in identified types of basal ganglia neurons. *J Neurosci* 17:204–215.

Grant SG, O'Dell TJ, Karl KA, Stein PL, Soriano P, Kandel ER (1992) Impaired long-term potentiation, spatial learning, and hippocampal development in fyn mutant mice. *Science* 258:1903–1910.

Gulyas AI, Megias M, Emri Z, Freund TF (1999) Total number and ratio of excitatory and inhibitory synapses converging onto sin-gle interneurons of different types in the CA1 area of the rat hippocampus. *J Neurosci* 19:10082–10097.

Gunther U, Benson J, Benke D, Fritschy JM, Reyes G, Knoflach F, Crestani F, Aguzzi A, Arigoni M, Lang Y, et al. (1995) Benzodiazepine-insensitive mice generated by targeted disruption of the gamma 2 subunit gene of gamma-aminobutyric acid type A receptors. *Proc Natl Acad Sci USA* 92:7749–7753.

Gutierrez R (2003) The GABAergic phenotype of the "glutamatergic" granule cells of the dentate gyrus. *Prog Neurobiol* 71:337–358.

Halasy K, Somogyi P (1993) Subdivisions in the multiple GABAergic innervation of granule cells in the dentate gyrus of the rat hippocampus. *Eur J Neurosci* 5:411–429.

Hanley JG, Khatri L, Hanson PI, Ziff EB (2002) NSF ATPase and alpha-/beta-SNAPs disassemble the AMPA receptor-PICK1 complex. *Neuron* 34:53–67.

Hanson PI, Roth R, Morisaki H, Jahn R, Heuser JE (1997) Structure and conformational changes in NSF and its membrane receptor complexes visualized by quick-freeze/deep-etch electron microscopy. *Cell* 90:523–535.

Hilfiker S, Pieribone VA, Czernik AJ, Kao HT, Augustine GJ, Greengard P (1999) Synapsins as regulators of neurotransmitter release. *Philos Trans R Soc Lond B Biol Sci* 354:269–279.

Hoffman DA, Sprengel R, Sakmann B (2002) Molecular dissection of hippocampal theta-burst pairing potentiation. *Proc Natl Acad Sci USA* 99:7740–7745.

Hosie AM, Dunne EL, Harvey RJ, Smart TG (2003) Zinc-mediated inhibition of GABA(A) receptors: discrete binding sites underlie subtype specificity. *Nat Neurosci* 6:362–369.

Hsia AY, Salin PA, Castillo PE, Aiba A, Abeliovich A, Tonegawa S, Nicoll RA (1995) Evidence against a role for metabotropic glutamate receptors in mossy fiber LTP: the use of mutant mice and pharmacological antagonists. *Neuropharmacology* 34:1567–1572.

Hsu FC, Zhang GJ, Raol YS, Valentino RJ, Coulter DA, Brooks-Kayal AR (2003) Repeated neonatal handling with maternal separation permanently alters hippocampal GABA_A receptors and behavioral stress responses. *Proc Natl Acad Sci USA* 100:12213–12218.

Huerta PT, Sun LD, Wilson MA, Tonegawa S (2000) Formation of temporal memory requires NMDA receptors within CA1 pyramidal neurons. *Neuron* 25:473–480.

Ikeda K, Araki K, Takayama C, Inoue Y, Yagi T, Aizawa S, Mishina M (1995) Reduced spontaneous activity of mice defective in the epsilon 4 subunit of the NMDA receptor channel. *Brain Res Mol Brain Res* 33:61–71.

Ito I, Futai K, Katagiri H, Watanabe M, Sakimura K, Mishina M, Sugiyama H (1997) Synapse-selective impairment of NMDA receptor functions in mice lacking NMDA receptor epsilon 1 or epsilon 2 subunit. *J Physiol* 500:401–408.

Jensen K, Chiu CS, Sokolova I, Lester HA, Mody I (2003a) GABA transporter-1 (GAT1)-deficient mice: differential tonic activation of GABA_A versus GABA_B receptors in the hippocampus. *J Neurophysiol* 90:2690–2701.

Jensen V, Kaiser KM, Borchardt T, Adelmann G, Rozov A, Burnashev N, Brix C, Frotscher M, Andersen P, Hvalby Ø, Sakmann B, Seeburg PH, Sprengel R (2003b) A juvenile form of postsynaptic hippocampal long-term potentiation in mice deficient for the AMPA receptor subunit GluR-A. *J Physiol* 553:843–856.

Ji D, Lape R, Dani JA (2001) Timing and location of nicotinic activity enhances or depresses hippocampal synaptic plasticity. *Neuron* 31:131–141.

Jia Z, Agopyan N, Miu P, Xiong Z, Henderson J, Gerlai R, Taverna FA, Velumian A, MacDonald J, Carlen P, Abramow-Newerly W, Roder J (1996) Enhanced LTP in mice deficient in the AMPA receptor GluR2. *Neuron* 17:945–956.

Kadotani H, Hirano T, Masugi M, Nakamura K, Nakao K, Katsuki M, Nakanishi S (1996) Motor discoordination results from combined gene disruption of the NMDA receptor NR2A and NR2C subunits, but not from single disruption of the NR2A or NR2C subunit. *J Neurosci* 16:7859–7867.

Kaila K, Lamsa K, Smirnov S, Taira T, Voipio J (1997) Long-lasting GABA-mediated depolarization evoked by high-frequency stimulation in pyramidal neurons of rat hippocampal slice is attributable to a network-driven, bicarbonate-dependent K^+ transient. *J Neurosci* 17:7662–7672.

Kawakami R, Shinohara Y, Kato Y, Sugiyama H, Shigemoto R, Ito I (2003) Asymmetrical allocation of NMDA receptor epsilon2 subunits in hippocampal circuitry. *Science* 300:990–994.

Keinanen K, Wisden W, Sommer B, Werner P, Herb A, Verdoorn TA, Sakmann B, Seeburg PH (1990) A family of AMPA-selective glutamate receptors. *Science* 249:556–560.

Kerner JA, Standaert DG, Penney JB Jr, Young AB, Landwehrmeyer GB (1997) Expression of group one metabotropic glutamate receptor subunit mRNAs in neurochemically identified neurons in the rat neostriatum, neocortex, and hippocampus. *Brain Res Mol Brain Res* 48:259–269.

Kew JN, Koester A, Moreau JL, Jenck F, Ouagazzal AM, Mutel V, Richards JG, Trube G, Fischer G, Montkowski A, Hundt W, Reinscheid RK, Pauly-Evers M, Kemp JA, Bluethmann H (2000) Functional consequences of reduction in NMDA receptor glycine affinity in mice carrying targeted point mutations in the glycine binding site. *J Neurosci* 20:4037–4049.

Khiroug L, Giniatullin R, Klein RC, Fayuk D, Yakel JL (2003) Functional mapping and Ca^{2+} regulation of nicotinic acetylcholine receptor channels in rat hippocampal CA1 neurons. *J Neurosci* 23:9024–9031.

Kim CH, Chung HJ, Lee HK, Huganir RL (2001) Interaction of the AMPA receptor subunit GluR2/3 with PDZ domains regulates hippocampal long-term depression. *Proc Natl Acad Sci USA* 98:11725–11730.

Kimura F (2000) Cholinergic modulation of cortical function: a hypothetical role in shifting the dynamics in cortical network. *Neurosci Res* 38:19–26.

Kittler JT, Moss SJ (2003) Modulation of GABAA receptor activity by phosphorylation and receptor trafficking: implications for the efficacy of synaptic inhibition. *Curr Opin Neurobiol* 13:341–347.

Kiyama Y, Manabe T, Sakimura K, Kawakami F, Mori H, Mishina M (1998) Increased thresholds for long-term potentiation and contextual learning in mice lacking the NMDA-type glutamate receptor epsilon1 subunit. *J Neurosci* 18:6704–6712.

Klausberger T, Roberts JD, Somogyi P (2002) Cell type- and input-specific differences in the number and subtypes of synaptic GABA(A) receptors in the hippocampus. *J Neurosci* 22:2513–2521.

Kneussel M, Brandstatter JH, Laube B, Stahl S, Muller U, Betz H (1999) Loss of postsynaptic GABA(A) receptor clustering in gephyrin-deficient mice. *J Neurosci* 19:9289–9297.

Köhr G, Jensen V, Koester HJ, Mihaljevic AL, Utvik JK, Kvello A, Ottersen OP, Seeburg PH, Sprengel R, Hvalby O (2003)

Intracellular domains of NMDA receptor subtypes are determinants for long-term potentiation induction. *J Neurosci* 23:10791–10799.

Kolleker A, Zhu JJ, Schupp BJ, Qin Y, Mack V, Borchardt T, Köhr G, Malinow R, Seeburg PH, Osten P (2003) Glutamatergic plasticity by synaptic delivery of GluR-B(long)-containing AMPA receptors. *Neuron* 40:1199–1212.

Kornau HC, Schenker LT, Kennedy MB, Seeburg PH (1995) Domain interaction between NMDA receptor subunits and the postsynaptic density protein PSD-95. *Science* 269:1737–1740.

Korpi ER, Grunder G, Luddens H (2002) Drug interactions at GABA(A) receptors. *Prog Neurobiol* 67:113–159.

Krestel HE, Shimshek DR, Jensen V, Nevian T, Kim J, Geng Y, Bast T, Depaulis A, Schonig K, Schwenk F, Bujard H, Hvalby O, Sprengel R, Seeburg PH (2004) A genetic switch for epilepsy in adult mice. *J Neurosci* 24:10568–10578.

Krupp JJ, Vissel B, Thomas CG, Heinemann SF, Westbrook GL (1999) Interactions of calmodulin and alpha-actinin with the NR1 subunit modulate Ca^{2+}-dependent inactivation of NMDA receptors. *J Neurosci* 19:1165–1178.

Kulik A, Vida I, Lujan R, Haas CA, Lopez-Bendito G, Shigemoto R, Frotscher M (2003) Subcellular localization of metabotropic GABA(B) receptor subunits GABA(B1a/b) and GABA(B2) in the rat hippocampus. *J Neurosci* 23:11026–11035.

Kullmann DM, Ruiz A, Rusakov DM, Scott R, Semyanov A, Walker MC (2005) Presynaptic, extrasynaptic and axonal $GABA_A$ receptors in the CNS: where and why? *Prog Biophys Mol Biol* 87:33–46.

Kutsuwada T, Sakimura K, Manabe T, Takayama C, Katakura N, Kushiya E, Natsume R, Watanabe M, Inoue Y, Yagi T, Aizawa S, Arakawa M, Takahashi T, Nakamura Y, Mori H, Mishina M (1996) Impairment of suckling response, trigeminal neuronal pattern formation, and hippocampal LTD in NMDA receptor epsilon 2 subunit mutant mice. *Neuron* 16:333–344.

Laezza F, Doherty JJ, Dingledine R (1999) Long-term depression in hippocampal interneurons: joint requirement for pre- and postsynaptic events. *Science* 285:1411–1414.

Laurie DJ, Seeburg PH (1994) Regional and developmental heterogeneity in splicing of the rat brain NMDAR1 mRNA. *J Neurosci* 14:3180–3194.

Lee HK, Takamiya K, Han JS, Man H, Kim CH, Rumbaugh G, Yu S, Ding L, He C, Petralia RS, Wenthold RJ, Gallagher M, Huganir RL (2003) Phosphorylation of the AMPA receptor GluR1 subunit is required for synaptic plasticity and retention of spatial memory. *Cell* 112:631–643.

Lee SH, Liu L, Wang YT, Sheng M (2002) Clathrin adaptor AP2 and NSF interact with overlapping sites of GluR2 and play distinct roles in AMPA receptor trafficking and hippocampal LTD. *Neuron* 36:661–674.

Lei S, McBain CJ (2002) Distinct NMDA receptors provide differential modes of transmission at mossy fiber–interneuron synapses. *Neuron* 33:921–933.

Lerma J (2003) Roles and rules of kainate receptors in synaptic transmission. *Nat Rev Neurosci* 4:481–495.

Letts VA (2005) Stargazer—a mouse to seize! *Epilepsy Curr* 5:161–165.

Levey AI, Edmunds SM, Koliatsos V, Wiley RG, Heilman CJ (1995) Expression of m1-m4 muscarinic acetylcholine receptor proteins in rat hippocampus and regulation by cholinergic innervation. *J Neurosci* 15:4077–4092.

Levi S, Grady RM, Henry MD, Campbell KP, Sanes JR, Craig AM

(2002) Dystroglycan is selectively associated with inhibitory GABAergic synapses but is dispensable for their differentiation. *J Neurosci* 22:4274–4285.

Levi S, Logan SM, Tovar KR, Craig AM (2004) Gephyrin is critical for glycine receptor clustering but not for the formation of functional GABAergic synapses in hippocampal neurons. *J Neurosci* 24:207–217.

Levin ED, Bradley A, Addy N, Sigurani N (2002) Hippocampal alpha 7 and alpha 4 beta 2 nicotinic receptors and working memory. *Neuroscience* 109:757–765.

Li L, Chin LS, Shupliakov O, Brodin L, Sihra TS, Hvalby O, Jensen V, Zheng D, McNamara JO, Greengard P, et al. (1995) Impairment of synaptic vesicle clustering and of synaptic transmission, and increased seizure propensity, in synapsin I-deficient mice. *Proc Natl Acad Sci USA* 92:9235–9239.

Lisman J, Schulman H, Cline H (2002) The molecular basis of CaMKII function in synaptic and behavioural memory. *Nat Rev Neurosci* 3:175–190.

Liu L, Wong TP, Pozza MF, Lingenhoehl K, Wang Y, Sheng M, Auberson YP, Wang YT (2004) Role of NMDA receptor subtypes in governing the direction of hippocampal synaptic plasticity. *Science* 304:1021–1024.

Liu Q, Kawai H, Berg DK (2001) Beta-amyloid peptide blocks the response of alpha 7-containing nicotinic receptors on hippocampal neurons. *Proc Natl Acad Sci USA* 98:4734–4739.

Lujan R, Nusser Z, Roberts JD, Shigemoto R, Somogyi P (1996) Perisynaptic location of metabotropic glutamate receptors mGluR1 and mGluR5 on dendrites and dendritic spines in the rat hippocampus. *Eur J Neurosci* 8:1488–1500.

Maccaferri G, Roberts JD, Szucs P, Cottingham CA, Somogyi P (2000) Cell surface domain specific postsynaptic currents evoked by identified GABAergic neurones in rat hippocampus in vitro. *J Physiol* 524:91–116.

Mack V, Burnashev N, Kaiser KM, Rozov A, Jensen V, Hvalby O, Seeburg PH, Sakmann B, Sprengel R (2001) Conditional restoration of hippocampal synaptic potentiation in GluR-A deficient mice. *Science* 292:2501–2504.

Magee JC, Cook EP (2000) Somatic EPSP amplitude is independent of synapse location in hippocampal pyramidal neurons. *Nat Neurosci* 3:895–903.

Mahmoudi M, Kang MH, Tillakaratne N, Tobin AJ, Olsen RW (1997) Chronic intermittent ethanol treatment in rats increases GABA(A) receptor alpha4-subunit expression: possible relevance to alcohol dependence. *J Neurochem* 68:2485–2492.

Malinow R, Malenka RC (2002) AMPA receptor trafficking and synaptic plasticity. *Annu Rev Neurosci* 25:103–126.

Marino MJ, Rouse ST, Levey AI, Potter LT, Conn PJ (1998) Activation of the genetically defined m1 muscarinic receptor potentiates *N*-methyl-D-aspartate (NMDA) receptor currents in hippocampal pyramidal cells. *Proc Natl Acad Sci USA* 95: 11465–11470.

May AP, Whiteheart SW, Weis WI (2001) Unraveling the mechanism of the vesicle transport ATPase NSF, the N-ethylmaleimide-sensitive factor. *J Biol Chem* 276:21991–21994.

McHugh TJ, Blum KI, Tsien JZ, Tonegawa S, Wilson MA (1996) Impaired hippocampal representation of space in CA1-specific NMDAR1 knockout mice. *Cell* 87:1339–1349.

Megias M, Emri Z, Freund TF, Gulyas AI (2001) Total number and distribution of inhibitory and excitatory synapses on hippocampal CA1 pyramidal cells. *Neuroscience* 102:527–540.

Meir A, Ginsburg S, Butkevich A, Kachalsky SG, Kaiserman I, Ahdut

R, Demirgoren S, Rahamimoff R (1999) Ion channels in presynaptic nerve terminals and control of transmitter release. *Physiol Rev* 79:1019–1088.

Meng Y, Zhang Y, Jia Z (2003) Synaptic transmission and plasticity in the absence of AMPA glutamate receptor GluR2 and GluR3. *Neuron* 39:163–176.

Migaud M, Charlesworth P, Dempster M, Webster LC, Watabe AM, Makhinson M, He Y, Ramsay MF, Morris RG, Morrison JH, O'Dell TJ, Grant SG (1998) Enhanced long-term potentiation and impaired learning in mice with mutant postsynaptic density-95 protein. *Nature* 396:433–439.

Mihalek RM, Banerjee PK, Korpi ER, Quinlan JJ, Firestone LL, Mi ZP, Lagenaur C, Tretter V, Sieghart W, Anagnostaras SG, Sage JR, Fanselow MS, Guidotti A, Spigelman I, Li Z, DeLorey TM, Olsen RW, Homanics GE (1999) Attenuated sensitivity to neuroactive steroids in gamma-aminobutyrate type A receptor delta subunit knockout mice. *Proc Natl Acad Sci USA* 96:12905–12910.

Mohn AR, Gainetdinov RR, Caron MG, Koller BH (1999) Mice with reduced NMDA receptor expression display behaviors related to schizophrenia. *Cell* 98:427–436.

Monyer H, Seeburg PH, Wisden W (1991) Glutamate-operated channels: developmentally early and mature forms arise by alternative splicing. *Neuron* 6:799–810.

Monyer H, Burnashev N, Laurie DJ, Sakmann B, Seeburg PH (1994) Developmental and regional expression in the rat brain and functional properties of four NMDA receptors. *Neuron* 12:529–540.

Mori H, Manabe T, Watanabe M, Satoh Y, Suzuki N, Toki S, Nakamura K, Yagi T, Kushiya E, Takahashi T, Inoue Y, Sakimura K, Mishina M (1998) Role of the carboxy-terminal region of the GluR epsilon2 subunit in synaptic localization of the NMDA receptor channel. *Neuron* 21:571–580.

Morris RG, Anderson E, Lynch GS, Baudry M (1986) Selective impairment of learning and blockade of long-term potentiation by an *N*-methyl-D-aspartate receptor antagonist, AP5. *Nature* 319:774–776.

Mott DD, Li Q, Okazaki MM, Turner DA, Lewis DV (1999) GABA$_B$-receptor-mediated currents in interneurons of the dentate-hilus border. *J Neurophysiol* 82:1438–1450.

Mulle C, Sailer A, Perez-Otano I, Dickinson-Anson H, Castillo PE, Bureau I, Maron C, Gage FH, Mann JR, Bettler B, Heinemann SF (1998) Altered synaptic physiology and reduced susceptibility to kainate-induced seizures in GluR6-deficient mice. *Nature* 392:601–605.

Mulle C, Sailer A, Swanson GT, Brana C, O'Gorman S, Bettler B, Heinemann SF (2000) Subunit composition of kainate receptors in hippocampal interneurons. *Neuron* 28:475–484.

Nakagawa T, Cheng Y, Ramm E, Sheng M, Walz T (2005) Structure and different conformational states of native AMPA receptor complexes. *Nature* 433:545–549.

Nakazawa K, Quirk MC, Chitwood RA, Watanabe M, Yeckel MF, Sun LD, Kato A, Carr CA, Johnston D, Wilson MA, Tonegawa S (2002) Requirement for hippocampal CA3 NMDA receptors in associative memory recall. *Science* 297:211–218.

Nakazawa K, Sun LD, Quirk MC, Rondi-Reig L, Wilson MA, Tonegawa S (2003) Hippocampal CA3 NMDA receptors are crucial for memory acquisition of one-time experience. *Neuron* 38:305–315.

Nehring RB, Horikawa HP, El Far O, Kneussel M, Brandstatter JH, Stamm S, Wischmeyer E, Betz H, Karschin A (2000) The metabotropic GABA$_B$ receptor directly interacts with the activating transcription factor 4. *J Biol Chem* 275:35185–35191.

Nishi T, Forgac M (2002) The vacuolar (H$^+$)-ATPases—nature's most versatile proton pumps. *Nat Rev Mol Cell Biol* 3:94–103.

Nusser Z (1999) A new approach to estimate the number, density and variability of receptors at central synapses. *Eur J Neurosci* 11:745–752.

Nusser Z, Sieghart W, Benke D, Fritschy JM, Somogyi P (1996) Differential synaptic localization of two major gamma-aminobutyric acid type A receptor alpha subunits on hippocampal pyramidal cells. *Proc Natl Acad Sci USA* 93:11939–11944.

Nusser Z, Hajos N, Somogyi P, Mody I (1998a) Increased number of synaptic GABA(A) receptors underlies potentiation at hippocampal inhibitory synapses. *Nature* 395:172–177.

Nusser Z, Lujan R, Laube G, Roberts JD, Molnar E, Somogyi P (1998b) Cell type and pathway dependence of synaptic AMPA receptor number and variability in the hippocampus. *Neuron* 21:545–559.

Nyiri G, Freund TF, Somogyi P (2001) Input-dependent synaptic targeting of alpha(2)-subunit-containing GABA(A) receptors in synapses of hippocampal pyramidal cells of the rat. *Eur J Neurosci* 13:428–442.

O'Brien RJ, Xu D, Petralia RS, Steward O, Huganir RL, Worley P (1999) Synaptic clustering of AMPA receptors by the extracellular immediate-early gene product Narp. *Neuron* 23:309–323.

Ohishi H, Shigemoto R, Nakanishi S, Mizuno N (1993) Distribution of the mRNA for a metabotropic glutamate receptor (mGluR3) in the rat brain: an in situ hybridization study. *J Comp Neurol* 335:252–266.

Ohishi H, Akazawa C, Shigemoto R, Nakanishi S, Mizuno N (1995) Distributions of the mRNAs for L-2-amino-4-phosphonobutyrate-sensitive metabotropic glutamate receptors, mGluR4 and mGluR7, in the rat brain. *J Comp Neurol* 360:555–570.

Okabe S, Collin C, Auerbach JM, Meiri N, Bengzon J, Kennedy MB, Segal M, McKay RD (1998) Hippocampal synaptic plasticity in mice overexpressing an embryonic subunit of the NMDA receptor. *J Neurosci* 18:4177–4188.

Orr-Urtreger A, Broide RS, Kasten MR, Dang H, Dani JA, Beaudet AL, Patrick JW (2000) Mice homozygous for the L250T mutation in the alpha7 nicotinic acetylcholine receptor show increased neuronal apoptosis and die within 1 day of birth. *J Neurochem* 74:2154–2166.

Osten P, Khatri L, Perez JL, Köhr G, Giese G, Daly C, Schulz TW, Wensky A, Lee LM, Ziff EB (2000) Mutagenesis reveals a role for ABP/GRIP binding to GluR2 in synaptic surface accumulation of the AMPA receptor. *Neuron* 27:313–325.

Pagano A, Rovelli G, Mosbacher J, Lohmann T, Duthey B, Stauffer D, Ristig D, Schuler V, Meigel I, Lampert C, Stein T, Prezeau L, Blahos J, Pin J, Froestl W, Kuhn R, Heid J, Kaupmann K, Bettler B (2001) C-terminal interaction is essential for surface trafficking but not for heteromeric assembly of GABA(b) receptors. *J Neurosci* 21:1189–1202.

Papp E, Leinekugel X, Henze DA, Lee J, Buzsaki G (2001) The apical shaft of CA1 pyramidal cells is under GABAergic interneuronal control. *Neuroscience* 102:715–721.

Paternain AV, Herrera MT, Nieto MA, Lerma J (2000) GluR5 and GluR6 kainate receptor subunits coexist in hippocampal neurons and coassemble to form functional receptors. *J Neurosci* 20:196–205.

Pawelzik H, Hughes DI, Thomson AM (2002) Physiological and morphological diversity of immunocytochemically defined parvalbumin- and cholecystokinin-positive interneurones in CA1 of the adult rat hippocampus. *J Comp Neurol* 443:346–367.

Pawlak V, Jensen V, Schupp BJ, Kvello A, Hvalby O, Seeburg PH, Köhr G (2005a) Frequency-dependent impairment of hippocampal LTP from NMDA receptors with reduced calcium permeability. *Eur J Neurosci* 22:476–484.

Pawlak V, Schupp BJ, Single FN, Seeburg PH, Köhr G (2005b) Impaired synaptic scaling in mouse hippocampal neurones expressing NMDA receptors with reduced calcium permeability. *J Physiol* 562:771–783.

Paylor R, Nguyen M, Crawley JN, Patrick J, Beaudet A, Orr-Urtreger A (1998) Alpha7 nicotinic receptor subunits are not necessary for hippocampal-dependent learning or sensorimotor gating: a behavioral characterization of Acra7-deficient mice. *Learn Mem* 5:302–316.

Peng Z, Hauer B, Mihalek RM, Homanics GE, Sieghart W, Olsen RW, Houser CR (2002) GABA(A) receptor changes in delta subunit-deficient mice: altered expression of alpha4 and gamma2 subunits in the forebrain. *J Comp Neurol* 446:179–197.

Persohn E, Malherbe P, Richards JG (1992) Comparative molecular neuroanatomy of cloned GABA$_A$ receptor subunits in the rat CNS. *J Comp Neurol* 326:193–216.

Petralia RS, Wenthold RJ (1992) Light and electron immunocytochemical localization of AMPA-selective glutamate receptors in the rat brain. *J Comp Neurol* 318:329–354.

Petralia RS, Esteban JA, Wang YX, Partridge JG, Zhao HM, Wenthold RJ, Malinow R (1999) Selective acquisition of AMPA receptors over postnatal development suggests a molecular basis for silent synapses. *Nat Neurosci* 2:31–36.

Pieribone VA, Porton B, Rendon B, Feng J, Greengard P, Kao HT (2002) Expression of synapsin III in nerve terminals and neurogenic regions of the adult brain. *J Comp Neurol* 454:105–114.

Pirker S, Schwarzer C, Wieselthaler A, Sieghart W, Sperk G (2000) GABA(A) receptors: immunocytochemical distribution of 13 subunits in the adult rat brain. *Neuroscience* 101:815–850.

Poncer JC, McKinney RA, Gahwiler BH, Thompson SM (2000) Differential control of GABA release at synapses from distinct interneurons in rat hippocampus. *J Physiol* 528 (Pt 1):123–130.

Powell CM, Schoch S, Monteggia L, Barrot M, Matos MF, Feldmann N, Südhof TC, Nestler EJ (2004) The presynaptic active zone protein RIM1alpha is critical for normal learning and memory. *Neuron* 42:143–153.

Priel A, Kolleker A, Ayalon G, Gillor M, Osten P, Stern-Bach Y (2005) Stargazin reduces desensitization and slows deactivation of the AMPA-type glutamate receptors. *J Neurosci* 25:2682–2686.

Prosser HM, Gill CH, Hirst WD, Grau E, Robbins M, Calver A, Soffin EM, Farmer CE, Lanneau C, Gray J, Schenck E, Warmerdam BS, Clapham C, Reavill C, Rogers DC, Stean T, Upton N, Humphreys K, Randall A, Geppert M, Davies CH, Pangalos MN (2001) Epileptogenesis and enhanced prepulse inhibition in GABA(B1)-deficient mice. *Mol Cell Neurosci* 17:1059–1070.

Rampon C, Jiang CH, Dong H, Tang YP, Lockhart DJ, Schultz PG, Tsien JZ, Hu Y (2000) Effects of environmental enrichment on gene expression in the brain. *Proc Natl Acad Sci USA* 97:12880–12884.

Reim K, Mansour M, Varoqueaux F, McMahon HT, Südhof TC, Brose N, Rosenmund C (2001) Complexins regulate a late step in Ca^{2+}-dependent neurotransmitter release. *Cell* 104:71–81.

Reisel D, Bannerman DM, Schmitt WB, Deacon RM, Flint J, Borchardt T, Seeburg PH, Rawlins JN (2002) Spatial memory dissociations in mice lacking GluR1. *Nat Neurosci* 5:868–873.

Richmond JE, Weimer RM, Jorgensen EM (2001) An open form of syntaxin bypasses the requirement for UNC-13 in vesicle priming. *Nature* 412:338–341.

Riedel G, Platt B, Micheau J (2003) Glutamate receptor function in learning and memory. *Behav Brain Res* 140:1–47.

Rizo J, Südhof TC (2002) Snares and Munc18 in synaptic vesicle fusion. *Nat Rev Neurosci* 3:641–653.

Rosahl TW, Geppert M, Spillane D, Herz J, Hammer RE, Malenka RC, Südhof TC (1993) Short-term synaptic plasticity is altered in mice lacking synapsin I. *Cell* 75:661–670.

Rosahl TW, Spillane D, Missler M, Herz J, Selig DK, Wolff JR, Hammer RE, Malenka RC, Südhof TC (1995) Essential functions of synapsins I and II in synaptic vesicle regulation. *Nature* 375:488–493.

Rouach N, Byrd K, Petralia RS, Elias GM, Adesnik H, Tomita S, Karimzadegan S, Kealey C, Bredt DS, Nicoll RA (2005) TARP gamma-8 controls hippocampal AMPA receptor number, distribution and synaptic plasticity. *Nat Neurosci* 8:1525–1533.

Rudolph U, Mohler H (2004) Analysis of GABA$_A$ receptor function and dissection of the pharmacology of benzodiazepines and general anesthetics through mouse genetics. *Annu Rev Pharmacol Toxicol* 44:475–498.

Ruiz A, Fabian-Fine R, Scott R, Walker MC, Rusakov DA, Kullmann DM (2003) GABA$_A$ receptors at hippocampal mossy fibers. *Neuron* 39:961–973.

Sailer A, Swanson GT, Perez-Otano I, O'Leary L, Malkmus SA, Dyck RH, Dickinson-Anson H, Schiffer HH, Maron C, Yaksh TL, Gage FH, O'Gorman S, Heinemann SF (1999) Generation and analysis of GluR5(Q636R) kainate receptor mutant mice. *J Neurosci* 19:8757–8764.

Sakimura K, Kutsuwada T, Ito I, Manabe T, Takayama C, Kushiya E, Yagi T, Aizawa S, Inoue Y, Sugiyama H, et al. (1995) Reduced hippocampal LTP and spatial learning in mice lacking NMDA receptor epsilon 1 subunit. *Nature* 373:151–155.

Sans N, Vissel B, Petralia RS, Wang YX, Chang K, Royle GA, Wang CY, O'Gorman S, Heinemann SF, Wenthold RJ (2003) Aberrant formation of glutamate receptor complexes in hippocampal neurons of mice lacking the GluR2 AMPA receptor subunit. *J Neurosci* 23:9367–9373.

Sansig G, Bushell TJ, Clarke VR, Rozov A, Burnashev N, Portet C, Gasparini F, Schmutz M, Klebs K, Shigemoto R, Flor PJ, Kuhn R, Knoepfel T, Schroeder M, Hampson DR, Collett VJ, Zhang C, Duvoisin RM, Collingridge GL, van Der Putten H (2001) Increased seizure susceptibility in mice lacking metabotropic glutamate receptor 7. *J Neurosci* 21:8734–8745.

Schlüter OM, Schnell E, Verhage M, Tzonopoulos T, Nicoll RA, Janz R, Malenka RC, Geppert M, Südhof TC (1999) Rabphilin knock-out mice reveal that rabphilin is not required for rab3 function in regulating neurotransmitter release. *J Neurosci* 19:5834–5846.

Schlüter OM, Schmitz F, Jahn R, Rosenmund C, Südhof TC (2004) A complete genetic analysis of neuronal Rab3 function. *J Neurosci* 24:6629–6637.

Schmid SL, McNiven MA, De Camilli P (1998) Dynamin and its partners: a progress report. *Curr Opin Cell Biol* 10:504–512.

Schmitt WB, Arianpour R, Deacon RM, Seeburg PH, Sprengel R, Rawlins JN, Bannerman DM (2004a) The role of hippocampal glutamate receptor-A-dependent synaptic plasticity in conditional learning: the importance of spatiotemporal discontiguity. *J Neurosci* 24:9277–9282.

Schmitt WB, Deacon RM, Reisel D, Sprengel R, Seeburg PH, Rawlins JN, Bannerman DM (2004b) Spatial reference memory in GluR-A-deficient mice using a novel hippocampal-dependent paddling pool escape task. *Hippocampus* 14:216–223.

Schmitt WB, Sprengel R, Mack V, Draft RW, Seeburg PH, Deacon RM, Rawlins JN, Bannerman DM (2005) Restoration of spatial working memory by genetic rescue of GluR-A-deficient mice. *Nat Neurosci* 8:270–272.

Schneggenburger R, Neher E (2000) Intracellular calcium dependence of transmitter release rates at a fast central synapse. *Nature* 406:889–893.

Schoch S, Deak F, Konigstorfer A, Mozhayeva M, Sara Y, Südhof TC, Kavalali ET (2001) SNARE function analyzed in synaptobrevin/VAMP knockout mice. *Science* 294:1117–1122.

Schoch S, Castillo PE, Jo T, Mukherjee K, Geppert M, Wang Y, Schmitz F, Malenka RC, Südhof TC (2002) RIM1alpha forms a protein scaffold for regulating neurotransmitter release at the active zone. *Nature* 415:321–326.

Schuler V, Luscher C, Blanchet C, Klix N, Sansig G, Klebs K, Schmutz M, Heid J, Gentry C, Urban L, Fox A, Spooren W, Jaton AL, Vigouret J, Pozza M, Kelly PH, Mosbacher J, Froestl W, Kaslin E, Korn R, Bischoff S, Kaupmann K, van der Putten H, Bettler B (2001) Epilepsy, hyperalgesia, impaired memory, and loss of pre- and postsynaptic GABA(B) responses in mice lacking GABA(B(1)). *Neuron* 31:47–58.

Schulz TW, Nakagawa T, Licznerski P, Pawlak V, Kolleker A, Rozov A, Kim J, Dittgen T, Kohr G, Sheng M, Seeburg PH, Osten P (2004) Actin/alpha-actinin-dependent transport of AMPA receptors in dendritic spines: role of the PDZ-LIM protein RIL. *J Neurosci* 24:8584–8594.

Schweizer C, Balsiger S, Bluethmann H, Mansuy IM, Fritschy JM, Mohler H, Luscher B (2003) The gamma 2 subunit of GABA(A) receptors is required for maintenance of receptors at mature synapses. *Mol Cell Neurosci* 24:442–450.

Seagar M, Leveque C, Charvin N, Marqueze B, Martin-Moutot N, Boudier JA, Boudier JL, Shoji-Kasai Y, Sato K, Takahashi M (1999) Interactions between proteins implicated in exocytosis and voltage-gated calcium channels. *Philos Trans R Soc Lond B Biol Sci* 354:289–297.

Seeburg PH, Higuchi M, Sprengel R (1998) RNA editing of brain glutamate receptor channels: mechanism and physiology. Brain Res Brain Res Rev 26:217–229.

Sheng M, Pak DT (2000) Ligand-gated ion channel interactions with cytoskeletal and signaling proteins. *Annu Rev Physiol* 62:755–778.

Sheng M, Sala C (2001) PDZ domains and the organization of supramolecular complexes. *Annu Rev Neurosci* 24:1–29.

Shigemoto R, Nakanishi S, Mizuno N (1992) Distribution of the mRNA for a metabotropic glutamate receptor (mGluR1) in the central nervous system: an in situ hybridization study in adult and developing rat. *J Comp Neurol* 322:121–135.

Shigemoto R, Kinoshita A, Wada E, Nomura S, Ohishi H, Takada M, Flor PJ, Neki A, Abe T, Nakanishi S, Mizuno N (1997) Differential presynaptic localization of metabotropic glutamate receptor subtypes in the rat hippocampus. *J Neurosci* 17:7503–7522.

Shimizu E, Tang YP, Rampon C, Tsien JZ (2000) NMDA receptor-dependent synaptic reinforcement as a crucial process for memory consolidation. *Science* 290:1170–1174.

Shimshek DR, Bus T, Kim J, Mihaljevic A, Mack V, Seeburg PH, Sprengel R, Schaefer AT (2005) Enhanced odor discrimination and impaired olfactory memory by spatially controlled switch of AMPA receptors. *PLoS Biol* 3:e354.

Shimshek DR, Jensen V, Celikel T, Geng Y, Schupp B, Bus T, Mack V,

Marx V, Hvalby Ø, Seeburg PH, Sprengel R (2006) Forebrain-specific glutamate receptor B deletion impairs spatial memory but not hippocampal field long-term potentiation. *J Neurosci* 26:8428–8440.

Silva AJ, Paylor R, Wehner JM, Tonegawa S (1992a) Impaired spatial learning in alpha-calcium-calmodulin kinase II mutant mice. *Science* 257:206–211.

Silva AJ, Stevens CF, Tonegawa S, Wang Y (1992b) Deficient hippocampal long-term potentiation in alpha-calcium-calmodulin kinase II mutant mice. *Science* 257:201–206.

Silva AJ, Rosahl TW, Chapman PF, Marowitz Z, Friedman E, Frankland PW, Cestari V, Cioffi D, Südhof TC, Bourtchuladze R (1996) Impaired learning in mice with abnormal short-lived plasticity. *Curr Biol* 6:1509–1518.

Single FN, Rozov A, Burnashev N, Zimmermann F, Hanley DF, Forrest D, Curran T, Jensen V, Hvalby O, Sprengel R, Seeburg PH (2000) Dysfunctions in mice by NMDA receptor point mutations NR1(N598Q) and NR1(N598R). *J Neurosci* 20:2558–2566.

Slepnev VI, De Camilli P (2000) Accessory factors in clathrin-dependent synaptic vesicle endocytosis. *Nat Rev Neurosci* 1:161–172.

Smith SS, Gong QH, Hsu FC, Markowitz RS, ffrench-Mullen JM, Li X (1998a) GABA(A) receptor alpha4 subunit suppression prevents withdrawal properties of an endogenous steroid. *Nature* 392:926–930.

Smith SS, Gong QH, Li X, Moran MH, Bitran D, Frye CA, Hsu FC (1998b) Withdrawal from 3alpha-OH-5alpha-pregnan-20-one using a pseudopregnancy model alters the kinetics of hippocampal GABA$_A$-gated current and increases the GABA$_A$ receptor alpha4 subunit in association with increased anxiety. *J Neurosci* 18:5275–5284.

Sommer B, Keinanen K, Verdoorn TA, Wisden W, Burnashev N, Herb A, Kohler M, Takagi T, Sakmann B, Seeburg PH (1990) Flip and flop: a cell-specific functional switch in glutamate-operated channels of the CNS. *Science* 249:1580–1585.

Somogyi P, Fritschy JM, Benke D, Roberts JD, Sieghart W (1996) The gamma 2 subunit of the GABA$_A$ receptor is concentrated in synaptic junctions containing the alpha 1 and beta 2/3 subunits in hippocampus, cerebellum and globus pallidus. *Neuropharmacology* 35:1425–1444.

Song I, Huganir RL (2002) Regulation of AMPA receptors during synaptic plasticity. *Trends Neurosci* 25:578–588.

Sperk G, Schwarzer C, Tsunashima K, Fuchs K, Sieghart W (1997) GABA(A) receptor subunits in the rat hippocampus. I. Immunocytochemical distribution of 13 subunits. *Neuroscience* 80:987–1000.

Sprengel R, Suchanek B, Amico C, Brusa R, Burnashev N, Rozov A, Hvalby O, Jensen V, Paulsen O, Andersen P, Kim JJ, Thompson RF, Sun W, Webster LC, Grant SG, Eilers J, Konnerth A, Li J, McNamara JO, Seeburg PH (1998) Importance of the intracellular domain of NR2 subunits for NMDA receptor function in vivo. *Cell* 92:279–289.

Standaert DG, Landwehrmeyer GB, Kerner JA, Penney JB Jr, Young AB (1996) Expression of NMDAR2D glutamate receptor subunit mRNA in neurochemically identified interneurons in the rat neostriatum, neocortex and hippocampus. *Brain Res Mol Brain Res* 42:89–102.

Stell BM, Brickley SG, Tang CY, Farrant M, Mody I (2003) Neuroactive steroids reduce neuronal excitability by selectively enhancing tonic inhibition mediated by delta subunit-containing GABA$_A$ receptors. *Proc Natl Acad Sci USA* 100:14439–14444.

Stowell JN, Craig AM (1999) Axon/dendrite targeting of

metabotropic glutamate receptors by their cytoplasmic carboxy-terminal domains. *Neuron* 22:525–536.

Sucher NJ, Akbarian S, Chi CL, Leclerc CL, Awobuluyi M, Deitcher DL, Wu MK, Yuan JP, Jones EG, Lipton SA (1995) Developmental and regional expression pattern of a novel NMDA receptor-like subunit (NMDAR-L) in the rodent brain. *J Neurosci* 15:6509–6520.

Südhof TC (2004) The synaptic vesicle cycle. *Annu Rev Neurosci* 27:509–547.

Südhof TC, Czernik AJ, Kao HT, Takei K, Johnston PA, Horiuchi A, Kanazir SD, Wagner MA, Perin MS, De Camilli P, Greengard P (1989) Synapsins: mosaics of shared and individual domains in a family of synaptic vesicle phosphoproteins. *Science* 245:1474–1480.

Sundstrom-Poromaa I, Smith DH, Gong QH, Sabado TN, Li X, Light A, Wiedmann M, Williams K, Smith SS (2002) Hormonally regulated alpha(4)beta(2)delta GABA(A) receptors are a target for alcohol. *Nat Neurosci* 5:721–722.

Sur C, Fresu L, Howell O, McKernan RM, Atack JR (1999) Autoradiographic localization of alpha5 subunit-containing GABA$_A$ receptors in rat brain. *Brain Res* 822:265–270.

Takei Y, Harada A, Takeda S, Kobayashi K, Terada S, Noda T, Takahashi T, Hirokawa N (1995) Synapsin I deficiency results in the structural change in the presynaptic terminals in the murine nervous system. *J Cell Biol* 131:1789–1800.

Tamaru Y, Nomura S, Mizuno N, Shigemoto R (2001) Distribution of metabotropic glutamate receptor mGluR3 in the mouse CNS: differential location relative to pre- and postsynaptic sites. *Neuroscience* 106:481–503.

Tang YP, Shimizu E, Dube GR, Rampon C, Kerchner GA, Zhuo M, Liu G, Tsien JZ (1999) Genetic enhancement of learning and memory in mice. *Nature* 401:63–69.

Terashima A, Cotton L, Dev KK, Meyer G, Zaman S, Duprat F, Henley JM, Collingridge GL, Isaac JT (2004) Regulation of synaptic strength and AMPA receptor subunit composition by PICK1. *J Neurosci* 24:5381–5390.

Thomson AM, Bannister AP, Hughes DI, Pawelzik H (2000) Differential sensitivity to zolpidem of IPSPs activated by morphologically identified CA1 interneurons in slices of rat hippocampus. *Eur J Neurosci* 12:425–436.

Tomita S, Chen L, Kawasaki Y, Petralia RS, Wenthold RJ, Nicoll RA, Bredt DS (2003) Functional studies and distribution define a family of transmembrane AMPA receptor regulatory proteins. *J Cell Biol* 161:805–816.

Tomita S, Adesnik H, Sekiguchi M, Zhang W, Wada K, Howe JR, Nicoll RA, Bredt DS (2005) Stargazin modulates AMPA receptor gating and trafficking by distinct domains. *Nature* 435:1052–1058.

Torres GE, Gainetdinov RR, Caron MG (2003) Plasma membrane monoamine transporters: structure, regulation and function. *Nat Rev Neurosci* 4:13–25.

Toth K, McBain CJ (1998) Afferent-specific innervation of two distinct AMPA receptor subtypes on single hippocampal interneurons. *Nat Neurosci* 1:572–578.

Tovar KR, Westbrook GL (1999) The incorporation of NMDA receptors with a distinct subunit composition at nascent hippocampal synapses in vitro. *J Neurosci* 19:4180–4188.

Towers SK, Gloveli T, Traub RD, Driver J, Engel D, Fradley R, Rosahl TW, Maubach K, Buhl EH, Whittington MA (2004) Alpha5 subunit-containing GABA$_A$ receptors affect the dynamic range of kainate-induced hippocampal gamma frequency oscillations in vitro. *J Physiol* 559:721–728.

Tsien JZ, Chen DF, Gerber D, Tom C, Mercer EH, Anderson DJ, Mayford M, Kandel ER, Tonegawa S (1996a) Subregion- and cell type-restricted gene knockout in mouse brain. *Cell* 87:1317–1326.

Tsien JZ, Huerta PT, Tonegawa S (1996b) The essential role of hippocampal CA1 NMDA receptor-dependent synaptic plasticity in spatial memory. *Cell* 87:1327–1338.

Turetsky D, Garringer E, Patneau DK (2005) Stargazin modulates native AMPA receptor functional properties by two distinct mechanisms. *J Neurosci* 25:7438–7448.

Turrigiano GG, Nelson SB (2004) Homeostatic plasticity in the developing nervous system. *Nat Rev Neurosci* 5:97–107.

Tzavara ET, Bymaster FP, Felder CC, Wade M, Gomeza J, Wess J, McKinzie DL, Nomikos GG (2003) Dysregulated hippocampal acetylcholine neurotransmission and impaired cognition in M2, M4 and M2/M4 muscarinic receptor knockout mice. *Mol Psychiatry* 8:673–679.

Vandenberghe W, Nicoll RA, Bredt DS (2005) Stargazin is an AMPA receptor auxiliary subunit. *Proc Natl Acad Sci USA* 102:485–490.

Varoqueaux F, Sigler A, Rhee JS, Brose N, Enk C, Reim K, Rosenmund C (2002) Total arrest of spontaneous and evoked synaptic transmission but normal synaptogenesis in the absence of Munc13-mediated vesicle priming. *Proc Natl Acad Sci USA* 99:9037–9042.

Vekovischeva OY, Aitta-Aho T, Echenko O, Kankaanpaa A, Seppala T, Honkanen A, Sprengel R, Korpi ER (2004) Reduced aggression in AMPA-type glutamate receptor GluR-A subunit-deficient mice. *Genes Brain Behav* 3:253–265.

Verhage M, Maia AS, Plomp JJ, Brussaard AB, Heeroma JH, Vermeer H, Toonen RF, Hammer RE, van den Berg TK, Missler M, Geuze HJ, Südhof TC (2000) Synaptic assembly of the brain in the absence of neurotransmitter secretion. *Science* 287:864–869.

Vignes M, Collingridge GL (1997) The synaptic activation of kainate receptors. *Nature* 388:179–182.

Vilaro MT, Palacios JM, Mengod G (1990) Localization of m5 muscarinic receptor mRNA in rat brain examined by in situ hybridization histochemistry. *Neurosci Lett* 114:154–159.

Vissel B, Royle GA, Christie BR, Schiffer HH, Ghetti A, Tritto T, Perez-Otano I, Radcliffe RA, Seamans J, Sejnowski T, Wehner JM, Collins AC, O'Gorman S, Heinemann SF (2001) The role of RNA editing of kainate receptors in synaptic plasticity and seizures. *Neuron* 29:217–227.

Vogt KE, Nicoll RA (1999) Glutamate and gamma-aminobutyric acid mediate a heterosynaptic depression at mossy fiber synapses in the hippocampus. *Proc Natl Acad Sci USA* 96:1118–1122.

Walker MC, Ruiz A, Kullmann DM (2001) Monosynaptic GABAergic signaling from dentate to CA3 with a pharmacological and physiological profile typical of mossy fiber synapses. *Neuron* 29:703–715.

Wallner M, Hanchar HJ, Olsen RW (2003) Ethanol enhances alpha 4 beta 3 delta and alpha 6 beta 3 delta gamma-aminobutyric acid type A receptors at low concentrations known to affect humans. *Proc Natl Acad Sci USA* 100:15218–15223.

Washbourne P, Thompson PM, Carta M, Costa ET, Mathews JR, Lopez-Bendito G, Molnar Z, Becher MW, Valenzuela CF, Partridge LD, Wilson MC (2002) Genetic ablation of the t-SNARE SNAP-25 distinguishes mechanisms of neuroexocytosis. *Nat Neurosci* 5:19–26.

Watt AJ, Sjostrom PJ, Hausser M, Nelson SB, Turrigiano GG (2004) A proportional but slower NMDA potentiation follows AMPA potentiation in LTP. *Nat Neurosci* 7:518–524.

Wei W, Zhang N, Peng Z, Houser CR, Mody I (2003) Perisynaptic localization of delta subunit-containing GABA(A) receptors and their activation by GABA spillover in the mouse dentate gyrus. *J Neurosci* 23:10650–10661.

Werner P, Voigt M, Keinanen K, Wisden W, Seeburg PH (1991) Cloning of a putative high-affinity kainate receptor expressed predominantly in hippocampal CA3 cells. *Nature* 351:742–744.

Wess J (2004) Muscarinic acetylcholine receptor knockout mice: novel phenotypes and clinical implications. *Annu Rev Pharmacol Toxicol* 44:423–450.

White JH, McIllhinney RA, Wise A, Ciruela F, Chan WY, Emson PC, Billinton A, Marshall FH (2000) The GABA$_B$ receptor interacts directly with the related transcription factors CREB2 and ATFx. *Proc Natl Acad Sci USA* 97:13967–13972.

Wisden W, Seeburg PH (1993) A complex mosaic of high-affinity kainate receptors in rat brain. *J Neurosci* 13:3582–3598.

Wisden W, Laurie DJ, Monyer H, Seeburg PH (1992) The distribution of 13 GABA$_A$ receptor subunit mRNAs in the rat brain. I. Telencephalon, diencephalon, mesencephalon. *J Neurosci* 12:1040–1062.

Wisden W, Seeburg PH, Monyer H (2000) AMPA, kainate and NMDA ionotropic glutamate receptor expression—an in situ hybridization atlas. In: *Handbook of chemical neuroanatomy: glutamate* (Ottersen OPaS-M J, ed), pp 99–143. Amsterdam: Elsevier.

Wohlfarth KM, Bianchi MT, Macdonald RL (2002) Enhanced neurosteroid potentiation of ternary GABA(A) receptors containing the delta subunit. *J Neurosci* 22:1541–1549.

Xiao B, Tu JC, Worley PF (2000) Homer: a link between neural activity and glutamate receptor function. *Curr Opin Neurobiol* 10:370–374.

Yan J, Zhang Y, Jia Z, Taverna FA, McDonald RJ, Muller RU, Roder JC (2002) Place-cell impairment in glutamate receptor 2 mutant mice. *J Neurosci* 22:RC204.

Yokoi M, Kobayashi K, Manabe T, Takahashi T, Sakaguchi I, Katsuura G, Shigemoto R, Ohishi H, Nomura S, Nakamura K, Nakao K, Katsuki M, Nakanishi S (1996) Impairment of hippocampal mossy fiber LTD in mice lacking mGluR2. *Science* 273:645–647.

Zamanillo D, Sprengel R, Hvalby O, Jensen V, Burnashev N, Rozov A, Kaiser KM, Koster HJ, Borchardt T, Worley P, Lubke J, Frotscher M, Kelly PH, Sommer B, Andersen P, Seeburg PH, Sakmann B (1999) Importance of AMPA receptors for hippocampal synaptic plasticity but not for spatial learning. *Science* 284:1805–1811.

Zhang S, Ehlers MD, Bernhardt JP, Su CT, Huganir RL (1998) Calmodulin mediates calcium-dependent inactivation of *N*-methyl-D-aspartate receptors. *Neuron* 21:443–453.

Zhu JJ, Esteban JA, Hayashi Y, Malinow R (2000) Postnatal synaptic potentiation: delivery of GluR4-containing AMPA receptors by spontaneous activity. *Nat Neurosci* 3:1098–1106.

Zoli M, Lena C, Picciotto MR, Changeux JP (1998) Identification of four classes of brain nicotinic receptors using beta2 mutant mice. *J Neurosci* 18:4461–4472.

8 ▦ Eberhard Buhl and Miles Whittington

Local Circuits

▦ 8.1 Overview

Local circuits play a critical role in determining the pattern of output from discrete brain regions receiving multiple inputs over time. Individual neurons have been proposed to act as integrators of multiple afferent inputs and/or coincidence detectors for these inputs depending on the compartmental organization of intrinsic membrane conductance and the type of synaptic input received. However, within a brain region, it is common to find the pattern of inputs, and subsequent outputs, of a subpopulation of neurons affecting the behavior of the population as a whole. This property of discrete brain regions is governed by the organization of local circuit connections between homogeneous and heterogeneous cell types. The aim of this chapter is to demonstrate the basic principles involved in local circuits in general and to review evidence for the organization of local circuits in the hippocampus.

8.1.1 Neuronal Classification Issues

Hippocampal neurons are divided into two major classes: principal cells (which form the major output pathway from hippocampal subregions) and interneurons (which are thought to be mainly local-circuit neurons). Interneurons are considerably less abundant ($< 10\%$) than spiny principal neurons, such as granule and mossy cells in the dentate gyrus and pyramidal neurons in the CA1 and CA3 areas. As yet (and in contrast to the neocortex), there is relatively little evidence that hippocampal principal neurons fall into many distinct subclasses. However, despite their relatively small numbers, recent technical and conceptual progress has indicated an astonishing variety of interneuron classes (for review see Freund and Buzsaki, 1996). Apart from highlighting the diversity of interneuronal subtypes, these data have also revealed an equally bewildering complexity of interneuronal organiza-

tion. Some "interneurons," for example, show properties that are traditionally associated with principal, projection neurons. Certain classes of hippocampal interneurons establish a commissural axon collateral or even project to extrahippocampal targets (Toth and Freund 1992), and others have been shown to have dendritic spines (Gulyas et al., 1992). Thus, some degree of caution is warranted when using the term local-circuit neuron and the associated morphological parameters as a synonym for interneuron. Conversely, virtually all excitatory hippocampal projection neurons have a local axonal arbor and could therefore be also considered bona fide local-circuit neurons.

Problems also arise when attempting to establish a more functionally oriented operational definition of interneurons. Although traditionally interneurons have been viewed as subserving an inhibitory function, recent anatomical studies indicate that the interneurons that selectively innervate other interneurons may have a net disinhibitory effect on principal cells (for review see Freund and Buzsaki, 1996). Moreover, γ-aminobutyric acid (GABA)ergic inhibitory postsynaptic potentials (IPSPs) may be depolarizing, for example during early development (Cherubini et al. 1991). GABAergic interneurons may also have pacemaker-like properties that are generally not associated with an inhibitory function.

Hippocampal interneurons can be defined operationally as GABAergic nonprincipal cells (Buckmaster and Soltesz 1996). Within this catch-all definition various attempts have been made to subclassify hippocampal interneurons based on their anatomical, electrophysiological, or neurochemical properties, including the following.

1. Dendritic morphology
2. Laminar position
3. Neuropeptide content
4. Type of calcium-binding proteins expressed
5. Efferent connectivity

6. Intrinsic conductance and firing properties
7. Participation in specific circuits

A number of these classification schemes have their undisputed merits, often facilitating the discrimination of interneurons into nonoverlapping subclasses; however, this is not always possible owing to common properties shared by otherwise distinct interneurons. For example, with respect to useful classification schemes, several extensive quantitative electron microscopic studies have provided compelling evidence that hippocampal interneurons show striking differences in their efferent connectivity properties (e.g., Gulyas et al., 1993a). However, combining this property with others in the above list leads to classification difficulties: Basket and axo-axonic (chandelier) cells both contain parvalbumin (Kosaka et al., 1987) but show clear-cut differences with respect to their efferent target profile. In addition, attempts to classify hippocampal interneurons based on their membrane and firing properties also cause problems (e.g., Lacaille and Williams, 1990; Mott et al, 1997). In short, it has, as yet, proved impossible to find a set of physiological parameters that allows a meaningful classification scheme of hippocampal interneurons to be established. For the future, the current inadequacy of this approach could be addressed by either finding more suitable criteria or, ideally, adopting a multiparametric, and therefore integrated, approach to refine the existing classification schemes, similar to efforts being made in neocortical areas (Gupta et al., 2000).

8.1.2 Input Specificity of Extrinsic Afferents

All hippocampal subfields receive an abundance of extrinsic afferents, which can be grouped into three broad classes: (1) glutamatergic inputs (e.g., originating in the entorhinal cortex and other ipsilateral and contralateral hippocampal subregions); (2) the septo-hippocampal GABAergic projection; and (3) several pathways from brain stem and forebrain nuclei, releasing neurotransmitters that are often referred to as "neuromodulators," among them acetylcholine, dopamine, serotonin, and noradrenaline (norepinephrine).

As far as excitatory, glutamatergic afferent pathways are concerned, it appears that most of them show a high degree of laminar selectivity. Entorhinal afferents target the distal apical dendrites of granule and pyramidal cells, whereas commissural/associational fibers innervate the proximal dendrites of granule cells and the apical and basal dendrites of pyramidal neurons in the strata radiatum and oriens of the CA3 and CA1 subfields. In addition, submammillary and thalamic nucleus reuniens pathways also show a high degree of laminar specificity. This laminar specificity of inputs can have powerful effects on shaping any consequent output from the target population.

Hippocampal principal cells show a marked distribution pattern of intrinsic conductance. In general, conductance that favors slower postsynaptic responses (e.g., I_h- and voltage-operated calcium channels) is preferentially located on distal dendritic compartments (Magee, 1998; Wei et al., 2001). The distribution of such conductance has profound effects on the integrative and coincidence-detection abilities of target neurons, suggesting that inputs with different laminar profiles are handled differently by neurons in the target regions. In addition, the high degree of laminar specificity of glutamatergic input to hippocampal subregions is also accompanied by specifity in interneuron targets. The axon domains of interneurons targeted by a specific pathway often match remarkably to the axon domains of that specific pathway (see Figs. 8–2 and 8–5, later in the chapter). This suggests that where compartment-specific excitatory inputs are present a specific feedforward inhibitory local circuit is also co-activated to control those compartments (see also Section 8.1.3). Thus, the architecture exists to provide specific target region responses to specific inputs at both the cellular compartmental level and local circuit levels.

With respect to target cell selectivity, there are, as yet, no data that suggest any clear biases toward particular target neurons for glutamatergic pathways. In contrast, the GABAergic septal projection has no obvious laminar innervation pattern (Freund and Antal, 1988) but does have a precise target cell preference. Synapses are formed exclusively with GABAergic interneurons, among them subpopulations co-localizing parvalbumin, calbindin, calretinin, somatostatin, and cholecystokinin (CCK) (Freund and Buzsaki, 1996). Interestingly, the cholinergic afferents, also forming part of the septo-hippocampal pathway, do not appear to have any particular target cell or laminar preference. Cholinergic axons branch profusely in all hippocampal layers and establish synaptic contacts with both principal cells and interneurons. This widespread, nonspecific influence over target areas is also seen to some extent for other neuromodulatory inputs. Noradrenergic afferents from the locus coeruleus do not appear to have a particular target cell preference but are particularly dense in areas that receive mossy fiber input (i.e., in the hilus of the dentate gyrus and stratum lucidum of the CA3 area). One branch of the serotoninergic raphe-hippocampal projection also shows this lack of specificity. Most transmitter-containing boutons in this pathway (> 75%) do not appear to make synaptic specializations and show no obvious association with particular target cells or a domain-specific innervation pattern (Oleskevich et al., 1991). Less specific data are available for dopaminergic and noradrenergic projections to the hippocampus. In general, although most hippocampal neurons express dopamine receptors, mesohippocampal projections are predominantly to area CA1. Terminals are found in all fields from the stratum oriens to the molecular layer (Gasbarri et al., 1997), with projections from the ventral tegmental area favoring the temporal hippocampus and nigral projections favoring septal CA1 fields (Gasbarri et al., 1994). In contrast, noradrenergic fibers from the locus coeruleus project mainly to the dentate gyrus and stratum lacunosum-moleculare (Swanson & Hartman, 1975; Samson et al., 1990).

Dense axonal varicosities are seen in the inner molecular layer, granule cell layer, and hilus (Ishida et al., 2000).

8.1.3 Subcellular Domain Specificity in Hippocampal Circuits

The pattern of co-lamination of specific extrinsic pathway inputs and their preferred interneuronal targets suggests a general pattern of organization whereby different interneurons control the activity of different principal cell compartments. Evidence for this division of labor by interneuron subtypes can also be found when considering other interneuron subtypes. Axo-axonic cells show remarkably high-target specificity for axon initial segments (Somogyi et al., 1985; Buhl et al., 1994b; Martinez et al., 1996). Conversely, basket cells clearly favor somata and proximal dendritic shafts of their postsynaptic targets (Gulyas et al., 1993; Halasy and Somogyi, 1993; Han et al., 1993). Thus, it appears that despite the spatial mixing of postsynaptic target domains at least some GABAergic cells maintain a remarkable degree of specificity for particular membrane compartments. It is interesting, however, to note that domain specificity and postsynaptic target cell selectivity are not necessarily linked. Although hippocampal basket cells appear to be invariably domain-specific, an individual basket cell may provide divergent innervation to both principal cells as well as other interneurons (Sik et al., 1995; Cobb et al., 1997).

8.1.4 Patterns of Local Circuit Connectivity

The previous two sections dealt predominantly with the pattern of input to local hippocampal circuits. These patterns involve two elements: the input profile directly onto local principal neurons and the concurrent activation of interneurons generating a feedforward inhibitory signal (Fig. 8–1A). Feedforward inhibition serves to impose a temporal framework on a target area on the basis of inputs received. The extra delay associated with an additional synapse in the circuit ensures that the feedforward inhibitory synaptic event does not impinge on the initial, direct extrinsic synaptic event in principal neurons. However, further extrinsic influence of the target principal cells is reduced for a time equal to the effective period of the feedforward inhibitory synaptic potential. Some interneurons receive input only from extrinsic afferents and can therefore participate only in feedforward inhibition. Examples are cells associated with the perforant path in the molecular layer of the dentate gyrus and neurogliaform cells in area CA1 (Han et al., 1993; Vida et al., 1998). Feedforward inhibition can account for most of the input from extrinsic sources. For example, the mossy fiber axons in area CA3 make roughly 10 times as many contacts with CA3 interneurons as with the far more numerous CA3 principal cells (Acsady et al., 1998).

If principal neurons fire, a number of interneurons receive synaptic excitation. Such interneurons include basket cells, bistratified cells, and oriens and lacunosum-moleculare cells. The strength of excitatory synaptic innervation is such that there is a high probability that the target interneuron will fire an action potential (see Section 8.3). In turn, interneurons target local principal cells, thus providing a feedback inhibitory circuit (Fig. 8–1B). As with feedforward inhibition, these local feedback circuits can account for most of the local output from principal neurons. In area CA1, excitatory neurons have a strong preference for interneurons as targets (e.g., Gulyas et al., 1998). Thus, generation of an output action potential from a hippocampal subregion is followed rapidly by a period of marked local inhibition. Many interneurons can be involved in both feedforward and feedback inhibition (e.g., Buzsaki, 1983; Frotscher et al., 1984), providing a functional link between afferent input patterns and any resulting output from the target area.

In addition to circuits involving both principal excitatory neurons and inhibitory interneurons, there are many examples of interneuron–interneuron synaptic interactions (see Sections 8.2.6 and 8.3.5). Most interneurons that target principal cells, such as basket and bistratified cells, also target other interneurons. There is evidence of a broad heterogeneity of interneuron–interneuron connections, with single presynaptic interneurons innervating other interneurons with different postsynaptic targets (e.g., the distal dendritic or perisomatic compartments of pyramidal cells) (Tamas et al., 1998). Unlike feedforward and feedback inhibition, this mutual inhibition (Fig. 8–1D) can be relatively weak. For example, CA1 basket cells are 25 times more likely to form synapses with principal cells than are other basket cells. However, there are also distinct subclasses of interneurons that appear to target other interneurons exclusively (Freund and Buzsaki, 1996). Networks of such interneurons, coupled with interneurons that have principal cells as targets, massively enrich the dynamics of local circuit responses to an afferent input. In particular, recurrent pathways provide a mechanism by which rhythmic patterns of activity can be j2generated in interneuron circuits and projected onto principal cells, thus generating network oscillatory activity (Whittington et al., 1995) (see Chapter 11).

The occurrence of recurrent connections is not limited to interneurons. Recurrent excitation is also seen in hippocampal local circuits (Fig. 8–1C). In the hippocampus there are probably few, if any, neurons without local axon collaterals synapsing on neighboring neurons. In general, principal neurons recurrently excite other local (or neighboring) principal neurons as well as interneurons. Only dentate granule cells in rodents appear to be wired differently (see Section 8.2.1).

8.1.5 Circuit Specific Receptor Distribution

The basic principles of connectivity for interneurons described above also have a correlate in the types of GABA receptor expressed at specific target sites. Thus, receptors that

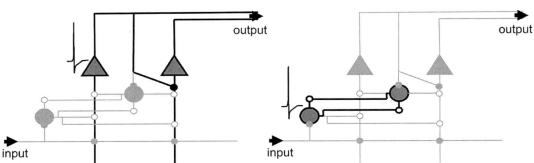

A. Feedforward inhibition

output

input

B. Feedback inhibition

output

input

C. Recurrent excitation

output

input

D. Mutual inhibition

output

input

Figure 8–1. Basic local circuit interactions. *A.* Feedforward inhibition. Axon collaterals from excitatory afferent fibers contact local interneurons. The additional synaptic delay compared to direct afferent excitation onto principal cells provides a time-dependent sequence of excitation and inhibition from single afferent inputs. *B.* Feedback inhibition. Axon collaterals from local principal cells contact local interneurons, providing a period of inhibition of principal cell activity following the generation of an output. Interneuron populations involved in *A* and *B* are not always mutually exclusive.

C. Recurrent excitation. Axon collaterals from local principal cells also contact other local principal cells, providing an excitatory mechanism for concerted, temporally coordinated population output. *D.* Mutual inhibition. Some interneuron subtypes contact other interneurons as well as principal cells, and some interneurons contact other interneurons exclusively. This pattern of connectivity can serve to impart spatiotemporally coordinated patterns of excitation and inhibition in the local circuit leading to rhythm generation. Filled circles, excitatory synapses; open circles, inhibitory synapses.

contain α5 subunits are enriched in the dendritic regions of the hippocampal subfields and therefore are associated with distinct presynaptic sources, such as the class of dendrite-targeting bistratified cells (Sperk et al., 1997; Thomson et al., 2000). Conversely, α1 and α2 subunits containing GABA$_A$ receptors predominate in the perisomatic domain of pyramidal neurons (Nusser et al., 1996; Nyiri et al., 2001). Those receptor complexes with an α2 subunit are primarily found on the axon initial segment and are, by default, associated with presynaptic terminals of axo-axonic cells, which provide the near-exclusive innervation of this neuronal compartment. The somata of pyramidal neurons, the postsynaptic target of basket cells, are decorated with both α1 and α2 subunit-containing GABA$_A$ receptors (Nusser et al., 1996). Interestingly, there is an even greater refinement of the input-specific recep-

tor distribution, as α1-containing receptors are matched with the terminals of parvalbumin-positive basket cells, whereas those with an α2 subunit are associated with synapses established by CCK-positive basket cells (Nyiri et al., 2001).

Apart from the domain-specific distribution of GABA$_A$ receptor α subunits, there is also evidence of remarkably selective expression across cell classes. Immunocytochemical double-labeling studies have revealed that all parvalbumin- and most NPY-positive interneurons express GABA$_A$ receptor α1 subunits, whereas calbindin-, vasoactiveinhibitory peptide (VIP)-, and CCK-containing neurons are immunonegative for α1 (Gao and Fritschy, 1994). In view of the different molecular pharmacology of GABA$_A$ receptors containing, for example, α1, α2, or α5 subunits, it is thus likely that specific inhibitory microcircuits are differentially modulated by those allosteric modulators of GABA$_A$ receptors that show a subunit-dependent pharmacological profile. Indeed, paired recordings from identified interneurons in the CA1 area have shown that IPSPs mediated by bistratified cells were not enhanced by zolpidem, a benzodiazepine type 1 agonist requiring an α1 subunit. However, they were powerfully enhanced by diazepam, which is consistent with evidence that these synapses are associated with α5 subunit–containing GABA$_A$ receptors (Thomson et al., 2000). Conversely, and as predicted, zolpidem potentiated the IPSPs mediated by fast-spiking basket cells.

Some classes of glutamate receptors are also distributed nonrandomly. Although the GluR1 subunit of α-amino-3-hydroxy-5-methyl-4-isoxazolepropionate (AMPA) receptors seems fairly evenly dispersed (Molnar et al., 1993), GluR2 subunits are lacking in interneurons (Leranth et al., 1996), giving interneuronal AMPA receptors a significant permeability for calcium (Burnashev et al., 1992) (see Chapters 6, 7, and 10). Metabotropic glutamate receptors also show a highly specific distribution. For example, mGluR1a-containing receptors are enriched in somatostatin-containing O-LM cells (Baude et al., 1993). These cells, along with other horizontal interneurons with cell bodies in the stratum oriens, appear to be the only class of hippocampal interneurons that exclusively mediate feedback inhibition (Blasco-Ibanez and Freund, 1995; Maccaferri and McBain, 1995).

Just as for GABA$_A$ and glutamate receptors, there is a similar degree of specificity in the expression of receptors that mediate responses of ascending modulatory fiber tracts, among them the cholinergic and serotoninergic systems. With respect to the latter, the subpopulation of GABAergic CCK-positive basket cells express high levels of ionotropic serotonin (5HT)-3 receptors (Morales et al., 1998). Likewise, metabotropic 5HT-2 receptors are enriched in GABAergic interneurons (Morilak et al., 1994). A similar picture is beginning to emerge with respect to the distribution of cholinergic receptor subtypes. For example, fast postsynaptic nicotinic responses have been recorded in GABAergic interneurons but are absent in pyramidal neurons (Jones and Yakel, 1997; Alkondon et al., 1998; Frazier et al., 1998), suggesting that nicotinic cholinergic responses are mediated indirectly via changes in interneuronal activity. However, more recent evidence has shown that nicotinic receptors on glutamatergic terminals may serve to modulate plastic changes at excitatory synapses (Fabian-Fine et al., 2001; Ge and Danni, 2005). Muscarinic acetylcholine receptors may also show a high degree of specificity in their expression patterns. Postsynaptic m2 receptors, for example, are predominantly found in a subset of GABAergic interneurons, whereas at the presynaptic level m2 receptors are enriched in the perisomatic terminals of basket and axo-axonic cells (Hajos et al., 1998).

As yet, too little is known about the precise cellular and subcellular distribution of most hippocampal neurotransmitter receptor systems to extract any general functional and/or organizational principles. The examples listed above provide no more than a sketchy picture. Hopefully, with the use of single-cell polymerase chain reaction (PCR) and subunit-specific antisera, a complete description may disclose clearer rules that govern the cell type-specific and/or circuit-specific distribution of receptor proteins.

8.1.6 Convergence and Divergence

In common with neocortical areas, the hippocampal formation is characterized by a high degree of neuronal interconnectivity. This is due to a multitude of converging inputs and diverging outputs; that is, an individual neuron is generally targeted by multiple afferents (convergence), whereas the efferent output of a single neuron contacts multiple postsynaptic target neurons (divergence). A hippocampal neuron may receive several thousand synaptic contacts that originate from distant brain areas (e.g., the septum or entorhinal cortex) or, conversely, arise from neighboring excitatory and/or inhibitory local-circuit neurons (Buhl et al., 1994a; Freund and Buzsaki 1996). In turn, hippocampal principal and interneurons give rise to extensive axonal systems that arborize locally and/or project to distant, extrahippocampal targets.

Using light-microscopic bouton counts and correlated electron microscopy, it is possible to determine the degree of divergence of individual hippocampal neurons (Halasy et al., 1996). Such estimates indicate that most hippocampal interneurons contact well in excess of 500 postsynaptic target neurons. In addition, it has been estimated that approximately 25 basket cells may innervate a single pyramidal neuron (Buhl et al., 1994a). This massive divergence of inhibitory axons and convergence of multiple inhibitory neuronal inputs onto single pyramidal cells underpins the ability of GABAergic neurons to synchronize hippocampal population activity.

8.2 Dentate Gyrus

Granule cells are the principal neuronal type of the dentate gyrus. Their sole efferent projection, the mossy fiber pathway, forms the second link of the so-called tri-synaptic loop by targeting CA3 pyramidal cells. Granule cells also form connections with interneurons, mossy cells (excitatory neurons in the hilus) and, in some epilepsy models, other granule cells (Dashtipour et al., 2002). Thus, within the dentate gyrus, granule cells may function as elements in circuits generating feedforward and feedback inhibition as well as homo- and heterogeneous recurrent excitatory circuits.

8.2.1 Inputs to the Dentate Gyrus

There is, as yet, little evidence for target cell specificity of excitatory inputs to the dentate granule cells. However, there is abundant evidence for subcellular domain specificity. The main perforant path input to the dentate gyrus from entorhinal stellate cells targets the distal apical dendrites of granule cells, whereas commissural/associational fibers innervate the

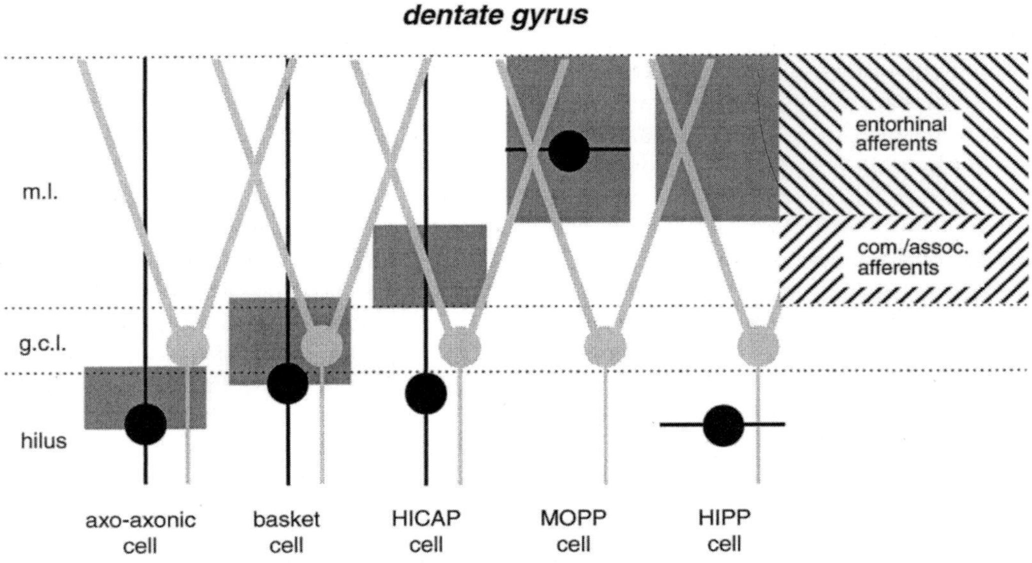

dentate gyrus

Figure 8–2. Basic organization of interneuron output fields in the dentate gyrus. Subcellular domain specificity of dendrite-targeting interneurons co-organizes with afferent inputs. M.l., molecular layer; G.c.l., granule cell layer; HICAP, hilar commissural/associa-tion pathway-associated interneuron; MOPP, molecular layer perforant path-associated interneuron; HIPP, hilar perforant path-associated interneuron. Shaded regions mark the axonal arbors for each cell type.

proximal dendrites (Blackstad 1958; Buhl and Dann, 1991; Deller et al., 1996). This target domain specificity is precisely reflected in the preferred interneuron targets for these dentate gyrus inputs (Fig. 8–2). MOPP (molecular layer perforant path-associated) cells receive excitatory inputs only from the perforant path projection; there is no recurrent feedback from innervated granule cells. HIPP (hilar perforant path-associated) cells also receive inputs from the perforant path, whereas HICAP (hilar commisural/association pathway-associated) cells receive external inputs from the commissural/association pathway (Han et al., 1993).

Other afferent input pathways also show some degree of specificity. The submammillary projection forms a dense plexus of axons in the border regions of the granule and molecular layer (Magloczky et al., 1994). In addition, the noradrenergic inputs from the locus coeruleus appear to target areas receiving mossy fiber input—the hilus and stratum lucidum of area CA3 (Loy et al., 1980; Oleskevich et al., 1989). In terms of neuronal subtypes, the serotoninergic raphe–hippocampal projection demonstrates the highest degree of target cell specificity. One part forms large synaptic boutons that form synapses predominantly with GABAergic interneurons, avoiding principal cells (Halasy et al., 1992). Within this group of interneurons there is specificity for distinct subsets.

The serotoninergic input preferentially targets calbindin-, calretinin-, somatostatin-, and neuropeptide Y-containing cells (i.e., those with an efferent target profile for the dendritic domain of principal neurons) (Miettinen and Freund, 1992). In contrast, the other part of the raphe projection conforms to the notion of modulatory inputs exerting a diffuse action (as with septal projections). Most transmitter-containing boutons in this part of the raphe projection (> 75%) do not appear to make synaptic specializations and show no obvious domain-specific innervation patterns or association with particular target cells (Oleskevich et al., 1991).

8.2.2 Granule Cell Projection to Area CA3

Granule cell axons aggregate in a distinct bundle of unmyelinated axons above the CA3 pyramidal cell layer, termed the stratum lucidum because of its characteristic light-microscopic appearance. Here they form three distinct types of synaptic terminal: the large en passant mossy boutons (4–10 μm), filopodial extensions of large mossy boutons (0.5-2.0 μm), and smaller en passant-type terminals (0.5–2.0 μm) (Acsady et al., 1998). The characteristic mossy terminals exclusively innervate hilar mossy cells and CA3 pyramidal neurons, forming a multitude (30–40) of synaptic junctions (release sites) with a single thorny excrescence on each innervated CA3 or hilar neuron (Chicurel and Harris, 1992). Conversely, filopodial extensions and en passant-type terminals selectively target hilar and CA3 area interneurons (Acsady et al., 1998). The total number of mossy terminals along the trajectory of completely labeled granule cell axons is relatively small (10-18), and it has been suggested that a single granule cell may contact no more than 11 to 15 CA3 pyramidal cells and a somewhat smaller number of hilar mossy cells (Acsady et al., 1998). Thus, in contrast to other cortical areas, there appears to be only a modest degree of excitatory convergence and divergence in the mossy fiber output. Moreover, due to the low firing probability of granule cells in vivo (Jung and McNaughton, 1993) the statistical likelihood of coincident activity among afferent inputs to a single target neuron seems relatively low. In addition, single spike transmission at the mossy fiber synapse is also rare, whereas transmission in response to spike trains in granule cells is robust (Geiger and Jonas, 2000; Henze et al., 2002).

8.2.3 Granule Cell–Interneuron Connections

In the CA3 area granule axons do not appear to display a preference for particular subtypes of GABAergic interneurons (Acsady et al., 1998). Thus, they make contact with substance P receptor-containing interneurons, interneurons positive for mGluR1a (a marker for somatostatin-containing interneurons with a dendritic innervation pattern, among them O-LM cells in the CA areas), and parvalbumin-labeled interneurons, which innervate the perisomatic region of their target cells. They do, however, contact, via en passant or filopodial terminals, interneurons in considerably larger numbers than pyramidal neurons; and it has been estimated that, compared to other cortical principal cells, granule cells innervate GABAergic targets ~10 times more frequently. The smaller mossy terminals on interneurons typically establish no more than a single synaptic release site (Acsady et al., 1998). Therefore, the substantially greater degree of mossy fiber convergence onto GABAergic neurons appears to be counterbalanced by a comparatively lower strength of unitary connections. It must be emphasized, however, that in general the absolute strength (in terms of amplitude and/or conductance) and kinetics of unitary granule cell-to-interneuron connections are comparable to pyramidal-to-interneuron connections in other hippocampal regions (Miles, 1990; Scharfman et al, 1990; Gulyas et al., 1993a,b; Buhl et al., 1994a,b; Geiger et al., 1997; Ali and Thomson, 1998; Ali et al., 1998).

As yet, relatively little is known with respect to putative differences in the innervation of dentate interneurons. Such differences are apparent in the hippocampal CA1 area (Ali and Thomson, 1998; Ali et al., 1998); and based on their dendritic architecture it seems reasonable to assume that certain subtypes of dentate gyrus interneurons, such as those with their dendritic arbor restricted to the outer two-thirds of the molecular layer (MOPP cells) (Han et al., 1993), are unlikely to receive a significant degree of recurrent excitatory granule cell input. In contrast, others, such as a class of interneurons that have their dendrites largely confined to the hilar region (HIPP cells) (Han et al., 1993), are predisposed to mediate recurrent input from granule cell collaterals. Indeed, their neurochemical equivalent, mGluR1a-containing neurons, have been shown to receive granule cell synapses, whereas it has been demonstrated in the CA1 area that their counterparts, mGluR1a/somatostatin-containing O-LM cells, are exclusively innervated by recurrent collaterals of CA1 pyramidal neurons (Blasco-Ibanez and Freund, 1995; Maccaferri and McBain, 1995).

8.2.4 Interneuron–Granule Cell Connections

Dentate interneurons all release the amino acid transmitter GABA. However, beyond this unifying characteristic, they constitute a heterogeneous class of neurons. Dentate interneurons differ with respect to their content of neuropeptides, calcium-binding proteins, and somatodendritic architecture as well as their axonal arborization pattern (Freund and Buzsaki, 1996). The latter feature in particular has been a useful guide to subdividing hippocampal interneurons into distinct subclasses.

The advent of intracellular labeling techniques has facilitated the near-complete visualization of interneurons, revealing axonal arbors with highly complex but distinct ramification patterns. As in all other hippocampal areas, several classes of GABAergic interneurons target distinct domains of their postsynaptic target neurons. Thus, axo-axonic cells, frequently referred to as chandelier cells, have an absolute target preference for the initial segment of granule and mossy cells (Somogyi et al., 1985; Han et al., 1993; Halasy and Somogyi, 1993; Buhl et al., 1994b). A specific example of this target preference for granule cells is shown in Figure 8–3C. In contrast, basket cells direct their efferent output toward the somata (78%) and proximal dendrites (22%) of granule cells (Halasy and Somogyi, 1993). Whereas these two types of interneuron appear to account for most of the inhibitory synapses in the perisomatic region, the axonal arbors of several other interneuron classes occupy distinct strata in the dentate molecular layer, innervating either proximal or distal segments of postsynaptic dendrites (Halasy and Somogyi, 1993; Han et al., 1993). Interestingly, as we have seen (Fig. 8–2), the target zones of these GABAergic axons overlap with the laminar distribution of the major excitatory pathways. Axons of the HICAP cells co-stratify with the commissural/associational afferents in the inner third of the dentate molecular layer, as demonstrated in Figure 8–4 (lower neuron), whereas two additional classes of dendrite-targeting neuron, HIPP and MOPP cells, innervate the outer two-thirds of the molecular layer, co-laminating with the perforant path input, as shown in Figure 8–4 (Han et al., 1993). It thus appears that distinct types of neuron have evolved that selectively and locally modulate the dendritic integration of a distinct set of glutamatergic afferents. Interestingly, this division of labor is even more refined, as those interneuron classes with overlapping terminal fields, such as HICAP and axo-axonic cells (Fig. 8–3), are further specialized to participate in feedforward or feedback inhibitory microcircuits, respectively (Han et al., 1993). However, other types of dendrite-targeting neurons show no apparent laminar preference (Soriano et al., 1993).

Although only a small number of dentate interneurons, such as somatostatin-positive cells, have a long-range commissural projection (Bakst et al., 1986; Schwerdtfeger and Buhl, 1986; Sik et al., 1997), virtually all of those that do have extensive axonal arbors (Han et al., 1993; Buckmaster and

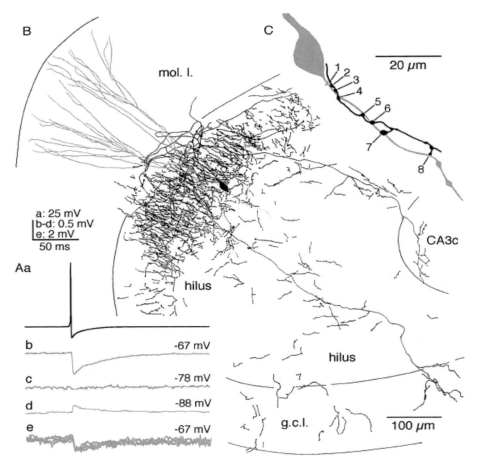

Figure 8–3. Pattern of axo-axonic cell axonal arborization. *A.* Action potential in an axo-axonic cell (*Aa*) generates a short-latency IPSP in a granule cell (*Ab*) with reversal potential around -80 mV (*Ac–e*). *B.* Axon of the axo-axonic cell innervates the granule cell layer, the hilus, and the tip of area CA3c. *C.* Location of eight synaptic junctions on the initial axonal segments of a granule cell whose responses are shown in *Ab-e.* (*Source*: Adapted from Buhl et al., 1994a, with permission.)

Schwartzkroin, 1995a,b; Sik et al., 1997). Individual axons have been shown to ramify extensively, filling both dentate blades and extending in excess of 3 mm along the septo-temporal axis (Sik et al., 1997). Although it appears that interneurons generally establish more than a single synaptic junction with a target neuron, the total number of release sites appears to be relatively small. In one instance, correlated light and electron microscopic analysis of a synaptically connected axo-axonic-to-granule cell pair revealed a total of eight sites of membrane apposition with an equivalent number of synaptic release sites that mediated the unitary interaction (Buhl et al., 1994a), with other light microscopic estimates being in a similar range. Because the granule cell axon initial segment received an additional 40 unlabeled synapses, it is—in view of the virtually exclusive innervation of this target domain by axo-axonic cells—reasonable to assume a convergence factor in the range of six. Clearly, however, there are too few data to extract any general rules as, for example, in one instance 36 VIP-positive boutons originating from a single axon collateral were counted on a single spiny substance P-positive dendrite in the hilus (Sik et al., 1997).

The relatively low number of interneurons and the modest number of release sites that characterize unitary connections are in stark contrast to estimates of the total bouton number established by individual GABAergic axons, ranging from approximately 10,000 to 75,000 (Sik et al., 1997). Accordingly, these data suggest a large degree of synaptic divergence, with individual interneurons occupying a large volume fraction of an entire hippocampus, perhaps in the range of 25%, and innervating up to 10,000 postsynaptic target neurons. Conversely, unitary inhibitory interactions appear to be relatively weak (Scharfman et al., 1990; Buhl et al., 1994a). Electron microscopic studies of individual biocytin-labeled axons consistently show a greater number and/or density of unlabeled inhibitory terminals converging on postsynaptic target structures, suggesting that several neurons of a given type converge on a postsynaptic neuron. It therefore appears that at least some of the GABAergic circuitry in the dentate gyrus is laid out to affect information processing at highly specific sites, such as dendritic segments, but generally at the level of neuronal populations it simultaneously affects several thousands of target cells.

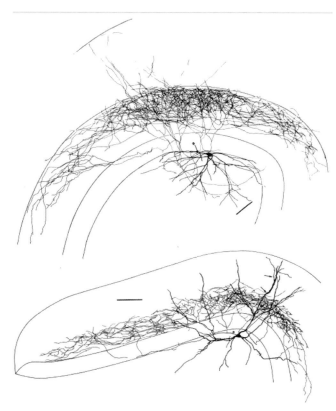

Figure 8–4. Domain specificity of axons in the dentate gyrus. Upper neuron: Reconstruction of a HIPP cell illustrating axonal fields closely associated with the distal granule cell dendritic termination zone for perforant path inputs from the entorhinal cortex. Bar = 0.1 mm. Lower neuron: Reconstruction of a HICAP cell demonstrating an axonal field distribution different from that of the HIPP cell. In this case the HICAP cell axonal field was associated with the proximal dendritic termination zone associated with commissural and associational pathways. Bar = 0.1 mm. (*Source*: Adapted from Han et al., 1993, with permission.)

8.2.5 Granule Cell–Local Excitatory Neuron Connections

Apart from dentate and CA3 interneurons, granule cells also innervate hilar mossy cells, both with large mossy terminals, impinging on mossy cell thorny excrescences as well as smaller terminals, contacting conventional spines on mossy cell dendrites (Frotscher et al., 1991; Acsady et al., 1998). However, in contrast to principal cells in other hippocampal and cortical areas, granule cells in rodents do not establish recurrent excitatory feedback to themselves, perhaps owing to the spatial segregation of granule cell dendrites (rodent granule cells lack basal dendrites) and their axons, which do not enter the molecular layer. Only certain pathological conditions, such as temporal lobe epilepsy, favor aberrant sprouting of mossy fibers into the dentate molecular layer and the de novo formation of recurrent feedback loops. Interestingly, in adult rhesus monkeys and humans a sizable proportion of granule cells extend basal dendrites into the hilar region, thereby pro-

viding the spatial proximity of dendrites and recurrent axons that might be expected to encourage monosynaptic granule cell–granule cell synapses (Seress and Mrzljak, 1987; Buhl and Dann, 1991). However, whether and to what extent primate granule cells are interconnected—and if so, what consequences it would have for their processing capabilities—remains to be established. Moreover, it is, as yet, unclear whether there is an archetypical mammalian blueprint for the dentate gyrus microcircuit and whether primates or rodents conform more closely to this ancestral blueprint.

8.2.6. Interneuron–Interneuron Connections

With the notable exception of axo-axonic cells, which exclusively innervate excitatory principal cells, the other interneuron types described above appear to have no particularly bias for a specific type of target neuron, innervating both principal neurons and interneurons (Sik et al., 1997). Immunocytochemical data, however, suggest an additional class of interneurons that are specialized to innervate other interneurons. A subpopulation of VIP-positive nonprincipal cells innervate substance P receptor-immunopositive hilar interneurons as their major postsynaptic target, and an additional subclass of VIP neurons with a projection to the molecular layer innervate several types of GABAergic neurons (Hajos et al., 1996). The functional role of these interneuron-targeting interneurons, which may include disinhibition or the synchronization of GABAergic networks, awaits experimental investigation.

8.3 Areas CA3 and CA1

The cornu ammonis is usually delineated into areas CA3 and CA1, with some researchers also distinguishing area CA2 (between area CA3 and CA1) (see Chapter 3). In the classic hippocampal trisynaptic circuit, activity is projected from the dentate gyrus (see Section 8.2) to CA3 and then from CA3 via Schaffer collaterals to CA1. However, direct input to areas CA3 and CA1 also originate from the entorhinal cortex, nucleus reuniens, and neuromodulatory regions (see below).

8.3.1 Inputs to CA3 and CA1

With one exception, the stratum radiatum giant cells (Gulyas et al., 1998), the principal neurons in the hippocampal subfields, constitute a relatively homogeneous population of glutamate-releasing pyramid-shaped neurons. In the CA1 and CA3 areas pyramidal neurons bear numerous spines, with estimates being as high as 30,000 (Bannister and Larkman, 1995; Trommald et al., 1995), and most of these spines receive a single excitatory synapse. Although single-cell-labeling studies indicate that all pyramidal neurons have a local axonal arbor, most excitatory synapses in the hippocampal subfields are of extraneous origin, arriving from a multitude of sources, such as a different hippocampal subfield, the contralateral hippocampus, the entorhinal cortex, the submammillary body (Magloczky et al., 1994), and the nucleus reuniens thalami (Wouterlood et al., 1990). More diffuse neuromodulatory inputs are seen from septal cholinergic axons (Frotscher and Lenrath, 1985; Lenrath and Frotsher, 1987) and interneuron-targeting raphe axons (Freund et al., 1990).

In contrast to the mossy fiber synapse(s) on the thorny excrescences of CA3 pyramidal neurons, the amplitude of unitary excitatory inputs to area CA1 is weak (< 2 mV) (Miles and Wong, 1986; Sayer et al., 1990; Malinow, 1991) and well below spike threshold. Although there are, as yet, no accurate estimates of the number of release sites at unitary connections established by an afferent excitatory axon, a wealth of indirect evidence suggests that the number of contact sites is small (see Chapters 3 and 6). First, the trajectory of incoming axons is often perpendicular to that of pyramidal dendrites, not dissimilar to the geometrical arrangement of parallel fibers and cerebellar Purkinje cells, thus decreasing the statistical likelihood of synaptic encounters on an individual target cell. Second, so-called single-fiber stimulation experiments generally yield low-amplitude responses, which are commensurate with the release of relatively few quanta of transmitter. These experiments involving paired recordings of CA3-to-CA1 pyramidal pairs (i.e., activation of a single Schaffer collateral) have revealed small-amplitude unitary excitatory responses, with quantal analysis providing evidence that the low quantal content was due to a small number of synaptic release sites rather than a low release probability (Sayer et al., 1990; Larkman et al., 1991; Malinow, 1991; Bolshakov and Siegelbaum, 1995). Synaptic CA3–CA1 responses have been attributed to as little as a single release site (e.g., Turner et al., 1997). Ultimately, however, correlated physiological and electron microscopic approaches are needed to resolve this important issue.

8.3.2 Pyramidal Cell–Interneuron Connections

Local connections between pyramidal neurons and interneurons form the physiological substrate for feedback inhibition in the hippocampal network. The efficacy of recurrent inhibition can be readily demonstrated, as action potentials in CA3 pyramidal neurons can frequently elicit IPSPs in neighboring pyramidal cells. These IPSPs are generated by the local network of inhibitory cells, which in turn have been synaptically activated by the excitatory feedback of the presynaptic pyramidal neuron. Accordingly, both $GABA_A$ and AMPA/kainate receptor antagonists are effective in abolishing disynaptic IPSPs (Miles, 1990). Apart from demonstrating the presence of inhibitory local feedback circuits, these data show that excitatory postsynaptic potentials (EPSPs) evoked by individual pyramidal neurons must be sufficiently strong to trigger action potentials reliably in postsynaptic interneurons. More direct evidence in support of this notion has been obtained with intracellular recordings of synaptically coupled pyramidal cell-to-interneuron pairs (Miles, 1990). These data show

that in such unitary interactions the probability of spike transduction can be as high as 60%, with mean EPSP amplitudes varying between 0.2 and 4.0 mV (Miles, 1990; Gulyas et al., 1993b). Similar values were reported for the CA1 area (Buhl et al., 1994a; Ali and Thomson, 1998; Ali et al., 1998). Multidisciplinary studies using paired recordings and post hoc correlated light and electron microscopic analysis demonstrate that pyramidal cell-to-interneuron connections in the CA3 and CA1 regions are generally established by one presynaptic bouton establishing no more than a single synaptic junction (Gulyas et al., 1993b; Buhl et al., 1994a). Quantal analysis of such interactions revealed a relatively high release probability (0.76) and, not surprisingly in view of the presumed small number of release sites, a sizable quantal amplitude (0.70 mV). Thus, it appears that a small number of synaptic junctions with a large quantal amplitude and a low failure rate, perhaps boosted by active dendritic conductance (Traub and Miles, 1995; Martina et al., 2000), is sufficient to guarantee relatively reliable spike transmission at pyramidal-to-interneuron connections.

Using paired recordings in conjunction with intracellular labeling techniques, at least three classes of interneurons have been conclusively identified as postsynaptic targets of local axon collaterals of pyramidal neurons: basket, bistratified, and O-LM cells (Gulyas et al., 1993b; Buhl et al., 1994a; Ali and Thomson, 1998; Ali et al., 1998). At least in the CA1 area, the overall probability of obtaining such a connection with paired recordings is substantially higher than that for pyramidal cell pairs. Moreover, there are marked differences depending on the type of postsynaptic interneuron. Thus, the probability of obtaining a pyramidal-to-basket cell connection is in the range of 1:22; that of finding a pyramidal-to-bistratified cell pair is 1:7; and pyramidal cell-to-O-LM cell interactions are most readily encountered (1:3) (Ali et al., 1998). Although, as a general rule, physiological estimates from paired recordings are prone to some degree of experimental bias, these differences appear to be sufficiently clear-cut to suggest not only that pyramidal neurons in the CA1 area have a marked target preference for inhibitory interneurons, but that there is a distinct bias toward favoring different subclasses of interneurons.

Hippocampal interneurons receive fewer excitatory synapses than principal neurons, with the numbers varying considerably depending on the class of cell (Gulyas et al., 1999). Parvalbumin-positive cells with a perisomatic efferent target profile (axo-axonic and basket cells) receive, on average, approximately 15,000 excitatory synapses, whereas the group of dendrite-targeting calbindin-positive interneurons (e.g., bistratified cells) receive in the range of 2600 excitatory inputs. The class of interneuron-targeting calretinin-positive interneurons are targeted by even fewer, in the order of 1700 excitatory synapses (Gulyas et al., 1999). Because it is unknown how many of the excitatory inputs to interneurons are from neighboring pyramidal neurons, it is not possible to calculate convergence factors for feedforward and recurrent pyramidal cells inputs. However, even if the proportion of recurrent inputs were as low as 10%, it (e.g., in the case of parvalbumin-positive cells) suggests that approximately 1500 neighboring pyramidal cells converge on a single interneuron. Accordingly, this conservative estimate suggests that the concomitant activity of no more than 1% of the local pyramidal cell population, with an average quantal amplitude of 0.7 mV, would be required to elicit 10 mV recurrent EPSPs in an interneuron. Thus, it seems likely that only a small fraction of feedforward and/or recurrent excitatory inputs is required to be simultaneously active (see below) to drive interneurons to their firing threshold.

It appears to be a general rule that EPSPs on hippocampal interneurons, regardless of whether they originate locally or in a different (hippocampal) brain area, have faster kinetic properties than excitatory inputs on principal neurons (Miles, 1990; Lacaille, 1991; Gulyas et al., 1993b; Buhl et al., 1994a, 1996; Ali and Thomson, 1998; Ali et al., 1998). There are several reasons for this: First, interneurons have comparatively short membrane time constants, in part due to their expression of Kv3 potassium channel subtypes (Lien and Jonas, 2003); second, active dendritic conductance may counterbalance the electrotonic slowing of synaptic potentials; third, the molecular composition of interneuronal AMPA receptors endows them with faster single-channel kinetics (Geiger et al. 1997); fourth, the contribution of an NMDA receptor-mediated component, which would slow EPSP kinetics, appears to be relatively small (Buhl et al., 1996). It is conceivable that all these factors act in unison to accelerate spiking in interneurons and thereby minimize the delay of disynaptic IPSPs, also explaining the well known observation that recurrent inhibition is effective in curtailing EPSPs evoked using electrical stimulation of afferent fibers. Moreover, fast EPSPs in interneurons improve the precision of spike timing by decreasing the temporal jitter of action potentials, a factor that is of considerable importance for the network activity during inhibition-based brain rhythms.

Excitatory unitary interactions in the adult hippocampus may show both frequency-dependent depression and facilitation of the postsynaptic response magnitude; that is, during repetitive presynaptic activity, successive action potentials elicit EPSPs with a gradually decremental or incremental amplitude (Miles and Wong, 1986; Miles, 1990; Deuchars and Thomson, 1996; Ali and Thomson, 1998; Ali et al., 1998). In general, unitary EPSPs in interneurons of the CA3 area show a greater tendency to facilitate, perhaps related to the greater propensity of CA3 neurons to fire bursts of action potentials. Moreover, evidence suggests that short-term plasticity of unitary excitatory connections may be target-dependent (i.e., determined by the postsynaptic neuron) (Ali and Thomson, 1998; Ali et al., 1998). The finding is particularly intriguing because what in essence is considered a presynaptic phenomenon is determined by the type of postsynaptic neuron. Thus, upon repetitive activation, the unitary responses evoked by CA1 pyramidal cells in CA1 basket and bistratified cells invariably exhibit gradual depression of their amplitudes, whereas those evoked in O-LM cells strongly facilitate (Ali and Thomson, 1998; Ali et al., 1998). The biophysical proper-

ties of the target cell may also affect the integration of unitary synaptic potentials, determining, for example, whether successive events will show response summation, thereby leading to an overall amplitude increase of the compound potential despite the fact that the input may show frequency-dependent depression. Because of their brief membrane time constants, unitary EPSPs in hippocampal interneurons generally show modest, if any, response summation, even with brief interevent intervals, whereas EPSPs evoked in pyramidal cells exhibit an incremental increase of the compound potential (Miles, 1990). Accordingly, pyramidal cells are often viewed as integrators (i.e., their output reflects the sum of inputs), whereas interneurons have been termed coincidence detectors, as their activation is strongly dependent on the temporal coherence of their inputs, showing only a significant degree of response summation with (near) synchronous inputs (Konig et al., 1996).

8.3.3 Interneuron–Pyramidal Cell Connections

As is the case in the dentate gyrus, a variety of intracellular labeling studies have provided evidence that GABAergic interneurons in the CA1 and CA3 regions are morphologically diverse and can be classified with respect to their laminar position, somatodendritic morphology, and most importantly efferent connectivity (Gulyas et al., 1993a,b; Buhl et al., 1994a,b, 1995; McBain et al., 1994; Sik et al., 1994, 1995; Halasy et al., 1996; Vida et al., 1998; Vida and Frotscher, 2000; but see Parra et al., 1998). A general scheme for interneuronal connectivity is illustrated in Figure 8–5 (compare with Fig. 8–2). Although there are region-specific variations, it appears that the fundamental principles in the organization of interneuron microcircuitry are similar in all hippocampal regions and indeed in all cortical areas (Somogyi et al., 1998). Thus, axoaxonic and basket cells in the CA1 and CA3 subfields target the perisomatic domain, with the former almost exclusively innervating the axon initial segment of principal cells and the latter forming synapses on somata and proximal dendrites (Gulyas et al., 1993a,b; Buhl et al., 1994a,b, 1995). Likewise, several classes of dendrite-targeting interneurons have their axonal arbor co-laminating with afferent excitatory inputs. The axons of bistratified cells in the CA1 area co-stratify with the Schaffer collateral/commissural input (Buhl et al., 1994b). The remarkable delineation of axonal fields between perisomatic targeting (basket cell) and dendrite targeting (e.g., bistratified) interneurons is illustrated in Figure 8–6. O–LM cells in both hippocampal subfields selectively innervate the perforant path termination zone in the stratum lacunosum-moleculare (Gulyas et al., 1993a,b; McBain et al., 1994); and mossy fiber-associated interneurons have their axons restricted to the stratum lucidum of the CA3 region and, as the name suggests, have been proposed to modulate selectively the granule cell output to the CA3 region (Vida and Frotscher, 2000). As in the dentate gyrus, more than a single type of interneuron may be associated with a particular pathway, such as OL-M cells and perforant-path associated interneurons at the stratum radia-

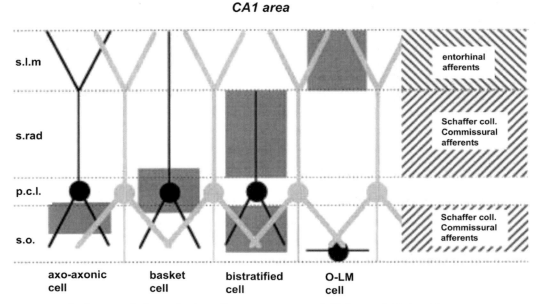

Figure 8–5. Basic anatomical organization of interneuron output fields in area CA1. As with the dentate gyrus, dendrite-targeting interneurons show a great deal of specificity when associating with termination fields for afferent inputs of differing anatomical origin. S.l.m., stratum lacunosum moeculare; S.rad., stratum radiatum; Pc.l., pyramidal cell layer; S.o., stratum oriens; O-LM cell, oriens-lacunosum moleculare cell.

Figure 8–6. Compartmental target specificity for interneurons in area CA1. Left-hand neuron: Axonal and dendritic arborizations of a bistratified neuron demonstrating the near absence of input to perisomatic compartments but dense arborization in the stratum radiatum and the stratum oriens (associated with Schaffer collateral commissural afferents). Right-hand neuron: Axonal and dendritic arborizations for a basket cell illustrating the high precision of axons for the perisomatic compartments and complete absence of projections to dendritic fields. Bar = 0.1 mm.

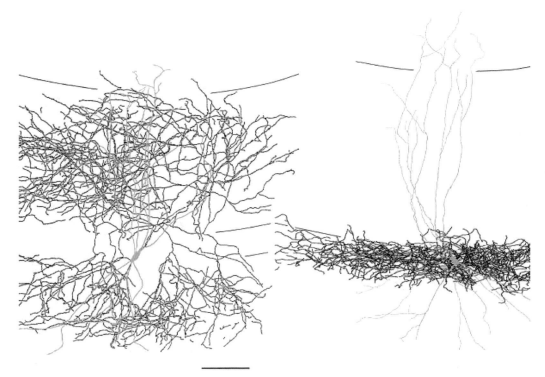

tum/lacunosum-moleculare border (Vida et al., 1998). However, their dendritic architecture suggests that interneurons with a similar efferent target profile may be preferentially involved in either feedforward or recurrent inhibitory microcircuits. Indeed, for O-LM cells compelling anatomical and physiological data show that they exclusively mediate recurrent inhibition onto pyramidal cells (Blasco-Ibanez and Freund, 1995; Maccaferri and McBain, 1995). Again, as in the dentate gyrus, there may be input selectivity for at least some of those interneurons involved in feedforward inhibitory circuits. For example, in view of their dendritic architecture, bistratified cells presumably receive commissural/associational afferents and are less likely to process a significant proportion of direct entorhinal input (Halasy et al., 1996).

Interneurons in the CA3 and CA1 subfields have axonal arbors of varying size. Neurogliaform and O-LM cells have the most compact axonal arbors (Gulyas et al., 1993a,b; Sik et al., 1995; Ali and Thomson, 1998; Vida et al., 1998), generally spanning less than 1 mm, whereas axo-axonic, basket, bistratified, and trilaminar cells have considerably larger axonal trees, with in vivo estimates for basket cell axon arbors being in the range of 1 mm, approximately 2 mm for a bistratified cell, and about 2.5 mm for a trilaminar interneuron (Sik et al., 1995). The available evidence suggests that axonal arbors tend to be relatively symmetrical in all hippocampal planes. Moreover, apart from having extensive local axonal arbors, several types of hippocampal interneuron have extra-areal projections. Axons of perforant path-associated interneurons in the CA1 area cross the hippocampal fissure and spread into the outer molecular layer of the dentate gyrus (Vida et al., 1998). Back-projecting cells in the CA1 region appear to have even larger axonal arbors, extending throughout all hippocampal subfields (Sik et al., 1994); and a subset of GABAergic calbindin-positive interneurons with an as yet unknown morphology project to the medial septum (Toth and Freund, 1992).

Electron microscopic data show that individual terminal boutons of most hippocampal interneurons usually establish a single synaptic junction per bouton, although occasionally a double junction is seen (Buhl et al., 1994a,b, 1995; Halasy et al., 1996; Vida et al., 1998). Thus, light-microscopic bouton counts are generally thought to be a reasonable approximation of the total number of synaptic contact sites established by a single inhibitory axon. Such estimates for a variety of interneurons labeled in vitro, among them basket, axo-axonic, neurogliaformand bistratified cells as well as Schaffer collateral and perforant path-associated interneurons, are consistently above 5000 and can be as high as ~13,000 (Gulyas et al., 1993a,b) (Halasy et al., 1996, Miles et al., 1996; Vida et al., 1998). Not surprisingly, in vivo estimates are substantially higher, approximately twofold, with basket cell axons having bouton counts up to 12,000 (Sik et al., 1995). Likewise, bouton counts for individual bistratified, trilaminar, and O-LM-cells were in the range of 15,000 (Sik et al., 1995). However, despite the large total number of boutons per axon, relatively few are associated with individual postsynaptic target neurons, providing further anatomical evidence for the divergent nature of inhibition (see Section 8.1.6). Correlated light and electron microscopic analysis of unitary inhibitory interactions revealed that hippocampal basket cells establish 2 to 12 synaptic junctions, whereas dendrite-targeting interneurons (e.g., bistratified cells) form 5 to 17 contacts with an individual pyramidal neuron (Buhl et al., 1994a,b; Miles et al., 1996; Tamas et al., 1997). Although there are relatively few published examples with electron microscopic counts of unitary release site numbers, several light microscopic estimates obtained from O-LM, bistratified, Schaffer collateral-associated, and axo-axonic cells confirm the above data (Gulyas et al., 1993a,b; Vida et al., 1998; Maccaferri et al., 2000). Thus, it seems reasonable to assume that the efferent output of most hippocampal interneurons distributes onto approximately 1000 to 2000 target neurons.

Connectivity estimates of hippocampal neurons have been obtained with paired recordings. On average, CA1 basket cells contact approximately 22% of pyramidal neurons within the confines of their axonal arbor, with the connection probability dropping from 54% for immediate neighbors to 5% for longer-range connections (Ali et al., 1999). Although there is an inevitable experimental bias with this approach, earlier quantitative anatomical data showed a surprising degree of agreement with estimates obtained from paired recording. Calculations based on pyramidal cell and basket cell terminal densities, taking an average number of synaptic release sites into account, suggest that CA1 basket cells contact approximately 28% of nearby target cells, with the connection probability plummeting to 4% toward the peripheral extent of the axonal arbor (Halasy et al., 1996).

Although it is probable that thousands of pyramidal cells converge on each inhibitory interneuron, for a number of reasons the convergence factors in the reciprocal direction are substantially smaller. First, as pyramidal cells are innervated by many classes of GABAergic neurons, each subpopulation supplies no more than a fraction of the total GABAergic input. Accordingly, cell class-specific convergence factors are inversely related to the number of interneuron types. Second, pyramidal cells receive fewer inhibitory than excitatory inputs, although the exact ratio is unknown. Although there are currently no data on the number of inhibitory inputs onto dendrites, electron microscopic estimates suggest that pyramidal cell somata receive in the range of 120 synapses and axon initial segments in the range of 100 to 200 (Kosaka 1980; Buhl et al., 1994). Third, unitary inhibitory interactions are generally mediated by several synaptic release sites, as illustrated in Figure 8–7. Accordingly, current estimates suggest that approximately 25 basket cells and even fewer axo-axonic cells (2–10), converge on a single pyramidal neuron (Li et al., 1992; Buhl et al., 1994). It therefore follows that, in contrast to presynaptic pyramidal cell input, a disproportionately large fraction of inhibitory neurons (at least 10%) must be active during neuronal population activity. Rhythmic network oscil-

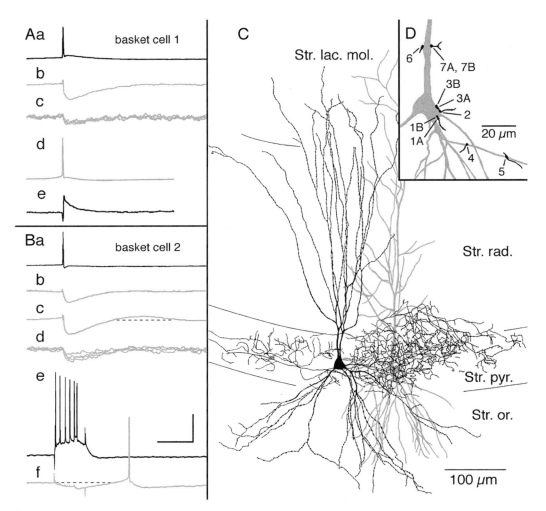

Figure 8–7. Basket cell morphology and effects on principal cells in area CA1. *A.* Single action potentials in basket cells (*Aa,d*) elicit short latency IPSPs in principal cells. Average of > 100 single IPSPs is shown in *Ab*, but individual IPSPs showed a great deal of amplitude variability (*Ac*). Hyperpolarization of pyramidal cells resulted in depolarizing IPSPs with a reversal potential, indicating a chloride-mediated event (*Ae*). *B.* Some IPSPs were followed by a distinct depolarizing membrane potential episode (*Bc*) that was sufficient to generate action potentials (*Be,f*). *C.* Axonal and dendritic fields of a single basket cell overlaid with a single target pyramidal neuron. Axon collaterals were limited to the perisomatic region. *D.* Expanded view of the pyramidal neuron somatic region showing 10 inhibitory synaptic connections. (*Source*: Adapted from Buhl et al., 1994a, with permission.)

lations, for example, require sustained GABAergic input from a specific source, such as fast perisomatic inhibition originating from basket or axo-axonic cells. Indeed, simultaneous multielectrode recordings of pyramidal cells and interneurons during rhythmic electroencephalographic (EEG) activity in the intact, behaving animal show that at least some interneurons fire considerably and consistently faster than neighboring pyramidal neurons, whereas others (e.g., the so-called anti-theta cells) may actually decrease their firing rate (Freund and Buzsaki, 1996).

Currently, our appreciation of the amazing morphological, neurochemical, and physiological complexity of GABAergic interneurons at the reductionist level contrasts with our relative lack of understanding of their functional role in the hippocampal network as a whole. There is a modest amount of

data illustrating the behavior of identified interneurons in the intact, behaving animal, showing, for example, phase-locked discharge of basket cells and O-LM cells during theta EEG activity (Buzsaki et al., 1983; Skaggs et al., 1996; Klausberger et al., 2003). A number of studies have attempted to address the functional role of interneurons at the cellular level. Paired interneuron-to-pyramidal cell recordings have revealed that all unitary inhibitory interactions have relatively fast kinetics and are (as yet without exception) mediated by GABA$_A$ receptors (Miles and Wong, 1983; Lacaille et al., 1987; Buhl et al., 1994a; 1995; Ouardouz and Lacaille, 1997; Vida et al., 1998; Thomson et al., 2000). In addition, the activation of GABA$_B$ receptors may either require high-frequency tetanic stimulation of a unitary inhibitory connection or, alternatively, the concomitant activation of multiple GABAergic inputs (Mody et al., 1994; Thomson and Destexhe, 1999). Although this may suggest overall uniformity in function, it is also clear that unitary hippocampal interactions differ with respect to the molecular composition and associated pharmacological properties of differentially distributed and domain-specific GABA$_A$ receptor subunits (Thomson et al., 2000). IPSPs evoked by fast-spiking basket cells are more potentiated by the α1 subunit-selective benzodiazepine zolpidem than are IPSPs elicited by regular-spiking basket cells. It has been proposed that fast-spiking basket cells are parvalbumin-positive and associated with postsynaptic receptors carrying an α1 subunit. Conversely, regular spiking basket cells may be the electrophysiological signature of CCK-positive basket cells and target perisomatic synapses with a predominance of GABA$_A$ receptors containing α2 subunits (Thomson et al., 2000). In addition, bistratified cells may be associated with dendritically located α5 subunits, and indeed bistratified cell-mediated unitary IPSPs are diazepam-sensitive but not zolpidem-sensitive (Thomson et al., 2000). Recent data from transgenic animals indicate that the molecular heterogeneity of GABA$_A$ receptors is indeed reflected in different functional roles, such as anxiety (Low et al., 2000). Moreover, work in intact animals suggests that neuroactive steroids may act as endogenous modulators to regulate the function of GABA$_A$ receptors with different subunit compositions differentially (Smith et al., 1998).

Apart from differences in their molecular pharmacology, the function of GABA$_A$ receptors may differ with their subcellular location. Because of the shunt and/or membrane polarization resulting from the opening of GABA$_A$ receptor channels, other domain-specific conductance may also be affected. Thus, unitary interactions mediated by dendrite-targeting interneurons, such as bistratified and O-LM cells, have slower kinetics and smaller amplitudes/conductance levels when measured at the level of the cell body. Some of this effect has been attributed to dendritic filtering (Buhl et al., 1994a,b; Miles and Freund, 1996; Maccaferri et al., 2000). Although there are, as yet, no compelling hippocampal data to demonstrate differences in the local versus somatic integration of compartmentalized excitatory and inhibitory inputs, there is at least evidence suggesting that domain-specific GABAergic inputs interact with local conductance. In the hippocampal CA3 area, microstimulation experiments have revealed that inhibitory inputs onto the dendrites of pyramidal neurons are effective in suppressing calcium-dependent spikes, and perisomatic inhibitory cells inhibit the repetitive discharge of sodium-dependent action potentials (Miles et al., 1996). However, the local interaction of unitary IPSPs and voltage-gated conductance can be even more complex. Basket and axo-axonic cells (i.e., interneurons with a perisomatic innervation pattern) have been shown to interact with intrinsic subthreshold membrane oscillations (Cobb et al., 1996). By resetting their phase, repetitive IPSPs originating from a single presynaptic interneuron are effective in phase-locking subthreshold oscillations, with the entrainment of oscillatory activity being most effective in the theta frequency band.

Moreover, as pyramidal neurons have a propensity to fire during the most depolarized part of the oscillatory waveform (Buhl et al., 1995), rhythmic unitary IPSPs are therefore also strikingly effective in pacing the discharge of postsynaptic pyramidal neurons—without, however, necessarily affecting the neuronal firing rate (Cobb et al., 1997). These authors demonstrated that the output from an individual interneuron not only may pace spontaneous action potential generation in multiple pyramidal cells but also synchronize these paced outputs, as shown in Figure 8–8. In view of the widespread divergence of basket and axo-axonic cell axons, it is reasonable to assume that the temporally coherent discharge of relatively few interneurons with a perisomatic termination pattern is sufficient to synchronize hippocampal population activity. Although they do not prove a causal relation, in vivo studies

Figure 8–8. Single IPSPs can synchronize ongoing pyramidal cell outputs. *A.* Overlaid responses from two concurrently recorded principal cells (PC1, PC2) receiving a single IPSP at the time illustrated by the arrow. Rebound from the IPSP generates action potentials in a time-dependent manner such that both pyramidal cells discharge within a small time window. *B.* Entrainment of theta-frequency pyramidal cell output by successive IPSPs from a single interneuron (*Bi*). Two pyramidal cells (PC1, PC2) were concurrently recorded and action potentials elicited in a single interneuron at times indicated by the arrows.. Cross correlations between the two pyramidal cells are shown before interneuron firing (*Bii*) and during (right-hand side) single, repetitive interneuron firing (*Biii*). (*Source*: From Cobb et al., 1995, with permission.)

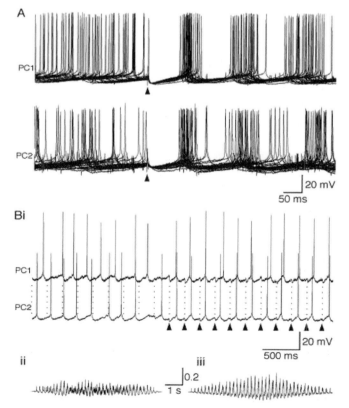

are clearly consistent with this notion, as they demonstrate a close temporal correlation of interneuron and principal cell activity during theta and gamma EEG activity (Bragin et al., 1995; Ylinen et al., 1995).

8.3.4 Pyramid–Pyramid Local Connections

In contrast to the dentate gyrus, principal neurons in the CA1 and CA3 subfields are interconnected with recurrent excitatory axon collaterals, thus increasing the computational complexity of local information processing. Pyramidal cells in the CA3 area are not only the source of major efferent fiber tracts, such as the Schaffer collateral pathway, they also give rise to several local axon collaterals, which emanate from the main axon in the stratum oriens. Axonal side branches branch further, with most of them remaining in the stratum oriens and the remainder penetrating the pyramidal cell layer and arborizing in the stratum radiatum (Gulyas et al., 1993a,b; Sik et al., 1993; Li et al., 1994). The terminal arbors in the CA3 area are generally large, frequently occupying several millimeters in the transverse and septo-temporal axis, indicating a large degree of divergence. Bouton counts of individual axons suggest that the number of hippocampal synaptic terminals is in the range of 10,000 to 60,000, with a sizable proportion remaining in the CA3 area. Quantitative studies suggest that CA3 pyramidal cells contact at least some of their postsynaptic targets randomly (i.e., in proportion to their occurrence in the neuropil) (Sik et al., 1993). Although there are no anatomical studies to provide reliable estimates with respect to pyramidal-to-pyramidal cell convergence, divergence, and number of synaptic release sites, physiological data provide evidence that CA3 pyramidal cells may be synaptically interconnected (Miles and Wong, 1986; Miles et al., 1996), with the connection probability of neighboring neurons being in the range of 2% (Miles and Wong, 1986). In general, unitary pyramidal-to-pyramidal cell EPSPs have small amplitudes, ranging between 1 and 2 mV, which fluctuate in amplitude and show apparent postsynaptic response failures, suggesting that they may be mediated by a small number of release sites (Miles and Wong, 1986). Thus, only a small proportion of unitary EPSPs (4%) are of sufficient strength to trigger action potentials in a postsynaptic neuron. Interestingly, however, when presynaptic pyramidal cells fire a salvo of several action potentials so as to mimic their physiological burst firing pattern, postsynaptic responses show a substantial degree of augmentation, and the incidence of burst-to-spike transduction can be as high as 35% (Miles and Wong, 1986). Indeed, experiments in disinhibited slices show that a single CA3 pyramidal neuron can trigger synchronous population discharges (Miles and Wong, 1983). Thus, despite the connection probability being relatively low, there is a sufficient degree of divergence and convergence to allow rapid, reliable synchronization of network activity.

As in area CA3, pyramidal neurons in the CA1 area emit local axon collaterals. The latter, however, establish smaller local axonal arbors and remain confined to the strata oriens and alveus, where they establish synaptic contacts with neigh-boring pyramidal cells and interneurons (Buhl et al., 1994a,b; Deuchars and Thomson, 1996; Ali and Thomson, 1998; Ali et al., 1998). The degree of pyramidal cell interconnectivity is approximately 1% and thus markedly lower than in the CA3 area (Deuchars and Thomson, 1996), which may also explain why the isolated CA1 area is less prone to develop seizure-like activity in the presence of GABA$_A$ receptor antagonists. Unitary responses tend to be relatively small (0.17–1.5 mV) and show paired-pulse depression, suggesting that a small number of synaptic release sites with a high release probability underlies the modest unitary responses. Indeed, correlated light and electron microscopic analysis of a single pyramidal-to-pyramidal cell pair showed that a unitary EPSP with a mean amplitude of 1.5 mV was mediated by a total of two synaptic release sites (Deuchars and Thomson, 1986). Both synaptic contacts were established on two third-order basal dendrites, suggesting that despite some degree of dendritic filtering even relatively distal excitatory quantal inputs can evoke measurable somatic responses.

8.3.5 Interneuron–Interneuron Connections

Reciprocally connected GABAergic interneurons comprise one of the key substrates for the generation of gamma frequency network oscillations. This finding has underscored the pivotal role of GABAergic neurons for the generation of EEG rhythms (Whittington et al., 1995). In principle, GABAergic inputs on hippocampal GABAergic neurons can be subdivided into three major categories.

- Extrinsic sources, particularly the septo-hippocampal GABAergic projection
- Output of interneurons, such as basket cells, which innervate principal cells and other interneurons in approximately random proportions
- Several subpopulations of interneurons that appear to have special, exclusive innervation of other interneurons

Regarding the septo-hippocampal GABAergic input, combined immunocytochemical and tracing studies have shown that, in contrast to the cholinergic input, this projection is highly selective in terms of targeting GABAergic interneurons, albeit with no apparent preference for particular subtypes (see Section 8.1.2) (Freund and Antal, 1988; Miettinen and Freund, 1992). The earlier in vivo observation that stimulation of the medial septum facilitates granule cell activity (Bilkey and Goddard, 1985) can be most parsimoniously explained by the inhibition of inhibitory interneurons (i.e., a disinhibitory mechanism). More direct evidence in support of this notion was obtained with a series of elegant in vitro experiments using a combined septo-hippocampal slice preparation (Toth et al., 1997), demonstrating a disinhibitory effect of septal stimulation on CA3 pyramidal cell activity. Thus, theta frequency activity in the medial septum diagonal band complex is likely to entrain hippocampal population activity by rhythmically releasing pyramidal neurons from a background of tonic inhibitory activity, thereby allowing them to fire while inhibition is maximally suppressed.

In contrast to the septal GABAergic projection, many interneurons in areas CA3 and CA1 target specific subcellular domains, but they appear to have no apparent specificity for innervating either principal cells or interneurons, contacting them in what has been referred to as a "quasi-random" fashion (i.e., based on the statistical distribution of postsynaptic elements in the neuropil) (Freund and Buzsaki, 1996). In the case of parvalbumin-positive basket cells, it has been estimated that they contact not only approximately 1500 pyramidal cells (see above) but also a proportionally smaller number (in the range of 60) parvalbumin-positive neurons (Sik et al., 1995). These anatomical data are corroborated by paired recordings of synaptically coupled and anatomically identified interneurons, revealing their divergent output to both excitatory and inhibitory neurons (Cobb et al., 1997; Ali et al., 1999). In addition, these studies not only demonstrate directly that basket cells are interconnected, they established the existence of synaptic coupling across interneuronal classes, such as between basket cells and trilaminar interneurons. Thus, the efferent output of basket cells not only directly (i.e., monosynaptically) affect inhibitory and excitatory hippocampal neurons, the output is likely to occur almost synchronously in all target neurons, an assumption with important implications for their putative role in hippocampal rhythmogenesis. Experimental findings and computational simulations provide compelling evidence for a synchronizing role of perisomatic fast IPSPs during gamma frequency network oscillations (Whittington et al., 1995; Wang and Buzsaki, 1996; Traub et al., 1997; Fisahn et al., 1998). It follows that the discharge of interneurons such as basket cells, with a widely divergent output, is phase-locked with the population rhythm, as they are the source of the phasic IPSPs (Andersen and Eccles, 1962). Indeed, in the awake rat the firing of putative interneurons is phase-locked to the underlying gamma rhythm (Bragin et al., 1995), and the discharge of identified basket cells was found to be temporally correlated with both gamma and theta activity (Ylinen et al., 1995). Despite the importance of GABAergic mechanisms for the generation of synchronous network behavior, it should be stressed that other synaptic as well as nonsynaptic factors, such as fast excitation and electrical coupling (see below), appear to have different but equally important roles in hippocampal rhythmogenesis (Traub et al., 1996, 2000; Fisahn et al., 1998; for a comprehensive review see Traub et al., 1999).

Unlike basket cells, a second major group of GABAergic interneurons, comprising at least three neurochemically distinct subclasses, exclusively innervate other GABAergic interneurons (for detailed review, see Freund and Buzsaki, 1996). These cells demonstrate that, in addition to subcellular domain specificity, interneurons may exhibit a high degree of target cell selectivity. The three subtypes are (1) a class of calretinin-positive neuron that innervates calbindin-positive dendrite-targeting cells, CCK/VIP-positive basket cells, and other calretinin-positive cells (Gulyas et al., 1996); (2) an interneuron-selective GABAergic cell that contains VIP and contacts calbindin-positive cells; and (3) a group of VIP-positive interneurons that show a preference for the soma-tostatin/mGluR-positive class of O-LM cells (Acsady et al., 1996a,b). It thus appears that distinct subsets of GABAergic interneurons selectively modulate the activity of several other types of interneuron, such as O-LM cells, which in turn have an efferent projection to the termination zone of entorhinal afferents in the stratum lacunosum-moleculare. Although a number of suggestions have been made as to their functional relevance there are, as yet, no experimental or modeling data to attribute specific functional roles to interneuron-selective interneurons during hippocampal information processing.

8.3.6 Gap Junction Connections

As already mentioned, during oscillatory network activity at gamma frequency, fast perisomatic IPSPs have a major role in pacing and synchronizing population activity. In view of their kinetics, however, experimental and computational data suggest that the upper limit of fast inhibition-based rhythms may not exceed ~80 Hz. Yet, in awake animals hippocampal sharp waves are accompanied by a high-frequency (~200 Hz) EEG oscillation with a high degree of spatiotemporal coherence (Buzsaki et al., 1992; Ylinen et al., 1995). As this ultrafast rhythm, frequently referred to as "ripples," is unlikely to be generated by phasic inhibition, it seems likely that a fundamentally different synchronizing mechanism is at work. Indeed, hippocampal slices maintain a fast ripple-like oscillatory activity pattern that remains after blockade of synaptic transmission but is abolished by a variety of gap junction uncoupling agents (Draguhn et al., 1998). Interestingly, gap junction blockers are also effective in abolishing pharmacologically induced gamma oscillations (Traub et al., 2000). It therefore appears that gap junction-mediated electrical coupling may have a strong role in the synchronization of gamma frequency oscillations as well as the generation of ultrafast neuronal population activity.

Gap junctions are the morphological correlate of electrical synapses, and anatomical studies have clearly demonstrated their presence in the adult mammalian hippocampus (Kosaka, 1983; Fukuda and Kosaka, 2000). Interestingly, however, these data have so far provided evidence for gap junctions only between the dendrites of GABAergic interneurons. There is compelling evidence for electrically coupled interneurons in the neocortex; and, intriguingly, these data also point to specific coupling between members of the same neuronal class (Galarreta and Hestrin, 1999; Gibson et al., 1999; Tamas et al., 2000). This may also apply for the hippocampus, where gap junctions have been identified between the dendrites of parvalbumin- and calretinin-positive interneurons (Gulyas et al., 1996; Fukuda and Kosaka, 2000), although these findings do not rule out the occurrence of heterologous connections.

Modeling studies have suggested that parameter heterogeneity in interneuronal circuits (e.g., differences in firing rates and/or kinetics of inhibitory conductance) destabilizes synchronous population activity (Wang and Buzsaki, 1996; White et al. 1998). However, when interneurons in such networks are interconnected with both chemical and electrical synapses (i.e., GABAergic synapses and gap junctions), their conjoint action tends to improve population coherence (White et al., 1998). Indeed, data from connexin36-deficient mice (a recently cloned neuronal gap junction-forming protein) (Condorelli et al., 1998) not only showed that GABAergic interneurons are electrically "uncoupled," they demonstrated that the presumed lack of gap junctions between interneurons results in impaired gamma frequency oscillatory network activity (Hormuzdi et al., 2001). With respect to the underlying mechanism, recordings of neocortical basket cell pairs showed an apparent synergistic effect of concurrent synaptic and nonsynaptic communication between interneurons (Fig. 8–9). With both mechanisms in place, action potential generation in one interneuron produced a biphasic membrane potential change in the coupled neuron: initial transient depolarization followed by IPSP-mediated hyperpolarization. Repeated action potential generation provided a powerful subthreshold membrane potential oscillation that influenced spike firing (Tamas et al., 2000).

Although this mechanism may account for establishing synchrony in the interneuronal network at gamma frequencies, it is unlikely to explain the generation of ultrafast ripple activity. Modeling studies suggest that when pyramidal cells are coupled by gap junctions in soma or dendrites the somatodendritic compartment, in conjunction with the gap junction, acts as a low-pass filter. The effect is to slow the kinetics of spikelets to such an extent that it is difficult, based on our current understanding of the biophysical properties of pyramidal neurons, to explain the emergence of ultrafast synchronous network activity (Draguhn et al., 1998; Traub and Bibbig, 2000). Moreover, despite numerous electron microscopic studies, there is, as yet, no ultrastructural evidence of gap junctions between the somatodendritic domain of hippocampal pyramidal neurons. However, putative axo-axonal gap junctions between pyramidal cells can allow spikes to produce either a spikelet in the postjunctional axon or, if above threshold, an action potential that may antidromically invade the parent cell body and/or rapidly propagate (provided there is a sufficient degree of interconnectivity) through the axonal plexus, thereby prompting the generation of coherent, ultrafast oscillatory activity as an emergent property of the axonal pyramidal network (Traub et al., 1999). These simulations indicate that as few as 2.5 to 3.0 gap junctions per axon may be sufficient, perhaps explaining why possible axo-axonal gap junctions have also gone unnoticed by anatomists. Indeed, intracellular labeling studies using time-lapse confocal microscopy have shown dye coupling between axons of hippocampal pyramidal neurons, thus providing experimental evidence for this notion (Schmitz et al., 2001). Moreover, electrophysiological studies have revealed the occurrence of spikelets in principal neurons following, for example, the antidromic activation of CA1 pyramidal cell axons (Kandel and Spencer, 1961; Taylor and Dudek, 1982; Schmitz et al., 2001). Ultimately, however, a more direct approach—such as paired recordings in conjunction with post hoc correlated

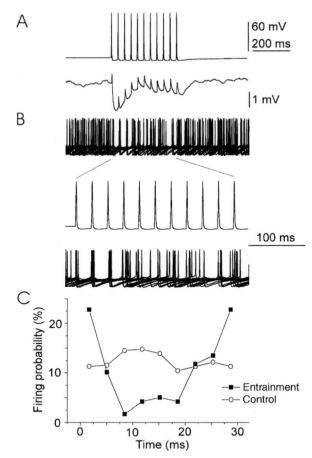

Figure 8–9. Synchrony via both gap junctional and IPSP-mediated interactions. *A.* Trains of presynaptic action potentials in one interneuron (top trace) generate a decrementing IPSP and spikelets in a connected interneuron (lower trace). *B.* Presynaptic action potential generation reduced the postsynaptic firing frequency and synchronized these action potentials with those from the presynaptic cell (bottom trace). *C.* Temporal correlation of postsynaptic firing probability in the postsynaptic cell during one action potential cycle in the presynaptic cell. Control condition is with no drive to either cell pair. Entrainment condition is as illustrated in *B.* (*Source*: Adapted from Tamas et al., 2000, with permission).

electron microscopy of the sites of interaction—is needed to resolve this intriguing issue.

8.4 Summary

Local circuits in the hippocampus are comprised of excitatory connections from principal cells to interneurons and mainly inhibitory interneuronal connections onto principal cells. A smaller number of connections are made up of mutual inhibitory interneuronal interconnectivity and recurrent excitatory connectivity between principal cells. The pattern of local connectivity is diverse and represents a rich tapestry of prospective strategies for modifying initial responses to inputs and post hoc responses to continued input activity on the basis of previously generated outputs.

The diverse profile of anatomical, pharmacological, and electrophysiological properties of local circuit connections can, to some extent, be reduced to a few basic properties. First, afferent activity invariably co-activates not only local principal cells but also local inhibitory interneurons. This organizing principle offers a mechanism by which any initial input can organize the response to any subsequent input, with the specific temporal profile being a consequence of the kinetics of interneuronal synaptic postsynaptic responses and their compartmental localization onto principal cells. Second, efferent activity also co-activates local inhibitory interneurons. There is some (but by no means complete) overlap between interneurons receiving feedforward and feedback signals. This organizing principle allows local circuits to modify responses to afferent activity further on the basis of whether an output is generated. Third, interconnectivity within either principal cell populations or local interneuron populations provides a mechanism by which spatially discrete patterns of input (and subsequent output) may influence populations of neurons outside the active area.

Taken together these three principles provide a form of architecture that seems unsuited to the classic notion of point-to-point neuronal communication. Instead, time appears to play a more critical role in governing neuronal output than space: Activation of feedforward circuits favors responses to inputs after a period of quiescence (governed by the duration of influence of feedforward inhibitory postsynaptic potentials). Activation of feedback circuits provides a further temporal constraint on subsequent outputs, effectively providing a short-term "history" of a local circuit's output. Convergence, divergence, and recurrent connectivity effectively spread these temporal influences spatially within the target neuronal population. If one considers the property of "bias" in principal neuronal responses to input (i.e., differences in afferent excitatory synaptic weights and/or tonic membrane potential heterogeneity), local circuit architecture can be seen to serve as an ideal mechanism by which to "read out" this bias as a specific pattern of outputs.

Local circuits of the type described in this chapter therefore provide a substrate for converting blanket (relatively unstructured) inputs into specific spatiotemporal profiles of output on the basis of the history of each principal neuron in the target population. Thus, a deeper insight into the role of the hippocampus as a region involved in aspects of learning and memory can be obtained by taking into account the organization of local patterns of neuronal interconnectivity.

ACKNOWLEDGMENTS

This work was conceived, and the first draft entirely written, by the late E.H. Buhl. Professor Buhl died during the revision of this chapter, and we dedicate it to his memory.

REFERENCES

Acsady L, Arabadzisz D, Freund TF (1996a) Correlated morphological and neurochemical features identify different subsets of vasoactive intestinal polypeptide-immunoreactive interneurons in rat hippocampus. *Neuroscience* 73:299–315.

Acsady L, Gorcs TJ, Freund TF (1996b) Different populations of vasoactive intestinal polypeptide-immunoreactive interneurons are specialized to control pyramidal cells or interneurons in the hippocampus. *Neuroscience* 73:317–334.

Acsady L, Kamondi A, Sik A, Freund T, Buzsaki G (1998) GABAergic cells are the major postsynaptic targets of mossy fibers in the rat hippocampus. *J Neurosci* 18:3386–3403.

Ali AB, Thomson AM (1998) Facilitating pyramid to horizontal oriens-alveus interneurone inputs: dual intracellular recordings in slices of rat hippocampus. *J Physiol (Lond)* 507:185–199.

Ali AB, Deuchars J, Pawelzik H, Thomson AM (1998) CA1 pyramidal to basket and bistratified cell EPSPs: dual intracellular recordings in rat hippocampal slices. *J Physiol (Lond)* 507:201–217.

Ali AB, Bannister AP, Thomson AM (1999) IPSPs elicited in CA1 pyramidal cells by putative basket cells in slices of adult rat hippocampus. *Eur J Neurosci* 11:1741–1753.

Alkondon M, Pereira EFR, Albuquerque EX (1998) alpha-Bungarotoxin- and methyl lycaconitine-sensitive nicotinic receptors mediate fast synaptic transmission in interneurons of rat hippocampal slices. *Brain Res* 810:257–263.

Andersen P, Eccles JC (1962) Inhibitory phasing of neuronal discharge. *Nature* 195:645–647.

Bakst I, Avendano C, Morrison JH, Amaral DG (1986) An experimental analysis of the origins of somatostatin-like immunoreactivity in the dentate gyrus of the rat. *J Neurosci* 6:1452–1462.

Bannister NJ, Larkman AU (1995) Dendritic morphology of CA1 pyramidal neurones from the rat hippocampus. II. Spine distributions. *J Comp Neurol* 360:161–171.

Baude A, Nusser Z, Roberts JDB, Mulvihill E, McIlhinney RAJ, Somogyi P (1993) The metabotropic glutamate receptor (mGluR1a) is concentrated at perisynaptic membrane of neuronal subpopulations as detected by immunogold reaction. *Neuron* 11:771–787.

Bilkey DK, Goddard GV (1985) Medial septal facilitation of hippocampal granule cell activity is mediated by inhibition of inhibitory interneurones. *Brain Res* 361:99–106.

Blackstad TW (1958) On the termination of some afferents to the hippocampus and fascia dentata: an experimental study in the rat. *Acta Anat (Basel)* 35:202–214.

Blasco-Ibanez JM, Freund TF (1995) Synaptic input of horizontal interneurons in stratum oriens of the hippocampal CA1 subfield: structural basis of feed-back activation. *Eur J Neurosci* 7:2170–2180.

Bolshakov VY, Siegelbaum SA (1995) Regulation of hippocampal transmitter release during development and long-term potentiation. *Science* 269:1730–1734.

Bragin A, Jando G, Nadasdy Z, Hetke J, Wise K, Buzsaki G (1995) Gamma (40–100 Hz) oscillation in the hippocampus of the behaving rat. *J Neurosci* 15:47–60.

Buckmaster PS, Schwartzkroin PA (1995a) Physiological and morphological heterogeneity of dentate gyrus-hilus interneurons in the gerbil hippocampus in vivo. *Eur J Neurosci* 7:1393–1402.

Buckmaster PS, Schwartzkroin PA (1995b) Interneurons and inhibition in the dentate gyrus of the rat in vivo. *J Neurosci* 15:774–789.

Buckmaster PS, Soltesz I (1996) Neurobiology of hippocampal interneurons: a workshop review. *Hippocampus* 6:330–339.

Buhl EH, Dann JF (1991) Cytoarchitecture, neuronal composition, and entorhinal afferents of the flying fox hippocampus. *Hippocampus* 1:131–152.

Buhl EH, Halasy K, Somogyi P (1994a) Diverse sources of hippocampal unitary inhibitory postsynaptic potentials and the number of synaptic release sites. *Nature* 368:823–828.

Buhl EH, Han Z-S, Lorinczi Z, Stezhka VV, Karnup SV, Somogyi P (1994b) Physiological properties of anatomically identified axo-axonic cells in the rat hippocampus. *J Neurophysiol* 71:1289–1307.

Buhl EH, Cobb SR, Halasy K, Somogyi P (1995) Properties of unitary IPSPs evoked by anatomically identified basket cells in the rat hippocampus. *Eur J Neurosci* 7:1989–2004.

Buhl EH, Szilagyi T, Halasy K, Somogyi P (1996) Physiological properties of anatomically identified basket and bistratified cells in the CA1 area of the rat hippocampus in vitro. *Hippocampus* 6:294–305.

Burnashev N, Schoepfer R, Monyer H, Ruppersberg JP, Gunther W, Seeburg PH, Sakmann B (1992) Control by asparagine residues of calcium permeability and magnesium blockade in the NMDA receptor. *Science* 257:1415–1419.

Buzsaki G, Leung L-WS, Vanderwolf CH (1983) Cellular bases of hippocampal EEG in the behaving rat. *Brain Res Rev* 6:139–171.

Buzsaki G, Horvath Z, Urioste R, Hetke J, Wise K (1992) High-frequency network oscillation in the hippocampus. *Science* 256:1025–1027.

Cherubini E, Gaiarsa JL, Ben-Ari Y (1991) GABA: an excitatory transmitter in early postnatal life. *Trends Neurosci* 14:515–519.

Chicurel ME, Harris KM (1992) Three-dimensional analysis of the structure and composition of CA3 branched dendritic spines and their synaptic relationships with mossy fiber boutons in the rat hippocampus. *J Comp Neurol* 325:169–182.

Cobb SR, Buhl EH, Halasy K, Paulsen O, Somogyi P (1996) Synchronization of neuronal activity in hippocampus by individual GABAergic interneurons. *Nature* 378:75–78.

Cobb SR, Halasy K, Vida I, Nyiri G, Tamas G, Buhl EH, Somogyi P (1997) Synaptic effects of identified interneurons innervating both interneurons and pyramidal cells in the rat hippocampus. *Neuroscience* 79:629–648.

Condorelli DF, Parenti R, Spinella F, Salinaro AT, Belluardo N, Cardile V, Cicirata F (1998) Coning of a new gap junction gene (C×36) highly expressed in mammalian brain neurons. *Eur J Neurosci* 10:1202–1208.

Dashtipour K, Yan XX, Dinh TT, Okazaki MM, Nadler JV, Ribak CE (2002) Quantitative and morphological analysis of dentate granule cells with recurrent basal dendrites from normal and epileptic rats. *Hippocampus* 12:235–244.

Deller T, Martinez A, Nitsch R, Frotscher M (1996) A novel entorhinal projection to the rat dentate gyrus: direct innervation of proximal dendrites and cell bodies of granule cells and GABAergic neurons. *J Neurosci* 16:3322–3333.

Deuchars J, Thomson AM (1996) CA1 pyramid-pyramid connections in rat hippocampus in vitro: dual intracellular recordings with biocytin filling. *Neuroscience* 74:1009–1018.

Draguhn A, Traub RD, Schmitz D, Jefferys JGR (1998) Electrical coupling underlies high-frequency oscillations in the hippocampus in vitro. *Nature* 394:189–192.

Fabian-Fine R, Skehel P, Errington ML, Davies HA, Sher E, Stewart MG, Fine A (2001) Ultrastructural distribution of the alpha7 nicotinic receptor subunit in rat hippocampus. *J Neurosci* 21:7993–8003.

Fisahn A, Pike FG, Buhl EH, Paulsen O (1998) Cholinergic induction of network oscillations at 40 Hz in the hippocampus in vitro. *Nature* 394:186–189.

Frazier CJ, Rollins YD, Breese CR, Leonard S, Freedman R, Dunwiddie TV (1998) Acetylcholine activates an alpha-bungarotoxin-sensitive nicotinic current in rat hippocampal interneurons, but not pyramidal cells. *J Neurosci* 18:1187–1195.

Freund TF, Antal M (1988) GABA-containing neurons in the septum control inhibitory interneurons in the hippocampus. *Nature* 336:170–173.

Freund TF, Buzsaki G (1996) Interneurons of the hippocampus. *Hippocampus* 6:347–470.

Freund TF, Gulyas AI, Acsady L, Gorcs L, Toth K (1990) Serotonergic control of the hippocampus via local inhibitory interneurons. *Proc Natl Acad Sci USA* 87:8501–8505.

Frotscher M, Leranth C (1985) Cholinergic innervation of the rat hippocampus as revealed by choline acetyltransferase immunocytochemistry: a combined light and electron microscopic study. *J Comp Neurol* 239:237–246.

Frotscher M, Leranth C, Lubbers K, Oertel WH (1984) Commissural afferents innervate glutamate decarboxylase immunoreactive non-pyramidal neurons in the guinea pig hippocampus. *Neurosci Lett* 46:137–143.

Frotscher M, Seress L, Schwerdtfeger WK, Buhl E (1991) The mossy cells of the fascia dentata: a comparative study of their fine structure and synaptic connections in rodents and primates. *J Comp Neurol* 312:145–163.

Fukuda T, Kosaka T (2000) Gap junctions linking the dendritic network of GABAergic interneurons in the hippocampus. *J Neurosci* 20:1519–1528.

Galarreta M, Hestrin S (1999) A network of fast-spiking cells in the neocortex connected by electrical synapses. *Nature* 402:72–75.

Gao B, Fritschy JM (1994) Selective allocation of GABA$_A$ receptors containing the a1 subunit to neurochemically distinct subpopulations of rat hippocampal interneurons. *Eur J Neurosci* 6:837–853.

Gasbarri A, Verney C, Innocenzi R, Campana E, Pacitti C (1994) Mesolimbic dopaminergic neurons innervating the hippocampal formation in the rat: a combined retrograde tracing and immunohistochemical study. *Brain Res* 668:71–79.

Gasbarri A, Sulli A, Packard MG (1997) The dopaminergic mesencephalic projections to the hippocampal formation in the rat. *Prog Neuropsychopharmacol Biol Psychiatry* 21:1–22.

Ge S, Dani JA (2005) Nicotinic acetylcholine receptors at glutamate synapses facilitate long-term depression or potentiation. *J Neurosci* 25:6084–6091.

Geiger JR, Jonas P (2000) Dynamic control of presynaptic Ca(2+) inflow by fast-inactivating K(+) channels in hippocampal mossy fiber boutons. *Neuron* 28:927–939.

Geiger JRP, Lubke J, Roth A, Frotscher M, Jonas P (1997) Submillisecond AMPA receptor-mediated signaling at a principal neuron-interneuron synapse. *Neuron* 18:1009–1023.

Gibson JR, Beierlein M, Connors BW (1999) Two networks of electrically coupled inhibitory neurons in neocortex. *Nature* 402:75–79.

Gulyas AI, Miettinen R, Jacobowitz DM, Freund TF (1992) Calretinin is present in non-pyramidal cells of the rat hippocampus. I. A new type of neuron specifically associated with the mossy fibre system. *Neuroscience* 48:1–27.

Gulyas AI, Miles R, Hajos N, Freund TF (1993a) Precision and variability in postsynaptic target selection of inhibitory cells in the hippocampal CA3 region. *Eur J Neurosci* 5:1729–1751.

Gulyas AI, Miles R, Sik A, Toth K, Tamamaki N, Freund TF (1993b) Hippocampal pyramidal cells excite inhibitory neurons through a single release site. *Nature* 366:683–687.

Gulyas AI, Hajos N, Freund TF (1996) Interneurons containing calretinin are specialized to control other interneurons in the rat hippocampus. *J Neurosci* 16:3397–3411.

Gulyas AI, Toth K, McBain CJ, Freund TF (1998) Stratum radiatum giant cells: a type of principal cell in the rat hippocampus. *Eur J Neurosci* 10:3813–3822.

Gulyas AI, Megias M, Emri Z, Freund TF (1999) Total number and ratio of excitatory and inhibitory synapses converging onto single interneurons of different types in the CA1 area of the rat hippocampus. *J Neurosci* 19:10082–10097.

Gupta A, Wang Y, Markram H (2000) Organizing principles for a diversity of GABAergic interneurons and synapses in the neocortex. *Science* 287:273–278.

Hajos N, Acsady L, Freund TF (1996) Target selectivity and neurochemical characteristics of VIP-immunoreactive interneurons in the rat dentate gyrus. *Eur J Neurosci* 8:1415–1431.

Hajos N, Papp EC, Acsady L, Levey AI, Freund TF (1998) Distinct interneuron types express M2 muscarinic receptor immunoreactivity on their dendrites or axon terminals in the hippocampus. *Neuroscience* 82:355–376.

Halasy K, Somogyi P (1993) Subdivisions in the multiple GABAergic innervation of granule cells in the dentate gyrus of the rat hippocampus. *Eur J Neurosci* 5:411–429.

Halasy K, Miettinen R, Szabat E, Freund TF (1992) GABAergic interneurons are the major postsynaptic targets of median raphe afferents in the rat dentate gyrus. *Eur J Neurosci* 4:144–153.

Halasy K, Buhl EH, Lorinczi Z, Tamas G, Somogyi P (1996) Synaptic target selectivity and input of GABAergic basket and bistratified interneurons in the CA1 area of the rat hippocampus. *Hippocampus* 6:306–329.

Han ZS, Buhl EH, Lorinczi Z, Somogyi P (1993) A high degree of spatial selectivity in the axonal and dendritic domains of physiologically identified local-circuit neurons in the dentate gyrus of the rat hippocampus. *Eur J Neurosci* 5:395–410.

Henze DA, Wittner L, Buzsaki G (2002) Single granule cells reliably discharge targets in the hippocampal CA3 network. *Nat Neurosci* 5:790–795

Hormuzdi SG, Pais I, LeBeau FEN, Towers SK, Rozov A, Buhl EH, Whittington MA, Monyer H (2001) Impaired electrical signaling disrupts gamma frequency oscillations in connexin 36 deficient mice. *Neuron* 31:487–495.

Ishida Y, Shirokawa T, Miyaishi O, Komatsu Y, Isobe K (2000) Age-dependent changes in projections from locus coeruleus to hippocampus dentate gyrus and frontal cortex. *Eur J Neurosci* 12:1263–1270.

Jones S, Yakel JL (1997) Functional nicotinic ACh receptors on interneurones in the rat hippocampus. *J Physiol (Lond)* 504:603–610.

Jung MW, McNaughton BL (1993) Spatial selectivity of unit activity in the hippocampal granular layer. *Hippocampus* 3:165–182.

Kandel ER, Spencer WA (1961) Electophysiological properties of an archicortical neuron. *Ann NY Acad Sci* 94;570–603.

Klausberger T, Magill PJ, Marton LF, Roberts JD, Cobden PM, Buzsaki G, Somogyi P (2003) Brain-state and cell-type-specific firing of hippocampal interneurons in vivo. *Nature* 421:844–848.

Konig P, Engel AK, Singer W (1996) Integrator or coincidence detector? The role of the cortical neuron revisited. *Trends Neurosci* 19:130–137.

Kosaka T (1980) The axon initial segment as a synaptic site: ultrastructure and synaptology of the initial segment of the pyramidal cell in the rat hippocampus (CA3 region). *J Neurocytol* 9:861–882.

Kosaka T (1983) Gap junctions between non-pyramidal cell dendrites in the rat hippocampus (CA1 and CA3 regions). *Brain Res* 271:157–161.

Kosaka T, Katsumaru H, Hama K, Wu J-Y, Heizmann CW (1987) GABAergic neurons containing the Ca^{2+}-binding protein parvalbumin in the rat hippocampus and dentate gyrus. *Brain Res* 419:119–130.

Lacaille J-C (1991) Postsynaptic potentials mediated by excitatory and inhibitory amino acids in interneurons of stratum pyramidale of the CA1 region of rat hippocampal slices in vitro. *J Neurophysiol* 66:1441–1454.

Lacaille J-C, Williams S (1990) Membrane properties of interneurons in stratum oriens-alveus of the CA1 region of rat hippocampus in vitro. *Neuroscience* 36:349–359.

Lacaille J-C, Mueller AL, Kunkel DD, Schwartzkroin PA (1987) Local circuit interactions between oriens/alveus interneurons and CA1 pyramidal cells in hippocampal slices: electrophysiology and morphology. *J Neurosci* 7:1979–1993.

Larkman A, Stratford K, Jack J (1991) Quantal analysis of excitatory synaptic action and depression in hippocampal slices. *Nature* 350:344–347.

Leranth C, Frotscher M (1987) Cholinergic innervation of hippocampal GAD- and somatostatin-immunoreactive commissural neurons. *J Comp Neurol* 261:33–47.

Leranth C, Szeidemann Z, Hsu M, Buzsaki G (1996) AMPA receptors in the rat and primate hippocampus: a possible absence of GluR2/3 subunits in most interneurons. *Neuroscience* 70:631–652.

Li X-G, Somogyi P, Tepper JM, Buzsaki G (1992) Axonal and dendritic arborization of an intracellularly labeled chandelier cell in the CA1 region of rat hippocampus. *Exp Brain Res* 90:519–525.

Li X-G, Somogyi P, Ylinen A, Buzsaki G (1994) The hippocampal CA3 network: an in vivo intracellular labeling study. *J Comp Neurol* 339:181–208.

Lien CC, Jonas P (2003) Kv3 potassium conductance is necessary and kinetically optimized for high-frequency action potential generation in hippocampal interneurons. *J Neurosci* 23:2055–2068.

Low K, Crestani F, Keist R, Benke D, Brunig I, Benson JA, Fritschy JM, Rulicke T, Bluethmann H, Mohler H, Rudolph U (2000) Molecular and neuronal substrate for the selective attenuation of anxiety. *Science* 290:131–134.

Loy R, Koziell DA, Lindsey JD, Moore RY (1980) Noradrenergic innervation of the adult rat hippocampal formation. *J Comp Neurol* 189:699–710.

Maccaferri G, McBain CJ (1995) Passive propagation of LTD to stratum oriens-alveus inhibitory neurons modulates the temporoammonic input to the hippocampal CA1 region. *Neuron* 15:137–145.

Maccaferri G, Roberts JDB, Szucs P, Cottingham CA, Somogyi P (2000) Cell surface domain specific postsynaptic currents evoked by identified GABAergic neurones in rat hippocampus in vitro. *J Physiol (Lond)* 524:91–116.

Magee JC (1998) Dendritic hyperpolarisation-activated currents modify the integrative properties of hippocampal CA1 pyramidal neurons. *J Neurosci* 18:7613–7624.

Magloczky Z, Acsady L, Freund TF (1994) Principal cells are the postsynaptic targets of supramammillary afferents in the hippocampus of the rat. *Hippocampus* 4:322–334.

Malinow R (1991) Transmission between pairs of hippocampal slice neurons: quantal levels, oscillations, and LTP. *Science* 252:722–724.

Martina M, Vida I, Jonas P (2000) Distal initiation and active propagation of action potentials in interneuron dendrites. *Science* 287:295–300.

Martinez A, Lubke J, Del Rio JA, Soriano E, Frotscher M (1996) Regional variability and postsynaptic targets of chandelier cells in the hippocampal formation of the rat. *J Comp Neurol* 376:28–44.

McBain CJ, DiChiara TJ, Kauer JA (1994) Activation of metabotropic glutamate receptors differentially affects two classes of hippocampal interneurons and potentiates excitatory synaptic transmission. *J Neurosci* 14:4433–4445.

Miettinen R, Freund TF (1992) Convergence and segregation of septal and median raphe inputs onto different subsets of hippocampal inhibitory interneurons. *Brain Res* 594:263–272.

Miles R (1990) Synaptic excitation of inhibitory cells by single CA3 hippocampal pyramidal cells of the guinea-pig in vitro. *J Physiol (Lond)* 428:61–77.

Miles R, Wong RKS (1983) Single neurones can initiate synchronized population discharge in the hippocampus. *Nature* 306:371–373.

Miles R, Wong RKS (1986) Excitatory synaptic interactions between CA3 neurones in the guinea-pig hippocampus. *J Physiol (Lond)* 373:397–418.

Miles R, Toth K, Gulyas AI, Hajos N, Freund TF (1996) Differences between somatic and dendritic inhibition in the hippocampus. *Neuron* 16:815–823.

Molnar E, Baude A, Richmond SA, Patel PB, Somogyi P, McIlhinney RAJ (1993) Biochemical and immunocytochemical characterization of antipeptide antibodies to a cloned GluR1 glutamate receptor subunit: cellular and subcellular distribution in the rat forebrain. *Neuroscience* 53:307–326.

Morales R, Battenberg E, Bloom FE (1998) Distribution of neurons expressing immunoreactivity for the 5HT(3) receptor subtype in the rat brain and spinal cord. *J Comp Neurol* 402:385–401.

Morilak DA, Somogyi P, Lujan-Miras R, Ciaranello RD (1994) Neurons expressing 5-HT2 receptors in the rat brain: neurochemical identification of cell types by immunocytochemistry. *Neuropsychopharmacology* 11:157–166.

Mott DD, Turner DA, Okazaki NM, Lewis DV (1997) Interneurons of the dentate-hilus border of the rat dentate gyrus: morphological and electrophysiological heterogeneity. *J Neurosci* 17:3990–4005.

Nusser Z, Sieghart W, Benke D, Fritschy J-M, Somogyi P (1996) Differential synaptic localization of two major γ-aminobutyric acid type A receptor a subunits on hippocampal pyramidal cells. *Proc Natl Acad Sci USA* 93:11939–11944.

Nyiri G, Freund TF, Somogyi P (2001) Input-dependent synaptic targeting of α2-subunit-containing GABA$_A$ receptors in synapses of hippocampal pyramidal cells of the rat. *Eur J Neurosci* 13:428–442.

Oleskevich S, Descarries L, Lacaille J-C (1989) Quantified distribution of the noradrenaline innervation in the hippocampus of adult rat. *J Neurosci* 9:3803–3815.

Oleskevich S, Descarries L, Watkins KC, Seguela P, Daszuta A (1991) Ultrastructural features of the serotonin innervation in adult rat hippocampus: an immunocytochemical description in single and serial thin sections. *Neuroscience* 42:777–791.

Ouardouz M, Lacaille J-C (1997) Properties of unitary IPSCs in hippocampal pyramidal cells originating from different types of interneurons in young rats. *J Neurophysiol* 77:1939–1949.

Parra P, Gulyas AI, Miles R (1998) How many subtypes of inhibitory cells in the hippocampus? *Neuron* 20:983–993.

Samson Y, Wu JJ, Friedman AH, Davis JN (1990) Catecholaminergic innervation of the hippocampus in the cynomolgus monkey. *J Comp Neurol* 298:250–263.

Sayer RJ, Friedlander MJ, Redman SJ (1990) The time course and amplitude of EPSPs evoked at synapses between pairs of CA3/CA1 neurons in the hippocampal slice. *J Neurosci* 10:826–836.

Scharfman HE, Kunkel DD, Schwartzkroin PA (1990) Synaptic connections of dentate granule cells and hilar neurons: results of paired intracellular recordings and intracellular horseradish peroxidase injections. *Neuroscience* 37:693–707.

Schmitz D, Schuchmann S, Fisahn A, Draguhn A, Buhl EH, Petrasch-Parwez RE, Dermietzel R, Heinemann U, Traub RD (2001) Axo-axonal coupling: a new mechanism for ultrafast neuronal communication. *Neuron* 31:669–671.

Schwerdtfeger WK, Buhl E (1986) Various types of non-pyramidal hippocampal neurons project to the septem and contralateral hippocampus. *Brain Res* 386:146–154.

Seress L, Mrzljak L (1987) Basal dendrites of granule cells are normal features of the fetal and adult dentate gyrus of both monkey and human hippocampal formations. *Brain Res* 405:169–174.

Sik A, Tamamaki N, Freund TF (1993) Complete axon arborization of a single CA3 pyramidal cell in the rat hippocampus, and its relationship with postsynaptic parvalbumin-containing interneurons. *Eur J Neurosci* 5:1719–1728.

Sik A, Ylinen A, Penttonen M, Buzsaki G (1994) Inhibitory CA1-CA3-hilar region feedback in the hippocampus. *Science* 265:1722–1724.

Sik A, Penttonen M, Ylinen A, Buzsaki G (1995) Hippocampal CA1 interneurons: an in vivo intracellular labeling study. *J Neurosci* 15:6651–6665.

Sik A, Penttonen M, Buzsaki G (1997) Interneurons in the hippocampal dentate gyrus: an in vivo intracellular study. *Eur J Neurosci* 9:573–588.

Skaggs WE, McNaughton BL, Wilson MA, Barnes CA (1996) Theta phase precession in hippocampal neuronal populations and the compression of temporal sequences. *Hippocampus* 6:149–172.

Smith SS, Gong QH, Hsu FC, Markowitz RS, ffrenchMullen JMH, Li HS (1998) GABA(A) receptor alpha 4 subunit suppression prevents withdrawal properties of an endogenous steroid. *Nature* 392:926–930.

Somogyi P, Freund TF, Hodgson AJ, Somogyi J, Beroukas D, Chubb IW (1985) Identified axo-axonic cells are immunoreactive for GABA in the hippocampus and visual cortex of the cat. *Brain Res* 332:143–149.

Somogyi P, Tamas G, Lujan R, Buhl EH (1998) Salient features of synaptic organisation in the cerebral cortex. *Brain Res Rev* 26:113–135.

Soriano E, Martinez A, Farinas I, Fortscher M (1993) Chandelier cells in the hippocampal formation of the rat: the entorhinal area and subicular complex. *J Comp Neurol* 337:151–167.

Sperk G, Schwarzer C, Tsunashima K, Fuchs K, Sieghart W (1997) GABA$_A$ receptor subunits in the rat hippocampus. 1. Immunocytochemical distribution of 13 subunits. *Neuroscience* 80:987–1000.

Swanson LW, Hartman BK (1975) The central noradrenergic system: an immunofluorescence study of the location of the cell bodies and their efferent connections in the rat utilizing dopamine-beta-hydroxylase. *J Comp Neurol* 163:467–507.

Tamas G, Buhl EH, Somogyi P (1997) Fast IPSPs elicited via multiple synaptic release sites by different types of GABAergic neurone in the cat visual cortex. *J Physiol (Lond)* 500:715–738.

Tamas G, Somogyi P, Buhl EH (1998) Differentially interconnected networks of GABAergic interneurons in the visual cortex of the cat. *J Neurosci* 18:4255–4270.

Tamas G, Buhl EH, Lorincz A, Somogyi P (2000) Proximally targeted GABAergic synapses and gap junctions synchronize cortical interneurons. *Nat Neurosci* 3:366–371.

Taylor CP, Dudek (1982) A physiological test for electrotonic coupling between CA1 pyramidal cells in rat hippocampal slices. *Brain Res* 235:351–357.

Thomson AM, Destexhe A (1999) Dual intracellular recordings and computational models of slow inhibitory postsynaptic potentials in rat neocortical and hippocampal slices. *Neuroscience* 92:1193–1215.

Thomson AM, Bannister AP, Hughes DI, Pawelzik H (2000) Differential sensitivity to zolpidem of IPSPs activated by morphologically identified CA1 interneurons in slices of rat hippocampus. *Eur J Neurosci* 12:425–436.

Toth K, Freund TF (1992) Calbindin D28k-containing nonpyramidal cells in the rat hippocampus: their immunoreactivity for GABA and projection to the medial septum. *Neuroscience* 49:793–805.

Toth K, Freund TF, Miles R (1997) Disinhibition of rat hippocampal pyramidal cells by GABAergic afferents from the septum. *J Physiol (Lond)* 500:463–474.

Traub RD, Bibbig A (2000) A model of high-frequency ripples in the hippocampus based on synaptic coupling plus axon-axon gap junctions between pyramidal neurons. *J Neurosci* 20:2086–2093.

Traub RD, Miles R (1995) Pyramidal cell to inhibitory cell spike transduction explicable by active dendritic conductances in inhibitory cell. *J Comput Neurosci* 2:291–298.

Traub RD, Whittington MA, Colling SB, Buzsaki G, Jefferys JGR (1996) Analysis of gamma rhythms in the rat hippocampus in vitro and in vivo. *J Physiol (Lond)* 493:471–484.

Traub RD, Jefferys JGR, Whittington MA (1997) Simulation of gamma rhythms in networks of interneurons and pyramidal cells. *J Comput Neurosci* 4:141–150.

Traub RD, Schmitz D, Jefferys JGR, Draguhn A (1999) High-frequency population oscillations are predicted to occur in hippocampal pyramidal neuronal networks interconnected by axoaxonal gap junctions. *Neuroscience* 92:407–426.

Traub RD, Bibbig A, Fisahn A, LeBeau FEN, Whittington MA, Buhl EH (2000) A model of gamma-frequency network oscillations induced in the rat CA3 region by carbachol in vitro. *Eur J Neurosci* 12:4093–4106.

Trommald M, Jensen V, Andersen P (1995) Analysis of dendritic spines in rat CA1 pyramidal cells intracellularly filled with a fluorescent dye. *J Comp Neurol* 353:260–274.

Turner DA, Chen Y, Isaac JT, West M, Wheal HV (1997) Excitatory synaptic site heterogeneity during paired pulse plasticity in CA1 pyramidal cells in rat hippocampus in vitro. *J Physiol (Lond)* 500:441–461.

Vida I, Frotscher M (2000) A hippocampal interneuron associated with the mossy fiber system. *Proc Natl Acad Sci USA* 97:1275–1280.

Vida I, Halasy K, Szinyei C, Somogyi P, Buhl EH (1998) Unitary IPSPs evoked by interneurons at the stratum radiatum stratum lacunosum-moleculare border in the CA1 area of the rat hippocampus in vitro. *J Physiol (Lond)* 506:755–773.

Wang X-J, Buzsaki G (1996) Gamma oscillation by synaptic inhibition in a hippocampal interneuronal network model. *J Neurosci* 16:6402–6413.

Wei DS, Mei YA, Bagal A, Yao JP, Thompson SM, Tang CM (2001) Compartmentalised and binary behaviour of terminal dendrites in hippocampal pyramidal neurons. *Science* 293:2272–2275.

White JA, Chow CC, Ritt J, Soto-Trevino C, Kopell N (1998) Synchronization and oscillatory dynamics in heterogeneous, mutually inhibited neurons. *J Comput Neurosci* 5:5–16.

Whittington MA, Traub RD, Jefferys JGR (1995) Synchronized oscillations in interneuron networks driven by metabotropic glutamate receptor activation. *Nature* 373:612–615.

Wouterlood FG, Saldana E, Witter MP (1990) Projection from the nucleus reuniens thalami to the hippocampal region: light and electron microscopic tracing study in the rat with the anterograde tracer Phaseolus vulgaris-leucoagglutinin. *J Comp Neurol* 296:179–203.

Ylinen A, Soltesz I, Bragin A, Penttonen M, Sik A, Buzsaki G (1995) Intracellular correlates of hippocampal theta rhythm in identified pyramidal cells, granule cells, and basket cells. *Hippocampus* 5:78–90.

9 ▦ Elizabeth Gould

Structural Plasticity

9.1 Overview

The hippocampal formation has been described as a relatively late-developing brain region. Rather than having a fixed, immutable structure, as might be implied by the earlier anatomical and physiological chapters, it is in fact known to undergo several structural changes throughout life that are traditionally described as "developmental". Numerous reports have demonstrated that the hippocampal formation is capable not only of substantial reorganization when damaged but also dramatic structural change when intact. It appears to undergo dynamic modifications continually in the form of dendritic extension and retraction as well as synapse formation and elimination.

Perhaps the most basic of all structural changes is the addition of new neurons, a phenomenon known as neurogenesis. Although this process was once believed to be restricted to the embryonic or early postnatal period, neurogenesis is now recognized to be a substantial process in some regions of the adult brain. In fact, the dentate gyrus of the rat adds thousands of new neurons every day throughout adulthood (Cameron and McKay, 2001), raising intriguing questions about the regulation and functional significance of this phenomenon.

The incorporation of new neurons into preexisting circuitry results in a cascade of structural changes that further increase the structural plasticity of this region. For example, new neurons elaborate axons and dendrites (Hastings and Gould, 1999; Markakis and Gage, 1999; Cameron and McKay, 2001) and undergo synaptogenesis (Kaplan and Hinds, 1977; Markakis and Gage, 1999). These progressive events are typically followed by a series of regressive phenomena, such as cell death (Gould et al., 1999a, 2001; Dayer et al., 2003), which likely involves process retraction and synapse elimination. Coincident with the growing acceptance of adult neurogenesis as a significant phenomenon in the mammalian brain,

numerous studies have identified factors and conditions that regulate its occurrence. This information has suggested possible functions for adult-generated neurons.

This chapter begins by discussing the types of structural plasticity in the hippocampal formation and then concentrates on the evidence revealing that new neurons are formed in the dentate gyrus throughout life. It then reviews the literature related to the modulation of neurogenesis in the dentate gyrus by hormones and by experience and finally focuses on the role these new cells may play in hippocampal function. The possibility that new cells participate in certain types of learning and in the modulation of anxiety and stress responses is explored. Some recent evidence suggesting unusual properties of immature neurons is considered in light of the hypothesis that a continual influx of these unique cells to hippocampal circuitry has important functional consequences.

9.2 Dendritic and Synaptic Plasticity in the Hippocampal Formation

9.2.1 Naturally Occurring Structural Plasticity

For more than a century, neuroanatomists have speculated about the capacity of the adult brain to change its structure (see Stanisch and Nitsch, 2002 for review). Evidence accumulated over the past several decades has identified the hippocampus as a region with a large degree of structural plasticity. These studies together indicate that the fine, and sometimes even the gross, structure of the hippocampal formation is constantly changing under normal conditions. Far from being a structurally static region, the hippocampal formation is a dynamic area whose synapses and dendrites are undergoing continuous rearrangement.

9.2.2 Hormones and Dendritic Architecture

Ovarian Steroids

A continual fluctuation in the numbers of dendritic spines on the pyramidal cells of the CA1 region has been reported in adult female rats and monkeys. This fluctuation occurs over a period of hours to days and is controlled by the levels of circulating ovarian steroids (Woolley et al., 1990b, 1997; Shors et al., 2001a; Hao et al., 2003; Cooke and Woolley, 2005). When ovarian steroids are at a high level, the number of dendritic spines is high. When the hormones are low, the number of spines is low. These changes in the number of dendritic spines are paralleled by changes in the number of excitatory synapses in this region (Woolley and McEwen, 1992; Woolley et al., 1996). The extent to which these structural changes reflect functional changes remains a matter of debate (Woolley, 1998). For example, conflicting literature exists on the influence of estrogen on behaviors associated with the hippocampus. Some reports indicate that estrogen improves performance on hippocampus-dependent tasks (Daniel et al., 1997; Gibbs, 1999; Daniel and Dohanich, 2001; Li et al., 2004; Sandstrom and Williams, 2004); and in some of these studies, the time course of behavioral improvement corresponds to changes in dendritic spines. Other reports have failed to demonstrate improvements in hippocampus-dependent tasks with estrogen treatment or across the estrous cycle (Berry et al., 1997; Warren and Juraska, 1997; Chesler and Juraska, 2000). Thus, the relation between behavior and dendritic spine number in the hippocampus remains unclear.

It is worth noting, however, that continuous estrous cycles, a common hormonal profile for female laboratory rodents, are probably uncommon in rodents living in the wild. A more likely endocrine profile would include postpubertal pregnancy followed by bouts of lactation, single estrous cycles just after weaning, and subsequent pregnancy. Thus, the relevance of estrogen-associated changes in dendritic spines on hippocampal function may lie in events such as pregnancy and the postpartum period (see Woolley, 1998, 1999 for commentary).

Adrenal Steroids

High levels of circulating glucocorticoids have been associated with atrophy of dendrites in the CA3 region. Chronic treatment with corticosterone, the main glucocorticoid in rodents, decreases the complexity and size of the apical dendritic tree of CA3 pyramidal neurons (Woolley et al., 1990a). Although it is possible that these changes are an impending sign of cell death, which has been reported with chronic elevated glucocorticoids (Sapolsky et al., 1985), it has been suggested that retraction of dendrites may play an adaptive role in protecting the hippocampus from excessive glutamate (Luine et al., 1994).

9.2.3 Experience and Dendritic Architecture

Stress

Dendritic architecture in the hippocampus is also influenced by experience. Chronic stress has generally been shown to have negative effects on the structure of dendrites in the hippocampus. As observed with chronic glucocorticoid treatment, the dendritic tree of the CA3 pyramidal neurons in adult male rats and tree shrews decreases in size following repeated restraint stress (Watanabe et al., 1992; Magarinos et al., 1996; McEwen, 1999). These effects appear to be reversible in unstressed conditions. In addition, changes in the dendritic tree with stress and recovery parallel performance on tasks that require the hippocampus (Luine et al., 1994).

Acute stress has also been shown to alter the number of dendritic spines on CA1 pyramidal cells of adult rats, but this effect seems to be dependent on the sex of the animal and, in the case of females, the stage of estrous. Brief, intermittent tail shocks have been shown to increase the number of dendritic spines on pyramidal cells of males (Shors et al., 2001a). By contrast, female rats showed the opposite effect—a decrease in the number of dendritic spines on pyramidal cells when shocked during diestrus but not when shocked during estrus (Shors et al., 2001a). Although it remains unclear what the functional significance of these effects is, it is worth noting that opposite effects of stress on learning have been reported in males and females (Wood et al., 2001). These behavioral effects appear to parallel the changes in dendritic spines suggesting a functional relation.

Environmental Complexity and Learning

Beginning with the early work of Rosenzweig and Diamond (Rosenzweig et al., 1962; reviewed in Will et al., 2004), a large body of literature has amassed regarding the effects of living in an enriched laboratory environment on brain structure. These studies have demonstrated repeatedly that, compared to laboratory control animals, animals living in enriched environments during either development or adulthood have larger brains along multiple measures. Most of this work has focused on the neocortex, but the effects are generally similar in the hippocampus. Studies have demonstrated that living in enriched environments increases the size of the dendritic tree (Juraska et al., 1985; Faherty et al., 2003), the number of dendritic spines (Moser et al., 1994), and the number of synapses (Altschuler, 1979; Briones et al., 2005) in the hippocampus compared to controls. Other studies have shown that rearing in an enriched environment is associated with improved performance on hippocampus-dependent learning tasks (Juraska et al., 1984; van Praag et al., 2000; Teather et al., 2002).

Enriched laboratory environments typically included a multitude of stimuli that increase stress, physical activity, and learning. Numerous studies have sought to identify the specific experiential cues that mediate the brain changes; but to date, questions remain. Several studies appear to have ruled out stress as a chief mediator of the effects of the enriched environment on the hippocampus either by demonstrating comparable stress hormone levels between groups or differential effects on brain structure following specific stressors. Some studies have suggested that physical activity is a contributing factor to the changes in hippocampal structure associated with living in an enriched environment. For instance, Eadie et al. (2005) reported an increased density of dendritic spine density on dentate granule cells in rodents that had access to a running wheel (but see Faherty et al., 2003). This finding is similar to that reported for animals living in enriched environments (Faherty et al., 2003). The extent to which changes in hippocampal structure induced by living in a complex environment are the result of one particular cue versus a constellation of cues remains unknown. The contribution of learning and synaptic plasticity to changes in hippocampal structure has also been investigated.

Several studies have reported structural changes in the hippocampus as a result of learning, or long-term potentiation (LTP), a form of synaptic plasticity often associated with learning. These effects of learning and LTP range from changes in the shape of dendritic spines (reviewed by Yuste and Bonhoeffer, 2001), increases in spine number (Moser et al., 1994; Trommald et al., 1996; O'Malley et al., 2000; Leuner et al., 2003), and changes in the number and distribution of synapses along dendrites (Chang et al., 1991; Rusakov et al., 1997; Andersen and Soleng, 1998; Toni et al., 1999). These findings mirror some of the changes associated with living in enriched environments. However, the extent to which these changes contribute to learning remains unknown.

9.2.4 Structural Plasticity Following Damage

Perhaps not surprisingly, given the large degree of structural change that can occur in the intact hippocampal formation even in the adult animal, this region also has a remarkable capacity for regeneration after injury. During the early 1970s, Raisman and Field (1973) reported evidence for extensive, predictable reorganization of synaptic connections in the septal nuclei following transection of the fimbria. This seminal study set the stage for work designed to explore related structures, and shortly thereafter similar results were observed for the deafferented hippocampus. Since then, the phenomenon of axonal sprouting has been examined extensively following transection of perforant path axons. After this manipulation, nondamaged axons sprout and occupy the now devoid target spaces in a layer-specific manner (Lynch et al., 1976; Scheff et al., 1977; Deller and Frotscher, 1997; Frotscher et al., 1997). This remarkable phenomenon has had a large impact on neuroscience as it provided definitive evidence that regeneration in the adult brain was possible—a phenomenon suggested by the work of Ramon y Cajal and other early neuroanatomists (Stahnisch and Nitsch, 2002). The therapeutic implications of this work are clear: If the mechanisms underlying sprouting

could be discovered, it might be possible to harness them in the service of brain repair. The phenomenon is not specific to just one set of axons in the hippocampus: Uninjured axons that sprout when hippocampal afferents are severed include commissural and crossed entorhinal afferents (Deller and Frotscher, 1997), cholinergic septo-hippocampal fibers (Forster et al., 1997), serotonergic axons (Zhou et al., 1995), and noradrenergic fibers (Peterson, 1994). Other axons however, including perforant path fibers, do not appear to sprout.

In some studies, structural regeneration has been associated with functional recovery. Time-dependent changes in open field activity after unilateral entorhinal lesions are correlated with the growth of the crossed pathway from the contralateral entorhinal region (Steward et al., 1977). Whereas animals with unilateral entorhinal lesions are sometimes unable to perform hippocampus-dependent tasks shortly after the damage has occurred, recovery of function has been noted following regeneration of sprouted axons (Leonard et al., 1995). This is particularly intriguing given the fact that it is often a different population of cells whose axons repopulate the absent target sites after the lesion. However, it is not absolutely clear that axonal regeneration is the cause of functional recovery, even if it takes place over the same time period. For example, studies by Ramirez and Stein (1984) indicated that sectioning the dorsal psalterium (through which the growing entorhinal fibers of the crossed pathway ordinarily travel) does not alter the time course of functional recovery seen after unilateral entorhinal lesions. Other mechanisms have been associated with functional recovery after axotomy, including hyperactivity of the remaining axons (Gage et al., 1983a) and the supersensitivity of postsynaptic neurotransmitter receptors (Patel et al., 1996). In some cases, these additional mechanisms appear to subside once axonal ingrowth is complete (Gage et al., 1983b).

Other examples of structural plasticity in the hippocampal formation have been observed in studies using animal models of disease states such as epilepsy and stroke. In these cases, many cells in the hippocampal formation die. With time following seizure or stroke, there is considerable structural reorganization in the form of axon sprouting, which could be viewed as regenerative (Sloviter, 1999). Studies examining human brains of epileptic individuals and those with Alzheimer's disease have detected evidence of structural reorganization (Cotman et al., 1990; Nadler, 2003). The extent to which these compensatory structural changes slow functional deterioration remains unknown. In addition, it is possible that experience can enhance or potentially exacerbate damage-induced reorganization (Icanco and Greenough, 2000).

The brain is protected from mechanical injury by the skull and from chemical injury by the blood-brain barrier. Thus, it is not obvious that the regenerative capacity inherent to the hippocampus evolved to correct brain damage, particularly that which occurs in old age. However, axonal sprouting and synaptogenesis may be developmental phenomena that are reinstated in the presence of certain environmental cues (e.g., the formation of a large number of target sites following cell death). Alternatively, or in addition, axonal sprouting and synaptogenesis may be occurring under normal circumstances at a low level, and the magnitude of their occurrence increases with damage-associated cues. Given the large amount of evidence suggesting that the hippocampus is structurally plastic under normal conditions, the latter possibility seems especially likely.

9.2.5 Transplantation

The remarkable plasticity of the hippocampus has also been demonstrated through experiments designed to induce regrowth of the damaged hippocampus via transplantation. Studies have shown that the hippocampus of adult rats incorporates fetal tissue from various brain regions (Bjorklund and Stenevi, 1984; Bjorklund and Gage, 1985). These studies have demonstrated much greater growth and survival of transplanted tissue when the host hippocampus has been damaged either directly or via axotomy or fimbria-fornix destruction (Low et al., 1982; Gage and Bjorklund, 1986). Grafting of subcortical noradrenergic or cholinergic fetal tissue into the denervated adult hippocampus results in ingrowth of the transplanted tissue into the unoccupied target areas (Nilsson et al., 1988), restoration of neurotransmitter levels (Bjorklund et al., 1990; Kalen et al., 1991), emergence of relatively normal electrophysiological responses (Buzsaki et al., 1987), and at least partial recovery of function (Low et al., 1982). However, there appears to be an advantage of homotypic tissue in terms of restoring a denervated area; cholinergic fetal transplants are more likely to restore the structural, biochemical, and behavioral deficits associated with selective cholinergic lesions than nonspecific lesions affecting numerous afferent types (Leanza et al., 1998). These studies suggest possible approaches for treatment of human conditions associated with diminished hippocampal function. However, there are serious limitations to this approach. Apart from the concern of immune rejection (Lawrence et al., 1990), the grafted tissue is rarely incorporated completely, and its survival and continued efficacy are not guaranteed. These limitations, coupled with the recognition that certain parts of the brain support neurogenesis even during adulthood, have led to the development of transplant strategies using fetal stem cells.

Transplantation of expanded neural stem cells into the damaged hippocampus has revealed successful incorporation of new neurons into the CA fields. These studies have shown that new neurons can arise from progenitors, migrate to their appropriate locations where they form long distance axons, make appropriate connections, and exihibit normal electrophysiological responses (Englund et al., 2002). Studies suggest that the hippocampus, particularly the dentate gyrus, is conducive to the acceptance of neural stem cell transplants because the environment of this brain region supports neurogenesis under normal conditions (Fricker et al., 1999). The field of transplantation research has elucidated the capacity of the hippocampus to reorganize structurally when provided

with an exogenous source of afferents or progenitor cells. Future studies using information gleaned from investigations of naturally occurring adult neurogenesis may facilitate the successful replacement of damaged neurons and complete recovery of function. This approach, however, may be useful only under certain conditions where the primary neuropathological hallmark is cell death, such as occurs with stroke. Other conditions, such as Alzheimer's disease, which result in the accumulation of abnormal proteins and the formation of senile plaques and neurofibrillary tangles, may be less amenable to transplantation.

9.3 Adult Neurogenesis

The first evidence for adult neurogenesis in the intact mammalian brain was published more than 40 years ago by Joseph Altman and colleagues (Altman, 1962, 1963, 1969; Altman and Das, 1965a,b). Over the ensuing decades, the findings were corroborated (Kaplan and Hinds, 1977; Kaplan, 1981; Kaplan and Bell, 1984; but see Rakic 1985), but only during the last decade has the phenomenon received intensive scrutiny and investigation by the neuroscience community (Boxes 9–1 and 9–2). The dentate gyrus is one of two brain regions in which adult neurogenesis has been widely recognized (Box 9–2), and the basic steps in the process of forming new neurons in this area are well understood.

In the dentate gyrus, new cells originate from progenitor or precursor cells located in the dentate gyrus itself. These cells have the capacity to proliferate and are more restricted in their progeny than stem cells. The progenitor cells have some characteristics of astroglia (Seri et al., 2001) and are primarily concentrated in the subgranular zone, the region between the granule cell layer and the hilus. The subgranular zone is not a distinct layer but, rather, a sporadic collection of progenitor cell clusters lining the deep aspect of the granule cell layer. Cells in this region divide, presumably asymmetrically, to produce some daughter cells that retain the ability to divide and other cells that become either neurons or glia. The new cells migrate the short distance to the granule cell layer and differentiate into neurons (Fig. 9–1).

Adult neurogenesis has been observed in the hippocampus of virtually every mammalian species examined, including mice, voles, rats, cats, rabbits, guinea pigs, tree shrews, marmosets, macaques, and humans (Altman and Das, 1965a,b; Gould et al., 1997, 1998, 1999b; Kaplan and Hinds, 1977; Eriksson et al., 1998; Galea and McEwen, 1999; Kornack and Rakic, 1999). There is some debate about the relative significance of this phenomenon across vertebrate species, and the argument has been made that an inverse relation exists between the amount of adult neurogenesis and cognitive complexity (Rakic, 1985a,b). However, the robustness of adult neurogenesis in the brains of adult avians (Nottebohm, 2002), creatures with extensive cognitive capabilities, argues against this interpretation. Although it is difficult to assess the relative

Given the magnitude of new neuron addition to the dentate gyrus, the fact that early neuroanatomists did not report evidence for structural change in this intensively studied brain region is puzzling. If ~9000 new cells are added to the dentate gyrus every day and a significant proportion of these cells extend axons, elaborate dendrites, and undergo synaptogenesis, evidence of massive structural change should have been noted. There are probably several reasons for this major oversight.

First, there is stability during the turnover. Neuron number in the dentate gyrus appears to be tightly regulated. In addition to massive cell production, neurite extension, and synaptogenesis, there is massive cell death, neurite retraction, and synapse elimination. Traditional histological methods would generally have failed to reveal these dynamic processes because they do not result in changes in the size or shape of the brain region or in the number of cells, dendritic elements, or synapses.

Second, because the prevailing view has been that structural change is a developmental, not adult, phenomenon, evidence for an adult change may have been interpreted otherwise. One possible example of this may be seen with descriptions of mossy fiber terminals in the CA3 region. Detailed neuroanatomical descriptions of the specialized synapses of mossy fibers on CA3 pyramidal cells, called "thorny excrescences," have described numerous morphological types of these terminals. Previously, these various types of terminal were presented as evidence that mossy fiber synapses were unusually complex. Given our current understanding of neurogenesis in the region, it seems reasonable to consider the possibility that these various types of synapse reflect different maturational stages of connections formed by newly generated granule cells. Structural variability in the adult hippocampus may reflect the dynamic changes occurring.

Figure 9–1. Adult neurogenesis in the dentate gyrus. *1.* Precursor cells, expressing the characteristics of astrocytes, reside in the subgranular zone (SGZ). *2.* Precursor cells divide asymmetrically at a rate that is modifiable by neural activity and experience. *3.* Following division, one cell remains in the SGZ and retains the capacity to proliferate, and the other cell enters the granule cell layer (GCL) of the dentate gyrus. Most of the newly born cells that enter the granule cell layer acquire neuronal characteristics.

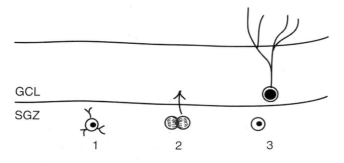

Around the time of the initial reports of adult neurogenesis in the dentate gyrus and olfactory bulb (Altman, 1962, 1969; Altman and Das, 1965a,b), Altman reported similar evidence for new neurons in the neocortex of adult rats and cats (Altman, 1962, 1963). This article was corroborated by a later study claiming new cells with ultrastructural characteristics of neurons in the neocortex of adult rats (Kaplan, 1981). This work was met with skepticism, as were the findings in the dentate gyrus and olfactory bulb (Rakic, 1985a,b; Kaplan, 2001). With the application of a different set of techniques (see Box 9–3), adult neurogenesis was rediscovered in the dentate gyrus and olfactory bulb during the 1990s and is now a relatively well established phenomenon. Both of these regions have been termed "neurogenic" in that they are widely believed to support adult neurogenesis. However, the case for the neocortex, as well as other brain regions, remains unresolved. Several studies have reported positive evidence in the form of BrdU-labeled cells with neuronal staining characteristics in the neocortex (Gould et al., 1999c, 2001; Bernier et al., 2002; Dayer et al., 2005), striatum (Bedard et al., 2002; Dayer et al., 2005), substantia nigra (Zhao et al., 2003), amygdala (Bernier et al., 2002; Fowler et al., 2005), and hypothalamus (Rankin et al., 2003; Fowler et al., 2005; Xu et al., 2005). Numerous other studies employing the same general methodologies reported no evidence for adult neurogenesis in these regions or evidence only for adult neurogenesis following damage (Magavi et al., 2000; Benraiss et al., 2001; Kornack and Rakic, 2001; Koketsu et al., 2003; Kodama et al., 2004; Yoshimi et al., 2005). The reasons for these discrepancies remain unclear, although they may be related to the fact that in the positive reports the relative number of new neurons reported in each of these regions is much lower than that reported in the olfactory bulb and dentate gyrus (see Gould et al., 2001 for a quantitative comparison of double-labeled cells between dentate gyrus and neocortex). If the phenomenon exists but at a much lower rate, it is possible that slight technical differences could make the difference between detecting and failing to detect a small number of new neurons. Alternatively, it is possible that the reports of adult neurogenesis outside the hippocampus and olfactory bulb are examples of false positives—new cells incorrectly identified as neurons or developmentally generated neurons incorrectly identified as new (Rakic, 2002). Future experimentation and the use of more definitive techniques should resolve these issues.

numbers of new neurons across species given that different methodologies are often utilized and there may be species differences in the efficacy of certain techniques, it seems clear that rodents exhibit a substantial amount of adult neurogenesis in the dentate gyrus.

In the rat dentate gyrus, the evidence that new cells differentiate into neurons is strong. New cells have been shown to receive synaptic input (Kaplan and Hinds, 1977; Markakis and

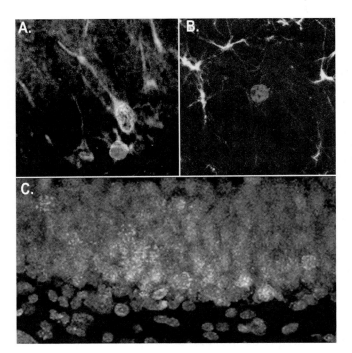

Figure 9–2. Most cells generated in the dentate gyrus of adults express neuronal characteristics. *A.* Photomicrograph of a BrdU-positive cell (red) in the adult rat dentate gyrus, expressing TUJ-1 (green), a marker of immature and mature neurons. *B.* Photomicrograph of a BrdU-positive cell (red) in the adult rat dentate gyrus, not expressing the astrocytic protein GFAP (green). *C.* Photomicrograph of a segment of dentate gyrus granule cell layer, triple-labeled with Hoechst, a DNA dye (blue), BrdU (red), and NeuN (green). Many but not all BrdU-positive cells express NeuN, a marker of mature neurons.

Gage, 1999), extend axons into the CA3 region (Stanfield and Trice, 1988; Hastings and Gould, 1999; Markakis and Gage, 1999), and express several biochemical markers of granule neurons, including NeuN, NSE, calbindin, MAP-2, and Tuj1 (Kuhn et al., 1996; Gould et al., 2001) (Fig. 9–2, see color insert; Box 9–3). Adult-generated cells in the mouse dentate gyrus have been shown to generate action potentials and exhibit other electrophysiological characteristics associated with granule cells (van Praag et al., 2002). Some newly generated cells in the dentate gyrus of adult rats may have the functional properties of inhibitory neurons (Liu et al., 2003). Although these findings suggest that two subpopulations of new neurons exist in this brain region (one with excitatory properties and the other with inhibitory properties), an alternative possibility is that new neurons temporarily exhibit characteristics of inhibitory neurons as part of a natural process of maturation.

9.3.1 Turnover of Dentate Gyrus Granule Cells

Several thousand new neurons are generated in the hippocampus every day in the young adult rat (Cameron and McKay, 2001) (Box 9–4). Although this number declines with age during adulthood, the phenomenon of adult neurogenesis appears to remain robust until animals become aged (Kuhn et al., 1996; Cameron and McKay, 1999). The addition of such a

large number of new neurons during adulthood raises the issue of whether the hippocampal formation continues to grow throughout life. It is now known that, alongside neurogenesis, there is substantial death of granule cells, especially of newborn neurons in adult rodents and primates under control conditions (Gould et al., 2001; Dayer et al., 2003). This cell death may offset the continual addition of new cells, resulting in a near-static total population of neurons (Box 9–1). The presence of pyknotic or degenerating cells in the dentate gyrus supports this view.

Several questions arise in connection with adult neurogenesis. First, do the new cells replace neurons that were born during development, or might they selectively replace those born during adulthood? Evidence suggests that both of these possibilities may be the case. Cells generated during the first postnatal week of life as well as those generated during adulthood decrease in number with time following mitosis (Dayer et al., 2003). However, most of the dying cells appear to be those that have been produced during adulthood. Pyknotic cells in the dentate gyrus are located primarily in the subgranular zone or deep in the granule cell layer, regions that contain progenitor cells and immature neurons. In addition, BrdU- and ^{3}H-thymidine-labeling studies in adults suggest that the originally labeled population expands owing to mitosis and then drops off in number. Coincident with the decrease in labeled cell number is the appearance of BrdU-labeled pyknotic cells (Gould et al., 2001). However, in the intact brain, environmental factors have been shown to influence the survival of adult-generated granule cells. This raises the issue of whether information on the turnover of newly produced granule cells is confounded by the abnormal conditions under which laboratory control animals exist. Thus, the natural lifespan of adult-generated neurons in the dentate gyrus remains unknown.

9.3.2 Hormones and Adult Neurogenesis

A separate set of questions concerning neurogenesis has to do with its regulation. One potential regulatory mechanism is endocrine, as the hippocampal formation is known to be richly endowed with hormone receptors. Many cell types in the hippocampal formation contain hormone receptors and, as discussed above, this area responds to experimental hormone manipulations during adulthood with dramatic structural changes (McEwen, 1999). Several studies have shown that the production of new neurons in the dentate gyrus is sensitive to the levels of circulating steroid hormones. This regulation can be in a negative direction, with the net effect being a decrease in the number of immature granule neurons, or in a positive direction, with the net effect being an increase in the number of new neurons.

Negative Regulation: Glucocorticoids

Several studies have indicated that glucocorticoids inhibit the production of new neurons by decreasing the proliferation of granule cell precursors. During development and adulthood,

Box 9–3
Methods for Visualizing New Neurons

To show that a new neuron has been produced in the adult brain, cell division and differentiation of the progeny into neurons must be demonstrated. The traditional method for demonstrating mitosis in the brain is ^{3}H-thymidine autoradiography. For in vivo studies, this technique requires injecting ^{3}H-thymidine into live animals (usually intraperitoneally) and then examining the brains at various survival times after injection. ^{3}H-thymidine is taken up by cells that are undergoing DNA synthesis in preparation for division. ^{3}H-thymidine can be used as a marker of proliferating cells (at short survival times) and their daughter cells (at longer survival times). ^{3}H-thymidine is a powerful method, but it has drawbacks, including lack of compatibility with stereological methods for cell counting and inability to determine with certainty whether new cells are co-labeled with cell type-specific markers.

A newer method, labeling with the thymidine analogue bromodeoxyuridine (BrdU), has been used more recently to investigate adult neurogenesis. BrdU is also incorporated into cells during S phase and can be used to label proliferating cells or their progeny. BrdU can be visualized using immunohistochemistry and has the advantage of being amenable to stereological estimates of the total number of new cells and the unequivocal demonstration that new cells are co-labeled with cell type-specific markers.

Evidence that new cells have differentiated into neurons can be achieved by combining ^{3}H-thymidine or BrdU with the following.

1. Electron microscopy: ^{3}H-thymidine autoradiography has been combined with electron microscopy to demonstrate synapses on cell bodies and dendrites of new cells in the dentate gyrus (Kaplan and Bell, 1984). BrdU labeling is less compatible with electron microscopic methods due to the harsh pretreatments necessary for staining.

2. Retrograde tracing: ^{3}H-thymidine autoradiography and BrdU labeling have been combined with retrograde tracer injections to show that new cells in the dentate gyrus extend axons into the CA3 region (Stanfield and Trice, 1988; Hastings and Gould, 1999; Markakis and Gage, 1999). This method is particularly useful when combined with BrdU because confocal microscopy can be used to verify double labeling in orthogonal planes.

3. Immunohistochemistry for neuronal markers: ^{3}H-thymidine autoradiography and BrdU labeling have been combined with immunolabeling for cell type-specific markers. These studies have shown that most cells made in the dentate gyrus of adult animals express neuronal markers (Kuhn et al., 1996; Cameron and McKay, 2001; Gould et al., 2001). This method is particularly useful when combined with BrdU because confocal microscopy can be used to assess double labeling throughout the extent of the cell.

4. Electrophysiology: There is evidence that new cells have the electrophysiological characteristics of neurons. This has been gained by identifying new cells with BrdU staining after electrophysiological characterization (Liu et al., 2003), by labeling new cells with GFP-tagged retrovirus (van Praag et al., 2002), and by recording from cells that are likely to be adult-generated on the basis of their location in the granule cell layer and staining for markers of immature neurons (Wang et al., 2000, Snyder et al., 2001). All of these approaches have revealed that new cells produced in the dentate gyrus during adulthood have the electrophysiological properties of neurons (see also Schmidt-Hieber et al., 2004 for the electrophysiological signature of newly born cells).

treating rat pups with corticosterone decreases the production of new granule cells (Gould et al., 1991; Cameron and Gould, 1994; Ambrogini et al., 2002). During adulthood, removal of circulating adrenal steroids by adrenalectomy increases the proliferation of granule cell precursors and ultimately the production of new neurons (Gould et al., 1992; Cameron and Gould, 1994). This phenomenon also occurs in aged animals in which granule cell production has diminished. Removal of adrenal steroids restores young adult levels of cell proliferation in the dentate gyrus of old rats (Cameron and McKay, 1999; Montaron et al., 2005).

The levels of circulating glucocorticoids change at various times of development and with experience, presenting the possibility that glucocorticoid inhibition of cell proliferation may reflect naturally occurring processes relevant to hippocampal function. A good example may be in observed in the dentate gyrus of the meadow vole. Meadow voles are seasonal breeders, and the breeding season is associated with higher levels of circulating glucocorticoids in females; cell proliferation is suppressed at this time (Galea and McEwen, 1999).

Positive Regulation: Estrogen

The ovarian steroid estradiol has a positive effect on the production of new cells in the dentate gyrus of adult rats (Tanapat et al., 1999, 2005; Banasr et al., 2001; Ormerod et al., 2003). Removal of estrogen by ovariectomy decreases the pro-

Box 9–4
Methodological Issues Related
to the BrdU Technique

The introduction of BrdU labeling has significantly advanced our understanding of adult neurogenesis. However, it has become clear that our understanding of this technique was based on erroneous assumptions derived from earlier developmental studies and thus, the phenomenon of neurogenesis continues to be underestimated and, perhaps, misinterpreted. Cameron and McKay (2001) have shown that the modal dose of BrdU for studies of adult neurogenesis (50 mg/kg) labels fewer than 50% of the total cells in S phase. In contrast, when used during development, this dose appears to label all cells in S phase. Although BrdU is a small molecule, differences in metabolism or blood-brain barrier (BBB) permeability prevent the adult animal from incorporating it at the same rate as the developing animal. Higher doses of BrdU (up to 600 mg/kg) label more proliferating cells, do not label nonspecifically, and are not toxic to the cells or animals. Using higher doses of BrdU, it appears that approximately 9000 new cells are generated every day in the dentate gyrus of the young adult rat. Divisions of the progenitor cells are presumed to be asymmetrical. Thus, ~4500 new cells are produced daily; and approximately 80% of these cells (~3600) exhibit characteristics of immature neurons. Over the course of 1 month (30 days), the number of immature neurons generated would be ~108,000. Estimates of the number of granule cells in the adult rat range from 1.5 million to 2.0 million. Given these numbers, a conservative estimate of the percentage of immature neurons produced in a month of a young adult rat's life is about 5%.

These findings have two important implications. First, the number of new neurons produced during adulthood is substantially higher than was originally predicted. Second, studies using nonsaturating doses of BrdU to investigate the effects of experimental manipulations on neurogenesis may be detecting changes in BrdU availability (e.g., due to alterations in blood flow or changes in the BBB) in contrast to changes in the actual number of new cells (Gould and Gross, 2002).

liferation of new cells, and replacement of estradiol to ovariectomized animals restores the rate of cell proliferation. Moreover, a natural fluctuation in the proliferation of granule cell precursors is evident across the estrous cycle; cell proliferation is highest during proestrus, the time of maximal estrogen levels. The stimulation of cell proliferation by estrogen results in a sex difference that favors females in the production of immature neurons. However, estrogen-related increases in the production of new cells are transient: By a few weeks after BrdU injection, no difference in the number of new cells can be detected. As with estrogen-related differences in spine density, similar differences in new neuron production may be confounded by the manner in which laboratory animals are housed. Estrogen may further increase the production of new neurons by enhancing their survival (Ormerod et al., 2004).

9.3.3. Experience and Adult Neurogenesis

A second major regulatory factor governing neurogenesis is experience. Environmental experience takes many forms: sensory and motor experience, changing cognitive demands, and stress.

Negative Regulation: Stress

The catabolic actions of stress and stress hormones have long been recognized. A major component of the "fight or flight" reaction is the mobilization of energy stores to facilitate reaction to imminent danger (Selye, 1976). This response inhibits costly processes (e.g., growth) that are only important for the future. It should come as no surprise, then, that stress inhibits the production of new granule cells during development and in adulthood (Gould and Tanapat, 1999). This phenomenon has been demonstrated in three mammalian species using a range of stressors. Exposure of postnatal and adult rats to the odors of natural predators, electric shock, or restraint decreases the rate of cell proliferation in the dentate gyrus (Tanapat et al., 2001; Malberg and Duman, 2003; Pham et al., 2003; Westenbroek et al., 2004). Similar studies have been carried out in adult marmosets and adult and aged tree shrews and marmosets using stress paradigms of resident-intruder (Gould et al., 1998) and social subordination (Gould et al., 1997; Czeh et al., 2001; Simon et al., 2005). In all cases, stress has been shown to decrease the proliferation of granule cell precursors and ultimately the production of immature neurons in the dentate gyrus. This effect appears to be region-specific in that changes in the number of BrdU-labeled cells were not observed in the subventricular zone (another site of neurogenesis) following stress.

Interestingly, prenatal stress has a persistent impact on the later production of granule cells. In both rodents and monkeys, prenatal stress results in persistent dampening of the proliferation of granule cell precursors during adulthood (in rats: Lemaire et al., 2000) and the late juvenile period (in monkeys: Coe et al., 2003). Furthermore, the postnatal stress of maternal separation results in persistent suppression of cell proliferation and immature neuron production in adult rats (Mirescu et al., 2004). Adult rats subjected to maternal separation early in life not only exhibit impaired neurogenesis but they also exhibit no changes in adult neurogenesis when exposed to stress during adulthood. As indicated earlier, exposure to predator odor decreases adult neurogenesis in control animals (this effect is absent in maternally separated animals). Prenatal and early postnatal stress are associated with persistent changes in the hypothalamic-pituitary-adrenal (HPA) axis, including the development of an inefficient shut-down mechanism for glucocorticoids. These findings present the possibility that new cell production is persistently inhibited in animals exposed to early life stressors because these animals either experience higher than normal levels of glucocorticoids or are hypersensitive to normal levels of these hormones. Indeed, lowering glucocorticoid levels below control values by adrenalectomy and low-dose corticosterone replacement has been shown to restore the levels of cell production in the dentate gyrus of maternally separated animals to control values (Mirescu et al., 2004). This is likely due to the fact that maternal separation results in lowered levels of corticosteroid-binding globulin, which modulates the amount of free corticosterone that enters the brain.

Collectively, these findings support the view that the production of immature neurons in the dentate gyrus varies depending on exposure to stressful experiences. In fact, the pool of immature neurons in the dentate gyrus may be an important substrate by which stress exerts long-lasting effects on hippocampal function. However, to understand the potential impact of stress on hippocampal structure and function, it may be necessary to examine these issues in animals living in more natural environments. Animals living in laboratory-controlled conditions appear to lose a larger proportion of adult-generated cells than those living in more complex environments (Kempermann et al., 1998; Nilsson et al., 1999; Tanapat et al., 2001). Thus far, the effects of chronic stress while living in naturalistic, relatively complex environments have not been explored.

Positive Regulation: Environmental Complexity, Learning, and Physical Activity

The first evidence that environmental complexity influences new hippocampal neurons in the adult was published by Barnea and Nottebohm (1994). This study showed that black-capped chickadees living in the wild maintained a higher number of new hippocampal neurons than those living in captivity. Work done on rodents also indicates a greater amount of cell proliferation and neurogenesis in the hippocampus of animals living in the wild compared to those living in the laboratory (Amrein et al., 2004a,b).

Adult neurogenesis as well as the entire volume of the hippocampal formation also changes over the seasons in some vertebrates. For example, the volume of the avian hippocampal formation fluctuates across the seasons in seed-caching birds such as the black-capped chickadee (Clayton, 1995, 1998; Smulders et al., 2000) and may be related to behaviors specific to these animals (see Chapter 13). Indeed, the lack of a change in the volume of this structure in birds that do not store food seasonally supports this view (Lee et al., 2001). This volumetric difference seems to be attributable to changes in the number of hippocampal neurons, with peak numbers occurring in the fall. Although sex differences in hippocampal volume have been reported in some species of food-storing mammals, such as gray squirrels, no seasonal changes have yet been observed (Lavenex et al., 2000). It may be that the phenomenon does not occur in mammals, or that naturally living species that occupy ecological niches with large changes in seasonal temperature and food availability need to be studied more closely.

Similar findings linking adult neurogenesis to experience were reported in the mouse and rat using an "enriched environment" paradigm; juvenile, young adult, and old rodents living in enriched environments maintained more new granule cells than those living in standard, deprived laboratory cages (Kempermann et al., 1997, 1998, 2002; Nilsson et al., 1999; Brown et al., 2003). These studies may indicate that standard control animals, be they birds living in aviaries or rodents living in laboratory cages, are living in an extremely deprived state (Box 9–5). Given the elaborate social and cognitive abilities of primates, it is likely that monkeys living in standard laboratory cages are experiencing an even more deprived set of experiences than less complex vertebrates.

There are many variables that differ between living in the wild and living in captivity or, in captivity, between living in an enriched environment and living in a standard laboratory cage. Among them are stress, social interaction, physical activity, and learning. In addition to reporting that birds living in complex environments have more new hippocampal neurons, a seasonal difference in new neuron number correlates with a seasonal difference in seed caching and retrieval. Because these behaviors are likely to include spatial navigation, a function attributed to the hippocampal formation (see Chapter 13), a causative link between learning and new neurons has been proposed. It has been shown that the number of new hippocampal neurons in the avian hippocampus can be increased by engaging birds in learning tasks that involve this

---

Box 9–5
Environmental Enrichment Versus Environmental Deprivation

Numerous studies have investigated structural changes in the hippocampal formation associated with rearing or living in "enriched environments." These studies have found several differences in the cortex, hippocampus, and other brain regions of animals living in the more complex environment compared to what is observed in animals living in standard laboratory cages (Rosenzweig et al., 1962; Icanco and Greenough, 2000; van Praag et al., 2000). In the case of rodents, the enriched environment typically consists of a larger living space, more conspecifics, toys, tunnels, exercise equipment, and often a more varied diet than the controls. Living in this type of environment enhances performance on certain hippocampus-dependent learning tasks and increases the hippocampal volume, number of dendrites of hippocampal neurons, number of glial cells, and number of new granule cells compared to controls. The most commonly applied interpretation of these findings is that hippocampal structure and function are responsive to environmental complexity. A converse interpretation is that they are deprivation effects; that is, the brain and behavior of control animals in the standard cages are abnormal because of the absence of normal stimulation. This puzzle could be solved by providing evidence for differences in animals living in super-complex versus complex environments.

brain region (Patel et al., 1997; Clayton, 1998). Studies have shown a similar phenomenon in rodents; learning tasks thought to depend on the integrity of the hippocampal formation enhance the number of new granule cells (Gould et al., 1999a; Ambrogini et al., 2000; Lemaire et al., 2000; Dobrossy et al., 2003; Leuner et al., 2004; Hairston et al., 2005; Olariu et al., 2005), whereas other types of learning may not have such an effect. For example, trace but not delay eyeblink conditioning increases the number of new granule cells in the dentate gyrus (Gould et al., 1999a; Leuner et al., 2004). This increase in the number of new neurons persists until at least 2 months after mitosis (Leuner et al., 2004) suggesting that the trophic effects of learning on new cells are not fleeting. Early training on tasks that require the hippocampal formation also enhances the number of new neurons, provided that learning has occurred; a significant correlation exists between the number of BrdU-labeled cells in the dentate gyrus and the percentage of conditioned responses in animals that have not yet fully acquired the conditioning task (Leuner et al., 2004). However, some studies have failed to find a significant increase in the number of new neurons following hippocampus-dependent learning (van Praag et al., 1999b; Snyder et al., 2005; Van der Borght et al., 2005), whereas others have reported decreased numbers of newly generated cells with learning (Dobrossy et al., 2003; Olariu et al., 2005; Pham et al., 2005). The reasons for these discrepancies remain unresolved; possible factors include variations in learning paradigms, different time courses between labeling new cells and training, and species and sex differences (reviewed by Abrous et al., 2005).

Because the hippocampus-dependent versions of the watermaze and eyeblink conditioning take more trials to acquire than the hippocampus-independent versions of these same tasks, it is possible that new cells respond especially to tasks that are more difficult. Although no study has yet matched the task difficulty of hippocampus-dependent and hippocampus-independent learning paradigms and examined new cell numbers, it is potentially instructive that place learning in the standard reference memory version of the watermaze is considerably easier (in terms of number of trials required to reach the criterion) than delay eyeblink conditioning. Thus, a simple relation to task difficulty—where this is operationally defined in terms of time or extent of training required for learning—does not seem to prevail.

Unlike the unsettled case for a link between learning and neurogenesis, there is now unambiguous evidence that physical activity increases cell proliferation and ultimately the production of new neurons in the dentate gyrus of adult rodents. Numerous studies have demonstrated that voluntary activity in a running wheel increases adult neurogenesis in rats and mice (van Praag et al., 1999ab; Fabel et al., 2003; Rhodes et al., 2003; Farmer et al., 2004; Holmes et al., 2004; Naylor et al., 2004; Persson et al., 2004; Bjornebekk et al., 2005). Even forced exercise, via running on a treadmill, has been shown to induce this effect (Trejo et al., 2001; Kim et al., 2004). This robust phenomenon is particularly surprising in light of the

fact that running causes activation of the HPA axis (Droste et al., 2003).

Although voluntary running might be considered a "positive stressor" (Selye, 1976), forced running is likely to have a more aversive component. Yet, both types of experience ultimately enhance adult neurogenesis. A few studies have demonstrated that high levels of running inhibit adult neurogenesis, but these negative effects appear to be specific to certain strains of animals (Naylor et al., 2004). The ability of this stimulus to override the negative actions of glucocorticoids is intriguing, and future experimentation is necessary to elucidate the mechanisms that enable running-induced neurogenesis despite activation of the HPA axis. It should be noted that there is an obvious hedonic component to running in rodents. Rodents are highly motivated to run and do so without additional incentives. In addition, rodents accustomed to running exhibit physiological and behavioral symptoms of withdrawal when access to a running wheel is denied. The extent to which these findings can be generalized to other animals that do not have an internal drive to run remains to be determined.

Some work suggests that the increase in neurogenesis associated with running leads to enhanced LTP as well as improved performance on hippocampus-dependent learning tasks (van Praag et al., 1999b). Although this evidence suggests a positive correlation between adult neurogenesis and learning, it is important to emphasize that running also alters other neural parameters in the hippocampus (Eadie et al., 2005). Thus, like the case for stress and enriched environments, changes in adult neurogenesis may contribute to altered hippocampal function, but they may not be the only cellular mediators of these effects.

Individual Differences in Adult Neurogenesis

Individual differences in the acquisition of learning tasks abound, even among animals of the same strain housed under the same conditions. Differences in the rate of acquisition of the trace eyeblink conditioned response are correlated positively with the number of new neurons in the dentate gyrus (Leuner et al., 2004).

Individual differences also exist in reaction to novelty. Rats that are highly reactive to novelty exhibit lower levels of cell proliferation, and therefore of neurogenesis or survival, in the dentate gyrus than their less reactive counterparts (Lemaire et al., 1999). Moreover, individual differences in aggressive behavior exist and appear to correlate with the rate of adult neurogenesis. When adult rodents are group-housed in a relatively large, complex enclosure, a dominance hierarchy forms. Dominant animals, characterized by the amount of offensive or aggressive behavior displayed, have substantially more new neurons than subordinate animals. Once the dominance hierarchy is formed, the difference in the number of new neurons persists regardless of whether animals continue to live in the complex environment (Kozorovitskiy and Gould, 2004). These results again raise the issue of whether the natural expression of structural plasticity in a given species is thwarted under artificial laboratory conditions. Differences in cell proliferation in the hippocampus of mountain chickadees depending on their dominance status have also been reported. Subordinate chickadees make fewer new cells in the hippocampus than dominant chickadees (Pravosudov and Omanska, 2005), again suggesting that individual experiences may increase variability on this measure.

9.3.4 Neurogenesis Following Damage

Another question raised by the phenomenon of neurogenesis is whether the ongoing processes of cell death and cell proliferation in the dentate gyrus are causally linked. There are several grounds to suspect that they are. First, endocrine manipulations that alter survival of granule cells also affect the production of new cells in a direction that tends to keep the total number of cells constant. For example, removal of circulating adrenal steroids by adrenalectomy results in massive death of granule cells (Sloviter et al., 1989; Gould et al., 1990) as well as enhanced proliferation of granule cell precursors (Gould et al., 1992; Cameron and Gould, 1994). Second, a specific lesion of the granule cell layer, by mechanical or excitotoxic means, results in a compensatory increase in the proliferation of granule cell precursors and ultimately the production of new neurons (Gould and Tanapat, 1997). Third, experimental conditions associated with granule cell death, such as ischemia and seizures, result in increased granule cell neurogenesis (Parent et al., 1997; Scott et al., 2000; Jim

et al., 2001; Kee et al., 2001; Kokaia and Lindvall, 2003; Scharfman, 2004). Damage-induced neurogenesis can also be observed in the CA fields of the hippocampal formation; ischemic damage induces the production of new hippocampal pyramidal cells, cells not normally thought to undergo adult neurogenesis (Rietze et al., 2000; Nakatomi et al., 2002). The extent to which damage-induced neurogenesis contributes to functional recovery remains unknown (Scharfman, 2004), but some evidence suggests that neurogenesis is upregulated in neurodegenerative conditions such as Alzheimer's disease (Jim et al., 2004) and Parkinson's disease (Yoshimi et al., 2005). One report suggested that there is a functional relation between regenerative adult neurogenesis and recovery insofar as blocking cell proliferation with irradiation prevents the formation of new synapses after ischemia (Wang et al., 2005).

Damage-induced neurogenesis may occur via at least two, not mutually exclusive, mechanisms.

1. Dying neurons send signals to progenitors to divide at a faster rate.
2. Death of mature neurons releases progenitor cells from inhibition by eliminating a neurogenesis-inhibitory signal.

Both of these mechanisms have been identified in other systems (Hastings and Gould, 2003) (Fig. 9–3), but the relevance of these results to the adult hippocampal formation remains unknown.

Figure 9–3. Cell proliferation is enhanced with neuronal damage: alternative mechanisms. *A*. In the intact adult brain, differentiated neurons do not affect the rate of cell proliferation; however, dying neurons can release molecules that stimulate nearby precursors to divide. *B*. In the intact adult brain, differentiated neurons release molecules that suppress cell proliferation. Neuronal death removes this inhibition, permitting a higher rate of cell proliferation after damage.

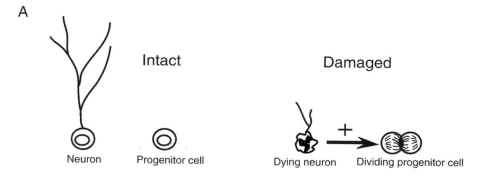

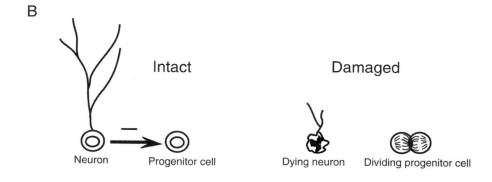

9.3.5 Unusual Features of Adult-Generated Neurons

All cells are not created equal. Not only are there the well known differences between different cell types, there are also developmental differences between individual cells of a common cell type. The granule cell layer consists of neurons ranging in age from hours to years. Although many thousands of new neurons are added to the dentate gyrus every day, this is a relatively small proportion of the large number of mature granule neurons produced during development and that survive through to adulthood (the total number of granule neurons is approximately one to two million in the adult rat). For the newly born cells to have an impact on adult hippocampal function, they must have unique functional properties that empower them in the face of the numerical superiority of mature granule cells. Growing evidence suggests that the newly born cells may be functionally stronger.

Structural Characteristics of Adult-Generated Neurons

Adult-generated neurons are likely to have structural characteristics that differ from developmentally generated neurons. These structural differences may enable a relatively small number of immature neurons to exert a disproportionate effect on hippocampal physiology. For example, adult-generated granule cells are capable of undergoing rapid structural change, as evidenced by the fact that they have axons in the distal CA3 within 4 to 10 days after mitosis (Hastings and Gould, 1999). This suggests a great capacity to form new connections under the appropriate environmental conditions. Retrograde tracer studies have also suggested differences in the axon terminal fields of granule neurons produced at different developmental time points. Some granule cells produced during development have axons that diverge longitudinally in the CA3 region, whereas no such adult-generated granule cells have been observed (Hastings et al., 2002). Detailed information about the sequence of synaptogenesis onto newly generated granule cells in the dentate gyrus is not yet available. However, because adult-generated granule cells are produced in the deep part of the granule cell layer, their dendritic trees do not extend as far into the molecular layer as those generated during development. This presents the possibility that adult-generated granule cells, because of their location in the layer, receive a different proportion of synaptic inputs from various sources. Clearly, more research is needed to determine the extent to which cells produced at different time points form different types of circuits in the hippocampal formation.

Functional Characteristics of Adult-Generated Neurons

Immature neurons have electrophysiological characteristics which differ from those of mature neurons. For example, developing neurons have been shown to exhibit giant depo-larizing potentials and respond to γ-aminobutyric acid (GABA) with depolarization instead of hyperpolarization. These data from hippocampal slices taken at different stages of development raise the possibility that adult-generated cells are transiently developmental in nature, at least for a short time after their generation. Indeed, it has been reported that immature granule cells in the dentate gyrus of the adult rat have more robust LTP than mature granule cells (Wang et al., 2000; Schmidt-Hieber et al., 2004). Moreover, this enhanced LTP cannot be inhibited by GABA agonists, unlike LTP elicited from mature granule cells (Snyder et al., 2001; Schmidt-Hieber et al., 2004). These findings support the view that a relatively small population of immature granule cells could exert a substantial functional influence over the hippocampal formation. However, research into this issue remains in its infancy; and much work is needed to determine the functional characteristics of new neurons in the dentate gyrus.

9.4 Possible Functions of New Neurons

The daily production of thousands of new granule cells and their incorporation into the existing circuitry are costly in terms of energy expenditure. It is likely that these new cells are not produced merely to replace older cells that die because a substantial amount of cell death occurring in this region involves the adult-generated population. The most intuitive explanation for the continual influx of new cells is that it provides an important mechanism for some aspect of the function of the dentate gyrus that cannot be obtained with a structure comprising mature neurons exclusively.

9.4.1 A Possible Role in Learning?

The existence of a large pool of immature neurons in a brain region that is important for certain types of learning and memory raises the possibility that these new cells participate in these functions. Although most theories of learning do not involve new neurons, many ideas about hippocampal function are compatible with such a possibility. Chapter 13 discusses the wide range of current theories of hippocampal function. One theory is that the hippocampal formation acts to associate discontiguous events (i.e., stimuli that are separated by space or time) (Wallenstein et al., 1998). A continual influx of new neurons accompanied by rapid synapse formation could play a role in connecting stimuli separated spatially or temporally. A widely held view is that the hippocampal formation plays a temporary role in storing new memories. This theory is consistent with data showing that recent, but not remote, memories for certain information are eliminated by lesioning the hippocampal formation (Kim et al., 1995; Zola and Squire, 2001). A rapidly changing population of adult-generated neurons with unique functional properties may serve as a substrate for this temporary role of the hippocampal formation in information storage. Neurons produced during adulthood might play a role in memory processing for a short time after their generation. The new cells might degenerate or undergo changes in connectivity, gene expression, or both around the time the hippocampal formation no longer plays a role in the storage of that particular memory. A temporary role for adult-generated granule neurons in learning has been suggested in canaries, in which seasonal changes in song correlate with the transient recruitment of more new neurons into the relevant circuitry (Barnea and Nottebohm, 1996; Nottebohm, 2002). However, a problem with taking this view of hippocampal memory is that it requires a cellular rather than a distributed synaptic view of memory storage. Neural network models of memory formation (see Chapter 14) support the distributed perspective. In addition, a temporary role for new neurons in learning implies that the new cells would persist only for as long as the hippocampus remains necessary for retention of that information. The observation that learning enhances the number of new neurons for at least 2 months (Leuner et al., 2004)—well beyond the time when the rodent hippocampal formation is necessary for the maintenance of those memories—argues against a clear role for new neurons in the temporary aspects of information storage.

Thus, although several theories of hippocampal learning are consistent with a possible role for new neurons, there are many details to be worked out. Do any data exist to support such a possibility? There is now some evidence for a positive correlation between the number of new hippocampal neurons and learning. For example, many factors and conditions that increase the number of new granule neurons have been shown to be associated with improved performance on hippocampus-dependent tasks, although the causal relation remains unproven (Gould et al., 1999a). Examples of factors that enhance both the number of new neurons and hippocampus-dependent learning are estrogen treatment and living in an enriched environment. Similarly, situations that decrease the number of new hippocampal neurons, such as glucocorticoids and stress, are associated with impaired performance on these tasks.

However, some recent studies have found either no relation between learning and the number of new neurons or, in fact, an inverse relation. With regard to the first case, aging is associated with a decline in new cell production in the hippocampus, and yet this decrease does not appear to be always associated with impaired performance on hippocampus-dependent tasks (Merrill et al., 2003). With regard to the second case, chronic stress has been shown to inhibit neurogenesis persistently in tree shrews; yet, this experience is associated with improved, not impaired, performance on a specific spatial navigation learning task (Bartolomucci et al., 2002). Do these negative findings indicate that new neurons are not involved in learning? Perhaps, but they may indicate that modulation of the rate at which new neurons accumulate affects hippocampal function only under certain conditions. Because stress, aging, and environmental complexity influence multiple brain measures in addition to neurogenesis, it is possible that changes in the new neuron number relate to learn-

ing only when imposed upon a particular neural background and under certain learning circumstances. For example, a decline in the new neuron number may fail to correlate with learning impairment because other age-associated changes dominate hippocampal function, such as diminished numbers of synapses (Morrison and Hof, 2002). When examining data related to the issue of adult neurogenesis and learning, it is important to note that new cells are likely to require some time for integration into the existing circuitry. Dendrites must be grown and functional synaptic connections formed on them; axons must grow and find their targets. Thus, acute changes in cell proliferation are not likely to influence hippocampal function until a certain amount of time has passed. Chronic changes in cell proliferation are those most likely to have functional consequences because their effects may be additive. This point is well illustrated by considering the acute and chronic effects of stress. Acute stress and chronic stress diminish the proliferation of granule cell precursors in the dentate gyrus. However, acute stress has been shown (with certain paradigms) to enhance learning, whereas chronic stress typically impairs learning (McEwen, 1999; Shors, 2001).

A direct link between new neurons and learning remains controversial. Thus far, two approaches have been used to deplete new cells: antimitotic agents and irradiation. Focal irradiation has been shown to decrease the number of new neurons almost completely, whereas treatment with the antimitotic agent methylazoxymethanol acetate (MAM) for 2 weeks has been shown to diminish the pool of new neurons by about 80% (Shors et al., 2000b, 2002; Bruel-Jungerman et al., 2005). The first obvious question is whether the depletion of new neurons produced during adulthood would be sufficient to influence hippocampal function. Cameron and McKay (2001) have shown that approximately 9000 new cells are produced every day in the rat dentate gyrus. If we assume that cell division in this population is asymmetrical, a maximum of 4500 new cells would be available to differentiate into neurons. Of this population, about 80% express markers of immature neurons (3600). Assuming a 30-day month, with approximately 108,000 immature neurons generated during this time, complete depletion would eliminate about 100,800 immature neurons (> 5% of the total number of granule cells, which is about 1.5–2.0 million). Although this is not a proportionately large number, if, as indicated above, the granule cells produced during adulthood are functionally different—less likely to be inhibited by GABA and more likely to display synaptic plasticity—they could be especially influential. Despite the fact that involvement of new neurons in learning is plausible, the available evidence supporting this view is incomplete and mixed.

Treatment with the antimitotic agent MAM has been shown to impair performance on trace eyeblink conditioning (Shors et al., 2001b). Delay eyeblink conditioning, the hippocampus-independent version of the same task, is unaffected by MAM treatment. Replenishment of immature neurons after cessation of MAM treatment results in the recovery of hippocampal function as indexed by normal trace eyeblink conditioning. Additional studies have shown that focal irradiation (which stops cell proliferation and hence neurogenesis) of the hippocampal formation of adult rodents impairs performance of a place recognition task in a T maze but not of an object recognition task (Madsen et al., 2003); it also impairs performance in a spatial version of the Barnes maze (Raber et al., 2004). In addition, a role for new neurons in enhanced learning associated with living in an enriched environment has been reported, using MAM to decrease the production of neurons (Bruel-Jungerman et al., 2005). These results are surprising given that studies of behavioral changes following lesions of the hippocampus rarely uncover a learning impairment unless a large percentage of the total hippocampal formation is destroyed (Moser et al., 1995). This again raises the issue of whether the increased efficacy of adult-generated neurons compared to their developmentally generated counterparts imparts a relatively small number of new neurons with substantial power to influence hippocampal function.

It is important to note that contradictory data exist. One study revealed that other forms of hippocampus-dependent learning tasks are insensitive to manipulations that decrease the number of new neurons. For example, spatial learning in a watermaze is not impaired by MAM treatment or irradiation (Shors et al., 2002; Snyder et al., 2005). Moreover, a simple form of contextual fear conditioning (a learning paradigm that involves the hippocampal formation) (Fanselow, 2000) is unaffected by MAM treatment (Shors et al., 2002). Because both spatial learning and context fear conditioning are both much more rapidly acquired than trace eyeblink conditioning, the possibility that new cells are important only for training on difficult tasks arises, as previously indicated. This suggests that either new dentate granule cells participate in only certain types of hippocampus-dependent learning (e.g., those that involve associating stimuli separated in time) or that some action of the drug other than its effects on neuron production is impairing trace eyeblink learning. However, the results from irradiation studies suggest that spatial memory, if not learning, is affected by depletion of new neurons. Prevention of neurogenesis results in an inability to retain spatial information pertaining to watermaze learning, whereas learning itself remains unaffected (Snyder et al., 2005).

All methods utilized thus far to block adult neurogenesis in the dentate gyrus are likely to have some nonspecific effects. MAM is a nonspecific antimitotic agent (sometimes used for chemotherapy). Impairment of hippocampus-dependent learning could be the result of the generalized toxic effects of the drug. The efficacy of MAM appears to vary across studies, with some investigators reporting larger depletions in new neuron number than others (compare Shors et al., 2000 and Bruel-Jungerman et al., 2005 with Dupret et al., 2005). In addition, variability in the degree to which the drug is reported to be toxic at doses sufficient to block neurogenesis exists (compare Shors et al., 2000 and Bruel-Jungerman et al., 2005 with Dupret et al., 2005). The reasons for these differences remain unknown but may be related to the overall health of the animals at the start of the study and the degree to which they experience stress during treatment. However, there is general agreement across groups that at high doses MAM is generally toxic. Nonspecific effects of treatment are also a feature of irradiation. Although the possibility that spurious changes, in contrast to specific effects on adult neurogenesis, contribute to the learning deficits with MAM treatment cannot be completely ruled out, there is some evidence to suggest this is not the case. The same regimen of MAM treatment that produces learning impairment does not cause weight loss, liver damage, or structural changes to the brain (including the hippocampus and cerebellum) (Shors et al, 2000; Bruel-Jungerman et al., 2005). In addition, MAM treatment does not prevent the hippocampus from having some normal electrophysiological responses, including induction of LTP in the CA1 region.

Collectively, these findings suggest that new neurons may play a role in certain types of learning but not others. Definitive information awaits the development of better methods for controlling neuronal proliferation and survival in the absence of nonspecific effects that are functionally deleterious. Transgenic mice designed to knock out new neurons during specific times of adulthood would be useful tools for investigating the possible role of new neurons in learning. If these animals exhibit normal learning and memory on a multitude of tasks, the function of new neurons will remain a completely open question. One possibility is that the new neurons participate in learning but only in a redundant fashion. That is, the new neurons may be necessary for learning only when other aspects of hippocampal function are compromised (e.g., following irradiation or treatment with an antimitotic agent).

9.4.2 A Possible Role in Endocrine Regulation?

In addition to its widely recognized role as a brain region involved in learning and memory, the hippocampal formation plays a less publicized role in the regulation of endocrine function. As indicated earlier, the hippocampal formation is known to have a relatively high concentration of steroid hormone receptors, in particular adrenal steroid receptors (McEwen, 1999). The hippocampal formation has been linked functionally to regulation of the HPA axis. In particular, it is purported to play a role in limiting the levels of circulating glucocorticoids following stress. For example, lesions of the hippocampal formation prevent the efficient shut-off of the HPA axis and the return of glucocorticoid levels to their basal state (Herman et al., 1995).

Research into the effects of early stressors on the development of the HPA axis and adult neurogenesis has revealed potential links between adult-generated neurons and hippocampal neuroendocrine function. That is, prenatal and postnatal stress have been shown to result in persistent changes in the HPA axis in the form of inefficient shut-off of the stress response during adulthood. Early stressors have additionally been shown to diminish cell proliferation in an acute manner and to dampen permanently the production of new neurons even during adulthood (Lemaire et al., 2000; Coe et al., 2003). These findings raise the as yet untested possibility that adult-generated neurons play an important role in regulating the HPA axis. Studies designed to examine the effects of specific depletion of adult-generated neurons on the shut-off of the stress response might reveal evidence that would add support to this view.

Observations of individuals suffering from psychiatric conditions, such as depression and posttraumatic stress disorder, have revealed signs of HPA axis dysregulation and diminished hippocampal volume in magnetic resonance imaging (MRI) studies (Vythilingam et al., 2002). Although the mechanisms that underlie diminished hippocampal volume in these conditions are unknown, it is possible that persistently decreased neurogenesis plays a role. Interestingly, the psychiatric conditions are also associated with impaired learning, but the mechanisms that underlie these cognitive changes remain unknown.

9.4.3 A Possible Role in the Etiology and Treatment of Depression?

A growing body of evidence points to a role for new granule neurons in the etiology of depression. This idea grew out of three findings: (1) hippocampal volume is smaller in depressed patients; (2) stress, which predisposes individuals to develop depression, inhibits hippocampal neurogenesis; and (3) antidepressants enhance hippocampal neurogenesis. These observations have led to the suggestion that some of the symptoms associated with depression may result from a persistent decrease in new neuron formation. This idea has been tested more directly in a study examining the effects of focal irradiation on the behavioral effects of antidepressants in mice (Santarelli et al., 2003). Prevention of an antidepressant-induced increase in adult neurogenesis blocks the ability of this therapy to alter behavioral signs of anxiety. These findings suggest that the efficacy of antidepressants may depend on their ability to restore neurogenesis to normal levels. To establish these links more conclusively, evidence that the hippocampus does indeed participate in the symptomatology of depression would be necessary. Furthermore, confirmation that diminished hippocampal volume—which has not been reported in all studies of depressed patients and is extremely small even when it has been established (about a 5% reduction)—is the result of reduced neurogenesis seems critical.

ACKNOWLEDGMENTS

Special thanks go to the editors for constructive criticism on several drafts of the manuscript. Also, my thanks go to past and present members of my laboratory for their hard work and dedication, especially Yevgenia Kozorovitskiy for help with the chapter and providing figures. Finally, thanks to the NIH and NARSAD for funding some of the research described this chapter.

REFERENCES

Abrous DN, Koehl M, LeMoal M (2005) Adult neurogenesis: from precursors to network and physiology. *Physiol Rev* 85:523–569.

Altman J (1962) Are new neurons formed in the brains of adult mammals? *Science* 135:1127–1128.

Altman J (1963) Autoradiographic investigation of cell proliferation in the brains of rats and cats. *Anat Rec* 145:573–591.

Altman J (1969) Autoradiographic and histological studies of postnatal neurogenesis. IV. Cell proliferation and migration in the anterior forebrain, with special reference to persisting neurogenesis in the olfactory bulb. *J Comp Neurol* 137:433–457.

Altman J, Das GD (1965a) Autoradiographic and histological evidence of postnatal hippocampal neurogenesis in rats. *J Comp Neurol* 124:319–335.

Altman J, Das GD (1965b) Post-natal origin of microneurones in the rat brain. *Nature* 207:953–956.

Altschuler RA (1979) Morphometry of the effect of increased experience and training on synaptic density in area CA3 of the rat hippocampus. *J Histochem Cytochem* 27:1548–1550.

Ambrogini P, Cuppini R, Cuppini C, Ciaroni S, Cecchini T, Ferri P, Sartini S, Del Grade P (2000) Spatial learning affects immature granule cell survival in adult rat dentate gyrus. *Neurosci Lett* 286:21–24.

Ambrogini P, Orsini L, Mancini C, Ferri P, Barbanti I, Cuppini R (2002) Persistently high corticosterone levels but not normal circadian fluctuations of the hormone affect cell proliferation in the adult rat dentate gyrus. *Neuroendocrinology* 76:366–372.

Amrein I, Slomianka L, Lipp HP (2004a) Granule cell number, cell death and cell proliferation in the dentate gyrus of wild-living rodents. *Eur J Neurosci* 20:3342–3350.

Amrein I, Slomianka L, Poletaeva II, Bologova NV, Lipp HP (2004b) Marked species and age-dependent differences in cell proliferation and neurogenesis in the hippocampus of wild-living rodents. *Hippocampus* 14:1000–1010.

Andersen P, Soleng AF (1998) Long-term potentiation and spatial training are both associated with the generation of new excitatory synapses. *Brain Res Rev* 26:353–359.

Banasr M, Hery M, Brezun JM, Daszuta A (2001) Serotonin mediates oestrogen stimulation of cell proliferation in the adult dentate gyrus. *Eur J Neurosci* 14:1417–1424.

Barnea A, Nottebohm F (1994) Seasonal recruitment of hippocampal neurons in adult free-ranging black-capped chickadees. *Proc Natl Acad Sci USA* 91:11217–11221.

Barnea A, Nottebohm F (1996) Recruitment and replacement of hippocampal neurons in young and adult chickadees: an addition to the theory of hippocampal learning. *Proc Natl Acad Sci USA* 93:714–718.

Bartolomucci A, de Biurrun G, Czeh B, van Kampen M, Fuchs E (2002) Selective enhancement of spatial learning under chronic psychosocial stress. *Eur J Neurosci* 15:1863–1866.

Bedard A, Cossette M, Levesque M, Parent A (2002) Proliferating cells can differentiate into neurons in the striatum of normal adult monkey. *Neurosci Lett* 328:213–216.

Benraiss A, Chmielnicki E, Lerner K, Roh D, Goldman SA (2001) Adenoviral brain-derived neurotrophic factor induces both neostriatal and olfactory neuronal recruitment from endogenous progenitor cells in the adult forebrain. *J Neurosci* 21:6718–6731.

Bernier PJ, Bedard A, Vinet J, Levesque M, Parent A (2002) Newly generated neurons in the amygdala and adjoining cortex of adult primates. *Proc Natl Acad Sci USA* 99:11464–11469.

Berry B, McMahan R, Gallagher M (1997) Spatial learning and memory at defined points of the estrous cycle: effects on performance of a hippocampal-dependent task. *Behav Neurosci* 111:267–274.

Bjorklund A, Gage FH (1985) Neural grafting in animal models of neurodegenerative diseases. *Ann NY Acad Sci* 457:53–81.

Bjorklund A, Stenevi U (1984) Intracerebral neural implants: neuronal replacement and reconstruction of damaged circuitries. *Annu Rev Neurosci* 7:279–308.

Bjorklund A, Nilsson OG, Kalen P (1990) Reafferentation of the subcortically denervated hippocampus as a model for transplant-induced functional recovery in the CNS. *Prog Brain Res* 83:411–426.

Bjornebekk A, Mathe AA, Brene S (2005) The antidepressant effect of running is associated with increased hippocampal cell proliferation. *Int J Neuropsychopharmacol* 8:1–12.

Briones TL, Suh E, Jozsa L, Rogozinska M, Woods J, Wadowska M (2005) Changes in number of synapses and mitochondria in presynaptic terminals in the dentate gyrus following cerebral ischemia and rehabilitation training. *Brain Res* 1033:51–57.

Brown J, Cooper-Kuhn CM, Kempermann G, Van Praag H, Winkler J, Gage FH, Kuhn HG (2003) Enriched environment and physical activity stimulate hippocampal but not olfactory bulb neurogenesis. *Eur J Neurosci* 17:2042–2046.

Bruel-Jungerman E, Laroche S, Rampon C (2005) New neurons in the dentate gyrus are involved in the expression of enhanced long-term memory following environmental enrichment. *Eur J Neurosci* 21:513–521.

Buzsaki G, Czopf J, Kondakor I, Bjorklund A, Gage FH (1987) Cellular activity of intracerebrally transplanted fetal hippocampus during behavior. *Neuroscience* 22:871–883.

Cameron HA, Gould E (1994) Adult neurogenesis is regulated by adrenal steroids in the dentate gyrus. *Neuroscience* 61:203–209.

Cameron HA, McKay RD (1999) Restoring production of hippocampal neurons in old age. *Nat Neurosci* 2:894–897.

Cameron HA, McKay RD (2001) Adult neurogenesis produces a large pool of new granule cells in the dentate gyrus. *J Comp Neurol* 435:406–417.

Chang PL, Isaacs KR, Greenough WT (1991) Synapse formation occurs in association with the induction of long-term potentiation in two-year-old rat hippocampus in vitro. *Neurobiol Aging* 12:517–522.

Chesler EJ, Juraska JM (2000) Acute administration of estrogen and progesterone impairs the acquisition of the spatial Morris watermaze in ovariectomized rats. *Horm Behav* 28:234–242.

Clayton NS (1995) The neuroethological development of food-storing memory: a case of use it, or lose it! *Behav Brain Res* 70:95–102.

Clayton NS (1998) Memory and the hippocampus in food-storing birds: a comparative approach. *Neuropharmacology* 37:441–452.

Coe CL, Kramer M, Czeh B, Gould E, Reeves AJ, Kirschbaum C, Fuchs E (2003) Prenatal stress diminishes neurogenesis in the dentate gyrus of juvenile rhesus monkeys. *Biol Psychiatry* 54:1025–1034.

Cooke BM, Woolley CS (2005) Gonadal hormone modulation of dendrites in the mammalian CNS. *J Neurobiol* 64:34–46.

Cotman CW, Geddes JW, Kahle JS (1990) Axon sprouting in the rodent and Alzheimer's disease brain: a reactivation of developmental mechanisms? *Prog Brain Res* 83:427–434.

Czeh B, Michaelis T, Watanabe T, Frahm J, de Biurrun G, van Kampen M, Bartolomucci A, Fuchs E (2001) Stress-induced changes in cerebral metabolites, hippocampal volume, and cell proliferation are prevented by antidepressant treatment with tianeptine. *Proc Natl Acad Sci USA* 98:12796–12801.

Daniel JM, Dohanich GP (2001) Acetylcholine mediates the estrogen-induced increase in NMDA receptor binding in CA1 of the hippocampus and the associated improvement in working memory. *J Neurosci* 21:6949–6956.

Daniel JM, Fader AJ, Spencer AL, Dohanich GP (1997) Estrogen enhances performance of female rats during acquisition of a radial arm maze. *Horm Behav* 32:217–225.

Dayer AG, Ford AA, Cleaver KM, Yassaee M, Cameron HA (2003) Short-term and long-term survival of new neurons in the rat dentate gyrus. *J Comp Neurol* 460:563–572.

Dayer AG, Cleaver KM, Abouantoun T, Cameron HA (2005) New GABAergic interneurons in the adult neocortex and striatum are generated from different precursors. *J Cell Biol* 168:415–427.

Deller T, Frotscher M (1997) Lesion-induced plasticity of central neurons: sprouting of single fibers in the rat hippocampus after unilateral entorhinal cortex lesion. *Prog Neurobiol* 53:687–727.

Dobrossy MD, Drapeau E, Aurousseau C, LeMoal M, Piazza PV, Abrous DN (2003) Differential effects of learning on neurogenesis: learning increases or decreases the number of newly born cells depending on their birth date. *Mol Psychiatry* 8:974–982.

Droste SK, Gesing A, Ulbricht S, Muller MB, Linthorst ACE, Reul JM (2003) Effects of long-term voluntary exercise on the mouse hypothalamic-pituitary-adrenocortical axis. *Endocrinology* 144:301–3023.

Dupret D, Montaron MF, Drapeau E, Aurousseau C, Le Moal M, Piazza PV, Abrous DN (2005) Methylazoxymethanol acetate does not fully block cell genesis in the young and aged dentate gyrus. *Eur J Neurosci* 22:778–783.

Eadie BD, Redila VA, Christie BR (2005) Voluntary exercise alters the cytoarchitecture of the adult dentate gyrus by increasing cellular proliferation, dendritic complexity, and spine density. *J Comp Neurol* 486:39–47.

Englund U, Bjorklund A, Wictorin K, Lindvall O, Kokaia M (2002) Grafted neural stem cells develop into functional pyramidal neurons and integrate into host cortical circuitry. *Proc Natl Acad Sci* 99:17089–17094.

Eriksson PS, Perfilieva E, Bjork-Eriksson T, Alborn AM, Nordborg C, Peterson DA, Gage FH (1998) Neurogenesis in the adult human hippocampus. *Nat Med* 4:1313–1317.

Fabel K, Fabel K, Palmer TD (2003) VEGF is necessary for exercise-induced neurogenesis. *Eur J Neurosci* 18:2803–2812.

Faherty CJ, Kerley D, Smeyne RJ (2003) A Golgi-Cox morphological analysis of neuronal changes induced by environmental enrichment. *Dev Brain Res* 141:55–61.

Fanselow MS (2000) Contextual fear, gestalt memories, and the hippocampus. *Behav Brain Res* 110:73–71.

Farmer J, Zhao X, Gage FH, Christie BR (2004) Effects of voluntary exercise on synaptic plasticity and gene expression in the dentate gyrus of adult male Sprague-Dawley rats in vivo. *Neuroscience* 124:71–79.

Forster E, Naumann T, Deller T, Straube A, Nitsch R, Frotscher M (1997) Cholinergic sprouting in the rat fascia dentata after entorhinal lesion is not linked to early changes in neurotrophin messenger RNA expression. *Neuroscience* 80:731–739.

Fowler CD, Johnaon F, Wang Z (2005) Estrogen regulation of cell proliferation and distribution of estrogen receptor-alpha in the brains of adult female prairie and meadow voles. *J Comp Neurol* 489:166–179.

Fricker RA, Carpenter MK, Winkler C, Greco C, Gates MA, Bjorklund A (1999) Site-specific migration and neuronal differentiation of human neural progenitor cells after transplantation in the adult rat brain. *J Neurosci* 19:5990–6005.

Frotscher M, Heimrich B, Deller T (1997) Sprouting in the hippocampus is layer-specific. *Trends Neurosci* 20:218–223.

Gage FH, Bjorklund A (1986) Enhanced graft survival in the hippocampus following selective denervation. *Neuroscience* 17:89–98.

Gage FH, Bjorklund A, Stenevi U (1983a) Local regulation of compensatory noradrenergic hyperactivity in the partially denervated hippocampus. *Nature* 303:819–821.

Gage FH, Bjorklund A, Stenevi U (1983b) Reinnervation of the partially deafferented hippocampus by compensatory collateral sprouting from spared cholinergic and noradrenergic afferents. *Brain Res* 268:27–37.

Galea LA, McEwen BS (1999) Sex and seasonal differences in the rate of cell proliferation in the dentate gyrus of adult wild meadow voles. *Neuroscience* 89:955–964.

Gibbs RB (1999) Estrogen replacement enhances acquisition of a spatial memory task and reduces deficits associated with hippocampal muscarinic receptor inhibition. *Horm Behav* 36:222–233.

Gould E, Gross CG (2002) Adult neurogenesis: some progress and problems. *J Neurosci* 22:619–623.

Gould E, Tanapat P (1997) Lesion-induced proliferation of neuronal progenitors in the dentate gyrus of the adult rat. *Neuroscience* 80:427–436.

Gould E, Tanapat P (1999) Stress and hippocampal neurogenesis. *Biol Psychiatry* 46:1472–1479.

Gould E, Woolley CS, McEwen BS (1990) Short-term glucocorticoid manipulations affect neuronal morphology and survival in the adult dentate gyrus. *Neuroscience* 37:367–375.

Gould E, Woolley CS, Cameron HA, Daniels DC, McEwen BS (1991) Adrenal steroids regulate postnatal development of the rat dentate gyrus. II. Effects of glucocorticoids and mineralocorticoids on cell birth. *J Comp Neurol* 313:486–493.

Gould E, Cameron HA, Daniels DC, Woolley CS, McEwen BS (1992) Adrenal hormones suppress cell division in the adult rat dentate gyrus. *J Neurosci* 12:3642–3650.

Gould E, McEwen BS, Tanapat P, Galea LA, Fuchs E (1997) Neurogenesis in the dentate gyrus of the adult tree shrew is regulated by psychosocial stress and NMDA receptor activation. *J Neurosci* 17:2492–2498.

Gould E, Tanapat P, McEwen BS, Flugge G, Fuchs E (1998) Proliferation of granule cell precursors in the dentate gyrus of adult monkeys is diminished by stress. *Proc Natl Acad Sci USA* 95:3168–3171.

Gould E, Beylin A, Tanapat P, Reeves A, Shors TJ (1999a) Learning enhances adult neurogenesis in the hippocampal formation. *Nat Neurosci* 2:260–265.

Gould E, Reeves AJ, Fallah M, Tanapat P, Gross CG, Fuchs E (1999b) Hippocampal neurogenesis in adult Old World primates. *Proc Natl Acad Sci USA* 96:5263–5267.

Gould E, Reeves AJ, Graziano MS, Gross CG (1999c) Neurogenesis in the neocortex of adult primates. *Science* 286:548–552.

Gould E, Vail N, Wagers M, Gross CG (2001) Adult-generated hippocampal and neocortical neurons in macaques have a transient existence. *Proc Natl Acad Sci USA* 98:10910–10917.

Hairston IS, Little MT, Scanlon MD, Barakat MT, Palmer TD, Sapolsky RM, Heller HC (2005) Sleep restriction suppresses neurogenesis induced by hippocampus-dependent learning. *J Neurophysiol* 94:4224–4233.

Hao J, Janssen WG, Tang Y, Roberts JA, McKay H, Lasley B, Allen PB, Greengard P, Rapp PR, Kordower JH, Hof PR, Morrison JH (2003) Estrogen increases the number of spinophilin-immunoreactive spines in the hippocampus of young and aged female rhesus monkeys. *J Comp Neurol* 465:540–550.

Hastings NB, Gould E (1999) Rapid extension of axons into the CA3 region by adult-generated granule cells. *J Comp Neurol* 413:146–154.

Hastings NB, Gould E (2003) Neurons inhibit neurogenesis. *Nat Med* 9:264–266.

Hastings NB, Seth MI, Tanapat P, Rydel TA, Gould E (2002) Granule neurons generated during development extend divergent axon collaterals to hippocampal area CA3. *J Comp Neurol* 452:324–333.

Herman JP, Cullinan WE, Morano MI, Akil H, Watson SJ (1995) Contribution of the ventral subiculum to inhibitory regulation of the hypothalamo-pituitary-adrenocortical axis. *J Neuroendocrinol* 7:475–482.

Holmes MM, Galea LA, Mistlberger RE, Kempermann G (2004) Adult hippocampal neurogenesis and voluntary running activity: circadian and dose-dependent effects. *J Neurosci Res* 76:216–222.

Icanco TL, Greenough WT (2000) Physiological consequences of morphologically detectable synaptic plasticity: potential uses for examining recovery following damage. *Neuropharmacology* 39:765–776.

Jim K, Minami M, Lan JQ, Mao XO, Batteur S, Simon RP, Greenberg DA (2001) Neurogenesis in the dentate subgranular zone and rostral subventricular zone after focal cerebral ischemia in the rat. *Proc Natl Acad Sci USA* 98:4710–4715.

Jim K, Peel AL, Mao XO, Xie L, Cottrell BA, Henshall DC, Greenberg DA (2004) Increased hippocampal neurogenesis in Alzheimer's disease. *Proc Natl Acad Sci USA* 101:343–347.

Juraska JM, Henderson C, Muller J (1984) Differential rearing experience, gender, and radial maze performance. *Dev Psychobiol* 17:209–215.

Juraska JM, Fitch JM, Henderson C, Rivers N (1985) Sex differences in the dendritic branching of dentate granule cells following differential experience. *Brain Res* 333:73–80.

Kalen P, Cenci MA, Lindvall O, Bjorklund A (1991) Host brain regulation of fetal locus coeruleus neurons grafted to the hippocampus in 6-hydroxydopamine-treated rats: an intracerebral microdialysis study. *Eur J Neurosci* 3:905–918.

Kaplan MS (1981) Neurogenesis in the 3-month old rat visual cortex *J Comp Neurol* 195:323–338.

Kaplan MS (2001) Environmental complexity stimulates visual cortex neurogenesis: death of a dogma and a research career. *Trends Neurosci* 24:617–620.

Kaplan MS, Bell DH (1984) Mitotic neuroblasts in the 9-day old and 11- month old rodent hippocampus. *J Neurosci* 4:1429–1441.

Kaplan MS, Hinds JW (1977) Neurogenesis in the adult rat: electron microscopic analysis of light radioautographs. *Science* 197:1092–1094.

Kee NJ, Preston E, Wojtowicz JM (2001) Enhanced neurogenesis after transient global ischemia in the dentate gyrus of the rat. *Exp Brain Res* 136:313–320.

Kempermann G, Kuhn HG, Gage FH (1997) More hippocampal neurons in adult mice living in an enriched environment. *Nature* 386:493–495.

Kempermann G, Kuhn HG, Gage FH (1998) Experience-induced neurogenesis in the senescent dentate gyrus. *J Neurosci* 18:3206–3212.

Kempermann G, Gast D, Gage FH (2002) Neuroplasticity in old age: sustained fivefold induction of hippocampal neurogenesis by long-term environmental enrichment. *Ann Neurol* 52:135–143.

Kim JJ, Clark RE, Thompson RF (1995) Hippocampectomy impairs the memory of recently, but not remotely acquired, trace eyeblink conditioned responses. *Behav Neurosci* 109:195–203.

Kim Y-P, Kim H, Shin MS, Chang H-K, Jang M-H, Shin MC, Lee SJ, Lee HH, Yoon JH, Jeong IG, Kim CJ (2004) Age-dependence of the effect of treadmill exercise on cell proliferation in the dentate gyrus of rats. *Neurosci Lett* 355:152–154.

Kodama M, Fujioka T, Duman RS (2004) Chronic olanzapine or fluoxetine administration increases cell proliferation in hippocampus and prefrontal cortex of adult rat. *Biol Psychiatry* 56:570–580.

Kokaia Z, Lindvall O (2003) Neurogenesis after ischaemic brain insults. *Curr Opin Neurobiol* 13:127–132.

Koketsu D, Mikami A, Miyamoto Y, Hisatsune T (2003) Nonrenewal of neurons in the cerebral cortex of adult macaque monkeys. *J Neurosci* 23:937–942.

Kornack DR, Rakic P (1999) Continuation of neurogenesis in the hippocampus of the adult macaque monkeys. *Proc Natl Acad Sci USA* 96:5768–5773.

Kornack DR, Rakic P (2001) Cell proliferation without neurogenesis in the adult primate neocortex. *Science* 294:2127–2130.

Kozorovitskiy Y, Gould E (2004) Dominance hierarchy influences adult neurogenesis in the dentate gyrus. *J Neurosci* 24:6755–6759.

Kuhn HG, Dickinson-Anson H, Gage FH (1996) Neurogenesis in the dentate gyrus of the adult rat: age-related decrease of neuronal progenitor proliferation. *J Neurosci* 16:2027–2033.

Lavenex P, Steele MA, Jacobs LF (2000) Sex differences, but no seasonal variations in the hippocampus of food-caching squirrels: a stereological study. *J Comp Neurol* 425:152–166.

Lawrence JM, Morris RJ, Wilson DJ, Raisman G (1990) Mechanisms of allograft rejection in the rat brain. *Neuroscience* 37:431–462.

Leanza G, Martinez-Serrano A, Bjorklund A (1998) Amelioration of spatial navigation and short-term memory deficits by grafts of foetal basal forebrain tissue placed into the hippocampus and cortex of rats with selective cholinergic lesions. *Eur J Neurosci* 10:2353–2370.

Lee DW, Smith GT, Tramontin AD, Soma KK, Brenowitz EA, Clayton NS (2001) Hippocampal volume does not change seasonally in a non food-storing songbird. *Neuroreport* 12:1925–1928.

Lemaire V, Aurousseau C, Le Moal M, Abrous DN (1999) Behavioural trait of reactivity to novelty is related to hippocampal neurogenesis. *Eur J Neurosci* 11:4006–4014.

Lemaire V, Koehl M, Le Moal M, Abrous DN (2000) Prenatal stress produces learning deficits associated with an inhibition of neurogenesis in the hippocampus. *Proc Natl Acad Sci USA* 97:11032–11037.

Leonard BW, Amaral DG, Squire LR, Zola-Morgan S (1995) Transient memory impairment in monkeys with bilateral lesions of the entorhinal cortex. *J Neurosci* 15:5637–5659.

Leuner B, Falduto J, Shors TJ (2003) Associative memory formation increases the observation of dendritic spines in the hippocampus. *J Neurosci* 23:659–665.

Leuner B, Mendolia-Loffredo S, Kozorovitskiy Y, Samburg D, Gould E, Shors TJ (2004) Learning enhances the survival of new neurons beyond the time when the hippocampus is required for memory. *J Neurosci* 24:7477–7481.

Li C, Brake WG, Romeo RD, Dunlop JC, Gordon M, Buzescu R, Magarinos AM, Allen PB, Greengard P, Luine V, McEwen BS (2004) Estrogen alters hippocampal dendritic spine shape and enhances synaptic protein immunoreactivity and spatial memory in female mice. *Proc Natl Acad Sci USA* 101:2185–2190.

Liu S, Wang J, Zhu D, Fu Y, Lukowiak K, Lu YM (2003) Generation of functional inhibitory neurons in the adult rat hippocampus. *J Neurosci* 23:732–736.

Low WC, Lewis PR, Bunch ST, Dunnett SB, Thomas SR, Iversen SD, Bjorklund A, Stenevi U (1982) Function recovery following neural transplantation of embryonic septal nuclei in adult rats with septohippocampal lesions. *Nature* 300:260–262.

Luine V, Villegas M, Martinez C, McEwen BS (1994) Repeated stress causes reversible impairments of spatial memory performance. *Brain Res* 639:167–170.

Lynch G, Gall C, Rose G, Cotman C (1976) Changes in the distribution of the dentate gyrus associational system following unilateral or bilateral entorhinal lesions in the adult rat. *Brain Res* 110:57–71.

Madsen TM, Kristjansen PEG, Bolwig TG, Wortwein G (2003) Arrested neuronal proliferation and impaired hippocampal function following fractionated brain irradiation in the adult rat. *Neuroscience* 119:635–642.

Magarinos AM, McEwen BS, Flugge G, Fuchs E (1996) Chronic psychosocial stress causes apical dendritic atrophy of hippocampal CA3 pyramidal neurons in subordinate tree shrews. *J Neurosci* 16:3534–3540.

Magavi SS, Leavitt BR, Macklis JD (2000) Induction of neurogenesis in the neocortex of adult mice. *Nature* 405:951–955.

Malberg JE, Duman RS (2003) Cell proliferation in adult hippocampus is decreased by inescapable stress: reversal by fluoxetine treatment. *Neuropsychopharmacology* 28:1562–1571.

Markakis E, Gage F (1999) Adult-generated neurons in the dentate gyrus send axonal projections to field CA3 and are surrounded by synaptic vesicles. *J Comp Neurol* 406:449–460.

McEwen BS (1999) Stress and hippocampal plasticity. *Annu Rev Neurosci* 22:105–122.

Merrill DA, Karim R, Darraq M, Chiba AA, Tuszynski MH (2003) Hippocampal cell genesis does not correlate with spatial learning ability in aged rats. *J Comp Neurol* 459:201–207.

Mirescu C, Peters JD, Gould E (2004) Early life experience alters response of adult neurogenesis to stress. *Nat Neurosci* 7:841–846.

Montaron MF, Drapeau E, Dupret D, Kitchener P, Aurousseau C, Le Moal M, Piazza PV, Abrous DN (2006) Lifelong corticosterone level determines age-related decline in neurogenesis and memory. *Neurobiol Aging* 27:645–654.

Morrison JH, Hof PR (2002) Selective vulnerability of corticocortical and hippocampal circuits in aging and Alzheimer's disease. *Prog Brain Res* 136:467–486.

Moser MB, Trommald M, Andersen P (1994) An increase in dendritic spine density on hippocampal CA1 pyramidal cells following spatial learning in adult rats suggests the formation of new synapses. *Proc Natl Acad Sci USA* 91:12673–12675.

Moser MB, Moser EI, Forrest E, Andersen P, Morris RG (1995) Spatial learning with a minislab in the dorsal hippocampus. *Proc Natl Acad Sci USA* 92:9697–9701.

Nadler JV (2003) The recurrent mossy fiber pathway of the epileptic brain. *Neurochem Res* 28:1649–1658.

Nakatomi H, Kuriu T, Okabe S, Yamamoto S, Hatano O, Kawahara N, Tamura A, Kirino T, Nakafuku M (2002) Regeneration of hippocampal pyramidal neurons after ischemic brain injury by recruitment of endogenous neural progenitors. *Cell* 110: 429–441.

Naylor AS, Persson AI, Eriksson PS, Jonsdottir IH, Thorlin T (2004) Extended voluntary running inhibits exercise induced adult hippocampal progenitor proliferation in the spontaneously hypertensive rat. *J Neurophysiol* 93:2406–2414.

Nilsson M, Perfilieva E, Johansson U, Orwar O, Eriksson PS (1999) Enriched environment increases neurogenesis in the adult rat dentate gyrus and improves spatial memory. *J Neurobiol* 39: 569–578.

Nilsson OG, Brundin P, WIdner H, Strecker RE, Bjorklund A (1988) Human fetal basal forebrain neurons grafted to the denervated rat hippocampus produce an organotypic cholinergic reinnervation pattern. *Brain Res* 456:193–198.

Nottebohm F (2002) Neuronal replacement in adult brain. *Brain Res Bull* 57:737–749.

Olariu A, Shore LE, Brewer MD, Cameron HA (2005) A natural form of learning can increase and decrease survival of new neurons in the dentate gyrus. *Hippocampus* 15:750–762.

O'Malley A, O'Connell C, Murphy KJ, Regan CM (2000) Transient spine density increases in the mid-molecular layer of hippocampal dentate gyrus accompany consolidation of a spatial learning task in the rodent. *Neuroscience* 99:229–232.

Ormerod BK, Lee TT, Galea LA (2003) Estradiol initially enhances but subsequently suppresses (via adrenal steroids) granule cell proliferation in the dentate gyrus of adult female rats. *J Neurobiol* 55:247–260.

Ormerod BK, Lee TT, Galea LA (2004) Estradiol enhances neurogenesis in the dentate gyri of adult male meadow voles by increasing the survival of young granule neurons. *Neuroscience* 128:645–654.

Parent JM, Yu TW, Leibowitz RT, Geschwind DH, Sloviter RS, Lowenstein DH (1997) Dentate granule cell neurogenesis is increased by seizures and contributes to aberrant network reorganization in the adult rat hippocampus. *J Neurosci* 17: 3727–3728.

Patel SN, Clayton NS, Krebs JR (1997) Spatial learning induces neurogenesis in the avian brain. *Behav Brain Res* 89:115–128.

Patel TD, Azmitia EC, Zhou FC (1996) Increased 5-HT1A receptor immunoreactivity in the rat hippocampus following 5,7-dihydroxytryptamine lesions in the cingulum bundle and fimbria-fornix. *Behav Brain Res* 73:319–323.

Persson AI, Naylor AS, Jonsdottir IH, Nyberg F, Eriksson PS, Thorlin T (2004) Differential regulation of hippocampal cell proliferation by opioid receptor antagonists in running and non-running spontaneously hypertensive rats. *Eur J Neurosci* 19:1847–1855.

Peterson GM (1994) Sprouting of central noradrenergic fibers in the dentate gyrus following combined lesions of its entorhinal and septal afferents. *Hippocampus* 4:635–648.

Pham K, Nacher J, Hof PR, McEwen BS (2003) Repeated restraint stress suppresses neurogenesis and induces biphasic PSA-NCAM expression in the adult rat dentate gyrus. *Eur J Neurosci* 17:879–886.

Pravosudov VV, Omanska A (2005) Dominance-related changes in spatial memory are associated with changes in hippocampal cell proliferation rates in mountain chickadees. *J Neurobiol* 62:31–41.

Raber J, Rola R, LeFevour A, Morhardt D, Curley J, Mizumatsu S, VandenBerg SR, Fike JR (2004) Radiation-induced cognitive impairments are associated with changes in indicators of hippocampal neurogenesis. *Radiat Res* 162:39–47.

Raisman G, Field P (1973) A quantitative investigation of the development of collateral reinnervation after partial deafferentation of the septal nuclei. *Brain Res* 50:241–264.

Rakic P (2002) Adult neurogenesis in mammals: an identity crisis. *J Neurosci* 22:614–618.

Rakic P (1985a) Limits of neurogenesis in primates. *Science* 227: 1054–1056.

Rakic P (1985b) DNA synthesis and cell division in the adult primate brain. *Ann NY Acad Sci* 457:193–211.

Ramirez JJ, Stein DG (1984) Sparing and recovery of spatial alternation performance after entorhinal cortex lesions in rats. *Behav Brain Res* 13:53–61.

Rankin SL, Partlow GD, McCurdy RD, Giles ED, Fisher KR (2003) Postnatal neurogenesis in the vasopressin and oxytocin-containing nucleus of the pig hypothalamus. *Brain Res* 971: 189–196.

Rhodes JS, van Praag H, Garland T, Gage FH (2003) Exercise increases hippocampal neurogenesis to high levels but does not improve spatial learning in mice bred for increased voluntary wheel-running. *Behav Neurosci* 117:1006–1016.

Rietze R, Poulin P, Weiss S (2000) Mitotically active cells that generate neurons and astrocytes are present in multiple regions of the adult mouse hippocampus. *J Comp Neurol* 424:397–408.

Rosenzweig MR, Krech D, Bennett EL, Diamond MC (1962) Effects of environmental complexity and training on brain chemistry and anatomy: a replication and extension. *J Comp Physiol Psychol* 55:429–437.

Rusakov DA, Richter-Levin G, Stewart MG, Bliss TV (1997) Reduction in spine density associated with long-term potentiation in the dentate gyrus suggests a spine fusion-and-branching model of potentiation. *Hippocampus* 7:489–500.

Sandstrom NJ, Williams CL (2004) Spatial memory retention is enhanced by acute and continuous estradiol replacement. *Horm Behav* 45:128–135.

Santarelli L, Saxe M, Gross C, Surget A, Battaglia F, Dulawa S, Weisstaub N, Lee J, Duman R, Arancio O, Belzung C, Hen R (2003) Requirement of hippocampal neurogenesis for the behavioral effects of antidepressants. *Science* 301:805–809.

Sapolsky RM, Krey LC, McEwen BS (1985) Prolonged glucocorticoid exposure reduces hippocampal neuron number: implications for aging. *J Neurosci* 5:1222–1227.

Scharfman HE (2004) Functional implications of seizure-induced neurogenesis. *Adv Exp Med Biol* 548:192–212.

Scheff S, Benardo I, Cotman C (1977) Progressive brain damage accelerates axon sprouting in the adult rat. *Science* 197:795–797.

Schmidt-Hieber C, Jonas P, Bischofberger J (2004) Enhanced synaptic plasticity in newly generated granule cells in the adult hippocampus. *Nature* 429:184–187.

Scott BW, Wojtowicz JM, Burnham WM (2000) Neurogenesis in the dentate gyrus of the rat following electroconvulsive shock seizures. *Exp Neurol* 165:231–236.

Seri B, Garcia-Verdugo JM, McEwen BS, Alvarez-Buylla A (2001) Astrocytes give rise to new neurons in the adult mammalian hippocampus. *J Neurosci* 21:7153–7160.

Selye H (1976) *The stress of life.* New York: McGraw-Hill.

Shors TJ (2001) Acute stress rapidly and persistently enhances memory formation in the male rat. *Neurobiol Learn Mem* 75:10–29.

Shors TJ, Chua C, Falduto J (2001a) Sex differences and opposite effects of stress on dendritic spine density in the male versus female hippocampus. *J Neurosci* 21:6292–6297.

Shors TJ, Miesegaes G, Beylin A, Zhao M, Rydel T, Gould E (2001b) Neurogenesis in the adult is involved in the formation of trace memories. *Nature* 410:372–376.

Shors TJ, Townsend DA, Zhao M, Kozorovitskiy Y, Gould E (2002) Neurogenesis may relate to some but not all types of hippocampal-dependent learning. *Hippocampus* 12:578–584

Simon M, Czeh B, Fuchs E (2005) Age-dependent susceptibility of adult hippocampal cell proliferation to chronic psychosocial stress. *Brain Res* 1049:244–248.

Sloviter RS (1999) Status epilepticus-induced neuronal injury and network reorganization. *Epilepsia* 1:S34–S39.

Sloviter RS, Valiquette G, Abrams GM, Ronk EC, Sollas AL, Paul LA, Neubort S (1989) Selective loss of hippocampal granule cells in the mature rat brain after adrenalectomy. *Science* 243:535–538.

Smulders TV, Shiflett MW, Sperling AJ, DeVoogd TJ (2000) Seasonal changes in neuron numbers in the hippocampal formation of a food-hoarding bird: the black-capped chickadee. *J Neurobiol* 44:414–422.

Snyder JS, Kee N, Wojtowicz JM (2001) Effects of adult neurogenesis on adult synaptic plasticity in the rat dentate gyrus. *J Neurophysiol* 85:2423–2431.

Snyder JS, Hong NS, McDonald RJ, Wojtowicz JM (2005) A role for adult neurogenesis in spatial long-term memory. *Neuroscience* 130:843–852.

Stahnisch FW, Nitsch R (2002) Santiago Ramon y Cajal's concept of neuronal plasticity: the ambiguity lives on. *Trends Neurosci* 25:589–591.

Stanfield BB, Trice JE (1988) Evidence that granule cells generated in the dentate gyrus of adult rats extend axonal projections. *Exp Brain Res* 72:399–406.

Steward O, Loesche J, Horton WC (1977) Behavioral correlates of denervation and reinnervation of the hippocampal formation of the rat: open field activity and cue utilization following bilateral entorhinal cortex lesions. *Brain Res Bull* 2:41–48

Tanapat P, Hastings NB, Reeves AJ, Gould E (1999) Estrogen stimulates a transient increase in the number of new neurons in the dentate gyrus of the adult female rat. *J Neurosci* 19:5792–5801.

Tanapat P, Hastings NB, Rydel TA, Galea LA, Gould E (2001) Exposure to fox odor inhibits cell proliferation in the hippocampus of adult rats via an adrenal hormone-dependent mechanism. *J Comp Neurol* 437:496–504.

Tanapat P, Hastings NB, Gould E (2005) Ovarian steroids influence cell proliferation in the dentate gyrus of the adult female rat in a dose- and time-dependent manner. *J Comp Neurol* 481:252–265.

Teather LA, Magnusson JE, Chow CM, Wurtman RJ (2002) Environmental conditions influence hippocampus-dependent behaviours and brain levels of amyloid precursor protein in rats. *Eur J Neurosci* 16:2405–2415.

Toni N, Buchs PA, Nikonenko I, Bron CR, Muller D (1999) LTP promotes formation of multiple spine synapses between a single axon terminal and a dendrite. *Nature* 402:421–425.

Trejo JL, Carro E, Torres-Aleman I (2001) Circulating IGF-1 mediates exercise-induced increases in the number of new neurons in the adult hippocampus. *J Neurosci* 21:1628–1634.

Trommald M, Hulleberg G, Andersen P (1996) Long-term potentiation is associated with new excitatory spine synapses on rat dentate granule cells. *Learn Mem* 3:218–228.

Van der Borght K, Wallinga AE, Luiten PG, Eggen BJ, Van der Zee EA (2005) Morris watermaze learning in two rat strains increases the expression of the polysialylated form of the neural cell adhesion molecule in the dentate gyrus but has no effect on hippocampal neurogenesis. *Behav Neurosci* 119:926–932.

Van Praag H, Christie BR, Sejnowski TJ, Gage FH (1999a) Running enhances neurogenesis, learning, and long-term potentiation in mice. *Proc Natl Acad Sci USA* 96:13427–13431.

Van Praag H, Kempermann G, Gage FH (1999b) Running increases cell proliferation and neurogenesis in the adult mouse dentate gyrus. *Nat Neurosci* 2:266–270.

Van Praag H, Kempermann G, Gage FH (2000) Neural consequences of environmental enrichment. *Nat Rev Neurosci* 1:191–198.

Van Praag H, Schinder AF, Christis BR, Toni N, Palmer N, Gage FH (2002) Functional neurogenesis in the adult hippocampus. *Nature* 415:1030–1034.

Vythilingam M, Heim C, Newport J, Miller AH, Anderson E, Bronen R, Brummer M, Staib L, Vermetten E, Charney DS, Nemeroff CB, Bremner JD (2002) Childhood trauma associated with smaller hippocampal volume in women with major depression. *Am J Psychiatry* 159:2072–2080.

Wallenstein GV, Eichenbaum H, Hasselmo ME (1998) The hippocampus as an associator of discontiguous events. *Trends Neurosci* 21:317–323.

Wang S, Scott BW, Wojtowicz JM (2000) Heterogeneous properties of dentate granule neurons in the adult rat. *J Neurobiol* 42:248–257.

Wang S, Kee N, Preston E, Wojtowicz JM (2005) Electrophysiological correlates of neural plasticity compensating for ischemia-induced damage in the hippocampus. *Exp Brain Res* 165:250–260.

Warren SG, Juraska JM (1997) Spatial and nonspatial learning across the rat estrous cycle. *Behav Neurosci* 111:259–266.

Watanabe Y, Gould E, McEwen BS (1992) Stress induces atrophy of apical dendrites of hippocampal CA3 pyramidal neurons. *Brain Res* 588:341–345.

Westenbroek C, Den Boer JA, Veenhuis M, Ter Horst G (2004) Chronic stress and social housing differentially affect neurogenesis in male and female rats. *Brain Res Bull* 64:303–308.

Will B, Galani R, Kelche C, Rosenzweig MR (2004) Recovery from brain injury in animals; relative efficacy of environmental enrichment, physical exercise or formal training (1990–2002). *Prog Neurobiol* 72:167–182

Wood GE, Beylin AV, Shors TJ (2001) The contribution of adrenal and reproductive hormones to the opposing effects of stress on trace conditioning in males versus females. *Behav Neurosci* 115:175–187.

Woolley CS (1998) Estrogen-mediated structural and functional synaptic plasticity in the female rat hippocampus. *Horm Behav* 34:140–148.

Woolley CS, Gould E, McEwen BS (1990a) Exposure to excess glucocorticoids alters dendritic morphology of adult hippocampal pyramidal neurons. *Brain Res* 531:225–231.

Woolley CS, Gould E, Frankfurt M, McEwen BS (1990b) Naturally occurring fluctuation in dendritic spine density on adult hippocampal pyramidal neurons. *J Neurosci* 10:4035–4039.

Woolley CS, McEwen BS (1992) Estradiol mediates fluctuation in hippocampal synapse density during the estrous cycle in the adult rat. *J Neurosci* 12:2549–2554.

Woolley CS, Wenzel HJ, Schwartzkroin PA (1996) Estradiol increases the frequency of multiple synapse boutons in the hippocampal CA1 region of the adult female rat. *J Comp Neurol* 373:108–117.

Woolley CS, Weiland NG, McEwen BS, Schwartzkroin PA (1997) Estradiol increases the sensitivity of hippocampal CA1 pyramidal cells to NMDA receptor-mediated synaptic input: correlation with dendritic spine density. *J Neurosci* 17:1848–1859.

Woolley CS (1999) Effects of estrogen in the CNS. *Curr Opin Neurobiol* 9:349–354.

Xu Y, Tamamaki N, Noda T, Kimura K, Itokazu Y, Matsumoto N, Dezawa M, Ide C (2005) Neurogenesis in the ependymal layer of the adult rat 3rd ventricle. *Exp Neurol* 192:251–264.

Yoshimi K, Ren YR, Seki T, Yamada M, Ooizumi H, Onodera M, Saito Y, Murayama S, Okano H, Mizuno Y, Mochizuki H (2005) Possibility for neurogenesis in substantia nigra of parkinsonian brain. *Ann Neurol* 58:31–40.

Yuste R, Bonhoeffer T (2001) Morphological changes in dendritic spines associated with long-term synaptic plasticity. *Annu Rev Neurosci* 24:1071–1089.

Zhao M, Momma S, Delfani K, Carlen M, Cassidy RM, Johansson CB, Brismar H, Shupliakov O, Frisen J, Janson AM (2003) Evidence for neurogenesis in the adult mammalian substantia nigra. *Proc Natl Acad Sci USA* 100:7925–7930.

Zhou FC, Azmitia EC, Bledsoe S (1995) Rapid serotonergic fiber sprouting in response to ibotenic acid lesion in the striatum and hippocampus. *Dev Brain Res* 84:89–98.

Zola SM, Squire LR (2001) Relationship between magnitude of damage to the hippocampus and impaired recognition memory in monkeys. *Hippocampus* 11:92–98.

10 ▦ Tim Bliss, Graham Collingridge, and Richard Morris

Synaptic Plasticity in the Hippocampus

▦
10.1 Overview

Of all the properties of hippocampal synapses, perhaps the most beguiling and consequential, and certainly the most enthusiastically studied, is their ability to respond to specific patterns of activation with long-lasting increases or decreases in synaptic efficacy. Although it is now clear that synaptic plasticity is a property of many, perhaps most, excitatory synapses in the brain, much of what is known about long-term potentiation (LTP) and long-term depression (LTD) has been worked out in the structure where they were discovered. When it comes to synaptic plasticity, the hippocampus is the *fons et origo*, the onlie begetter, the home team.

The chapter opens with a brief historical account of the first two decades of research into LTP and LTD. During this period, from 1966 to the mid-1980s, the major characteristics of LTP, including its persistence, input specificity, and associativity, were established, the critical role of the *N*-methyl-D-aspartate (NMDA) receptor in the induction of LTP identified, and the first steps taken to link LTP to hippocampus-dependent learning. At the end of this period, it was clear that at most hippocampal synapses the conditions required for the induction of LTP are identical to the conditions required for the activation of the NMDA receptor, and that the cellular event that triggers the induction of LTP is the influx of Ca^{2+} through the activated NMDA receptor. We then, in Section 10.2, begin our survey of synaptic plasticity in the hippocampus with a discussion of the various short-term forms of plasticity that hippocampal synapses share with most if not all synapses: paired-pulse facilitation and depression and post-tetanic potentiation. We devote the next two sections, 10.3 and 10.4, to the mechanisms supporting the induction and expression of NMDA receptor-dependent LTP, the form of LTP displayed by, for example, perforant path-granule cell synapses and by commissural and Schaffer collateral synapses on CA1 pyramidal cells. Section 10.3 covers the properties of LTP, the proto-

cols that produce it, and the role of the NMDA receptor. Other aspects of NMDA receptor-dependent synaptic plasticity in the hippocampus are introduced, including EPSP-spike (E-S) potentiation, synaptic scaling, and metaplasticity. In the next section, 10.4, we turn to the mechanisms that support the expression of LTP. In contrast to the consensus that exists concerning the NMDA receptor-dependent events that mediate the induction of LTP, the mechanisms underlying its expression—that is, the pre- or postsynaptic changes that directly result in an increase in synaptic efficacy—are more complex and less well understood. Attention has mostly focused on postsynaptic changes involving the phosphorylation or insertion of AMPA receptor subunits. We assess the evidence that presynaptic changes also contribute to the increase in synaptic efficacy during the first few hours after induction. The study of morphological changes goes back to the very early days of LTP research, and it has often been proposed that a growth in the number or size of synapses is a correlate of LTP. Modern optical techniques allow spine growth to be imaged in real time, and there is evidence that this may occur in LTP. Additional mechanisms, involving gene transcription and protein synthesis, are required to sustain LTP for longer periods, giving rise to the distinction between early LTP (E-LTP) and protein synthesis-dependent late LTP (L-LTP). Late LTP, like early LTP, is input-specific, which raises the question of how somatically generated transcripts and proteins are targeted specifically to recently activated inputs, a discussion that leads to the idea of synaptic tagging.

Around the time that the NMDA receptor was being hailed for the elegant molecular explanation it offered for input specificity and associativity, examples of activity-dependent plasticity that did not require the NMDA receptor were being uncovered. In particular, the mossy fiber projection from granule cells to CA3 pyramidal cells supports a very different form of LTP that is not blocked by NMDA receptor antagonists. Both the induction and expression of mossy fiber LTP appear to be predominantly presynaptic. The discussion of mossy fiber LTP receives its own section, 10.5, and is followed, in 10.6, by a survey of neuromodulatory systems that affect LTP, such as the cholinergic input, catecholamines, and neurotrophins. In section 10.7 we explore the world of long-term depression, and the "depotentiation" of LTP. Although more difficult to obtain than LTP, and more difficult in adult than juvenile animals, a substantial literature, both in vitro and in vitro, supports the idea that LTD has both NMDA receptor-dependent and NMDA receptor-independent forms. Synaptic plasticity is not confined to excitatory connections between principal neurons; in Section 10.8 we examine the evidence for LTP and LTD at excitatory synapses onto interneurons and inhibitory synapses made by interneurons. Next, in section 10.9, we turn to synaptic plasticity in development, and in the aging animal, and discuss how LTP and LTD are affected in animal models of cognitive decline.

Finally, what's it all for? Why do hippocampal synapses display these striking forms of plasticity, and does the intact animal exploit them to acquire and store memories? In Section 10.10 we survey and assess the evidence relating to this central question. The readers will probably not be surprised to learn that we are able to provide only partial answers.

10.1.1 LTP: The First Two Decades

The term "synaptic plasticity" was introduced by the Polish psychologist Jerzy Konorski to describe the persistent, activity-driven changes in synaptic efficacy that he assumed, in common with most neuroscientists since Santiago Ramon y Cajal, to be the basis of information storage in the brain (Konorski, 1948). A formal hypothesis embodying this idea was advanced by the Canadian psychologist Donald Hebb in 1949. According to Hebb's celebrated postulate (Hebb, 1949),

> When an axon of cell A is near enough to excite a cell B and repeatedly or persistently takes part in firing it, some growth process or metabolic change takes place in one or both cells such that A's efficiency, as one of the cells firing B, is increased.

Nearly 25 years were to pass before the first description of a Hebb-like synapse in the mammalian brain. In 1973, Tim Bliss and Terje Lømo reported that long-lasting changes in synaptic efficacy at perforant path-granule cell synapses in the hippocampus could be induced by brief tetanic stimulation (Bliss and Lømo, 1973). The discovery of what has come to be known as "long-term potentiation" (or LTP) emerged from experiments that Per Andersen and Lømo, then a PhD student, were conducting at the University of Oslo during the mid-1960s on the phenomenon of frequency potentiation in excitatory hippocampal pathways. Working with anesthetized rabbits, Andersen had earlier observed that field potentials evoked by stimulation at frequencies of 1 Hz or less were stable, whereas the response to successive stimuli grew steadily larger when the stimulus frequency was stepped up to 5 to 10 Hz (Andersen, 1960). While exploring this phenomenon in the dentate gyrus, Lømo noticed that after episodes of high-

frequency stimulation of the perforant path lasting a few seconds the responses evoked by subsequent stimuli could remain enhanced for many tens of minutes. He reported his observations at the 1966 meeting of the Scandinavian Physiological Society in Åbo, Finland (Lømo, 1966). In 1968, Lømo and Bliss, a postdoctoral fellow from the National Institute for Medical Research in London with an interest in the neural basis of learning, embarked on a systematic investigation of what they at first called long-lasting potentiation (later renamed long-term potentiation by Graham Goddard) (Douglas and Goddard, 1975), a name that stuck no doubt because its acronym, LTP, tripped more lightly off the tongue than LLP. Bliss and Lømo delivered test stimuli at intervals of 2 to 3 seconds to the perforant path on each side of the brain and recorded the evoked response from either the granule cell layer of the dentate gyrus or the synaptic terminal region in the molecular layer. Tetanic stimulation of 100 Hz for 3 to 4 seconds or, more usually, 15 Hz for 10 to 20 seconds was given to the perforant path on one side, the other acting as a nontetanized control. An example of the potentiation they observed following repeated episodes of tetanic stimulation is shown in Figure 10-1A. In many cases, potentiation of the field EPSP (fEPSP) was accompanied by an increase in the amplitude and a decrease in the latency of the population spike (see traces in Fig. 10-1A) (for an introduction to field potentials and their interpretation, see Chapter 2, Box 2–1). The potentiation was apparent within 30 to 60 seconds of the tetanus and could be followed, with little decrement, for several hours.

A more extensive account by Bliss and Lømo of the background to their experiments can be found at http://www.ergito.com/main-lcd.jsp:bcs=EXP.13.8; other recollections of the early days of LTP by Andersen, Bliss, Lømo, Graham Collingridge, Gary Lynch, Bruce McNaughton, and Richard Morris are gathered in *LTP: Enhancing Neuroscience for 30 Years* (Oxford: Oxford University Press; 2004. Reprinted from Bliss et al., 2003).

Subsequently, Bliss and Tony Gardner-Medwin (1973) found that tetanus-induced potentiation could persist for many days in the unanesthetized rabbit with chronically implanted electrodes (Fig. 10–1B). Potentiation was not seen with low-intensity tetanization but required a stimulation strength that exceeded a threshold approximately equal to that required to activate a population spike. Analysis of input-output curves suggested that only the synaptic inputs that had actually been tetanized were potentiated, a phenomenon called "input specificity" (Bliss et al., 1973). Direct proof was delivered some years later following the introduction of the hippocampal slice preparation, which made it easier to activate two separate pathways converging on the same population of cells. LTP of the fEPSP was induced in the tetanized pathway, whereas the response evoked in the second, untetanized pathway remained at baseline levels (Andersen et al. 1977). In some cases, LTP of the population spike occurred without a corresponding change in the fEPSP (Bliss and Lømo, 1973). This result implies the existence of a second component of LTP,

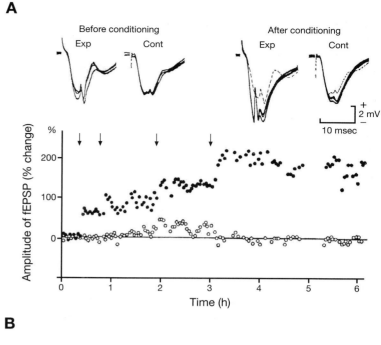

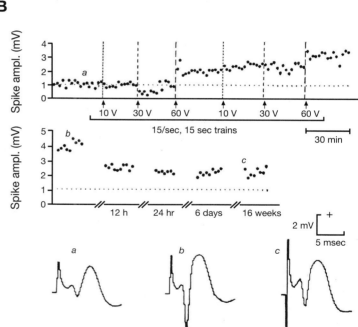

Figure 10–1. Tetanic stimulation induces long-lasting potentiation in the dentate gyrus of the intact rabbit. *A*. Brief tetanic stimulation (arrows) of the perforant path induces a rapid, persistent increase in the amplitude of the field EPSP. Further episodes of tetanic stimulation (15 Hz for 15 seconds) produce more potentiation until eventually, as illustrated in Figure 10–2A, the response saturates. The sample responses above reveal that the amplitude of the population spike is also potentiated and its latency reduced. (*Source*: Bliss and Lømo, 1973.) *B*. Potentiation of the population spike lasting for many weeks in a freely moving rabbit with chronically implanted electrodes given high-frequency trains of increasing stimulus intensity. Note the lack of effect of weak trains. The upper and lower part of the figure are continuous. Following the second train at 60 V, the response was monitored for 45 minutes and the animal then returned to its home cage. Twelve hours later, potentiation had declined to about half its maximum value and remained at that level for the following 16 weeks. The traces at the bottom of the panel were obtained at times indicated by a–c in the spike amplitude plots. (*Source*: Bliss and Gardner-Medwin, 1973.)

reflecting an increase in the coupling between the synaptic response and the population spike. The effect was subsequently given the name EPSP-spike (E-S) potentiation (Andersen et al., 1980).

Other important early contributions to the study of LTP in the intact animal came from the laboratory of Graham Goddard in Halifax, Nova Scotia. These studies established that briefer, more physiologically plausible tetani (7 stimuli at 400 Hz) could produce LTP in the perforant path of the anesthetized rat (Douglas and Goddard, 1975) and formalized the notion of *cooperativity* between afferent fibers to explain the existence of an intensity threshold for LTP induction

(McNaughton et al., 1978). Goddard and his colleagues, principally Rob Douglas, Carol Barnes, and Bruce McNaughton, were also the first to find a way to block the induction of LTP—by delivering a coincident high-frequency train to the commissural input to the dentate gyrus (Douglas et al., 1982). Because commissural stimulation suppressed the firing of granule cells, this last result suggested that the "locus of control" for induction was postsynaptic. From Goddard's laboratory too came the first description of the property of *associativity*, whereby a weak input could be potentiated if its activation coincided with a tetanus to another input (McNaughton et al., 1978). Around the same time, associativity was also documented in the weak pathway made by contralateral perforant path fibers to the molecular layer of the dentate gyrus (Levy and Steward, 1979).

The experiments described so far were all carried out on intact animals. Introduction of the living brain slice as a physiological preparation by Henry McIlwain during the 1960s (see Chapter 2) stimulated the development of the transverse hippocampal slice preparation in the Oslo laboratory (Skrede and Westgaard, 1971). This preparation allows ready access to all pathways of the dentate gyrus and hippocampus, provides mechanical stability for intracellular recording, and makes possible rapid pharmacological manipulation of the extracellular environment (see Chapter 5). Not surprisingly, it has achieved enormous popularity with investigators of synaptic function. Using this preparation, LTP was revealed at two other hippocampal pathways: the mossy fiber projection to CA3 pyramidal cells and the interleaved commissural and Schaffer collateral fibers from CA3 to CA1 pyramidal cells (Schwartzkroin and Wester, 1975). We refer to these fibers as the Schaffer-commissural projection. As we have seen, the transverse slice also allowed the *input specificity* of LTP to be demonstrated in a more direct way than had been possible in the dentate gyrus in vivo (Andersen et al., 1977; Lynch et al., 1977).

In contrast to in vivo preparations where the dentate gyrus offers the most stable recording conditions, the region most commonly studied in vitro has been area CA1. This is partly because LTP in the dentate gyrus in vitro is difficult to obtain without reducing tonic inhibition by perfusing a $GABA_A$ receptor antagonist (Wigström and Gustafsson, 1983) and perhaps partly because of a feeling of unease engendered by the fact that in the slice preparation the perforant path fibers are unattached to their parent cell bodies. It is well to remember that the hippocampal slice is a heavily reduced preparation. Although it makes possible a range of physiological and pharmacological experiments that would not otherwise be feasible, a full understanding of the mechanisms and significance of hippocampal synaptic plasticity cannot be reached by in vitro studies alone.

Experimental analysis of the properties and mechanisms of LTP has concentrated on the Hebbian form of synaptic plasticity exhibited by the perforant path projection to granule cells of the dentate gyrus and by Schaffer-commissural afferents to area CA1. It is this "classical" form of LTP that we discuss in most detail. Tetanic stimulation of both these pathways results in a rapid, persistent increase in synaptic responses, whether recorded intracellularly or extracellularly. LTP can be followed for many hours in both the slice preparation and the anesthetized animal and for days, weeks, or months in animals with implanted electrodes. LTP generally decays to baseline over a period of several days in rats with electrodes chronically implanted in the dentate gyrus, though potentiation lasting more than a year has been reported (Abraham, 2003).

Two important clues to the mechanisms underlying the induction of LTP were discovered in 1983. The first clue was provided by Graham Collingridge and colleagues, who showed that D-2-amino-5-phosphonopentanoic acid (D-AP5), a highly specific antagonist of the NMDA subtype of glutamate receptor that had been developed by Jeff Watkins and coworkers (Davies et al., 1981), blocks the induction of LTP in area CA1 while having little or no effect on synaptic responses recorded at low rates of stimulation (Collingridge et al., 1983). Then Gary Lynch and his collaborators reported that injection of a calcium chelator, ethyleneglycol-bis-(β-aminoethylether)-N,N,N′,N′,-tetraacetic acid (EGTA), into CA1 pyramidal cells blocks the induction of LTP (Lynch et al., 1983). This experiment confirmed the critical importance of the postsynaptic cell in the induction process and established an essential role for calcium.

As discussed in Chapter 6, excitatory synapses express up to four types of postsynaptic glutamate receptor: α-amino-3-hydroxy-5-methyl-4-isoxazolepropionate (AMPA), kainate, NMDA, and metabotropic glutamate (mGlu) receptors. The excitatory postsynaptic currents (EPSCs) evoked at low rates of stimulation are largely mediated by activation of AMPA receptors (Davies and Collingridge, 1989). NMDA receptors contribute only a small component of these EPSCs but are critical for synaptic plasticity. Two unexpected properties of the NMDA receptor were identified during the 1980s. First, the NMDA channel is unusual for a ligand-conducted ionophore in that its conductance is both ligand- and voltage-dependent. At near-resting membrane potentials, the channel is blocked by Mg^{2+}, and substantial depolarization is required to drive Mg^{2+} from the channel (Ault et al., 1980; Mayer et al., 1984; Nowak et al., 1984). Thus, activation of the NMDA channel requires the temporal coincidence of activity in presynaptic terminals to release transmitter plus adequate depolarization of the postsynaptic membrane. The properties of cooperativity, input specificity, and associativity follow directly from the dual ligand and voltage dependence of the NMDA receptor. As a result of these properties, the NMDA receptor can be thought of as a molecular coincidence detector, endowing pyramidal and granule cells with the capacity to detect coincident activity at multiple excitatory inputs. Second, the ionophore of the activated NMDA receptor is permeable to Ca^{2+} ions (MacDermott et al., 1986; Jahr and Stevens, 1987; Ascher and Nowak, 1988). This led to the idea that the trigger for the cellular processes leading to LTP is the entry of Ca^{2+} ions through the ionophore associated with the NMDA receptor and the subsequent activation of Ca^{2+}-dependent enzymes in the dendritic spine.

Thus, by the second half of the 1980s studies had matured to the point where a simple, compelling molecular explanation could be given for three defining properties of LTP: cooperativity, input specificity, and associativity. The hypothesis that the necessary and sufficient conditions for inducing LTP are just those required to activate the NMDA receptor received further support in 1986. Holger Wigström, Bengt Gustafsson, and others showed that even low-frequency stimuli could induce LTP in single CA1 pyramidal cells if each stimulus was given in conjunction with a strong depolarizing pulse (Wigström et al., 1986). This dramatic result showed that the induction of LTP did not absolutely depend on the strong, high-frequency trains that had been largely used up until then and the artificial nature of which had called into question the physiological relevance of LTP; on the contrary, weak low-frequency stimulation was equally effective provided the target cell was sufficiently depolarized by neighboring activity. The realization of the Hebbian nature of the induction of LTP took root at the same time as Richard Morris and his colleagues were demonstrating that animals without the capacity for hippocampal LTP owing to blockade of the NMDA receptor were severely impaired in the acquisition and retention of spatial learning in the watermaze (Morris et al., 1986). The mid-1980s was thus a time when LTP seemed well on the way to gaining acceptance as a physiological mechanism underlying the cognitive faculties of learning and memory and mark an appropriate point at which to bring this brief historical survey to a conclusion.

10.2 Transient Activity-dependent Plasticity in Hippocampal Synapses

10.2.1 Short-term Activity-dependent Changes in Synaptic Efficacy in the Hippocampal Formation

Synaptic transmission at the level of the single synapse is an inherently stochastic process (see Box 10–1; see also Chapter 6, Box 6–1) that can be modulated by prior activity in the presynaptic or postsynaptic neuron and by a wide variety of neuromodulators acting both pre- and postsynaptically. Some of the activity-dependent changes in synaptic efficacy that occur in the hippocampal formation, such as facilitation and depression, augmentation, and (post-tetanic) potentiation, are relatively short-lasting. It is with these short-lived types of plasticity that we begin our discussion (reviewed by Zucker and Regehr, 2002) (see Chapter 6–2).

10.2.2 Single Stimuli in Hippocampal Pathways Produce Two Transient Aftereffects: Facilitation and Depression

The aftereffects on synaptic transmission of a single stimulus can be tested by delivering a second stimulus at a variable time after the first. When pairs of stimuli are delivered to the perforant path, the amplitude of the second response recorded in the molecular layer of the dentate gyrus in vivo is typically facilitated at interstimulus intervals of less than 200 to 300 ms and depressed at longer intervals of up to a few seconds (McNaughton, 1980, 1982). Similar effects are seen at Schaffer-commissural synapses in area CA1 (Andersen, 1960). Paired-pulse facilitation and depression were first studied in the neuromuscular junction and appear to be a common feature of all chemically transmitting synapses (Magleby, 1979; Nicholls et al., 2001).

Facilitation

Facilitation can be attributed to the transient increase in the concentration of intraterminal calcium produced by an invading action potential. The concentration declines to basal values over a few hundred milliseconds, but the calcium influx at the time of the second stimulus adds to the residual calcium from the first, resulting in an enhanced calcium concentration and hence to an increase in the probability of release (Wu and Saggau, 1994). The magnitude of facilitation is inversely related to the initial probability of release. Analysis of elementary (quantal) synaptic events suggests that facilitation is largely due to presynaptic mechanisms (Zucker and Regehr, 2002). Note, however, that a postsynaptic component of facilitation has been described in both cortical pyramidal cells (Rozov and Burnashev, 1999) and CA1 pyramidal neurons (Bagal et al., 2005). A widely used test for discriminating presynaptic from postsynaptic mechanisms in LTP was introduced by McNaughton (1982), based on the fact that the higher the probability of release, the less scope there is for presynaptically mediated facilitation, and so the smaller is the observed degree of paired-pulse facilitation. A reduction in paired-pulse facilitation following the expression of LTP is therefore often taken as evidence for an increase in the probability of release. Initial studies found that whereas paired-pulse facilitation was decreased in post-tetanic potentiation (PTP), there was no change in LTP, implying that the expression mechanism was more likely to be postsynaptic (see Fig. 10–10A). As with most tests for the locus of expression of LTP, the paired-pulse facilitation test is suggestive but not conclusive: For example, no change in facilitation would be observed if LTP resulted from recruitment of a population of silent boutons (that is, boutons with zero probability of release before the induction of LTP) that, following induction, assumed a distribution of release probabilities similar to that of the population activated before induction. (See below and Box 10–1 for a discussion of this and other tests to determine the locus of expression of LTP.)

Depression

Transient depression of synaptic efficacy also occurs to the second of a pair of stimuli. To a large extent, this can be explained by a process of vesicle depletion, although receptor desensitization may also make a contribution. Evidence that transmitter depletion contributes to depression comes from the observation that in situations where transmitter release is artificially reduced, as when extracellular calcium concentration is lowered, depression is attenuated. This allows the full time course of facilitation to be revealed. Transmitter released by an action potential can also dampen the response produced by a subsequent stimulus via negative feedback involving activation of presynaptic glutamate receptors. In a similar manner, presynaptic $GABA_B$ autoreceptors on inhibitory terminals are thought to be responsible for the reduced inhibition that underlies the effectiveness of primed burst stimulation in

Pitfalls of Paired-Pulse Facilitation and Quantal Analysis as Techniques for Studying the Locus of Change in Synaptic Plasticity

PAIRED-PULSE FACILITATION

Paired-pulse facilitation (PPF) is due to an activity-dependent presynaptic modulation of transmitter release (Zucker and Regehr, 2002). It reflects the fact that at many synapses, such as those made by Schaffer commissural axons, an invading action potential has a greater chance of evoking exocytosis of neurotransmitter when it arrives within a few tens of milliseconds of a preceding action potential. When studying PPF, two stimuli are delivered with an interval of, say, 50 ms, and the amplitude of the first and second synaptic responses are compared. The amplitude of the second response relative to the first (facilitation ratio) is then a reflection of the increase in the probability of transmitter release (Pr). Facilitation is a function of the mean Pr of the synapses under study. Clearly if Pr is at or close to 1, there is little or no scope for facilitation. The standard argument, first advanced in the context of LTP by McNaughton (1982), is that modulation of synaptic efficacy due to a change in Pr is reflected in a converse change in facilitation; that is, an increase in Pr results in a decrease in facilitation and vice versa. During the first few minutes after a tetanus, the rapidly declining phases of PTP and short-term potentiation (STP) are mirrored by a decrease in facilitation; this is as expected for PTP, which is presynaptically mediated (see Section 10.2.3) and suggests that the early kinase-independent phenomenon of STP is also presynaptic. Thereafter, during LTP, facilitation is at baseline levels, arguing against a presynaptic change in LTP (see Fig. 10–11A). However, the evidence provided by a PPF analysis is suggestive rather than conclusive, and a change in PPF is not a wholly reliable guide to a presynaptic locus. To take a hypothetical example, suppose PPF increases after the induction of LTD. The conventional interpretation would be that this reflects a reduction in Pr. However, there are plausible postsynaptic changes that could give rise to an increase in PPF. Thus, if LTD involves the internalization of receptors, and the probability of internalization is dependent on the binding of transmitter, receptors at those synapses with the highest Pr would be internalized first. In this model, the mean Pr of the remaining active synapses would steadily fall, and PPF would increase as a result of a purely postsynaptic change. Evidence for this model is found in mGluR-dependent LTD (see Section 10.7.5)

QUANTAL ANALYSIS

When the quantal variable n, the number of release sites, is large (e.g., when stimulating many Schaffer-commissural fibers) the stochastic nature of neurotransmitter release is seen as trial-by-trial fluctuations in the amplitude of the evoked synaptic response. A measure of this variability is the coefficient of variance (CV = SD/mean), which is sensitive to changes in Pr and n but also, in some circumstances, to postsynaptic factors (Auger and Marty, 2000). For example, if during LTP Pr tends toward 1 (i.e., fewer failures), there is less variability due to trial-by-trial fluctuations in neurotransmitter release, and CV decreases. In the case of minimal stimulation, where one or at most a few axons are stimulated, there may be random failures of response due to the failure of the invading action potential to cause exocytosis of transmitter. A decrease in failures is classically equated with an increase in Pr and vice versa.

When a package of neurotransmitter is released, it evokes a postsynaptic response, the size of which is referred to as the quantal amplitude (q). The magnitude of this response varies from trial to trial as a result of the stochastic nature of postsynaptic channel opening and fluctuations in the amount of L-glutamate released. When a single release site is activated ($n = 1$), the variability in the magnitude of successful responses is due solely to this intra-site quantal variance. When multiple sites are activated ($n > 1$) there is an additional variance due to the between-site variation in quantal size. This inter-site variability could be large, reflecting, for example, differences in receptor number and electrotonic distance from the recording site.

The study of the relative contributions of n, Pr, and q to changes in synaptic efficacy is the subject of quantal analysis. Typically, quantal analysis involves collecting many responses to plot an amplitude frequency histogram. The mean amplitude of an evoked synaptic response is simply $n.Pr.q$. The spacing between peaks in the histogram provides an estimate of q. A change in q alters the interpeak spacing without altering the amplitudes of the peaks, whereas a change in n or Pr modifies the amplitudes of the peaks but not the spacing between them

Although these approaches are powerful in theory, they are often difficult to interpret in practice. There are many reasons for this situation, which can be considered in two main categories. The first major problem is the difficulty of making accurate measurements. This requires high quality voltage-clamp recordings, so events are measured (as far as possible) at

(Continued)

the same membrane voltage. It also requires the elimination of as many confounding variables (e.g., voltage-dependent conductances that may be imperfectly clamped, and synaptic inhibition) as is practical. Assuming that this has been achieved, a remaining major problem is that unitary EPSCs in hippocampal neurons are very small. As a result, it is difficult to distinguish all of the EPSCs above the background noise. Consequently, estimates of the frequency and amplitude distributions of miniature EPSCs can be inaccurate, and small evoked EPSCs may be misclassified as failures. The technically demanding technique of dendritic recording close to the site of synaptic activation improves the signal-to-noise ratio; using this approach it has been shown that EPSCs at Schaffer commissural synapses can be generated by fewer than five AMPA receptors (Isaac et al., 1998). These very small responses would probably be undetectable with standard somatic recording techniques and so would be misclassified as failures. A second problem is that quantal variance (both inter- and intra-site) is often large, making it difficult to construct clean histograms for quantal analysis.

The second class of problem is how to interpret the parameters that are altered during LTP or LTD. The classical interpretation is that changes in n or Pr are due to presynaptic changes, and changes, in q are due to postsynaptic changes. However, even at the neuromuscular junction where quantal analysis was invented and the application used to most powerful effect, it was recognized that these parameters could be interpreted in different ways. For example, an increase in q could be due to more neurotransmitter contained in a synaptic vesicle. In hippocampal neurons, LTP is often associated with a decrease in the failure rate (Malinow and Tsien, 1990). This was initially interpreted in the classical tradition as an increase in Pr. However, the failure rate is determined by the product of Pr and n, the number of competent synaptic sites. In was subsequently postulated (Kullmann, 1994) and then demonstrated (Isaac et al., 1995; Liao et al., 1995) that a decrease in failures may be due to the unsilencing of silent synapses (see Fig. 10–21A). The idea is that a stimulated afferent fiber may fail to generate a response either because $Pr = 0$ or because there are no postsynaptic receptors to which transmitter can bind. By awakening these synapses, LTP adds new synaptic sites (n) to the equation. There has been much debate as to whether the increase in n is presynaptic (more functional release sites) or postsynaptic (more synapses with functional receptors), as discussed in Section 10.4; but either way, this alters radically the interpretation of changes in failure rates. The unsilencing of silent synapses during LTP and, conversely, the silencing of synapses during LTD is now a widely documented phenomenon (see Sections 10.4 and 10.7) and needs to be taken into account during any interpretation of analyses of the quantal parameters of LTP. For example, alterations in the frequency of spontaneous mini-EPSCs could reflect changes in Pr and/or n, where changes in n reflect pre- or postsynaptic unsilencing of silent synapses.

Alterations in n, whether pre- or postsynaptic, can also explain changes in PPF, as in the hypothetical example given above in which a postsynaptic change gives rise to a change in PPF. Conversely, presynaptic changes could occur without a change in PPF (e.g., if LTP were achieved by unsilencing of a population of new release sites with a similar distribution of Pr to existing sites). Therefore changes in each of the basic electrophysiological parameters of neurotransmission (n, Pr, q, PPF) can have more than one, radically different interpretation.

inducing LTP (Davies et al., 1991) (see Section 10.3.1 and Fig. 10–6).

Facilitation and depression necessarily interact. The conditions for facilitation are set in place by the arrival of an action potential at the presynaptic terminal and are independent of whether transmitter release occurs. The same is not true for depression, which is a consequence of transmitter release. Thus, if a pair of action potentials invades the terminal within a few tens of milliseconds, the response to the second action potential is determined by both facilitation and inhibition if the first action potential resulted in transmitter release but is influenced by facilitation alone if the first action potential fails to release transmitter. On the other hand, where release probability is relatively high, thus limiting the scope for facilitation, depression may predominate at all intervals; this appears to be the case in vitro at synapses of the medial but, interestingly, not the lateral perforant path (McNaughton, 1980; Allen et al., 2000). Another consequence of the interplay between facilitation and depression is the difficulty of predicting how the induction of LTP affects a cell's response to bursts of stimuli. The increased response to single test stimuli conventionally used to monitor synaptic efficacy in LTP experiments is not necessarily a useful predictor of the response that a postsynaptic cell might make to a burst of afferent impulses. For example, an increase in the probability of release as the result of the induction of LTP might, because of paired-pulse depression, lead to a reduction in the probability of release to the second or following stimuli in the burst (Lisman, 1997). However, although Markram and Tsodyks (1996) reported effects of this kind at potentiated synapses in visual cortex,

Selig et al. (1999) did not find a similar redistribution of synaptic efficacy when bursts of stimuli were delivered to potentiated hippocampal synapses; instead, the response to each stimulus of the burst was potentiated.

Paired-pulse facilitation and depression of the population spike can give useful information about feedforward and feedback inhibitory circuits in the hippocampus. If the first of a pair of stimuli is strong enough to evoke a sizable population spike, a brief period of intense $GABA_A$-mediated feedback inhibition lasting 10 to 20 ms is generated, during which time a second stimulus of equal or lesser intensity does not evoke a population spike; this gives way to a much longer period of spike facilitation that can be explained by suppression of feedforward inhibition mediated by presynaptic $GABA_B$ autoreceptors; this effect peaks at an interstimulus interval of 100 to 200 ms and can last for 1000 ms or longer (Davies et al., 1991).

10.2.3 Post-tetanic Potentiation Is the Sum of Two Exponential Components: Augmentation and Potentiation

Repetitive stimulation of peripheral and central synapses brings into play another transient facilitatory process called post-tetanic potentiation (PTP). At perforant path synapses, a weak high-frequency train leads to a substantial elevation of test responses immediately after the train, which declines back to baseline within a few minutes (Fig. 10–2A). With longer stimulus trains, PTP is superimposed on a background of LTP, and this complicates the analysis of the time course of both phenomena. When suitable controls are conducted, PTP is seen to be the sum of two exponential processes known as *augmentation* and *potentiation* that in the medial perforant path have time constants of 7 s and 2 to 3 minutes, respectively (McNaughton, 1982). The concentration of Ca^{2+} in terminal boutons rises during PTP, suggesting that, like facilitation, it is a presynaptic process (Wu and Saggau, 1994; Tang and Zucker, 1997).

10.3 NMDA Receptor-dependent Long-term Potentiation: Properties and Determinants

We begin by discussing the varieties of stimulus protocol that lead to the induction of NMDA receptor-dependent LTP and then explore more fully its properties and characteristics.

10.3.1 Long-term Potentiation: Tetanic Stimulation Induces a Persistent Increase in Synaptic Efficacy

Whether conducted in vivo or in vitro, a typical experiment on LTP takes the following form. The animal or brain slice is prepared, electrodes are located at the appropriate sites for stimulating and recording, and observations are made to ensure that electrophysiological responses are stable, via a computer-based system that calculates various measures of field potentials, EPSPs or EPSCs, as appropriate (Bortolotto et al., 2002). Once this preliminary work is complete, the experiment proper progresses through three phases. In the first phase baseline responses are elicited using low-frequency test pulses (e.g., at 30-second intervals) for a period sufficient to ensure stability (the duration of which depends on the type of experiment to be performed but typically is in the range of 10–60 minutes). Sometimes an input-output curve is obtained in which the strength of the stimulation is systematically varied to provide information on the relation between the fiber volley (reflecting the number of fibers activated), the synaptic component of the evoked response (the fEPSP), and the population spike (reflecting the number of cells discharged). The second phase is brief but critical: It is the point at which the stimulated pathway is tetanized or, in the case of most intracellular recordings, the moment when afferent stimulation is paired with postsynaptic depolarization. Common tetanization protocols include one or more trains of pulses at 100 Hz for 1 second per train or patterns consisting of shorter trains arranged in a pattern that contains a theta frequency component (see below). The third phase involves a return to low-frequency stimulation at the same frequency and intensity as was used to measure the baseline; data for further input-output curves may be collected at intervals after tetanization.

In a typical LTP experiment, the response is dramatically amplified following the tetanus. The initial slope of the EPSP rises more steeply, the onset latency of the population spike (if present) is reduced, and its amplitude is often enhanced several-fold. So startling is the transformation that Bliss and Marina Lynch (1988) were moved to confess "no matter how often one has witnessed the phenomenon, it is impossible not to retain a sense of amazement that such modest stimulation can produce so immediate, so profound and so persistent an effect." The basic phenomenon of LTP is easily elicited and gratifyingly immediate.

It is a common convention to refer to synaptic potentiation as LTP if the potentiated response is maintained without appreciable downward drift for longer than 30 to 60 minutes. This covers only the early phase of LTP, however, and allows the experimenter to say nothing about later phases. In field potential studies, three phases of potentiation can be defined on the basis of susceptibility to drugs. As discussed in more detail below, LTP decays to baseline over a period of 3 to 5 hours when induction takes place in the presence of inhibitors of gene transcription or protein synthesis. Frey and coworkers assigned the name "late LTP" (L-LTP) to the persistent, protein synthesis-dependent phase of LTP; the protein synthesis-independent phase was termed "early LTP" (E-LTP) (Frey et al., 1993). A third, earlier phase that survives protein kinase inhibitors and decays to baseline usually within 30-60 minutes is referred to as "short-term potentiation" (STP).

Originally observed in anesthetized rabbits, hippocampal LTP has since been described in numerous vertebrate species, including rats, guinea pigs, mice, and chicks (Margrie et al.,

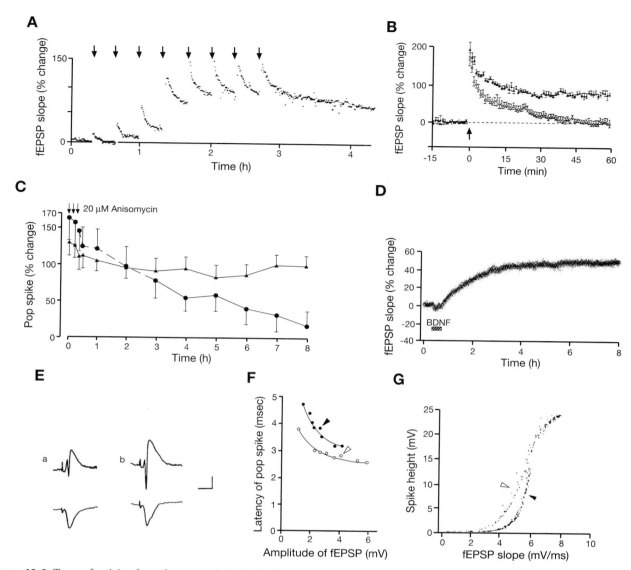

Figure 10–2. Types of activity-dependent potentiation in the hippocampus. *A.* Post-tetanic potentiation (PTP), lasting for a few minutes, is always induced in the dentate gyrus of the intact animal, even when longer-lasting forms of potentiation are saturated by repeated tetanization. Tetani of increasing intensity were given; note that at the lowest intensitiy LTP is not induced though PTP is still present. (*Source:* Bliss et al., 1983) *B.* Short-term potentiation (STP) in area CA1 in vitro. In the presence of a broad-spectrum protein kinase inhibitor, tetanus-induced potentiation returns to baseline within 30 to 60 minutes (open triangles). After initial PTP, LTP in control medium (filled triangles) persists without further decrement for 60 minutes. (*Source:* Malenka et al., 1989.) *C.* The protein synthesis inhibitor anisomycin curtails the duration of LTP. The amplitude of the population spike in area CA1 in vitro was monitored after tetanic stimulation in control medium (triangles) or in the presence of anisomycin (circles). E-LTP, defined as the component of LTP that is protein synthesis-independent, returns to baseline within 5 to 8 hours. Late LTP is the more persistent component that is blocked by protein synthesis inhibitors. (*Source:* Frey et al., 1988.) *D.* Transient exposure to brain-derived neurotrophic factor (BDNF) induces a slow-onset late LTP in the dentate gyrus of the anesthetized rat. (*Source:* Bramham and Messaoudi, 2005.) *E.* LTP of the population spike without potentiation of the fEPSP. Field potentials recorded in the pyramidal cell layer (upper traces) and stratum radiatum (lower traces) of area CA1 before (left) and 25 minures after the induction of LTP by an orthodromic/antidromic pairing protocol. Calibrationz: 10 ms, 2 mV. (*Source:* Jester et al., 1995.) *F.* The latency of the population spike plotted as a function of the amplitude of the EPSP before (solid circles) and 8 hours after (open circles) induction of LTP by tetanic stimulation of the perforant path (same experiment as in Figure 10–1A). The curve was plotted from responses evoked by a series of stimuli generated at different stimulus strengths. Note that an fEPSP of a given amplitude evokes a population spike with a shorter latency after the induction of LTP than before, demonstrating that LTP consists not only of an increase in the synaptic drive but enhancement of the coupling between synaptic input and cell firing. This latter component is called EPSP-spike (E-S) potentiation. (*Source:* Bliss and Lømo, 1973.) *G.* Another experiment in which E-S curves were generated before and after the induction of LTP. Here, the amplitude of the population spike is plotted against the EPSP. The curve shifts to the left, reflecting E-S potentiation. (*Source:* Bliss et al., 1983.) In F, G points indicated by filled and open arrow heads were obtained before and after induction of LTP respectively.

1998), macaque monkeys (Urban et al., 1996), and humans (Beck et al., 2000; reviewed by Cooke and Bliss, 2006).

Long-term potentiation has been subjected to more intense study in the hippocampal formation (particularly the dentate gyrus and CA1 and CA3 pyramidal subfields) than elsewhere in the brain. In addition to the synapses of the tri-synaptic loop (i.e., perforant path to granule cells; mossy fibers to CA3 cells; Schaffer collaterals to CA1 cells), LTP has been observed at associational connections between CA3 cells, the perforant path projections to area CA3 (Do et al., 2002) and area CA1 (Colbert and Levy, 1993), the projections from CA1 to the subiculum (O'Mara et al., 2000), in some but not all excitatory connections onto hippocampal interneurons (Lamsa et al., 2005) and even at synaptic connections made by hippocampal CA1 neurons on a class of macroglia-like cells (Ge et al., 2006). However, the fact that LTP has been observed in birds and reptiles lacking a laminated hippocampal formation raises the possibility that its discovery in the mammalian hippocampus was fortuitous. Although the laminated structure of the hippocampus makes it particularly convenient for the study of LTP, there is no reason to suppose that hippocampal synapses occupy a privileged position in the hierarchy of plasticity. LTP has been described in many other brain regions (Racine et al., 1983), including cerebellum (Crépel and Jaillard, 1991), amygdala (Chapman et al., 1990) , sensory cortex (Artola and Singer, 1987), motor cortex (Sakamoto et al., 1987), prefrontal cortex (Laroche et al., 1990), and nucleus accumbens (Kombian and Malenka, 1994). Long-term changes in synaptic efficacy have also been found in sympathetic ganglia (Brown and McAfee, 1982) and in the nociceptive circuitry of the spinal cord (Ikeda et al., 2003).

A Wide Range of Stimulus Protocols Can Induce LTP

LTP can be induced by a broad range of stimulus parameters. As first noted by Bliss and Gardner-Medwin (1973) in their study of LTP in awake rabbits, the stimulus intensity during the tetanus must be sufficiently strong. In a systematic study of this effect, McNaughton et al. (1978) gradually increased the intensity of tetanization to reveal that LTP occurred only above what they termed the "cooperativity" threshold. PTP was observed at lower intensities with the response amplitude declining to baseline between successive tetanizations (see example in Fig. 10–2A). Their supposition was that some minimum number of afferent fibers had to be activated for LTP to occur and that thereafter the magnitude of LTP could increase until an asymptote was reached. However, it is now known that activation of some minimum number of fibers is neither a necessary nor a sufficient condition for inducing LTP. Although not indisputably established, it is likely that LTP can be induced by activating a single axon if a target cell of that axon is sufficiently depolarized. In the behaving animal, therefore, there may be circumstances in which individual synapses can be independently potentiated. Nevertheless, cooperativity serves as a reminder that a threshold for LTP, whether expressed in terms of the number of activated axons

or in terms of local dendritic depolarization, does exist and has important consequences for network behavior. First, network stability is less at risk from unrestricted increases in excitatory drive; second, the cooperativity threshold may act as filter, restricting access to long-term storage to those neural signals with a sufficiently high information content.

The magnitude and duration of LTP is also a function of tetanus intensity. If a tetanus that is suprathreshold for LTP is repeated, it may induce a further increment of LTP when repeated some time later (Bliss and Lømo, 1973), suggesting that at the level of the single synapse LTP may be incremental rather than all-or-none. Eventually, however, LTP becomes saturated, and tetanic stimulation produces no further effect. Clearly, the response to identical episodes of tetanic stimulation depends on the history of the network, and this has given rise to the concept of metaplasticity (see below). The maximal level of synaptic efficacy a given pathway can reach is not necessarily attained when LTP is apparently saturated. In the first place, PTP can transiently elevate the response above the existing level. Furthermore, if an interval of several hours is allowed to elapse after saturating tetanic stimulation, additional potentiation can be elicited with a further tetanus, even if there has been no decrement in the response during the intervening period (Frey et al., 1995).

The stimulus patterns used to elicit LTP have varied widely among laboratories, ranging from brief trains at 400 Hz (Douglas and Goddard, 1975) to single stimuli of high intensity repeated at 1 Hz in the presence of picrotoxin (Abraham et al., 1986). Probably the most commonly used protocol is a single train of 100 Hz for 1 second. Two other widely used protocols are primed-burst stimulation (PBS) and theta-burst stimulation (TBS), in which the common feature is an interval of 200 ms, either between a priming stimulus and a brief burst of stimuli in the case of PBS (Larson and Lynch, 1986), or between a succession of brief trains in TBS (Rose and Dunwiddie, 1986). It may not be coincidental that 200 ms is close to the periodicity of the theta rhythm (an endogenous hippocamapal rhythm generated during movement—see Chapter 11). In most cases, it is probably true to say that the choice of protocol favored by a particular laboratory relies more on tradition than any clearly demonstrated superiority. In a parametric study of induction protocols in which theta-burst stimulation was compared with simple trains of high-frequency stimulation, Hernandez et al. (2005) concluded that the major factor controlling the magnitude of LTP is the number of stimuli in a train rather than the pattern of stimulation. High-frequency trains can be used to induce LTP in cell populations or single cells. In the latter case, two other protocols for inducing LTP are available: pairing, and spike timing. With the former, single stimuli repeated at low frequency are paired with depolarizing pulses that induce brisk firing of the recorded cell (Abraham et al., 1986; Kelso et al., 1986). With spike timing-dependent potentiation (STDP), the pairing is between the afferent stimulus and a brief depolarizing pulse that fires the target cell only once. The latter protocol allows the timing between pre- and postsynaptic firing to be controlled with some precision and has led to the important observation that LTP occurs only when the presynaptic impulse precedes the firing of the target cell; when the opposite relation obtains, the result is LTD rather than LTP (Bi and Poo, 1998) (see Section 10.3.8).

The reason for the effectiveness of the prime-burst or theta-burst procedure has been clarified (Davies et al., 1991). The priming stimulus (or initial brief train) activates feedforward GABA interneurons, leading to GABA$_A$- and GABA$_B$-mediated hyperpolarization in the pyramidal cell but, importantly, also to activation of presynaptic GABA$_B$ autoreceptors. The latter produce a transient reduction in GABA release that is maximal at around 100 to 200 ms. Thus the second train produces much less GABA-mediated hyperpolarization with consequent enhancement of the voltage-dependent NMDA receptor-mediated current. Minimal patterns of stimulation of this kind are far more likely to occur naturally than the longer trains of tens or hundreds of stimuli (e.g., 100 Hz for 1 second) that are frequently used for reasons of convenience and custom. Hippocampal pyramidal neurons can and do fire in high-frequency bursts, although it remains to be established whether LTP is induced by naturally occurring patterns of activity in the freely moving animal (Buzsaki, 1987) (see Chapter 8, Section 8.4 for a further discussion of this point).

10.3.2 Time Course of LTP: Rapid Onset and Variable Duration

How quickly after a tetanus is LTP induced? The time course of the onset of LTP is difficult to measure because it is confounded by the extremely rapid onset of PTP. By studying PTP in isolation using trains subthreshold for LTP or in the presence of AP5, which blocks the induction of LTP without affecting PTP, and by making the assumption that LTP and PTP are independent processes, it is possible to dissect out the two processes (McNaughton, 1980; Gustafsson et al., 1989). In CA1 in vitro, LTP begins within 2 to 3 seconds of the tetanus, peaks within 30 seconds, and then declines for 10 to 20 minutes to a lower, more stable value. In the dentate gyrus, LTP takes longer (1–2 minutes) to reach its peak (Hanse and Gustafsson, 1992). Estimates are confounded, however, by the possibility that onset kinetics are modulated by the test stimuli given to sample synaptic responses.

How long does LTP last? This is a question of obvious significance but one to which no simple answer can be given. A short answer is that LTP shows variable persistence. The duration of the effect depends on the parameters of the tetanus, the type of preparation, and the region of the hippocampus. In both hippocampal slices and anesthetized animals, the maximal duration of LTP is obviously limited to the lifetime of the preparation. In the intact animal, time constants as short as a few days (Racine et al., 1983) and as long as 73 days (Doyère and Laroche, 1992) to more than a year (Abraham, 2003) have been reported for the dentate gyrus. Fewer experiments have been carried out in area CA1 in vivo, but it

has been claimed that LTP in this region is sometimes nondecremental (Staubli and Lynch, 1987). Later, we discuss mechanisms responsible for modulating the persistence of LTP. Intriguingly, the decay of LTP may be an active process, as in the dentate gyrus LTP is prolonged if an NMDA receptor antagonist is given after induction (Villarreal et al., 2001).

Can all excitatory synapses onto principal cells in the hippocampus be potentiated? Not all attempts to induce LTP between pairs of cells using a pairing induction protocol or between a presumed single axon and a target cell have been successful. However, this may reflect an unhealthy or dialyzed cell or an inappropriate stimulus protocol for that synapse. Based on results of attempting to induce LTP by a pairing protocol using minimal stimulation to activate one or at most a few synapses in area CA1, Petersen et al. (1998) estimated that between 45% and 75% of excitatory synapses in area CA1 can be potentiated, a proportion low enough to raise suspicions that not all such synapses are potentiable. A similar conclusion was reached by Debanne et al. (1999), working with pairs of interconnected cells in organotypic hippocampal cultures. In their sample, 24% of unitary EPSPs (a term here used to cover the multiple connections that a CA3 cell in organotypic culture may make with a target CA3 or CA1 cell) could not be potentiated. Unpotentiable connections may represent synapses at which LTP has been saturated and that might therefore be more susceptible to LTD-inducing stimulation, but 63% of nonpotentiable connections in the experiments of Debanne et al. (1999) could not be depressed either. These studies suggest that there is a small proportion of excitatory synapses on hippocampal pyramidal cells, perhaps 10% to 20% of the total, that do not exhibit synaptic plasticity.

10.3.3 Three Distinct Temporal Components of Potentiation: STP, Early LTP, Late LTP

Broad-spectrum protein kinase inhibitors curtail the duration of potentiation to an hour or so (e.g., Lovinger et al., 1987; Malenka et al., 1989; Malinow et al., 1989 Matthies and Reymann, 1993; see also reviews by Soderling and Derkach, 2000; Lisman et al., 2002; Nguyen and Woo, 2003) (Fig 10–2B and Section 10.4.3). In the presence of protein synthesis inhibitors such as emetine or anisomycin, or transcription inhibitors such as actinomycin, the potentiated response in area CA1 of hippocampal slices returns to baseline within 5 to 6 hours (Frey et al., 1988) (Fig. 10–2C). From these findings emerged the defining characteristics of early and late LTP (E-LTP and L-LTP) as protein kinase-dependent and protein synthesis-dependent, respectively. Note that this leaves a component of LTP, usually lasting less than an hour, referred to as short-term potentiation (STP). STP is NMDA receptor-dependent but depends neither on protein synthesis nor, in general, on protein kinase activity (Fig. 10–2B). Weak stimulus trains sometimes produce E-LTP without L-LTP, but no stimulus protocols have been identified that produce L-LTP without the preceding phase of E-LTP. However, as as we shall

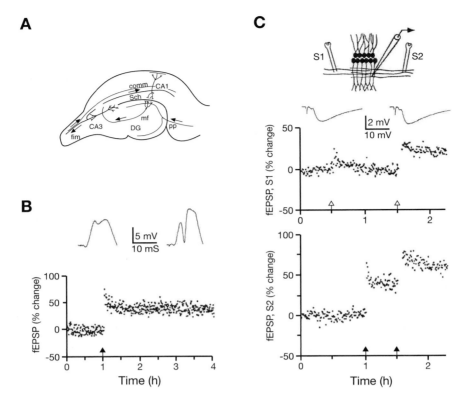

Figure 10–3. Induction properties of LTP: coooperativity, input specificity, and associativity. *A.* Diagram of a transverse section through hippocampus showing principal excitatory connections. *B.* LTP induced by a tetanus (250 Hz for 200 ms) to the perforant path in an anesthetized rat. Field responses recorded in the granule cell layer before and after the induction of LTP are shown above. *C.* Input specificity and associativity demonstrated using a two-pathway protocol in area CA1 in vitro. Stimulating electrodes S1 and S2 are placed in the stratum radiatum on either side of a recording electrode to excite two independent sets of axons. The slope of the fEPSP evoked by test stimuli to S1 and S2 are plotted in the two panels below the diagram of the recording arrangement. The intensity of the tetanus delivered via S1 is set below the cooperativity threshold for LTP, so only PTP is elicited (upper panel). At 1 hour a strong tetanus is given to S2, inducing robust LTP. Note that the response to S1 is unchanged: LTP is input-specific. However, when a weak tetanus to S1, which by itself is ineffective, is combined with a strong tetanus to S1, LTP is induced in both inputs. This is the property of associativity. (*Source*: Bliss and Collingridge, 1993.)

see in Section 10.4.9, late-onset, protein synthesis-dependent potentiation can be induced by applying activators of PKA to area CAI, or brain-derived neurotrophic factor (BDNF) to the dentate gyrus (Fig. 10–2D).

10.3.4 Input-Specificity of LTP: Potentiation Occurs Only at Active Synapses

Compelling evidence for input specificity was first obtained in area CA1 of the hippocampal slice in experiments using two stimulating electrodes positioned to activate two sets of fibers converging on the same cell population (Andersen et al., 1977; Lynch et al., 1977). Tetanization of either pathway resulted in potentiation specific to that pathway. This outcome is true whether one stimulating pathway is in the stratum oriens and the other in the stratum radiatum, or both pathways are in the same stratum. The two-pathway design, which has made an important contribution to physiological studies of LTP, exploits the fact that most fibers travel at an angle to the plane of the slice. Thus, stimulating electrodes positioned on either side of the target neuron (in single-cell studies) or of a population of neurons (in field recordings) activate a nonoverlapping set of axons projecting to the same target cell(s) (Fig. 10–4).

Input specificity at the relatively crude level of two-pathway experiments does not imply specificity at the level of single synapses. To demonstrate the latter, it will be necessary to monitor the activation of neighboring synapses. Optical methods offer the best chance of achieving this, but the relevant experiments have not yet been done. Even so, experiments can be conducted to investigate whether the expression of LTP is restricted to the synapses at which it is induced. Two ingenious electrophysiological studies, one by Haley et al. (1996) and the other by Engert and Bonhoeffer (1997), suggest that synapse specificity breaks down within a radius of a few tens of microns of a site of potentiation, regardless of whether synapses are on the same target cell or are active at the time of potentiation.

A

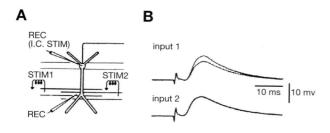

B

C

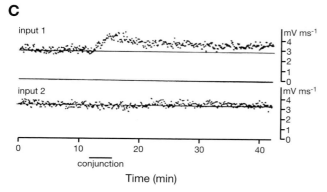

Figure 10–4. LTP as a Hebbian mechanism. The repeated pairing of single stimuli with depolarization of the membrane potential is sufficient to induce LTP. *A.* Experimental arrangement, with two independent afferent pathways and an intracellular electrode to record evoked EPSPs and through which current can be passed to depolarize the membrane potential. *B.* Examples of EPSPs before and after the induction of LTP in input 1. Note that there is no change in input 2. *C.* Plots of the response evoked by test stimuli delivered alternately at an interval of 3.5 seconds to S1 and S2. During the period indicated by the bar ("conjunction"), the stimulus to S1 was followed 7 ms later by a 400-ms depolarizing pulse that elicited a burst of cell firing. The pairing of single stimuli and depolarization induced an increase in the EPSP that reached a maximum within 20 to 30 pairings and persisted, with some initial decay, for the rest of the recording session. The response to the second pathway was unaffected. (*Source*: Wigström et al., 1986.)

10.3.5 Associativity: Induction of LTP Is Influenced by Activity at Other Synapses

Associativity, a defining property of LTP, was discovered by McNaughton et al. (1978), and independently by Levy and Steward (1979) who introduced the term in the context of LTP. In both cases, interactions between two afferent pathways in the dentate gyrus of the anesthetized rat were examined. McNaughton and his colleagues compared cooperativity in the medial and lateral perforant path projections to the ipsilateral dentate gyrus; they found that when weak tetani were given simultaneously to the medial and lateral branches of the perforant path, LTP was induced in both pathways, though each tetanus, when given separately, was below the cooperativity threshold. Levy and Steward investigated the properties of the crossed perforant path. The latter is a weak projection containing few axons that projects from the entorhinal cortex

to the molecular layer of the contralateral dentate gyrus. Tetanic stimulation of the weak crossed pathway was incapable of inducing LTP when given alone; but if given at the same time as a tetanus to the strong ipsilateral perforant pathway, LTP was induced in both ipsilateral and contralateral pathways (see Fig. 10–17A). This experiment demonstrated that activity at one input has the potential for promoting plasticity at another active input—in other words that LTP is associative. Levy and Steward argued that the asociative property of LTP was a desirable feature of "memory elements in the hippocampal formation." These two sets of experiments also made it clear that the distinction between cooperativity and associativity is essentially semantic. Cooperativity can be thought of as an associative interaction between the afferent fibers accessible to a single stimulating electrode. Associativity was subsequently observed at the intracellular level in the hippocampal slice using a two-pathway design (Barrionuevo and Brown, 1983).

These early experiments did not distinguish between associative interactions occurring presynaptically and postsynaptically. One possibility was that cooperativity and associativity reflected the requirement for sufficient depolarization of the target cells. As already noted, experiments demonstrating that inhibition of granule cells by commissural afferents could suppress the induction of LTP, suggested to Goddard and his colleagues that the postsynaptic cell provided the "locus of control" for LTP (Douglas et al., 1982). In 1986 Wigström, Gustafsson and their coworkers (Wigström et al., 1986), and independently two other groups (Kelso et al., 1986; Sastry et al., 1986), confirmed in spectacular fashion that LTP in area CA1 could be induced by the simple expedient of repeatedly pairing single stimuli to Schaffer-commissural fibers with a depolarizing pulse generating multiple spikes in the impaled cell (Fig. 10-4). The explanation for the efficacy of this procedure became clear when it was shown that it enabled NMDAR-mediated responses to be evoked by single stimuli (Collingridge et al., 1988). Pairing single stimuli with iontophoretic application of glutamate was similarly effective at inducing LTP (Hvalby et al., 1987). By varying the time between the stimulus and the onset of the depolarizing pulse, the time window for associative interaction could be studied. The maximum effect occured when the stimulus was given at the beginning of the 100-ms depolarizing pulse; the degree of potentiation declined to zero when the interval between this single stimulus and the onset of the depolarizing pulse was longer than 100 ms and no potentiation occurred if the afferent stimulus was given after the depolarizing pulse (Gustafsson et al., 1987). Extracellular experiments in the dentate gyrus (Levy and Steward, 1983) and in area CA1 (Gustafsson and Wigström, 1986; Kelso et al., 1986), using a two-pathway protocol with one "weak" and one "strong" input also showed that associative potentiation of the weak pathway requires near-coincidence of weak and strong inputs, with potentiation occurring if the weak immediately precedes the strong input but not if the strong precedes the weak input.

The timing requirements for coincident pre- and postsynaptic activity that emerged from these early experiments are somewhat less constrained than those that have more recently been characterized in the context of spike timing-dependent plasticity (STDP) (see Section 10.3.8).

Because of its potential for strengthening co-active inputs, the property of associativity lies at the heart of the role that LTP is likely to play in memory functions of the hippocampus. Note that cooperativity, associativity, and input specificity can all be explained on the assumption that the induction of LTP at a given synapse requires presynaptic activity with coincident activation of the postsynaptic neuron. This is very close to the criterion that Hebb proposed for the enhancement of synaptic strength in hypothetical neural circuits mediating associative conditioning (Hebb, 1949). Consequently, hippocampal synapses displaying associative LTP are often referred to as "Hebb synapses." In the next section we explore the Hebbian nature of LTP in more detail.

10.3.6 Requirement for Tight Coincidence of Presynaptic and Postsynaptic Activity Implies a Hebbian Induction Rule

There is convincing evidence that the induction of LTP in the Schaffer-commissural projection in area CA1 is indeed Hebbian in nature. In the first place, the postsynaptic cell plays an obligatory role in induction, as first revealed in experiments showing that LTP could be blocked by injecting the calcium chelator EGTA into the postsynaptic cell (Lynch et al., 1983) (Fig. 10–5B) or by hyperpolarizing the postsynaptic neuron (Malinow and Miller, 1986). In later work, Malenka et al. (1992) used a caged form of the calcium chelator 1,2-bis (aminophenoxy)ethane-$N,N,N',N',$-tetraacetic acid (BAPTA), in which BAPTA is bound as an inactive but photolabile

molecular complex, from which it can be rapidly released by a flash of ultraviolet light, to establish that the obligatory rise in calcium is confined to a window of less than 2.0 to 2.5 seconds following the tetanus. Second, as we have seen, LTP can be induced by the repeated conjunction of single (Wigström et al., 1986) or multiple (Kelso et al., 1986; Sastry et al., 1986) afferent volleys with strong depolarizing pulses applied through an intracellular electrode. In the latter experiments, the relatively long depolarizing pulses produced multiple spikes falling on either side of the single afferent stimulus. Later work by Magee and Johnston (1997), Bi and Poo (1998), and others established that LTP in the hippocampus, as in neocortex (Markram et al., 1997), can be induced by repeated pairing of an afferent stimulus with a single back-propagating action potential, provided the EPSP precedes the action potential by less than ~10 ms (STDP) (reviewed in Dan and Poo, 2004) (see Section 10.3.8).

Is Postsynaptic Spiking Necessary for LTP?

Hebb's postulate implies that the postsynaptic cell must fire for changes in synaptic weight to occur. There are several types of plasticity where this is not the case (for example, as we shall see, mossy fiber LTP, heterosynaptic LTP and LTD, mGluR-dependent LTD), and firing may not be necessary for LTP even at the canonical Hebbian synapse, the Schaffer-commissural projection to hippocampal CA1 pyramidal cells. Many protocols for inducing LTP in this pathway do fire the postsynaptic cell (for example, STDP and some though not all forms of pairing), but with tetanic stimulation the target cell may fire only to the first stimulus of the train or not at all (for review see Linden, 1999). Moreover, pairing-induced LTP is not blocked by intracellular injection of lidocaine derivatives such as QX-314 that block spiking (Kelso et al., 1986; Gustafs-

Figure 10–5. The induction of LTP requires activation of NMDA receptors and postsynaptic Ca^{2+} signaling. *A*. A plot of synaptic response versus time to show that the broad spectrum glutamate receptor antagonist γ-D-glutamylglycine (γDGG), applied to the synaptic region by microiontophoresis, depresses synaptic transmission and blocks induction of LTP. In contrast, D-2-amino-5-phosphonopentanoate (D-AP5) has no effect on pre-established LTP but blocks its induction. A single tetanus (100 Hz, 1 second) was delivered at the points indicated by arrows. The stimulus inten-

sity was reduced between the time-course plots shown in the upper and lower sections of the figure. (*Source*: Collingridge et al., 1983.) *B*. Intracellular recordings showing superimposed EPSPs before and after induction of LTP under control conditions (left) and the block of LTP induction when the intracellular electrode contained the Ca^{2+} buffer EGTA (right). Plots of the change in EPSP amplitude over time from a control and an EGTA-filled cell are also shown. A tetanus was delivered at the times indicated by small arrows. (*Source*: Lynch et al., 1983.)

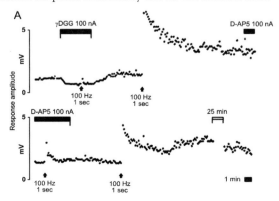
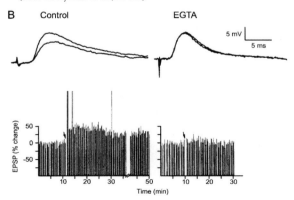

son et al., 1987). According to Thomas et al. (1998), intracellular QX-314 prevents LTP induced by low-frequency theta trains but has no effect on the efficacy of high-frequency trains. Primed burst stimulation can readily induce LTP in area CA1 in vitro at stimulus strengths that are below threshold for spike firing (Davies et al., 1991). In some circumstances, even low-frequency trains can induce LTP without firing the postsynaptic cell (Krasteniakov et al., 2004; but see Pike et al., 1999). LTP can also be induced by repetitive pulses of glutamate targeted by two-photon excitation of a caged precursor to a single spine, a protocol that does not fire the postsynaptic cell and is on the face of it entirely lacking in associative credentials (Matsuzaki et al., 2004). In contrast, STDP, which may or may not be the usual mechanism by which synaptic weights are modified in vivo, is defined by a requirement for postsynaptic spiking. Indeed, STDP is the very cynosure of Hebbian plasticity; not only does it require tight temporal contiguity of presynaptic and postsynaptic firing, but the back-propagating spike provides the associative signal that informs dendritic synapses that the postsynaptic cell has fired. However, even here, in Hebb's heartland, locally generated and spatially restricted spiking can, in distal dendrites, take the place of a back-propagating action potential (Golding et al., 2003). It seems safe to conclude that postsynaptic somatic action potentials are not an absolute requirement for LTP at Schaffer-commissural synapses, at least in vitro. Whether a strict Hebbian conjunction of pre- and postsynaptic spiking is the norm in vivo remains to be seen (Lisman and Spruston, 2005).

In summary, although it is experimentally possible to bypass the postsynaptic action potential, it may be that in a physiological context the only way that sufficient depolarization can be obtained is by postsynaptic firing, as postulated by Hebb. To the extent that it is the idea of sufficient depolarization, however produced, that is critical for NMDA receptor activation, the strict form of the Hebbian coincidence rule can be relaxed slightly without compromising its spirit: It is the coincidence, within a narrow time window of *firing* in the presynaptic cell with *sufficient depolarization* in the postsynaptic cell, that is the criterion for the induction of LTP. These considerations allow us to formulate a Hebbian induction rule for associative synaptic potentiation at excitatory synapses on CA1 pyramidal and dentate granule cells:

A synapse will be potentiated if, and only if, it is active at a time when its dendritic spine is sufficiently depolarized.

It is easy to see—and is an instructive exercise for the reader to confirm—that this rule accounts for the properties of cooperativity, input specificity, and associativity.

10.3.7 Molecular Basis for the Hebbian Induction Rule: Voltage Dependence of the NMDA Receptor Explains Cooperativity, Input Specificity, and Associativity

Perhaps the most remarkable advance to date in understanding the cellular mechanisms responsible for LTP has been

elucidation of the role of the NMDA receptor in its induction. The first indication of the importance of this subtype of glutamate receptor came in 1983, when it was found that a specific NMDA receptor antagonist, D(-)aminophosphopentanoic acid (D-AP5) (Davies et al., 1981), blocked induction of LTP in area CA1 of the hippocampal slice (Collingridge et al., 1983) (Fig. 10–5A). Because AP5 does not affect the response to single stimuli, the NMDA receptor is not involved in any obvious way in the mediation of synaptic transmission at low frequencies (see Chapter 6). Moreover, AP5 does not block LTP once it is induced, indicating that the effect of the drug is on the induction, rather than the expression, of LTP. The finding that blockade of the NMDA receptor suppresses the induction of LTP has been confirmed using other competitive NMDA antagonists (Harris et al, 1984), the use-dependent noncompetitive antagonist MK-801 (Coan et al., 1987) and the glycine site antagonist 7-chlorokynurenic acid (Bashir et al., 1990). Independent confirmation that the NMDA receptor is necessary for LTP has been provided by studies on genetically engineered mice. Particularly convincing evidence came from experiments in which the cre-lox technique was used to delete genes in a cell-type and region-specific way (see Section 10.10). Tsien et al. (1996), for example, created mice harboring a deletion of NMDAR1 (the obligatory subunit of the NMDA receptor) in area CA1 but not in the dentate gyrus. Slices from these animals showed no LTP in CA1 but normal LTP in the dentate gyrus. In site-directed mutagenesis experiments, Sprengel et al. (1998) created mice in which the intracellular carboxy terminus of the NMDA receptor was deleted. The inability of these mutants to display LTP despite unaltered Ca^{2+} current through the mutant receptor indicates that the NMDA receptor plays a further role in the genesis of LTP, downstream of its function as a Ca^{2+}-permeable ionophore.

An explanation of how NMDA receptors trigger the induction of LTP quickly followed the discovery of their critical role in the process. It was already known that NMDA receptor-mediated responses are potently blocked by Mg^{2+} in spinal cord neurons (Evans et al., 1977). In addition, MacDonald and Wojtowicz (1980) had discovered that, in contrast to all other known ligand-gated ion fluxes, NMDA receptor-mediated responses are strongly voltage-dependent. The key observation that made everything clear was the discovery in 1984 that the voltage dependence was caused by the Mg^{2+} block (Mayer et al., 1984; Nowak et al., 1984). At resting membrane potential, glutamate or other NMDA receptor ligands induce negligible inward current through the channel associated with the NMDA receptor. With increasing depolarization, Mg^{2+} ions are driven from the channel, and an inward current carried by Na^+ and Ca^{2+} develops.

It was quickly realized that the dual ligand and voltage dependence of the NMDA receptor response offers an elegant molecular mechanism for both the induction of LTP (Collingridge, 1985) and the properties of associativity and input specificity (Wigström and Gustafsson, 1985). Two conditions must be met for an NMDA receptor-mediated response to be generated: presynaptic activity to release glutamate and strong postsynaptic depolarization to relieve the Mg^{2+} block of the NMDA receptor channel. These are just the conditions that, as we saw in the previous section, are required for the induction of LTP. Because Ca^{2+} is required for the induction of LTP (Lynch et al., 1983), and because activated NMDA receptor channels, unlike most ionotropic AMPA receptor channels, are highly permeable to calcium (MacDermott et al., 1986; Jahr and Stevens, 1987, 1993), it seems reasonable to conclude that the trigger for the induction of LTP is the entry of calcium ions through the channel associated with the NMDA receptor.

Although activation of NMDA receptors is a necessary condition for the induction of a major component of LTP at Schaffer-commissural and perforant path synapses, it is not, or at least not always, a sufficient condition. NMDA alone can induce short-term potentiation Collingridge et al. (1983), but neither NMDA (Kauer et al., 1988) nor glutamate (Hvalby et al., 1987), when applied alone to hippocampal slices, readily induces long-lasting potentiation. This result does not sit easily with a purely postsynaptic model of the induction and expression of LTP but is consistent with models in which the expression of LTP is dependent, in part, on presynaptic mechanisms. Alternatively, other postsynaptic signaling pathways, such as mGluRs, may be necessary co-triggers. In addition, the way in which NMDA receptors are activated may be a critical factor, as more prolonged application of NMDA receptors tends to induce LTD or depotentiation, which could mask or obliterate any underlying potentiation. Photolysis of caged glutamate combined with depolarization does, however, produce long-lasting potentiation of the responses of single spines in organotypic culture to test pulses of uncaged glutamate (Bagal, et al., 2005). Thus, in this preparation, NMDA receptor activation is sufficient to induce a postsynaptic component of LTP.

Role of NMDAR subtypes in LTP.

There is evidence that specific NMDAR subtypes are involved in LTP. A role for NR2A-containing NMDARs was suggested in experiments in which the NR2A subunit was knocked out (Sakimura et al., 1995). These animals still exhibited LTP but its magnitude was reduced to approximately half of that seen in wildtypes. This may may reflect developmental consequences of the knockout but subsequent pharmacological experiments have also suggested a role for different NR2 subtypes in LTP. For example, LTP was found to be more sensitive to NR2A/2B selective antagonists, whilst LTD was more sensitive to NR2C/D selective antagonists (Hrabetova et al., 2000). This differential sensitivity suggested a role for NR2A and/ or NR2B receptors in LTP. Sorting out the relative roles of NR2A and NR2B-containing receptors has proved difficult and may be confounded by the existence of triheteromers that comprise both NR2A and NR2B subunits, in addition to the obligatory NR1 subunit. An NR2A selective antagonist, NVP-AAM077, inhibits LTP (Liu et al., 2004; Berberich et al., 2005). However, the selectivity of this compound versus the other

four subunits is rather narrow (Feng et al., 2004). NR2B antagonists are much more selective, but highly variable results have been reported ranging from complete block of LTP (Barria and Malinow, 2005) to no effect on LTP (Liu et al., 2004a). Further work is clearly required to establish the relative roles of the different NR2 subunits in LTP.

10.3.8 Spike Timing-dependent Plasticity (STDP)

Explicit in Hebb's postulate is the notion of causality: Presynaptic cell A must "repeatedly or persistently take part" in firing postsynaptic cell B. In a Hebb synapse, therefore, an increase in synaptic weight occurs only when the presynaptic cell fires shortly before the postsynaptic cell. If induction is mediated by the postsynaptic cell, this condition may be expressed as a requirement that the synaptically generated current should begin before, but overlap with, the firing of the postsynaptic cell. In practice, given the time course of excitatory EPSCs (and, in particular, of the NMDA receptor-mediated component of the EPSC), this interval may extend to a few tens of milliseconds. Early experiments on associative LTP using "weak" and "strong" inputs to the dentate gyrus suggested that LTP satisfies these requirements for temporal contiguity (Levy and Steward, 1983). The weak pathway was potentiated only if it was active within 20 ms of activation of the strong pathway. Moreover, if the order of activation was reversed, with the weak input stimulated up to 20 ms after the strong input, LTD was induced (Levy and Steward, 1983). As discussed above, other two-pathway studies using intracellular recording confirmed the importance of temporal contiguity in pre- and postsynaptic spiking for the induction of LTP (Gustafsson and Wigström, 1986; Kelso and Brown, 1986; reviewed in Bi and Poo, 2001).

In two of the conventional ways to induce LTP— tetanic stimulation and low frequency pairing of presynaptic stimuli with trains of postsynaptic spikes induced by a depolarizing pulse—the precise temporal relation between pre- and postsynaptic spiking is not straightforward. During a tetanus at 100 Hz, firing of the postsynaptic cell rapidly accommodates, and the number of coincident action potentials in pre- and postsynaptic cells is limited. During pairing, there is generally only one presynaptic spike and multiple firing of the postsynaptic cell. In 1994, Stuart and Sakmann demonstrated unequivocally that the action potential in cortical pyramidal cells propagates back into the dendritic tree (Stuart and Sakmann, 1994). This discovery identified an associative signal at the synapse that could link presynaptic and postsynaptic firing and initiated a period of intense study into the effects of varying the timing between presynaptic firing and the back-propagating action potential. The first synapses to be investigated were local excitatory connections between cortical pyramidal cells (Markram et al., 1997). Potentiation was achieved when the presynaptic spike preceded the postsynaptic spike, with maximal potentiation at near-zero intervals, and the degree of potentiation declining with longer intervals; at delays greater than 20 ms no effect was seen. When postsynaptic firing preceded presynaptic firing, the effect was reversed and LTD was induced; again the maximum effect was seen at the shortest post-pre intervals, declining to zero over 20 ms. STDP –the term was introduced by Song et al. (2000)– has also been extensively studied in the hippocampus (Bi and Poo, 1998; Debanne et al., 1998; reviewed by Bi and Poo, 2001 and Lisman and Spruston, 2005) (see Fig. 10–19C,D, below). In dissociated hippocampal cultures, the STDP function relating magnitude and direction of plasticity to the interval betweeen the pair of pre- and postsynaptic spikes is antisymmetrical (Fig. 10–19D), as it is in cortical pyramidal cells. In acute slices, however, the function is more symmetrical, with two intervals of depression flanking the region of potentiation (Nishiyama et al., 2000) (see Section 10.7.3).

The STDP function predicts the polarity and magnitude of change to a single pair of action potentials, one in the presynaptic cell and the other in the postsynaptic cell. How does the computation scale up when trains of spikes are considered? In the simplest case, any two trains in the two connected cells can be considered as sets of pairs, with each of the n_1 action potentials in one train paired with each of the n_2 action potentials in the other train, forming a total of $n_1 \times n_2$ pairs. The STDP function can be used to compute the effect on plasticity for each pair independently and the total effect calculated by summing the contribution to synaptic weight contributed by each pair. Providing the STDP function has a bias in favor of depression (i.e., the integral of the post-before-pre function exceeds that of the pre-before-post function), a stable network evolves in which inputs that are biased toward firing the postsynaptic cell are strengthened at the expense of those that are not (Song et al., 2000). However, experiments in the visual cortex suggest that spike pairs do not combine independently in this way, and that the first spike in a short train has a disproportionate effect on the outcome (Froemke and Dan, 2002). A model based on these findings proved more accurate than the independent model for predicting the polarity and magnitude of plasticity when naturally recorded spike trains were used as artificial stimuli for monosynaptically linked pairs of layer 2/3 neurons in cortical slices. However, it is not clear that either model can account for the fact that repeated pairing of single presynaptic spikes delivered during a depolarization-induced spike train in the postsynaptic cell invariably produces LTP.

Inhibitory synapses onto hippocampal pyramidal cells exhibit an atypical temporal window for STDP—whatever the order, provided the interneuron and target pyramidal cell fire within 20 ms of each other, the synapse is potentiated (see Section 10.8.2).

10.3.9 Ca²⁺ Signaling in LTP

Ca²⁺ Release from Ca²⁺ Stores Contributes to Induction of LTP

A major source of Ca²⁺ in neurons is via release from intracellular stores. A role for Ca²⁺ stores in synaptic plasticity is implicated by the finding that thapsigargin, which prevents the refilling of these stores, can block the induction but not the expression of LTP at CA1 synapses (Harvey and Collingridge, 1992). Ca²⁺ may be released from stores via the generation of inositol trisphosphate (IP3) and/or via Ca²⁺-induced Ca²⁺ release media by IP3 and/or ryanodine receptors, respectively. Evidence that Ca²⁺-induced Ca²⁺ release may be important was provided by the finding that dantrolene, an inhibitor of ryanodine receptors, blocks induction of LTP at these synapses (Obenaus et al., 1989). In support of this possibility, tetanic stimulation was shown to elicit a large NMDA receptor-dependent Ca²⁺ signal at synapses that was substantially inhibited by either thapsigargin or ryanodine (Alford et al., 1993). Collectively, these data suggest that Ca²⁺-induced Ca²⁺ release can greatly augment the Ca²⁺ signal that permeates NMDA receptors and may be involved in the induction of LTP. Such a signal may maintain the specificity of LTP, as NMDA receptor-triggered, store-derived Ca²⁺ signals can be observed within individual spines (Emptage et al., 1999). Conceivably, however, under certain circumstances sufficient Ca²⁺ may enter directly via NMDA receptors such that the boost from intracellular stores is not required. Also conceivably, Ca²⁺ release from intracellular stores may be induced by other mechanisms, for example via activation of voltage-gated Ca²⁺ channels, phospholipase C (PLC)-coupled receptors, or other Ca²⁺-permeable ligand-gated channels. Any of these paths could, in theory, induce NMDAR-dependent LTP without activating the normal induction trigger, the NMDA receptor itself. There is evidence that Ca²⁺ permeation through presynaptic kainate receptors can trigger Ca²⁺-induced Ca²⁺ release to induce an NMDA receptor-independent form of LTP at mossy fiber synapses on CA3 pyramidal cells (Lauri et al., 2003), as discussed in Section 10.5.3. Again, the extent to which Ca²⁺ release from intracellular stores is exploited by the hippocampus during NMDA receptor-dependent LTP in vivo is not known.

Ca²⁺ Entry via Voltage-gated Ca²⁺ Channels Enables NMDA Receptor-independent LTP

Although it is accepted that Ca²⁺ entry directly through the NMDAR channel is the trigger for NMDAR-dependent LTP, this pathway is not necessarily the only source of elevated intracellular Ca²⁺. In particular, depolarization during summated EPSPs leads to Ca²⁺ entry via voltage-gated Ca²⁺ channels (VGCCs). Because NMDA receptors provide much of the depolarization during a high-frequency synaptic response (Herron et al., 1986), this Ca²⁺ source is largely NMDAR-dependent (Alford et al., 1993). Determining the relative importance of the two NMDAR-dependent sources is not a trivial matter. In theory, the latter can be excluded in voltage-clamp experiments, but a perfect clamp of synapses located on dendritic spines is not achievable. Blocking VGCCs pharmacologically is also problematic as certain types are required for neurotransmitter release. An alternative strategy has been to activate VGCCs by intracellular depolarization, in the absence of evoked synaptic transmission. This generally does not induce LTP unless phosphatases are also blocked (Wyllie and Nicoll, 1994). The logical conclusion is that it may be possible to induce LTP if sufficient Ca^{2+} enters via VGCCs because it can access the sites that normally are reached only by the Ca^{2+}-permeating NMDARs. It follows, therefore, that under most conditions VGCCs are not required for the induction of NMDAR-dependent LTP. On the other hand, stronger induction protocols would promote the activation of VGCCs. Because the depolarization spreads to other regions of the cell, this could lead to partial breakdown in input specificity. It might also result in Ca^{2+} entry at the cell soma, where it could act as a nuclear signal. At the extreme, depolarization provided by AMPA receptors alone could result in Ca^{2+} entry and LTP that appears to be NMDAR-independent but in fact engages the same mechanisms as NMDAR-dependent LTP downstream of the NMDAR. Consistent with this notion, there is evidence that higher frequencies during tetanization (e.g., 200 Hz) promote NMDAR-independent LTP in the Schaffer-commissural pathway (Grover and Teyler, 1990). However, in this case the downstream signaling pathways may be also different, pointing to the existence of a truly NMDAR-independent form of LTP at these synapses (Cavus and Teyler, 1996). This LTP develops relatively slowly, is of small amplitude but is long-lasting, and is triggered by entry of Ca^{2+} through L-type calcium channels (Grover and Teyler, 1990). The L-type channel isoform has now been identified as $Ca_v1.2$, and mutant mice with inactivation of this isoform do not display NMDA receptor-independent LTP (Moosmang et al., 2005). Significantly, they are also severely impaired in a spatial discrimination task, demonstrating that NMDA receptor-independent LTP contributes to the neural processing of hippocampus-dependent learning and memory. Ca^{2+}-dependent mechanisms contributing to protein synthesis in the late form of NMDAR-independent LTP are discussed in Section 10.4.9.

10.3.10 Metabotropic Glutamate Receptors Contribute to Induction of NMDA Receptor-dependent LTP

Metabotropic glutamate receptors (mGluRs), by virtue of their coupling to G proteins, can affect various intracellular signaling pathways that might be involved in LTP. The first direct evidence that they may be activated during the induction of LTP followed the development of the first selective mGluR antagonist, α-methyl-4-carboxyphenylglycine (MCPG) (Eaton et al., 1993). MCPG had no effect on basal synaptic transmission or the expression of LTP but completely inhibited the induction of LTP in a fully reversible manner (Bashir et al., 1993). Unlike NMDAR antagonists, however, MCPG had no effect on STP. In complementary studies it was found that the selective activation of mGluRs with (1S,3R)-1-aminocyclopentane-1,3-dicarboxylic acid [(1S,3R)-ACPD] could induce LTP without the STP phase (Bortolotto and Collingridge, 1993). This "slow-onset" potentiation was not

prevented by an NMDAR antagonist, but it occluded NMDAR-dependent tetanus-induced LTP, suggesting convergence with the mechanisms underlying the expression of classical LTP. ACPD-induced slow-onset potentiation was blocked by thapsigargin. This observation provides a potential route by which ACPD may access NMDAR-dependent LTP, the point of convergence being the intracellular Ca^{2+} stores. Ca^{2+} release from these stores is normally triggered by Ca^{2+} permeating via NMDA receptors; but under certain circumstances, stored Ca^{2+} may be released by activation of mGluRs in the absence of NMDAR activation. Group I mGluRs (mGluR1 and mGluR5) couple to phospholipase C, leading to the liberation of IP3, which acts on IP3 receptors to trigger Ca^{2+} release from intracellular stores (see Chapter 6, Section 6. 3). Consistent with this hypothesis, (1S,3R)-ACPD activates and MCPG inhibits both mGluR1 and mGluR5. An unusual aspect of the action of (1S,3R)-ACPD in area CA1 is that it depends on intact connections from area CA3 (Bortolotto and Collingridge, 1995). A possible explanation is that (1S,3R)-ACPD excites CA3 pyramidal cells sufficiently to depolarize CA1 neurons, which in turn may lead to the sensitization of intracellular Ca^{2+} stores to the mGluR-triggered generation of IP3. Consistent with this hypothesis, modest depolarization of CA1 neurons greatly facilitates the Ca^{2+}- mobilizing response to group I mGluR agonists (Rae et al., 2000).

Several studies have attempted to replicate the original MCPG experiments, with variable results. One camp agreed that MCPG blocked induction of LTP (Riedel and Reymann, 1993; Sergueeva et al., 1993; Richter-Levin et al., 1994), whereas the second camp found no effect of this antagonist (Manzoni et al., 1994; Selig et al., 1995b; Thomas and O'Dell, 1995; Martin and Morris, 1997). The simplest conclusion to be drawn from these findings is that MCPG-sensitive mGluRs may be necessary for the induction of LTP under certain, but not all, experimental conditions. A possible resolution of the controversy emerged when it was discovered that the activation of mGluRs did not have to occur at the same time as the tetanus that activated NMDA receptors (Bortolotto et al., 1994). Thus, the induction of LTP in one pathway prevented MCPG from inhibiting the induction of more LTP in the same pathway. The initial conditioning tetanus did not have to induce LTP, as a tetanus delivered in the presence of an NMDAR antagonist still produced the conditioning. This led to the proposal that the activation of mGluRs sets a "molecular switch" that negates the need for subsequent activation of mGluRs for induction of LTP in that pathway. Once activated, the switch remains set for at least several hours unless it is turned off by a depotentiating stimulus. These observations suggest that the initial activation of mGluRs converts them to a constitutively active state, although how this switch is achieved is not known. The molecular switch is a form of metaplasticity, which may explain some of the controversy surrounding the effects of MCPG on the induction of NMDAR-dependent LTP. It is likely, however, that other experimental factors are also important (Thomas and O'Dell, 1995; reviewed by Anwyl, 1999).

With the development of various mGluR knockout mice and newer mGluR antagonists, with differing patterns of subtype selectivity, the role of mGluR subtypes in NMDAR-dependent LTP has been further investigated. However, no clear picture has yet emerged. At Schaffer-commissural synapses there are high levels of mGluR5 postsynaptically and mGluR7 presynaptically. Other subunits, including mGluR1, may be expressed at lower levels. The knockout of mGluR1 was reported either to inhibit (Aiba et al., 1994) or to have no effect (Conquet et al., 1994) on the induction of LTP. Surprisingly, although an initial study reported a small decrease in LTP in the mGlu5 knockout (Lu et al., 1997), no effect was found by the same group in a more detailed follow-up investigation (Jia et al., 1998). Interestingly, although LTP was normal in the mGluR7 knockout, there was a deficiency in STP (Bushell et al., 2002). This suggests that presynaptic mGluRs play a role in this initial presynaptic form of plasticity, although developmental consequences of the loss of mGluR7 cannot be discounted. Perhaps most perplexing was the finding that LY341495, a compound that can be used at high concentrations to block all known mGluRs (mGluR1-8), had no effect on LTP (Fitzjohn et al., 1998). The difference between the effects of MCPG and LY341495, which can demonstrated in the same pathway, suggests that either MCPG is acting on some receptor other than mGlu1-8 or that the blanket inhibition of mGluRs has effects that are different from the selective inhibition of some subunits. Clearly, further work is required to clarify the roles of mGluRs in NMDAR-dependent LTP.

10.3.11 Role of GABA Receptors in the Induction of NMDAR-dependent LTP

It has been known for many years that blockade of GABA inhibition can greatly facilitate the induction of NMDAR-dependent LTP (Wigström and Gustafsson, 1983). The mech-

anism for this effect is well established. Normally, when an EPSP is evoked by stimulation of an afferent pathway, such as the Schaffer commissural projection, it is curtailed by a biphasic inhibitory postsynaptic potential (IPSP) comprising a rapid $GABA_A$ receptor-mediated component and a slower $GABA_B$ receptor-mediated component. The hyperpolarizing effect of the IPSP intensifies the Mg^{2+} block of NMDARs, and this greatly limits the extent to which NMDARs contribute to the synaptic response. This was first demonstrated by a simple pharmacological experiment. When $GABA_A$ receptors were blocked pharmacologically, an NMDAR-mediated synaptic response appeared during low-frequency stimulation in the presence of Mg^{2+} (Herron et al., 1985; Dingledine et al., 1986). Indeed, it is probably no coincidence that the kinetics of the $GABA_A$ receptor-mediated IPSP is such that this component of the biphasic IPSP coincides with the greater part of the NMDAR-mediated conductance.

Blockade of GABA inhibition is not simply a pharmacological curiosity but a key feature of LTP induction. This is shown by the remarkable efficacy of "priming" induction protocols, discussed above, in which a single stimulus precedes a brief high-frequency burst by about 200 ms. A primed burst containing typically four shocks (i.e., five shocks in total) can induce LTP. The potency of the burst derives from the fact that the priming stimulus (or the preceding burst during "theta" patterns) causes a substantial reduction in the GABA receptor-mediated IPSP. The mechanism of this effect has been established (Davies et al., 1991) (Fig. 10–6). Some of the GABA that is released in response to the priming stimulus feeds back to activate $GABA_B$ autoreceptors, which results in inhibition of subsequent GABA release. Thus, the priming stimulus releases a normal level of GABA, but the stimuli during the burst release considerably less GABA, which facilitates the synaptic activation of NMDA receptors on pyramidal neurons. The kinetics of the $GABA_B$ autoreceptor mechanism determines the optimal timing for priming; it has a latency of

Figure 10–6. $GABA_B$ autoreceptors regulate the induction of LTP. LTP plots show that the $GABA_B$ antagonist CGP35348 (1 mM) blocks induction of LTP induced by primed-burst stimulation (1 priming stimulus followed 200 ms later by 4 shocks at 100 Hz) (left panel). However, the antagonist is ineffective if experiments are performed in the presence of a $GABA_A$ antagonist (middle panel) or if

a tetanus (100 Hz, 1 second) is used (right panel). The open symbols plot control experiments, and the filled symbols plot experiments performed in the presence of CGP35348. The primed-burst stimulus or tetanus was delivered at the times indicated by arrows. The traces were obtained during baseline and 30 minutes following the priming/tetanus. (*Source*: Davies et al., 1996.)

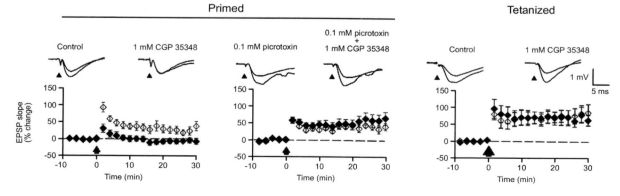

around 20 ms, a peak effect around 200 ms, and a duration of around 1 second (Davies et al., 1990). Thus, theta patterns of activity are tuned to the maximum depression of GABA inhibition by the autoreceptor mechanism. The importance of autoinhibition for the induction of LTP can be readily demonstrated. GABA$_B$ antagonists, applied at concentrations that prevent the GABA$_B$ autoreceptor from operating and thereby maintain GABA$_A$ receptor-mediated inhibition, completely prevent induction of LTP by priming stimulation. As one would predict for a mechanism that works by modulating GABA$_A$ receptor-mediated inhibition, GABA$_B$ antagonists do not block LTP induced in the presence of a GABA$_A$ receptor antagonist (Davies and Collingridge, 1993). They are also ineffective when tested against a conventional tetanus (e.g., 100 Hz for 1 second) as the GABA$_B$ autoreceptor mechanism operates for only a few stimuli. The system is finely tuned to suppress GABA inhibition during theta-type patterns of activity, which from a physiological perspective suggests that hippocampal synapses may be particularly susceptible to potentiation during exploration, locomotion, and other behavioral states that give rise to theta activity (see Chapter 11). The importance of the GABA$_B$ autoreceptor system is emphasized in the induction scheme for LTP illustrated in Figure 10–7.

Theoretically, many neurotransmitters and neuromodulators could interact with the LTP induction process via an effect on GABA inhibition. For example, it has been shown that endocannabinoids released from pyramidal neurons can depress GABA inhibition, which can result in the facilitation of LTP (see Section 10.3.12). In one series of experiments it was shown that LTP is associated with an endocannabinoid-mediated LTD of GABA inhibition in a narrow band surrounding the potentiated synapses (Chevaleyre and Castillo, 2004). The LTD of synaptic inhibition then promotes induction of LTP in this surround.

10.3.12 E-S Potentiation: A Component of LTP That Reflects Enhanced Coupling Between Synaptic Drive and Cell Firing

Characteristics of E-S Potentiation

Conventional synaptic LTP is characterized by a persistent increase in synaptic current and a proportionate increase in the amplitude of the population spike or, in single unit recordings, in the probability of the cell firing an action potential in response to the test stimulus. In these cases, potentiation of the population spike, or an increase in the probability of cell firing, is no more than would be predicted from the increase in the EPSP. Often, though, the increase is much greater. In extreme cases, spike potentiation can occur in the absence of EPSP potentiation (Bliss and Lømo, 1973). This property of hippocampal synapses was given the name EPSP-spike or E-S potentiation by Andersen et al. (1980). In general, E-S potentiation appears as a leftward shift of the curve obtained by plotting the amplitude or latency of the popula-

tion spike, or the probability of unit discharge, against the slope of the synaptic component (Bliss et al., 1973) (Fig. 10–2E-G). Although E-S potentiation is usually observed in conjunction with synaptic LTP, pure E-S potentiation has been obtained in area CA1 in vitro by combining low-frequency afferent stimulation with high-frequency antidromic trains (Jester et al., 1995; Nakanishi et al., 2001). Like synaptic LTP, E-S potentiation in area CA1 is NMDAR-dependent (Jester et al., 1995; Lu et al., 2000a; Daoudal et al., 2002); and the observation that the NMDAR antagonist D-AP5 blocks both spike and EPSP potentiation implies that this is also the case in the dentate gyrus in vivo (Errington et al., 1987). However, E-S potentiation and synaptic LTP are differently affected by drugs that modulate the monoaminergic input to the hippocampus. Depletion of noradrenaline (norepinephrine) reduces synaptic LTP in the dentate gyrus but leaves LTP of the population spike unaffected (Bliss et al., 1983; Munro et al., 2001).

Several groups have reported that E-S potentiation is input-specific when induced by tetanic stimulation in area CA1 in vitro (Andersen et al., 1980; Daoudal et al., 2002; Marder and Buonomano, 2003). However, this conclusion has been disputed by Jester et al. (2003), who found that input specificity was violated in more than half of their experiments in CA1 in vitro; there is also evidence for a lack of input specificity in the dentate gyrus in vivo (Abraham et al., 1985). Further experiments are needed to resolve this question. The persistence of E-S potentiation has not been explored in the freely moving animal.

Mechanisms of E-S Potentiation

Inhibitors of GABA$_A$ receptors block a substantial component of E-S potentiation produced by tetanic stimulation (Abraham et al., 1987; Chavez-Noriega et al., 1989; Daoudal et al., 2002; Marder and Buonomano, 2003; Staff and Spruston, 2003), suggesting that it reflects an increase in excitability brought about by a relative reduction in feedforward inhibition. Support for this hypothesis has been provided by Lu et al. (2000a), who found that E-S potentiation in CA1 neurons is accompanied by a tetanus-induced LTD of feedforward IPSPs; both E-S potentiation and LTD of IPSPs were abolished by NMDA antagonists, or by injecting the phosphatase calcineurin into pyramidal cells. This last result implies that the site of induction of E-S potentiation is the inhibitory synapse on the principal cell, not the excitatory input to the GABAergic interneuron. Nevertheless, the latter site may contribute to persistent reduction in feedforward inhibition and hence to E-S potentiation because tetanic stimulation can induce LTD at these synapses (Laezza et al., 1999) (see Section 10.8.1). Because the expression of E-S potentiation manifests as an increase in postsynaptic cell firing for a given synaptic input, the results of Lu et al. (2000a) imply that expression of this form of LTP, like its induction, is postsynaptic. However, this is unlikely to be the whole story. E-S potentiation has been induced by a pairing protocol, in which plasticity in

Induction

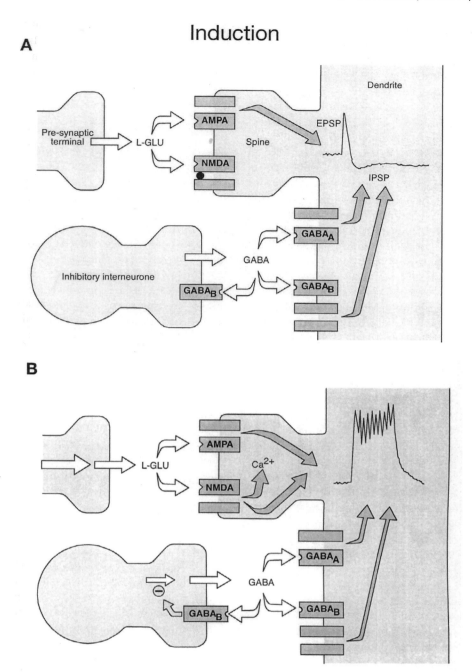

Figure 10–7. Activation of NMDA receptors, modulated by other ionotropic amino acid receptors, triggers the induction of LTP in principal cells of area CA1 and dentate gyrus. *A.* Low-frequency stimulation of Schaffer commissural axons evokes an EPSP that is mediated by L-glutamate acting on AMPA receptors. The EPSP is followed by a biphasic IPSP, produced by glutamatergic excitation of feedforward GABAergic interneurons. The early part of the IPSP is due to activation of $GABA_A$ receptors, which are permeable to Cl^- ions; the slow component of the IPSP reflects activation of $GABA_B$ receptors, indirectly coupled to K^+ channels. Because of its slow kinetics and the voltage-dependent block of its channel by Mg^{2+} ions, the NMDA receptor contributes little to the EPSP at low frequencies of stimulation. *B.* During high-frequency stimulation, the activated spines become strongly depolarized with the result that the Mg^{2+} block of the NMDA receptor channel is relieved, allowing Ca^{2+} to permeate through the receptor. Factors that contribute to sustained depolarization, including temporal summation of EPSPs and the accumulation of Cl^- in the spine and K^+ in the synaptic cleft, leading to depolarizing shifts in reversal potentials. Some protocols, in particular theta burst stimulation, depend for their efficacy on the suppression of inhibition mediated via $GABA_B$ autoreceptors on inhibitory terminals. The suppression of GABA release reaches a maximum around 200 ms after a priming stimulus, explaining the peculiar efficacy of priming and theta burst stimulation (see text). (*Source*: After Bliss and Collingridge (1993).

inhibitory circuits presumably does not occur (Marder and Buonomano, 2004). There is also a component of E-S potentiation that is not GABA$_A$ receptor-dependent; in the well documented study by Daoudal et al. (2002), this component amounted to 40% of the overall effect.

A novel interpretation of the idea that E-S potentiation reflects a persistent reduction in inhibitory input has come from an analysis of mGluR-dependent LTD of inhibitory transmission between interneurons and pyramidal cells in area CA1, touched on above (Chevaleyre and Castillo, 2003). This unusual form of heterosynaptic inhibitory LTD is mediated by the activation of group 1 mGluRs on CA1 pyramidal cells by high-frequency stimulation of Schaffer-commissural fibers. There is a consequent retrograde release of the cannabinoid 2-AG (Wilson and Nicoll, 2001), leading to the activation of endogenous CB1 receptors on the terminals of inhibitory axons projecting to the same pyramidal cell and, by unknown mechanisms, to a suppression of the release of inhibitory transmitter. The persistent disinhibition leads to E-S potentiation. Chevaleyre and Castillo carried out their experiments in a medium that blocked ionotropic glutamate receptors. High-frequency stimulation in the presence of NMDAR antagonists should therefore lead to E-S potentiation without synaptic potentiation. However, both in area CA1 in vitro (Collingridge et al., 1983) and in the dentate gyrus in vivo (Errington et al., 1987), AP5 blocks potentiation of both the population spike and the fEPSP. It remains to be established whether the retrograde release of 2-AG provides an explanation for E-S potentiation in area CA1 in vivo.

The input specificity of E-S potentiation, whether established in the presence of a GABA$_A$ receptor antagonist (Daoudal et al., 2002) or in normal bathing medium (Marder and Buonomano, 2003), is something of a puzzle, as an increase in excitability, or the tendency to fire an action potential, is most readily explained in terms of the conductances controlling the threshold of cell firing at the axon hillock. Regardless of whether E-S potentiation is due to local disinhibition, we may ask how local changes in the region of those inputs whose activity results in E-S potentiation can give rise to increased probability of cell firing at those inputs and not at others. A possible mechanism is upregulation of postsynaptic conductances that allow local spiking, as modeled by Wathey et al. (1992). High-threshold calcium channels are potential candidates (Chetkovich et al., 1991; Wathey et al., 1992). In their analysis of GABA$_A$ receptor-independent E-S potentiation in hippocampal and cortical layer V pyramidal cells, Debanne and colleagues found evidence that the effect depended on the activation of group I mGluRs by the activated fibers, leading by an unknown pathway to suppression of a local K conductance (Daoudal et al., 2002; Sourdet et al., 2003). Induction of LTP in CA1 pyramidal cells results in persistent enhancement of local dendritic excitability, ascribed to modulation of the potassium current I$_A$ (Frick et al., 2004) or in cultured neurons to the nonspecific cation current I$_h$ (Wang et al., 2003). An increase in dendritic excitability may lead to local calcium spikes and generation of somatic action

potentials (Larkum et al., 1999) or favor the shift of the action potential initiation site toward the dendrites. An increase in dendritic excitability could preserve the input specificity of E-S potentiation via the generation of local Ca^{2+} spikes, leading to somatic action potentials.

Bidirectional changes in the E-S relation have also been described (Daoudal et al., 2002; Wang et al., 2003). Like E-S potentiation, E-S depression is NMDAR-dependent and displays input specificity when monitored in the presence of picrotoxin (Daoudal et al., 2002).

E-S Potentiation: Functional Considerations

The functional consequences of E-S potentiation and depression have not been explored in any depth, and will depend on several factors about which there is currently little information, including the persistence of the effect in the behaving animal and the degree to which input specificity is maintained. Reactivation of a specific network of cells in which E-S potentiation has been induced by a particular input pattern will be facilitated when that pattern is re-presented. Input specificity would add the useful feature that only the original input pattern would be subject to such amplification. Clearly, an increase (or decrease) in excitability will also enhance or depress the ability of the network to communicate with downstream targets.

10.3.13 Metaplasticity: The Magnitude and Direction of Activity-dependent Changes in Synaptic Weight Are Influenced by Prior Activity

The fact that LTP eventually reaches an asymptotic level after repeated episodes of high-frequency stimulation demonstrates that plasticity itself depends on the prior history of synaptic activity. The term "metaplasticity" was coined by Abraham and colleagues to describe this concept (Abraham and Bear, 1996; Abraham and Tate, 1997). The essential feature of metaplasticity is a persistent change in the plastic properties of the synapse brought about by prior synaptic or neuromodulatory activity that may or may not itself alter synaptic function. In the case of saturation, the prior activity (that is, preceding strong high-frequency trains) induces LTP. However, low-intensity ("priming") trains, which themselves elicit no change in synaptic weight, can also inhibit the subsequent induction of LTP (Huang YY et al., 1992). This effect of priming trains can persist for 1 to 2 hours, is specific to the primed input, and is mediated by a mechanism that requires the activation of NMDA receptors. Similarly, low-frequency activation of NMDA receptors in Mg^{2+}-free medium can prevent induction of LTP (Coan et al., 1989). These studies demonstrate the need for an optimal level of NMDAR activation for the induction of LTP; persistent low levels of activation may oppose induction of LTP via metaplasticity. Activation of mGluR receptors appears to facilitate the subsequent induction of LTP (Cohen and Abraham, 1996) and, as discussed above, can modify the subsequent requirement for mGluR activation for LTP induction (Bortolotto et al., 1994). There is evidence that early stimuli in the long low-frequency trains used to induce of LTD (see Section 10.7) perform a priming function; they do not themselves induce LTD but enable the later stimuli in the train to do so by an NMDAR-dependent mechanism (Mockett et al., 2002). An example of state dependence, which can be regarded as a form of metaplasticity, is provided by the observation that LTD cannot be induced in newly unsilenced synapses for the first 30 minutes after unsilencing (Montgomery and Madison, 2002) (see Section 10.7.6). Another, extreme case of metaplasticity is exhibited by synapses made by mossy fibers on interneurons in stratum lucidum of area CA3, at these synapses, depending on prior activity, tetanic stimulation of mossy fibers can produce either LTP or LTD (Pelkey et al., 2005) (see Section 10.8.1) for the mechanism underlying this striking instance of bidirectional plasticity. A striking case of metaplasticity is exhibited by synapses made by mossy fibers on interneurons in stratum lucidum of area CA3; at these synapses, depending on prior activity, tetanic stimulation of mossy fibers can produce either LTP or LTD (Pelkey et al., 2005) (see Section 10.8.1)

Some years before the first experimental studies of metaplasticity, the idea had been explored by Bienenstock, Cooper, and Munro in a theoretical analysis of developmental plasticity in the kitten visual system (Bienenstock et al., 1982; Bear et al., 1987). In the Bienenstock, Cooper, and Munro (BCM) model, the rate of change in synaptic weight, f, is a function of postsynaptic activity; it is negative for low rates of activity and positive for high rates of activity, corresponding to LTD and LTP respectively (see Box 10–2). The critical new feature of the BCM formulation is that the threshold for LTP, θ, is not static but is itself a function of the average activity of the cell. For maintained high rates of activity, the threshold slides to the right, facilitating the subsequent induction of LTD, whereas for low rates of activity, the threshold moves to the left, encouraging the induction of LTP. An element of homeostasis is thereby introduced to the system, preventing runaway potentiation and allowing situations in which activity is low to regain synaptic strength when the input is restored. The BCM model accounts for several features of metaplasticity in the hippocampus. The facilitation of LTD (depotentiation) after induction of LTP is one example (to our knowledge, there are no data on the converse prediction that LTP should be easier to obtain after induction of LTD); saturation of LTP is another. Other aspects are not so easily explained by the BCM model, such as the fact that metaplastic effects commonly persist for only an hour or two, and the essentially homosynaptic nature of metaplasticity in the hippocampus. In the BCM theory, θ is a global threshold applicable to all synapses and is a function only of postsynaptic activity, which itself reflects the integrated activity of all inputs to the cell. Yet metaplastic effects in the hippocampus are for the most part input-specific and do not seem to be much affected by heterosynaptic activity (Abraham and Tate, 1997).

The BCM rule is not the only synaptic learning rule with built-in homeostasis; other models are based on covariance rules proposed by Stent (1973), Sejnowski (1977), Singer (1990), and Friedlander et al. (1993) among others. Thus, although we tend to regard plasticity as a mechanim for driving changes in synaptic function, these formal sets of rules, as well as the phenomenon of metaplasticity, remind us that plasticity can also be the engine of stability. If LTD is easier to induce after LTP (and vice versa) the strength of connections will tend to stabilize around a mean. Similar adjustments in cell excitability are discussed in Section 10.3.14.

The patterns of synaptic activity that lead to metaplasticity are in many cases comparable to those that induce LTP or LTD. In some forms of metaplasticity the NMDA receptor plays an essential role, presumably reflecting the plasticity of NMDA receptor-mediated responses themselves (see Section 10.4), whereas in others, such as that mediated by the molecular switch (Section 10.3.10), metabotropic glutamate receptors are involved. It is likely, then, that the cellular correlates of metaplasticity overlap with those of LTP and LTD, and the point has been made, with some justice, that biochemical correlates of metaplasticity may be mistaken for biochemical correlates of LTP or LTD (Abraham and Tate, 1997).

A possible candidate for the molecular basis of metaplasticity is the NMDA receptor. The 2B subunit of the NMDA receptor is phosphorylated in LTP, an effect that in the anesthetized animal peaks between 2 and 5 hours after induction (Rosenblum et al., 1996; Rostas et al., 1996). In freely-moving animals, LTP in the dentate gyrus is associated with an increase in NR1 and NR2B levels that are still present 48 hours after induction (Williams et al., 2003). Phosphorylation of NR2B in expression systems enhances NMDAR-mediated currents by increasing the open time of the channel. This has little effect on the largely AMPA receptor-mediated synaptic responses (and thus cannot be the mechanism for LTP itself), but it does have consequences for subsequent attempts to induce plasticity. On the face of it, phosphorylation of NR2B and the increased receptor subunit levels constitute a positive feedback system. However, based on the assumption that both LTD and LTP are triggered by increases in intracellular Ca^{2+}, with the threshold for LTD being lower than that for LTP, both types of plasticity are facilitated by the increase in NMDAR-mediated Ca^{2+} current. The entire BCM curve, including θ, is shifted to the left; at low frequencies LTD is facilitated, and at intermediate and higher frequencies LTP is facilitated. Just this combination of effects is seen in the visual cortex following enhanced NMDAR function driven by sensory deprivation (Philpot et al., 2003). Another hint that changes in NMDA receptor function may underlie the expression of metaplasticity comes from the finding that low-intensity trains of the sort that impair the subsequent induction of LTP in area CA1 also induce LTD of the NMDAR-mediated component of the evoked response (Selig et al., 1995a).

Whatever the mechanisms by which changes in activity lead to metaplasticity, there is evidence that it may be affected by a variety of neuromodulators including corticosteroids, estrogen, catecholamines, acetylcholine, and serotonin. In general, these modulators lead to an increase in the threshold

Box 10–2
Synaptic Plasticity and the BCM Curve

The BCM function was introduced by Bienenstock, Cooper, and Munro (Bienenstock et al., 1982) to provide a mathematical description of activity-dependent changes in synaptic weight in the developing visual system (see Bear, 1996, for its application to hippocampal plasticity). The BCM function, f, is a function of c, the firing rate of the postsynaptic cell; it changes sign at a value of c called the threshold, θ; this itself is a function of c and the variable $<c>$ (the mean rate of postsynaptic activity, measured over minutes or hours). Thus f is a function of both c and $<c>$. In the BCM theory, the rate of change of synaptic efficacy, m_j, at the jth synapse on a cell, is given by the equation

$$dm_j/dt = f(c,<c>)d_j$$

where d_j is the rate of activity at the jth synapse. Note that the value of the BCM function, f, is determined only by the state of the postsynaptic cell. Synaptic plasticity—the rate of change of synaptic weights—is a product of f and afferent activity, d_j.

The function f is shown graphically in Box Fig. 10–2A. Note that an active synapse will be potentiated if it is active when $c > \theta$. This is likely to happen only when the cell is driven at high frequency, as with tetanic stimulation (Box Fig. 10–2B) or its postsynaptic state is manipulated, as by application of AP5 (Box Fig. 10–2C) or by depolarization (Box Fig. 10–2D). If a synapse is activated alone at low frequency, c is less than θ, and efficacy will be depressed. In general, θ is a nonlinear function of $<c>$; see Bear et al. (1987) for a discussion of the case where $\theta = <c>$. The magnitude of the change in synaptic weight is proportional to d_j, the rate of afferent activity; and there is no change when afferent activity is not driven ($d_j = 0$). Note also that the BCM formulation bequeaths inherent stability to the network: When $<c>$ is high, the threshold shifts to the right, so synaptic weights tend to be reduced, and postsynaptic activity is correspondingly dampened; and when the mean afferent activity is low, θ shifts to the left, synaptic weights increase, and activity is restored to the network. This prevents synaptic weights from increasing explosively when activity is high or decreasing to zero when activity is low.

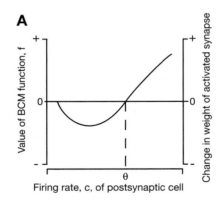

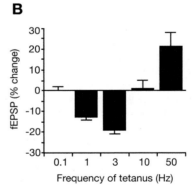

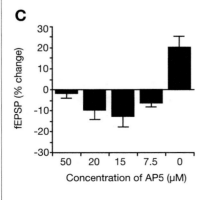

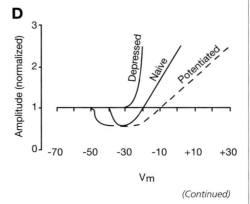

(Continued)

The curve relating tetanus frequency to the magnitude and polarity of the change in synaptic efficacy is sometimes interpreted as if it is a direct illustration of the function, f, in the BCM theory. However, although the two sets of curves have a similar form, passing from negative values to positive values at a modifiable threshold, the changes in synaptic efficacy are a function of postsynaptic firing rate in BCM theory and of presynaptic activity along a restricted set of afferent fibers in experimental investigations of bidirectional plasticity. The two descriptions approach congruence if presynaptic activity in the stimulated afferent(s) is the main determinant of cell firing; this may be the case in vitro where spontaneous activity is low, but is not the case in general. Reversal from LTD to LTP can also be achieved in single cells by manipulating the membrane potential; in strongly depolarized cells, brief trains induce LTP, whereas the same trains given when the cell is weakly depolarized induce LTD (Cummings et al., 1996; Ngezahayo et al., 2000) (see Box Fig. 10–2D), confirming that the polarity of change is under the control of the postsynaptic cell. The reversal point for LTD/LTP (θ in the BCM curve) is a function of past activity. For example, the prior induction of LTP in vitro shifts the reversal point (in terms of membrane depolarization) to the right, whereas the prior induction of LTD shifts it to the left (Ngezahayo et al., 2000) (see Box Fig. 10–2D). Similarly, prolonged prior antidromic or heterosynaptic activity in the dentate gyrus of the freely moving rat raises the threshold for LTP (Abraham et al., 2001). In each case, synaptic weights are changed in a direction that restores the output of the cell toward a non-zero mean.

Box Fig. 10–1. Bienenstock, Cooper, and Munro (BCM) curve and bidirectional synaptic plasticity. *A.* The BCM function f is negative for low firing rates of the postsynaptic cell, crosses zero at a threshold value (θ) and is positive thereafter. Because changes in synaptic weight at a given synapse are given in the BCM theory by f.d, where d is the rate of afferent activity at that synapse, the curve for changes in synaptic weight has the same shape. (*Source:* After Bienenstock et al., 1982.) *B.* Bidirectional changes in synaptic weight can be achieved by manipulating the frequency of afferent stimulation. The total number of stimuli (900) was the same in each case. The result is consistent with the BCM theory, as changes in stimulus frequency affect the firing of the postsynaptic cell. (*Source:* Bear and Linden, 2001; after Dudek and Bear, 1992.) *C.* Pharmacological manipulation of the postsynaptic NMDA receptor with varying concentrations of AP5 elicit bidirectional plasticity. Afferent stimulation was the same in each case (600 stimuli at 20 Hz). In control medium, this protocol induced LTP. With weak to intermediate concentrations of AP5, sufficient to reduce the firing of the postsynaptic cell to afferent stimulation, LTD was induced. Finally, at a concentration of 50 μm, changes in synaptic weight were blocked. (*Source:* Bear and Linden, 2001; after Cummings et al., 1996.) *D.* Bidirectional changes in synaptic weight produced by pairing afferent stimulation with depolarizing pulses to the postsynaptic cell. In each case, 100 afferent stimuli were given at 2 Hz. The polarity and magnitude of the change in synaptic efficacy was determined by the membrane potential to which the postsynaptic cell was clamped during pairing. In naïve cells (not previously subjected to pairing), depolarization to −30 mV resulted in LTD, whereas depolarization to −10 mV or more led to LTP. Threshold (θ) was at − 20 mV. This experiment also revealed how prior activity can alter θ. Once LTD had been induced, θ shifted to the left; and pairing to −30 mV, which in the naïve cell had induced LTD, now resulted in no change. Conversely, if LTP was induced, it was subsequently possible to induce LTD at a more modest depolarizing potential, implying a rightward shift of θ (dotted line, not experimentally confirmed). (*Source:* Ngezahayo et al., 2000.)

for LTP and a decrease in the threshold for LTD (reviewed by Abraham and Tate, 1997).

Transgenic Mice Can Exhibit Shifts in the BCM Curve

An example of a genetic modification leading to a striking shift in the frequency dependence of synaptic plasticity is the transgenic mouse carrying a mutated form of CaMKII engineered by Mayford et al. (1995). By changing a single residue (threonine 286 to aspartate), the enzyme was rendered calcium-independent. The effect was to shift the curve relating the frequency of the conditioning train to the change in synaptic efficacy to the right in αCaMKII(T286D) animals relative to wild-type littermates; thus, protocols that in wild-type mice produced LTP led to LTD in the transgenic animals. A similar shift to the left of the frequency or BCM curve for synaptic plasticity occurs in other mutants, including an NR2B overexpressing transgenic mouse (Tang et al., 1999) and a calcineurin knockout (Zeng et al., 2001). In contrast, mice lacking the GluR2 subunit (Jia et al., 1996) or the postsynaptic density protein PSD95 (Migaud et al., 1998) showed a shift to the left of the frequency-response curve; thus, stimulus protocols that produced LTD in wild types induced LTP in the mutant animals. The shift in baseline θ exhibited by these and other mutants suggests that there may be two mechanistically distinct forms of metaplasticity: (1) homosynaptic (input-specific) metaplasticity lasting not more than a few hours and attributable to post-translational changes in, for example, NMDA receptors; and (2) a more persistent, generalized form of metaplasticity that regulates baseline θ and requires gene expression (Deisseroth et al., 1995; Abraham and Tate, 1997).

10.3.14 Synaptic Scaling and Long-term Changes in Intrinsic Excitabililty

A neural network in which Hebbian synapses provide the only mechanism for plasticity cannot sustain a state of dynamic stability in which the mean rate of activity remains constant, while the potential for modification of individual synapses is retained. In a Hebbian network, successful inputs are strengthened, becoming more successful, whereas unsuccessful inputs remain unsuccessful or are depressed; the network is ultimately driven to an invariant state where activity is controlled by a subset of maximally potentiated synapses. Several theoretical fixes to the problem of runaway excitation due to Hebbian positive feedback have been proposed. In the covariance rule proposed by Stent (1973), a synapse is potentiated when activity in the pre- and postsynaptic cells are in phase and depressed when they are out of phase. There is some experimental evidence for Stent's rule (Artola and Singer, 1993; Debanne et al., 1998). As we saw above, in the influential model proposed by Bienenstock et al. (1982) and extended and updated by Shouval et al. (2002), the magnitude and polarity of plastic changes are controlled by the overall activity of the network to maintain a constant mean firing rate (see also reviews by Abbott and Nelson, 2000 and Bi and Poo, 2001).

There is now considerable evidence that homeostatic mechanisms operate to maintain a constant mean level of firing in neural networks. Homeostasis is achieved by overall adjustments to synaptic weights, a process called "synaptic scaling." The phenomenon was first studied in cultured cortical networks. Addition of a GABA$_A$ antagonist to the culture medium produced an initial increase in spontaneous activity, but activity returned to control levels over the following 2 days (reviewed by Turrigiano and Nelson, 2004). In cultured hippocampal neurons, similarly, the GABA$_A$ antagonist picrotoxin produced a long-term reduction in surface AMPA receptors (Lissin et al., 1998). Homeostasis can also operate at the level of the single hippocampal pyramidal cell embedded in an active network of cultured hippocampal neurons. Overexpression of an inward-rectifier K channel resulted in an initial decrease in the firing rate of the transfected cell, but over time the firing rate was restored to control values by a homeostatic increase in synaptic drive (Burrone et al., 2002).

Finally, the increase in excitability of neurons in hippocampal cultures that is induced by prolonged blockade of activity appears to reflect an up regulation of synaptic AMPARs, driven by glial release of the cytokine tumor-necrosis factor-α (TNF-α) (Stellwagen and Malenka, 2006).

Activity-dependent changes in intrinsic excitability have also been documented in hippocampal, cortical, and cerebellar neurons (for review see Zhang and Linden, 2003). An important insight was gained when two groups reported that persistent changes in local dendritic excitability accompany synaptic plasticity in CA1 pyramidal neurons. In one case, a theta-burst pairing protocol produced a long-lasting shift in the inactivation curve of the K$^+$ conductance I$_A$, leading to local boosting of synaptic responses and back-propagating spikes (Frick et al., 2004). In the other study, spike timing-dependent plasticity was accompanied by persistent changes in the cationic current I$_h$ (Wang et al., 2003). These findings imply that the throughput of synaptic information to the soma is enhanced not just from the tetanized region but also from distal synapses on the same dendrite.

Another intriguing finding comes from the behavioral literature. About 50% of CA1 pyramidal cells examined in slices from rabbits trained in a trace conditioning task (eyeblink conditioning using a tone as the conditioned stimulus and an airpuff as the unconditioned stimulus) exhibited a reduction in spike frequency adaption and spike after-hyperpolarization (Moyer et al., 1996). (Although these changes in excitability last several days, they cannot encode the memory for the conditioned response, which can last months). A similar reduction in after-hyperpolarization is seen in rat CA1 neurons after spatial training in the watermaze (Oh et al., 2003). Activity-dependent changes in excitability, in contrast to the synaptic scaling produced by prolonged hypo- or hyperactivity, are in general nonhomeostatic because they act in the same direction as synaptic changes. Note also that changes in local dendritic excitability introduce a potential for metaplasticity, as they may affect subsequent STDP. Exploration of long-term changes in excitability is at an early stage, and relatively little is known about the conductances responsible or the second messenger systems that modulate them.

Back-propagating Synaptic Plasticity and Long-range Cytoplasmic Signaling

Back-propagation of synaptic weight changes is the central feature of an efficient design for unsupervised learning in model neural networks (Rumelhart et al., 1986). There was, however, little evidence for back-propagation in biological nervous systems until the studies by Poo and his colleagues in hippocampal cultures (Fitzsimonds et al., 1997; Tao et al., 2000). LTP or LTD induced at a particular connection by spike pairing of presynaptic and postsynaptic neurons in the appropriate temporal conjunction—results in the spread of plasticity (of the same polarity) to other synapses onto the presynaptic neuron and to other synapses made by the presynaptic neuron. However, there is no spread to other connections made by or onto the postsynaptic neuron (Bi and Poo, 2001). Thus, LTP at a given synapse is propagated only to synapses made by or onto the presynaptic neuron. The presynaptic cell was voltage-clamped except when required to fire an action potential to induce the primary LTP; it is therefore likely that back-propagated changes are not activity-driven but involve some form of cytoplasmic long-range signaling. There are as yet no reports of back-propagating plasticity in hippocampal slices or in the hippocampus in vivo. However, in the developing retinotectal system of the tadpole, application of BDNF to the tectum (where axons of retinal ganglion cells terminate) results in potentiation of retinotectal synapses and a back-propagated increase in the number of glutamate receptors on dendrites of ganglion cells (Du and Poo, 2004).

10.4 NMDA Receptor-dependent LTP: Expression Mechanisms

10.4.1 From Induction to Expression of LTP

The various properties of LTP that we have summarized above arise from the complex interplay of biophysical and cell-biological mechanisms operating at the cellular and local circuit levels. In approaching this complexity, it is convenient to distinguish between the *induction* of LTP, which comprises the collection of short-lived events that trigger changes in synaptic weight but do not themselves affect it, and the *expression* of LTP, which includes all those mechanisms, whether presynaptic or postsynaptic, that directly enhance or, in the case of LTD, diminish synaptic efficacy. (Note that, in addition to expression, two other equivalent terms are found in the LTP literature: *persistence* and *maintenance*.) Thus, events associated with the activation of NMDA receptors, relief of the magnesium block, permeation of Ca^{2+} through the NMDA receptor, and activation of Ca^{2+}-dependent protein kinases can all be considered components of induction. Expression mechanisms include increases in the probability of transmitter release, phosphorylation of AMPA receptors and their insertion into the postsynaptic density.

10.4.2 STP Is a Transient Presynaptic Form of Plasticity

In an early experiment to probe for changes in postsynaptic sensitivity, it was observed that LTP was associated with a delayed increase in sensitivity to AMPAR agonists (Davies et al., 1989). This suggests that whereas E-LTP correlates in time with alterations in postsynaptic function, STP occurs without any such changes. The simplest interpretation of this result is that STP is presynaptic, a conclusion supported by a detailed paired-pulse facilitation analysis (Volianskis and Jensen, 2003). This study revealed a surprising property of STP: It decays in an activity-dependent manner. If afferent stimulation is discontinued after tetenization, STP appears at full

strength and decays with the same time course when afferent stimulation is resumed, even when the intervening period is as long as 6 hours. [As a result, it was proposed that STP may be more accurately referred to as a transient form of LTP (T-LTP); however, here we retain the more widely known term, STP.] In addition, it was found that the magnitude of STP was influenced by the frequency of afferent stimulation, such that higher frequencies favored larger STP. This finding may explain why the extent of STP observed in different experiments is highly variable. In particular, a brief high-frequency tetanus followed by a low rate of test stimulation (as typically used in field potential recordings) would favor the generation of a large-magnitude STP with slow decay, whereas an intermediate frequency of stimulation for both the induction and expression periods (as typically used during pairing experiments) militates against STP. This may explain why pairing induced potentiation generally lacks the STP component.

10.4.3 Early LTP Involves Multiple Protein Kinase-dependent Mechanisms

Many studies have presented evidence that protein kinases are involved in LTP (Fig. 10–8). Most of this work relates to the study of E-LTP. With few exceptions, STP is resistant to kinase inhibitors. The role of protein kinases in L-LTP is discussed later in this section.

Protein Kinase C

The first kinase to be implicated in LTP was protein kinase C (PKC) (Lovinger et al., 1987) (Fig. 10–9A). However, the inhibitors used in these initial studies were relatively nonspecific, so the effects observed may have been via actions on other kinases. Indeed, several reports have observed no effect of potent, more specific PKC inhibitors on LTP (see Muller et al., 1992; Bortolotto and Collingridge, 2000). On the other hand, a role for PKC has been proposed based on the use of peptide inhibitors applied intracellularly (Malinow et al., 1989). In addition, effects of more selective (though not totally specific) PKC inhibitors have been described under certain circumstances, for example during de-depression (the tetanus-induced restoration of the response in a pathway in which LTD has previously been induced) (Daw et al., 2000). The most likely explanation is that PKC is involved in some, but not all, aspects of E-LTP. Understanding the role of PKC in LTP is complicated by the existence of multiple isoforms; the Ca^{2+} and diacylglycerol-activated, conventional PKCs (cPKCs: α, βI, βII , γ); Ca^{2+}-independent, diacylglycerol-activated, novel PKCs (nPKCs: δ, ε, η, θ); and the Ca^{2+}-independent, diacylglycerol-independent atypical PKCs (aPKCs: ζ, ι). The spectrum of subtype selectivity of the various inhibitors is incomplete, and there is limited information available from knockout experiments. Elimination of the neuron-specific isoform PKCγ leads to inhibition of LTP, although not if the LTP is preceded by low-frequency stimulation (Abeliovich et al., 1993). This suggests that PKCγ may play a regulatory role

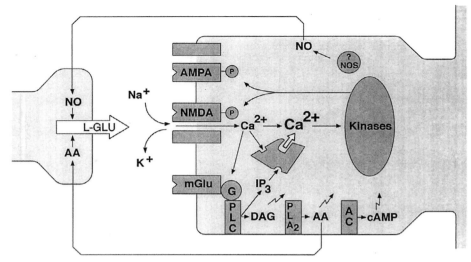

Figure 10–8. Signal transduction mechanisms in early LTP. The trigger for the induction of LTP is Ca²⁺ permeating through the NMDA receptor. This is amplified by Ca²⁺ release from Ca²⁺/IP3-sensitive stores. The amplified Ca²⁺ signal together with other activators of protein kinases (zigzag arrows) then leads to the phosphorylation of substrate proteins, including AMPA and NMDA receptors, and the insertion of AMPA receptors into the postsynaptic membrane (not shown). These post-translational processes contribute to E-LTP. Protein synthesis-dependent mechanisms at the synapse and by signals passing to the nucleus are responsible for L-LTP. Putative retrograde messengers, Nitric oxide (NO) and arachidonic acid (AA), that may stimulate presynaptic changes are also indicated. (*Source*: After Bliss and Collingridge, 1993.)

in the induction of LTP. Of great interest is the finding by Sacktor and colleagues that a peptide substrate inhibitor of PKMζ, the autonomously active catalytic domain of PKCζ, blocks the expression of pre-established L-LTP (Ling et al., 2002; Serrano et al., 2005; see Section 10.4.9). Bath application of the inhibitor at the time of the tetanus has no effect on E-LTP but blocks the development of L-LTP.

In other experiments phorbol esters have been used to activate PKC. This treatment leads to a potentiation of synaptic transmission which superficially resembles LTP (Malenka et al., 1986; Hu et al., 1987). However, the potentiation is reversible following washout of the phorbol ester and does not occlude with tetanus-induced LTP. Moreover, phorbol esters directly interact with other proteins, such as munc-13, a protein involved in neurotransmitter release, and so any effects of phorbol esters may be unrelated to activation of PKC (Kazanietz et al., 2000).

The trigger for the induction of PKC-dependent potentiation may be Ca²⁺ entering via NMDA receptors. An alternative route is via glutamate binding to group I mGluRs (mGluR1 and mGluR5), the activation of which leads to production of diacylglycerol and release of Ca²⁺ from intracellular stores— the two triggers for activation of cPKCs. In this context, potent PKC inhibitors prevent mGluR-mediated metaplasticity (Bortolotto and Collingridge, 2000).

CaMKII

Calcium/calmodulin-dependent protein kinase II (CaMKII) is a major component of the postsynaptic density, comprising 2% of its protein content (Lisman et al., 2002). The holoenzyme consists of dodecamers of α and β subunits. In its inactive state, the ATP binding site of the catalytic region of the enzyme is bound to an autoinhibitory domain in the regulatory region. When calcium-loaded calmodulin binds to a calmodulin-binding region in the 3′ region of the molecule, a conformational change occurs that separates the autoinhibitory domain from the ATP binding site and renders the enzyme active. Following a transient surge in calcium concentration, intramolecular autophosphorylation at threonine 286 can occur, producing a conformation that allows the enzyme to remain autonomously active when calcium levels fall, thereby endowing the enzyme with the properties of a molecular switch (Miller and Kennedy, 1986). Two isoforms of the calcium/calmodulin-dependent protein kinase II are present in the adult hippocampus, αCaMKII and βCaMKII, of which the dominant form in area CA1 is αCaMKII. There is a wealth of evidence to indicate that αCaMKII is required for and, when activated, capable of producing LTP in area CA1 of the adult animal (reviewed by Lisman et al., 2002). First, specific peptide inhibitors of αCaMKII, based on the autoinhibitory domain of the enzyme, which suppress both calcium-dependent and calcium-independent activity, block induction of LTP (Malinow et al., 1989) (Fig. 10–9B). Second, the membrane-permeable CaMKII inhibitors KN-62 and KN-93 block induction of LTP in a reversible manner (Ito et al., 1991). Third, LTP is impaired in αCaMKII⁻/⁻ mice (Silva et al., 1992b), although there may be a background effect contributing to this deficit (Hinds et al., 1998). Fourth, mice with a threonine to alanine point mutation at residue 286 that prevents autophosphorylation do not display LTP in area CA1 (Giese et al., 1998). In addition, LTP is associated with the dendritic accumulation of

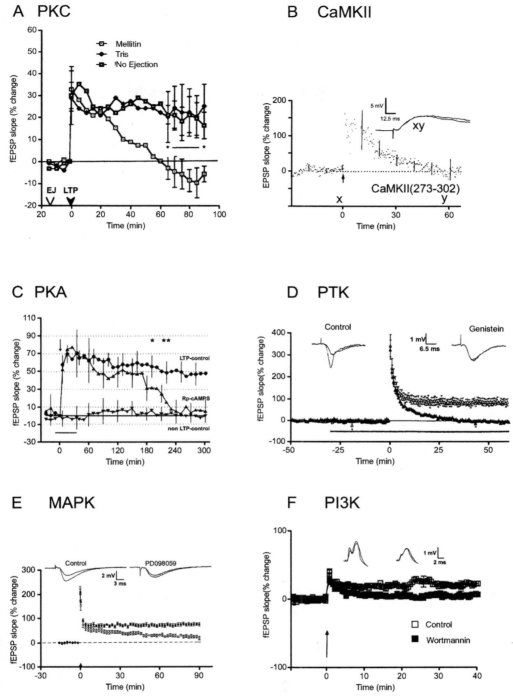

Figure 10–9. Role of protein kinases in the induction and expression of LTP. *A.* The PKC inhibitor mellitin, injected into the dentate gyrus in vivo 15 minutes prior to a tetanus, blocks E-LTP but spares STP. Similar findings were obtained with polymyxin B and H-7, implicating PKC as the kinase responsible. (*Source*: Lovinger et al., 1987.) In this and subsequent panels the slope of the fEPSP (or intracellular EPSP in *B*) is plotted versus time. Control experiments are also shown, except in *B*. In each case, a tetanus was delivered at t = 0. *B.* A peptide inhibitor of CaMKII [CaMKII(273-302)] loaded into CA1 neurons in vitro blocks E-LTP but not STP. Similar results were obtained using a peptide inhibitor of PKC. (*Source*: Malinow et al., 1989.) *C.* The PKA inhibitor Rp-cAMPS blocks L-LTP in the CA1 region of the hippocampus in vitro. STP and E-LTP are unaffected. (*Source*: Matthies and Reymann, 1993.) *D.* The tyrosine kinase inhibitor genistein blocks E-LTP but not STP at CA1 synapses in vitro. Similar results were obtained using lavendustin A. (*Source*: O'Dell et al., 1991a.) *E.* The MAPK inhibitor PD098059 blocks induction of E-LTP but not STP at CA1 synapses in vitro. (*Source*: English and Sweatt, 1997.) *F.* ICV application of the PI3K inhibitor wortmannin blocks induction of E-LTP at perforant path-granule cell synapses in vivo. (*Source*: Kelly et al., 2000.)

activated CaMKII and an associated phosphorylation of AMPARs (Fukunaga et al., 1995). Finally, CaMKII mimics and occludes the induction of LTP (Pettit et al., 1994). However, as compelling as the evidence is for involvement of CaMKII in LTP under some circumstances, the situation is not as straightforward as it may seem. Although there is general agreement that the induction of LTP is associated with a persistent (> 1 hour) phosphorylation of αCaMKII, there is disagreement about whether the increase in enzyme activity is transient (Lengyel et al., 2004) or persistent (Fukunaga et al., 1995). Also there is currently no direct evidence that a constitutively active form of CaMKII is involved in the maintenance of LTP. Inhibitors of CaMKII applied following the induction of LTP have no effect (Ito et al., 1991; Chen et al., 2001b). However, these inhibitors compete with the calmodulin binding site, and hence the Ca^{2+}/calmodulin-dependent activation of the enzyme, but do not affect the constitutively active form. Thus whilst persistent re-activation of the enzyme can be discounted as a mechanism it is possible that a constitutively active form of CaMKII maintains LTP. Specific membrane permeable inhibitors of the constitutively active form are required to test this possibility. What is clear however is that CaMKII is not ubiquitous in its involvement in NMDAR-dependent LTP. For example, in area CA1 at an early stage in development (P9) CaMKII inhibitors have no effect on the induction of LTP (Yasuda et al., 2003), and at an intermediate stage of development (P14) CaMKII forms one arm of a parallel kinase cascade (Wikström et al., 2003). Thus, the importance of CaMKII in LTP increases during development. Even in the adult animal, however, autophosphorylation of αCaMKII is not a general requirement for NMDAR-dependent LTP, since potentiation in the medial perforant path of the dentate gyrus is minimally affected in T286A mutant mice; in these mice autophosphorylation at residue 286 cannot occur (Cooke et al, 2006). However, as in juvenile CA1, there is evidence for involvement of CaMKII as part of a parallel pathway also involving PKA and MAPK (Cooke et al, 2006; see below). Finally, it should be noted that CaMKII is involved in metaplasticity in area CA1 (Bortolotto & Collingridge, 1998) and so biochemical changes that accompany LTP may relate to metaplasticity rather than the plasticity *per se* (see Abraham and Tate, 1997).

Protein Kinase A

Protein kinase A (PKA) is another kinase involved in LTP, and again its role is complex and not fully understood. In general, PKA inhibitors appear to block L-LTP but spare E-LTP (Matthies and Reymann, 1993; Huang and Kandel, 1994) (Fig. 10–9C) via an action in the postsynaptic neuron (Duffy and Nguyen, 2003). A similar conclusion has, in general, been reached on the basis of various genetic experiments in mice (Nguyen and Woo, 2003). However, LTP lasting many hours can be induced in the presence of PKA inhibitors (Bortolotto and Collingridge, 2000). Conversely, E-LTP is affected by PKA inhibitors in some cases (Huang and Kandel, 1994; Blitzer et

al., 1995; Otmakhova et al., 2000). It seems that the role of PKA is determined by a variety of factors, such as the strength and patterns of the high-frequency trains used to induce LTP. Typically, PKA inhibitors are more effective when strong induction protocols are used (Nguyen and Woo, 2003). They are also more effective early in development, before the CaMKII-dependent form of LTP is expressed (Yasuda et al., 2003). Interestingly, the sensitivity of E-LTP to PKA inhibitors is also dependent on the prior level of experience of the animal, such that environmental enrichment results in a larger LTP with the additional component being selectively sensitive to PKA inhibition (Duffy et al., 2001).

Transient bath application of the constitutively active cAMP analogue Sp-cAMPS can produce a persistent, slow-onset enhancement of synaptic transmission in area CA1 that occludes with tetanus-induced LTP (Frey et al., 1993). However, like the PKA-dependent component of tetanus-induced LTP, this is not invariably observed. For example, in one study cAMP analogues did not affect basal transmission but reversed LTD, implicating PKA in de-depression (Kameyama et al., 1998). Intriguingly, there is a strong strain difference in the ability of mice to express cAMP-induced facilitation (Nguyen et al., 2000).

These various observations suggest that the role of PKA is probably to modulate, rather than directly mediate, NMDAR-dependent LTP. One idea is that PKA gates the activity of the pathway leading from activation of CaMKII to the expression of early LTP (Blitzer et al., 1995) via inhibition of the protein phosphatase 1 (PP1), which dephosphorylates CaMKII at ser831 and ser845 (Blitzer et al., 1998). Whether LTP-inducing stimuli induce an increase in the level of cAMP is disputed (Chetkovich and Sweatt, 1993; Blitzer et al., 1995; Pokorska et al., 2003). If there is no increase, constitutive levels of cAMP must be adequate to maintain the gate in its open state.

Tyrosine Kinases

Initial pharmacological evidence, using relatively nonspecific PTK inhibitors, suggested that protein tyrosine kinases (PTKs) are necessary for E-LTP (O'Dell et al., 1991a Fig. 10–9D). Various nonreceptor tyrosine kinases are expressed in the central nervous system, including src and the src family members fyn and lyn. Genetic elimination of fyn resulted in a deficit in LTP (O'Dell et al., 1991a). Although this knockout was associated with gross structural changes in the dentate gyrus, a successful rescue experiment suggested that the LTP deficit reflected the loss of fyn in the adult, rather than impaired neuronal development (Kojima et al., 1997). The role of fyn appears to be developmentally regulated, as no LTP deficits are seen in animals at less than 14 weeks. Fyn probably acts as a regulatory molecule, as LTP can be induced in the fyn knockout when a strong induction protocol is used. One potential mechanism for how fyn regulates LTP is via phosphorylation of NMDARs (Rosenblum et al., 1996; Rostas et al., 1996) to increase their function. There is also evidence that src is involved in the induction of LTP via upregulation of the function of NMDARs (Lu et al., 1998). This pathway involves the focal adhesion kinase CAKβ/PyK2 upstream of src (Huang Y et al., 2001).

MAP Kinase

Of the several mitogen-associated protein (MAP) kinase cascades that carry extracellular signals to the nucleus, the two that have been extensively studied in the context of LTP are inititiated by the small G proteins Ras and Rap-1. They activate the MAP kinase kinase kinases Raf-1 and B-Raf, respectively, the first of the kinases in the three-kinase cascade. The two pathways converge on the second kinase, MEK (MAP kinase kinase), which in turn phosphorylates a pair of MAP kinases known as extracellular regulated kinases 1 and 2 (ERK1, or p44MAPK, and ERK2, or p42MAPK). The ERK/MAP kinase pathway can be positively regulated by PKA via the Rap-1, B-raf pathway and by PKC via the Ras, Raf-1 pathway. PKA can also inhibit the latter pathway. The convergence of initial pathways onto MEK during the second stage of the cascade, and the fact that MAPKs are the only known substrates for MEK has provided a target for pharmacological intervention. Three specific inhibitors are available—PD098059, U0126, SL327—the last of which can cross the blood-brain barrier.

English and Sweatt were the first to explore the role of the MAPK pathway in LTP. They found that LTP-inducing stimuli resulted in increased phosphorylation of ERK1, 2 (English and Sweatt, 1996) and that MEK inhibitors blocked both E-LTP and L-LTP in area CA1 of hippocampal slices (English and Sweatt, 1997) (Fig. 10–9E). However, MAPK seems to be involved in only some forms of LTP. For example, in one study MEK inhibitors blocked induction of a form of theta-induced LTP but did not affect pairing-induced or tetanus-induced LTP (Opazo et al., 2003). The reduction in E-LTP has also been questioned by Kelleher et al. (2004b), who found that LTP in a transgenic mouse expressing a dominant negative MEK was indistinguishable from E-LTP generated in normal mice in the presence of protein synthesis inhibitors; they concluded that the main substrates of the MAP kinase pathway were kinases regulating the protein translational machinery in dendrites.

Nevertheless, local targets that might underlie a contribution of the MAP kinase cascade to E-LTP have begun to be identified. Ras, the small G protein that activates the first kinases (Raf and B-Raf) in the MAP kinase cascade, is implicated in AMPA receptor trafficking in LTP, and another G protein, Rap, which activates a member of the ERK family, p38, is involved in the removal of AMPA receptors from synapses during LTD (Zhu et al., 2002). There is also evidence that MAP kinases interact with scaffolding proteins and with cytoskeletal proteins. A further suggestive finding is that activation of MAP kinase through PKA and PKC can downregulate a dendritic A-type K^+ channel in CA1 pyramidal neurons, leading to a reduction in the threshold for back-propagation

and potential enhancement of LTP (Yuan et al., 2002; reviewed by Sweatt, 2004).

PI3 Kinase

Phosphoinositide 3-kinase (PI3K) phosphorylates phosphatidylinositol 4,5-bisphosphate [PtdIns(4,5)P2, or PIP2] to produce phosphatidylinositol 3,4,5-trisphosphate [PtdIns(3,4,5)P3, or PIP3], which in turn can activate Ca^{2+}-independent isoforms of PKC (such as PKCγ), Akt/PKB, and phospholipase Cγ. PI3K was first implicated in NMDAR-dependent LTP in the dentate gyrus, where it was shown that the inhibitor wortmannin inhibited E-LTP but not STP at perforant path synapses (Kelly and Lynch, 2000) (Fig. 10–9F). Similarly, inhibition of E-LTP but not STP was observed at CA1 synapses using a different PI3K inhibitor, LY294002 (Raymond et al., 2002). In the dentate gyrus in vivo, this inhibitor blocked E-LTP induced by single but not multiple trains, suggesting that P13K is not an obligatory enzyme in LTP induction (Horwood et al., 2006). Interestingly, PI3K may be required specifically for the expression of LTP, as inhibition of the enzyme led to depression of preestablished LTP and, following washout of the inhibitor, recovery of LTP to its initial level (Sanna et al., 2002; but see Opazo et al., 2003). The downstream processes modulated by PI3K are not known but may involve both MAPK-dependent and MAPK-independent pathways (Opazo et al., 2003) that affect the surface expression of AMPARs (Man et al., 2003).

LTP Involves Multiple and Parallel Kinase Cascades

The principal message to emerge from studies investigating the role of kinases in NMDA receptor-dependent LTP is that several kinases are involved but none is obligatory. The situation is complicated by the fact that the kinase cascades underlying LTP change during development. In area CA1 of the adult animal, as we have seen, αCaMKII is required for the induction of LTP, and LTP can be induced in the presence of PKA inhibitors. Earlier, at postnatal day 9, the lead role is taken by PKA, as inhibitors of PKA, but not of αCaMKII, block induction of LTP (Yasuda et al., 2003; see Fig. 10–21C). The situation is made even more complex by the existence of parallel kinase cascades, as first identified at CA1 synapses in juvenile rats. Thus at 2 weeks of age, a combination of inhibitors is required to block the induction of LTP. Inhibitors of CaMKII, PKA, and PKC have no effect on induction when applied alone. Similarly, a PKA inhibitor plus a PKC inhibitor is ineffective. However, a CaMKII inhibitor applied together with either a PKA or a PKC inhibitor fully blocks the induction of LTP (Wikström et al., 2003). This suggests that two parallel kinase pathways, one involving CaMKII and the other involving both PKA and PKC, can each mediate LTP. As the animal matures, αCaMKII assumes the dominant role, and PKA and PKC become more modulatory in nature. The involvement of parallel kinase cascades is, however, not simply a developmental issue, since a similar parallel pathway has been observed in the medial perforant path in the dentate gyrus of adult mice (Cooke et al, 2006) and rats (Wu et al., 2006). Here we have a pathway that requires activation of CaMKII for one limb and PKA/MAPK for the other. Since both PKA and PKC can lead to activation of MAPK it is possible that in both juvenile CA1 and adult dentate gyrus the same two parallel pathways co-exist, one arm using CaMKII and the other PKA/PKC/MAPK.

10.4.4 Site of Expression of Early LTP: Experimental Approaches

LTP research during the 1990s was enlivened by intense debate as to whether NMDAR-dependent LTP is expressed presynaptically or postsynaptically. Many experiments relied on classical electrophysiological approaches, such as paired-pulse facilitation, failures analysis, or quantal analysis (see Box 10–1). Unfortunately, no clear consensus has emerged owing to the difficulty of obtaining accurate measurements coupled with an incomplete understanding of the quantal basis of synaptic transmission at central synapses (see Box 10–1).

Over the years considerable evidence has accumulated in favor of both presynaptic (Fig. 10–11) and postsynaptic (Fig. 10–12) mechanisms, and we examine the evidence for each in turn. First, though, we consider three experimental approaches that were designed to detect changes in transmitter release following the induction of LTP and that, by and large, failed to do so.

Differential Potentiation of AMPA and NMDA Receptor-Mediated Responses

An electrophysiological approach that has been used to address the locus of expression of LTP is based on a comparison of the relative potentiation of the AMPA and NMDA receptor-mediated components of synaptic transmission—the logic being that an increase in the probability of transmitter release (Pr) should affect both components equally, while a postsynaptic modification of the AMPA receptor should result in selective potentiation of the AMPA receptor-mediated component. This makes the assumption that an increase in L-glutamate would increase both synaptic components equally. This would not be the case if, for example, NMDA receptors were saturated, or nearer to being saturated, than AMPA receptors—an issue that still has not been fully resolved at hippocampal synapses (see Section 6.6.1). Conversely, a similar increase in both synaptic components could occur by a postsynaptic mechanism that affects both AMPA and NMDA receptor-mediated components of synaptic transmission. In addition to these theoretical caveats, there has been no experimental consensus with respect to whether LTP involves a specific increase in the AMPAR-mediated component. While one early study reported a selective increase in the AMPAR-mediated component (Kauer et al., 1988), others have reported an increase in both components, ranging from

a larger increase in the AMPAR-mediated component (Muller et al., 1988; Kullmann et al., 1996; Dozmorov et al., 2006) to a similar increase in both synaptic components (Clark and Collingridge, 1995; O'Connor et al., 1995). The lack of consensus plus the issues of interpretation mean that little can be concluded from these experiments regarding the locus of expression of LTP. Another conclusion to have emerged from these studies is that the NMDAR-mediated component of synaptic transmission is plastic. Interpretation of alterations in the NMDAR-mediated component of dual-component synaptic transmission is complicated by the voltage escape associated with the AMPAR-mediated component coupled with the voltage dependence of the NMDAR-mediated conductance. However, LTP has been observed by several groups following blockade of AMPAR-mediated synaptic transmission (Bashir et al., 1991; Berretta et al., 1991; O'Connor et al., 1994; Grosshans et al., 2002). Plasticity of the NMDAR-mediated response has obvious functional implications for metaplasticity (see Section 10.3.13).

Kinetics of Open Channel Blockers Do Not Indicate an Increase in Transmitter Release in LTP

Another approach has been to use open-channel blockers to estimate the probability of release, Pr. The potent noncompetitive NMDAR antagonist MK-801 blocks NMDA receptors once they have been activated by synaptically released L-glutamate, and once in the channel the receptor remains blocked during the lifetime of the experiment (Hessler et al., 1993; Rosenmund et al., 1993). During repetitive stimulation high-Pr synapses are therefore blocked more quickly than low-Pr synapses. It was found that LTP of AMPA receptor-mediated synaptic transmission was not associated with any change in the MK-801 blocking rate of NMDAR-mediated synaptic transmission (Manabe and Nicoll, 1994) (Fig. 10–10B). This was taken as evidence that LTP does not involve an increase in Pr. A more direct approach was to use an open-channel blocker of the AMPAR-mediated component. Philanthotoxin (PhTx) blocks GluR2-lacking, Ca^{2+}-permeable AMPA receptors in a use-dependent manner and so can be used to monitor Pr. LTP was not associated with any change in the PhTx blocking rate in the GluR2 knockout mouse (Mainen et al., 1998) (Fig. 10–10C), again indicating no change in Pr. Similar experiments could not be performed in wild-type animals owing to the presence of GluR2 subunits in the great majority of the AMPA receptors on principal neurons.

Electrogenic Uptake of Glutamate by Glia Reports an Increase in Extracellular Glutamate During PTP but Not During LTP

Yet another approach has been to use glial currents as a monitor of neurotransmitter release. Glial cells accumulate synaptically released L-glutamate by an electrogenic uptake carrier: An increase in neurotransmitter release should therefore generate a larger glial current. An increase in electrogenic current was

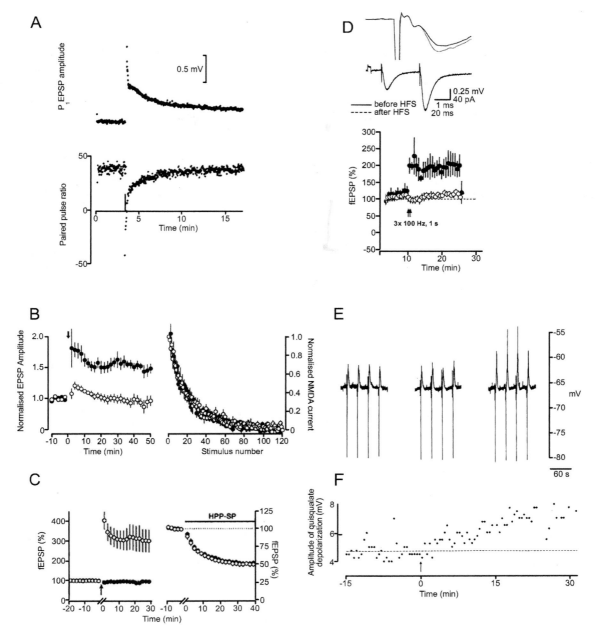

Figure 10–10. Evidence that LTP involves postsynaptic changes. *A.* LTP is not associated with a corresponding alteration in paired-pulse facilitation in the dentate gyrus in vivo. The upper plot shows the amplitude of the EPSP evoked by the first stimulus of the pair. The lower plot shows the amplitude of the second EPSP divided by that of the first EPSP for each pair to generate the paired-pulse ratio. Note that there was a decrease in the paired-pulse ratio only during the initial phase of PTP, lasting approximately 10 minutes. (*Source*: McNaughton, 1982.) *B.* LTP is not associated with changes in Pr at CA1 synapses in vitro, as assessed by measuring the rate of blockade of NMDA receptor-mediated currents by MK-801. LTP of AMPA receptor-mediated EPSCs was induced (at t = 0) in one input (filled symbols) but not in a control input (open symbols). AMPA receptors were then blocked and the neurons depolarized to reveal the NMDA receptor-mediated EPSC. MK-801 was applied and allowed to equilibrate before stimulation was commenced. Both inputs were blocked at the same rate, indicating that the average Pr at control and potentiated inputs was similar. (*Source*: Manabe and Nicoll, 1994.) *C.* LTP is not associated with changes in Pr at CA1 synapses in vitro, as assessed by measuring the rate of blockade of

AMPA receptor-mediated currents by spermine in the GluR2 knockout mouse. This experiment was conducted in a manner similar to that illustrated in *B* except AMPA receptor-mediated synaptic transmission was monitored throughout, and a spermine derivative (HPP-SP) was used to block the activated receptors. (*Source*: Mainen et al., 1998.) *D.* LTP is not associated with an alteration in L-glutamate release, as detected using glial transporter currents. LTP of fEPSPs is illustrated in the upper traces and in the time-course plot. The lower traces are glia-transporter currents in response to paired-pulse stimulation before and following the induction of LTP. Note that the records are superimposable, indicating no change in the glial current. (*Source*: Diamond et al., 1998.) *E.* LTP is associated with an increase in postsynaptic sensitivity to exogenous AMPA receptor activation. The upper records are depolarizations of a CA1 neuron in response to ionophoretic application of an AMPA receptor ligand (quisqualate) obtained before, immediately following, and 30 minutes following the induction of LTP (at t = 0). The graph plots the amplitude of these depolarizations with time. Note the gradual increase in postsynaptic sensitivity, with a time course that correlates with E-LTP. (*Source*: Davies et al., 1989.)

observed during PTP but not during LTP in area CA1, providing evidence against increased release as an expression mechanism for LTP (Diamond et al., 1998; Luscher et al., 1998) (Fig. 10–10D). An analogous result was obtained in area CA3. LTP at mossy fiber synapses, but not at associational-commissural synapses, was associated with a sustained increase in glial uptake current (Kamamura et al., 2004). This observation is consistent with other evidence that LTP at mossy fibers is maintained by presynaptic mechanisms (see Section 10.5) and suggests that LTP at associational-commissural synapses lacks a strong presynaptic component.

Evidence for Presynaptic and Postsynaptic Mechanisms in LTP

Disagreements among laboratories notwithstanding, these three approaches have generally been seen as providing evidence against presynaptic changes and hence as strengthening the case for a purely postsynaptic change. There is, nevertheless, as we discuss below, a corpus of data that provides evidence for both presynaptic and postsynaptic changes. Although there is a sufficient body of data to make a convincing case for presynaptic changes, relatively little insight has yet been gained into molecular mechanisms that support an increase in transmitter release. For the postsynaptic side, there are also direct experiments demonstrating changes in response to applied transmitter following induction of LTP. In addition, there is now a large and compelling set of data that gives detailed insights into how postsynaptic changes are brought about by posttranslational modifications of existing receptors and trafficking of receptors between the cytoplasm and extrasynaptic and synaptic membranes. A cautionary note should be entered here; almost all the work that has characterized the molecular substrate of postsynaptically mediated LTP and LTD has been carried out in in vitro preparations during the first hour or so of early LTP or LTD. The mechanisms that support the enduring changes seen in late LTP or LTD are more likely to be structural in nature, and such changes almost certainly involve both sides of the synapse.

10.4.5 E-LTP: Presynaptic Mechanisms of Expression

The induction of LTP in the dentate gyrus in vivo is associated with a persistent increase in the efflux of L-glutamate (Dolphin et al., 1982) (Fig. 10–11A). The increase is activity- and NMDA receptor-dependent and has been detected using both a push-pull perfusion technique (Errington et al., 1987, but see Aniksztejn et al., 1989) and a glutamate-sensitive electrode (Errington et al., 2003). There are several ways, not mutually exclusive, in which LTP could be expressed presynaptically. There could be an increase in the number of release sites, either within a presynaptic terminal or as a result of the formation of new terminals. Alternatively, there could be an increase in the number of vesicles released per impulse. Another possibility is an alteration in the amount of L-

glutamate stored in or released from each vesicle. Finally, there could be an increase in the probability that an action potential in an afferent fiber leads to transmitter release, either because of a more efficient conduction of the impulse to the terminal or because of a higher probability of release (Pr) in response to the invading action potential. The studies that have measured the gross amount of L-glutamate released cannot distinguish between these possibilities or other alterations that affect the extracellular concentration of L-glutamate. In this context, however, there is little evidence that the uptake or diffusion of L-glutamate is affected during LTP.

Several lines of evidence are consistent with an increase in the probablility of transmitter release. Using minimal stimulation to activate a putative single release site, Stevens and Wang (1994) showed that LTP in area CA1 was associated with a decrease in failure rate without change in potency (the mean amplitude of responses excluding failures) (Fig. 10–11B). Bolshakov and Siegelbaum (1995) also reported an increase in Pr in the same region in neonatal rats. These findings are subject to the usual caveats regarding interpretation of quantal observations (see Box 10–1), although it should be emphasized that these were not silent synapses.

Consistent with the idea of an increase in Pr, a few studies have detected a decrease in paired-pulse facilitation (PPF) during LTP (Schulz et al., 1994; Kleschevnikov et al., 1997). For example, in slices from P6 rats there is a large decrease in PPF that fully accounts for the LTP in most, but not all, neurons (Palmer et al., 2004) (see Fig. 10-21D). This alteration is not due to changes in fiber failures, suggesting that an increase in Pr is the most likely explanation. However, the effect was tightly regulated developmentally and was absent by P12. Moreover, many studies have not observed changes in PPF.

Direct evidence for a presynaptic mechanism in cultured hippocampal neurons was obtained by measuring exocytotic-endocytotic cycling with antibodies against the synaptic vesicle protein synaptotagmin (Malgaroli et al., 1995) (Fig. 10–11C). A novel mechanism proposed by Tsien and colleagues involves an LTP-dependent modification of the fusion pore such that more L-glutamate is released from a fused vesicle (Choi et al., 2000). Under basal conditions the amount of L-glutamate released may be so small as not to elicit a detectable AMPAR-mediated postsynaptic response. Glutamate concentration may, however, be high enough to activate NMDARs, thus providing a potential presynaptic explanation for silent synapses. LTP then modifies the release machinery to enable a greater amount of L-glutamate discharge from each fused vesicle. Another direct way of estimating the probability of glutamate release is to measure the rate of destaining of synaptic vesicles loaded with the steryl dye FM1-43. Activity-dependent destaining was more rapid following induction of LTP, an effect that was blocked by NMDA receptor antagonists (Fig. 10–11D). An intriguing example of presynaptic unsilencing has been provided by Ma et al. (1999), who showed that in hippocampal cultures treated with a cAMP analogue (a treatment that induces a late, protein synthesis-dependent form of LTP), there was a dramatic increase in the number of active boutons taking up the dye FM1-43 (Fig. 10–11E).

Long-term potentiation is associated with an increase in phosphorylation of the presynaptic protein GAP-43 (Routtenberg and Lovinger, 1985; Gianotti et al., 1992). Other studies examined glutamate-induced LTP in cultured hippocampal neurons and found an increase in presynaptic boutons associated with clusters of the presynaptic proteins synaptophysin (Antonova et al., 2001) and α-synuclein (Liu et al., 2004b).

Changes in Pr at single synapses following induction of LTP in pyramidal cells of areas CA1 and CA3 has been assessed using Ca^{2+} indicators to monitor synaptic events at single visualised spines in organotypic hippocampal cultures (Emptage et al., 2003; Fig. 10.11F). Emptage et al. argued that the probability of evoking a Ca^{2+} transient in the visualised spine, PCa, provides an accurate measure of the probability of transmitter release, Pr, at that synapse, since manipulations that reflect an increase in Pr, such as paired pulse facilitation, also result in an increase in PCa, whereas manipulations that decrease Pr, such as bath application of adenosine, lead to a decrease in PCa. In the majority of spines examined, induction of LTP by high-frequency stimulation was accompanied by an increase in PCa at the imaged spine, whereas in experiments in which LTP was blocked by D-AP5, or in which the threshold for LTP was not reached, no change in PCa was seen. The Ca^{2+} signal is NMDA receptor-dependent, but the extent to which the evoked Ca^{2+} transient in spines reflects Ca^{2+} entering through the NMDA receptor varies with cell type and preparation (Yuste and Denk, 1995; Kovalchuk et al., 2000; Sabatini et al., 2002). Ca^{2+} entering via the NMDA receptor following a single stimulus could not be resolved by Emptage et al. (2003), but the trigger signal was greatly amplified, and the event thus made visible, by calcium-induced calcium release from internal stores (Emptage et al., 1999). The indirect nature of the Ca^{2+} transient raises the possibility that the observed increase in PCa following LTP may reflect an increase in the coupling between the initial trigger Ca^{2+} and store release, rather than an increase in Pr. Failures, according to this account, would include not only failures of release but also failures of postsynaptic coupling, so that pCa gives an underestimate of Pr. In this view, the reason that pCa is increased in LTP is that enhanced AMPAR function leads to an increase in the EPSP at the spine, a consequent increase in trigger Ca^{2+} entering through the NMDA receptor, and hence to a reduction in the number of failures due to failed coupling. This interpretation is rendered unlikely by the observation that bath application of a low dose of the AMPAR antagonist CNQX, which greatly reduces the amplitude of the AMPAR-mediated EPSP recorded at the soma, has little if any effect on PCa (Emptage et al., 2003). Nevertheless, a more direct method of measuring Pr would be desirable. One promising approach is to transfect neurons with a glutamate-binding protein tagged with a pair of fluorophores that yield a fluorescence resonance energy transfer (FRET) signal when L-glutamate is released from the presynaptic terminal (Okumoto et al., 2005).

10.4.6 E-LTP: Postsynaptic Mechanisms of Expression

There is also direct evidence for postsynaptic alterations. Initial experiments compared the sensitivity of neurons, before and after the induction of LTP, to ligands that act on AMPA receptors. LTP was invariably associated with an NMDA receptor-dependent increase in AMPA receptor sensitivity (Davies et al., 1989) (Fig. 10–10E). The effect was not immediate but occurred after a short delay (a few minutes or tens of minutes depending on the precise experimental protocol used). Subsequent work has also detected an increase in sensitivity to exogenously applied AMPA receptor ligands (Montgomery et al., 2001). A more refined approach is to deliver L-glutamate locally by photolytic release of glutamate from a caged precursor. Under these conditions, a rapid NMDAR-dependent increase in sensitivity has been observed (Matsuzaki et al., 2004; Bagal et al., 2005).

Broadly speaking, there are three categories of postsynaptic mechanisms by which LTP can be expressed. The first is modification of the properties of the receptors already present at the synapse. The second is an increase in the number of receptors available at the synapse to respond to the synaptic release of L-glutamate. The third involves changes downstream of glutamate receptors, such as alterations in voltage-gated or leak channels to affect the spread of depolarization (e.g., Fan et al., 2005). Although there is evidence for alterations in voltage-gated ion channels, most emphasis has been on the glutamate receptors themselves. As discussed above, NMDA receptor-dependent LTP is expressed as changes in both AMPA receptor- and NMDA receptor-mediated synaptic transmission. Because synaptic responses evoked at resting membrane potentials by low-frequency stimulation are mediated predominantly by the activation of AMPA receptors (Herron et al. 1986), it is these receptors that have been at the center of attention.

Modification of Existing Receptors Contributes to LTP

The amount of current that passes through an AMPA receptor is determined by the probability of opening (Po) on binding L-glutamate, the mean open time, and the single-channel conductance (γ). Alterations in mean open time of AMPARs would be reflected as a change in the kinetics of EPSCs. Despite claims to the contrary (Kolta et al, 1998), it is usually accepted that the decay of AMPAR-mediated EPSCs is not changed by LTP. This is most clearly seen when dendritic recording is used to maximize the signal-to-noise of minimal EPSCs and to reduce the dendritic filtering that is unavoidable with somatic recording (Benke et al., 1998). Also, treatment with cyclothiazide, which inhibits both deactivation and desensitization to cause pronounced slowing of the EPSC, does not affect the expression of LTP (Rammes et al., 1999).

Electrophysiological experiments cannot easily distinguish between insertion of AMPA receptors, and changes in Po or γ. However, in a few cases γ has been estimated by nonstation-

A

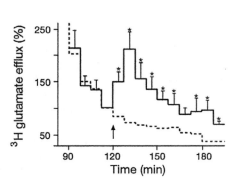

B

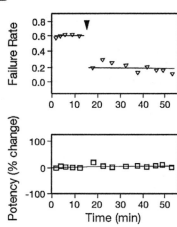

C

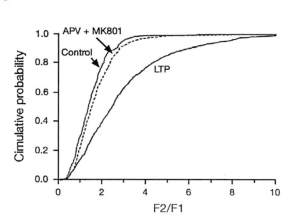

D

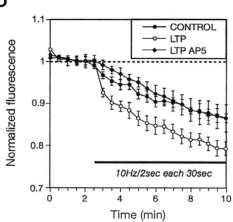

E

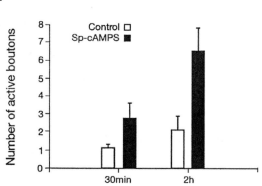

F

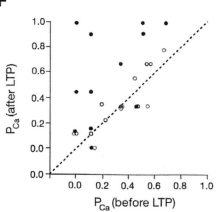

ary fluctuation analysis. At CA1 synapses of 2-week-old rats it was found that in most neurons γ increased sufficiently to account for LTP (Benke et al. 1998) (Fig. 10–12A). In other neurons γ did not change, suggesting that any postsynaptic change was due to an increase in N, the number of receptors, or Po. The simplest explanation for the increase in γ is a modification of receptors already present at the synapse, but it could theoretically be due to the exchange of lower for higher γ receptors at the synapse. The estimate of γ derived from nonstationary fluctuation analysis is the weighted mean of all subconductance states (Cull-Candy and Usowicz 1987; Jahr and Stevens, 1987). Because AMPA receptors can adopt multiple conductance states, it was suggested that LTP was due to an alteration in the relative time spent in these various states (Benke et al., 1998). Consistent with this idea, CaMKII-mediated phosphorylation of ser831 on GluR1 not only occurs during LTP (Barria et al., 1997a,b) but leads to an increase in precisely this parameter in HEK293 cells expressing GluR1 (Derkach et al., 1999). Furthermore, synaptic potentiation induced by postsynaptic application of a constitutive form of CaMKII is associated with an increase in γ (Poncer et al., 2002). Thus a simple scheme for the induction and expression of LTP is that Ca^{2+} entering via NMDA receptors triggers

CaMKII-dependent phosphorylation of GluR1 to increase the single-channel conductance of existing AMPA receptors. However, although this mechanism may occur, it cannot be the whole story, as CaMKII inhibitors applied alone fail to inhibit LTP at this stage of development (Wikström et al., 2003; Yasuda et al., 2003).

Insertion of AMPA Receptors Contributes to LTP

A popular hypothesis for the expression of LTP is an increase in the number of AMPA receptors available to respond to synaptically released L-glutamate. These receptors could be inserted from an intracellular compartment and/or diffuse laterally from extrasynaptic regions. In the simplest scenario, the new synaptic receptors would have conductance properties identical to those of the existing ones. Alternatively, the new receptors could have a different subunit composition, thereby conferring different conductance properties (i.e., single-channel conductance, rectification, Ca^{2+} permeability) to the potentiated synapses. Indeed, early in development (around the first week of life) LTP was observed in some neurons that was associated with a decrease in γ (Palmer et al., 2004), the simplest explanation of which is the insertion of

Figure 10–11. Evidence that LTP involves presynaptic changes. *A.* LTP in the dentate gyrus of the anesthetized rat is associated with an increase in the efflux of ^3H glutamate. At the beginning of the experiment a bolus of ^3H-glutamine was injected into the dentate gyrus. The dentate gyrus was perfused using a push-pull cannula; and perfusates were collected for the measurement of ^3H-glutamate, newly synthesized from ^3H-glutamine. In control animals, the concentration of ^3H-glutamate declined exponentially (dotted line). Field responses were recorded at the same time (not shown). In animals in which LTP was induced by high-frequency stimulation (arrow), the concentration of ^3H-glutamate was increased relative to control values for the following hour (solid line). Abscissa, time since injection of ^3H-glutamine; ordinate, ^3H-glutamate concentration normalized to its value in the collection interval immediately preceding the tetanus. (*Source:* Dolphin et al., 1982.) *B.* LTP at presumptive single synapses in area CA1 is associated with a decrease in failure rate (upper panel), with no change in the potency of the response (i.e., the amplitude of the evoked synaptic current for trials where a release event occurred) (lower panel). Responses were evoked by minimal stimulation to Schaffer-commissural axons in the acute hippocampal slice. (*Source:* Stevens and Wang, 1994.) *C.* Increase in synaptic activity visualized at single synapses in cultured hippocampal neurons following glutamate-induced LTP. Goat or rabbit antibodies recognizing the intraluminal domain of the vesicular protein synaptotagmin were used to measure vesicular cycling. Cultures were incubated with one of the antibodies for an hour. LTP was then induced by brief application of glutamate, and the second antibody then applied for a second hour. The degree of internalization of each antibody was measured using fluorescence-labeled anti-goat and anti-rabbit antibodies. The ratio of fluorescence during the second hour relative to the first (F2/F1) was measured in several hundred individual synapses. The shift to the right in the cumula-

tive distribution curve in potentiated cultures compared to control cultures or cultures in which LTP was blocked by NMDA receptor antagonists indicates a significant increase in vesicular cycling after induction of LTP. (*Source:* Malgaroli et al., 1995.) *D.* Visualization of increased transmitter release after LTP using the dye FM1-43. The rapidly recycling pool of vesicles in Schaffer-commissural terminals was loaded in vitro by exposing slices to FM1-43 in hypertonic ACSF to stimulate transmitter release. Activity-induced destaining was measured 30 minutes after reperfusion with ACSF by stimulating with 10 Hz, 2-second trains at 30-second intervals. The rate of destaining was accelerated in potentiated tissue (open circles), relative to tissue treated with AP5 to block LTP (filled diamonds) or to control tissue (filled circles). (*Source:* Stanton et al., 2005 with addition of control data courtesy of the authors.) *E.* A membrane-permeable analogue of cAMP induces an increase in the number of boutons taking up FM1-43 in CA3-CA1 neuronal cultures. The bars show the ratio of the number of stained boutons before and 30 minutes or 2 hours after exposure to the control solution (open bars) or solution containing Sp-cAMP. Exposure to cAMP itself can induce slow-onset late LTP (see Section 10.4.3). Both cAMP-induced LTP and the increase in the number of active boutons is protein synthesis-dependent. (*Source:* Ma et al., 1999.) *F.* Tetanus-induced LTP in organotypic hippocampal cultures is associated with an increase in the probability of obtaining a synaptically generated Ca^{2+} transient (p_{Ca}) in single visualized spines on pyramidal neurons. The graph plots p_{Ca} before and 30 minutes after the induction of LTP for a group of individual spines (filled circles). In other experiments (open circles), LTP was not induced either because no tetanus was given or induction was blocked by AP5. There was a significant increase in p_{Ca} in the group of tetanized spines from cells in which LTP was induced relative to control spines. (*Source:* Emptage et al., 2003.)

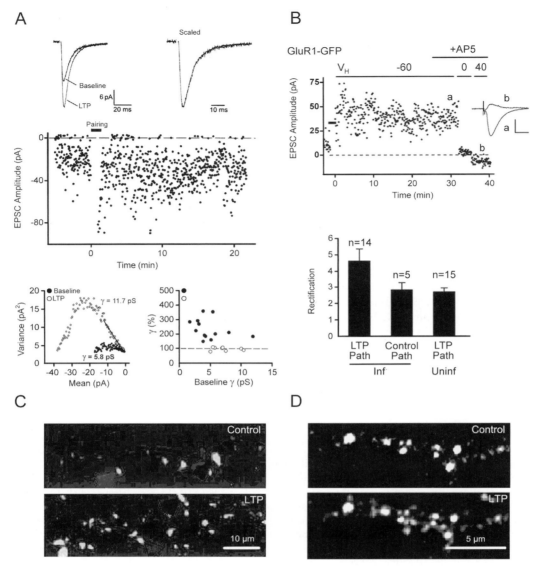

Figure 10–12. Postsynaptic mechanisms involved in the expression of LTP. *A.* LTP is associated with an increase in single-channel conductance (γ) of synaptic AMPA receptors at CA1 synapses in vitro. The traces are the mean amplitudes before and following induction of LTP superimposed (left) and expanded and peak-scaled (right). Note the lack of change in the shape of the potentiated EPSC. The graph plots the amplitude of EPSCs versus time before and following pairing induced LTP. The graph below (left) plots the variance of the decay phase of the EPSC versus the amplitude of each point on the EPSC decay. The initial slope of the plot provides an estimate of γ, which is this neuron approximately doubled following LTP. The graph (right) plots the change in γ associated with LTP against the baseline value of γ. Note that in most neurons γ increased (and this was sufficient to account for LTP), but in some neurons there was no change in γ. The latter neurons tended to have a higher baseline γ. (*Source*: Benke et al., 1998.) *B.* LTP involves the insertion of AMPA receptors at CA1 synapses in vitro, as determined using recombinant receptors with distinct electrophysiological properties. The graph plots EPSC amplitude versus time, and LTP was induced at t = 0. The rectification of the AMPA receptor-mediated EPSC was estimated by comparing its amplitude at positive and negative membrane potentials following blockade of NMDA receptors. LTP caused an increase in rectification in GluR1-transfected cells (Inf), indicating insertion of new GluR1 homomeric receptors. (*Source*: Hayashi

et al., 2000.) *C.* LTP in cultured neurons is associated with the insertion of native AMPA receptors, as assessed using a GluR1-specific antibody. AMPA receptors in cultured hippocampal neurons were labeled with a GluR1-specific antibody, and a nonfluorescent secondary antibody was then bound to them. LTP was induced by perfusion with glycine. The cultures were then challenged with GluR1 antibody, which bound to the newly inserted GluR1 receptors and were detected using a fluorescent secondary antibody. The panels show a representative portion of a dendrite from a control neuron (upper) and a neuron following glycine-induced LTP (lower). (*Source*: Lu et al., 2001.) *D.* LTP in cultured neurons is associated with the insertion of native AMPA receptors, as assessed using a pan-AMPA antibody. AMPA receptors in cultured hippocampal neurons were labeled with a GluR1-4-specific antibody, and their distribution visualized using a fluorescent secondary antibody. LTP was then induced by transient depolarization (3 × 1-second pulses of 50 mM K[+]). The cultures were then challenged with pan-AMPA antibody raised in a different species. This bound to newly inserted AMPA receptors, which were detected using a fluorescent secondary antibody directed against the second species. The panels show a representative portion of dendrite from a neuron before (upper) and following (lower) induction of LTP. Note the appearance of new clusters of AMPA receptors at sites that had previously lacked any detectable AMPA receptors. (*Source*: Pickard et al., 2001.)

new receptors with a lower γ than the existing population of receptors.

To address AMPA receptor movement in relation to LTP more directly, two complementary approaches have been used, each with its own relative advantages and disadvantages. In one approach, recombinant AMPA receptor subunits are constructed containing a reporter, such as green fluorescent protein (GFP). LTP in organotypic slice cultures was found to be associated with delivery of GFP-GluR1 to dendritic spines (Shi et al., 1999). However, because imaging could not determine whether these constructs were inserted into the plasma membrane, mutated receptors were used that had a distinct electrophysiological signature (Hayashi et al., 2000). The synaptic delivery of these receptors was then determined by alterations in the rectification properties of the synaptic currents (Fig. 10–12B). Based on these studies it is clear that recombinant AMPA receptors can be rapidly inserted into synapses during LTP in organotypic slices. Whether the recombinant receptors are inserted selectively into potentiated synapses and, if so, whether they fully account for the potentiated response remains to be established.

In the second method, antibodies that recognize extracellular epitopes of AMPA receptor subunits are used, in conjunction with protocols that induce NMDAR-dependent LTP in dissociated cultured hippocampal neurons. The alteration in native AMPA receptor distribution is determined using fluorescently conjugated secondary antibodies. Using this approach, insertion of native AMPA receptors during NMDAR-dependent LTP has been described (Lu et al., 2001; Pickard et al., 2001). These studies identified the insertion of GluR1-containing AMPA receptors into synapses that previously lacked GluR1 (Lu et al., 2001; Fig. 10–12C) via a PI3K-dependent process (Man et al., 2003). They also demonstrated insertion of AMPA receptors into anatomically "silent" synapses (synapses where AMPA receptors could not be detected on the cell surface) (Pickard et al., 2001; Fig. 10–12D). The use of AMPA receptor antibodies has also enabled the lateral mobility of AMPA receptors to be studied in the plasma membrane. Single-molecule fluorescence microscopy has revealed that there are both mobile and immobile receptors contained within spines and extrasynaptically (Tardin et al., 2003). Stimulation with L-glutamate increases synaptic AMPA receptor diffusion rates, raising the possibility that LTP involves the mobilization of extrasynaptic AMPA receptors and their targeting to the postsynaptic density. Consistent with this idea, there is evidence that following exocytosis AMPA receptors are diffusively distributed along dendrites before accumulating at synaptic sites (Passafaro et al., 2001).

Molecules that bind to AMPARs give clues to the molecular mechanisms involved in LTP. Understanding the molecular mechanisms of AMPA receptor synaptic trafficking during LTP has been greatly aided by the identification of proteins that bind directly to, and regulate the synaptic function of, AMPA receptors. Different proteins interact with the GluR1 and GluR2 subunits, and seem to play distinct roles in LTP

and LTD (see sections 10.3.7 and 10.7.3). From this has arisen the concept of the subunit-dependence of synaptic plasticity. In broad terms, the GluR1 subunit seems to play a major role in LTP whilst the GluR2 subunit is the more important in LTD. However, as we shall see, this is to simplify a complex situation.

GluR2 interactors: Evidence for rapid recycling and regulation of subunit composition of AMPARs at synapses. An initially surprising observation was that *N*-ethylmaleimide-sensitive fusion protein (NSF), an ATPase involved in membrane fusion events, binds directly to the GluR2 subunit (Nishimune et al., 1998; Osten et al., 1998; Song et al., 1998). Blockade of the GluR2-NSF interaction resulted in a rapid decrease in electrically evoked AMPAR-mediated synaptic transmission, suggesting that AMPA receptors can rapidly recycle at the synapse (Nishimune et al., 1998). Blockade of this interaction also led to internalisation of AMPARs, suggesting that NSF regulates the membrane insertion or stabilisation of synaptic AMPARs (Noel et al,, 1999, Luscher et al., 1999). These observations raised the possibility that modification of recyling rates could underlie LTP. Indeed, there is some evidence for a role of NSF and soluble NSF attachment proteins (SNAPs) in AMPA receptor insertion during LTP (Lledo et al., 1998).

A second region of the C-terminal tail of GluR2 is the site of interaction of the PDZ-containing proteins GRIP (glutamate receptor interacting protein), ABP (AMPA receptor binding protein), and PICK1 (protein interacting with C-kinase 1). ABP and GRIP contain multiple PDZ domains and probably serve to anchor AMPA receptors at both synaptic (Osten et al., 2000) and intracellular (Daw et al., 2000) locations. Some isoforms of ABP/GRIP are palmitoylated, which targets them to the synaptic membrane (Yamazaki et al., 2001; DeSouza et al., 2002). These molecules presumably also localize other proteins involved in the LTP process, close to AMPA receptors. For example, GRIP binds to an associated protein, GRASP-1, which is a neuronal RasGEF and so may link AMPA receptors to Ras signaling (Ye et al., 2000).

PICK1 can also bind PKCα, suggesting that one of its functions is to target PKC to phosphorylate AMPA receptors. Indeed, there is evidence that PICK1 may phosphorylate GluR2 on ser880 to inhibit the binding of AMPA receptors to ABP/GRIP (Matsuda et al., 1999), and this mechanism may be involved in the mobilization of AMPA receptors from their ABP/GRIP tethers. In the context of LTP, it has been proposed that PICK1-PKC phosphorylation of ser880 on GluR2 mobilizes AMPA receptors from intracellular sites during de-depression (i.e., reversal of LTD by an LTP induction protocol) (Daw et al., 2002). PICK1 is a particularly interesting molecule since it also regulates the GluR2 content of AMPA receptors at synapses (Terashima et al., 2004), raising the possibility that it may play a role in LTP by altering the conductance properties of synaptic AMPA receptors. Indeed, it has been found that LTP at CA1 synapses in two-week-old animals involves the rapid insertion of GluR2-lacking AMPARs followed by their replacement with GluR2-containing AMPARs, over a period of 20 minutes or so (Plant et al., 2006). The transient insertion of calcium permeable AMPARs may provide a signal, or tag, to mark recently potentiated synapses. Given that PICK1 is able to regulate the GluR2-content of AMPARs, and is the only molecule known to do this, it is a prime candidate for mediating this effect.

GluR1 interactors: A key role in LTP? There is evidence that GluR1 receptors are particularly important for synaptic delivery during LTP (Hayashi et al., 2000). Malinow and his colleagues have proposed that GluR1/GluR2 heteromers are inserted into the membrane during LTP, whilst GluR2/GluR3 heteromers are important for constitutive recycling of AMPA receptors at synapses (Shi et al., 2001). However, the mechanisms involved are unclear. Both spine delivery of GluR1 and LTP in organotypic slices requires activation of CaMKII, but deletion of ser831, the CaMKII phosphorylation site on the C-terminal tail of GluR1, did not prevent either of these effects (Hayashi et al., 2000). However, a point mutation on the PDZ domain at the extreme C-terminus of GluR1 (T887A) did prevent spine delivery and LTP suggesting that CaMKII may phosphorylate a protein that binds to this site. One such candidate is the membrane associated guanylate kinase (MAGUK) SAP97, which binds to GluR1 via its PDZ domain and has been implicated in trafficking to the synapse (Leonard et al., 1998). SAP97 enhances AMPAR-mediated synaptic transmission in cultured neurons, an effect mediated by a SAP97 splice variant containing a binding site for a GluR1 binding protein, 4.1, that has been implicated in linking AMPA receptors to the cytoskeleton (Rumbaugh et al., 2003). Overexpression of SAP97 leads to an enhancement of AMPAR-mediated transmission in hippocampal organotypic cultures that partially occludes with LTP (Nakagawa et al., 2004); the effect depends on the L27 domain of SAP97, which is involved in forming multimeric assemblies of SAP97, either with itself or other proteins containing a similar domain. Another pertinent finding is that CaMKII is able to phosphorylate SAP97 and this targets SAP97 to synapses (Mauceri et al., 2004), an effect that may explain the actions of CaMKII in driving AMPARs into synapses and into the PSD. Such a process may involve the motor protein myosin VI, since this forms a complex with both GluR1 and SAP97 (Wu et al., 2002). However, deletion of the entire PDZ domain of GluR1 does not prevent the induction of LTP in transgenic mice (Kim et al., 2005a). Further work is therefore required to establish the role of the PDZ domain of GluR1 in LTP.

There is also evidence for a role of PKA in driving GluR1-containing AMPARs into synapses (Esteban et al., 2003). Mutagenesis of ser845 has shown that this PKA site is required though its phosphorylation is not sufficient for LTP, suggesting that this is one stage in a multi-step process. One possibility is that PKA-dependent phosphorylation of ser845 is involved in the membrane targeting of AMPARs to extrasynaptic sites (Oh et al, 2006). PKC is also implicated in the trafficking of GluR1 and LTP, via phosphorylation of ser818 (Boehm et al, 2006).

Tarps add a new dimension. AMPA receptors also bind to stargazin, which in turn binds to PSD95 (Chen et al., 2000). Stargazin is one of a class of TARPs (transmembrane AMPAR regulatory proteins) that are involved in the recruitment of AMPA receptors from extrasynaptic to synaptic sites during LTP (Bredt and Nicoll, 2003). Consistent with this role of TARPS and PSD95, overexpression of PSD95 selectively enhances AMPAR-mediated synaptic transmission and occludes LTP (Stein et al., 2003; Ehrlich and Malinow, 2004). Indeed, the level of PSD95 at the synapse, which may be regulated by ubiquitination (Colledge et al., 2003) and palmitoylation (El Husseini et al., 2002), could directly determine the number of AMPA receptors at synapses. In addition, the interaction of AMPA receptors with TARPs is dynamically regulated both allosterically via ligand binding and through phosphorylation of TARPs (Chetkovich et al., 2002; Tomita et al., 2004).

In addition to regulating the number of AMPARs on the membrane surface, TARPs also increase the apparent affinity of AMPARs for glutamate. They slow the rate of both deactivation and desensitization and enhance γ, by increasing the prevalence of high conductance substates (Tomita et al, 2005). It has been estimated that TARPs increase the charge transfer of synaptic currents by approximately 30%.

The γ-8 TARP isoform is highly enriched in the hippocampus and the knockout of this protein leads to a profound loss of AMPAR subunits and a reduction in AMPAR-mediated EPSCs. LTP in knockout animals was greatly reduced, suggesting that TARPs are involved in synaptic plasticity (Rouach et al, 2005). TARPs can be phosphorylated by both CaMKII and PKC and dephosphorylated by PP1 and PP2B. Mutation of the target serines to alanine resulted in block of LTP, whilst conversely mutation of these residues to aspartic acid, to mimic phosphorylation, drove AMPARs to synapses and blocked LTD (Tomita et al, 2005). Thus, regulation of TARPs seems play a critical role in hippocampal synaptic plasticity.

In summary, a scheme is emerging whereby alterations in AMPA receptor number are controlled by protein–protein interactions and phosphorylation. The types of binding partners and kinases involved seem to vary depending on the AMPA receptor subunit and the stage of development. During LTP, AMPA receptors probably diffuse laterally in the synaptic membrane from extrasynaptic sites to the PSD to increase the number of receptors available to bind to synaptically released L-glutamate. This process may also be associated with insertion of AMPA receptors from an intracellular reservoir via exocytosis.

Locus of Expression of NMDAR-dependent LTP: a Site Inspection

What emerges from this summary of a large literature is that there is no clear consensus on the question of the locus of hippocampal LTP. Most camps were, and some remain today, highly entrenched in their view that LTP can be expressed only via their own favored mechanism. Objective analysis of all of the evidence, however, points to a multitude of expression mechanisms that may vary according to the component of LTP under investigation (i.e., STP, E-LTP, L-LTP), the developmental stage of the animal (see Fig. 10–21), and even the experimental approach used to tackle the problem. More recently, attention has focused on trying to understand the molecular mechanisms responsible for pre- and postsynaptic changes.

There are several indisputable facts. First, there is strong evidence in favor of both pre- and postsynaptic mechanisms, so NMDAR-dependent LTP can involve changes at both sides of the synapse. Second, there are pronounced differences in the signalling and expression mechanisms of LTP at different stages of development (see Section 10.9). Third, there is evidence that the various phases of LTP may involve different expression mechanisms. For example, the increase in sensitivity to AMPA receptor ligands correlates with E-LTP but not STP. Fourth, the type of LTP and its expression mechanism may depend on how it is induced; a tetanus causes repetitive activation of the presynaptic cell whereas pairing does not. We conclude therefore that LTP is expressed by alterations in either L-glutamate release and/or AMPA receptor function, the extent of each component depending on several factors, of which the list above is unlikely to be exhaustive.

10.4.7 Retrograde Signaling Is Required for Communication Between the Postsynaptic Site of Induction and the Presynaptic Terminal

We have seen that the trigger for the induction of LTP in the Schaffer-commissural and perforant pathways is the entry of calcium through activated NMDA channels located on the postsynaptic cell. Evidence from a variety of techniques and preparations points to a presynaptic component to the expression of LTP (Section 10.4.5). Early evidence for increased transmitter release in LTP led Bliss and Dolphin (1984) to postulate that a diffusible retrograde signal is released from the postsynaptic site of induction to interact with the presynaptic terminal and in some manner stimulate transmitter release. To date, there has been no unequivocal identification of a retrograde signaling molecule mediating LTP or LTD at hippocampal excitatory synapses. Most attention has focused on two candidates, the unsaturated membrane fatty acid arachidonic acid (AA) and the gas nitric oxide (NO) synthesized from L-arginine by nitric oxide synthase. Other potential retrograde messengers not considered further here that at one time had their champions include platelet-activating factor (Miller et al., 1992) and carbon monoxide (Stevens and Wang, 1993). Other potential diffusible messengers are brain-derived trophic factor (BDNF) (see Section 10.6.1) and an endogenous endocannabinoid, 2-AG, discussed above in the context of E-S potentiation (Section 10.3.12), which appears to act as a retrograde mediator of heterosynaptic LTD at inhibitory synapses in area CA1 (Chevaleyre and Castillo, 2003). Intersynaptic communication via membrane-spanning adhesion molecules is another way in which signals could be com-

municated in a retrograde direction (Murai and Pasquale, 2004). In this section we review the evidence for these various candidates. Before starting, we consider a set of criteria that a diffusible candidate messenger should satisfy. Note that a retrograde messenger is required only to generate the presynaptic component of LTP; this is designated LTP_{pre} in the following list.

- The cellular machinery for synthesis of the messenger exists in the postsynaptic cell.
- The synthesis of the messenger is upregulated by LTP-inducing stimuli.
- Postsynaptic injection of drugs that block synthesis inhibits LTP induction.
- The messenger is released into the extracellular compartment following induction of LTP_{pre}.
- Perfusion with extracellular scavengers small enough to access the synaptic cleft inhibit LTP_{pre}.
- A target molecule in the presynaptic terminal, positively linked to transmitter release, is activated by the messenger.
- Drugs that inhibit the link between messenger and exocytosis suppress LTP_{pre}.
- Exogenous application of the messenger induces LTP_{pre} or lowers the threshold for its induction.

No candidate retrograde messenger has yet been shown to satisfy all the criteria on this admittedly demanding list.

Arachidonic Acid

Arachidonic acid (AA) is produced by the action of a calcium-dependent enzyme, phospholipase A2, on membrane phospholipids. In 1987, Piomelli et al. (1987) suggested that AA, or one of its lipoxygenase metabolites, might serve as a synaptic retrograde messenger in LTP on the basis of experiments in *Aplysia* that identified lipoxygenase metabolites of arachidonic acid as a novel class of second messenger. A year later, Bockaert and his colleagues made the significant observation that activation of NMDA receptors in cultured striatal neurons led to the release of AA into the culture medium (Dumuis et al., 1988). The first evidence that the AA cascade played a role in LTP followed in the same year in a report that an inhibitor of AA production blocked chemically induced LTP in area CA1 and the dentate gyrus (Williams and Bliss, 1988). Subsequent studies, reviewed in Bliss et al. (1990), demonstrated that AA satisfies several of the criteria for a retrograde messenger: (1) LTP is accompanied by an increase in the concentration of AA in a postsynaptic membrane fraction and an increase in the extracellular concentration of AA; (2) inhibitors of phospholipase A_2 block induction of LTP; (3) the application of arachidonic acid to active hippocampal synapses causes delayed but persistent potentiation of evoked responses. Nevertheless, these results, although pointing to a role for arachidonic acid in LTP, do not compel the conclusion that it is a retrograde messenger; there are missing gaps in the evidence (Do extracellular scavengers of AA block induction? What is the presynaptic mode of action of AA that leads to an increase in transmitter release?). Moreover, some of the evidence can be explained by other known properties of AA, including inhibition of glutamate uptake into glia (Barbour et al., 1989) and its facilitatory action on NMDA currents (Miller et al., 1992). For these reasons, AA has fallen out of fashion as a candidate messenger for LTP. However, evidence that a 12-lipoxygenase metabolite of AA, 12(S)-HPETE, mediates the induction of mGluR-dependent LTD in area CA1 of young rats has been presented by Bolshakov and colleagues (Feinmark et al., 2003). It remains to be seen whether 12(S)-HPETE satisfies all the criteria for a retrograde messenger, including activity-dependent upregulation in the postsynaptic cell.

Nitric Oxide

Nitric oxide has had a more durable career as a candidate retrograde messenger than AA, though again the evidence remains incomplete. NO is a small membrane-permeable molecule with a short half-life—two desirable properties for a potential retrograde messenger. In neurons, NO is derived from L-arginine in a reaction catalyzed by nitric oxide synthase, of which two isoforms, nNOS and eNOS, are expressed in dendrites of hippocampal neurons. Like AA, NO is released from cultured neurons exposed to NMDA (Garthwaite et al., 1988). The target of NO is soluble guanylyl cyclase, which activates cyclic guanosine monophosphate (cGMP), one substrate for which is protein kinase G (PKG). Little is known of the effector molecules linked to this second messenger system in hippocampal synaptic terminals (see review by Hawkins et al., 1998).

Attempts to block induction of LTP with inhibitors of nitric oxide synthase have met with variable success. In vitro (Cummings et al., 1994) and in vivo (Bannerman et al., 1994) experiments failed to confirm initial reports that inhibition of NO synthase blocked the induction of LTP (Bohme et al., 1991; Schuman and Madison, 1991; Haley et al., 1992). In experiments in hippocampal slices, inhibition of LTP by NO synthesis inhibitors was seen at room temperatures but not at higher, more physiological temperatures (Williams et al., 1989). There is also disagreement about whether the application of NO, in combination with weak synaptic activation, produces LTP; two groups reported that it did (O'Dell et al., 1991b; Bon and Garthwaite, 2003), whereas a third found that it did not (Murphy et al., 1994). However, the latter finding, based on the release of NO by flash photolysis from an inactive caged precursor, has been shown to reflect an interaction between NO and ultraviolet light, leading to artifactual inhibition of NMDA receptor currents (Hopper et al., 2004). Knockout by homologous recombination of either of the two genes encoding the two isoforms of NO in hippocampal neurons fails to block LTP. However, LTP is compromised, though not abolished, in a double knockout of both genes (Son et al., 1996).

Evidence linking postsynaptically generated NO to enhanced transmitter release has emerged from a study on cultured hippocampal neurons, in which NO released by synaptic stimulation led to accelerated vesicle endocytosis via a cGMP-dependent pathway (Micheva et al., 2003). An interesting insight from this work is that NO acts only on stimulated terminals, consistent with the possibility that it could selectively affect neighboring active terminals, in addition to the terminal(s) whose activity was responsible for evoking its release from postsynaptic cell(s). The observed changes were blocked by NMDA receptor antagonists, establishing the likelihood that NO was produced postsynaptically and was thus acting as a genuine diffusible retrograde messenger. There is also evidence that NO affects vesicle recycling in LTD (see Section 10.7.4), suggesting that the direction of change is determined by the interaction of NO with presynaptic factors (see Section 10.4.9 for discussion of a potentially similar role played by somatically generated plasticity factors in their interaction with synaptic tags that are set either for LTD or LTP).

In a provocative study, Madison and Schuman (1994) made the intriguing observation that intracellular injection of NO synthase inhibitors blocked LTP when it was induced by pairing of single stimuli with depolarization of the impaled cell but not when it was induced by high-frequency trains. Their explanation of this dissociation is as follows. When pairing is used to induce LTP, the paired cell itself is the sole source of the putative retrograde messenger. If it is NO (or a messenger downstream of NO synthesis), intracellular application of an NO synthase inhibitor would be expected to block LTP, as observed. However, when LTP is induced by a tetanus, the surrounding cells are subject to LTP and themselves make and release the putative retrograde messenger. This could act on the single cell in which NO synthesis has been shut down. Thus, aided and abetted by its neighbors, terminals afferent to this cell can share in the potentiation induced by the high-frequency train. However, this ingenious interpretation is at odds with earlier, well established reports that maneuvers that block LTP at the level of the single cell, such as intracellular injections of calcium chelators (Lynch et al., 1983) or hyperpolarization (Kelso et al., 1986; Malinow and Miller, 1986), block both pairing-induced and tetanus-induced LTP in pyramidal cells. Little further work has been done on this aspect of hippocampal NO signaling, and there for the moment the story rests.

10.4.8 Membrane Spanning Molecules Contribute to Signaling Between Presynaptic and Postsynaptic Sides of the Synapse

The retrograde messengers we have considered so far are diffusible substances released from the postsynaptic spine to act in ways that are still somewhat mysterious to affect transmitter release. Another way in which communication can be effected between the two sides of the synapse is via the various classes of membrane-spanning molecules that have partners on the opposite side. In this section we summarize the little that is known about the way in which these interneuronal interactions are regulated by activity and the consequent effects on synaptic function.

Ephrins and Eph Receptors

Members of the large Eph family of receptor tyrosine kinases and their ephrin ligands play important roles in axon guidance, migration, and boundary determination in neural development (Wilkinson, 2001). Evidence is emerging that Eph receptors and ephrins are involved in the synaptic processes leading to LTP and LTD (reviewed by Murai and Pasquale, 2004) (see Section 10.5.3 for a discussion of their role in mossy fiber LTP). Eph receptors bind to ephrins via their extracellular domains and in doing so trigger reciprocal signaling pathways inititiated via the carboxy cytoplasmic regions of both Eph receptors and ephrins, a capability that for Eph receptors is referred to as forward signaling and for ephrins as reverse signaling. EphB2, a member of one of the two major subfamilies of Eph receptors, interacts with NMDA receptors and also, via a PDZ binding domain, with the AMPA receptor scaffolding protein GRIP. These interactions are presumably the route by which Eph receptors become responsive to synaptic activity, and they also provide a route for modulating synaptic function (Henderson et al., 2001). This possibility is reinforced by the demonstration by Grunwald et al. (2004) that ephrinB ligands are required for full expression of LTP and LTD at CA3-CA1 synapses. In both sets of studies, the functionality of the Eph receptor/ephrin partnership was unimpaired by removing the cytoplasmic tail of the Eph receptor, suggesting that reverse signaling by ephrins is the active route to LTP and LTD (Grunwald et al., 2004).

Another potentially important role for Eph receptors and their ephrin partners is in the regulation of spine morphology. EphA4 receptors are expressed on spines of cultured hippocampal pyramidal cells and can be targeted by ephrinA3, which is strongly expressed on the astroglia that envelop spines. This interaction leads to the retraction of spines (Murai et al., 2003). In this way Eph receptors and ephrin interactions could provide a mechanism for structural changes underlying synaptic plasticity.

Cell Adhesion Molecules

Cell adhesion molecules (CAMs) comprise a large class of diverse membrane-spanning molecules with extracellular ligand-binding domains that are important for cell-cell recognition during neural development and are potential candidates for both anterograde and retrograde transsynaptic signaling. CAMs expressed by neurons fall into four broad types: integrins, cadherins, immunoglobulin superfamily CAMs, and neuroligins and their ligands neurexins (reviewed by Benson et al., 2000 and Yamagata et al., 2003). CAMs, via their extracellular domains, can bind to the same members of the family (homophilic binding) or to other members (heterophilic binding). The C terminal region of many CAMs is associated directly or via accessory proteins to the actin cytoskeleton and can potentially initiate changes in the morphology of the spine or bouton in which they are embedded. In this section

we briefly review the evidence for the involvement of immunoglobulin superfamily members, cadherins, integrins, and neuroligins in LTP.

Immunoglobulin Superfamily Members. Mice treated with antibodies to the immunoglobulin superfamily member NCAM and mice with a targeted deletion of NCAM show reduced LTP in area CA1 and in the mossy fiber projection to area CA3 (Benson et al., 2000). PSA-NCAM, a form of NCAM carrying multiple copies of polysialic acid linked to the fifth immunoglobulin domain on the extracellular part of the molecule, has also been implicated in LTP. Enzymatic removal of PSA from NCAM inhibits LTP in area CA1 (Muller et al., 1996). Similarly, LTP is impaired in area CA1 in a knockout mouse lacking one of the two polysialyltransferases that link PSA to NCAM. However, in this mouse, LTP is normal in area CA3, suggesting that whereas PSA-NCAM is required for LTP in area CA1, NCAM itself is needed to support LTP in the mossy fiber projection (Cremer et al., 1998). The roles of two other members of the NCAM family, L1 and Thy-1, in hippocampal synaptic plasticity have also been examined. LTP in a Thy-1 knockout mouse was normal in area CA1 but impaired in the dentate gyrus in vivo; performance on the Morris watermaze was unaffected (Nosten-Bertrand et al., 1996; Errington et al., 1997). There is disagreement about whether L1 plays a role in LTP. In an in vitro study using functional antibodies against L1, Lüthi et al. (1994) saw reduced LTP in area CA1, but Bliss et al. (2000) found no effect on LTP in area CA1 in vitro or in the dentate gyrus in vivo in an L1 knockout mouse.

Cadherins. Cadherins are an extensive family of cell adhesion molecules with cytoplasmic signaling domains that are linked to the actin cytoskeleton through two accessory proteins: β.catenin, which binds to cadherin, and α-catenin, which binds to both β.catenin and actin. Cadherin dimers form strongly adhesive homophilic partnerships with similar cadherin dimers on the other side of the synapse. Interestingly, although both E- and N-cadherins are strongly expressed in the hippocampus, N-cadherins are found only at excitatory synapses (Huntley, 2002). The importance of cadherins in the induction of LTP is beginning to emerge from studies using inhibitors, targeted mutations, and confocal microscopy. Tetanus-induced LTP in area CA1 is reduced by peptide blockers of N-cadherin (Tang et al., 1998). Late, delayed-onset LTP, induced in hippocampal slices by bath application of a membrane-permeable cAMP analogue, is accompanied by a rise in synaptic puncta containing both N-cadherins and the presynaptic marker synaptophysin (Bozdagi et al., 2000). Conversely, cAMP-induced LTP is abolished by bath application of blocking antibodies against the dimerization and homophilic interaction domains of N-cadherins (Bozdagi et al., 2000).

The effect on spine morphology of blocking N-cadherin in cultured hippocampal neurons was investigated by Togashi et al. (2002), who found that over a period of 2 days or more spines became longer and more filopodia-like. The same effect was observed in mutant mice lacking α-catenin, suggesting that cadherin signaling through actin is required for spine shortening. There is some information on how synaptic activity modulates N-cadherin function. Strong synaptic activation can change the conformation of N-cadherin (Tanaka et al., 2000), and Murase et al. (2002) have made the significant observation that β.catenin is rapidly (within 30 minutes) translocated from dendrite to spine in an NMDAR-dependent manner following synaptic activity. Finally, tyrosine dephosphorylation of β.catenin promotes its movement into the spine, providing a potential point for regulation by synaptic activity via a calcium-dependent tyrosine phosphatase (Murase et al., 2002).

Integrins. Integrins are heterodimeric glycoproteins formed from α. and β.subunits; each comprises a single membrane-spanning domain linking the ligand-binding extracellular domain to a cytoplasmic tail that is connected to actin via the accessory proteins α-actinin, talin, and vinculin (Benson et al., 2000). There are multiple forms of each subunit, a number of which have been identified in hippocampal pyramidal neurons, including α3, α5, α8, and β8 (Chan et al., 2003), The primary extracellular ligands of integrins are matrix proteins, but integrins also participate in cell-cell adhesion through binding to cadherins and members of the immunoglobulin superfamily of cell adhesion molecules. Their role in the stabilization of LTP has been explored by Lynch, Gall, and colleagues (reviewed in Gall and Lynch, 2004). Broad-spectrum peptide inhibitors of integrins attenuate the magnitude and duration of LTP and can reverse LTP if given within a few minutes after induction (Staubli et al., 1998). In a survey of mice with heterozygous deletions of α3, α5, or α8 integrin (homozygous deletions are lethal), Chan et al. found that LTP was attenuated only in the α3 mutants. Complete suppression of LTP and a deficit in watermaze performance was only seen in mice heterozyous for all three integrins (Chan et al., 2003).

Neuroligins and Neurexins. Neuroligins and their ligands neurexins are brain-specific cell adhesion molecules, with multiple forms arising from differential splicing. Neurexins are localized presynaptically, and members of the β subgroup make heterophilic connections with postsynaptic neuroligins. The intracellular C-termini of neuroligins bind to the PDZ region of the postsynaptic protein PSD-95, and the C-termini of neurexins are linked to another PDZ-containing protein, CASK. As Benson et al. (2000) pointed out, these interactions make neuroligins and neurexins potentially well suited for intercellular signaling. Their involvement in LTP has yet to be explored.

Summary

It is evident from this brief survey of the large, diverse families of neural cell adhesion molecules that there is still much to learn about their role in synaptic plasticity. Disruption of

intercellular interactions has little effect on baseline transmission but, as we have seen, can impair the magnitude and duration of LTP. A major gap in our knowledge is how synaptic activity is signaled to and detected by CAMs. It seems likely that the major contribution of CAMs is as mediators of structural changes, where they can ensure that pre- and postsynaptic changes can be kept in register. However, the potential for two-way signaling, from cytoplasm to cell adhesion molecule and vice versa, remains a highly attractive mechanism for conveying information across the synapse that is only now beginning to be explored.

10.4.9 Late LTP: Persistent Potentiation Requires Gene Transcription and Protein Synthesis

Late LTP (L-LTP) is defined as the temporal component of LTP that is abolished by protein synthesis inhibitors or by transcriptional blockers. Because no stimulus protocol has been found that produces L-LTP without the preceding early LTP, the time course of L-LTP must be estimated by a subtraction process. This reveals slow-onset potentiation rising from baseline to reach a plateau after 1 to 2 hours. The slowly growing L-LTP induced by BDNF (Fig. 10–2D) or cAMP analogues has a similar time course.

In principle, persistent changes in synaptic efficacy could occur through self-perpetuating renewal of posttranslational changes (Crick, 1984; reviewed by Routtenberg and Rekart, 2005). Indeed, Kandel and colleagues found evidence for such a mechanism in the translational regulator CPEB (cytoplasmic polyadenylation element-binding protein), a protein with prion-like self-perpetuating properties that is involved in long-lasting facilitation in *Aplysia* (Si et al., 2003). However, the same year that Crick's proposal was published, the first evidence appeared that protein synthesis was indeed essential if LTP in the hippocampus was to persist for more than a few hours. Krug et al. (1984) infused the protein synthesis inhibitor anisomycin into the lateral ventricles of freely moving rats and found that the potentiated fEPSP in the dentate gyrus slowly declined to baseline over 3 to 5 hours. The baseline response was not affected in control experiments. This result appeared to establish an upper limit for the duration of posttranslational changes. A similar result was obtained in the anesthetized rat (Otani and Abraham, 1989) and in area CA1 in the hippocampal slice (Frey et al., 1988) (Fig. 10–2C). Transcriptional inhibitors such as actinomycin also block L-LTP in area CA1 in vitro (Nguyen et al., 1994) and in the dentate gyrus in vivo (Frey et al., 1996; but see Otani et al., 1989). Mossy fiber L-LTP, too, as discussed in Section 10.5, is dependent on protein synthesis and gene transcription (Huang et al., 1994). In addition, the slowly growing L-LTP elicited by cAMP analogues (Nguyen et al., 1994) or by BDNF (Kang and Schuman, 1996; Messaoudi et al., 2002) (see Section 10.6.1) is susceptible to translational and transcriptional inhibitors. Thus, all forms of L-LTP that have been identified in the hippocampus require protein synthesis. Persistent LTD induced by mGluR agonists or by paired-pulse low-frequency stimulation is also rapidly blocked by protein synthesis inhibitors (see Section 10.7.4).

The rapid effect of translational inhibitors suggests that the initial phase of L-LTP is dependent on protein synthesis from preexisting mRNA in the dendrites of potentiated synapses (see below). In fact, despite an earlier negative report (Frey et al., 1989), there is persuasive evidence that isolated dendrites can support L-LTP (Vickers et al., 2005). Moreover, local dendritic application of a protein synthesis inhibitor reduces L-LTP in intact slices (Bradshaw et al., 2003). Nevertheless, dendritic protein synthesis cannot be the whole story, given the impairment of L-LTP by transcriptional inhibitors. The effect of transcriptional inhibitors is delayed, beginning 1 to 2 hours after induction. The delay is consistent with a model in which a signal from stimulated synapses is transported to the nucleus, where it triggers transcription of new mRNA species. The products of transcription, whether mRNA transcripts themselves or the proteins they encode, are delivered to dendrites to stabilize LTP at potentiated synapses.

We consider in more detail below the evidence that the initial phase of L-LTP is supported by dendritic protein synthesis. We then discuss the role of transcription in generating the persistent late phase, which leads to a description of the two (somatopetal and somatofugal) signaling trade routes and the largely unidentified molecular cargoes that are exchanged between soma and dendrite. Finally, we consider the concept of synaptic tagging and the surprising answers this gives to the perplexing question of how a dendritic flow of "plasticity molecules" generated by transcription is restricted to potentiated synapses to preserve the input specificity of LTP. Comprehensive reviews of the ways in which translation and transcription may be regulated to achieve persistent L-LTP can be found in Kelleher et al. (2004a) and West et al. (2002).

Time Window for Blocking Induction of Late LTP by Protein Synthesis Inhibitors

An important and somewhat puzzling feature of the block of L-LTP by protein synthesis or transcriptional inhibitors, both in vitro and in vivo, is that the drugs are effective when given during or immediately after induction of LTP (Otani et al., 1989; Nguyen et al., 1994) but are ineffective once LTP has become established. The existence of this time window implies that the synthesis of the proteins necessary to support L-LTP occurs at the time of or soon after the tetanus and that thereafter new protein synthesis is not required, even though expression of L-LTP can take some hours to reach its maximum and is then maintained at that level. A similar profile is seen in behavioral experiments when protein synthesis inhibitors are given around the time of one-trial learning; short-term memory is unaffected by the inhibitors, and long-term memory is blocked (Squire and Barondes, 1972). As we shall see later when considering the synaptic tag experiments of Frey and Morris (1997), there are circumstances in which L-LTP can be induced in the presence of protein synthesis inhibitors. We also note here that the reconsolidation of

memories after retrieval may open up another window of protein synthesis dependence in the hippocampus (Alberini, 2005).

It is not known if there are proteins that are expressed only in the context of synaptic plasticity and in no other circumstance, but is important to distinguish between synthesis of proteins that are related to the changes in synaptic strength and synthesis of general housekeeping proteins that reflect and service overall changes in neural activity (see discussion in Sanes and Lichtman, 1999). These two possibilities cannot be distinguished on the basis of a general blockade of protein synthesis. However, the fact that translational and transcriptional inhibitors are effective only during a narrow temporal window around the time of induction, well before L-LTP is established, implies that proteins synthesized during that time are not predominantly housekeeping genes.

Does protein synthesis in presynaptic neurons contribute to L-LTP? In the transverse hipppocampal slice, axons projecting to granule cells are severed from their cell bodies in the entorhinal cortex. The fact that L-LTP can be induced in the dentate gyrus in vitro (Balschun et al., 1999) therefore demonstrates that presynaptic gene transcription is not a requirement for L-LTP in the perforant path. Presynaptic protein synthesis, however, cannot be excluded on this evidence alone, and an LTP-associated increase in a number of presynaptic proteins has been reported following the induction of LTP in perforant path-granule cell synapses (Kelly et al., 2000). Whether these changes are necessary for the full expression of L-LTP is not known.

Dendritic Protein Synthesis Plays a Role in the Initial Phase of Late LTP

Proteins required for L-LTP could be all be generated in the soma and transported to where they are required. However, there is increasing evidence that this is not what happens and that dendritic protein synthesis plays an important role in generating the initial phase of late LTP. Local protein synthesis has the conceptual merit of providing an immediate solution to the problem of input specificity at the metabolic cost of transporting a population of mRNAs to the far reaches of the dendritic tree. It would, on the face of it, make the cell's life a good deal easier if the machinery for late as well as early LTP were located at the synapse, and there are good reasons for supposing that protein synthesis does in fact occur in dendrites. It has long been known that ribosomes and other elements of the protein synthetic machinery are positioned subsynaptically at many hippocampal synapses (Steward, 1983; reviewed by Steward and Schuman, 2001), and ultrastructural studies have shown that polyribosomes redistribute from dendrites to the base of dendritic spines with enlarged postsynaptic densities following the induction of LTP (Ostroff et al., 2002). An estimated 400 mRNA species are found in hippocampal dendrites (Eberwine et al., 2001), including components of the translation machinery as well as mRNAs for several proteins known to play a role in the induction or expression of LTP, among them αCaMKII, PKMζ arc/arg3.1, BNDF and its receptor trkB, and AMPA receptor subunits GluR1 and GluR2 (Martin and Kosik, 2002; Martin, 2004). The demonstration that isolated dendrites of CA1 pyramidal cells can support BDNF-induced LTP and mGluR-dependent LTD provides direct evidence that dendritic protein synthesis is sufficient to support persistent synaptic plasticity (Kang and Schuman, 1996; Hüber et al., 2000); in both cases the effects are blocked by protein synthesis inhibitors. Tetanus-induced LTP lasting a number of hours also occurs in isolated dendrites, and its decay is hastened by protein synthesis inhibitors (Frey et al., 1989). These experiments demonstrate that translation of existing dendritic mRNA can support a component of L-LTP that extends well beyond the duration of E-LTP. Evidence that local protein synthesis is necessary for the full expression of L-LTP in intact cells has come from experiments in which local perfusion of the protein synthesis inhibitor emetine selectively depressed L-LTP in the perfused region without affecting its time course at distant synapses (Bradshaw et al., 2003). Overall, these observations strongly suggest that local protein synthesis plays an important part in the early stabilization of LTP or, to put it another way, in the passage from early to late LTP.

Transcription and Translation of New mRNAs: Dialogue Between Synapse and Nucleus

What is the evidence that the conversion from early to late LTP requires gene transcription and/or somatic protein synthesis? First, as we have seen, transcriptional blockers such as actinomycin block L-LTP in area CA1 in vitro (Nguyen et al., 1994; Frey et al., 1996; Kelleher et al., 2004b) and in the dentate gyrus in vivo (Frey et al., 1996; but see Otani et al., 1989). Second, upregulation of immediate early genes such as c-*fos*, *zif268*, and *arc/arg3.1* reveal a correlation between transcription and LTP induction (reviewed by Kuhl and Skehel (1998). The absence of L-LTP in the dentate gyrus of a mutant mouse with targeted inactivation of the immediate early gene and transcription factor zif268 confirms a causal role for gene transcription in the induction of L-LTP (Jones et al., 2001), as does the impairment of L-LTP when the same region is infused with antisense mRNA to *arc/arg3.1* (Guzowski et al., 2000). Finally, experiments on synaptic tagging, described below, make it clear that a global signal, presumed to originate from the soma, is made available to the whole cell following the induction of L-LTP. As we shall see, this signal can be intercepted and utilized for the purposes of stabilizing LTP at other synapses that may have been activated up to 1 to 2 hours earlier or later than the pathway whose strong activation led to the initiation of transcription. Local protein synthesis alone cannot account for the observation that plasticity can be modulated in this associative manner by a geographically distant pathway; there has to be a transcriptional or translational signal from the soma that either supplies the required stabilizing proteins or transcripts or stimulates local protein synthesis to do so. Thus, it is difficult to avoid the conclusion that protein synthesis at both the local and global levels is involved in the conversion of early to late LTP.

Signaling to Nucleus

A major route for activity-dependent protein synthesis proceeds via long-range activation of nuclear transcription factors, including members of the CREB family of proteins which bind to cAMP response elements (CREs) in the regulatory regions of target genes to initiate transcription. What is the signal, and how is it conveyed to the nucleus? We have seen that calcium influx through the NMDA receptor is the trigger for NMDAR-mediated LTP; and it is therefore no surprise that calcium, particularly when bound to calmodulin, is a key player in signaling to the nucleus (reviewed by Lonze and Ginty, 2002). There is disagreement, however, about how this is achieved. One possibility is that calcium is released from the endoplasmic reticulum as a traveling wave proceeding from dendrite to soma, where it binds to nuclear calmodulin to activate target kinases (Hardingham et al., 2001). A second possibility is that calcium/calmodulin translocates from synapse to nucleus (Deisseroth et al., 1998); and a third, discussed below, is that Ca^{2+} enters the nucleus via voltage-gated calcium channels in the somatic plasma membrane.

A principal target for nuclear calcium/calmodulin is CaMKIV, a member of the calcium/calmodulin-dependent kinase family whose location is predominantly nuclear (Lonze and Ginty, 2002). Activation of CaMKIV by phosphorylation at ser133 allows it to bind an accessory CRE-binding protein (CBP) and initiate transcription. Other Ca^{2+}-activated signaling pathways are also recruited, including the Ras/MAP kinase and PKA pathways (for reviews see Roberson et al., 1999; Lonze and Ginty, 2002; Sweatt, 2004).

The MAP kinase signaling cascade can be triggered by a wide variety of stimuli, including extracellular ligands binding to receptor tyrosine kinases and G protein-coupled receptors, and by synaptic activity leading to calcium entry through ionotropic glutamate receptors or voltage-gated calcium channels. We have seen in Section 10.4.3 that the MAP kinase cascade regulates both early LTP and late LTP via substrate proteins that control translation, probably at dendritic sites (reviewed by Sweatt, 2001b; Thomas and Huganir, 2004). Here, we are concerned with its role in establishing L-LTP by stimulating gene expression in the nucleus. Synaptic activity leads to the phosphorylation of ERK1, 2 in both dendrites and soma. As with the calmodulin signal, the mechanism by which the activated ERK signal is translocated to the nucleus is not known. Although phospho-ERK does not phosphorylate CREB, inhibition of MEK, the kinase that phosphorylates ERK, prevents phosphorylation of CREB on ser133. There must therefore be intermediate kinase(s) that are substrates for phospho-ERK and allow it control over CREB phosphorylation; these intermediates are thought to be members of the RSK or MSK families of nuclear kinases (Lonze and Ginty, 2002; Thomas and Huganir, 2004) (see below).

Another route from synapse to soma is via the activation of G protein-coupled receptors, such as D1/D5 dopamine receptors. Late LTP in area CA1 is blocked by dopamine antagonists (Frey et al., 1990) and facilitated by D1/D5 agonists, although the report by Huang and Kandel (1995) that stimulation of dopamine receptors can induce late potentiation in an activity-independent manner has been disputed by Mockett et al. (2004). Dopamine receptor activation leads to upregulation of cAMP and presumptive translocation of activated PKA to the soma, where it can directly phosphorylate CREB on ser133 (Lonze and Ginty, 2002).

Action Potential Signaling as a Form of Synapse-to-Nucleus Signaling

As Adams and Dudek (2005) have pointed out, there are two problems with the concept of synapse-to-soma signaling that are often overlooked. First, how does the signal generated by one or a few potentiated synapses (in the limit, a single synapse) located at any position on the dendritic tree reach a concentration in the nucleus that allows activation of transcription factors? Second, transcription of immediate early genes such as c-*fos* and *zif268* begins within a few minutes of LTP induction. How does the signal reach the soma so quickly? Adams and Dudek (2005) suggested that both problems can be circumvented if the signal is generated not at the synapse but by somatic action potentials. Because action potential(s) generally (though not always, see Section 10.3.6) occur during the induction of LTP, the nuclear signal could in principle be generated by Ca^{2+} entering through somatic voltage-gated channels. Such a mechanism would provide an economical solution to both the problems noted above. A number of observations are consistent with the hypothesis. Antidromically driven action potentials can induce expression of immediate early genes, and antidromic stimulation of CA1 axons converts E-LTP to L-LTP, suggesting that action potentials can induce expression of soma-to-synapse plasticity factors (Dudek and Fields, 2002). Moreover, it is well established that the synaptic activation of NMDA receptors during high-frequency stimulation can drive somatic action potentials and so provide a rapid NMDAR-dependent signal from synapse to soma (Herron et al, 1986). Furthermore, synaptic activation of NMDA receptors can lead to somatic Ca^{2+} entry via L-type voltage-gated Ca^{2+} channels (Alford et al, 1993). In addition, strong induction protocols that induce NMDAR-independent L-LTP in area CA1 also lead to a large somatic Ca^{2+} signal that is blocked by L-type Ca^{2+} channel inhibitors (Raymond and Redman, 2006). Note that the somatic Ca^{2+} hypothesis predicts an absolute requirement for postsynaptic action potentials to secure L-LTP by this route.

The Nuclear Transcription Factor CREB Is a Target for Several Kinases

CREB is activated by phosphorylation on ser133. Not all active kinases can directly phosphorylate CREB on this residue: PKA

can, MAPK cannot. Unexpectedly, however, it was found that MEK inhibitors completely block the increase in CREB phosphorylation caused by bath application of the cAMP activator forskolin, thus establishing that ERK1, 2 acts downstream of the PKA cascade (Roberson et al., 1999). The activation of PKA by cAMP leads to activation of the GTPases Rap-1 and B-raf and thence to phosphorylation of MEK. The kinase intermediaries linking MAPK to CREB in the L-LTP pathway in vivo are probably members of the RSK and/or MSK kinase families. A second arm of the MAP kinase cascade is activated by ligand binding to metabotropic glutamate receptors, activating PLC and leading to the release of diacyl glycerol and activation of PKC. PKC activates Ras/Raf-1, the first links in the three-kinase MAP cascade, leading to phosphorylation of MEK. BDNF, acting on its receptor TrkB, also uses the Ras/Raf-1 pathway, again converging on MEK, as does acetylcholine (ACh) acting on muscarinic receptors (Sweatt 2004). Thus, many of the extracellular stimuli (ACh, BDNF, glutamate) that are known to cause CREB phosphorylation on ser133 and thence gene expression, are funneled through the Ras/Raf-1 arm of the MAPK pathway (Sweatt, 2001a, b).

Our discussion of signaling pathways in L-LTP has so far avoided the question of how specific genes are targeted by different stimuli if the same signal cascades are engaged in each case. It is likely that different combinations of kinases are activated by different stimuli and that expression of specific target genes is achieved by combinatorial selection from the cell's portfolio of transcription factors. For example, transcription of the immediate early gene c-*fos* can be triggered by any one of several stimuli (growth factors, neuromodulators, neurotransmitters), all of which lead to phosphorylation of CREB on serine 133. Neurotransmitters, but not growth factors or neuromodulators, increase calcium levels, either directly through opening calcium permeable receptor channels (e.g., the NMDA receptor) or indirectly through depolarization-gated opening of L-type voltage-sensitive calcium channels. High Ca^{2+} levels can lead to phosphorylation of another transcription factor, calcium response factor (CRF), and to phosphorylation of CREB at ser141 and ser143; phosphorylation at the latter two serine residues reduces the ability of ser133 phospho-CREB to bind to CBP. The combination of these two transcription factors (CRF and CREB phosphorylated at ser141 and ser143 but unassociated with CBP) directs the stimulus-dependent transcription of BDNF (West et al., 2002). Similarly, activation of at least two transcription factors, CREB and Elk1, is required to drive expression of the immediate early gene *zif268* (Davis et al., 2000).

The LTP connection was taken a step further when CREB phosphorylation induced by tetanic stimulation was also shown to be blocked by MEK inhibitors, both in CA1 in vitro and in the dentate gyrus in vivo (Impey et al., 1998; Davis et al., 2000). In the latter case, upregulation of *zif268*, one of the target genes of CREB, was also suppressed. While CREB is rapidly phosphorylated in a Ca^{2+} dependent manner by stimuli that induce LTP, it is also the case that CREB is activated by patterns of synaptic activity that do not elicit potentiation

(Deisseroth et al., 1966). Thus, CREB phosphorylation may be required for the transcription of genes encoding effector proteins whose role is to sustain synaptic activity in general, rather than specifically to promote synaptic plasticity. Initial studies of genetically hypomorphic CREB mice supported the idea that CREB was important for LTP as well as for hippocampus-dependent memory (Bourtchuladze et al., 1994). Later work on CREB knockout mice failed to detect a robust effect on LTP, though there remained the possibility that this result could be explained by the upregulation of other members of the CREB family. However, Balschun et al. (2003) generated a mouse in which expression of all CREB isoforms was either absent or limited, and found no effect on L-LTP. The role of CREB in generating L-LTP cannot therefore be regarded as securely established.

What are the target genes for CREB? Some of them at least are transcription factors—the immediate early genes such as c-*fos* and *zif268* and others of unknown function such as *arc/arg3.1*. An upper limit on the number of genes that might be activated by CREB can be estimated from genes containing CRE sequences in their promoter regions (Lonze and Ginty, 2002). More than 80 have been identified, coding for: neurotransmitters and peptides ($n = 35$), growth factors and their receptors ($n = 7$), structure-related proteins ($n = 4$), proteins involved in cellular metabolism ($n = 16$), transcription factors ($n = 13$), signal transduction proteins ($n = 8$). The presence of transcription factors opens up the potential for a second wave of target genes.

Markers of LTP: Immediate Early Genes
zif268, c-fos, and *arc/arg3.1*

Long-term potentiation is associated with the rapid, transient expression of several transcription factors, including c-*fos*, *cJun*, *krox 20*, and *zif268*, of which c-*fos* and *zif268* have been the most intensively studied (Dragunow, 1996; Lanahan and Worley, 1998). These and other genes, such as *arc/arg 3.1* and *homer1a*, which encode for proteins that contribute to synaptic scaffolding complexes, are members of a group of genes known as immediate early genes (IEGs) whose transcription is upregulated by activity without the need for prior protein synthesis. Enhanced mRNA expression for both c-*fos* and *zif268* (a member of the krox family of transcription factors; synonyms are *krox24*, *egr1*, and *NGF1*) occurs within minutes of induction and peaks around 30 minutes after induction, returning to baseline levels (which in the dentate gyrus is very low for *zif268*, c-*fos*, and *arg/arc3.1*) within 2 to 4 hours. Expression of the corresponding proteins lags by 1 to 2 hours. Transient upregulation of IEGs is a marker for LTP in the dentate gyrus in the sense that whenever a stimulus is sufficiently strong to induce L-LTP immediate early gene expression is triggered. Moreover, maneuvers that block induction of LTP also block the enhanced expression of immediate early genes (Wisden et al., 1990; Dragunow, 1996). As we have seen, L-LTP is not expressed in the dentate gyrus of mice with a targeted

inactivation of *zif268*, indicating that *zif268* is required for L-LTP, though it is not necessary for E-LTP (Jones et al., 2001). However, enhanced expression of transcription factors such as *zif268* and c-*fos* can be induced by procedures that do not induce LTP, such as nonsynaptic excitation of neurons by antidromic stimulation. The mechanical disturbance involved in cutting a hippocampal slice can also induce long-lasting upregulation of IEG expression in the dentate gyrus (French et al., 2001). In these cases, upregulation of IEGs is not sufficient to induce LTP, possibly because synaptic tags have not been set. Note too that although *zif268* and other immediate early genes can be activated by seizure activity in all areas of the hippocampus they are not readily switched on by LTP-inducing stimulation in area CA1, in contrast to their robust upregulation in the dentate gyrus (French et al., 2001). On the other hand, there is an increase in the number of pyramidal neurons in area CA1 expressing *arc/arg3.1* mRNA following exposure to a novel environment (Guzowski et al., 1999). Until the reasons for these puzzling and intriguing discrepancies between the pyramidal and granule cell fields are resolved, the use of IEG expression as a marker for the induction of L-LTP is probably justified only in the dentate gyrus.

Beyond Immediate Early Genes:
Effector Genes that Promote Late LTP

The identities of effector genes that are activated either in the first round of gene expression by constitutively active transcription factors such as CREB, or in the subsequent round by IEG transcription factors such c-fos and zif268 are still largely unknown. Some clues can be gathered from the fact that not all IEGs encode for transcription factors, and several of those that are not transcription factors are targeted to dendrites, either as mRNA (arc/arg3.1, homer, αCaMKII) or as protein (BDNF). Transcription of *Arc/arg3.1* is itself regulated by zif268, and by another member of the egr family of transcription factors, egr3 (Li et al., 2005). Differential screens for genes up- or downregulated by the induction of late LTP in the dentate gyrus of the freely moving animal have yielded lists of a dozen or so transcripts that are upregulated 75 minutes after LTP induction in the freely moving rat (Matsuo et al., 2000) or 1.5 to 7.0 hours after induction in the anesthetized rat (Hevroni et al., 1998). These plasticity-related genes are in each case a subset of a considerably larger group of genes whose expression is stimulated by seizure activity. Another differential display study followed the time course of the regulation of a transcript for A kinase anchoring protein (AKAP-150). Unusually for an activity-regulated transcript, AKAP mRNA was not altered by seizures but was markedly affected by LTP-inducing stimulation, exhibiting an initial decrease at 1 hour and climbing to a peak increase at around 6 hours before falling back to baseline by 24 hours after induction (Génin et al., 2003). Using probes for specific transcripts at different times after induction Thomas et al. (1994) were able to follow the time course of tetanus-induced changes in mRNA for a number of serine/threonine protein kinases in the dentate gyrus; αCaMKII, and PKCγ showed transient increases, and increases in ERK2 and B-Raf were seen only at 24 hours. A finding that suggests a direct link to synaptic function was reported by Nayak et al. (1998): LTP in isolated CA1 dendrites is associated with a PKA- and transcription-dependent increase in the synthesis of AMPA receptors. Study of the identification and functional characterization of effector proteins that sustain maintenance of L-LTP, and the nature of their interaction with the putative synaptic tag, is likely to prove a challenging and fertile field for future research. Meanwhile, a systematic study of transcriptional changes related to LTP and their time courses has now become feasible through the use of DNA microarray screening (Lein et al., 2004 Lee et al., 2005; Wibrand et al., 2006).

Return Pathway: Signaling from Nucleus to Synapse and the Synaptic Tag Hypothesis

How are somatically generated transcripts and/or proteins delivered to the appropriate synapses? Frey and Morris (1997) considered a number of possibilities, of which conceptually the simplest was the idea that a potentiated synapse sets a marker or tag that is recognized by the mRNA or protein products that are transported into dendrites from the soma. This tag must have a lifetime at least long enough to engage with the newly generated mRNA or proteins. Transcriptional inhibitors given at the time of induction can take 2 hours or more to begin to affect LTP (Kelleher et al., 2004a; but see Barco et al., 2002 for a case where the transcriptional inhibitor actinomycin also acts rapidly). The relative delay in the action of transcriptional inhibitors presumably reflects the time taken for a signal to pass from synapse to nucleus for transcription first of IEGs and then of genes encoding effector proteins, followed by transport of mRNA and/or proteins into dendrites and their postulated capture by tagged spines. Frey and Morris speculated that the setting of the tag itself might be protein synthesis-independent. If this were the case, a tetanus to one pathway should still generate L-LTP even in the presence of a protein synthesis inhibitor if a second pathway was tetanized within a time window of 1 to 2 hours on either side of the tetanus to the first pathway. The tag would be set in the first pathway, notwithstanding the presence of the protein synthesis inhibitor, and would capture the plasticity-related proteins generated by the second pathway. These predictions were confirmed (Frey and Morris, 1997). (Note that the conversion of E-LTP to late L-LTP begins before the protein synthesis inhibitor has been washed out, which suggests that both the tag and the plasticity factor interacting with the tag are proteins rather than mRNA transcripts). Equally arresting was the demonstration that E-LTP, produced by a tetanus that by itself was too weak to produce L-LTP, could be converted to L-LTP by a preceding or subsequent strong tetanus given to a second pathway within a similar time window. Again, this result can be explained if the weak tetanus was below threshold for triggering local or somatic protein synthesis but nevertheless was able to set a tag that could capture the new proteins synthesized as a result of the strong tetanus to the second pathway.

Late LTD is also associated with the setting of a tag (Kauderer and Kandel, 2000). Sajikumar and Frey (2004a) presented evidence that it is the tag, rather than the plasticity factors, that determines the direction of change; thus, LTD-inducing stimuli generate an LTD-specific tag and LTP-inducing stimuli an LTP-specific tag (but see below for evidence that PKMζ is an LTP-specific plasticity factor). Although the tag normally has a lifetime of 1 to 2 hours, it can be canceled prematurely if depotentiation is induced by low-frequency stimulation delivered a few minutes after LTP induction (Sajikumar and Frey, 2004b). When tags are set on two pathways, they compete for the available supply of plasticity-related proteins, leading to a process of "competitive maintenance" in which potentiation at one pathway occurs at the expense of a reduction in potentiation at another (Fonseca et al., 2004).

Although the identity of the tag (or tags) is unknown, candidate tags must satisfy the following criteria (Barco et al., 2002; Kelleher et al., 2004a): (1) tags are generated by an activity-dependent, NMDAR-dependent, but protein synthesis-independent process; (2) they have a lifetime of 1 to 2 hours but are susceptible to cancelation by low-frequency trains within the first few minutes of being set; (3) at least two tags can be set, one induced by activity patterns that produce early or late LTP and the other by activity leading to early or late LTD; (4) tags are input-specific; (5) tags interact with proteins generated by de novo nuclear transcription (the process of "synaptic capture") to trigger the conversion of early to late LTP or early to late LTD. What clues to the identity of the tag do these criteria offer? The rapid, reversible, protein synthesis-independent setting of the tag points toward a protein kinase, possibly PKA (Barco et al., 2002), as candidate tags for LTP and protein phosphatases for LTD (Frey and Morris, 1998a; Kelleher et al., 2004a). The possibilities are much broader than this, however; any class of synaptic molecule whose phosphorylation state, configuration, or concentration is altered as a result of NMDAR-mediated events is in principle a candidate tag. Finally, it is worth emphasizing that a tag can be set without inducing L-LTP; so although the setting of a tag may or may not be a necessary precursor for induction of late LTP or late LTD, it is clearly not sufficient.

The Frey and Morris experiments revealed a complex pattern of temporal and spatial associativity in hippocampal synaptic plasticity, which they encapsulated by reference to the notion of "flashbulb" memory. A cell is continually bombarded with events of moderate significance to the organism; at inputs activated by these events, tags are set for an hour or two and then expire (whether tags decay over their lifetime or behave as molecular switches with on and off modes is unknown). When an event of major significance occurs, equivalent to a strong tetanus, late LTP is induced not only in

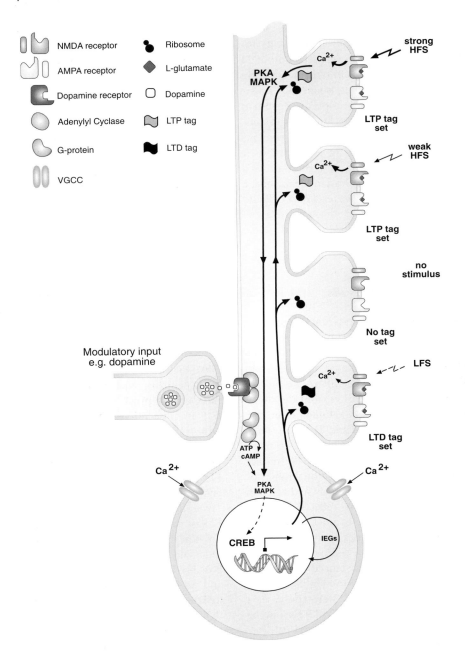

Figure 10–13. Signaling pathways involved in the genesis of late LTP. In this scheme, LTP induced by strong tetanic stimulation is represented by the distal synapse (top right). The large, rapid increase in Ca²⁺ stimulates local changes, leading to phosphorylation of receptors and other proteins (see Fig. 10–8); it also activates synapse-to-soma signaling cascades that may involve translocation of Ca²⁺/calmodulin, PKA and MAPK. At the same time, a synaptic tag is set to identify the synapse as having been recently activated. Weaker stimulation, leading only to early LTP, does not trigger a synapse-to-soma signal but does set a tag. Unstimulated synapses are left in molecular peace, whereas synapses receiving prolonged low-frequency stimulation (LFS) set an LTD tag and may generate similar nuclear signals (not shown). Additional dendrite-to-nucleus and soma-to-nucleus signals may be contributed by modulatory inputs such as dopaminergic innervation and by Ca²⁺ entering the soma through voltage-gated Ca²⁺ channels as a result of action potentials generated during activity. The targets of synapse-to-soma signaling are transcription factors, including CREB. Phosphorylation of CREB leads to the transcription of a number of genes that contain CRE (cAMP response elements) domains in their regulatory regions, among which are the early immediate genes such as *arc/arg3.1*, *homer*, *c-fos*, and *zif268*, some of which are themselves transcription factors. The return leg of the signaling system carries transcripts (e.g., mRNA for arc/arg3.1 and PKMζ) and unidentified proteins from the nucleus into dendrites. According to the tag hypothesis (see text), the soma-to-dendrite messengers are intercepted or captured by the tag, the nature of which has not been identified, and this triggers the changes that lead to late LTP (for an LTP tag) or late LTD (for an LTD tag).

that pathway, but via tagging and synaptic capture, with all other pathways carrying information about events of minor significance occurring an hour or two on either side of the significant event. We can speculate with Frey and Morris that through the tagging mechanism these secondary events acquire the same mnemonic potential as the major event and provide the contextual information that allows us to remember, for example, where we were and what we were doing on 9/11. A cartoon of some of the concepts we have been discussing in this section on late LTP is presented in Figure 10–13.

The Duration of Late LTP Is Regulated by the NMDA Receptor

We have seen that the expression of L-LTP depends on de novo protein synthesis around the time of induction, give or take a few hours during which a prior or later setting of the synaptic tag can engage with newly synthesized proteins. Thereafter, LTP proceeds without benefit of further de novo protein synthesis. Surprisingly, among the various largely uncharacterized posttranslational molecules and mechanisms that sustain the expression of LTP is the protein indelibly associated with its induction, the NMDA receptor. The time course of LTP in the dentate gyrus of the freely moving rat is prolonged by many days if the NMDAR antagonist CPP is infused after the tetanus (Villarreal et al., 2001). Infusion can be delayed for 2 days after induction and still rescue the decay of protein synthesis-dependent LTP. This startling result demonstrates that long after induction NMDAR-dependent signaling continues to control the fate of the potentiated synapse perhaps via the block of NMDAR-dependent depotentiation. Here is another area ripe for further investigation.

PKMζ maintains LTP

In the search for molecules that mediate the long-term persistence of LTP an interesting candidate has emerged in PKMζ (see Section 10.4.3). This member of the PKC family was identified as the only isoform that was activated 30 min after the induction of NMDAR-dependent LTP (Sacktor et al., 1993). PKMζ is a constitutively active catalytic fragment of the atypical PKCζ, which can be produced by proteolytic cleavage by proteases, such a calpain, or by synthesis from mRNA encoding just this fragment. Subsequent work showed that LTP involves the *de novo* synthesis of PKMζ (Hernandez et al., 2003). Interestingly, PKMζ appears to be both necessary and sufficient for L-LTP since PKMζ mimics and occludes LTP and since inhibition of PKMζ either by chelerythrine, which in low concentrations is selective for the ζ isoform, or by transfection with a dominant negative inhibitor, PKMζ-K281W, blocks LTP (Ling et al., 2002). The dominant negative inhibitor also blocked induction of E-LTP which led to the suggestion that PKMζ enzymatically cleaved from PKCζ, perhaps by the actions of calpain, may mediate the early protein synthesis–independent phase of LTP. However, a subsequent

study using a myristoylated form of a ζ-pseudosubstrate inhibitory peptide (termed ZIP), that binds to PKMζ and reconstitutes the autoinhibition in the absence of the PKCζ autoregulatory domain, blocked induction of L-LTP but not E-LTP (Serrano et al., 2005). Indeed, there is evidence that PKMζ is a plasticity factor that specifically targets synapses exhibiting a tag for LTP. In tagging experiments in which two independent pathways were given weak and strong tetani offset by 30 min, ZIP reversed L-LTP in both pathways. But when a strong tetanus to one pathway was given in conjunction with a weak LTD-inducing protocol to the other, ZIP reversed the maintenance of L-LTP but not of L-LTD; conversely, when a strong LTD inducing protocol to one pathway was paired with a weak tetanus to the other, the maintenance of L-LTP but again not of L-LTD was disrupted (Sajikumar et al., 2005). Note that this result is on the face of it inconsistent with the suggestion by Sajikumar and Frey (2004b) that newly transcribed plasticity factors are 'process-independent', with the direction of change being determined solely by local LTP- or LTD-specific tags.

The mechanism by which PKMζ-dependent L-LTP is maintained appears to be an increase in AMPAR number, since potentiation of synaptic transmission induced by PKMζ increased the amplitude, but not the frequency, of AMPAR-mediated mEPSCs and had no effect on their kinetics, or on mean single channel conductance, γ, the latter estimated using non-stationary fluctuation analysis (Ling et al., 2006). Interestingly, application of either chelerythrine or ZIP is able to reverse pre-established LTP (Ling et al., 2002) when applied 1 hour or later post-induction, though in another study chelerythrine given 30 min after induction did not block E-LTP (Bortolotto and Collingridge, 2000), suggesting that PKM is specifically involved in the maintenance of L-LTP. Perhaps most amazingly ZIP is able to reverse completely the potentiated response at perforant path synapses when injected 22 h following the establishment of LTP in the dentate gyrus of freely-moving rats, paving the way for an exploration of the role of LTP maintenance in memory (Pastalkova et al., 2006; see Section 10.10.4).

10.4.10 Structural Remodeling and Growth of Spines Can Be Stimulated by Induction of LTP

The idea that changes in synaptic efficacy could be embodied in changes in synaptic number or in remodeling of synaptic morphology predates the discovery of LTP by many decades and appears explicitly in the writings of Ramon y Cajal, William James, and Donald Hebb, among others. More spines, larger spines, and wider spine necks have all borne the burden of theories of memory, with the implicit assumption that appropriate changes occur also in the presynaptic partner. What is the status of these enduring theories today, and specifically do they provide a mechanism for the expression of LTP? The evidence is not straightforward, and disagreements among laboratories are as vigorous in this area as in many others (reviewed by Harris, 1999; Yuste and Bonhoeffer, 2001;

Nimchinsky et al., 2002; Kasai et al., 2003; Tashiro and Yuste, 2003; Lemphrect and Le Doux, 2004).

Spine numbers, even in adult animals, are not set in stone: Many experimental and indeed physiological situations are associated with dramatic changes in spine number. For example, spine densities in CA1 pyramidal neurons (but, interestingly, not in CA3 pyramidal cells or granule cells) vary by up to 30% during the estrus cycle in female rats (Woolley et al., 1990). Allowing adult rats a daily opportunity to explore a complex environment leads to an increase in spine density in CA1 pyramidal cells (Moser et al., 1994); and in organotypic cultures spines are rapidly retracted following bath application of botulinum toxin, which suppresses all transmitter release (McKinney et al., 1999). The physiologist engaged in cutting hippocampal slices no doubt prefers not to dwell too deeply on a report that CA1 neurons in slices from the adult rat contain 40% to 50% more synapses than similar cells in perfused and fixed tissue (Kirov et al., 1999). Comfort can perhaps be taken from the remarkable stability of spines in rat visual cortex when imaged over a period of many months (Grutzendler et al., 2002), although in mouse barrel cortex a more dynamic picture is seen, with only half of the imaged spines remaining stable over a period of a month (Trachtenberg et al., 2002).

Ultrastructural Changes Associated with LTP

The first investigation of tetanus-induced changes in spine morphology was published in 1975 (Van Harreveld and Fifkova, 1975). In this and subsequent studies, Fifkova and her colleagues reported an increase in spine area and the width of the spine neck in the outer part of the molecular layer of the dentate gyrus following tetanic stimulation of the perforant path. No changes were seen in spines in the unstimulated inner molecular layer. A problem with this work is that no recordings were made of evoked responses, so it is not possible to be sure that LTP was in fact induced. Further studies, notably by Desmond and Levy in the dentate gyrus, and by Lynch and his colleagues in area CA1, followed soon thereafter (Lee et al., 1980; Desmond and Levy, 1983; reviewed by Yuste and Bonhoeffer, 2001). Although Desmond and Levy found no consistent changes in spine density, they documented an increase in the length of the PSD following LTP induction (Desmond and Levy, 1986a) and an increase in cup-shaped spines (Desmond and Levy, 1986b). These observations supported the conclusion reached by Fifkova et al. (1997) that LTP is associated with changes in the morphology and ultrastructural organization of existing spines, rather than the generation of new spines. In area CA1, Lynch's group also saw no change in spine density but detected a substantial increase (35%) in the number of synapses—presumed inhibitory—on dendritic shafts (Lee et al., 1980). Technical advances in electron microscopy, including the introduction of the disector technique for unbiased stereological sampling and the use of serial sectioning to obtain authentic three-dimensional structural information, have strengthened the view that LTP is not associated with an overall change in spine density, either in the dentate gyrus 6 hours after tetanus in vivo (Popov et al., 2004; see Trommald et al., 1996 for a counter claim) or in area CA1 in vitro (2 hours after tetanus (Sorra and Harris, 1998). As we shall see below, this does not exclude the possibility that there are increases in the frequency of certain forms of spine at the expense of others.

In an influential series of studies, Geinisman documented an increase in the number of synapses with perforated and segmented PSDs in axospinous synapses in the dentate gyrus after daily episodes of tetanization for 4 days (Geinisman et al., 1991, 1993). Geinisman and colleagues proposed that these changes marked stages in the transformation of spines with single macular, or continuous, PSDs to potentiated spines with fully segmented PSDs, allowing two independent sites for synaptic transmission: a "spine splitting" model in which single boutons make multiple synapses on single dendrites. However, Harris et al. (2003) presented electron microscopic (EM) evidence that spine splitting is unlikely to occur in the adult hippocampus, as the gap between two spines is invariably filled with axons and dendrites. They concluded that the extra spine is more likely to represent new growth. However, even in potentiated tissue, instances where a single bouton makes contact with a pair of neighboring spines on the same dendrite comprise less than 3% of all synapses on hippocampal pyramidal cells and so are unlikely to provide a structural basis for more than a fraction of the potentiated response.

An ingenious method of labeling active synapses for EM was developed by Buchs and Muller (1996) based on the transient increase in the concentration of calcium that occurs in spines following tetanic stimulation. The method depends on precipitating calcium in smooth endoplasmic reticulum (SER) and rendering it electron-dense. Buchs and Muller noted an increase in the proportion of spines that contained perforated PSDs when synapses were labeled 30 minutes after the induction of LTP, compared to the proportion in labeled spines in naïve tissue or in spines examined 5 minutes after LTP induction. In a follow-up study using serial section EM, Toni et al. (1999) observed a delayed but persistent LTP-associated increase in the proportion of boutons making synapses on more than one spine (multiple synapse boutons); the proportion remained at its baseline value of around 6% for the first 30 minutes after tetanus, then rose to 15% at 45 to 120 minutes after tetanus (Fig. 10–14A). Moreover, in 66% of the latter cases, the two spines arose from the same dendrite, compared to 11% in tissue fixed 5 minutes after the tetanus. The method allows analysis only of the small proportion (15%) of spines that contain SER. Nevertheless, these striking observations suggest that LTP is expressed as an increase in the number of effective synapses, with input specificity conserved by the partitioning of tetanized boutons to allow for two release sites. This is similar to the spine-splitting model proposed by Geinisman; whether multiple spine synapses make up too small a proportion of the total to account fully for LTP, as maintained by Harris et al. (2003), remains for future work to determine.

Serial section EM allows construction of three-dimensional images of synapses in control and potentiated tissue, which is often the only way to resolve the ambiguities that can arise with two-dimensional sampling. Sorra and Harris (1998) examined synapses in tissue from area CA1 prepared 2 hours after the induction of LTP in vitro. No change in the density or size of spines was found. However, in the absence of any marker for potentiated synapses, it remained possible that an enlargement of potentiated spines was balanced by a decrease in the size of unstimulated spines. This drawback was addressed in further experiments from the same laboratory that focussed on a subpopulation of spines containing polyribosomes, the macromolecular complexes that contain the machinery for protein synthesis. Given the extensive evidence for local protein synthesis during LTP, could polyribosomes be used as a marker for potentiated synapses? Harris and her colleagues found that the proportion of spines containing polyribosomes was appreciably enhanced, from 12% to 39%, after LTP induction in area CA1 (Ostroff et al., 2002). Moreover, the surface area of the postsynaptic density in polyribosome-associated spines was greater in potentiated tissue than in control tissue, whereas for spines without polyribosomes the size of the PSD was unchanged (Fig. 10.14B). This result is consistent with a model in which potentiation is driven by synaptic enlargement. The situation is different in the dentate gyrus, however, where a decrease in polyribosome frequency occurs after LTP induction (Desmond and Levy, 1990).

Another three-dimensional EM study analyzed spines in the dentate gyrus 6 hours after the induction of LTP in vivo (Popov et al., 2004). Again, no overall change in spine density was seen, although in this case there was an increase in the proportion of synapses on thin spines and reductions in the number of stubby spines and spines on dendritic shafts (Fig. 10.14C). There was also a significant increase in the volume of thin and mushroom spines and an increase in the area of their PSDs. The picture that emerges from the EM studies considered thus far is that LTP is associated not with an overall increase in spine density but, rather, an increase in the size of certain subpopulations of spines.

Longitudinal Studies: Imaging Spines Before and After Induction of LTP

In addition to the problem of labeling potentiated synapses, an inherent limitation of electron microscopy is that it is not possible to image the same structure at multiple time points, so time-dependent changes have to be compared in different preparations. The advent of laser scanning confocal microscopy has improved the resolution of light microscopy to a level where synaptic stuctures (boutons and dendritic spines) can be visualized in living tissue, so the same spine, bouton, or length of dendrite can be measured before and at various times after

the induction of LTP (Hosokawa et al, 1995; Emptage et al., 2003; Matsuzaki et al., 2004), as discussed below.

Two other studies provide evidence that new spines can be formed after the induction of LTP in area CA1 in vitro. Maletic-Savatic et al. (1999) transfected CA1 pyramidal cells in organotypic culture with green fluorescent protein and used two-photon confocal microscopy to image synaptic structures. Within a few minutes of applying localized tetanic stimulation, they saw a rapid growth of filopodia-like structures emanating from the dendrite; filopodia were not seen in regions of the dendrite distant from the stimulating electrode and were not produced by low-frequency stimulation. Moreover, filopodial growth was blocked by AP5. A small proportion of induced filopodia developed bulbous heads within an hour of the tetanus, suggesting that the induced filopodia are precursors to new dendritic spines.

Engert and Bonhoeffer (1999) used two-photon microscopy to image dendrites and spines of dye-filled CA1 pyramidal cells in organotypic cultures and a local perfusion technique to restrict synaptic activity to a small volume (approximately 30 μm in diameter). Within 20 to 40 minutes of the tetanus new spines began to form in the activated volume at an average frequency of 0.06 spines/μm of dendrite (relative to a basal spine density of 0.40 spines/μm) (Fig. 10–14D). New spines were not formed elsewhere, and their appearance was blocked if the tetanus was given in the presence of AP5. The dramatic images obtained by Engert and Bonhoeffer are reminiscent of the tetanus-induced appearance of multiple synapse boutons on single dendrites described by Toni et al. (1999). Note, however, that the formation of new spines, in contrast to the near-immediate induction of LTP, was delayed by at least 20 minutes.

On the face of it, the studies described above make a strong case that new spines contribute to the expression of LTP in organotypic cultures and in acute slices. However, they are inconsistent with other confocal studies in area CA1 in which new spines were not observed, either after the induction of chemically induced LTP (Hosokawa et al., 1995) or after tetanus-induced LTP at visualized single spines (Emptage et al., 2003; Matsuzaki et al., 2004). Transformation of the spine from one displaying a continuous PSD to a perforated or segmented PSD would remain undetectable, as possibly would spine splitting; but the genesis of a new spine is well within the resolution of the technique. These discrepancies are unlikely to reflect differences in the time points chosen for study. Emptage et al. (2003) collected their data 30 to 60 minutes after tetanus, whereas Matsuzaki et al. (2004), using two-photon photolysis of caged glutamate, routinely extended their period of observation to 100 minutes after tetanus, spanning the period of 20 to 60 minutes during which the new spines charted by Engert and Bonhoeffer (1999) and by Toni et al. (1999) were being born. Once generated, the new spines survived for at least 2 hours in both sets of experiments and so should have been detected, if present in any number, by Sorra and Harris (1998), whose EM study in CA1 in vitro was car-

A

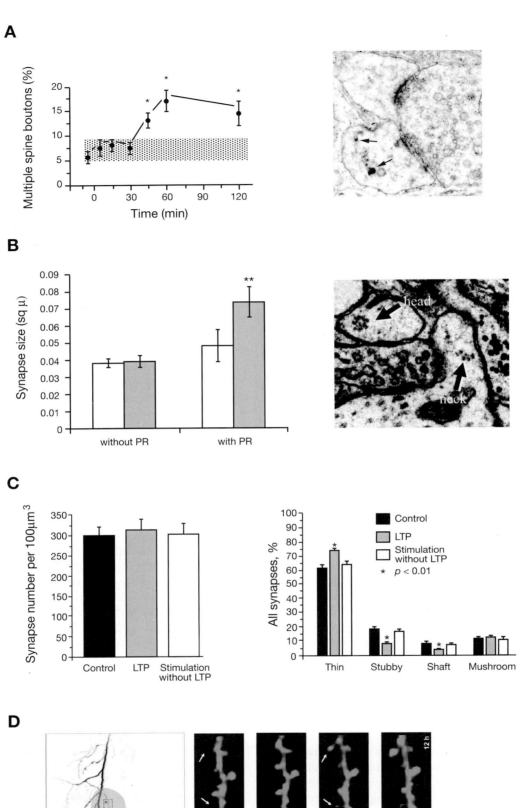

B

C

D

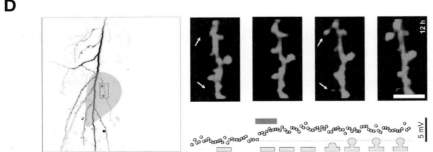

ried out 2 hours after tetanus (see below). The experiments of Matsuzaki et al. (2004) provided the first evidence of an increase in spine size in longitudinal studies LTP was induced by repetitive focal photolyis of caged glutamate in low Mg^{2+} to allow activation of both AMPA and NMDA receptors. Only small spines showed a persistent increase in size after the induction of LTP, and spine enlargement was accompanied by an increase in sensitivity to uncaged glutamate.

Despite two decades of work on structural changes associated with LTP, it is still not possible to reach a definitive conclusion on such basic questions as whether synaptogenesis plays a role in LTP or whether morphological changes in existing spines and boutons contribute to the enhanced response. In different preparations and at different times, there is evidence for one or other or both types of change. However, even where there is compelling evidence that such changes can occur, there is often no demonstrated causal link with LTP. Thus, when new spines have been observed, it has not been demonstrated that they contribute to the enhanced response (Engert and Bonhoeffer, 1999; Maletic-Savatic et al., 1999; Toni et al., 1999); moreover, the delayed time course of synaptogenesis rules out any contribution to the first 20-30 minutes of LTP. The experiments of Matzusaki et al. (2004) provide the strongest evidence that morphological changes are causally linked to LTP because the increase in spine size occurred immediately, was blocked by the same drugs that block the induction of LTP, and was associated with an increase in the response to uncaged glutamate. These experiments are also partly consistent with the LTP-associated increases in the volume of thin and mushroom spines observed by Popov et al. (2004) in their serial section EM analysis of LTP in the dentate gyrus. Matzusaki et al. (2004) speculated that large spines are

the repositories of previously stored information and are protected from further change. However, this prediction is not supported by the data of Popov et al. (2004), which shows an increase in the size of the largest subset of mushroom spines following the induction of LTP.

Alterations in the Cytoskeleton Contribute to LTP and LTD

Dendritic spines are not static structures; rather, their shape is determined from moment to moment by the dynamics of their actin cytoskeleton, as dramatically demonstrated in cultured neurons transfected with actin-GFP (Fischer et al., 1998; Matus, 2005). There is a growing body of evidence that activity-dependent regulation of actin polymerization and the consequent changes in synaptic morphology contribute to the expression of synaptic plasticity. At low concentrations, latrunculin A, an inhibitor of actin polymerization, blocks late but not early LTP in area CA1 in vitro (Krucker et al., 2003); a similar result has been reported in the dentate gyrus of the freely moving rat (Fukazawa et al., 2003). In the latter study, induction of LTP resulted in an NMDAR-dependent increase in F-actin (the polymerized form of actin) that was restricted to synapses of the tetanized pathway. The increase in F-actin was of rapid onset (< 20 minutes) and could be detected in tissue from animals killed as long as 5 weeks after the induction of LTP. An EM analysis also revealed significantly increased F-actin in spines in potentiated tissue; the F-actin content was appreciably greater in large spines, consistent with a model in which actin drives enlargement of the spine. F-actin is polymerized from globular G-actin monomers. Okamoto et al. (2004) used a fluorescence resonance energy

Figure 10–14. Morphological changes associated with LTP. *A.* LTP is accompanied by a delayed increase in the proportion of synapses in which the presynaptic bouton makes contact with more than one spine on a single dendrite. The graph plots the proportion of multiple spine boutons in the overall population of tetanized synapses as a function of time after the induction of LTP (5 to 120 minutes). A Ca^{2+} precipitation technique was used to label tetanized spines (arrowheads in the electron micrograph). (*Source*: Toni et al., 1999.) *B.* Spine growth following the induction of LTP is restricted to those spines that contain polyribosomes (PR), indicated by arrows in the electon micrograph. Analysis of three-dimensionsal reconstructions showed that the mean area of the postsynaptic density in spines lacking polyribosomes was the same before (open bars) and 2 hours after (gray bars) induction of LTP, whereas spines that contained polyribsomes were significantly larger after induction. LTP was also associated with a redistribution of polyribosomes from dendritic shafts to spines. (*Source*: Harris et al., 2003; adapted from Ostroff et al., 2002.) *C.* Spine density is not affected by the induction of LTP (left), but there are changes in the distribution of spine types (right), with an increase in the proportion of thin spines and a decrease in the proportion of stubby and shaft spines. Data were obtained from three-dimensional electron microscopic (EM) recon-

structions of dendritic segments from the medial molecular layer of the dentate gyrus. Three groups of rats were analyzed: controls (unstimulated, black bars), those with LTP (6 hours after induction of LTP by tetanic stimulation of the perforant path in anesthetized animals, gray bars), and animals that received the same total number of stimuli but in a pattern that did not induce LTP (white bars). (*Source*: Popov et al., 2004.) *D.* High-frequency stimulation leads to the appearance of new spines in the potentiated region of CA1 cells in organotypic cultures. Slice cultures were maintained in a solution containing Cd^{2+} and low Ca^{2+} to prevent transmitter release. A cell was impaled with a recording pipette containing fluorescent dye, and a small region of its dendritic tree was made competent for synaptic transmission by local perfusion of a solution containing normal ACSF. In the example shown in the left-hand panel, the extent of the perfused area is indicated by shading, with the pipette tip at the lower end. LTP was induced by pairing (see plot of EPSP amplitude, lower right). The two-photon confocal images on the right were obtained 10 minutes before and 0.5, 1, and 12 hours after induction of LTP. The icons below indicate the times at which the two new spines (indicated by arrows) were visible. Note the delay, observed in all cases, between the induction of LTP and the appearance of the new spines. (*Source*: Engert and Bonhoeffer, 1997.)

transfer (FRET) strategy to estimate the ratio between soluble G-actin and polymerized F-actin in the dendritic spines of pyramidal cells in organotypic hippocampal cultures. Tetanic stimulation increased the F-actin/G-actin ratio, whereas prolonged low-frequency trains caused a decrease in the ratio. These changes were correlated with increases and decreases in spine width, suggesting a model in which bidirectional, activity-dependent changes in F-actin control synaptic efficacy through changes in synaptic morphology. Because the size of the presynaptic bouton is closely matched to the size of the spine (Harris and Stevens, 1989), there must be a corresponding change in the presynaptic side. Evidence for an activity-dependent increase in the size and number of presynaptic boutons was uncovered by Colicos et al. (2001) in a study on dissociated hippocampal neurons transfected with GFP-actin. As we saw above, the EM evidence is more consistent with an increase in the size than the number of synapses during LTP. Which of the possible models (no change in spine size or number, or changes in one or both) more accurately describes the activity-driven changes that may occur in vivo is another goal for future research.

10.5 LTP at Mossy Fiber Synapses

In this section we consider the very different form that LTP takes at the largest synapses in the hippocampus, indeed, among the largest in the mammalian brain—the synapses made by granule cell axons (the mossy fibers) on CA3 pyramidal cells. These synapses also support LTD, a topic that is covered in see Section 10.7. Mossy fibers make most of their connections not on CA3 pyramidal cells but on inhibitory interneurons in the hilus and stratum radiatum. We discuss plasticity at these connections in Section 10.8.

10.5.1 Mossy Fiber Synapses Display Striking Short-term Plasticity

Mossy fiber boutons make giant, interdigitating synapses at complex spines (Cajal's "thorny excrescences") on the proximal dendrites of CA3 pyramidal cells. Giant synapses contain up to 35 release sites (Henze et al., 2000) and show a greater degree of short-term plasticity (paired-pulse facilitation and frequency potentiation during repetitive stimulation) than associational-commissural (A/C) synapses linking ipsilateral and contralateral CA3 pyramidal cells (Salin et al., 1996). These properties are mediated, at least in part, by synaptically released glutamate acting on presynaptic kainate receptors that are positively linked to transmitter release (Lauri et al., 2001; Schmitz et al., 2001). In addition, at mossy fiber synapses in vitro, PTP of several hundred percent can be elicited by long tetani (Langdon et al., 1995); in the anesthetized rat, in contrast, PTP is typically not seen with similar tetanus protocols (Derrick and Martinez, 1994b).

10.5.2 Basic Characteristics of NMDA Receptor-independent LTP at Mossy Fiber Synapses

Long-term potentiation in the mossy fiber projection was first documented by Schwartzkroin and Wester (1975). A striking feature of this form of LTP is its immunity to NMDA receptor antagonists (Harris and Cotman, 1985) (Fig. 10–15A), consistent with the relatively sparse distribution of NMDA receptors in stratum lucidum, the mossy fiber terminal zone (Monaghan and Cotman, 1885). (Note that synaptically evoked NMDAR-mediated currents can nevertheless be recorded from CA3 cells following mossy fiber stimulation, a property that has been exploited to provide evidence for a presynaptic expression mechanism in mossy fiber LTP (Weisskopf and Nicoll, 1995) (see below). Although there is wide agreement that the expression of mossy fiber LTP is presynaptically mediated, there has been a persistent and unresolved debate about whether the induction of LTP in this pathway is triggered by presynaptic or postsynaptic processes—a curious reversal of the controversies that invigorate discussion on induction and expression in other regions of the hippocampus. Mossy fiber LTP in vitro shows input specificity (Zalutsky and Nicoll, 1992) and associativity (Schmitz et al., 2003). In addition, associativity between mossy fiber and A/C fibers has been reported both in vivo (Derrick and Martinez, 1994b) and in vitro (Kobayashi and Poo, 2004); in the latter case, induction of LTP in A/C synapses could be boosted by trains to a single mossy fiber. Cooperativity (see Section 10.1.1) has been reported in vivo (Derrick and Martinez, 1994b) but is not seen in vitro (Zalutsky and Nicoll, 1992).

The duration of mossy fiber LTP has not been studied in the freely moving animal, but with multiple trains at 100 Hz LTP lasting for several hours has been recorded in vivo (Henze et al., 2000). Most of what follows is based on a survey of the much larger slice literature, but the in vivo data should be borne in mind when considering the functional consequences of mossy fiber plasticity.

10.5.3 Induction Mechanisms of Mossy Fiber LTP

A Continuing Controversy: The Locus of Induction of Mossy Fiber LTP

The Hebbian characteristics of LTP in the Schaffer-commissural and perforant path projections arise from the voltage-dependent properties of the NMDA receptor. It is a matter of continuing controversy as to whether induction is also Hebbian in the mossy fiber projection. The most straightforward way of settling the issue would be to establish whether postsynaptic maneuvers, such as injection of a Ca^{2+} chelator into the target cell or voltage-clamping the cell at hyperpolarized potentials, blocks induction of LTP. Both experiments have been done, and different groups have come up with different answers. According to Johnston and colleagues, mossy fiber LTP is blocked by hyperpolarizing the CA3 pyramidal

A
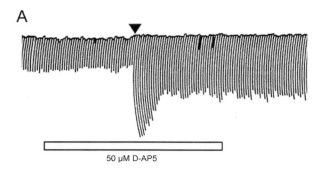
50 µM D-AP5

B
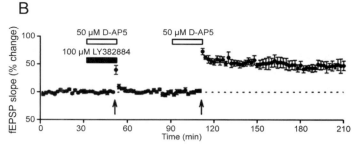

C
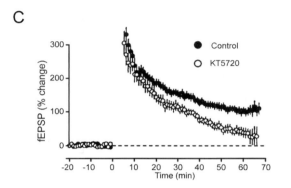

D
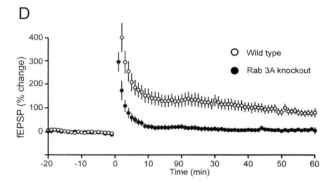

Figure 10–15. Properties of mossy fiber LTP. *A.* Mossy fiber LTP in vitro is readily induced during blockade of NMDA receptors. The graph plots fEPSP amplitude vs time and shows that a tetanus (delivered at the time indicated by the arrowhead) induced LTP in the presence of D-APS (applied for 35 min. Mean baseline amplitude of fEPSPs was 0.4 mV. (*Source*: Harris and Cotman, 1986.) *B.* The induction of mossy fiber LTP in vitro can be prevented by kainate receptor antagonists. The graph plots fEPSP amplitude versus time and shows that the GluR5-containing kainate receptor antagonist LY382884 blocks the induction of mossy fiber LTP in a

reversible manner. A tetanus (100 Hz, 1 second, test intensity) was delivered in the presence of D-APV at the times indicated by arrows. (*Source*: Bortolotto et al., 1999.) *C.* Inhibition of PKA prevents the full expression of mossy fiber LTP in vitro. The graph plots fEPSP versus time to show the effects of the PKA inhibitor KT5720 and control experiments. A tetanus was delivered at t = 0. (*Source*: Weisskopf et al., 1994.) *D.* Mossy fiber LTP in vitro is absent in the Rab 3A knockout. The effects of a tetanus (t = 0) on fEPSPs is compared for Rab 3A knockout and wild-type mice. (*Source*: Castillo et al., 1997a.)

neuron (Jaffe and Johnston, 1990) or by injecting the calcium chelator BAPTA (Williams and Johnston, 1989). A report by Zalutsky and Nicoll (1990), working with guinea pig rather than rat hippocampus, disputed both these findings; induction of LTP was insensitive to membrane potential and to intracellular injections of BAPTA. LTP in the A/C projection, however, was blocked by BAPTA. Because these synapses are located more distally on CA3 cells than the complex spines on which mossy fibers terminate, Zalutsky and Nicoll argued that the concentration of BAPTA was likely to have been sufficient to chelate free Ca^{2+} in complex spines. They concluded that the induction of mossy fiber LTP was not controlled postsynaptically and was therefore non-Hebbian (Nicoll and Schmitz, 2005).

A subsequent in vitro study offered a partial resolution of the controversy (Urban and Barrionuevo, 1996). Brief trains of high-frequency stimulation (B-HFS) (typically 8 stimuli at 100 Hz, repeated eight times at 5-second intervals), as normally used by Johnston and his colleagues, led to a Hebbian

form of mossy fiber LTP, the induction of which was blocked by a number of postsynaptic maneuvers, including hyperpolarization, internal perfusion with BAPTA, and iontropic glutamate receptor blockade with kynurenate (which prevents synaptically evoked depolarization). In contrast, long trains of high-frequency stimulation (L-HFS) (typically 100 stimuli at 100 Hz, repeated three times at 10-second intervals), as favored by Nicoll and his colleagues, produced a non-Hebbian form of LTP that was not affected by hyperpolarization, kynurenate, or BAPTA.

Johnston's laboratory reentered the arena in 1999, reporting that B-HFS and L-HFS were associated with an increase in dendritic Ca^{2+} concentration; moreover, induction of both forms of LTP could be blocked by postsynaptic injection of BAPTA (Yeckel et al., 1999). However, the source of the increase in Ca^{2+} was different in the two cases. LTP induced by brief trains was associated with an influx of Ca^{2+} through voltage-gated Ca^{2+} channels because, as shown earlier (Urban and Barrionuevo, 1996), it could be blocked by kynurenate, by hyperpolarization, and by Ca^{2+} channel blockers (Kapur et al., 1998). LTP and the rise in dendritic Ca^{2+} induced by long trains was insensitive to membrane potential and to kynurenate (confirming the observation of Zalutsky and Nicoll, 1990) but could be blocked by mGluR1 antagonists and by agents such as ryanodine and thapsigargin, which compromise release of Ca^{2+} from internal stores. These results suggest that a build-up of glutamate in the synaptic cleft leads to activation of type 1 mGluRs, stimulation of PLC, and a consequent IP3-induced release of Ca^{2+} from internal stores. Both forms of LTP could be blocked by an inhibitor of PKA, indicating that elevation of Ca^{2+} by the two routes converges on a PKA-dependent pathway to drive the expression of LTP. However, Mellor and Nicoll (2001) were unable to confirm these results and so the impasse remains unresolved. We are left with the unsatisfactory conclusion that in certain not precisely defined conditions the induction of mossy fiber LTP requires involvement of the postsynaptic cell, whereas in others, equally imprecisely characterized, it does not. It is notable, however, that a number of subsequent studies have emphasized the importance of the postsynaptic cell in the induction (and in one case the expression) of mossy fiber plasticity. Thus, a protocol in which LTP was induced by pairing mossy fiber stimulation with *hyper*polarization of the CA3 neuron was developed by Sokolov et al. (2003). In contrast, Lei et al. (2003) reported that pairing low-frequency stimulation with sustained depolarization of the target CA3 cell led to a form of mossy fiber LTD in which expression as well as induction is postsynaptically driven.

Finally, in experiments that introduced a new dimension to mossy fiber plasticity, Contractor et al. (2002) established that the ephrin–EphB receptor tyrosine kinase signaling system (see Section 10.4.8) plays a critical role in the induction of LTP. The native B-ephrin ligand is expressed in the presynaptic membrane where it can potentially engage with the postsynaptic EphB receptor. Postsynaptic injection of antibodies that compromise protein–protein interaction domains on the intracellular C terminus of the EphB receptor blocks the induction of LTP, as does bath perfusion with a soluble form of B-ephrin. These experiments offer strong evidence for a postsynaptic involvement in the induction of mossy fiber LTP. They also provide a potential mechanism for retrograde transsynaptic signaling by which the presynaptic terminal can be informed about critical postsynaptic induction events. The reduction of mossy fiber LTP in NCAM knockout mice provides another indication of the potential importance of transsynaptic signaling at these synapses (Benson et al., 2000).

Role of Kainate Receptors in the Induction of Mossy Fiber LTP

Kainate receptors are located both presynaptically and postsynaptically at mossy fiber synapses. The presynaptic kainate receptors regulate L-glutamate release (Vignes and Collingridge, 1997), and the postsynaptic kainate receptors contribute a slow component to the synaptic current gener-

ated by stimulation of mossy fibers (Castillo et al., 1997b; Vignes and Collingridge, 1997) (see Chapter 6, Section 6.3). The role of kainate receptors in the induction of mossy fiber LTP has provided another opportunity for lively disagreement. In the first study to use a specific kainate receptor antagonist, Bortolotto et al. (1999) reported that induction of mossy fiber LTP was blocked by LY382884 (Fig. 10–15B). Mossy fiber LTP was also blocked by CNQX and kynurenate, reagents that block both AMPA and kainate receptors. Their results were challenged by Nicoll and colleagues, who pointed to previous experiments of theirs and others in which CNQX and kynurenate had failed to block induction of mossy fiber LTP (see exchange of letters between Nicoll et al. and Bortolotto et al. in *Nature* 2000;406:957). Subsequently, Collingridge's group reported that the kainate receptor antagonist LY382884 acted presynaptically to reduce transmitter release from mossy fiber terminals and that this effect occluded mossy fiber LTP (Lauri et al., 2001). In this view, tetanic stimulation led to activation of presynaptic kainate receptors containing GluR5 subunits (the target of LY382884) and thence by a Ca^{2+}-dependent pathway to a persistent increase in transmitter release. A possible reconciliation of the two positions has emerged from later studies by the two groups. Lauri et al. (2003) found that the requirement for kainate receptor activation could be negated if the extracellular Ca^{2+} concentration was increased from 2 mM to 4 mM (the level normally employed in Nicoll's laboratory). Lauri and colleagues suggested that, at this concentration, sufficient Ca^{2+} entered via L-type Ca^{2+} channels to compensate for the block of kainate receptors. However, this cannot be the entire explanation because Schmitz et al (2003) failed to block mossy fiber LTP with LY382884 even in the presence of 2 mM Ca^{2+}. Hence, it appears that multiple factors determine the role of kainate receptors in mossy fiber LTP.

Nicoll's group ascribed a role for presynaptic kainate receptors in mediating associative induction properties, in which neighboring mossy fiber or associational/commissural activity can lower the threshold for induction of mossy fiber LTP (Schmitz et al., 2003). Independent support for a critical role of presynaptic kainate receptors in mossy fiber plasticity has also come from the demonstration that LTP is absent in a knockout mouse lacking a functional GluR6 subunit (Contractor et al., 2001). Somewhat unfortunately for the prospects of reconciliation, the same study showed that mossy fiber LTP was unimpaired in mice lacking the GluR5 subunit. However, these results are not necessarily incompatible with the studies using LY382884 because, first, GluR6 is probably necessary for targeting kainate receptors and, second, there may be compensatory upregulation of other kainate receptor subunits in the knockout (Kerchner et al., 2002a). Furthermore, more recently developed antagonists of GluR5-containing kainate receptors, such as UBP296, also block the induction of mossy fiber LTP (More et al., 2004). The actions of GluR5 antagonists can therefore safely be attributed to their ability to inhibit this subunit. Given that LY382884 inhibits GluR5-containing heteromeric kainate receptors, the most likely explanation for the discordant results is that the presynaptic kainate receptor may, but does not invariably, contain the GluR5 subunit.

Role of mGluRs in the Induction of Mossy Fiber LTP

As we saw in Section 10.3.10, one of the many controversies that enliven the study of hippocampal plasticity concerns the role of metabotropic glutamate receptors in LTP. In the case of mossy fiber LTP, it has been claimed that mGluR antagonists (Bashir et al., 1993), or the targeted deletion of mGluR1 (Conquet et al., 1994), severely impairs induction of LTP at mossy fiber synapses. However, both these findings have been disputed (Hsia et al., 1995; Selig et al., 1995b). In a subsequent study, it was reported that antagonism of both ionotropic and group 1 metabotropic receptors is required before LTP induced by long high-frequency trains (L-HFS) is blocked (Yeckel et al., 1999). Clearly, further work is needed to elucidate the involvement of mGluRs in mossy fiber LTP.

Mossy Fiber LTP Requires Activation of the cAMP/PKA Pathway

There is convincing evidence that the cAMP and cAMP-dependent protein kinase (PKA) pathway is involved in the generation of mossy fiber LTP. First, bath application of PKA inhibitors blocks the induction of mossy fiber LTP (Huang and Kandel, 1994; Weisskopf et al., 1994) (Fig. 10–15C). Second, bath application of membrane-permeable cAMP analogues or of forskolin, an activator of adenylyl cyclase, induces a form of LTP that occludes with tetanus-induced LTP (Huang and Kandel, 1994; Weisskopf et al., 1994). Third, mutant mice with a targeted deletion of type I adenylyl cyclase show impaired mossy fiber LTP (Wu Z-L et al., 1995). These observations do not directly address the question of pre- versus postsynaptic locus of induction or expression. Forskolin-induced LTP is probably expressed presynaptically for the following reasons: First, there is a reduction in paired-pulse facilitation (Huang and Kandel, 1994; Weisskopf et al., 1994); second, there is no change in the response evoked by iontophoretic glutamate (Weisskopf et al., 1994); and third, there is an increase in the coefficient of variation of synaptic responses, indicative of a presynaptic change (Weisskopf et al., 1994) (see Box 10.1). However, postsynaptic involvement of the PKA signal cascade in mossy fiber LTP has also been suggested by reports that injection of a cAMP analogue into the postsynaptic cell can facilitate induction of LTP (Hopkins and Johnston, 1988) and, conversely, that postsynaptic injection of a PKA peptide inhibitor can impair induction (Yeckel et al., 1999).

Role of Opioid Peptides in Mossy Fiber Plasticity

Mossy fiber terminals, like the terminals of the lateral perforant path, co-release the opioid peptides enkephalin and dynorphin in a frequency-dependent manner. The involve-ment of opioid peptides in mossy fiber LTP is yet another area of dispute, with opioid receptor antagonists reportedly blocking mossy fiber LTP in vivo (Derrick and Martinez, 1994a, 1996) but not in vitro (Salin et al., 1995). In vivo, mossy fiber LTP can be induced by a combination of strong activation of A/C fibers, low frequency mossy fiber activation, and injection of μ receptor agonists. Any combination of two of these procedures yields mossy fiber LTD rather than LTP (Derrick and Martinez, 1996).

Role of Zinc in Mossy Fiber LTP

Vesicles in mossy fiber glutamatergic terminals sequester large amounts of Zn^{2+} (Haug, 1967; Danscher et al., 1976; reviewed by Frederickson and Danscher, 1990). There is good evidence that Zn^{2+} can be released from mossy fibers during synaptic stimulation, where it may be co-released with L-glutamate (Assaf and Chung, 1984; Howell et al., 1984; Quinta-Ferreira and Matias, 2004). Zn^{2+} can modulate the function of a variety of ligand-gated and voltage-gated ions channels (Harrison and Gibbons, 1994), via which it may modulate synaptic plasticity. For example, Zn^{2+} inhibits NMDA receptors, providing a route by which it could affect the induction of NMDAR-dependent LTP (Xie and Smart, 1994; Ueno et al., 2002). There is also a body of evidence suggesting that Zn^{2+} is involved (Weiss et al., 1989). For example, a variety of Zn^{2+} chelators can inhibit the induction of mossy fiber LTP (Budde et al., 1997; Lu et al., 2000b; Li et al., 2001), as can chronic deficiency of dietary zinc (Lu et al., 2000b). Conversely, exogenous application of Zn^{2+} can induce long-lasting potentiation of mossy fiber transmission (Li et al., 2001). Mossy fiber LTP seems to require the entry of Zn^{2+} from the extracellular space into the postsynaptic neuron, entering via Ca^{2+}-permeable AMPA or kainate receptors or via voltage-gated ion channels (Li et al., 2001; Jia et al., 2002). Its target in the postsynaptic cell is not known.

LTP at Connections Between Mossy Fibers and Interneurons

In addition to the large excitatory synapses made by mossy fibers on CA3 pyramidal cells, at least two kinds of connections to inhibitory interneurons in the stratum lucidum have been described (see Chapter 4). LTP at these synapses is considered in Section 10.8.1.

10.5.4 Expression of Mossy Fiber LTP Is Presynaptic

There is general agreement that the locus of expression of mossy fiber LTP is presynaptic, in contrast to the long-running dispute concerning its locus of induction. Evidence for a presynaptic locus of expression was first presented by Zalutsky and Nicoll (1990), who found that paired-pulse facilitation (PPF) of responses evoked by mossy fiber stimulation was reduced after induction of LTP. However interpretation of this result as evidence of a presynaptic change is itself based on the assumption that PPF is wholly presynaptic, a claim for which there is no incontrovertible evidence in the mossy fiber pathway and that cannot be taken for granted (see Box 10–1). However, related evidence for a presynaptic locus has come from the demonstration that presynaptic kainate receptors mediate a component of synaptic facilitation that occludes with mossy fiber LTP (Lauri et al., 2001).

Further support for a presynaptic locus of expression has emerged from a comparison of the decay constant of NMDAR-mediated currents in the presence of the activity-dependent blocker MK801 in potentiated and nonpotentiated synapses. Potentiated mossy fiber synapses show a more rapid block than nonpotentiated mossy synapses, in contrast to A/C synapses where the decay rate is unaffected by potentiation (Weisskopf and Nicoll, 1995). This result implies an increase in mean Pr following the induction of LTP (see Section 10.4.4), which could be achieved by an increase in Pr at preexisting release sites or by activation of silent synapses with a mean Pr higher than that of the pretetanus population. Activation of silent synapses could occur by the insertion of receptor clusters or by the awakening of previously silent release sites. In cultured granule cells making autaptic synapses onto themselves, there is evidence that the latter is more likely to be the case (Tong et al., 1996). The existence of NMDAR-independent LTP at granule cell autapses establishes that the CA3 pyramidal cell is not an obligatory component of the LTP machinery at granule cell terminal boutons. As discussed is section 10.4.4, Kawamura et al. (2003), using an optical method to detect glutamate-induced glial depolarization, also reached the conclusion that LTP at mossy fiber synapses, but not at A/C synapses, was associated with an increase in glutamate release.

Quantal analysis has been applied to mossy fiber LTP in slices (Xiang et al., 1994) and in a culture system (Lopez-Garcia et al., 1996); in both studies there was an increase in the coefficient of variation and a reduction in failures at initially nonsilent connections, indicating a presynaptic locus for the expression of LTP (but see Yamamoto et al., 1992). Confocal imaging of excitatory postsynaptic calcium transients (EPSCaTs) at single complex spines is also consistent with a presynaptic locus of expression. LTP is accompanied by an increase in the number of active release sites and/or an increase in Pr at already active sites (Reid et al., 2004).

Some insight has been gained into the mechanisms underlying expression of mossy fiber LTP. Thus, mossy fiber LTP is absent in mice lacking the synaptic vesicle protein Rab3a (Castillo et al, 1997a) (Fig. 10–15D) and the GTP-dependent Rab3a binding partner RIM1α (Castillo et al, 2002). RIM1α is located at the active zone and is a substrate for PKA. Therefore LTP could involve a PKA-dependent interaction between Rab3a and RIM1α to enhance transmitter release. Surprisingly, however, forskolin-induced potentiation, which occludes with mossy fiber LTP, is not affected in either knockout. Therefore, the relation between PKA-dependent signaling and the role of these two proteins in mossy fiber LTP is unclear.

Another possible mechanism was suggested by the finding that mossy fiber LTP occludes the facilitation of synaptic

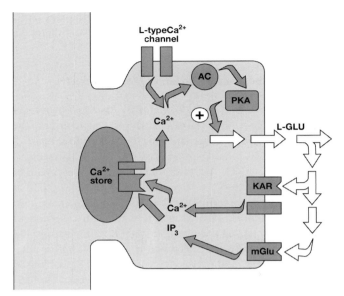

Figure 10–16. Mechanisms involved in the expression of mossy fiber LTP. Synaptically released L-glutamate can feed back onto presynaptic receptors. Under certain circumstances, at least, this may involve kainate receptors, group I mGlu receptors, and Ca^{2+}-induced Ca^{2+} release. A possible scheme to link these components is illustrated, which involves convergence of Ca^{2+} and IP3 at the ryanodine receptor. Ca^{2+} entry via voltage-gated Ca^{2+} channels can provide an alternative source of Ca^{2+}. Increases in Ca^{2+} stimulate adenylyl cyclase (AC) to activate PKA, and this modifies L-glutamate release. Other mechanisms, including a postsynaptic component, could also be involved in mossy fiber LTP.

transmission induced by depolarization with K^+ (Lauri et al, 2001). This suggests that mossy fiber LTP may alter an ion channel to affect the resting membrane potential of mossy fiber boutons. One candidate is the hyperpolarization-activated cation channel Ih (Mellor et al., 2002, but see Chevaleyre and Castillo, 2002). Thus, a wide range of evidence indicates a presynaptic locus of expression for mossy fiber LTP (Fig. 10–16).

10.5.5 E-LTP and L-LTP at Mossy Fiber Synapses Can Be Distinguished by the Effects of Protein Synthesis Inhibitors

Repeated long trains of high-frequency stimulation result in L-LTP lasting undiminished for 6 hours or more at mossy fiber synapses in vitro (Urban and Barrionuevo, 1996). In the presence of transcriptional and translational inhibitors, potentiation is initially similar, but responses decline to baseline levels over the following 3 to 4 hours (Huang YY et al., 1994). As is the case elsewhere in the hippocampus, mossy fiber LTP can therefore be subdivided into L-LTP, requiring gene expression and protein synthesis, and E-LTP, which is independent of protein synthesis. The cAMP-dependent protein kinase cascade is implicated in both early and late mossy fiber LTP. PKA inhibitors block both phases, and bath application of forskolin, an activator of adenylyl cyclase, induces both early protein synthesis-independent and late protein synthesis-dependent potentiation. Moreover, early tetanus-induced LTP occludes forskolin-induced LTP and vice versa (Huang YY et al., 1994; Weisskopf et al., 1994). Early LTP is associated with a conspicuous reduction in paired-pulse facilitation (Zalutsky and Nicoll, 1990); interestingly, this effect attenuates over time, suggesting a switch to mechanisms of potentiation that do not depend on an increase in Pr at individual release sites but, instead, require either postsynaptic changes or an increase in the number of synapses or active zones (Huang and Kandel, 1994).

10.5.6 Summary

Despite its independence of the NMDA receptor, it is evident that LTP at mossy fiber synapses requires an increase in intracellular Ca^{2+}; but whether the critical compartment is the presynaptic terminal or the postsynaptic spine remains unresolved and may depend on the pattern of the plasticity-inducing stimulation. What is clear is that the increase in Ca^{2+} is not achieved by activation of NMDA receptors. Instead, increases in Ca^{2+} are achieved by a variety of alternative routes, including the opening of voltage-dependent Ca^{2+} channels following depolarization (caused by the presynaptic action potential in the case of the presynaptic terminal and by binding of glutamate to postsynaptic AMPA receptors in the case of the postsynaptic cell) and the binding of glutamate to type I mGluRs, leading to release of Ca^{2+} from intracellular stores. The finding that kainate receptor antagonists, and philanthotoxin which blocks Ca^{2+} permeation, can block mossy fiber LTP under similar experimental conditions raises the possibility that Ca^{2+} entry through these receptors may also regulate plasticity at mossy fiber synapses.

Finally, little is known about the role of mossy fiber LTP in the behaving animal. The long (1 second) trains at 100 Hz that are required to produce robust mossy fiber LTP are not likely to be mimicked by granule cells in vivo, and it remains to be established that naturally occurring patterns of granule cell activity lead to LTP at mossy fiber synapses.

10.6 LTP Can Be Modulated by Other Neurotransmitters, Neuromodulators, and Effectors and by Endogenous and Circadian Rhythms

The degree and duration of LTP produced by a standard induction protocol is influenced by a multitude of factors in addition to the frequency and duration of the tetanus. We have already discussed the effects of prior activity (metaplasticity) and the critical role of inhibitory circuits in setting the threshold for LTP. A good example of the importance of inhibition is seen in the dentate gyrus of the hippocampal slice, where LTP usually cannnot be elicited at all unless the slice is perfused with a $GABA_A$ antagonist. We now examine the role of some of the more important of the many other neuro-

transmitters and neuromodulators that can affect the threshold for induction or the magnitude and/or duration of LTP. We also consider cyclical influences on LTP, including sleep and circadian rythms. In this section also we discuss the evidence that newborn granule cells in the dentate gyrus contribute to synaptic plasticity.

10.6.1 Modulation by Other Neurotransmitters and Neuromodulators

Acetylcholine

Both the early literature (reviewed in Segal and Auerbach, 1997) and more recent studies support the conclusion that the septal cholinergic input can facilitate the induction of hippocampal LTP. Evidence includes (1) inhibition of LTP by broad-spectrum muscarinic antagonists and (2) reduction in the threshold for LTP by muscarinic agonists or by stimulation of the septum. A revealing study in the freely moving rat demonstrates that these effects depend on the behavioral state of the animal (Leung et al., 2003). Basal LTP in the immobile or sleeping rat is not affected by muscarinic antagonists; but if tetanic stimulation is delivered to the Schaffer-commissural projection when the animal is generating cholinergically driven theta activity as it moves around its environment, an enhanced level of LTP is induced in area CA1. Pretreatment with the muscarinic antagonist scopolamine reduced the level of LTP to near-baseline levels, as did injection into the medial septum of the neurotoxin immunoglobulin G (IgG)-saporin, directed against cholinergic neurons. These experiments demonstrate that LTP can be modulated by an endogenous, behaviorally driven cholinergic input from the septum. The effect is probably mediated by high-affinity postsynaptic M2 receptors (Segal and Auerbach, 1997). It is notable that afferent cholinergic fibers and M2 receptors are both present at higher density in the stratum oriens than in the stratum radiatum of area CA1. Activation of muscarinic receptors in the hippocampus leads to G protein-mediated block of a number of K^+ channels, including I_{AHP}, I_M, and I_L, as well as enhanced NMDA receptor function (Segal and Auerbach, 1997). Interestingly, direct potentiation of the NMDA receptor conductance occurs at lower concentrations of ACh than that usually required to block K^+ channels (Harvey et al., 1993). Any or all of these effects may contribute to the positive modulation of LTP induction by ACh acting on muscarinic receptors.

Monoamines

Norepinephrine (Noradrenaline). Noradrenergic innervation of the hippocampus originates primarily from neurons in the locus coeruleus (see Chapter 8, Section 8.1.2). In the first study of the role of monamines in LTP, Bliss et al. (1983) investigated the effects of the depletion of norepinephrine and serotonin. Depletion of norepinephrine was achieved by injecting the neurotoxin 6-hydroxydopamine (6-OHDA) into the locus coeruleus, leading to a reduction in the magnitude of LTP of the fEPSP in the dentate gyrus (Bliss et al., 1983).

Curiously, LTP of the population spike was not affected, a result mirrored in a study showing that β-adrenergic receptor antagonists block LTP of the fEPSP but not of the population spike in the dentate gyrus (Munro et al., 2001, but see Stanton and Sarvey, 1985). There is also evidence that norepinephrine can promote late LTP: Stimulation of adrenergic neurons in the locus coeruleus by injection of glutamate produces a delayed protein synthesis-dependent potentiation of perforant path-evoked responses in the dentate gyrus (Walling and Harley, 2004). A similar pattern of results is seen in area CA1. Depletion of norepinephrine or bath application of β-adrenergic receptor antagonists blocks LTP, and bath application of norepinephrine lowers the threshold for the induction of LTP (Izumi and Zorumski, 1999). Enhancement or reduction of LTP by drugs that respectively stimulate or block β-adenergic receptors has also been reported in the mossy fiber projection (Hopkins and Johnston, 1988). Because β-adrenergic receptors are positively linked to adenlyate cyclase, the mechanism of action of norepinephrine is likely to be similar to that of dopamine, leading (via an increase in cAMP) to activation of PKA.

Serotonin. The modulatory effects of serotonin (5-hydroxytryptamine, 5-HT) on LTP have been relatively less studied, and there is little consensus among studies. Selective depletion of serotonin reduced the magnitude of LTP in the dentate gyrus in vivo (Bliss et al., 1983), but this result was not replicated in an in vitro study (Stanton and Sarvey, 1985). At commissural-associational synapses in area CA3 in vitro, bath application of 5-HT was reported to inhibit LTP (Villani and Johnston, 1993), whereas depletion of serotonin in area CA1 was without effect (Stanton and Sarvey, 1985). The role of serotonin receptor subclasses in LTP has received some attention. Injection of ondansetron, a selective antagonist of 5-HT3 receptors, significantly enhanced the magnitude of LTP in area CA1 in the freely moving rat, probably by suppressing the excitability of interneurons mediating feedforward inhibition (Staubli and Xu, 1995). Support for the notion that the predominant effect of 5-HT is to suppress LTP comes from studies showing that the 5-HT uptake inhibitor fluvoxamine reduces LTP via activation of 5-HT1A receptors (Kojima et al., 2003), whereas injection of a 5-HT4 receptor agonist into the lateral ventricle inhibited LTP, an effect that was blocked by a selective 5-HT4 antagonist (Kulla and Manahan-Vaughan, 2002). The cellular distribution of the relevant 5-HT receptors and the downstream signaling pathways by which 5-HT exerts its effects on LTP remain largely unexplored.

Dopamine. Dopaminergic projections to the hippocampus (primarily to the hilus and stratum radiatum lacunosum) originate in the ventral tegmental area (VTA) and substantia nigra (Scattton et al., 1980; Gasbarri et al., 1997). There is persuasive evidence that dopamine plays an important modulatory role in the induction of protein synthesis-dependent L-LTP in area CA1 (reviewed by Lisman and Grace, 2005). Knockout of the D1 dopamine receptor produces mice that lack L-LTP while displaying normal E-LTP (Matthies et al.,

1997). Bath-applied dopaminergic antagonists similarly block L-LTP when given during, but not after, a strong tetanus applied to induce L-LTP (Frey et al., 1990). Moreover, bath-applied phosphodiesterase inhibitors, which prolong the action of cAMP and so enhance the action of the principal downstream effector of dopamine, protein kinase A, can convert E-LTP into L-LTP (Navakkode et al., 2004). Stimulation of the dopamine receptor-mediated signaling cascade with D1/D5 dopamine receptor agonists or with the cAMP activator forskolin induces protein sythesis-dependent late potentiation that occludes with L-LTP in area CA1 in vitro (Frey et al., 1993; Huang and Kandel, 1995; but see Mockett et al., 2004). Thus, in area CA1, dopamine receptor activation appears to be both necessary and sufficient for the induction of L-LTP. This is not, of course, to say that the release of dopamine or of any other neuromodulator is the primary cause of NMDAR-dependent LTP. D1/D5 agonists can lower the threshold for input-specific tetanus-induced LTP in vitro (Otmakhova and Lisman, 1996) and in vivo (Kusuki et al., 1997). When bath applied at high doses, it can under some circumstances produce L-LTP nonspecifically at many synapses; but this cannot be what happens in the context of input-specific L-LTP. Here, its action may be, rather, to convert or consolidate E-LTP into L-LTP by facilitating gene expression via enhanced PKA activity. Dopamine exerts its effects through activation of PKA, which as we have seen is intimately involved in the dendrite-to-nucleus signaling that triggers gene transcription, and in local dendritic protein synthesis (see Section 10.4.9). In this model, then, dopamine, via cAMP and PKA, is directly involved in the synthesis of plasticity-related proteins (Navakkode et al., 2004). An intriguing aspect of dopamine signaling in area CA1 is that it drives the enhancement of LTP in novel environments (Li et al., 2003; see Lisman and Grace, 2005 for a model of how the hippocampal-VTA loop controls entry of novel experiences into long-term memory). Interestingly, noradrenergic rather than dopaminergic signaling appears to be responsible for novelty-dependent modulation of LTP in the dentate gyrus (Straube et al., 2003).

Brain-derived Neurotrophic Factor

There is abundant evidence that the neurotrophic peptide, brain-derived neurotrophic factor (BDNF), is released as a result of synaptic activity at hippocampal synapses. Extracellular BDNF can act on its receptor trkB, a member of the tropomyosin-related family of receptor tyrosine kinases, to enhance synaptic efficacy at excitatory synapses and diminish efficacy at inhibitory synapses (for reviews, see Schinder and Poo, 2000 and Ernfors and Bramham, 2003). BDNF can probably be released from both pre- and postsynaptic sites at hippocampal synapses and act on populations of pre- and/or postsynaptic trkB receptors whose numbers are regulated by activity. At Schaffer-commissural synapses in area CA1, BDNF can act as a potent excitatory transmitter (Kafitz et al., 1999).

BDNF appears to play a critical role in the induction of LTP. LTP is impaired in BDNF-null mice (Korte et al., 1995), and the deficit can be rescued in vitro by BDNF administered directly (Patterson et al., 1996) or by viral transfection (Korte et al., 1996). BDNF can also produce LTP. Bath application of BDNF to hippocampal slices induces slow-onset, protein synthesis-dependent LTP in area CA1 (Kang and Schuman, 1995), whereas in the dentate gyrus repeated pairing of weak synaptic stimulation with focal dendritic application of BDNF leads to rapid-onset LTP that occludes with tetanus-induced LTP (Kovalchuk et al., 2002). This form of LTP satisfies the criterion for postsynaptic induction, as it is blocked by postsynaptic injection of calcium chelators. A late-onset, transcription-dependent potentiation of synaptic transmission has also been described in the dentate gyrus of the anesthetized rat following transient perfusion with BDNF (Messaoudi et al., 2002) (Fig. 10–2D). The synaptic response climbs gradually after perfusion and persists for many hours thereafter. BDNF-induced late LTP occludes with late tetanus-induced LTP; but in contrast to the rapid-onset LTP observed in the dentate gyrus in vitro, it is not NMDAR-dependent. However, because it leads to CREB phosphorylation via activation of ERK1/2 and upregulation of immediate early genes in granule cells, bath application of BDNF activates, at least in part, the normal late LTP-inducing machinery in the postsynaptic cell downstream from the NMDA receptor (Ying et al., 2002). Changes in CREB phosphorylation in the entorhinal cortex, where the perforant path projection to the dentate gyrus originates, suggests there may also be presynaptic involvement (Gooney et al., 2004).

Little information is available on whether the expression of BDNF-induced LTP is pre- and/or postsynaptically mediated in the hippocampus. In hippocampal cultures, neurotrophin-induced potentiation lasting 10 to 15 minutes carries the hallmarks of a presynaptic mechanism: reduced paired-pulse facilitation, increased mini-EPSP frequency without an increase in amplitude, a reduction in the coefficient of variation, and comparable enhancement of both AMPAR- and NMDA-mediated responses (Schinder and Poo, 2000). Whether endogenous BDNF acts as a retrograde messenger released from the postsynaptic cell to act on presynaptic TrkB receptors remains to be established. A presynaptic component of LTP induced at Schaffer-commissural synapses on CA1 pyramidal cells by theta-burst stimulation requires BDNF. However, analysis of two mutant lines—one expressing a mutant form of BDNF in both CA3 and CA1 cells and the other only in CA1 cells—disclosed an impairment of theta-burst LTP only in the former mutant, suggesting that the source of BDNF is in presynaptic neurons (Zakharenko et al., 2003). In other systems, however, such as the neuromuscular junction, there is clear evidence that BDNF acts as a retrograde messenger (Schinder and Poo, 2000).

Cytokines

A variety of cytokines have been found to interact with LTP. For example, interleukin-1β (IL-1β) reduces mossy fiber LTP (Katsuki et al., 1990) and NMDA receptor-dependent LTP in area CA1 and the dentate gyrus (Bellinger et al., 1993; Cunningham et al., 1996). It has been suggested that endogenous levels of IL-1β are elevated in response to stress, infection, the amyloid peptide Aβ, and aging, and that this may partly account for the neurodegeneration and cognitive deficits sometimes observed in such circumstances (Murray and Lynch, 1998; Minogue et al., 2003). The mechanism by which IL-1β exerts its effects is not fully established but may involve activation of c-Jun N-terminal kinase (JNK) and p38MAPK as well as caspase-1 and NKκB (Vereker et al., 2000a,b; Curran et al., 2003; Kelly et al., 2003). Il-1β also seems to stimulate superoxide dismutase to increase reactive oxygen species (Vereker et al., 2001). In addition to a role in pathology, however, studies with an IL-1 receptor antagonist and an IL-1 receptor knockout have suggested that IL-1 may be required for the induction of LTP under physiological conditions (Avital et al., 2003; Ross et al., 2003; Maher et al., 2005).

Other interleukins, such as IL-2, IL-6, IL-8, and IL-18, also inhibit the induction of LTP (Tancredi et al., 1990; Bellinger et al., 1995; Li et al., 1997; Curran and O'Connor, 2001; Xiong et al., 2003). However, certain interleukins have complex interactions in their regulation of LTP. For example, IL-10 blocks the inhibitory effect of IL-1β on LTP (Kelly et al., 2001). Other cytokines that have been reported to inhibit LTP include the interferons (D'Arcangelo et al., 1991; Mendoza-Fernandez et al., 2000) and tumor necrosis factor alpha (TNFα) (Tancredi et al., 1992). TNFα inhibits early LTP, but not late LTP, via activation of a p38MAPK cascade (Butler et al., 2004) and may mediate its actions via an effect on the trafficking of AMPA receptors (Beattie et al., 2002)

Corticosteroids

The effects of stress on hippocampal plasticity were first explored by Foy et al. (1987). Rats were subjected to mild inescapable stress by confining them in a restraining tube for 30 minutes. Hippocampal slices cut from the brains of animals killed immediately afterward displayed significant impairment in LTP relative to control animals. It later became apparent that an important factor is whether the stress is avoidable; slices from animals that were given shocks but had control over the termination of the shock showed greater LTP than an unshocked group, whereas those that had no control over termination showed less LTP (Shors et al., 1989). Hippocampus-dependent learning is also modulated by stress (see Chapter 15). Later it is was found that mild stress can facilitate the induction of LTD (Xu et al., 1997; Manahan-Vaughan, 2000).

In rodents, stress is associated with an increased plasma concentration of the adrenal hormone corticosterone, The hippocampus is richly endowed with the two types of corticosteroid receptor: the high-affinity mineralocorticoid (or type 1) receptor and the low-affinity glucocorticoid (type II) receptor. Activation of mineralocorticoid receptors promote LTP, whereas high corticosterone levels activate the glucocorticoid receptor, which is the primary mediator of stress-induced impairment of LTP and spatial learning. Thus, there is an inverted-U relationship between the plasma concentration of corticosterone and its effects on LTP and learning. At low concentrations of corticosterone (as occurs following adrenalectomy) the occupancy of mineralocorticoid receptors is low, whereas at high levels (as during severe stress) the glucocorticoid receptors are fully occupied; both conditions are associated with a reduction of LTP, promotion of LTD, and impaired learning. Consequently, LTP and learning are maximal at intermediate levels of circulating corticosterone (Diamond et al., 1992; Kim and Diamond, 2002). It is an oversimplification, however, to assume that corticosterone is the only mediator of the effects of stress on LTP and behavior; in fact, corticosterone is neither necessary nor sufficient for these effects to occur. For example, stress can still suppress LTP in rats deprived of corticosterone by adrenalectomy, and lesions of the amygdala block the stress-induced impairment of LTP even though corticosterone levels remained high in lesioned animals (Kim and Diamond, 2002; Kim et al., 2005c). Priming stimuli delivered to the basolateral amygdala has a biphasic effect on LTP in the dentate gyrus in vivo, enhancing LTP at short priming-tetanus intervals and suppressing LTP if given an hour before the tetanus to the perforant path. The mechanisms by which activity in the amgygdala is able to block LTP in the hippocampus have yet to be worked out, but these findings reflect the intimate manner in which hippocampal plasticity is modulated by the amygdala's view of a stress-filled world (Kim et al., 2005c).

There is evidence that stress engages some of the same signaling pathways that are involved in synaptic plasticity. For example, phosphorylation of the MAP kinase signaling molecules ERK1/2 is markedly increased by stress, and the inhibitory effects of stress on learning and LTP can be blocked by inhibitors of ERK1/2 phosphorylation (Yang et al., 2004). This raises the possibility that the reduction in tetanus-induced LTP during stress reflects potentiation caused by stress itself, pushing the affected synapses toward saturation. However, neither applied corticosterone nor stress has been reported to enhance baseline levels of hippocampal evoked responses. Because NMDA receptor antagonists given at the time of the stressful experience can block the subsequent reduction in LTP, it is likely that the impairment of LTP is due to a metaplastic effect mediated by NMDA receptor activation rather than to saturation of LTP (Abraham, 2004).

Hippocampal regulation of the hypothalamic-pituitary-adrenal axis is discussed in Chapter 15.

10.6.2 Cyclical Influences Modulate Induction of LTP

Sex Hormones and LTP

During proestrus in female rats, when levels of estrogens reach a peak, the number of spines on CA1 pyramdal cells is as much as 30% higher than during estrus (Woolley et al., 1990) (see Chapter 9). Are there corresponding change in the magnitude of LTP and/or LTD during the estrus cycle? There have been two reports that LTP in area CA1 of female rats with chronically implanted electrodes is enhanced during proestrus

(Warren et al., 1995; Good et al., 1999). Subsequent experiments have largely been conducted on ovariectomized animals where the total absence of estrogen has not always led to the reduction in LTP that the experiments in normally cycling animals might have predicted. For example, Day and Good (2005) saw no change in LTP following ovariectomy but did observe impaired LTD that was reversed by chronic estrogen replacement. Whether these estrogen-induced effects on synaptic plasticity are an indirect result of changes in spine numbers or reflect an action of the hormone on signaling pathways or protein synthesis remains to be seen. Puberty in male rats is associated with a bias toward LTD (Hebbard et al., 2003). The effect of pregnancy on LTP does not appear to have been specifically examined, although a greater flexibility in behavior in the watermaze has been noted (Bodensteiner et al., 2006).

Sleep, Circadian Rhythms, and LTP

Sleep is necessary for normal cognitive processing. In particular, it seems likely that during sleep the brain sorts newly acquired information to determine what needs to be committed to long-term storage and then assimilates it with previously learned experiences. The brain is therefore performing complex cognitive processing during sleep that is probably crucial for the consolidation of memories. Several groups have wondered if LTP is modulated during sleep, and in particular during dreaming in REM sleep. Our memory for dreams is surprisingly tenuous, given the vividness of the dreaming experience. Can this be linked to suppression of LTP during REM sleep? It seems not. In the dentate gyrus, the magnitude of LTP induced during REM sleep is similar to that obtained during the alert state (Bramham and Srebro, 1989), although there is a significant reduction in magnitude during slow-wave sleep (Leonard et al., 1987).

Other studies have found that sleep deprivation (12–72 hours) can impair the ability to induce LTP (Campbell et al. 2002; Davis et al. 2003; McDermott et al. 2003; Kim et al., 2005b), possibly because of the stress that is associated with sleep deprivation. However, even when precautions are taken to minimize stress, short periods (4 hours) of REM sleep deprivation result in selective impairment in the maintenance of L-LTP in the perforant path (Romcy-Pereira and Pavlides, 2004).

A clue to what sleep might be doing has been obtained by mapping plasticity using the expression of the immediate early gere *zif268* (Ribeiro et al. 2002). The induction of LTP in the perforant path, which is associated with a rapid increase in the expression of *zif268*, also leads to upregulation of *zif268* expression during subsequent episodes of REM sleep in extrahippocampal regions, predominantly in the amygdala, entorhinal, and auditory cortices during the first REM sleep episode and the somatosensory and motor cerebral cortices as REM sleep recurs. These observations support the hypothesis that sleep enables the spread of memory traces from hippocampus to the cerebral cortex.

Exercise promotes LTP at CA1 synapses: LTP is greater when induced in walking rats than in awake but immobile animals or during slow-wave or REM sleep (Leung et al., 2003). The enhanced synaptic plasticity in walking animals is promoted by the septal cholinergic input to the hippocampus.

The pyramidal and granule cell subfields respond differently to night–day variations. In the dentate gyrus, LTP is significantly greater when induced during the dark, active stage of the rat's diurnal cycle (Harris and Teyler, 1983; Dana and Martinez, 1984), consistent with the reduction in LTP observed during slow-wave sleep and perhaps reflecting the greater baseline fEPSPs obtained in the dark (Barnes et al., 1977). In CA1, in contrast, LTP is greater during the light, behaviorally inactive stage. The reasons for this difference and its functional significance are unknown.

Hibernation

The temperature of hibernating animals can fall to a value at which synaptic transmission fails. As temperature rises on arousal from hibernation, the magnitude of LTP is greater than in control animals maintained at the same temperature (Spangenberger et al., 1995). This no doubt provides a welcome boost to its cognitive faculties at a generally trying time for the hamster.

10.6.3 Neurogenesis and LTP

Neurogenesis proceeds at a truly astonishing rate in the dentate gyrus of adult animals (see Chapter 9). In the rat, approximately 9000 new granule cells are born each day. (Box 9–1), approaching 1% of the total number of granule cells in the each dentate gyrus (Section 3.4.1). Performance in some (but not all) hippocampus-dependent tasks (e.g., trace eyeblink conditioning) is blocked by administration of methylazoxymethanol, a toxin that kills dividing cells (Shors et al., 2001). One explanation for this observation is that newborn granule cells are necessary for encoding the learned task. What is the physiological evidence that would support such a conclusion? First, although most newborn cells die, those that survive are incorporated into the neural network of the dentate gyrus, sending axons toward the stratum pyramidale of area CA3 (Hastings and Gould, 1999; Markakis and Gage, 1999) and extending dendrites into the molecular layer where they make synaptic contact with axons of the perforant path (Song et al., 2002). Second, neurogenesis and LTP are enhanced by running (van Praag et al., 1999). Third, immature granule cells have a lower threshold for LTP than do adult cells (Schmidt-Hieber et al., 2004). The reason for this seems to be the much higher input resistance of immature cells (leading to greater depolarization for a given synaptic current) and the expression by immature cells of T-type Ca^{2+} channels that support Ca^{2+} spikes following relatively small depolarizations. These characteristics lead, on the one hand, to greater relief of the Mg^{2+} block of the NMDA receptor and, on the other, to enhanced Ca^{2+} entry, both of which promote the induction of LTP (Schmidt-Hieber et al., 2004). However, there is clearly some way to go before we can conclude that neurogenesis contributes to the cellular basis of learning. Among the basic questions that await answers are (1) what is the lifetime of newborn cells that mature into fully connected members of the adult granule cell network, (2) how does the hippocampus maintain a stable representation of stored events in the face of a continuing turnover of granule cells, and (3) why is adult neurogenesis confined to the dentate gyrus and olfactory bulb. As Schinder and Gage (2004) have pointed out, the tool needed to establish a causal role for neurogenesis in learning is a genetic model in which neurogenesis can be turned on and off at will.

10.7 Long-term Depression and Depotentiation: Properties and Mechanisms

10.7.1 Overview

If activity-dependent plasticity operated only to enhance synaptic weights, saturation of synaptic efficacy would eventually ensue. A neural net composed of Hebbian synapses all of whose synaptic weights were maximal would be incapable of learning. Although many, if not all, potentiated synapses may eventually decay to baseline through the passage of time, an activity-driven mechanism to allow erasure, or depotentiation, of LTP would enhance the computational flexibility of the network. An additional mechanism permitting activity-dependent LTD from baseline values of synaptic efficacy, and independent of LTP, so-called de novo LTD, would further enhance the flexibility of the system and increase its storage capacity (Dayan and Willshaw, 1991). Another important consideration is the balance of excitation and inhibition that determines the overall stability of the network. Unbridled potentiation would carry the danger of disrupting this balance and driving the system to instability and seizure. The homeostatic checks and balances that the hippocampus deploys at both the cell and network levels to guard against runaway excitation are described in Section 10.3.14; in this light, both the homosynaptic properties of LTD and depotentiation, and the heterosynaptic depression that in some cases accompanies the induction of LTP, may be considered additional weapons in the network's homeostatic armory.

A word on nomenclature: In what follows, by LTD we mean de novo LTD. The depression of a potentiated response we refer to as depotentiation, and the repotentiation of a depressed response as de-depression. It is important to keep these terms distinct because, as we shall see, they embody different mechanisms. Depotentiation, for example, is true reversal or erasure of LTP, not the superposition of depression on a still potentiated background.

Heterosynaptic forms of LTD and depotentiation provided the first indication that, in addition to LTP, hippocampal synapses could support long-term, activity-dependent reductions in synaptic efficacy (Lynch et al., 1977; Levy and Steward, 1979) (Fig. 10–17A,B). Later work also established that during the first few minutes after its induction (but not at later times) LTP could be "destabilized" (depotentiated) by low-frequency stimulation (Barrionuevo et al., 1980; Staubli and Lynch, 1990; Fujii et al., 1991) (Fig. 10–17B). Further progress was slow, largely because of the lack of a reliable protocol for inducing LTD. The discovery by Dudek and Bear (1992) that prolonged trains of low-frequency stimulation (LFS), typically 900 stimuli at 1 Hz, induced both homosynaptic LTD and homosynaptic depotentiation in hippocampal slices from juvenile rats provided a major impetus to research (Fig. 10–17D, Fig. 10–19A). Progress in studying LTD in the adult animal, however, whether in vivo or in vitro, is still hampered by the lack of effective stimulus protocol(s) that produce LTD most of the time in most laboratories. This has led to speculation that de novo LTD is a form of synaptic plasticity whose major role lies in the sculpting and pruning of synaptic connections during development of the nervous system. Nevertheless, to prevent network saturation and to preserve an overall mean level of excitability in the network, the conclusion seems unavoidable that mechanisms to decrease synaptic weights must also be available to the fully developed hippocampus.

Initial uncertainties about whether the induction of LTD in area CA1 was NMDAR-dependent (Dudek and Bear, 1992) or mGluR-dependent (Bashir et al., 1993) were resolved when Oliet et al. (1997) showed that it was possible to obtain either result by manipulating the induction protocol, thus confirming the existence of two independent forms of homosynaptic LTD. In both area CA1 and the dentate gyrus, mGluR-dependent LTD is reliably induced at all ages by exposure to the group 1 agonist DHPG (Palmer et al., 1997) (Fig. 10-17E) or by low-frequency trains of *pairs* of pulses at an appropriate inter-pulse interval (Kemp et al., 2000) (see Section 10.7.5). A third form of LTD has been reported at mossy fiber synapses early in postnatal development that requires neither NMDA nor mGlu receptors (Domenici et al., 1998).

The two major forms of LTD have different developmental profiles: In vitro, both NMDAR- and mGlu receptor-dependent LTD occur in area CA1 in the neonate, giving way to predominantly mGluR-LTD in the adult (Kemp et al., 2000). Pharmacological blockade of the uptake of L-glutamate facilitates induction of NMDAR-dependent LTD in perirhinal cortex (Massey et al., 2004) and in area CA1 (Yang et al., 2005). This suggests that mechanisms exist for NMDAR-dependent LTD but that normal uptake processes limit their deployment. Because uptake mechanisms are strongly temperature-dependent, they are likely to be more effective in vivo than in vitro, where experiments are rarely performed at physiological temperatures. This might be one reason why LTD is often not observed in vivo. However, NMDAR-dependent LTD can be induced in area CA1 of the adult rat in vivo by low-frequency trains of paired-pulse stimuli with a brief 25 msec interpulse interval (Thiels et al., 1994; Doyère et al., 1996; Thiels et al., 2002).

The molecular mechanisms responsible for the expression of NMDAR-dependent LTD have been extensively studied; induction is postsynaptic, and postsynaptic components of expression include dephosphorylation of GluR1 subunits and internalization of GluR2-containing AMPA receptors. Expression of mGluR-LTD appears to involve both presynaptic and postsynaptic components.

In this section, we deal first with homosynaptic forms of synaptic depression and then go on to examine heterosynaptic LTD and depotentiation. Different hippocampal subfields display substantial differences in the types of homosynaptic and heterosynaptic LTD and depotentiation they can sustain. Although the number of in vivo studies on LTD is growing, most of the experiments have been conducted on hippocampal slices from young animals in area CA1, and the text necessarily reflects this bias. Separate sections are devoted to LTD and depotentiation in the mossy fiber projection (see Section 10.7.8) and LTD at connections to and from interneurons (see Section 10.8). For a wide-ranging review of LTD and depotentiation see Kemp and Bashir (2001); mGluR-dependent LTD has been reviewed by Bashir (2003).

10.7.2 NMDAR-dependent LTD: Properties and Characteristics

In Vitro Studies

The first report that LTD could be achieved with low-frequency stimulation (LFS) (e.g., 100 stimuli at 1 Hz) was published by Dunwiddie and Lynch (1978). However, it was not until several years later when Dudek and Bear (1992) (Fig. 10–17D) found that prolonged trains of LFS reliably produced LTD in young animals that experimental interest in LTD began to accelerate. LTD is routinely obtained with the Bear-Dudek protocol (typically 900 stimuli at 1Hz) only when slices are prepared from juvenile rats (Dudek and Bear, 1993; O'Dell and Kandel, 1994; Wang and Alger, 1995). LTD induced with this protocol is long-lasting, input-specific, NMDAR-dependent, apparently saturable, and reversible by tetanic stimulation ("dedepression") (Dudek and Bear, 1992).

Dudek and Bear went on to develop the notion of graded bidirectional synaptic modifiability (Dudek and Bear, 1993) (Fig. 10–19A). In this model, with appropriate high- or low-frequency stimulation, a synapse could be potentiated, depotentiated, depressed, or de-depressed, thus allowing its efficacy to be set anywhere within a range of approximately ± 50% of its base level. The difficulty often encountered of depotentiating a pathway once LTP has been stabilized in the adult animal implies that there are temporal constraints on bidirectionality. A proposed molecular basis for bidirectionality is discussed below. [An alternative hypothesis to graded bidirectional changes is that a modifiable synapse can switch only between three digital levels: resting, potentiated, and depressed. Electrophysiological evidence in favor of a binary all-or-none model of LTP at single synapses was presented by Petersen et al. (1998), but confirmatory studies have not been published.

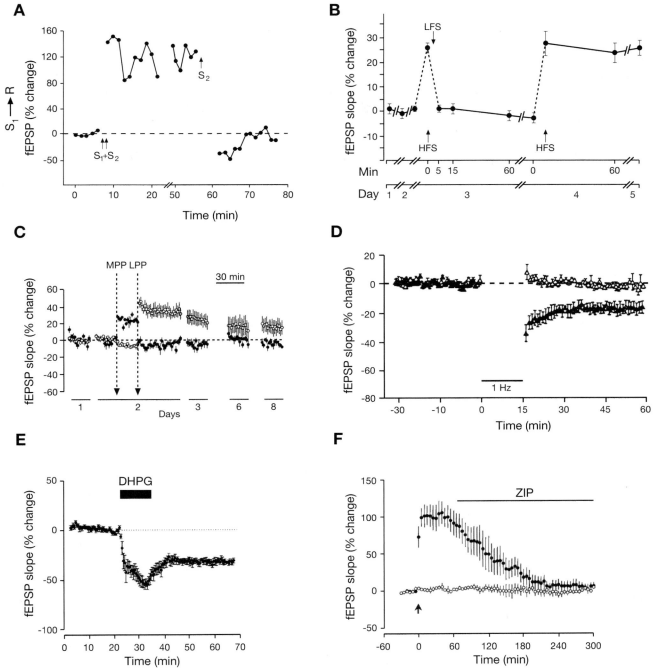

Figure 10–17. Types of hippocampal long-term homosynaptic and heterosynaptic depression. *A.* Heterosynaptic depotentiation of crossed perforant path responses ($S_1 \rightarrow R$) in the anesthetized rat. The graph plots the amplitude of fEPSPs evoked in the dentate gyrus of an anesthetized rat by test stimuli (S_1) to the contralateral perforant path. LTP of the contralateral input is induced only by associative tetanization of both ipsilateral and contralateral inputs (double arrow, $S_1 + S_2$). The potentiated contralateral response was then heterosynaptically depotentiated by a tetanus to the ipsilateral pathway (S_2). A subsequent combined tetanus restored the potentiated response (not shown). (*Source*: Levy and Steward, 1979.) *B.* Persistent homosynaptic depotentiation in a freely moving rat. Low-frequency trains (1 Hz for 100 to 250 seconds) given 10 to 15 minutes after the induction of LTP in area CA1 caused a rapid return to baseline. A second tetanus delivered 24 hours later, when the response was still at baseline, led to the reinstatement of LTP.

(*Source*: Staubli and Lynch, 1990.) *C.* Heterosynaptic depotentiation of the medial perforant path in the freely moving rat after tetanic stimulation of the lateral perforant path. The response remains depotentiated over the following days. (*Source*: Doyère et al., 1997.) *D.* Prolonged low-frequency stimulation (1 Hz for 15 min) induces LTD in area CA1 in vitro. This is the protocol now most commonly used to induce LTD. It is most effective in young animals. (*Source*: Dudek and Bear, 1992.) *E.* LTD induced in area CA1 in vitro by bath application of the type 1 mGluR agonist DHPG. The perfusion fluid contained picrotoxin and AP5; hence, under these conditions the effect is NMDA receptor-independent. Synaptic responses were recorded using a grease gap technique (*Source*: Palmer et al., 1997.) *F.* ZIP, a membrane permeable substrate inhibitor of PKMζ, reverses LTP in area CA1 in vitro when applied 60 min after induction (filled circles) without affecting the nontetanized control pathway (open circles) (*Source*: Ling et al., 2002).

Optical studies of transmission at single visualized synapses probably offer the best approach to the issue.]

When LTP is saturated and then depotentiated by LFS, it can subsequently be reinstated from the depotentiated level by high-frequency stimulation. This experiment demonstrates that depotentiation is not simply a superposition of LTD on a continuing but now hidden LTP because if that were the case LTP would remain saturated and thus be incapable of enhancement. Rather, depotentiation is genuine erasure of LTP, returning the pathway to a state in which LTP can again be elicited (Dudek and Bear, 1992, 1993). However, LTD and depotentiation are not the same phenomenon (in the sense that they are generated by a common mechanism) because different phosphatases are involved in the two cases (Lee et al., 2000) (see Fig. 10–19B); and in cortex at least, induction is controlled by different NMDA receptor subunits (NR2B for LTD and NR2A for depotentiation) (Massey et al., 2004). Moreover, in knockout mice lacking the Aα catalytic subunit of calcineurin, LTD can be elicited but depotentiation cannot (Zhuo et al., 1999). The limited time window for depotentiation following the induction of LTP also suggests that it is mechanistically different from LTD, which can be induced, in principle, at any time in naïve synapses.

In Vivo Studies

In general, in vivo experiments confirm that it is considerably more difficult to obtain LTD and depotentiation in the intact adult rat than in younger animals. Nevertheless, both LTD and depotentiation can be induced with low-frequency trains in area CA1 of the intact animal, although modifications of the standard protocol are often necessary. There is also evidence that susceptibility to LTD is strain-specific, with Wistar and Sprague-Dawley rats showing a lower threshold for LTD than hooded Listers (Manahan-Vaughan, 2000). The standard 900 pulses/1Hz protocol has been successfully used by some (Heynen et al., 1996; Manahan-Vaughan, 1997), whereas others have found it necessary to use trains at higher frequencies (2–5 Hz) (Doyle et al., 1997) or paired-pulse trains consisting of pairs of stimuli at 0.5 Hz, with a 25-ms interpulse interval chosen to maximize paired-pulse depression (Thiels et al., 1994; Doyère et al., 1996). The incidence of LTD is greater in freely moving animals if they are subjected to mild stress (Xu et al., 1997). LTD has been particularly elusive in the dentate gyrus (Errington et al., 1995; Abraham et al., 1996) where in the freely moving rat it has been elicited only under conditions of stress or following perfusion with mGluR agonists (reviewed by Braunewell and Manahan-Vaughan, 2001). It is, of course, possible that the optimal patterns of activity for inducing LTD in the dentate gyrus have yet to be identified. Depotentiation in the intact animal is discussed below.

How long is the "long" in long-term depression? Homosynaptic LTD can persist for days in chronically implanted animals (Doyère et al., 1996), and depotentiation has been followed for more than 24 hours (Kulla et al., 1999). Heterosynaptic depression can also last for days (Abraham et al., 1994; Doyère et al., 1997) (Fig. 10–17C). A late, protein synthesis-dependent component of LTD has been described for NMDAR-dependent LTD in area CA1, induced by low-frequency stimulation both in vivo (Manahan-Vaughan et al. m 2000) and in hippocampal slice cultures (Kauderer and Kandel, 2000). An early protein synthesis-dependent phase of mGluR-dependent LTD is seen in acute slices (Hüber et al., 2000). An experimentally useful equivalence has been established between LTD induced by the mGluR group 1 agonist DHPG and by a low-frequency paired-pulse protocol; these two stimulus protocols both produce long-lasting, protein synthesis-dependent forms of LTD that when saturated mutually occlude each other, strongly suggesting a shared mechanism (Hüber et al., 2001).

10.7.3 NMDAR-dependent LTD: Induction Mechanisms

Long-term depression is defined as NMDAR-dependent if it is blocked by D-AP5 or other NMDA antagonists. There is convincing evidence that the induction of NMDAR-dependent LTD requires a rise in postsynaptic Ca^{2+} and that the polarity of the change in synaptic efficacy is determined by the amplitude and time course of the Ca^{2+} transient. First, the induction of LTD can be prevented by dialyzing CA1 pyramidal cells with a Ca^{2+} chelator (Mulkey and Malenka, 1992). Second, lowering external Ca^{2+} transforms a protocol that normally induces LTP into one that produces LTD (Mulkey and Malenka, 1992). Third, Cummings et al. (1996) manipulated Ca^{2+} entry into the postsynaptic cell in a number of ways, including the application of low doses of AP5 to limit Ca^{2+} entry during the tetanus, which again converted LTP to LTD. These observations indicate that the level of the increase in intracellular Ca^{2+} is a critical parameter in determining the direction of change in synaptic strength. They provide support for an influential scheme proposed by Lisman (1989) that exploits the fact that certain protein phosphatases have a higher affinity for Ca^{2+} than most protein kinases. This suggests a potential mechanism whereby low elevations of Ca^{2+} activate protein phosphatases to yield LTD, whereas higher concentrations activate protein kinases to yield LTP. In Lisman's scheme, activated protein kinases, in particular autophosphorylated αCaMKII, enhance synaptic efficacy by phosphorylating receptor subunits, while this process is reversed by activation of phosphatases. Phosphorylation of AMPA receptors is known to increase AMPA receptor-mediated currents, which could account at least in part for the increase in synaptic efficacy in LTP (see Section 10.4). Phosphorylated CaMKII is a substrate for a protein phosphatase (PP1) but PP1 is not itself Ca^{2+}-sensitive. To account for LTD, Lisman therefore invoked a phosphatase cascade that begins with activation of the Ca^{2+}-sensitive protein phosphatase calcineurin (also known as protein phosphatase 2B, or PP2B). Activated calcineurin then dephosphorylates a phosphoprotein called inhibitor 1 (I1), which in its activated state inhibits PP1. Activation of calcineurin thus leads to the activation of PP1 by disinhibition, allowing CaMKII to be dephosphorylated. A critical feature of this scheme is that calcineurin has a higher sensitivity for Ca^{2+} than CaMKII, consistent with the hypothesis that small increases in intracellular Ca^{2+} lead to LTD and larger increases to LTP. Note also that the scheme provides for a feedback, or gating, mechanism in which the PKA/inhibitor 1 pathway counteracts the effects of the calcineurin pathway when Ca^{2+} levels rise to levels that lead to autophosphorylation of CaMKII and LTP (Lisman, 1989; Blitzer et al., 1998).

As is the case for LTP, there is evidence that specific NMDAR subtypes are involved in LTD. A requirement for the NR2B-containing NMDARs was suggested by a knockout of this subunit (Kutsuwada et al., 1996). These animals lacked LTD but had major developmental problems and died young. Several groups have subsequently used NR2B subtype-specific NMDAR antagonists, such as ifenprodil and its more selective derivatives Ro-25-6981 and CP-101,606, to investigate the role of this subunit more directly, but no clear picture has yet emerged. Thus, at one extreme LTD is reported to be enhanced by NR2B inhibitors (Hendricson et al., 2002) and at the other blocked by these compounds (Liu et al., 2004a) Other pharmacological evidence has instead provided evidence for a role of NR2C and/or NR2D receptors in LTD (Hrabetova et al., 2000). There is also evidence that NR2D receptors can mediate a very slow component of the synaptic response at hippocampal synapses (Lozovaya et al., 2004). The very slow kinetics of this channel coupled with its low sensitivity to Mg^{2+} means that the NR2D component of the NMDAR-mediated EPSC will summate effectively at the low frequencies of stimulation that are typically used to induce LTD. Presumably, the relative roles of the different NR2 subunits in LTD is determined by a variety of factors. Interestingly, in this context, Pro-BDNF has been shown to facilitate LTD via activation of p75 leading to up-regulation of NR2B receptors (Woo et al., 2005).

Support for the Lisman hypothesis has come from experiments by Malenka and colleagues, who found that LTD was blocked by injecting specific inhibitors of PP1 and calcineurin into CA1 neurons (Mulkey et al., 1993, 1994). On the other hand, a study of transgenic mice expressing an inducible calcineurin inhibitor failed to confirm the importance of calcineurin for LTD; although LTP was enhanced, LTD was not affected (Malleret et al., 2001), suggesting either that the inhibitors were acting on another phosphatase or that another high-affinity phosphatase can take over the role normally played by calcineurin. Overall, there is good evidence that the amplitude and kinetics of the synaptically evoked Ca^{2+} transient is critical for setting the sign of synaptic change. As predicted by the model, lower Ca^{2+} charge transfer through the NMDA receptor channel is associated with LTD and higher transfer with LTP (Cho et al., 2001; Wu et al., 2001).

Depolarizing pulses delivered to the postsynaptic cell to draw Ca^{2+} into the cell via L-type Ca^{2+} channels is itself suffi-

cient to induce persistent LTD (Cummings et al., 1996). This approach was taken further by Yang et al. (1999), who used graduated photolysis of a caged Ca^{2+} compound, DM-EGTA, to control the level and rate of rise of cytosolic calcium. These studies made the important point that the rate of rise and the magnitude of the Ca^{2+} transient are jointly involved in determining the polarity of the change in synaptic efficacy. Large, rapid rises in Ca^{2+} invariably produced persistent potentiation, whereas small, prolonged increases always induced persistent depression. In both cases calcium-induced plasticity occluded activity-induced LTP or LTD, suggesting a convergence of cellular mechanisms. The importance of the prolonged duration of the Ca^{2+} transient for the induction of LTD in area CA1 has been further underlined in experiments by Mizuno et al. (2001); pharmacological manipulations were used to control the magnitude of the Ca^{2+} transient produced by 1 Hz stimulation, but under no circumstances were trains of less than 200 stimuli successful in inducing LTD. A model of the probable signaling cascades involved in NMDAR-dependent LTD is shown in Figure 10–18A.

Spike Timing-dependent Induction of LTD

As we saw in Section 10.3, when plasticity is induced by conjoint presynaptic stimulation and a back-propagating spike in the postsynaptic neuron, it is the interval between the onset of the two events that determines the sign of the persistent change. In hippocampal slices, potentiation results when the EPSP precedes the back-propagating action potential (AP) in CA1 pyramidal neurons by 0 to 10 ms (Magee and Johnston, 1997). This result was confirmed in experiments on pairs of connected hippocampal neurons in organotypic culture (Debanne et al., 1998) (Fig. 10–19C) or in dissociated culture (Bi and Poo, 1998) (Fig. 10–19D). Moreover, LTD was induced if the order was reversed, with the back-propagating AP preceding the EPSP, extending to the hippocampus a pattern first established in neocortical neurons (Markram et al., 1997). The pattern of excitation and inhibition is more complex in hippocampal slices (Nishiyama et al., 2000). Potentiation results when the onset of the EPSP and back-propagating AP occur within 10 ms of each other, irrespective of order. Symmetrically placed on either side of the window of potentiation are two 20-ms intervals, between −10 and − 30 ms (AP preceding EPSP) and 10 and 30 ms (EPSP preceding AP), within which paired activity results in homosynaptic LTD. The latter is probably explained by the recruitment of feedforward inhibition (Bi and Rubin, 2005). Furthermore, in contrast to the usual absence of heterosynaptic depression in area CA1 following tetanus-induced LTP, heterosynaptic depression occupied the same intervals and displayed the same magnitude as homosynaptic depression; notably absent, however, was any indication of heterosynaptic LTP.

Spike timing-dependent LTD is also NMDAR-dependent, but it is far from clear how it relates to conventional LTD induced by prolonged low-frequency stimulation (Lisman and Spruston, 2005). The rules of induction are very different,

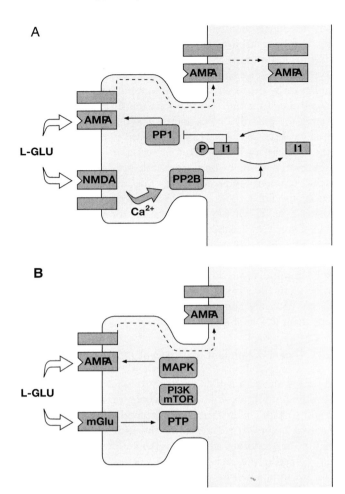

Figure 10–18. Mechanisms involved in the induction of LTD. *A.* NMDA receptor-dependent LTD. The entry of Ca^{2+} via NMDA receptors leads to activation of calcineurin (PP2B). This inhibits inhibitor-1 (I1), which in turn results in activation of protein phosphatase 1 (PP1). This leads to the internalization of AMPARs, probably after they have moved laterally away from the synapse. *B.* mGluR-dependent LTD. Activation of mGlu receptors, in particular mGlu5, also leads to removal of AMPARs from synapses. Here the signaling mechanisms involve protein tyrosine phosphatases (PTPs), mTOR, PI3K and MAPKs. How these enzymes interact is not known. See text for further details.

and it is possible that their expression mechanisms are different too. Do they occlude? Is spike timing-dependent LTD blocked by the same sub type selective NMDA receptor antagonists as conventional LTD? What is the age dependence of spike timing-dependent LTD? What are the relative roles of conventional LTD and spike timing-dependent LTD in the behaving animal? These are questions for future research.

10.7.4 NMDAR-dependent LTD: Expression Mechanisms

In their characterization of two forms of LTD referred to above, Oliet et al. (1997) concluded that NMDAR-dependent

LTD, which was accompanied by a decrease in quantal size, is probably mediated by a postsynaptic mechanism; mGluR-dependent LTD, in contrast, is more likely to be presynaptically expressed (see below). Subsequently, dephosphorylation of AMPA receptor subunits and internalization of both AMPA and NMDA receptors have emerged as mechanisms contributing to the early expression of NMDAR-dependent LTD. There is also evidence for a presynaptic component of expression.

Presynaptic Expression Mechanisms

NMDAR-mediated and AMPAR-mediated currents are equally downregulated in LTD (Xiao et al., 1995), a finding that is compatible with a reduction in transmitter release or with internalization of both receptor types. The evidence for downregulation of AMPA receptors is strong and, together with other evidence for postsynaptic changes discussed above, makes an overwhelming case for a postsynaptic contribution to NMDAR-dependent LTP. However, this does not exclude a presynaptic contribution. Evidence for presynaptic involvement in the expression of NMDAR-dependent LTD has emerged from imaging studies of vesicular turnover using the fluorescent styryl dye FM1-43 (Stanton et al., 2001, 2003). The rate of release from a rapidly releasing pool of vesicles was significantly less after the induction of LTD than it was before induction. The effect was NMDAR-dependent and required NO release and activation of presynaptic cGMP, raising the possibility that NO is acting as a retrograde messenger (see Section 10.4.7).

Postsynaptic Expression Mechanisms

A unitary mechanism for bidirectional changes in synaptic efficacy has obvious attractions (Dudek and Bear, 1993). However, an illuminating study on the phosphorylation of GluR1 residues in LTP and LTD, although confirming the view that depotentiation is a reversal of LTP, suggests that LTP and LTD involve phosphorylation and dephosphorylation at different residues on GluR1 (Lee et al., 2000). In this scheme (Fig. 10–19B), AMPA receptors in the baseline state are phosphorylated at serine residue 845. High-frequency stimulation leads to activation of CaMKII and phosphorylation of ser831, a state associated with increased single-channel conductance of the receptor (Derkach et al., 1999). Depotentiation by low-frequency stimulation reverses this process by activation of protein phosphatases PP1 and PP2A. Low-frequency stimulation in the naïve slice activates the same okadaic acid-sensitive protein phosphatases, but in this condition it is ser845 that is dephosphorylated, leading to a subunit that is phosphorylated at neither serine residue. High-frequency stimulation in this state activates PKA to rephosphorylate the receptor on ser845 and restore it to its baseline state. Continued high-frequency stimulation would then progress to activation of αCaMKII via phosphorylation of S831 and hence to LTP. Note that this scheme cannot explain the relative immunity to depotentia-

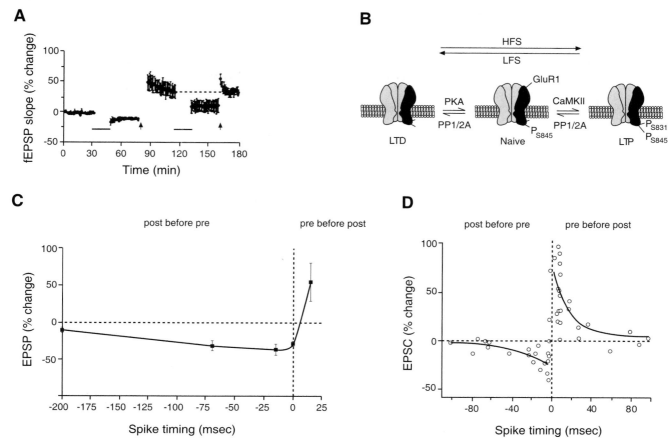

Figure 10–19. Bidirectional plasticiy. *A*. Bidirectional plasticiy in area CA1 in vivo. LTD induced by low-frequency stimulation (LFS) (1 Hz for 15 minutes) (bar) followed by induction of LTP by high-frequency stimulation (HFS) (100 Hz for 1 second) (arrow), partial depotentiation by LFS, and repotentiation by HFS. (*Source*: Heynen et al., 1996.) *B*. Model of changes in the phosphorylation state of the GluR1 subunit of the AMPA receptor that underlie NMDA receptor-dependent early LTP, depotentiation, early LTD and dedepression. In the naïve state, the receptor is phosphorylated at serine 845 (S845). E-LTP is expressed via αCaMKII-mediated phosphorylation of serine 831. Depotentiation involves the dephosphorylation of S831 via protein phosphatases PP1 and/or PP2A. Early LTD involves dephosphorylation of S845, again by PP1/PP2A, and dedepression after LTD brings the receptor back to the naïve

state via PKA-mediated phosphorylation of serine845. (*Source*: Lee et al., 2000.) *C, D*. Two examples of bidirectional spike timing-dependent synaptic plasticity (STDP). *C*. STDP elicited by activating pairs of interconnected CA3 cells in organotypic cultures. LTP was induced if an action potential in the presynaptic cell was repeatedly evoked 15 ms before an action potential in the postsynaptic cell; at zero delay or when the postsynaptic spike preceded the presynaptic spike by 15 to 70 ms, LTD was induced. (*Source*: After Debanne et al., 1998.) *D*. STDP in pairs of interconnected pyramidal cells in dissociated hippocampal cultures. Again, LTP is induced if the presynaptic cell fires shortly before the postsynaptic cell, and LTD ensues if the timing is reversed. Each circle represents a single pairing experiment. (*Source*: Bi and Poo, 1998.)

tion once LTP has become stabilized, perhaps by protein synthesis-dependent mechanisms. Subsequent studies have shown that results from the intact animal are compatible with the model. Similar post-translational changes in GluR1 phosphorylation levels on ser845 occur in visual cortex following monocular deprivation (Bear, 2003) and transgenic animals with point mutations on serine residues 831 and 845 (rendering them nonphosphorylatable) exhibit impaired spatial memory, deficits in LTP, and complete suppression of NMDAR-dependent LTD (Lee et al., 2000). The latter result must be reconciled with the evidence for a protein synthesis-dependent component of this form of LTD, discussed below (Kauderer and Kandel, 2000).

A number of techniques have been used to demonstrate downregulation of both AMPA and NMDA receptors in NMDAR-dependent LTD. They include photolytic uncaging of caged glutamate (Kandler et al., 1998; Rammes et al., 2003), iontophoresis of NMDA (Montgomery and Madison, 2002), and immunocytochemical estimates of both AMPA and NMDA populations in tissue from animals in which LTD was induced in vivo (Heynen et al., 2000). The use of antibodies that recognize extracellular epitopes of AMPA receptors on living neurons (Collingridge et al., 2004) has allowed direct demonstration of AMPA receptor internalization during LTD in cultured hippocampal neurons (Beattie et al., 2000). Subsequent studies using pHluorin-GluR2 have suggested that internalization occurs at extrasynaptic sites and that this precedes removal of AMPA receptors from the synapse (Ashby et al., 2004). The simplest model therefore is one in which endocytosis at an extrasynaptic site is followed by lateral diffusion of AMPA receptors from synaptic to extrasynaptic locations.

Many of the proteins that control the cycling of GluR2 between cytoplasm and synaptic membrane have been identified, and details of their modes of action are beginning to emerge (Collingridge et al., 2004). The concept of subunit-dependent regulation of synaptic plasticity arose from the finding that NSF binds selectively to the GluR2 subunit of AMPA receptors (Nishimune et al., 1998; Osten et al., 1998; Song et al., 1998). Of note were the observations that blockade of the GluR2 interaction with NSF leads to a run-down in AMPAR-mediated synaptic transmission (Nishimune et al., 1998; Song et al., 1998), a reduction in the surface expression of AMPA receptors (Lüscher et al., 1999; Noel et al; 1999), and occlusion with NMDAR-dependent LTD (Lüscher et al., 1999; Lüthi et al., 1999). It was subsequently discovered that AP2 binds to a region of GluR2 that overlaps with the NSF site (Lee et al., 2002). Selective block of the GluR2 interaction with NSF caused a run-down in synaptic transmission, and selective block of the GluR2 interaction with AP2 resulted in suppression LTD. This suggests a mechanism whereby NSF is normally bound to GluR2 subunits to stabilize AMPA receptors at the synapse. However, in response to an LTD-inducing stimulus, AP2 exchanges with NSF, and this initiates clathrin-dependent endocytosis (Collingridge et al., 2004). This scheme requires a mechanism to initiate the exchange of NSF for AP2. One possibility is that Ca^{2+} entry during the induction of LTD interacts with the neuronal Ca^{2+} sensor hippocalcin (Burgoyne, 2004). On binding Ca^{2+}, hippocalcin undergoes a conformational change to expose a myristoylated region that can target the molecule to the plasma membrane. It also binds both AP2 and GluR2 subunits in a Ca^{2+}-dependent manner (Palmer et al, 2005). Thus, hippocalcin is well placed to actively promote the exchange of NSF for AP2. Consistent with this idea, a dominant negative form of hippocalcin blocks induction of NMDAR-dependent LTD (Palmer et al, 2005). Thus, hippocalcin is a strong contender for the role of Ca^{2+} sensor in LTD. It is likely, however, that other Ca^{2+}-sensing proteins are also involved in the induction of LTD, and the full mechanistic details have yet to be elucidated.

Scaffolding proteins such as GRIP/ABP (Dong et al., 1997; Srivastava and Ziff, 1999) and the PKC-targeting protein PICK (Dev et al., 1999; Xia et al., 1999) also bind to the C terminal tail of the GluR2 subunit, where they may tether AMPA receptors at the plasma membrane or at intracellular sites. There is evidence that PICK1 is directly involved in LTD (Kim et al., 2001). The proposal is that GRIP/ABP normally anchors AMPA receptors at the synapse. However, LTD leads to activation of PICK1, which phosphorylates GluR2 subunits, causing them to dissociate from GRIP/ABP so they can be removed from the synapse. Indeed, it has been shown that PICK1 binds Ca^{2+}, facilitating its interaction with AMPA receptors (Hanley

and Henley, 2005). Furthermore, a Ca^{2+}-insensitive PICK1 mutant blocks NMDA-induced internalization of AMPA receptors, implicating this interaction in LTD. However, another idea is that GRIP/ABP binds the GluR2 subunit to maintain a store of AMPA receptors intracellularly (Daw et al., 2000). In this scheme, when PICK1 phosphorylates GluR2 it untethers AMPA receptors and so provides a pool near the synapse, ready for membrane insertion. It is possible that these diametrically opposed roles of PICK1, via its interaction with GRIP/ABP, can both operate under different conditions. Considerable work still needs to be done to understand the relation between the various proteins involved in AMPA receptor trafficking and LTD.

Although the role of the GluR2 subunit in LTD is well established, it is not the only mechanism that supports NMDAR-dependent LTD in the hippocampus. This is shown by studies using knockouts, where NMDAR-dependent LTD has been observed in both the GluR2 knockout and the GluR2/GluR3 double knockout (Jia et al., 1996; Meng et al., 2003). Moreover, as we have seen, the dephosphorylation of ser845 of GluR1 can also result in LTD (Kameyama et al., 1998), suggesting that there are multiple mechanisms for the induction of LTD. Further studies are required to understand the relative contributions of these various mechanisms to LTD in wild-type animals in vivo.

A Protein Synthesis-dependent Phase of NMDAR-dependent LTD

Three investigations published in 2000 established that NMDAR-dependent LTD can sustain a late, protein-dependent phase. Different preparations were used in each of these studies: organotypic cultures (Kauderer and Kandel, 2000), acute slices (Hüber et al., 2000), and freely moving rats (Manahan-Vaughan et al., 2000). In all three preparations, late LTD lasting several hours could be induced by prolonged low-frequency stimulation, and in each case it was blocked by protein synthesis inhibitors. However, only in organotypic culture was late LTD blocked by transcriptional inhibitors. Local protein synthesis may therefore provide the message captured by the tags set by LTD-inducing stimulation (Kauderer and Kandel, 2000; Sajikumar and Frey, 2004b) (see Section 10.4.9).

10.7.5 mGluR-dependent LTD

mGluR-dependent LTD Induced by Synaptic Activity

Homosynaptic LTD using low-frequency stimulation is blocked by NMDA receptor antagonists (Dudek and Bear, 1992; Mulkey and Malenka, 1992). Before long, however, it was shown that certain forms of LTD and depotentiation were prevented by mGluR antagonists rather than by NMDA antagonists (Bashir et al, 1993; Bashir and Collingridge, 1994; Bolshakov and Siegelbaum, 1994; Yang et al., 1994), thereby demonstrating two mechanistically distinct forms of synaptic depression. Both types were pathway-specific The mechanistically distinct nature of these two forms of LTD was confirmed by the lack of occlusion between the two (Oliet et al., 1997; Palmer et al, 1997). Oliet et al. (1997) also observed a decrease in the quantal size of miniature EPSCs without a change in miniature frequency in NMDAR-dependent LTD, suggesting a postsynaptic expression mechanism. In contrast, in mGluR-LTD there was a reduction in miniature frequency, with no change in quantal size, suggesting a presynaptic expression mechanism. Finally, induction of mGluR-dependent LTD did not erase LTP, as was the case with depotentiation produced by the stimulus protocol that produced NMDAR-dependent LTD but, rather, was superimposed on LTP. These experiments confirmed the existence of two distinct types of LTD at Schaffer-commissural–CA1 pyramidal synapses with distinct induction and expression mechanisms.

Low-frequency trains to Schaffer-commissural fibers in slices from neonatal rats induce a form of mGluR-dependent LTD that is blocked by postsynaptic injection of calcium chelators but is, at least in part, expressed as an increase in transmitter release (Bolshakov and Siegelbaum, 1994)—a combination that immediately suggests the need for a retrograde messenger (see Section 10.4.7). Strong, if incomplete, evidence that a lipoxygenase metabolite of arachidonic acid, 12(S)HPETE, may be the retrograde messenger in this case has been presented by Feinmark et al. (2003).

A study by Kemp et al. (2000) illustrates the complexity of LTD induction mechanisms. The effects of two protocols in area CA1 were compared: trains of single stimuli at 1 Hz and trains of paired pulses also at 1 Hz. In slices from young animals, LTD produced by either protocol was blocked by AP5. Adult animals showed a shift toward mGluR-dependent LTD and in general required longer trains, but it remained possible, by varying the stimulus parameters, to obtain either mGluR-dependent or NMDAR-dependent LTD. Again, the two forms of LTD did not occlude, indicating the independence of the associated expression mechanisms. The mechanisms behind the age- and activity-related shift from NMDAR-mediated to mGluR-mediated LTD are unknown but may reflect the developmental regulation of receptor subtypes. Whatever the reasons, these observations make it clear that the precise details of activity-induced changes in synaptic efficacy depend on the fine temporal structure of the patterns of neural activity itself.

Although the paired-pulse protocol introduced by Kemp et al. (2000) (900 pairs at 1 Hz with an interpulse interval of 50 msec) generates mGluR-dependent LTD in area CA1 in vitro (see also Hüber et al., 2000), it has not been shown to be effective in vivo. The subtly different paired-pulse protocol formulated by Thiels et al. (1994), in which the interpulse interval is set at 25 ms to maximize inhibitory feedback, produces a depression that is NMDAR-dependent rather than mGluR-dependent (Thiels et al, 2002). Furthermore, although group I mGluR antagonists are generally more effective at blocking mGluR-dependent LTD in area CA1 in vitro, group II antago-nists depress the late component of LTD in vivo (Manahan-Vaughan, 1997).

mGluR-dependent LTD Induced by Exposure to mGluR Agonists

Brief exposure to the group I mGluR agonist dihydroxy-phenylglycine (DHPG) induces a reassuringly robust LTD in adult slice preparations in both area CA1 (Palmer et al., 1997) (Fig 10.17E) and the dentate gyrus (Camodeca et al., 1999). This form of LTD, probably mediated by mGluR5 receptors, is blocked by group I or broad-spectrum mGluR antagonists but not by NMDA receptor antagonists. Experiments to probe the induction site of mGluR-LTD point toward a postsynaptic locus of induction. Intracellular injection of a G protein inhibitor into CA1 pyramidal cells suppressed the ability of DHPG to induce LTD (Watabe et al., 2002). Intracellular injection of BAPTA, on the other hand, had no such effect (Fitzjohn et al., 2001b), suggesting a Ca^{2+}-insensitive induction process. The experiments of Hüber et al. (2000) led to the conclusion that mGluR-LTP depends on rapid activation of local postsynaptic protein synthesis. In the presence of the protein synthesis inhibitor anisomycin, the depression induced by DHPG quickly attenuates, and responses recover to baseline within 60 minutes (Hüber et al., 2000). LTD induced by mGluR agonists thus quickly becomes dependent on protein synthesis. Consistent with the rapid action of anisomycin, mGluR-induced LTD survived in an isolated in vitro preparation, from which both pre- and postsynaptic cell bodies had been removed by appropriate scalpel cuts. This result implies that local protein synthesis at synaptic sites is required early in the expression of mGluR-induced LTD. Given that protein synthetic machinery has not been described at presynaptic boutons, it seems safe to conclude that the induction of this early form of protein synthesis-dependent LTD is located in dendrites. Synaptically driven mGluR-dependent LTD induced by low-frequency trains of paired pulses was also blocked by anisomycin (Hüber et al., 2000).

There is less agreement concerning the locus of expression of this form of LTD. On the one hand there is evidence that it is presynaptically mediated because (1) there is no postsynaptic change in response to flash photolysis of caged glutamate (Rammes et al., 2003), (2) NMDA and AMPA receptor components of synaptic responses are equally depressed (Watabe et al., 2002), (3) paired-pulse facilitation is increased (Fitzjohn et al., 2001), and (4) DHPG produces a persistent decrease in the frequency of miniature EPSCs with no change in amplitude in tetrodotoxin-treated cultured hippocampal neurons (Fitzjohn et al., 2001b). However, there is also evidence that DHPG-induced LTD involves removal of both AMPA and NMDA receptors from synapses (Snyder et al., 2001). These disparate observations may be reconciled by the finding that mGluR-dependent LTD, induced by DHPG, is blocked by postsynaptically applied inhibitors of protein tyrosine phosphatases (PTPs) and of the actin cytoskeleton (Moult et al,

2006).These postsynaptic manipulations blocked the changes in paired-pulse facilitation and miniature frequency, suggesting a retrograde signaling process that is dependent on PTPs and the actin cytoskeleton. An alternative explanation is that AMPA receptors are removed to create silent synapses. If this occurs preferentially at high-Pr synapses owing to the requirement for activity to drive the movement, the changes in paired-pulse facilitation would simply reflect this postsynaptic alteration (see Box 10–1). The lack of change in the response to uncaged glutamate, which act on both spines and dendrites, can be reconciled with a postsynaptic model if, instead of being internalized, AMPA receptors diffuse laterally to extrasynaptic sites (Moult et al., 2006).

Signaling Pathways in mGluR-dependent LTD

DHPG-induced LTD has been widely used as a model to explore the signalling mechanisms involved in mGluR-dependent LTD. By definition, mGluRs are coupled to G-proteins, and as expected DHPG-induced LTD requires activation of G-proteins (Watabe et al., 2002; Huang CC et al., 2004). Since group I mGluRs are positively linked to PLC, and thereby the generation of diacylglycerol and IP3, it might have been anticipated that inhibitors of PKC and/or release of Ca^{2+} from stores would block mGluR-dependent LTD. However, a variety of potent PKC inhibitors and blockers of Ca^{2+} stores, applied alone or in combination, failed to affect DHPG-induced LTD (Camodeca et al., 1999; Schnabel et al., 2001). Furthermore, DHPG-induced LTD is insensitive to inhibitors of PKA (Camodeca et al., 1999; Schnabel et al., 2001), while inhibitors of CaMKII cause a modest enhancement of the effect (Schnabel et al., 1999). It has been suggested that DHPG-induced LTD is blocked by PTK inhibitors in the dentate gyrus (Camodeca et al., 1999) but this finding was not replicated in area CA1 (Moult et al., 2002), suggesting the possibility of regional differences. Whilst there is general agreement for a role of MAPK cascades, there is some contention as to whether the mechanism involves the Ras-activated ERKs (Gallagher et al., 2004) or the Rap-activated p38 MAPK (Rush et al., 2002; Huang CC et al., 2004). Finally, so far as kinases are concerned, there is evidence for a role of the PI3K-Akt-mTOR signalling pathway in DHPG-induced LTD (Hou and Klann, 2004). With respect to phosphatases, inhibitors of the ser/thr phosphatases that are involved in NMDAR-dependent LTD (PP1/PP2A and PP2B) do not inhibit DHPG-induced LTD; rather, PP1/PP2A inhibitors cause a small facilitation of the effect (Schnabel et al., 2001). However, inhibitors of tyrosine phosphatases completely eliminate DHPG-induced LTD (Moult et al., 2002; Huang CC and Hsu, 2006), a result that identifies a major signalling pathway for this robust form of LTD.

Less is known about the signalling pathways involved in synaptically-induced mGluR-dependent LTD. The report that the DHPG-induced and synaptically-induced forms mutually occlude each other suggests a common underlying pathway (Hüber et al., 2001), and, as we have seen, both are blocked by protein synthesis inhibitors (Hüber et al., 2000). However, unlike DHPG-induced LTD, synaptically-induced mGluR-dependent LTD appears also to be sensitive to PKC inhibitors (Oliet et al, 1997). Whether this reflects a heterogeneity in the synaptic forms is unknown.

How the various signalling components that have been identified in mGluR-dependent LTD (e.g., PI3K-Akt-mTOR, MAPKs, PTPs) interrelate is not known. What is clear, however, is that the signalling mechanisms involved in mGluR-induced LTD are very different from those involved in NMDAR-dependent LTD (see schemas in Fig. 10–18A and B).

10.7.6 Homosynaptic Depotentiation

Long-term potentiation in vitro can be reversed by low-frequency stimulation when it is given within a few minutes of the tetanus used to induce LTP (Barrionuevo et al., 1980; Staubli and Lynch, 1990; Fujii et al., 1991), a process sometimes referred to as destabilization of LTP. Destabilization is a specific example of the more general phenomenon of depotentiation, which refers to the reversal of LTP at any post-tetanus interval. Whereas destabilization is a robust phenomenon observed in all hippocampal pathways and at all ages, depotentiation at longer intervals after induction is less easily induced in adult animals.

In all hippocampal subfields and in both adult and juvenile animals, LTP can be depotentiated by a prolonged low-frequency train (e.g., 900 stimuli at 1 Hz) beginning immediately after induction. The time window for induction and the input specificity of depotentiation have been documented. The efficiency of the depotentiating train quickly declines after the LTP-inducing event; and many, though not all, in vitro studies suggest that depotentiation can be induced only if low-frequency stimulation is applied within minutes of LTP induction. A similar time window is seen in the dentate gyrus of the intact animal (Martin, 1998; Kulla et al., 1999; Straube and Frey, 2003). In area CA1 of the awake animal, however, Doyle et al. (1997), using 900 stimuli at 5 to 10 Hz, succeeded in depotentiating LTP at a range of intervals from 10 minutes to 24 hours after induction in area CA1. Lower stimulus frequencies were ineffective, and Doyle et al. were unable to induce LTD at any frequency. Another question is how long depotentiation lasts. In the dentate gyrus of the unanesthetized rat, depotentiation has been reported to persist for 24 hours (Kulla et al., 1999). This raises the question of the stability of the depotentiated response: Do depotentiated synapses, like their potentiated counterparts, retain the potential for reversed plasticity only during a limited time window after induction? In other words, is de-depression, like depotentiation, time-limited? The essence of "bidirectional plasticity" is that synaptic efficacy can be reset up and down at will, but this may be the case only within specific time windows. There is some evidence to suggest that, at least in area CA1, depotentiation appears to be input-specific (Bortolotto et al,

1994; Huang CC et al., 2001; but see Muller et al., 1995). However, in the dentate gyrus in vivo and at mossy fiber synapses, heterosynaptic effects become apparent (see below).

According to the model of early LTP and LTD expression proposed by Lee et al. (2000), potentiation occurs as a result of the phosphorylation of S831 on GluR1, leading to an increase in channel conductance (Derkach et al., 1999). Depotentiation results when this residue is dephosphorylated (Lee et al., 2000; Huang CC et al., 2001). Consistent with this idea, it has been shown that depotentiation can be, but is not invariably, accompanied by a decrease in single-channel conductance (Lüthi et al, 2004). Indeed, there is a precise relation between the type of LTP and depotentiation observed; when LTP is the result of an increase in single-channel conductance, the increase is reversed in depotentiation. However, in cases where there is no change in single-channel conductance during LTP, neither is there any change in this parameter during depotentiation. With the latter form of bidirectional plasticity, the most likely explanation is changes in the number of AMPA receptors expressed at synapses. Both the protein kinase (CaMKII) and protein phosphatases (PP1/2A) involved in these processes are calcium-dependent; and, adapting the Lisman hypothesis, strong, rapid increases should favor phosphorylation and potentiation, whereas prolonged, modest increases in calcium should favor dephosphorylation and depotentiation (Yang et al., 1999; Mizuno et al., 2001). There is disagreement about the pharmacology of depotentiation. Some authors have reported that AP5 blocks depotentiation in area CA1 in vitro (Fujii et al., 1991; Selig et al., 1995b; Huang CC et al., 2001; Lüthi et al., 2004), whereas others have found it is blocked by Gp 1/II mGluR antagonists, and not by NMDAR antagonists, in both area CA1 in acute slices (Bashir and Collingridge, 1994; Fitzjohn et al., 1998) and between pairs of CA3 pyramidal cells in organotypic hippocampal cultures (Montgomery and Madison, 2002). As with LTD, the data suggest that two forms of depotentiation exist: one depending on activation of NMDA receptors, and the other on mGluRs. The extent to which each form is accessed is likely to depend on the experimental conditions employed.

The extent to which different NR2 subunits are involved in the NMDA receptor-dependent form of depotentiation in the hippocampus is unknown. The possibility that there may be differences between depotentiation and LTD in this regard is however suggested by experiments performed in perirhinal cortex (Massey et al., 2004). Depotentiation was not affected by selective NR2B inhibitors whilst LTD, recorded in the presence of an uptake inhibitor, was fully blocked by these compounds. Conversely, a partially selective NR2A antagonist, NVP-AAM007, blocked depotentiation whilst having no effect on LTD.

An interesting twist to the depotentiation story was uncovered by Woo and Nguyen (2003). Multiple trains of tetanic stimulation not only produce maximal LTP but protect against depotentiation by low-frequency stimulation beginning 5 minutes after induction. Surprisingly, this rapidly mounted protection is provided through local protein synthesis. The protein synthesis blockers emetine and anisomycin block the protection and do so in slices in which a cut is made between the cell body layer and the recording and stimulating sites in the stratum radiatum of area CA1. The protection is input-specific, but within 40 minutes heterosynaptic protection against depotentiation is extended to synapses throughout the cell by a transcriptional-dependent process. These results are reminiscent of the finding of Huber et al. (2000) that mGluR-dependent LTD involves rapid local protein synthesis as well as the tagging experiments of Frey and Morris (1997) and Kauderer and Kandel (2000). In none of these cases have the effector molecules responsible or their mode of action yet been identified.

Depotentiation exhibits an intriguing form of state dependence in newly unsilenced connections between CA3 pyramidal cells in organotypic cultures. In this preparation, about 20% of connected cells are originally silent (that is, the postsynaptic cell does not respond to an action potential generated in the presynaptic cell) but can be made active by an LTP-inducing pairing protocol. For the first few minutes or so after unsilencing, these new functional connections are immune to re-silencing. After 30 minutes, the newly activated connections enter a state in which they can be depressed by low-frequency stimulation and after LTP induction can be depotentiated in the usual way by low-frequency stimulation (Montgomery and Madison, 2002).

We end this section with the reminder that a potent chemical activator of depotentiation, which appears to be effective at arbitrarily long intervals after induction, exists in the form of a membrane permeable inhibitor of the autonomously active PKC isoform PKMζ (Serrano et al., 2005; see Section 10.4.9).

10.7.7 Heterosynaptic LTD and Depotentiation: Activity in One Input Can Induce LTD in Another

Heterosynaptic LTD and depotentiation were the first forms of long-term activity-dependent depression to be discovered in the hippocampus. In two-pathway experiments in area CA1 of the hippocampal slice, Lynch et al. (1977) noticed that a strong tetanus to one pathway was sometimes accompanied by a depression of the population spike in the second, nontetanized pathway. However, even when present, heterosynaptic depression rarely lasted for more than a few minutes in slices from adult animals. Two years later, in a study in the dentate gyrus of the anesthetized rat, Levy and Steward (1979) showed that previously potentiated responses evoked by stimulation of the contralateral perforant path were depressed by tetanic stimulation of the ipsilateral perforant path (Fig. 10–17A). Depression could also be induced in the naïve contralateral pathway. The crossed perforant path thus exhibits both heterosynaptic LTD and heterosynaptic depotentiation.

More recently, heterosynaptic LTD in area CA1 has been documented in slices from young animals, induced by a tetanus (Scanziani et al., 1996; Nagase et al., 2003) or by low-frequency stimulation (Wasling et al., 2002) delivered to another pathway. Others have been able to elicit heterosynaptic depression only if the heterosynaptic pathway was first potentiated (heterosynaptic depotentiation) (Muller et al., 1995). Evidence that cytoplasmic Ca^{2+} is a trigger for heterosynaptic depression has been provided by a detailed study of spike timing-dependent plasticity in slices from 1-month-old rats (Nishiyama et al., 2000). When an LTD-inducing protocol was delivered to the first pathway (that is, when the afferent input was repeatedly paired with a back-propagating action potential, the latter preceding the former by ~20 ms), LTD was also induced in a second, unpaired pathway. The effect was blocked by injection of an antibody to the IP3 receptor, and it was not seen in IP3 receptor knockout mice (see also Nagase et al., 2003). Nishiyama et al. (2000) attributed the spread of LTD to the propagation of IP3 receptor-mediated Ca^{2+} waves propagating via the endoplasmic reticulum to neighboring synaptic sites. These experiments, together with the work of Daw et al. (2002), suggest that "input specificity in synaptic modification is not an intrinsic property ... but a dynamic variable linked to the pattern of long-range Ca^{2+} signaling in the postsynaptic dendrite" (Nishiyama et al., 2000). In complementary work, Daw et al. (2002) found that the input specificity of LTD was lost in the presence of an inhibitor of IP3, leading to heterosynaptic depression. This result is in line with the conclusions of Nishiyama et al. (2000), since a likely consequence of PI3 kinase inhibition is an increase in IP3 concentration.

A novel, unsuspected form of heterosynaptic depression has emerged as a result of the growing interest in the effects of cannabinoids and their receptors in the hippocampus. Tetanic stimulation of the Schaffer-commissural pathway in hippocampal slices induces a powerful and persistent depression of neighboring GABAergic terminals projecting to the same target CA1 pyramidal cells (Chevaleyre and Castillo, 2003). The effect relies on release of the cannabinoid diacylglycerol (2-AG) from postsynaptic cells; 2-AG binds to cannabinoid CB1 receptors on the terminals of GABAergic interneurons, leading by an unknown route to a reduction in transmitter release. The resulting disinhibition provides a potential mechanism for the phenomenon of E-S potentiation (see Section 10.3.12).This and other examples of cannabinoid-mediated synaptic plasticity are reviewed by Chevaleyre et al. (2006).

Heterosynaptic LTD and Depotentiation in the Medial and Lateral Perforant Path of the Intact Rat

The strongest body of in vivo evidence relating to heterosynaptic LTD and depotentiation has come from studies of the medial and lateral components of the ipsilateral perforant path (MPP and LPP, respectively) in the intact rat (Abraham and Goddard, 1983; Abraham et al., 1985, 1994l; Doyère et al., 1997) (Fig. 10–17B). Though accounts differ as to the relative ease of obtaining heterosynaptic effects in the two pathways,

there is evidence it can work in both directions. Tetanization of the LPP induces persistent LTD in naïve MPP responses and persistent and reversible depotentiation of potentiated MPP responses (Doyère et al., 1997) (Fig. 10–17C). Moreover, in contrast to homosynaptic depotentiation, there is no restricted time window for the induction of heterosynaptic depotentiation; in the freely moving animal, a tetanus to the LPP can depotentiate MPP responses several days after induction. Both heterosynaptic LTD and depotentiation can persist for days, though the depression is in general less persistent than homosynaptic LTP in the same pathways (Doyère et al., 1997). Doyère et al. were not able to produce heterosynaptic LTD in the LPP; but in Abraham's laboratory, tetanic stimulation of the MPP led to LTD that lasted for days in the LPP (Abraham et al., 1994).

Heterosynaptic depression and depotentiation in the dentate gyrus in vivo are largely confined to the fEPSP; Doyère et al. reported small but significant heterosynaptic depression of the population spike but little if any depotentation. A possible explanation for this seemingly anomalous result is that heterosynaptic depression is accompanied by heterosynaptic E-S potentiation (Abraham et al., 1985).

Heterosynaptic Associative LTD: A Rarely Observed Form of Synaptic Plasticity

Because the nontetanized pathway is not—or need not be—active at the time of induction, heterosynaptic LTD represents a mechanism for generalized synaptic depression. With associative heterosynaptic LTD, in contrast, it is only the synapses active at the time of induction that are depressed. Convincing examples of this form of LTD are rare, and it remains to be established if associative LTD exists in the hippocampus of the intact animal. A report by Stanton and Sejnowski (1989) that heterosynaptic associative LTD could be induced in area CA1 in vitro by pairing single stimuli to one pathway with out-of-phase brief high-frequency trains to a second pathway could not be replicated by Kerr and Abraham, (1993); or Paulsen et al., (1993). In a variant of this protocol, Christie and Abraham (1992) reported that the lateral perforant path in the dentate gyrus of the anesthetized rat can exhibit associative LTD if it has previously been "primed" by stimulation at theta frequency (Abraham and Goddard, 1983; Christie and Abraham, 1992). However, no evidence of priming was seen in area CA1 in the in vitro experiments of Paulsen et al. (1993), suggesting that the effect may be confined to the dentate gyrus or to the intact animal. A homosynaptic variant of the Stanton and Sejnowski protocol has been studied in organotypic hippocampal cultures (Debanne et al., 1994). Repeated pairing of a depolarizing pulse to an impaled CA1 neuron with a single stimulus delivered several hundred milliseconds later to Schaffer-commissural fibers resulted in prolonged depression in the stimulated pathway. The time window during which associative LTD could be obtained was fairly broad: Maximal depression was obtained with a pairing interval of 800 ms, but

1600 ms was almost as effective. The effect is associative because it required both afferent activity and strong depolarizing pulses to fire the postsynaptic cell, and it is input-specific because it was not observed in unstimulated inputs. Associative LTD in organotypic cultures is NMDAR-dependent and is blocked in cells dialyzed with Ca^{2+} chelators.

10.7.8 LTD and Depotentiation at Mossy Fiber–CA3 Pyramidal Cell Synapses

LTD at Mossy Fiber Synapses

Homosynaptic LTD can be induced at mossy fiber synapses in vitro by continuous low-frequency stimulation (1 Hz for 15 minutes), at least in young animals (Battistin and Cherubini, 1994; Kobayashi et al., 1996; Domenici et al., 1998; Tzounopoulos et al., 1998). However, homosynaptic LTD in mossy fibers appears to be more readily induced by low-intensity, high-frequency stimulation than by prolonged low-frequency stimulation, possibly reflecting a requirement for the frequency-dependent co-release of dynorphin from mossy fiber terminals. Release of dynorphin can also lead to transient heterosynaptic depression (Weisskopf et al., 1993). In the anesthetized rat, there is evidence that dynorphin acts postsynaptically to modulate both homosynaptic and heterosynaptic LTD (Derrick and Martinez, 1996).

As with mossy fiber LTP, NMDA receptor antagonists do not block mossy fiber LTD, though group II mGluR antagonists are effective (Kobayashi et al., 1996; Tzounopoulos et al., 1998; Chen et al., 2001a). Its induction is not affected by clamping the postsynaptic cell at a hyperpolarized membrane potential or by loading the cell with BAPTA (Kobayashi et al., 1996; Domenici et al., 1998). Given the controversy surrounding similar experiments addressing the mechanism of mossy fiber LTP, it may be premature to conclude that these results provide conclusive evidence for a presynaptic induction mechanism. Tzounopoulos et al. (1998) have presented evidence for a presynaptic model of mossy fiber LTD in which a decrease in the activity of PKA, triggered by a group II mGluR-mediated decrease in adenyl cyclase activity, leads to a persistent decrease in release probability at mossy fiber terminals. Two lines of knockout mice that lack presynaptic proteins are further pointers to a presynaptic expression mechanism for mossy fiber LTD: One lacks the predominantly presynaptic receptor mGluR2 (Yokoi et al., 1996) and shows impairment in LTD; the other, which shows enhanced LTD, lacks RIMα, an active zone protein that binds to Rab3a and is also a PKA substrate (Castillo et al., 2002).

A pairing-induced postsynaptic form of LTD has been uncovered in the mossy fiber projection to CA3 pyramidal cells. Postsynaptic depolarization combined with low-frequency (0.33 Hz) stimulation of mossy fibers causes persistent depression that depends on Ca^{2+} entry through L-type Ca^{2+} channels in proximal dendrites of CA3 pyramidal cells (Lei et al., 2003). That this is a novel form of mossy fiber LTD is con-

firmed by the fact that it does not occlude with LTD induced by low-frequency stimulation of mossy fibers.

Depotentiation at Mossy Fiber Synapses

Low-frequency stimulation applied immediately, but not 30 to 60 minutes, after a tetanus reverses mossy fiber LTP (Tzounopoulos et al., 1998; Chen et al., 2001a). Thus, as in area CA1 and the dentate gyrus, LTP in time becomes immune to depotentiation. Depotentiation is blocked by group II mGluR antagonists, and group II agonists can substitute for low-frequency stimulation in producing time-dependent depotentiation (Chen et al., 2001a). Low-frequency stimulation can induce heterosynaptic depotentiation in a neighboring mossy fiber pathway, perhaps as a result of glutamate spillover (Chen et al., 2001). In contrast to LTD, depotentiation can be readily elicited in adult animals (Huang CC and Hsu, 2001).

Chen et al. (2001a) have made the interesting observation that depotentiation in the mossy fiber pathway is not input-specific. A low-frequency train to a recently potentiated mossy fiber input leads to depotentiation of that input and of a second mossy fiber input, not exposed to low-frequency stimulation, that was potentiated at the same time as the first. This is in contrast to the input specificity of depotentiation that the same group found in area CA1 (Huang CC and Hsu, 2001). Another study (Huang et al., 2002) provided evidence of the involvement of presynaptic mGluR2 receptors in heterosynaptic depotentiation, activated perhaps by spillover from activated fibers. Although these experiments demonstrate the potential for erasing LTP in a nonspecific way in the mossy fiber pathway, it is important to emphasize once again that there is as yet no evidence that this occurs in the intact, behaving animal.

Mossy Fiber LTD Is Developmentally Regulated

In slices from young rats (less than 14 days after birth), another form of mossy fiber LTD has been observed that can be induced by high-frequency stimulation (100 Hz for 1 second) and is independent of both NMDA and metabotropic glutamate receptors (Battistin and Cherubini 1994). The induction of this form of LTD is blocked by postsynaptic injection of BAPTA, but its expression remains presynaptic (Domenici et al., 1998). Intriguingly, mGluR-dependent LTD induced by low-frequency stimulation and high-frequency-induced LTD do not occlude, suggesting that both induction and expression mechanisms are different in the two forms of LTD (see Section 10.9.1).

LTD: Roles and Rules in the Intact Animal

In the freely moving animal, mild stress promotes LTD and inhibits LTP, though the effect is short-lasting (Xu et al., 1997). Exploration of a novel environment, on the other hand, can promote partial or total depotentiation for an extended period. In one study, the effect was restricted to a time window of more than an hour but less than 24 hours after induction (Xu et al., 1998). In another study in which a tetanus protocol was adopted that produced a very long-lasting form of LTP, depotentiation could be induced several weeks (but not months) after induction by leaving rats for a few nights in a rodent Disney World with endless possibilities for exploration (Abraham et al., 2002).

What is the function of LTD and its partner depotentiation? Theoretical analysis of distributed neural nets suggests that a network whose synaptic elements are endowed with the property of bidirectional plasticity, including heterosynaptic plasticity, are more stable and have a larger storage capacity than networks where only potentiation (or depression) is possible (Willshaw and Dayan, 1990). It is usually presumed that if the encoding of memories and semantic knowledge is achieved by changes in synaptic weights these changes must be stable, but models where this is not the case have been proposed (Abraham and Robins, 2005). Such models are even more dependent on mechanisms allowing easy reversibility of changes in synaptic weights. What then is the role of LTD? Clearly depotentiation has the potential to disrupt memory circuits and cause active forgetting. What is the evidence that activity-dependent erasure is necessary for forgetting? To put it another way, what sorts of forgetting, if any, could not be explained by the gradual decay of LTP? After all, forgetting on demand is next to impossible.

One consequence of heterosynaptic LTD is to maintain relatively constant the net excitatory drive onto target cells. The observation that there is no increase in the mean firing rate of place cells following the induction of LTP is consistent with this ideas (McNaughton et al., 1984; Dragoi et al., 2003).

In the laboratory there are two very different ways of eliciting LTD: (1) with long low-frequency trains tuned to mGluR group I receptors or to NMDA receptors; and (2) by appropriate pairings of presynaptic and back-propagating postsynaptic spikes. There are several fundamental issues to be resolved here. How is the "tuning" realized mechanistically? Do the endogenous patterns of activity provide anything like 1 Hz/900 pulse regimens that are required to obtain sustained LTD? Does LTD or any of the other forms of persistent synaptic depression described in this section occur at all in the hippocampus of the freely moving, behaving animal? The nearest this question has come to receiving a positive answer comes from the experiments in behaving animals discussed above.

10.8 Synaptic Plasticity and Inhibitory Pathways

In addition to plasticity at glutamatergic synapses on glutamatergic principal cells, there is a growing body of data on plasticity at synapses where a GABAergic neuron comprises one or other side of the synaptic partnership (Bischofberger and Jonas, 2002; Lawrence and McBain, 2003). In this section we examine LTP and LTD at excitatory synapses onto interneurons and at inhibitory synapses made by interneurons onto excitatory and inhibitory neurons.

10.8.1 LTP and LTD at Glutamatergic Synapses on Interneurons

The subunit composition of AMPA and NMDA receptors on interneurons differ in detail from that found on pyramidal cells (see Chapter 5 and Chapter 6, Section 6.3). The dominant NMDA subunit is NR2B, the presence of which prolongs NMDAR-mediated currents (McBain et al., 1999). The AMPA receptor subunit GluR2, which in its edited form limits the calcium permeability of the AMPA receptor ion channel, is generally in low abundance at synapses on inhibitory interneurons, and AMPAR-mediated calcium fluxes are correspondingly higher (Lawrence and McBain, 2003). The distinct assemblage of glutamate receptor subtypes at interneuron synaptic membranes is reflected in the types of plasticity observed; high-frequency trains can, depending on the protocol or cell type, induce either no change, LTP (Maccaferri and McBain, 1996; Perez et al., 2001; Lapointe et al., 2003), or LTD (McMahon and Kauer, 1997). Induction of LTP at excitatory synapses on stratum oriens/alveus (OA) interneurons in stratum oriens is mGluR1-dependent and requires postsynaptic Ca^{2+} entry; expression appears to be presynaptic (Lapointe et al., 2003). There are no reports of long-term changes produced by low-frequency trains. However, LTD at feedforward excitatory synapses on CA1 interneurons can be induced by high-frequency stimulation, as first described at Schaffer-commissural inputs to interneurons in stratum radiatum of area CA1 (McMahon and Kauer, 1997). This form of LTD appears not to be input-specific. Functional suppression, via LTD, of excitatory feedforward synapses onto interneurons in stratum radiatum provides a potential mechanism for the phenomenon of E-S potentiation (see Section 10.3.12).

A pairing strategy (depolarizing pulses combined with theta-burst afferent stimulation) has been successfully employed to induce LTP of excitatory afferents to interneurons of stratum oriens in area CA1, but the same protocol is ineffective in the stratum radiatum (Perez et al., 2001). Thus, the magnitude and polarity of activity-induced plasticity at excitatory synapses on CA1 interneurons depends on the stimulus protocol, the location of the interneuron, and presumably the distribution of its receptor subunits.

Mossy fibers provide an interesting example of terminal-specific plasticity. As we have seen, both LTP and LTD are expressed presynaptically at mossy fiber–CA3 pyramidal cell synapses. Filopodial extensions of mossy fiber giant boutons and mossy fibers with en passant boutons make excitatory synapses on dendrites of CA3 interneurons. In stratum radiatum of area CA3, tetanic stimulation of mossy fibers induces LTD in interneurons expressing calcium-permeable AMPA

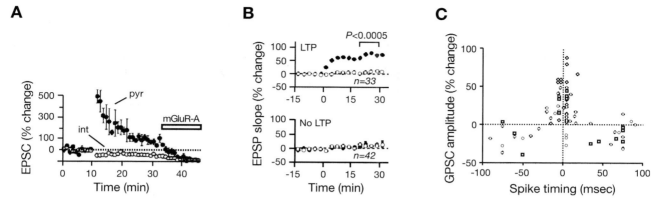

Figure 10–20. Synaptic plasticity of glutamatergic inputs to hippocampal interneurons and at GABAergic inputs from interneurons. *A.* Tetanic stimulation of mossy fibers produces LTP at CA3 pyramidal cells (pyr) (filled circles) but a mean depression in a population of interneurons (int) (open circles). Note that responses were blocked by an mGluR agonist (mGluR-A), consistent with activation of mossy fibers. (*Source*: Maccaferri et al., 1998.) *B.* With perforated patch recording, input-specific LTP can be induced by pairing in a subpopulation of small feedforward interneurons in the stratum radiatum of area CA1. EPSPs from Interneurons showing LTP are plotted in the upper panel (filled circles are responses from paired input, open circles from unpaired input); responses from non-potentating interneurons are pollted in the lower panel. (*Source*: Lamsa et al., 2005.) *C.* Potentiation of GABAergic postsynaptic currents (GPSCs) recorded in dissociated hippocampal cultures following repeated pairing of presynaptic and postsynaptic neurons. LTP of GABAergic transmission is input-specific; and unlike pairing-induced plasticity at glutamatergic synapses, it occurs 20 ms either side of coincident presynaptic and postsynaptic activity. The effect is caused by an L-type calcium channel-dependent local suppression of Cl^- transporter activity. The resulting decrease in the reversal potential for Cl^- results in an increase in the GPSC when the cell is clamped at a hyperpolarized potential. (*Source*: Woodin et al., 2003.)

receptors; and presynaptic mGluRs but not NMDARs are required for its induction (Maccaferri et al., 1998; Laezza et al., 1999) (Fig. 10–20A). In further work from McBain's group, tetanus-induced LTP was observed in stratum lucidum interneurons expressing Ca^{2+}-impermeable GluR2-containing AMPA receptors. The mechanism underlying LTD depends on whether there are calcium-permeable or calcium-impermeable AMPA receptors at that synapse; for both types of synapse, the locus of induction is postsynaptic, although the evidence points to presynaptic expression in the former case and postsynaptic expression in the latter (Lawrence and McBain, 2003). At the mossy fiber–basket cell connection in the dentate gyrus, LTP can be induced by high-frequency stimulation paired with depolarization of the basket cell; LTD is the outcome of tetanic stimulation without depolarisation. Analysis of the number of failures, coefficient of variation, and paired-pulse modulation indicate a presynaptic locus for LTD (Alle et al., 2001). A general conclusion from these studies is that the target cell controls the type and extent of plasticity at mossy fiber terminals.

An intriguing form of E-S potentiation (see Section 10.3.12) at interneurons in the molecular layer of the dentate gyrus has been reported by Ross and Soltesz (2001). Tetanic stimulation of the perforant path leads to a persistent decrease in membrane potential, which increases the probability of the interneuron firing to subsequent stimuli without affecting the amplitude of the EPSP. The effect requires activation of Ca^{2+}-permeable AMPA receptors and reflects downregulation in the activity of the electrogenic Na/K ATPase pump.

Two other examples of plasticity at excitatory synapses have been identified at hippocampal interneurons. Lamsa et al. (2005) observed LTP at feedforward excitatory synapses on a subset of interneurons (about half their sample of aspiny interneurons) in area CA1 using perforated patch recordings to preserve the cytoplasmic integrity of the cell. The authors suggest that LTP at this synapse is important for preserving the temporal fidelity of pyramidal cell firing (Fig. 10–20B). McBain and his colleagues have identified a metabotropic switch mediating bidirectional plasticity at synapses made by mossy fibers onto stratum lucidum interneurons (SLINs) (Pelkey et al., 2005). The switch is operated by mGluR7 receptors, which in the resting state are present on presynaptic terminals of mossy fiber-SLIN synapses. Intense activity (such as a high-frequency train) activates the receptors and triggers a sequence of events that leads to LTD, expressed as a reduction in transmitter release from mossy fiber–SLIN terminals. The resulting decrease in feedforward inhibition promotes the firing of CA3 pyramidal cells. Another consequence of the intense activation during the train is that mGluR7 receptors become internalized; now, without the feedback suppression of transmitter release that they control, the mossy fiber terminals onto SLINs display LTP when strongly activated, and feedforward inhibition is restored. By this remarkable metaplastic mechanism the balance of excitation and inhibition is maintained in the CA3 network. These two sets of results demonstrate a greater potential for plasticity in the inhibitory circuits of the hippocampus than has been generally assumed (McBain et al., 1999).

10.8.2 LTP and LTD at GABAergic Synapses

It might be expected that GABAergic synapses would not display plasticity because they lack the equivalent of the voltage-dependent NMDA receptor that for most excitatory synapses is an essential component of the inductive machinery. However, both LTP and LTD have been observed following tetanic stimulation of GABAergic afferents to pyramidal cells in area CA1, under conditions in which all ionotropic glutamate channels are blocked (Caillard et al., 1999; Shew et al., 2000). There is disagreement about whether the postsynaptic cell is (Shew et al., 2000) or is not (Caillard et al., 1999) involved in the induction of LTP, but the evidence points to a presynaptic locus of expression. These experiments were carried out on animals 2 weeks old or less. In a study on hippocampal slices from 4- to 5-week-old rats, tetanic stimulation resulted in LTD of GABAergic responses in CA1 pyramidal cells (Lu et al., 2000a). Here the effect appears to have been induced heterosynaptically by co-activation of convergent excitatory fibers, as induction was blocked by bath application of AP5 or by injecting a calcineurin inhibitor into the postsynaptic cell. A novel form of heterosynaptic LTD at inhibitory synapses in area CA1 has been discovered by Chevaleyre and Castillo (2003). Persistent reduction of evoked IPSCs was induced by brief high-frequency stimulation of Schaffer-commissural fibers, again under conditions in which ionotropic glutamate receptors were blocked. The effect was abolished by antagonists of group 1 mGluRs and cannabinoid CB1 receptors. Chevaleyre and Castillo (2003) concluded that the sequence of events underlying this form of plasticity begins with mGluR-mediated release of the endogenous agonist 2-AG from stimulated pyramidal cells followed by binding of 2-AG to CB1 receptors on the terminals of inhibitory boutons. For further discussion of the results of Lu et al. (2000a) and Chevaleyre and Castillo (2003) in the context of E-S potentiation, see Section 10.3.12.

Woodin et al. (2003) uncovered an unusual form of spike timing-dependent plasticity (STDP) (see Section 10.3.8) that is independent of the order of the pre- and postsynaptic activity at inhibitory synapses onto hippocampal pyramidal cells. Repeated pairings between the presynaptic action potential and the back-propagating dendritic spike at intervals up to 20 ms on either side of coincidence result in long-term reduction in the GABAergic IPSC. The effect is triggered by Ca^{2+} entry through L-type Ca^{2+} channels, leading to persistent downregulation of the K^+/Cl^- co-transporter, with a consequent buildup in the concentration of intracellular Cl^- and a depolarizing shift in the Cl^- equilibrium potential (Fig. 10–20C).

An unsuspected mechanism for potentiation of the GABAergic slow IPSC has been revealed in dendritic spines of CA1 pyramidal cells (Huang CS et al., 2005). The slow IPSC is mediated by $GABA_B$ receptors and the G protein-activated inwardly rectifying K^+ (GIRK) channel, both of which are located on spines as well as dendrites of CA1 neurons. Pairing of single stimuli with depolarization induces LTP of the slow IPSC that is both NMDAR-dependent and αCaMKII-dependent. Remarkably, the same induction mechanisms that lead to LTP of excitatory transmission also mediate potentiation of slow GABAergic responses in the same spines. Huang et al. speculate that the temporal window for coincidence detection is sharpened in spines equipped with the $GABA_B$/GIRK system because subsequent excitatory responses are held in check by the slow IPSC.

To conclude this section, we note that to date there have been no studies on plasticity at inhibitory synapses on granule cells or at inhibitory synapses on interneurons.

10.9 LTP and LTD in Development and Aging and in Animal Models of Cognitive Dysfunction

Long-term potentiation is often considered as if it were a unitary process. However, as documented elsewhere in the chapter, various factors can greatly influence the properties of LTP, such as the pathway under investigation, the phase of LTP being studied, and the methods used for its induction. Another critical factor is the age of the animal. It is likely that the predominant role for synaptic plasticity early in development is in the formation and refinement of synaptic connections. As animals develop, it can be assumed that LTP and other manifestations of plasticity are involved in modifying synaptic strength at existing synapses, but here too there could be age-dependent alterations in the underlying mechanisms. Juvenile forms of LTP may be less evident but may persist into adulthood in some circumstances, for example during reactive synaptogenesis in response to brain injury and in the dentate gyrus when newborn granule cells are incorporated into the network of mature granule cells (Schmidt-Hieber et al., 2004).

10.9.1 Hippocampal Synaptic Plasticity During Development

LTP and the Postnatal Hippocampus

Because they have been the most extensively investigated, more is known about age-dependent changes in LTP at CA1 synapses than elsewhere in the brain. Silent synapses—defined as synapses that have an NMDAR-mediated component of synaptic transmission but no detectable AMPAR-mediated component (Fig. 10–21A)—account for approximately 80% of CA3–CA1 connections during the first 2 days of postnatal life in the rat, decreasing dramatically over the next week or so (Durand et al., 1996) (Fig. 10–21B). By P5 to P6 they account for half this number and continue to decline steeply thereafter. The mechanism of LTP at these synapses involves the rapid unsilencing of silent synapses through the NMDAR-dependent appearance of AMPAR-mediated responses. The simplest mechanism to explain this is the rapid recruitment to the synapse of AMPA receptors, though presynaptic mechanisms have also been proposed (Kullmann, 2003). A reappraisal of the role of silent synapses may be needed following the observation that synapses are not initially silent; rather, the AMPAR-mediated component disappears as a result of the synaptic stimulation used to obtain baseline responses (Xiao et al., 2004). This activity-dependent silencing is developmentally regulated; it is evident at P3 to P12 but not at P29 to P32, which could account for the developmental profile of silent synapses. Whatever its origin and mechanisms, the unsilencing of silent synapses is best regarded as a juvenile form of LTP; the extent to which it is involved, if at all, during LTP in more mature animals or during reactive synaptogenesis is currently unknown.

NMDA receptors are likely to be the primary trigger for LTP induction throughout life but signaling molecules activated downstream of these receptors may change as the animal matures. We have already alluded in section 10.4.3 to the developmental switch in the kinase dependence of E-LTP that occurs between P7 and P8 when LTP is primarily PKA-dependent, and P27 when LTP acquires its adult dependence on CaMKII (Yasuda et al., 2003) (Fig. 10–21C).

Another study compared LTP mechanisms at CA1 synapses at two stages of development under otherwise identical conditions (Palmer et al., 2004). It was found that LTP involved two mechanisms at P6. The more prevalent form was exhibited by synapses that had an initially low Pr (and showed pronounced PPF); at these synapses LTP was expressed as an increase in Pr (and an associated decrease in PPF) (Fig. 10–21D). The second form displayed no significant change in Pr or PPF but was associated with a decrease in the mean unitary conductance of AMPA receptors. As noted earlier this can most simply be explained by the insertion of additional receptors but with lower single-channel conductance than preexisting receptors. By P12, neither of these mechanisms was present. Instead, LTP was associated with either an increase or no change in the mean unitary conductance, consistent with an increase in the single-channel conductance of preexisting AMPA receptors (or, alternatively, an exchange of high for low conductance receptors) and the insertion of additional receptors of the same unitary conductance as the preexisting receptors, respectively. Regardless of the precise underlying mechanisms, this study illustrates the diversity of LTP mechanisms that can exist at a single type of synapse. The coexistence of more than one mechanism in the same preparation adds further complexity and may reflect the heterogeneity of the developmental state of synapses at any one age.

LTD and the Postnatal Hippocampus

In addition to marked alterations in the properties and mechanisms of LTP during development, there are also significant changes in LTD. At Schaffer-commissural synapses, LTD is often induced by a prolonged period of low-frequency stimulation (e.g., 900 pulses at 1 Hz). As noted in Section 10.7, LTD is more readily induced in juvenile animals than in adults. However, NMDAR-dependent LTD can be induced in adults when glutamate uptake is blocked (Yang et al, 2005), as earlier

described at cortical synapses (Massey et al., 2004). This suggests that the mechanisms for LTD exist in adults but are less readily accessible. These differences in the ability to induce LTD presumably reflect age-related changes in induction mechanisms. For example, in very young animals it seems that mGluRs and voltage-gated Ca^{2+} channels are important triggers (Bolshakov and Siegelbaum, 1994). In juveniles and adults, both NMDAR- and mGluR-dependent forms of LTD may coexist, though the relative contributions of each form may change with age (Kemp et al., 2000).

Developmental shifts in the generation of LTD also occur at mossy fiber synapses, as noted in Section 10.7.8. Between the first and second week of life it is possible to induce two forms of LTD (Domenici et al, 1998). One form is induced by a high-frequency train and is independent of both NMDARs and mGluRs. The second form is induced by prolonged low-frequency stimulation and depends on activation of mGluRs. The high-frequency form of LTD, however, is replaced by LTP in rats more than 2 weeks of age (Battistin and Cherubini, 1994).

10.9.2 Synaptic Plasticity and the Aging Hippocampus

Changes in the molecular mechanisms of LTP are unlikely to change radically during norml aging: LTP induction, for example, still requires the activation of NMDA receptors (Barnes et al., 1996). However, during aging there are alterations in the LTP process that could contribute to a decline in cognitive function. In general, it can be concluded that aged rats have deficits in both the induction and maintenance of LTP; however, these deficits are complex and depend on the pathway under investigation and the experimental protocol (reviewed by Burke and Barnes, 2006). For example, in aged rats there is an increased rate of decay of LTP at perforant path–granule cell synapses that correlates with the rate of forgetting (Barnes, 1979). A similar deficit in the maintenance of LTP in the perforant path input to CA3 neurons has been reported (Dieguez and Barea-Rodriguez, 2004). There is also an increase in the induction threshold of LTP in aged rats at perforant path–granule cell synapses that is detectable with submaximal induction protocols (Barnes et al., 2000). At CA1 synapses, the primary deficit with aging seems to be a reduction in the magnitude of LTP, which may be explained by less depolarization during induction and presumably therefore less activation of NMDA receptors (Deupree et al., 1991; Moore et al., 1993; Rosenzweig et al., 1997; Tombaugh et al., 2002). Thus, it appears that a major factor in age-related changes in LTP is alterations in conditions affecting NMDA receptor function and its associated Ca^{2+} signaling. In turn, alterations in NMDA receptor-dependent plasticity seem to account for many of the alterations in the dynamics of neuronal assemblies that occur with aging. This is indicated by the findings that blockade of NMDA receptors in young rats results in ensemble dynamics that resemble those of old rats (Kentros et al., 1998; Ekstrom et al., 2001).

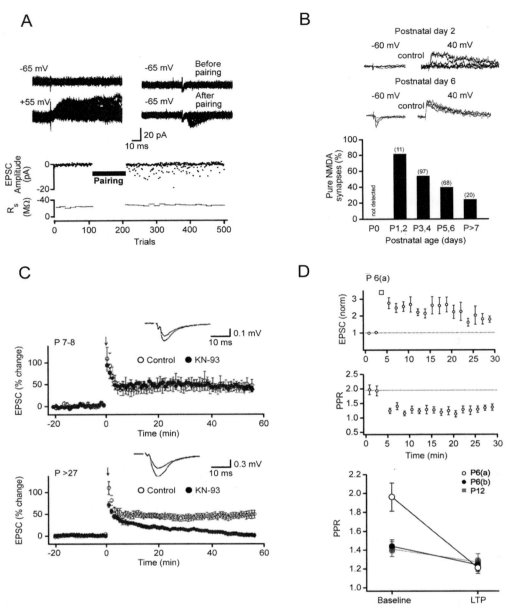

Figure 10–21. Developmental changes in LTP. *A.* Early in development there are silent synapses that display NMDA but not AMPA receptor-mediated EPSCs. These can be rapidly unsilenced by an LTP induction protocol. The traces (left-hand side) show only failures at a negative membrane potential but NMDA receptor-mediated synaptic responses at a positive holding potential. The traces (right-hand side) show only failures before but some AMPA receptor-mediated EPSCs after pairing-induced LTP. The graph plots the amplitude of EPSCs versus time. (*Source*: Liao et al., 1995.) *B.* The incidence of silent synapses dramatically decreases with development. The traces are EPSCs at negative and positive membrane potentials at postnatal day 2 (P2) and P6. At P2 the synapse is silent because only NMDA receptor-mediated responses are observed. At P6 the synapse is no longer silent because both AMPA and NMDA receptor-mediated responses are observed. The graph plots the incidence of silent synapses versus the developmental age

of the animal. Note the dramatic decrease in the incidence of silent synapses with age. (*Source*: Durand et al., 1996.) *C.* Sensitivity to the CaMKII inhibitor KN-93 increases with development. The upper graph shows that KN-93 has no effect on LTP at CA1 synapses in slices obtained from P7 to P8 rats. However, KN-93 blocked the induction of E-LTP in slices obtained from rats at P27 and later. (*Source*: Yasuda et al., 2003.) *D.* The expression mechanisms of LTP, assessed as changes in paired-pulse facilitation, alter during development. The upper graph plots the EPSC amplitude (upper) and paired-pulse ratio (lower) before and following pairing induced LTP (at the time depicted by open square) for a subclass of P6 neurons-termed P6(a). The lower graph plots the change in the paired-pulse ratio following LTP for this group of synapses and for another subclass of P6 neurons [P6(b)] and P12 neurons. Note the dramatic decrease in paired pulse facilitation that is specific for P6(a). (*Source*: Palmer et al., 2004.)

In aged animals it once again appears to be easier to induce LTD and depotentiation (Norris et al., 1996).

10.9.3 Animal Models of Cognitive Decline

Alzheimer's Disease

Memory loss is a prominent aspect of Alzheimer's disease (AD), and given the strong presumptive links between synaptic plasticity and memory, it is not surprising that several groups have asked whether synaptic plasticity is affected in rodent models of the disease (reviewed by Rowan et al., 2003).

The diagnostic, postmortem feature of Alzheimer's disease in humans is the deposition of amyloid plaque in structures of the temporal lobe (see Chapter 16). Whether plaque deposition is the cause or a consequence of the disease has not been resolved, but many believe that excessive levels of amyloid β (Aβ) is the primary cause of the disease. Aβ is a peptide fragment that is cleaved from the amyloid precursor protein (APP) by the action of secretases. In various familial forms of early-onset AD, there are mutations in APP that result in its misprocessing, leading to deposition of Aβ. Several mouse lines have been created that overexpress these mutant forms of APP. These mice display age-related cognitive deficits and amyloid plaque deposition. With respect to alterations in synaptic function, two main effects have been noted. In some, but not all, studies there is a decrease in LTP (Chapman et al., 1999; Moechars et al., 1999). In other studies the most dramatic effect is a decrease in basal synaptic transmission (Hsia et al., 1999; Larson et al., 1999; Fitzjohn et al., 2001a), which could indirectly affect LTP through the property of cooperativity (see Section 10.3.1). A decrease in LTP was also observed in a mouse that overexpressed an amyloidogenic fragment of the C-terminal of APP (Nalbantoglu et al., 1997). An alternative approach to investigating the role of APP in AD is to generate a mouse with null expression of APP. APP-null mice also display LTP deficits under some, but not all, conditions (Seabrook et al., 1999). In particular, no deficit was seen when GABA inhibition was blocked, suggesting that the effect on LTP is mediated via a relative increase in synaptic inhibition (Fitzjohn et al., 2001a). This raises the possibility that APP is required for normal functioning of GABA-mediated synaptic transmission.

A larger number of cases of familial AD have mutations in *PS1*, a component of the machinery involved in APP processing. Mice expressing *PS* mutations generally have enhanced LTP (Parent et al., 1999; Barrow et al., 2000; Zaman et al., 2000) possibly because Ca^{2+} homeostasis is affected (Schneider et al., 2001). In a conditional forebrain-specific *PS1* knockout mice there were no detectable changes in basal transmission or LTP (Yu et al., 2001), whereas in a mouse underexpressing *PS1* there was a deficit in LTP evoked with multiple tetani (Morton et al., 2002). In humans, the ApoE4 isoform of the lipid-shuttling protein apolipoprotein E (ApoE) is a risk factor for AD. A mouse with the ApoE gene knocked out showed near-normal LTP (Anderson et al., 1998)

even in the aged animal (Valastro et al, 2001), though a deficit in LTP has also been reported (Trommer et al., 2004). Interestingly, a knock-in mouse expressing human ApoE4 showed enhanced LTP when young (Kitamura et al., 2004); LTP dropped back to wild-type levels during adulthood and has not yet been examined in the aged knock-in mice.

The other major approach to investigating the role of Aβ in AD is to apply Aβ exogenously. In most such studies, Aβ has been found to impair LTP. For example, Aβ blocked both E-LTP and L-LTP without affecting baseline transmission in both the dentate gyrus and area CA1 in vitro (Lambert et al., 1998; Chen et al., 2000; Wang et al., 2002). Not all studies, however, have reported deficits in LTP following Aβ application. For example, LTP was enhanced in the perforant path input to dentate gyrus (Wu et al., 1995a). There is also generally a block of LTP in vivo, though L-LTP appears to be more sensitive than E-LTP (Cullen et al., 1997; Freir et al., 2001). At longer intervals after Aβ injection impairment of baseline transmission also becomes apparent (Cullen et al., 1996; Stephan et al., 2001), resembling the situation in several of the transgenic mouse studies.

Interestingly, studies with Aβ fragments suggest that the active forms responsible for the inhibition of LTP are soluble Aβ oligomers (Walsh et al., 2002). Other studies have addressed the mechanisms responsible for the Aβ impairment of LTP and have uncovered interactions of Aβ with the cholinergic system (Auld et al., 2002), in particular nicotinic receptors and the ERK2 MAPK cascade (Dineley et al., 2001), the GABA system (Sun and Alkon, 2002), NMDA receptors (Wu et al., 1995b), and CREB (Tong et al., 2001).

The first, partially effective, drugs used to treat AD were cholinesterase inhibitors, which exert their effect by potentiating cholinergic function in regions such as the hippocampus. Cholinergic systems facilitate NMDAR-dependent LTP, possibly in part by direct potentiation of the NMDA receptor conductance (see Section 10.6.1). It is feasible, therefore, that their cognitive enhancing effect at the early stages of AD is due to the facilitation of LTP. The next compound to be introduced into the clinic for the treatment of AD was memantine, which is a weak NMDA receptor antagonist (Parsons et al., 1999). It may seem paradoxical that an NMDA receptor antagonist can have cognitive enhancing properties. However, a plausible mechanism of action has been advanced based on studies on hippocampal LTP (Coan et al., 1989). It was found that bathing hippocampal slices in a Mg^{2+}-free medium resulted in the inhibition of LTP. However, if a concentration of AP5 was added to the slices that would ordinarily block LTP, LTP could be obtained. If, however, a higher concentration of AP5 was used, LTP was inhibited. These surprising findings were interpreted as follows. To induce LTP requires either no activation or perhaps a very low level of NMDA receptor activation during baseline stimulation but then a high degree of NMDA receptor activity briefly during a tetanus. When Mg^{2+} was omitted from the bathing medium, the baseline level of NMDA receptor activation both before and following the tetanus was greatly enhanced; this inhibited the LTP process, probably by preinduction and partial saturation of LTP. The addition of a standard concentration of AP5 substituted for Mg^{2+} and suppressed NMDA receptor activation. During the tetanus, however, the concentration was insufficient to block the induction of LTP given the absence of Mg^{2+}. That a higher concentration was effective demonstrates that it is NMDAR-dependent LTP that is recovered by AP5 treatment. What is the relevance of this to disease? In various pathological states, such as AD, the general dysfunction could lead to depolarization of neurons, for example due to problems with energy levels affecting glutamate uptake. Indeed, blocking glutamate uptake produces a similar NMDA receptor-dependent inhibition of LTP (Katagiri et al., 2001). Memantine is a weak, high voltage-dependent NMDA receptor antagonist (Parsons et al., 1993) that can also restore the ability of slices bathed in Mg^{2+}-free medium to undergo LTP (Frankiewiez and Parson), 1999). So its probable mechanism of action is to inhibit spurious activation of NMDA receptors in modestly depolarized cells; but during strong depolarization (e.g., during a tetanus) it is rapidly displaced from NMDA receptors. In this way it can facilitate LTP. In addition, its ability to inhibit tonic activation of NMDA receptors could endow it with neuroprotective properties (Danysz et al., 2000).

Down's Syndrome

The segmental trisomy mouse (Ts65Dn) has an extra chromosome 16 (corresponding to human chromosome 21) and has accordingly found use as a model for Down's syndrome. The Ts65Dn mouse shows learning impairments and a reduction in LTP at CA1 synapses in vitro (Siarey et al, 1997). In a subsequent study, a deficit was found in theta-burst LTP but not in tetanus-induced LTP; the deficit was rescued by blocking GABA inhibition (Costa and Grybko, 2005). A reduction in LTP in the dentate gyrus of the Ts65Dn mouse that was rescued by blockade of GABA inhibition has also been observed (Kleschevnikov et al, 2004). There is also a deficit in LTP in the Ts1Cje mouse model of Down's syndrome (Siarey et al, 2005). In this mouse both the cognitive deficits and the LTP deficits are less severe. Whereas LTP is reduced in mouse models of Down's syndrome, LTD is increased (Siarey et al., 1999, 2005). A mouse expressing most of human chromosome 21, in addition to both copies of the homologous mouse chromosome 16, shows learning deficits and a reduction in LTP in the dentate gyrus in vivo (O'Doherty et al., 2005). Thus, all mouse models of Down's syndrome so far studied have displayed alterations in LTP or LTD, consistent with the hypothesis that deficits in hippocampal synaptic plasticity may play a causative role in the cognitive deficits associated with the condition.

Huntington's Disease

Huntington's disease is a progressive neurodegenerative disorder associated with multiple CAG repeats in the gene encoding the protein huntingtin; it usually starts around the third to fifth decade of life. Neuronal loss is primarily in the striatum and cerebral cortex but can involve the hippocampus at later stages. However, before the onset of classical symptoms, patients often exhibit cognitive deficits. Studies in various mouse models of Huntington's disease have reported deficits in LTP at Schaffer–commissural synapses (Usdin et al., 1999; Hodgson et al., 1999; Murphy et al., 2000). Strikingly, and in contrast to control animals, slices from adult mutant mice readily displayed NMDA receptor-dependent LTD and depotentiation at Schaffer–commissural synapses (Murphy et al., 2000). Expression of the full-length mutated huntingtin in cell lines results in augmentation of NR2B containing NMDA receptors (Chen et al., 1999), which might explain the enhancement of LTD (see Section 10.7.3). Mossy fiber LTP is also reduced in a mouse model of Huntington's disease (Gibson et al., 2005). In this study a similar LTP deficit was observed in mice lacking complexin II, a protein that is reduced in Huntington's disease patients.

Schizophrenia

Schizophrenia is another developmentally regulated disorder that involves cognitive impairment as well as psychosis. There are good reasons to believe that schizophrenia involves pathological alterations in synaptic plasticity, in particular LTP-like processes. Thus, one of the best animal models of schizophrenia involves injection of phencyclidine (PCP). It is a curious coincidence that in the same year that the NMDA receptor was established as the trigger for LTP at Schaffer-commissural synapses (Collingridge et al., 1983), it was also shown that PCP and other dissociative anesthetics such as ketamine are potent blockers of NMDA receptors (Anis et al., 1983) and that PCP blocks induction of LTP at these synapses (Stringer et al, 1983). Since then, the glutamate hypothesis of schizophrenia has gained in popularity and is now the dominant hypothesis in the field. The general notion is that schizophrenia may involve impairment of NMDAR-dependent LTP in the hippocampus and other brain regions affected by the disease, thereby leading to impairment of LTP, cognitive dysfunction, and thought disturbances. Evidence to support the hypothesis that LTP may be affected in schizophrenia is starting to accumulate. For example, in the post-weaning social isolation model of schizophrenia there is a reduction in NMDAR-dependent LTP in the CA1 projection to the subiculum (Roberts and Greene, 2003). There are many ways in which NMDA receptor-dependent LTP could be directly or indirectly affected, and it seems likely that genetic and environmental influences can modify synaptic plasticity in various ways. For example, the schizophrenia-susceptibility gene *neuregulin-1* stimulates the internalization of GluR1-containing AMPA receptors and leads to depotentiation of NMDAR-dependent LTP (Kwon et al., 2005).

Diabetes and Other Diseases Associated with Potential Cognitive Deficits

Cognitive deficits associated with type I diabetes may also involve alterations in hippocampal synaptic plasticity. For example, there is an impairment of LTP at Schaffer–commissural synapses in nonobese diabetic rats and upregulation of NMDA receptors (Valastro et al., 2002). Similarly, rats treated with streptozotocin, a pancreatic beta cell toxin, have impaired LTP and enhanced LTD at Schaffer–commissural synapses (Artola et al., 2005). In contrast, LTP appeared normal at these synapses in Zucker diabetic fatty rats, a model of type II diabetes (Belanger et al., 2004).

Epilepsy

A link between epilepsy and LTP has long been suspected, but the evidence to date is not compelling. In two animal models of human temporal lobe epilepsy—kindling and pilocarpine-induced seizures—LTP is reduced, probably because synapses become potentiated during the seizures (Schubert et al., 2005). LTP is also impaired in slices prepared from human epileptic dentate gyrus relative to nonepileptic tissue (Beck et al., 2000). Kindling is induced in temporal lobe structures, most readily in the amygdala, by daily repetitions of brief high-frequency sinusoidal stimulation, typically at 60 Hz for 1 second. Initially, stimulation produces no behavioral effects, but eventually, after several daily repetitions, the same protocol leads to generalized convulsions (Goddard, 1967). Is there an LTP component to kindling? Cain (1989) noted several differences between LTP and the pathological processes elicited by kindling stimulation. Thus, the development of kindling may be delayed but is not blocked by NMDA receptor antagonists. During later stages of kindling, evoked responses are often diminished rather than enhanced. Moreover, repeated tetanic stimulation of afferent pathways of the kind that induces LTP does not elicit kindling. The kinetics of onset and persistence are also very different in the two cases; kindling requires several daily sessions to reach full expression and is then effectively permanent. LTP is induced within seconds or minutes but in most cases returns to baseline within days or weeks. Thus, it seems reasonable to conclude that the sorts of stimulation that lead to LTP are not in themselves epileptogenic, and that LTP lies at the benign end of the spectrum of activity-dependent changes in synaptic efficacy.

Synaptic Plasticity and the Enhancement or Suppression of Memory

Increasing confidence in the existence of a causal link between LTP and memory has encouraged the development of pharmaceutical approaches to the treatment of memory dysfunction based on targets such as glutamate receptors and transcription factors known to be important in LTP and/or LTD. Though still at a relatively early stage of development, these approaches hold great promise for the future (see reviews by Cooke and Bliss, 2005 and Lynch, 2006).

Summary

A common emerging theme is that a number of diseases involving cognitive deficits have altered hippocampal synaptic plasticity, in particular changes in NMDAR-dependent LTP and/or LTD. It seems likely, therefore, that synaptic plasticity in the brain of the type represented by LTP and LTD is disrupted in these diseases and contributes to the etiology of cognitive impairment. By extension, it seems likely that alterations in LTP and LTD in the hippocampus and other brain regions may be involved in other neurological and psychiatric disorders, including drug addiction (Hyman and Malenka, 2001) anxiety, depression, bipolar disorders, motoneuron disease, and Parkinson's disease.

10.10 Functional Implications of Hippocampal Synaptic Plasticity

What is the function of LTP? Is it a physiological phenomenon that engages the same neural mechanisms that are responsible for certain forms of learning and memory? Or is it a laboratory curiosity of no functional significance? A version of these questions was posed at the end of the first article on LTP (Bliss and Lomo, 1973), and the debate has been with us ever since. In this concluding section of the chapter, we turn to the functional significance of activity-dependent synaptic plasticity in relation to behavior.

10.10.1 Synaptic Plasticity and Memory Hypothesis

Most functional studies of LTP and LTD address their possible roles in learning, with the majority of studies focusing on NMDAR-dependent forms of plasticity. The aim of such research has been caricatured by Stevens (1998) in the question "Does LTP equal memory?" There are numerous qualifications to such a question. What type of LTP? What type of learning? What role for LTD and depotentiation? Is the persistence of LTP correlated with and responsible for the persistence of memory? These questions indicate that the debate has moved on from merely recognizing certain analogies between LTP and learning to specific ideas about how the mechanisms of induction and expression of synaptic plasticity relate to the multiple types and processes of memory that we now know to exist (see Chapter 13). These ideas share a common generic theme that has been called the "synaptic plasticity and memory" (SPM) hypothesis (Martin et al., 2000). The SPM hypothesis asserts that synaptic plasticity (1) occurs during ordinary brain activity, and (2) is responsible for memory formation, as follows (Martin et al., 2000).

> Activity-dependent synaptic plasticity is induced at appropriate synapses during memory formation, and is both necessary and sufficient for the information storage underlying the type of memory mediated by the brain area in which that plasticity is observed.

With respect to the hippocampus, this implies that some of the neural mechanisms of synaptic plasticity discussed above, such as alterations in AMPA receptor trafficking, should occur during hippocampus-dependent forms of learning and be necessary for that learning to occur.

Earlier in the chapter, it was pointed out that synaptic plasticity displays physiological properties that are highly suggestive of an information storage device, as many have asserted the hippocampus to be (McNaughton, 1983; Lynch and Baudry, 1984; Goelet et al., 1986; Morris et al., 1990; Bliss and Collingridge, 1993; Barnes, 1995; Jeffery, 1997; Shors and Matzel, 1997). Such classical properties include *associativity*, *input-specificity*, and *persistence*. These may be relevant to associative features of learning and memory, as follows. First, associative induction implies the capacity to relate a pattern of presynaptic neural activity with a pattern of postsynaptic activity, as in the association of ideas. Second, they are relevant to storage capacity because a synapse-specific mechanism endows the network with greater storage capacity than would changes in cell excitability. Third, to store information in the brain, some persistent change in the nervous system has to occur. Whether these changes necessarily have to last as long as memory is debatable. A qualification is that hippocampal-neocortical consolidation mechanisms may become engaged that would obviate the need for long-lasting persistence in the hippocampus, notwithstanding the fact that LTP in the dentate gyrus has been shown to last for more than a year in rodents (Abraham, 2003; Abraham and Robins, 2005).

The pioneering studies implicating LTP in memory were correlational. Barnes (1979) and Barnes and McNaughton (1985) observed, in the course of work on aging, that the persistence of LTP over time was statistically correlated with the rate of learning and/or the degree of retention of spatial memory in a circular arena task (see Chapter 13 for a description of this and other behavioral tasks). Similar correlations have been observed many times, another example arising in studies of the overexpression of human mutant amyloid precursor protein (hAPP) in a murine model of Alzheimer's disease (Hsiao et al., 1996). This is associated with an age-related decline in performance in a delayed spatial alternation task that is correlated with a corresponding decline in LTP, assessed in vivo and in vitro (Chapman et al., 1999). Lynch (2004) reviewed a number of other cases where similar correlations are observed.

However, it is far from clear that the physiological properties of synaptic plasticity are, in general, likely to be exactly homologous to, and thus correlated with, parameters of learning at the behavioral level. Some properties should be directly related. One example is that the mechanisms of "induction" of LTP and the "encoding" of memory should overlap. Other properties are less likely to be correlated because the overt manifestations of memory are not due solely to synaptic properties—they also depend on the properties of the network in which that plasticity is embedded (see Chapter 14). An example of mismatch is that the temporal contiguity requirements for presynaptic glutamate release and postsynaptic depolarization in the induction of NMDAR-dependent LTP (see Section 10.3) are temporally much tighter than those governing various forms of associative conditioning. This has sometimes been mentioned as a weakness of the SPM hypothesis (Diamond and Rose, 1994). Associative conditioning depends on the ability of the CS to predict the US (contingency); simply pairing—CS and US (contiguity)—is not sufficient if, for example, many additional unpaired CS and US presentations are also introduced. The studies of spike timing plasticity (see Section 10.3) illustrate the temporal contiguity requirements for LTP, but to date they say nothing about contingency. However, an investigation of amygdalar plasticity reveals that LTP and fear conditioning are indeed both sensitive to CS-US contingency (Bauer et al., 2001). A train of tetanic stimulation of thalamic afferents to the lateral amygdala in vitro was paired with a series of depolarizing current pulses to the postsynaptic neuron. This procedure was repeated 15 times at 20-second intervals, resulting in robust LTP. Intriguingly, the addition of unpaired depolarization 10 seconds after each pairing—analogous to unpaired US presentations—resulted in almost no LTP despite the preservation of contiguity. The mechanisms underlying this contingency phenomenon clearly operate over a time scale of at least 10 seconds. These findings illustrate that LTP, at least in the lateral amygdala, reflects a property of learning that might have been expected to arise only at the circuit level.

Synaptic plasticity does, of course, have distinct functions in different parts of the nervous system. In the amygdala, it has been implicated in conditioned fear (LeDoux, 2000), thereby reflecting a feature of the generic SPM hypothesis ("type of memory mediated by the brain area"). However, in the spinal cord, LTP-like changes have been implicated in hyperalgesia to painful stimuli (Fitzgerald, 2005). This illustrates one of the themes of this book—how principles that were first developed for the hippocampus have had a wider significance in neuroscience. LTP and LTD may also have other functions in the hippocampus. Proposals include the "plasticity/pathology continuum" hypothesis (McEachern and Shaw, 1996) and the notion that synaptic changes play a role in attentional rather than memory processes (Shors and Matzel, 1997). Distinguishing between these and alternative hypotheses about the functions of synaptic plasticity is not always easy, and exacting analytical studies are required.

Martin et al. (2000) proposed four criteria for a rigorous test of the SPM hypothesis: detectability, anterograde alteration, retrograde alteration, and mimicry. Broadly speaking, they correspond to correlation, necessity, and sufficiency. The first of these four criteria, *detectability*, states that, in association with the formation of memory lasting any length of time, LTP or LTD must occur at certain synapses in one or more brain areas and should, in principle, be detectable. The limited number of synapses that change with any one learning experience might make this criterion difficult to meet experimentally. The possibility of heterosynaptic LTD in conjunction with learning-induced potentiation poses a similar problem. The second criterion, *anterograde alteration*, asserts that blocking the mechanisms that induce or express changes in synaptic weights should have the anterograde effect of impairing new learning. The intervention may be achieved in various ways: physiologically, pharmacologically, or through molecular-genetic manipulation. The NMDA receptor has been a particular target, but there is a growing body of work examining interventions that affect the transition from protein synthesis-independent to protein synthesis-dependent forms of LTP and of memory. A separate aspect of necessity—our third criterion, *retrograde alteration*—is that altering the pattern of synaptic weights after learning has taken place should affect an animal's memory of past experience. This arises because altering the spatial distributon of synaptic weights within a distributed associative matrix such as the hippocampus should alter the associations retrieved from such a network. Finally, if changes in synaptic weight are the neural basis of trace storage, their artificial induction in a specific spatial pattern of weights should give rise to an "apparent" memory (mimicry) for a stimulus or event that did not, in practice, actually occur. Although this criterion may seem fanciful, particularly in the hippocampus, it is the ultimate "engineering" criterion that is most likely to convince skeptics of the functional importance of LTP. For reasons we shall come to, it may be easier to meet this criterion in brain areas such as the amygdala than in the hippocampus.

10.10.2 Detectability: Is Learning Associated with the Induction of LTP?

The SPM hypothesis requires that synaptic changes must occur during learning. The experimental design is ostensibly straightforward: Synaptic efficacy is compared before and after a variety of learning experiences. The prediction is that a persistent increase in synaptic efficacy should occur at appropriate synapses in association with certain types of learning. Types of learning that engage the hippocampal formation should be associated with synaptic potentiation, whereas other types of learning should not. What is less clear is whether such synaptic changes would be readily detectable in global measures such as fEPSPs.

Exploration-induced and Spatial Learning-induced Changes in Hippocampal Field Potentials and Transmitter Release

Considerable excitement surrounded the discovery of what appeared to be striking short-term modulation of perforant-path evoked EPSPs in the dentate gyrus during spatial exploration (Sharp et al., 1989; Green et al., 1990). Exploratory activity was accompanied by an increase in the dentate fEPSP and a decrease in both amplitude and latency of the population spike. However, Moser et al. (1993a) discovered that this unusual pattern of electrophysiological change during exploration is largely due to changes in brain temperature caused by associated muscular activity (Fig. 10–22A). Application of

radiant heat was sufficient to induce changes in fEPSPs. If during exploration the animal's brain was "temperature-clamped" by intermittent infrared heating, exploratory motor activity was no longer associated with changes in the fEPSP. Moser et al. (1993b, 1994) went on to work out the calibration functions relating brain temperature to fEPSP magnitude before placing animals in an environment containing six landmarks. A small temperature-independent component of the increase in fEPSP was observed that was correlated with exploration (Fig. 10–22B). This increased rapidly at the start of exploration and declined gradually to baseline over a short period (15 minutes). Further studies have shown exploratory behavior to be associated with the activation of immediate early genes (IEGs) such as c-*fos* (Gall et al., 1998) and *Arc* (Guzowski et al., 1999). Temperature controls have not, to our knowledge, been conducted in these studies, but these patterns of IEG activation are unlikely to be entirely due to activity-associated changes in brain temperature, as the spatial distribution of Arc expression in area CA1 over two exploration sessions is exquisitely sensitive to the spatial similarity of the two enclosures in which testing takes place (Guzowski et al., 1999).

Complementing these studies of fEPSPs in behaving animals have been studies comparing brain tissue (in vitro) from animals that have been exposed to a learning situation with tissue from animals that have been left unattended. For example, Green and Greenough (1986) saw enhanced fEPSPs in the dentate gyrus in response to perforant path stimulation in slices taken from adult animals that had been reared in complex environments. This study was particularly well controlled in showing no changes in antidromic potentials or presynaptic fiber volleys. However, it is possible that experience can alter neurogenesis in the dentate gyrus (see Chapter 9). Such changes could contribute to or account for the findings of Green and Greenough (1986); enhanced fEPSPs could reflect the creation of new neurons and synapses.

An increase in glutamate release has also been reported following both LTP (see Section 10.3) and watermaze learning (Richter-Levin et al., 1995; McGahon et al., 1996). Richter-Levin et al. (1997) trained rats in a spatial watermaze task for varying numbers of trials and then induced LTP in vivo on one side of the brain; finally, they examined veratridine-induced glutamate release in synaptosomes prepared from the hippocampus of the trained animals. Learning was associated with increased glutamate release. Tissue prepared from the hemisphere in which LTP had been induced showed a greater increase in glutamate release when taken from rats at an early stage of training than at a later stage. Thus, not only were both LTP and learning associated with an increase in glutamate release, but the learning-associated increase occluded the increase normally seen after LTP. This striking result would be in accord with the SPM hypothesis were it not for the further finding that the amount of perforant path-induced LTP in vivo was the same in both the undertrained and extensively trained groups. This is puzzling. That the magnitude of electrophysiologically induced LTP is unaffected by prior spatial learning is consistent with the idea that an individual learning experience may enhance only a small proportion of synapses in the dentate gyrus. However, if this is the case, why was the LTP seen after extensive learning not associated with an increase in glutamate release? Perhaps learning is associated with a shift in the relative expression of presynaptically mediated and postsynaptically mediated LTP.

One puzzle about detectability concerns the difficulty in oberving learning-associated synaptic changes in the hippocampus. Storage capacity could be one factor, particularly in a distributed-associative system such as the hippocampus; another could be that heterosynaptic depression (LTD) may occur at other synapses during learning, rendering field potentials an inappropriate way to investigate the issue. Heterosynaptic LTD might serve a normalizing or scaling function in a distributed associative memory system by ensuring that the sum of the synaptic weights on any given neuron remains roughly constant (Willshaw and Dayan, 1990) see Section 10.3.14; fEPSP amplitude would then remain unchanged. Given this, the issue might be better pursued in other brain structures or with other techniques.

Learning-related fEPSP Changes in Other Brain Areas

Vindicating this suspicion, the detectability criterion has been spectacularly upheld in studies of amygdala-dependent fear conditioning. Rogan et al. (1997) monitored evoked potentials elicited by an auditory CS in the lateral amygdala in vivo before and after auditory fear conditioning. Paired presentations of the auditory CS and foot shock resulted in increased freezing behavior and a parallel potentiation of the CS-evoked potential. Enhancement of electrically evoked responses was also found in brain slices taken from fear-conditioned rats (McKernan and Shinnick-Gallagher, 1997), and an increase in auditory evoked responses following tone fear conditioning has since been reported in freely moving mice (Tang et al., 2001, 2003). Learning-induced changes in evoked responses occlude electrically induced LTP, implying that the two processes engage common mechanisms (Tsvetkov et al., 2002; Schroeder and Shinnick-Gallagher, 2005); such changes can also be persistent, lasting at least 10 days in the latter case. A recent study offers further insights into the mechanisms of learning-related plasticity, providing more direct evidence that the learning-related changes are mechanistically similar to LTP (Rumpel et al., 2005). Using the rectification of AMPA receptor-mediated transmission as an index of mutated GluR1 subunit incorporation, as in the studies of LTP expression described above (see Section 10.4), tone-fear conditioning was shown to be associated with an increase in EPSCs associated with AMPA receptor trafficking in the pathway from the auditory thalamus to the amygdala in vitro (Fig. 10–22C). The change was greater when paired conditioning trials were used in which the tone preceded the fear-evoking shock by an optimum CS–US interval but much weaker after unpaired conditioning. Use of a "plasticity-block" vector (Malinow and Malenka, 2002) to interfere with AMPA receptor trafficking prevented the learning-associated rectification of AMPA-mediated transmission and, in separate experiments, learning itself. Intriguingly, plasticity had to be disturbed in only a small percentage of neurons (approximately 27%) for an effect to be observed, raising the possibility that combinatorial effects may be responsible for the learning of different CS-US pairings.

A phenomenon resembling LTP also occurs in the primary motor cortex (M1) following acquisition of a motor skill in rats. Rioult-Pedotti et al. (1998) trained rats to reach through a hole in a small plastic box with their preferred paw to retrieve food pellets. After a few days of training, recordings from brain slices revealed that EPSPs from layer II/III of the contralateral M1 of trained rats were substantially larger than those recorded in the ipilateral untrained hemisphere or in untrained animals (Fig. 10–22D). Similar LTP-like changes have since been observed in M1 following motor learning in vivo (Monfils and Teskey, 2004). In a follow-up study, repeated trains of either high- or low-frequency stimulation were delivered to saturate LTP or LTD, respectively (Rioult-Pedotti et al., 2000). Strikingly, the capacity for further LTP was reduced (and LTD enhanced) following motor learning despite the synaptic potentials being larger—reflecting no change in the synaptic plasticity range of the synapses affected by or involved in motor learning. This partial occlusion suggests that LTP and skill learning may engage similar neuronal mechanisms. However, a puzzle about these findings is that the increase in EPSPs is typically large (about 50%), and the spatial distribution of the weight changes and their information content are currently unknown. We argued above that, in the hippocampus at least, learning-related changes in EPSPs are likely to be extremely small. This may not be true in the motor cortex, but the result is surprising nonetheless. It is not clear whether such changes actually encode the learned skill—thus constituting a motor engram—or serve some other, less specific role in the information processing that accompanies motor learning. Would similar fEPSP increases be seen for each new skill that is learned? Alternatively, might such a large change occur only when the rodent motor cortex is engaged in skill learning for the first time?

Learning-induced changes in evoked responses have also been observed in several other brain areas. For example, increased fEPSPs have been observed in the piriform cortex in conjunction with olfactory learning (Roman et al., 2004; Sevelinges et al., 2004); and enhancement of LTP accompanied by facilitation of LTD has also been reported (Lebel et al., 2001). Lasting potentiation of transmission at the parallel fiber–Purkinje cell synapse of the cerebellum has been observed following auditory fear conditioning (Sacchetti et al., 2004), and induction of an LTP-like effect during learning has been observed in the connections of the fimbria to the lateral septum (Jaffard et al., 1996). Synaptic changes are also implicated in the experience-dependent reorganization of

A Exploration (STEM)   Heating only

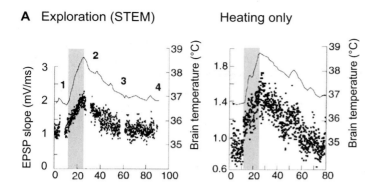

B Exploration, with heating subtracted

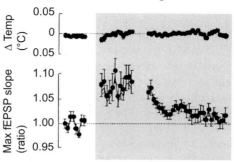

C AMPA receptor trafficking induced by learning

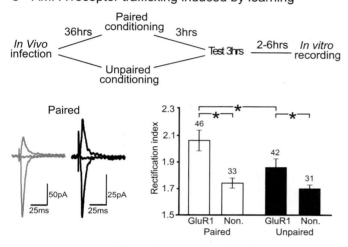

D Induction of LTP by motor learning

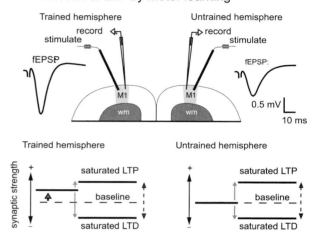

Figure 10–22. Detectability: induction of LTP-like changes in association with learning? *A, B.* Early studies that explored whether learning is associated with increased fEPSPs revealed some constraints on this approach. For example, novelty exploration is associated with an increase in both fEPSPs and brain temperature. Control studies established that in most cases the temperature change could explain some but not all of the change in fEPSPs that were at first thought to be due to learning-associated LTP induction. A short-lasting temperature-independent component can be detected. (*Source:* Moser et al., 1993a, 1994.) *C.* Fear conditioning in

the amygdala is associated with enhanced AMPA receptor trafficking, measured using rectification of AMPA receptor-mediated transmission as an index of mutated GluR1 subunit incorporation. See text for discussion. (*Source:* After Rumpel et al., 2005.) *D.* Motor learning restricted to one limb in rodents (food-pellet collecting) is associated with an increase in the size of fEPSPs in layer III of the contralateral motor cortex, and this increase occludes the extent of subsequent LTP induction relative to the opposite hemisphere. (*Source:* After Rioult-Pedotti et al., 1998, 2000.)

Associative Conditioning and Hippocampal fEPSPs

Despite the difficulty of detecting hippocampal LTP-like phenomena after spatial learning, lasting changes in population measures of hippocampal activity have been observed after certain forms of conditioning (see Weisz et al., 1984). For example, an increase in the slope of the CA1 fEPSP has been reported in rat hippocampal slices prepared after contextual fear conditioning (Sacchetti et al., 2001) and in freely moving mice after auditory fear conditioning (Tang et al., 2003) and

cortical representations (e.g., Weinberger, 2004), but a detailed treatment of this topic is beyond the scope of this book.

trace eyeblink conditioning (Gruart et al., 2006). In a follow-up to their original study, Sacchetti et al. (2002) found that, as in M1 and piriform cortex, learning results in partial occlusion of subsequent LTP only when assessed up to 1 day after training; the increase in fEPSPs was previously found to last for 7 days. Perhaps synapse formation occurs in tandem with the consolidation of existing memory trace, reestablishing the capacity for normal LTP after several days while preserving established changes in synaptic strength—although metaplastic chances might provide an alternative explanation (Abraham and Tate, 1997; cf. Moser, et al., 1993a; Lebel et al., 2001). Consistent with other early work of Moser et al. (1993b, 1994), mere exploration of a novel context without shock resulted in an increase in the evoked response and partial occlusion of LTP in slices prepared 10 minutes after exploration but not at later time points. These findings confirm that exploration alone is insufficient to cause lasting potentiation of hippocampal fEPSPs (Sacchetti et al., 2001).

The less than compelling literature on detectability in the hippocampus considered so far received a major boost from two papers published in 2006. In the first study, Gruart et al. (2006) implanted stimulating and recording electrodes in area CA1 of the mouse hippocampus, and monitored Schaffer-commissural responses while animals were trained in a trace eyeblink conditioning task, using an airpuff as the unconditioned stimulus, and a tone as the conditioned stimulus. Trace conditioning is a hippocampus-dependent form of classical conditioning in which a delay is imposed between the end of the CS and the onset of the US. Gruart et al found that the amplitude of the evoked fEPSP significantly increased as training progressed, and then declined as the conditioned response was extinguished. Both learning and the potentiation of the fEPSP were NMDAR-dependent, indicating that the potentiation was LTP rather than some other facilitatory process. In the second study, from Mark Bear's laboratory, Whitlock et al. (2006) used a hippocampus-dependent one-trial learning procedure to look for changes in fEPSPs using an array of 8 recording electrodes implanted in area CA1. In a first recording session baseline responses were collected. The animals were then trained in an inhibitory avoidance conditioning task, in which the rat forms an immediate aversion to the dark compartment of a two-compartment box after receiving a footshock there. Animals were then returned to the recording chamber. Across all trained animals, a significant potentiation of the fEPSP was seen in 27% of electrodes, detectable as soon as recording was begun 15 min after the footshock, and continuing at a stable level for 4 hours. A tetanus was then given to test for occlusion. LTP was significantly greater at non-potentiated than potentiated recording sites; this partial occlusion is powerful evidence that the potentiation observed was LTP. Whitlock et al. wondered if their failure to see LTP at more recording sites was a reflection that learning induces both LTP and LTD. They examined this possibility using an ingenious biochemical approach. LTP and LTD are associated with phosphorylation of AMPA receptors at different residues (see Section 10.7.4); using phospho-antibodies specific to the two sites they were able to obtain a phosphorylation index of the degree of LTP and LTD in hippocampal tissue from trained and control animals. The surprising finding was that training was associated with an increase in phosphorylation at ser831, the LTP-specific residue, but no change at ser845, the LTD specific residue. A question for future work is whether this result can be reconciled with the widely held assumption that stability in the hippocampal network requires LTP at some synapses to be balanced by LTD at others. One possibility is that other forms of persistent depression, such as heterosynaptic depotentiation and depression, which may have different biochemical signatures and which are easier to obtain in adults than de

novo LTD, provide the counterbalance. But perhaps the most provocative question to arise from this study is this: Given that some electrodes detect potentiation, why don't they all? The finding implies that synaptic weight changes are not uniformly distributed within the network, and suggests instead a "currant bun" model of memory, in which representations are stored in clusters of potentiated cells that are relatively far apart compared to the inter-electrode distance (250 μm) (see commentary by Bliss et al., 2006).

10.10.3 Anterograde Alteration: Do Manipulations That Block the Induction or Expression of Synaptic Plasticity Impair Learning?

The SPM hypothesis requires that any manipulations that limit or block the induction or expression of synaptic plasticity in the hippocampus should have corresponding effects on hippocampus-dependent learning. Meeting this second criterion has proved a particularly popular approach, with numerous pharmacological, molecular-genetic, and occlusion studies being conducted. Enhancement of LTP might also enhance learning, but this prediction is less straightforward because, as the BCM theory of metaplasticity implies (see Section 10.3.13), LTP and LTD exist in dynamic equilibrium. Disrupting this equilibrium might cause dysfunction, even if the agent of disruption is enhanced LTP. Moreover, perturbations that enhance LTP could arise for several reasons, only some of which would be expected to enhance learning.

Pharmacological Blockade of the NMDA Receptor Impairs Learning

Morris et al. (1986) showed that chronic intraventricular infusion of the NMDA antagonist D,L-AP5 blocked spatial but not visual discrimination learning in a watermaze (Fig. 10–23A). Later work established that this effect was due to the active D-isomer of AP5 (Davis et al., 1992) and that it occurs with acute intrahippocampal infusions of D-AP5 (Morris et al., 1989) and over a range of intrahippocampal drug concentrations comparable to those that impair hippocampal LTP in vivo and in vitro (Davis et al., 1992). Numerous studies have since found that competitive NMDA antagonists impair hippocampus-dependent learning. Learning paradigms used include spatial learning, T-maze alternation, certain types of olfactory learning, contextual fear-conditioning, social transmission of food preference, flavor-place paired associate learning (delayed reinforcement of low rates of response—DRL), and other operant tasks (Danysz et al., 1988; Tonkiss et al., 1988; Staubli et al., 1989; Tonkiss and Rawlins, 1991; Bolhuis and Reid, 1992; Cole et al., 1993; Lyford et al., 1993; Caramanos and Shapiro, 1994; Fanselow et al., 1994; Li et al., 1997; Steele and Morris, 1999; Lee and Kesner, 2002; Roberts and Shapiro, 2002; Day et al., 2003; Bast et al., 2005; for reviews see Danysz et al., 1995 and Lynch, 2004). These data strongly support the SPM hypothesis, but there are problems with the interpretation of these findings associated with sensorimotor side effects of NMDA antagonists and effects of these drugs on neuronal processes other than LTP.

In humans, administration of ketamine results in hallucinations. We cannot know what rats are seeing or smelling under the influence of an NMDA antagonist. However, sensorimotor disturbances are sometimes observed during watermaze training with diffuse NMDA receptor blockade, including falling off the platform during a "wet-dog" shake, thigmotaxis, and failure to climb onto the platform (Cain et al., 1996; Saucier et al., 1996). Motor disturbances induced by NMDA antagonists are also seen during other tasks. Such abnormalities could be due to diffusion of drug to the thalamus disrupting the normal transmission of somatosensory and visual information (Sillito, 1985; Salt, 1986; Salt and Eaton, 1989) or to the striatum causing motor disturbances such as flaccidity (Turski et al., 1990). Clearly, learning cannot proceed when animals can neither sense nor move properly, and equally obviously it would be fallacious to assert that the drug is having a *direct* effect on learning mechanisms per se. Many laboratories have noted that animals treated with noncompetitive NMDA antagonists (such as MK-801) show sensory inattention and motor stereotypies (Koek et al., 1988; Tricklebank et al., 1989; Keith and Rudy, 1990; Tiedtke et al., 1990; Mondadori and Weiskrantz, 1991; Danysz et al., 1995; Cain et al., 1996). At high doses, AP5-treated animals also display stereotypies, but these doses are substantially higher than those necessary to block LTP in vivo following regionally restricted infusion. These problems are much less apparent with acute intrahippocampal infusion.

Using peripheral injections of an NMDA antagonist, Cain et al. (1996) showed that the impairment of spatial learning in a watermaze is correlated with the degree of sensorimotor impairment. They asserted that the sensorimotor deficit is primary and the learning deficit merely secondary. Saucier and Cain (1995) also observed that the impairment in watermaze learning that normally occurs following intraperitoneal administration of a competitive NMDA antagonist disappears if the animals are given sufficient pretraining to prevent the drug-induced sensorimotor disturbances seen in experimentally naive animals. Their pretrained animals showed a clear block of LTP after drug treatment, no sensorimotor impairment, and normal rates of spatial learning.

Other data indicate, however, that a deficit in spatial learning can still be observed, relative to appropriate control groups, following nonspatial pretraining (Morris, 1989; Bannerman et al., 1995). Bannerman et al. (1995) discovered that the usual AP5-induced learning deficit all but disappeared in animals trained first as normal animals in one watermaze ("downstairs") before later being trained in a second watermaze ("upstairs") under the influence of the drug. However, if training in the downstairs watermaze was nonspatial in character, with sight of extramaze cues occluded, the normal AP5-induced deficit in spatial learning was seen dur-

ing the second task. Sensorimotor disturbances were equally reduced by both procedures. Bannerman et al. (1995) suggested that blocking NMDA receptors dissociated different components of spatial learning—impairing an animal's ability to learn the required strategy rather than the map of landmarks in the room in which the watermaze is situated. This explanation was apparently refuted by Hoh et al. (1999), who reported that watermaze "strategy learning" is unaffected by intraperitoneal administration of the NMDA antagonist CGS19755 during nonspatial pretraining at a dose that successfully blocks LTP in freely moving animals in both CA1 and the dentate gyrus. The drug-treated rats learned nonspatial strategies adequately and showed equivalent performance in subsequent spatial learning and spatial reversal relative to vehicle-treated control animals. Hoh et al. (1999) suggested that relative task difficulty may explain the different outcome of their study and that of Bannerman et al. (1995)—the latter study involved a larger pool and a smaller escape platform.

Using single-unit recording to study the effects of the NMDA antagonist 3-(2-carboxypiperazin-4-yl)propyl-1-phosphonic acid (CPP) on hippocampal place fields (see Chapter 11), Kentros et al. (1998) showed that previously established firing fields are unchanged, and new place fields are acquired normally when rats are placed in a new environment. These findings are inconsistent with a sensorimotor disturbance hypothesis. Kentros et al. went on to show that the new place fields are unstable over time, implicating LTP induction in the learning of a new spatial context. Temporal instability of place fields was also observed in transgenic mice with altered LTP (Rotenberg et al., 1996). This temporal instability could account for Bannerman et al.'s (1995) finding of poor learning by naive animals trained with one trial per day but not the observation that spatially pretrained AP5-treated animals learn normally in a new environment.

Poor spatial memory over time in the presence of NMDA receptor blockade is unlikely to be specific to novel environments but task-specific in other ways. Steele and Morris (1999) trained rats in a delayed matching-to-place (DMP) task in the watermaze. In this variant of the task, the platform is hidden in a different location each day and stays there for four trials. Normal rats show quite long escape latencies on trial 1 (when they do not know where the platform is hidden) but much shorter latencies on subsequent trials (when they do). Most of the "savings" in escape latency occur between trials 1 and 2, indicative of one-trial learning. Infusion of APV had no effect on performance at a short memory delay (15-second intertrial interval) but caused pronounced impairment at 20 minutes and 2 hours. This delay-dependent deficit occurred irrespective of whether the animals stayed in the training context throughout the memory delay or were returned to the room with their home cages and irrespective of whether the drug was infused chronically into the ventricle or acutely into the hippocampus. If the AP5-induced impairment of the DMP task were sensorimotor or attentional in

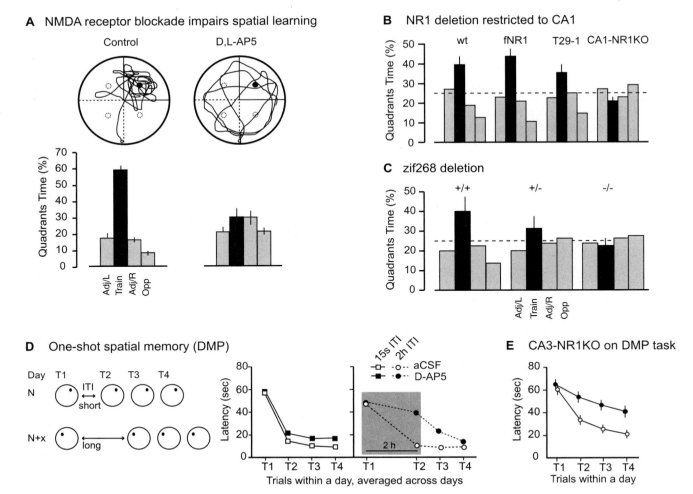

Figure 10–23. Anterograde alteration of LTP and memory. *A.* Chronic intraventricular infusion of the NMDA receptor antagonist D,L-AP5 blocks LTP induction in the dentate gyrus (not shown) and impairs spatial memory in a watermaze. Swim paths show focused searching in the target quadrant only by aCSF controls. Other experiments established that the drug spared simple visual discrimination learning. (*Source*: After Morris et al., 1986.) *B.* Cell-type and region-specific knockout of the NR1 subunit of the NMDA receptor in area CA1 of the hippocampus blocks LTP induction (not shown) and impairs spatial reference memory. (*Source*: After Tsien et al., 1996.) *C.* Knockout of the immediate early gene

zif-268 impairs LTP and long-term memory in the watermaze. Other experiments established that short-term memory was intact. (*Source*: After Jones et al., 2001.) *D.* One-shot learning in the watermaze can be studied using the DMP paradigm (see Figure 13–23 for explanation). Intrahippocampal D-AP5 infusion blocks memory of a one-time experience after 2 hours but leaves short-term (15 seconds) memory unaffected. (*Source*: After Steele and Morris, 1999.) *E.* Region-specific knockout of NR1 in area CA3 leaves spatial reference memory intact but impairs one-shot memory. (*Source*: After Nakazawa et al., 2003.)

nature, a deficit would be expected at all delays. The delay-dependent memory impairment is inconsistent with Kentros et al.'s (1998) proposal that temporal instability occurs only in a novel context.

In addition to addressing the potential sensorimotor side effects of AP5, the study by Steele and Morris (1999) indicated that rapid spatial learning remains sensitive to NMDA receptor blockade, even after pretraining. (The animals tested in this study received several days of "pretraining" on the DMP task prior to surgery and drug infusion). It may be significant that the DMP task requires the trial-unique encoding of novel locations, whereas the reference memory task involves the incremental learning of a single location over multiple trials. Consequently, the reference memory task may require little hippocampal synaptic plasticity in experienced animals, whereas substantial NMDAR-dependent plasticity might remain essential for one-trial encoding, even after extensive training. Consistent with this, selective impairment for rapid learning has been observed after several genetic interventions. Mice lacking the GluRI (GluR-A) subunit of the AMPA receptor, for example, have profound deficits in CA1 LTP, but acquisition of a watermaze reference memory task is normal; severe impairments are found in spatial working memory, however, such as T-maze nonmatching to place (see Chapter 7 for a detailed discussion). Similar results have also been obtained after targeting an entirely different component of the hippocampal circuitry—the recurrent collateral system of CA3. Mice with a CA3-specific knockout of the gene coding for the NR1 subunit of the NMDA receptor lack associative LTP in this subregion (although the direct entorhinal input to CA3 is probably also compromised), but the acquisition of a standard watermaze reference memory task remains unaffected, at least when all cues are present during retrieval (Nakazawa et al., 2002). Performance in a DMP version of the task, in contrast, is markedly impaired (Nakazawa et al., 2003). Molecular-genetic approaches are discussed below.

The NMDA receptor is implicated in the induction but not the expression of LTP (see Section 10.3). By analogy, one may predict that NMDA antagonists should impair the encoding of new memory "traces" (induction) but have no effect on memory retrieval (expression). Consistent with this idea, Staubli et al. (1989) found that administering AP5 to animals after they had been trained in odor discrimination learning had no effect on retention, although the drug did impair new learning. Entorhinal cortex lesions, on the other hand, cause rapid forgetting of olfactory information (Staubli et al., 1984). Likewise, Morris (1989) and Morris et al. (1990) found that APV had no effect on retention of a previously trained water-maze task, whereas lesions of the hippocampal formation were disruptive when given shortly after the end of training. Similar deficits in encoding but not retrieval were noted in the DMP task of Steele and Morris (1999). Using a one-trial paired-associate learning paradigm, Day et al. (2003) showed that intrahippocampal infusion of D-AP5 prior to the "sample" trial when two novel stimuli were paired for the first time caused subsequent choice performance in the memory "retrieval" trial to fall to chance. Delaying the infusion of D-AP5 by 20 minutes until after the sample trial, such that memory retrieval was also conducted with dorsal hippocampal NMDA receptors blocked, had no effect on memory. Both effects were seen at doses sufficient to block LTP in vivo. Similar recents were recently obtained in a purely spatial version of the task (Bast et al., 2005).

Long-term memory retention can, however, be impaired by the blockade of hippocampal NMDA receptors soon after, as well as during, learning (Izquierdo et al., 1993, 1998; Packard and Teather, 1997; McDonald et al., 2005). These findings suggest that the early stabilization of memory requires additional "offline" episodes of NMDA receptor activation after initial encoding. The involvement of NMDA receptors in systems consolidation and long-term information is less well understood. Shimizu et al. (2000) used the tTA and Cre/loxP systems to develop a mouse with an apparently CA1-specific (but see Fukaya et al., 2003) inducible deletion of the NMDA NR1 subunit. Deletion of this subunit by application of doxycycline 1 to 7 days after training on a watermaze reference memory task caused subsequent impairment in retention of the platform location. However, chronic blockade of hippocampal NMDA receptors during the days after spatial

training by either daily injections of CPP in rats (Villarreal et al., 2002) or intraventricular minipump infusions of D-AP5 in both rats and mice (Day and Langston, 2006) does not impair retention. In fact, Villarreal et al. (2002) reported enhancement of spatial memory after posttraining NMDA receptor antagonism, consistent with their additional finding that chronic NMDA receptor blockade prevents the decay of LTP that usually occurs over a period of several days. Modest enhancement of retention was also found by Day and Langston (2006). Perhaps the blockade of synaptic plasticity after training reduces retroactive interference from ongoing experience that might otherwise degrade the original memory (see also Rosenzweig et al., 2002).

Several studies have indicated that low doses of NMDA receptor antagonists can, paradoxically, enhance the learning of certain tasks, such as step-down inhibitory avoidance (Mondadori et al., 1989) and social learning (Lederer et al., 1993). These findings do not challenge the SPM hypothesis because the effects are observed at doses far too low to block LTP in vivo, and different mechanisms are likely to be involved in antagonist-induced facilitation of learning. For instance, the facilitation of inhibitory avoidance by low doses of NMDA antagonists is sensitive to pretreatment by steroids such as aldosterone or corticosterone, whereas the impaired inhibitory avoidance caused by high doses is steroid-insensitive (Mondadori and Weiskrantz, 1993; Mondadori et al., 1996). Work with the noncompetitive NMDA receptor antagonist memantine has also led to counterintuitive findings by virtue of its rapid on-and-off kinetics of channel blocking. At therapeutic doses, memantine does not impair learning or LTP, but it does limit neurotoxicity and so prevent impairments in cognitive function or their accumulation over time (Parsons et al., 1999).

Studies targeting the NMDA receptor are now complemented by many pharmacological manipulations directed at the diversity of receptors and intracellular signaling pathways that play a role in synaptic plasticity. To take just one example, there is considerable evidence that blockade or knockout of group I mGluRs, a class of receptor implicated in both LTP and LTD (see Section 10.3), can impair a variety of forms of memory, including spatial learning, contextual fear conditioning, and inhibitory avoidance (for reviews see Holscher et al., 1999; Riedel et al., 2003; Simonyi et al., 2005). For a fuller account of pharmacological interventions targeting sites other than the NMDA receptor, see Lynch (2004).

Targeted Disruption of the NMDA Receptor and Downstream Signal-transduction Pathways Impairs Hippocampus-dependent Learning

Some of the earliest uses of targeted molecular engineering in neuroscience were in relation to synaptic plasticity and learning in studies of downstream signal-transduction pathways (Silva et al., 1992a,b; Grant et al., 1995). These early studies revealed intriguing correlations between LTP and hippocampus-dependent learning. They set the pattern for a host of subsequent studies in which homologous recombination was used to delete genes in all cells of the body for the lifetime of the animal (Capecchi, 1989). The approach is often characterized by cell biological evidence that the deletion has been successful, followed by electrophysiological and behavioral analyses of the phenotype of the mutant progeny. The array of generally positive findings obtained from well over 100 relevant knockouts developed since 1992 lends general support to the SPM hypothesis (see Table 5 in Lynch (2004).

Numerous problems, however, were soon identified. For certain critically important proteins, there can be a catastrophic outcome such as embryonic or perinatal lethality. This occurred with an attempted deletion of the NR1 subtype of the NMDA receptor (Chen and Tonegawa, 1997), although deletion of the NR2A (ϵ1) subunit using conventional homologous recombination could be successfully carried forward to adults, and these mice showed a deficit in both hippocampal LTP and spatial learning (Sakimura et al., 1995). Other mutants display the opposite problem, a null phenotype, though it is hard to believe that key brain enzymes have no function. Either inappropriate behavioral assays have been used, or there has been compensation by other closely related genes (Grant et al., 1995). Another problem is interanimal variability; for example, it is puzzling that some slices from the αCaMKII mutants studied by Silva et al. (1992a) show normal LTP, whereas most show none unless parallel biochemical pathways can be activated in a probabilistic fashion. Hinds et al. (1998) reported a yet higher proportion of αCaMKII mutants showing normal LTP and suggested that the β enzyme may have been upregulated. Hinds et al.'s (1998) study involved animals cross-bred with C57/BL6 mice. The issue of genetic background is important: The embryonic stem cells most widely used to make mutants are derived from a specific strain of mice—the Sv129 strain; and when these mice are cross-bred with strains such as C57/BL6, a number of "flanking" genes derived from the 129 strain are still expressed alongside the mutated gene. Aspects of the resulting phenotype may reflect these flanking genes (Gerlai, 1996). Residual Sv129 genes have unpredictable effects and are undesirable because the Sv129 strain is notoriously poor at learning (Lipp and Wolfer, 1998). Recommendations about the desirability of back-crosses into more suitable strains (such as C57/BL6) were subsequently discussed in the gene-targeting community and a set of guidelines published (Anonymous, 1997).

Another issue is that many studies examine LTP only using in vitro brain slices. This is insufficient and a separate consideration concerns the value of looking at LTP in vivo. Nosten-Bertrand et al. (1996) found that *thy-1* mutants had normal LTP in area CA1 but no LTP in the dentate gyrus when measured in anesthetized animals in vivo. Further studies revealed, however, that normal LTP could be obtained in dentate slices when bicuculline was added to reduce inhibition, implying that the machinery for inducing LTP must still be present in *thy-1* mutants. When bicuculline was infused locally in vivo in

small quantities (to avoid seizure activity), the now disinhibited area of the dentate showed normal LTP. Errington et al. (1997) also found that LTP in freely moving *thy-1* mutants was compromised but not totally abolished, with a wide range of variability among individual animals. An important general message of the *thy-1* study for the field is that electrophysiological results in brain slices are not infallible predictors of what might happen to synaptic plasticity in the whole animal. The study also highlights the value of assessing both learning and LTP in the same animals.

A third problem when using mice to assess the SPM hypothesis has been the inappropriate interpretation of behavioral studies. Some studies using the watermaze with transgenic mice have used an apparatus that is too small to study spatial learning effectively (< 1.2 m) or failed to use posttraining probe tests. In a careful factor analysis of hundreds of experiments, Wolfer et al. (1998) statistically dissociated spatial learning in the watermaze from thigmotaxis and other species-specific swimming strategies. Emphasizing also the value of looking at LTP in vivo in association with behavioral studies, their work has played an important part in improving the analytical quality of modern studies.

Regionally specific mutants can now been made in which CRE recombinase is expressed downstream of specific promoters in one line of mice that, after crossing, target genes flanked with *loxP* sites in another. The resulting progeny enable the development of mutant strains in which a target gene is deleted (or mutated) in only one area of the brain. This approach was used to knock out the NR1 subunit of the NMDA receptor in area CA1 of the hippocampus only (Tsien et al., 1996; Mayford et al., 1997). The mice showed no LTP in area CA1, normal LTP in the dentate gyrus and neocortex, and learning impairment in the watermaze (Fig. 10–23B). Using multiple single-unit recording, McHugh et al. (1996) discovered that these mice had abnormal place fields and a reduction in the correlated firing of cells with overlapping place fields (see Chapter 11). Such regionally specific manipulations are beginning to allow the targeting of specific components of the hippocampal network. For example, Nakazawa et al. (2002) created a mouse in which the NR1 gene was deleted only in CA3, a manipulation that blocks NMDAR-dependent LTP at CA3 recurrent synapses but not NMDAR-independent potentiation in the mossy fiber input. These mice learned a watermaze reference memory task as well as the control animals. Retention was likewise unaffected when all extramaze cues were present, but performance deteriorated substantially when only partial cues were present (see Chapter 13, Fig. 13–21). These findings are consistent with a long-held view of CA3 as an autoassociative network capable of pattern completion—reconstruction of a complete output pattern from partial or degraded input (cf. Marr, 1971). According to this view, synaptic plasticity at recurrent synapses is necessary for the formation of a memory trace that can later be recalled in the presence of partial retrieval cues. In a follow-up study, the same mice were found to be impaired in one-trial place learning (see above), again supporting the notion of CA3 as a rapid autoassociative storage device (Nakazawa et al., 2003). Consistent with this finding, place cell recordings in area CA1 of these mice revealed a reduction in spatial tuning during early exploration of novel environments, implicating CA3 synaptic plasticity in the refinement of the spatial representation supported by the direct entorhinal input to CA1 (see Brun et al., 2002). The Cre-loxP system has now been used to target many components of the plasticity machinery in addition to the NMDA receptor (for reviews see Matynia et al., 2002; Lynch, 2004). For example, mice lacking the AMPA receptor GluRI (GluR-A) subunit show impairments in CA1 LTP and spatial working memory, although the acquisition of spatial reference memory is unaffected (Zamanillo et al., 1999; Reisel et al., 2002) (see Chapter 7). The impairments in LTP and memory can be rescued by adding a forebrain-specific GFP-tagged GluRI expression system to these mice, confirming the specificity of the impairment (Schmitt et al., 2005).

Region- and cell type-specific interventions are powerful, as they carry the potential to investigate gene function in specific cells, to manipulate pre- or postsynaptic sites of synapses independently, and to intervene in biochemical pathways for which there is no known ligand. The αCaMKII promoter has been useful in such experiments because it is not activated until around day 20, obviating certain developmental problems. The approach, however, is expensive as numerous lines have to be developed of which only some show useful expression patterns. Moreover, although achieving precise regional and cell-type specificity is advantageous over pharmacological manipulations, it does not yet allow the same precise temporal control as drugs. In the previous section, experiments were described in which animals were "normal" in one phase of an experiment but "treated" in another. This enabled dissociations between encoding and retrieval processes of memory to be addressed using highly selective anatagonists such as D-AP5. The corresponding way forward, using genetic interventions, is via conditional mutants in which inducible promoters are engineered to put gene activation (or inactivation) under experimental control. Use of the tetracycline transactivator systems, rtTA and tTA (see Box 7.1), provides one example of this approach (see Furth et al., 1994; Kistner et al., 1996). Inducible genetic interventions also finesse the complications of altered neuronal development that can occur with nonconditional knockouts (Lathe and Morris, 1994; Mayford et al., 1997) and can otherwise only be addressed using "rescue" experiments.

Using inducible techniques, Mayford et al. (1996) created a transgenic mouse in which overexpression of a constitutive CaMKII was under the control of tetracycline. This study built upon previous work using standard transgenic mice that overexpress the autophosphorylated form of CaMKII through a point mutation of Thr^{286} (Mayford et al., 1995). These animals had exhibited normal CA1 LTP in response to high-frequency stimulation at 100 Hz, but stimulation in the 5- to 10-Hz range (encompassing theta) preferentially resulted in

LTD rather than LTP—a shift of θ in the BCM function seen in Box Fig. 10–2A. Hippocampus-dependent learning was impaired: The mice showed impaired spatial learning using a Barnes maze (Bach et al., 1995). Mayford et al. (1996) replicated the learning impairments and deficits in LTP found by Bach et al. (1995) and Mayford et al. (1995), with suppression of the transgene by administration of doxycycline relieving the impairment of both learning and synaptic plasticity. Work by Giese et al. (1998) complemented these studies. Instead of using transgenic techniques, they introduced a point mutation (threonine to alanine) into the gene encoding αCaMKII to block autophosphorylation at residue 286, thereby preventing the transition of this kinase into a CaM-independent state without disrupting its CaM-dependent activity. LTP could not be elicited in area CA1 in the mutant mice across a range of stimulation frequencies, a slightly different profile to that shown by Mayford's transgenic mouse. Giese et al.'s mice also had profound deficits in spatial learning in the watermaze and showed altered dependence on extramaze versus intramaze cues in single-unit recording studies of place cells (Cho et al., 1998). Although this mutation is not inducible, temporal control can be achieved by combining pharmacological and molecular genetic techniques. Heterozygous Thr^{286} mutant mice have no deficit in contextual fear conditioning or LTP, but injection of a low dose of CPP that in wild type mice has no effect results in impairment of both learning and plasticity, suggesting that the NMDAR-dependent activation of αCaMKII is necessary for both processes (Ohno et al., 2001, 2002).

Other early studies to use the tTA technique were those of Mansuy et al. (1998a,b) and Winder et al. (1998). They reported that transgenic mice overexpressing a truncated form of the phosphatase calcineurin display normal early-LTP and short-term memory but defective late-LTP and long-term memory. However, evidence that the latter deficit was secondary to some other problem came from behavioral work showing that a change in training protocol could "rescue" the impaired long-term memory. This suggested that the deficit in these animals was more likely in the transition from short- to long-term memory than in the mechanisms underlying either on its own. Regulation of calcineurin overexpression using the rtTA technique was examined in animals tested in the watermaze (Mansuy et al., 1998b). In the latter study, animals completed training and were first tested with the transgene "off." They learned the platform location as indexed by good performance in a posttraining probe test. When the transgene was then turned "on," performance in a second probe test fell to chance; and when it was later turned "off" again, performance recovered. These results suggest that calcineurin constrains memory retrieval. The rtTA system has also been used to enhance the inhibition of calcineurin. Malleret et al. (2001) created a mouse with inducible overexpression of a C-terminal autoinhibitory domain that reduces calcineurin activity. Expression of the transgene facilitated LTP both in vivo and in vitro but did not affect LTD. Parallel enhancement of hippocampus-dependent memory was observed. Following an analogous strategy, a regulatory subunit of calcinuerin, CNB1, was deleted in a forebrain-specific manner, resulting in reduced calcineurin activity (Zeng et al., 2001). Although the mutation was not inducible, it did not become detectable until 5 weeks of age, obviating to some extent the possibility of developmental consequences. No enhancement of LTP was evident following a standard high-frequency tetanus, but an overall leftward shift in the function relating LTP/ LTD to tetanus frequency was observed together with impaired LTD. Perhaps for the latter reason, these mice did not show enhanced learning and memory. Performance in a watermaze reference memory task was normal, but acquisition of a task requiring the learning of multiple novel locations was impaired, as was performance in a radial-arm maze working memory task. These findings highlight the potential importance of decreases, as well as increases, in synaptic strength. Perhaps LTD-like mechanisms are particularly important in tasks that require flexible learning of new information in conjunction with rapid suppression of information that is no longer relevant (cf. Manahan-Vaughan and Braunewell, 1999; Kemp and Manahan-Vaughan, 2004).

Despite its power, the tTA system still requires several days for complete induction and repression, and advances in temporal control are eagerly awaited. A novel inducible system has since been developed based on fusion of a target protein with the ligand-binding domain of the estrogen receptor modified to bind tamoxifen instead of estrogen (Kida et al., 2002). Using this system, expression can be turned on and off within hours, but the range of potential target proteins is limited compared to the tTA approach. Another development is the increasing use of viral vector-mediated gene transfer. This approach enables the targeted and temporally controlled overexpression of transgenes following local transfection within a specific brain region. For example, the virus-mediated expression of calcium-permeable AMPA receptors in CA1 resulted in enhanced CA1 LTP in vitro and facilitated place learning and memory (Okada et al., 2003). However, dentate transfection impaired watermaze performance despite similar enhancememt of LTP, perhaps reflecting functional differences between these two subregions. The behavioral consequences of enhancing LTP are considered in more detail in the following section. In another study, intrahippocampal infusion of a viral vector conveying an inactive mutant form of CREB was found to block long-term, but not short-term, memory for socially transmitted food preference (Brightwell et al., 2005). Conversely, overexpression of CREB induced by intraamygdalar infusion of a viral vector results in enhancement of amygdala-dependent memory (Josselyn et al., 2001; Jasnow et al., 2005). Alternatively, the virus-mediated delivery of Cre can be used to trigger deletion of a target gene flanked by lox-P sites (e.g., Scammell et al., 2003). Using this technique, Rajji et al. (2006) were able to target deletion of the NR1 gene to area CA3 of the dorsal hippocampus, a manipulation that resulted in an impairment in the acquisi-

tion, but not the expression, of odor-context paired associate memory.

Good temporal control can also be achieved using antisense techniques. These methods lie somewhere between the genetic and pharmacological approaches, having some of advantages and disadvantages of both. Examples of their use include studies in which the expression of mRNA for two different potassium channels was reduced by repeated intracerebroventricular injections of oligodeoxyribonucleotides to reveal a dissociation between learning and plasticity. Antisense disruption of the presynaptic A-type potassium channel, Kv 1.4, eliminated both early and late phases of CA1 LTP without affecting LTP in the dentate gyrus in rats (Meiri et al., 1998). However, this antisense "knockdown" of plasticity had no effect on spatial learning. Given that threshold changes in the intensity of the tetanus required to induce LTP have been seen with some genetic manipulations (Kiyama et al., 1998), the fact that Meiri et al. (1998) used different intensities to induce LTP significantly strengthens their conclusion that CA1 LTP was successfully blocked in the antisense group. However, this study did not include in vivo observations, a range of tetanization frequencies (Mayford et al., 1995; Migaud et al., 1998), or information about the regional spread of the antisense oligo. The latter point is important, as LTP may have been monitored in an area along the longitudinal axis of the hippocampus that was affected by the oligo, whereas learning may have utilized neurons along the full length of this axis. It should be recognized, however, that antisense disruption of Kv 1.1, a different potassium channel that is highly localized in dendrites of CA3 neurons, had no effect on LTP in either the CA1 subfield or the dentate gyrus but did cause profound deficits in spatial learning (Meiri et al., 1997). Clearly, the longitudinal axis objection cannot apply here, and the significance of both these studies should be recognized. The antisense approach has also generated discrepancies between LTP and memory in the opposite direction (i.e., enhanced LTP associated with impaired memory) (Pineda et al., 2004), although such findings are potentially less troublesome for the synaptic plasticity and memory hypothesis, as discussed below. Other studies have reported parallel effects on both LTP and memory (Guzowski et al., 2000; Hou et al., 2004). In the former study, for example, antisense inhibition of the expression of hippocampal Arc protein (see Section 10.9) resulted in a deficit in long-term spatial memory in a watermaze reference memory task and impairment in the late maintenance of dentate LTP in vivo (Guzowski et al., 2000), consistent with a role for Arc in the long-term synaptic modifications postulated to underlie memory storage.

The development of methods for gene silencing does not end with the antisense approach. A more effective alternative to antisense knockdown is the RNA interference technique (RNAi). In a refinement of this technique, small interfering RNA (siRNA) sequences are targeted to a specific brain region by local elecroporation or by viral transfection, thereby offering excellent regional and temporal control (Akaneya et al.,

2005). Although highly promising, this approach has not yet been applied to studies of hippocampal synaptic plasticity and memory.

Do Treatments That Enhance LTP Also Enhance Memory?

As we discussed earlier, the circuit-level consequences of enhancing synaptic plasticity may be far from straightforward. Synaptic plasticity might normally be optimally tuned for the efficient encoding of information, such that any disturbance—even enhancement—has disruptive effects on memory. Nonetheless, many pharmacological and molecular-genetic manipulations do enhance both LTP and memory. Perhaps the best-known example of the pharmacological approach involves treatment with "ampakines," which decrease the rate of AMPA receptor desensitization and slow the deactivation of receptor currents after agonist application (Arai et al., 1994, 1996). Consequently, they facilitate the induction of hippocampal LTP (Staubli et al., 1994); and there is now a considerable body of evidence that they can enhance the encoding of memory in a variety of tasks (Lynch, 2006). A number of other compounds have also been reported to enhance both learning and hippocampal LTP (Cooke and Bliss, 2005).

Similarly, Manabe et al. (1998) reported that mice lacking the nociceptin/orphaninFQ receptor show enhanced LTP in area CA1 (possibly also due to a change in K^+ channel function) and both a modest but significant decrease in escape latency in the watermaze and enhanced memory consolidation in step-through avoidance learning. In a widely discussed study, Tang et al. (1999) showed that overexpression of the "juvenile" 2B subunit of the NMDA receptor both facilitated LTP across a range of induction frequencies and enhanced memory in novel object recognition, cue and context fear-conditioning, and the earliest stages of learning a watermaze. This pattern of results has since been observed following many other genetic interventions (e.g., Futatsugi et al., 1999; Madani et al., 1999; Routtenberg et al., 2000; Malleret et al., 2001; Nakamura et al., 2001; Jeon et al., 2003).

In contrast, Migaud et al. (1998) reported that a PSD-95 mutant that shows enhanced hippocampal LTP and decreased LTD across a range of induction frequencies displays profound impairment of watermaze performance. The finding of enhanced LTP and impaired spatial memory has since been reported in several other strains of mutant mice (Uetani et al., 2000; Zeng et al., 2001; Kaksonen et al., 2002; Cox et al., 2003; Vaillend et al., 2004), whereas other interventions result in normal (or near-normal) spatial memory despite enhancement of LTP (Jun et al., 1998; Gu et al., 2002; Cox et al., 2003; Pineda et al., 2004). However, impairment of other forms of memory were reported in some of these studies. In some cases, impaired behavioral performance might result from the dysfunction of extrahippocampal systems (Gerlai et al., 1998), but other factors may also be relevant. For instance, the PSD-95 mutant mice created by Migaud et al. (1998) exhibited a shift in θ_M of the BCM function well to the left of its optimal position for bidirectional plasticity. Perhaps it is this abnormality or simply a deficiency in LTD that underlies the learning problems evident in these animals.

Parallels Between Different Phases of LTP Expression and Memory Consolidation

There is considerable evidence that both hippocampus-dependent memories and increases in synaptic strength each undergo a period of consolidation in the minutes to hours following their formation (McGaugh, 2000). A variety of interventions can interfere with both memory consolidation and stabilization of LTP, including (1) disrupting the activity of a range of protein kinases (Izquierdo and Medina, 1997; Micheau and Riedel, 1999) such as CaMKII (Lisman et al., 2002; Colbran and Brown, 2004), MAPK/ERK (Kelleher et al., 2004a; Sweatt, 2004; Thomas and Huganir, 2004), tyrosine kinases (Purcell and Carew, 2003), PKA (Nguyen and Woo, 2003), and PKC (Sun and Alkon, 2005); (2) disrupting the expression of immediate early genes such as *Zif268* (Jones et al., 2000) (Fig. 10–23C) or *arc* (Guzowski et al., 2000); (3) temporary neuronal inactivation (e.g., Ambrogi Lorenzini et al., 1999; Florian and Roullet, 2004; Daumas et al., 2005); and (4) inhibition of macromolecular synthesis (for review see Davis and Squire, 1984; Frey and Morris, 1998a; Dudai and Morris, 2000). Growing evidence also supports a role for cell adhesion molecules in consolidation processes (Murase and Schuman, 1999; Benson et al., 2000; Gall and Lynch, 2004). Studies such as these offer broad support for the idea that lasting changes in synaptic strength underlie the formation of long-term memory.

For instance, late-LTP (i.e., LTP lasting around 4 hours or more), like cellular consolidation, requires synthesis of new proteins (for review see Frey and Morris, 1998a). As discussed in Section 10.4.9, application of protein synthesis inhibitors such as anisomycin prevents late-LTP. Importantly, however, the events leading to protein synthesis do not have to occur at exactly the same time as the stimulation that induces synaptic potentiation. Tetanization in the presence of a protein synthesis inhibitor still results in late-LTP if a strong tetanus is applied to a separate pathway up to 2 hours previously (Frey and Morris, 1997). Together with other findings, this result has led to the notion that a high-frequency tetanus sets "synaptic tags" that can capture plasticity proteins as they become available (Frey and Morris, 1997, 1998b). The same may be true of memory formation. Activation of neuromodulatory systems by novelty, reward, or punishment (Frey et al., 2001; Richter-Levin and Akirav, 2003; Lisman and Grace, 2005) may cause widespead upregulation of gene expression and protein synthesis via activation of cAMP-, PKA-, and CREB-dependent pathways. This would enable capture of proteins by synapses that have recently been potentiated and "tagged" or are about to be potentiated as a result of normal experience (Frey and Morris, 1998a). However, MAPK-mediated upregulation of translation—perhaps in dendrites—

might also be critical under some circumstances (Martin et al., 2000a; Steward and Schuman, 2003; Kelleher et al., 2004b) (see Section 10.4 for a discussion of dendritic protein synthesis). The interaction of specific synaptic signals with widespread transcriptional or translational upregulation may provide an explanation for the facilitated retention of memory for episodes occurring shortly before or after events of motivational importance, episodes that would otherwise be rapidly forgotten (cf. Seidenbecher et al., 1995).

Consistent with this scenario, a number of studies have suggested that activation of CREB is necessary for both the induction of hippocampal late-LTP and the formation of long-term memory (i.e., cellular consolidation) in mice and rats (Bourtchuladze et al., 1994; Bernabeu et al., 1997; Guzowski and McGaugh, 1997; Kogan et al., 2000; Pittenger et al., 2002; Brightwell et al., 2005; Wood et al., 2005). Barco et al. (2002) recently created a mouse in which a constitutively active form of CREB, VP16-CREB, is expressed in a forebrain-restricted and temporally regulated manner. In these animals, the threshold for late-LTP induction in the Schaffer-commissural to CA1 pyramidal cell pathway was reduced, such that a weak tetanus capable of inducing only a decremental early-LTP in normal mice induced late-LTP in VP16-CREB animals. These findings suggest that elevated CREB-mediated transcription in these animals leads to synthesis of a pool of proteins or mRNAs that can subsequently be captured by synapses tagged during weak tetanization, without the need for new transcription. A follow-up study implicates the overexpression of BDNF in this phenomenon (Barco et al., 2002). However, it is not yet known whether VP16-CREB mice exhibit enhanced long-term memory for weakly encoded information, consistent with their LTP phenotype.

Does Saturation of LTP or LTD Occlude the Encoding of New Memory Traces?

In studies of expression mechanisms for LTP, occlusion was often deployed as a tool to identify that LTP had been engaged. The same approach can be deployed in behavioral studies. It is important, however, to distinguish between the cumulative induction of LTP (or LTD) and the saturation of either process. Successive episodes of LTP may have a cumulative effect on synaptic strength, at least at a population level (cf. Petersen et al., 1998), but not saturate the plasticity available on the pathway being stimulated (Jeffery, 1997). Cumulative LTP may *enhance* neural throughput and so improve learning. Berger (1984) obtained just such a result in a study of nictitating membrane conditioning in rabbits, the original species in which LTP was discovered. In contrast, true saturation of LTP prior to behavioral training should *prevent* new learning because no further LTP would then be possible. Similar considerations would apply to saturation of LTD, which can be achieved with three successive trains of stimulus pairs (Thiels et al., 1998).

Research on the behavioral effects of LTP saturation reached an impasse in 1993 when a series of articles (Cain et al., 1993; Jeffery and Morris, 1993; Korol et al., 1993; Sutherland et al., 1993) reported an inability to replicate earlier findings indicating that saturation induced reversible occlusion of subsequent spatial learning (McNaughton et al., 1986; Castro et al., 1989). Jeffery and Morris (1993) and Korol et al. (1993) conducted exact replications of part of Castro et al.'s (1989) experiment. In neither study was any learning deficit observed. Reid and Stewart (1997) succeeded in replicating Castro et al.'s findings, including decay of the effect over time, but they used electroconvulsive seizures, which among other effects can cause indiscriminate induction of LTP rather than explicit saturation on a single pathway.

Bliss and Richter-Levin (1993) suggested several reasons the negative results might have been obtained: (1) cumulative LTP of perforant path terminals may not have reached a true state of saturation; (2) perforant path terminals may have been sufficiently saturated, but not those of other extrinsic or intrinsic hippocampal pathways that are also critical for learning (e.g., CA3-CA1 terminals); (3) appropriate saturation of the full septotemporal axis of the hippocampus may not have been achieved with stimulation at a single site in the angular bundle. Evidence for this third idea was presented by Barnes et al. (1994), who found upregulation of the immediate early gene *zif-268* restricted to the dorsal hippocampus after stimulation at one site in the angular bundle. They also noted differences in the sensitivity of various learning tasks to LTP saturation.

Moser et al. (1998) designed a study with these issues in mind. There were three key features: (1) use of an array of cross-bundle stimulation electrodes designed to maximally activate the perforant path, with the cathode switched frequently between active electrodes; (2) use of a separate "probe" stimulating electrode to test whether the asymptotic LTP induced by the electrode array was true saturation of LTP on that pathway; (3) use of animals given unilateral hippocampal lesions to reduce the amount of tissue to be potentiated. Subsequent to multiple high-frequency (HF) trains or control low-frequency (LF) stimulation, the rats were trained in a standard watermaze task. Controls learned normally. The HF group showed a bimodal distribution, with some animals learning where the platform was located and others failing to learn. When all animals were subsequently tested for induction of LTP from the probe site in the perforant path, the HF animals in which it was impossible to induce further LTP (i.e., the "saturated" subgroup) were the ones that had failed to learn the watermaze, whereas those in whom LTP could still be induced had learned a little about where the platform was located. Thus, true saturation of LTP in the perforant path does impair spatial learning. These findings vindicate the earlier claims of McNaughton et al. (1986) and Castro et al. (1989).

Despite these positive findings, there remains skepticism about the analytical potential of the occlusion approach. One concern is that repeated tetanization may result in acute pathological phenomena, such as seizure-like after-discharges, that would cause learning deficits (McEachern and Shaw, 1996). However, Moser et al. (1998) found no after-discharges during tetanization. Also, learning was impaired only in the animals with saturated LTP, despite all rats having received the same course of tetanic stimulation. A second point concerns homeostatic compensatory changes, such as altered inhibitory transmission, synapse formation, and reduced postsynaptic sensitivity. These compensatory changes were considered in a review article by Moser and Moser (1999) but primarily as factors contributing to the difficulty often experienced in saturating LTP. Even when LTP saturation is successful, it might still be argued that such changes, rather than saturation itself, are responsible for the learning impairment. A third area of disquiet is that LTP saturation does, of course, increase synaptic weight; a global increase in the efficacy of synaptic transmission might, on its own, disrupt normal hippocampal information processing. However, the number of studies reporting normal learning despite the induction of substantial LTP suggests that a cumulative increase in synaptic weight does not in itself disrupt the encoding of new information. In fact, Moser et al. (1998) found no correlation between the magnitude of LTP induced by cross-bundle tetanization and subsequent learning.

Moser et al.'s (1998) study is unlikely to be the last word. First, saturation itself is not well understood physiologically. Doing so could offer new insights into the maximum amounts of potentiation the hippocampus could sustain. Second, saturation might be achieved in other ways. It might also be realized by bilateral stimulation of the ventral hippocampal commissure to potentiate the commissural/associational pathway in CA3 and CA1 (Bliss and Richter-Levin, 1993). Another study has suggested that as little as a single LTP-inducing tetanus delivered to the Schaffer-commissural pathway can impair trace eyeblink conditioning (Gruart et al., 2006). A pharmacological, rather than an electrophysiological, approach should also be considered using drugs such as BDNF (Bramham and Messaoudi, 2005) or agonists of adenylate cyclase, protein kinase A, or mitogen-activated protein kinase (MAPK), to induce slow-onset but asymptotic synaptic potentiation. Multiple approaches are required to rigorously test this component of the SPM hypothesis.

10.10.4 Retrograde Alteration: Does Further Induction or Reversal of LTP Cause Forgetting?

If memory traces related to a recent learning experience are temporarily stored in the hippocampus, procedures that induce further LTP in the same network, or successfully erase LTP, should cause forgetting. Erasure might be achieved (1) using trains of suitable depotentiating (e.g., low frequency) stimulation or (2) applying drugs or enzyme inhibitors that interrupt expression of LTP when given shortly after its induction (e.g., kinase inhibitors).

Depotentiation can be induced using continuous trains of single pulses at 1 to 5 Hz (Barrionuevo et al., 1980; Stäubli and

Lynch, 1990; Bashir and Collingridge, 1994). Stäubli and Chun (1996) found that a few minutes of 5-Hz stimulation can depotentiate recently induced LTP in area CA1 in vitro. The efficacy of depotentiation declines rapidly as the interval between the tetanus and 5 Hz is increased, with little effect being obtained 30 minutes after LTP induction. Dentate LTP in vivo can also be reversed by 5-Hz stimulation when delivered up to a few minutes after tetanization, but later stimulation is ineffective (Martin, 1998; Kulla, 1999). Unfortunately, none of the protocols for inducing depotentiation has yet been tested for its ability to cause forgetting in behaving animals.

Xu et al. (1998) reported that exposing freely moving animals to a novel but nonstressful recording chamber can reverse recently induced LTP without affecting a control pathway. They speculated that exposure to novelty has the effect of erasing hitherto unconsolidated information (see also Manahan-Vaughan and Braunewell, 1999). Support for this interpretation is offered in a report (Izquierdo et al., 1999) in which exposure to novelty limited the ability of an animal to remember a one-trial inhibitory avoidance task carried out up to 1 hour previously. Exploration of novelty shortly before or long after the training trial was without effect. The effect appears to be NMDAR- and CaMKII-dependent.

Instead of erasing LTP, the induction of further LTP should alter the spatial distribution of synaptic weights in the distributed network of areas CA3 and CA1 and so prevent successful retrieval of information stored earlier. In an early study of this kind, McNaughton et al. (1986) trained rats to remember the location of an escape tunnel in a "Barnes arena" and then induced LTP in the dentate gyrus via chronically implanted electrodes in the angular bundle. Recently acquired reference memory was disrupted by LTP induction, whereas well established spatial memory was unaffected. Results consistent with these have been reported by Brun et al. (2001), who trained rats in a spatial reference memory task in the watermaze for 5 days, before also inducing LTP via stimulating electrodes straddling the angular bundle of the perforant path. In contrast to nonstimulated and low-frequency control groups, rats that had been subjected to high-frequency tetanization were completely unable to remember the platform location in a subsequent probe trial (Fig. 10–24B). Nevertheless, the same animals were able to learn a new platform location in a different watermaze environment as well as the controls, a result consistent with the finding reported by Otnaess et al. (1999) that pretraining eliminates the LTP saturation-induced deficit in new spatial reference learning (cf. Bannerman et al., 1995; Saucier and Cain, 1995).

In the study of Brun et al. (2001), a group of rats was tetanized in the presence of the NMDA receptor antagonist CPP. These animals remembered the platform location as well as the controls in a subsequent retention test (carried out in the absence of CPP). In conjunction with the intact ability of animals with asymptotic or near-asymptotic LTP to learn a new watermaze task, these results suggest that neither high-frequency tetanization nor LTP induction per se causes significant hippocampal dysfunction, and they add further credence to the notion that memories are stored as patterns of changes in synaptic strength, and that these patterns can be disrupted by the addition of tetanus-induced LTP that constitutes meaningless noise. This notion is further supported by the finding that LTP induction at CA3–CA1 synapses prevents

the recall of trace eyeblink conditioning (Gruart et al., 2006), although more widespread alteration of synaptic strengths is sometimes necessary to disrupt memory (Leung and Shen, 2006).

Finally, Pastalkova et al (2006) have shown that application of ZIP, a membrane permeable inhibitor of PKMζ that is thought to mediate the persistence of hippocampal LTP over

Figure 10–24. Retrograde alteration of LTP and memory. *A.* Depotentiation of LTP should erase memory. One way in this might be achieved is through experiences such as novelty exploration. Rats in which LTP had been recently induced showed persistent potentiation when placed in a familiar environment (top), but LTP was erased when they explored a novel room. The novelty acts in an analogous manner to "distraction." (*Source*: After Xu et al., 1998.) *B.* Alternatively, if memory traces involve a particular spatial distribution of synaptic potentiation, artificial induction of further LTP (black symbols) should make it difficult to retrieve the appropriate memory (1,2,3) later. *C.* When rats, soon after learning a spatial watermaze task, were given high-frequency stimulation to multiple

afferents of the perforant path that ordinarily induces LTP in the dentate gyrus, they were later unable to remember the location of the hidden platform, as shown in post-training probe tests (see Fig. 13(23 for explanation of behavioural task). Giving such stimulation in the presence of an NMDA antagonist had no effect on memory. (*Source*: After Brun et al., 1998). *D.* Application of ZIP (see text) reverses established LTP to baseline. *E.* Rats trained to avoid a zone on a rotating arena where they receive a footshock (place avoidance) take longer to enter this region as training progresses. Application of ZIP at the end of training abolishes this memory. (*Source*: Pastalkova et al, 2006).

A   Novel room exploration depotentiates LTP

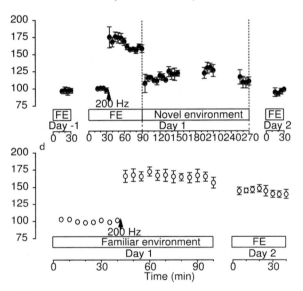

B   Retrograde alteration of synaptic weights

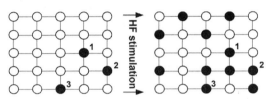

C   Tetanisation after learning impairs memory

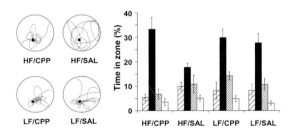

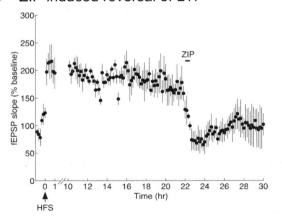

D   ZIP induced reversal of LTP

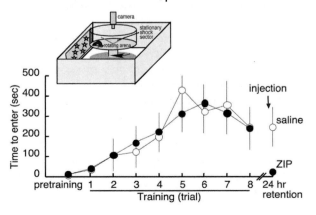

E   ZIP induced loss of place avoidance memory

time (see Section 10.4.9), causes both a reversal of LTP established 22 hrs earlier and a loss of place-avoidance memory (Fig 10-24D,E). With this striking new result, it seems that predictions of the retrograde alteration criterion are being upheld.

10.10.5 Mimicry

A key test of any hypothesis concerning memory encoding and storage must be a mimicry experiment, in which apparent memory is generated artificially without the usual requirement for a learning experience. This would constitute a critical test that changes in synaptic efficacy are *sufficient* for memory, rather than merely necessary.

Pairing of electrical stimulation in specific CS and US pathways to the amygdala should result in potentiation of interconnecting pathways. Subsequent behavioral testing might reveal that this LTP constitutes the "engineering" of an emotional memory. Such an experiment may be difficult in practice, and no such reports have yet appeared; nor have any reports of the artifical engineering of hippocampal memory been reported. However, several "detectability" studies have employed a methodology that might be regarded as a halfway house between detectability and mimicry. Studies in which sensory stimulation is replaced with electrical stimulation of a particular neural pathway, as a discriminative cue (Mouly et al., 2001; Roman et al., 2004) or a conditioned stimulus (Matthies et al., 1986; Laroche et al., 1989; Doyere and Laroche, 1992) fall into this category. In such experiments, posttraining LTP-like changes in evoked potentials are often found in response to stimulation of the same pathway that was stimulated during learning. The difficulty lies in ensuring that the electrical stimulation adequately mimics natural sensory stimulation, such that any learning-related changes in synaptic strength might plausibly be expected to occur—albeit perhaps in a more diffuse and sparse fashion—during "normal" learning. In this respect, studies involving stimulation of sensory pathways are arguably easier to interpret than studies in which, for instance, perforant path tetanization is used as a CS (Laroche et al., 1989; Doyere and Laroche, 1992). A range of other relevant studies examining the artificial induction of receptive field plasticity in the neocortex has been reported, but they lie outside the scope of this book (e.g., Talwar and Gerstein, 2001; Weinberger, 2004). Nonetheless, we are unaware of any study to date that adequately meets the mimicry criterion.

10.10.6 Synaptic Plasticity, Learning, and Memory: The Story So Far

In this chapter we have covered the more important advances in the field of synaptic plasticity that have emerged from neuroscience laboratories around the world over the last three decades as a result of the enormous interest generated by the discovery of LTP. That interest is driven, at heart, by the belief that in hippocampal LTP we have found a window into the synaptic basis of a central aspect of cognition—episodic memory. At the same time, the study of synaptic plasticity has led to a heightened appreciation of the richness and complexity of synaptic function. Synapses are simply more interesting when they are endowed with memory. The question remains, however, as to whether this avalanche of new knowledge about the physiology, pharmacology, and molecular and developmental biology of synapses has taught us anything fundamental about how the brain stores memories.

Many of the issues encountered in the last section are a product of the painful realization that although we now know a great deal about plasticity at the level of the individual neuron, and even the individual synapse, we know relatively little about how individual synapses integrate to influence the behavior of the single neuron. We know even less about how networks of neurons interact to encode and store information and about the processes of retrieval that allow memory to be expressed as changes in behavior. The problem of detectability discussed in Section 10.10.2 reflects our ignorance of hippocampal function at the network level. If LTP is so pervasive—estimates cited in Section 10.3.2 suggest that most synapses made by interconnected hippocampal pyramidal cells support LTP—why has it been so difficult to detect in the intact, learning animal? Does it reflect the sparseness of encoding, or is it that every instance of LTP is accompanied by LTD at other synapses, thus compromising the experimenter's ability to detect changes in field potential responses? A striking increase in the number of CA1 neurons expressing mRNA transcripts actiivity related gene *arc/arg3.1* has been detected while animals explore a new environment, and it has been possible to show that different but overlapping networks of *arc*-expressing cells are engaged when different environments are explored (Guzowski et al., 1999) (see also discussion in Chapter 13). This is a promising approach, but it does not allow us to make the unequivocal claim that LTP has been detected, as *arc* and other potential markers such as *zif268* and *homer* are not exclusively activated by LTP. In this respect, phospho specific antibodies directed to protein kinases that are phosphorylated on different residues in LTP and LTD (see section 10.4.6) should offer a powerful tool in the analysis of plasticity at the network level.

Estimates of correlated activity between populations of neurons is another promising approach to the question: Does LTP happen in real life? A suggestive example was offered by Mehta et al. (2000), who examined changes in the statistical coupling of cells as animals repeatedly moved through their adjacent place fields in a toroidal running maze. Each time the animal traversed the circular maze, entering the CA3 place field just before the CA1 place field, the CA3 place cell repeatedly fired immediately before the CA1 cell. After several circuits, the place field of the CA3 cell moved toward that of the CA1 cell. This is the result that would be predicted if the two cells were coupled and the strength of the connection between them had become strengthened. Is it LTP? Does this change in coupling reflect some gain in the animal's knowledge of the maze? Experiments on remapping of place cells when animals are put in a new environment suggest that NMDAR-mediated processes are required for the stability and fine tuning of the new mapping. These are promising but perhaps not compelling examples, an obvious difficulty being that changes in cell firing are an indirect measure of presumed changes in synaptic connectivity. Nevertheless, techniques for listening into the conversations between large ensembles of neurons offer one hope of establishing the role of synaptic potentiation in network behavior.

It is already possible to implant several multiunit recording assemblies into each of the hippocampal subfields and to record the activity of many tens of neurons in each subfield. Some of these neurons will be connected. Cross-correlational analysis of unit firing can pick out those that are and allow estimates to be made of the strength of the connection between them. The timing of monosynaptic connections between CA3 and CA1 neurons reduces the possibility that both cells are being driven by another cell. A protocol to detect LTP might be the following. Record simultaneously from many such pairs while the animal is learning a CA3/CA1-dependent task, and changes in the weights that connect at least some of the pairs should become apparent. Now depotentiate the potentiated pairs by stimulating the presynaptic neuron, via the appropriate electrode in the recording assembly, soon after the change is detected. Do that to enough pairs whose altered weights marks them as participating in the representation of the memory, and what has been learned, according to the SPM hypothesis, should be attenuated or lost. Now restore the synaptic weights to the pairs that have been depotentiated by tetanic stimulation, pair on pair, again using the presynaptic recording electrode as a stimulating electrode, and the memory should be recovered—a primitive form of mimicry. This is not, admittedly, the formation of a new memory but recovery of a lost memory by restoring synaptic strengths specifically to a subpopulation of the synapses that encoded the original representation of that memory. Achieving the stimulation specificity to achieve this project may be difficult, but thought experiments of this kind challenge us to consider what would be needed to test the SPM hypothesis with the appropriate rigor.

Although this and other experiments are for the future, they are within the bounds of what is technically feasible and make at least the point that the SPM hypothesis is potentially falsifiable. Before the role of the hippocampus in episodic memory was revealed in H.M. and before the Hebb synapse was made manifest in LTP, neuroscientists who thought about the neural basis of learning were faced with what must have seemed a series of unbridgeable chasms between the experience to be remembered and its representation and storage in the neural network, between the network and its constituent neurons, and between the neuron and its synapses, the ultimate units of information storage. The enormous advances in our knowledge of the mechanisms and functions of synaptic plasticity summarized in this chapter can give us some confi-

dence that we now have the conceptual and instrumental tools to tackle these obstacles. It is this sense of optimism that gives the field its vitality and excitement. If the field of consciousness has its easy and hard problems, so has LTP—with this difference: that its hard problem, the link between plasticity and memory, is solvable.

ACKNOWLEDGMENTS

T.V.P.B. thanks those who over the years gave him refuge to write: Susan and Robert Alain at Lac Laroche, Quebec and on the north Norfolk coast Julia Peyton-Jones at Southrepps and Mike and Eithne Doy at Cley. Wai Han Yau skillfully turned sketches and scans into figures. G.L.C. is grateful to Andy Doherty for help with preparing figures. R.G.M.M. thanks Stephen Martin for assistance with the text and Simon Rempel for providing material for one of the figures. The work of T.V.P.B., G.L.C., and R.G.M.M. has been supported for many years in whole or in part by the MRC. We acknowledge support also from the Human Frontiers Science Program and the EU.

REFERENCES

Abbott LF, Nelson SB (2000) Synaptic plasticity: taming the beast. *Nat Neurosci* 3(Suppl):1178–1183.

Abeliovich A, Chen C, Goda Y, Silva AJ, Stevens CF, Tonegawa S (1993) Modified hippocampal long-term potentiation in PKC gamma-mutant mice. *Cell* 75:1253–1262.

Abraham WC (2003) How long will long-term potentiation last? *Philos Trans R Soc Lond B Biol Sci* 358:735–744.

Abraham WC (2004) Stress-related phenomena. *Hippocampus* 14:675–676.

Abraham WC, Bear MF (1996) Metaplasticity: the plasticity of synaptic plasticity. *Trends Neurosci* 19:126–130.

Abraham WC, Mason-Parker SE, Bear MF, Webb S, Tate WP (2001) Heterosynaptic metaplasticity in the hippocampus in vivo: a BCM-like modifiable threshold for LTP. *Proc Natl Acad Sci USA* 98:10924–10929.

Abraham WC, Goddard GV (1983) Asymmetric relationships between homosynaptic long-term potentiation and heterosynaptic long-term depression. *Nature* 305:717–719.

Abraham WC, Robins A (2005) Memory retention: the synaptic stability versus plasticity dilemma. *Trends Neurosci* 28:73–78.

Abraham WC, Tate WP (1997) Metaplasticity: a new vista across the field of synaptic plasticity. *Prog Neurobiol* 52:303–323.

Abraham WC, Bliss TVP, Goddard GV (1985) Heterosynaptic changes accompany long-term but not short-term potentiation of the perforant path in the anaesthetized rat. *J Physiol* 363:335–349.

Abraham WC, Gustafsson B, Wigström H (1986) Single high-strength afferent volleys can produce long-term potentiation in the hippocampus in vitro. *Neurosci Lett* 70:217–222.

Abraham WC, Gustafsson B, Wigström H (1987) Hippocampal long-term potentiation involves an increase in synaptic excitation relative to inhibition. *Int J Neurosci* 35:128.

Abraham WC, Christie BR, Logan B, Lawlor P, Dragunow M (1994) Immediate early gene expression associated with the persistence of heterosynaptic long-term depression in the hippocampus. *Proc Natl Acad Sci USA* 91:10049–10053.

Abraham WC, Mason-Parker SE, Logan B (1996) Low-frequency stimulation does not readily cause long-term depression or depotentiation in the dentate gyrus of awake rats. *Brain Res* 722:217–221.

Abraham WC, Logan B, Greenwood JM, Dragunow M (2002) Induction and experience-dependent consolidation of stable long-term potentiation lasting months in the hippocampus. *J Neurosci* 22:9626–9634.

Adams JP, Dudek SM (2005) Late-phase long-term potentiation: getting to the nucleus. *Nat Rev Neurosci* 6:737–743.

Aiba A, Chen C, Herrup K, Rosenmund C, Stevens CF, Tonegawa S (1994) Reduced hippocampal long-term potentiation and context-specific deficit in associative learning in mGluR1 mutant mice. *Cell* 79:365–375.

Akaneya Y, Jiang B, Tsumoto T (2005) RNAi-induced gene silencing by local electroporation in targeting brain region. *J Neurophysiol* 93:594–602.

Alberini CM (2005) Mechanisms of memory stabilization: are consolidation and reconsolidation similar or distinct processes? *Trends Neurosci* 28:51–56.

Alford S, Frenguelli BG, Schofield JG, Collingridge GL (1993) Characterization of Ca^{2+} signals induced in hippocampal CA1 neurones by the synaptic activation of NMDA receptors. *J Physiol* 469:693–716.

Alle H, Jonas P, Geiger JRP (2001) PTP and LTP at a hippocampal mossy fiber–interneuron synapse. *Proc Natl Acad Sci USA* 98:14708–14713.

Allen PB, Hvalby O, Jensen V, Errington ML, Ramsay M, Chaudhry FA, Bliss TV, Storm-Mathisen J, Morris RG, Andersen P, Greengard P (2000) Protein phosphatase-1 regulation in the induction of long-term potentiation: heterogeneous molecular mechanisms. *J Neurosci* 20:3537–3543.

Ambrogi Lorenzini CG, Baldi E, Bucherelli C, Sacchetti B, Tassoni G (1999) Neural topography and chronology of memory consolidation: a review of functional inactivation findings. *Neurobiol Learn Mem* 71:1–18.

Andersen P (1960) Interhippocampal impulses. II. Apical dendritic activation of CA1 neurons. *Acta Physiol Scand* 48:178–208.

Andersen P, Sundberg SH, Sveen O, Wigström H (1977) Specific long-lasting potentiation of synaptic transmission in hippocampal slices. *Nature* 266:736–737.

Andersen P, Sundberg SH, Sveen O, Swann JW, Wigström H (1980) Possible mechanisms for long-lasting potentiation of synaptic transmission in hippocampal slices from guinea-pigs. *J Physiol* 302:463–482.

Anderson R, Barnes JC, Bliss TV, Cain DP, Cambon K, Davies HA, Errington ML, Fellows LA, Gray RA, Hoh T, Stewart M, Large CH, Higgins GA (1998) Behavioural, physiological and morphological analysis of a line of apolipoprotein E knockout mouse. *Neuroscience* 85:93–110.

Aniksztejn L, Roisin MP, Amsellem R, Ben-Ari Y (1989) Long-term potentiation is not associated with a sustained enhanced release of endogenous excitatory amino acids. *Neuroscience* 28:387–392.

Anis NA, Berry SC, Burton NR, Lodge D (1983) The dissociative anaesthetics, ketamine and phencyclidine, selectively reduce excitation of central mammalian neurones by *N*-methyl-aspartate. *Br J Pharmacol* 79:565–575.

Anonymous (1997) Mutant mice and neuroscience: recommendations concerning genetic background. *Neuron* 19:755–759.

Antonova I, Arancio O, Trillat AC, Wang HG, Zablow L, Udo H, Kandel ER, Hawkins RD (2001) Rapid increase in clusters of presynaptic proteins at onset of long-lasting potentiation. *Science* 294:1547–1450.

Anwyl R (1999) Metabotropic glutamate receptors: electrophysiological properties and role in plasticity. *Brain Res Rev* 29:83–120.

Arai A, Kessler M, Xiao P, Ambros-Ingerson J, Rogers G, Lynch G (1994) A centrally active drug that modulates AMPA receptor gated currents. *Brain Res* 638:343–346.

Arai A, Kessler M, Ambros-Ingerson J, Quan A, Yigiter E, Rogers G, Lynch G (1996) Effects of a centrally active benzoylpyrrolidine drug on AMPA receptor kinetics. *Neuroscience* 75:573–585.

Artola A, Singer W (1987) Long-term potentiation and NMDA receptors in rat visual cortex. *Nature* 330:649–652.

Artola A, Singer W (1993) Long-term depression of excitatory synaptic transmission and its relationship to long-term potentiation. *Trends Neurosci* 16:480–487.

Artola A, Kamal A, Ramakers GM, Biessels GJ, Gispen WH (2005) Diabetes mellitus concomitantly facilitates the induction of long-term depression and inhibits that of long-term potentiation in hippocampus. *Eur J Neurosci* 22:169–178.

Ascher P, Nowak L (1988) The role of divalent cations in the *N*-methyl-D-aspartate responses of mouse central neurones in culture. *J Physiol (Lond)* 399:247–266.

Ashby MC, De La Rue SA, Ralph GS, Uney J, Collingridge GL, Henley JM (2004) Removal of AMPA receptors (AMPARs) from synapses is preceded by transient endocytosis of extrasynaptic AMPARs. *J Neurosci* 24:5172–5176.

Assaf SY, Chung SH (1984) Release of endogenous Zn^{2+} from brain tissue during activity. *Nature* 308:734–746.

Auger C, Marty A (2000) Quantal currents at single-site central synapses. *J Physiol (Lond)* 526:3–11

Auld DS, Kornecook TJ, Bastianetto S, Quirion R (2002) Alzheimer's disease and the basal forebrain cholinergic system: relations to beta-amyloid peptides, cognition, and treatment strategies. *Prog Neurobiol* 68:209–245.

Ault B, Evans RH, Francis AA, Oakes DJ, Watkins JC (1980) Selective depression of excitatory amino acid induced depolarizations by magnesium ions in isolated spinal cord preparations. *J Physiol (Lond)* 307:413–428.

Avital A, Goshen I, Kamsler A, Segal M, Iverfeldt K, Richter-Levin G, Yirmiya R (2003) Impaired interleukin-1 signaling is associated with deficits in hippocampal memory processes and neural plasticity. *Hippocampus* 13:826–834.

Bach ME, Hawkins RD, Osman M, Kandel ER, Mayford M (1995) Impairment of spatial but not contextual memory in CaMKII mutant mice with a selective loss of hippocampal LTP in the range of the theta frequency. *Cell* 81:905–915.

Bagal AA, Kao JP, Tang CM, Thompson SM (2005) Long-term potentiation of exogenous glutamate responses at single dendritic spines. *Proc Natl Acad Sci USA* 102:14434–14439.

Balschun D, Wolfer D, Bertocchini F, Barone V, Conti A, Zuschratter W, Missiaen L, Lipp H-P, Frey JU, Sorrentino V (1999) Deletion of the ryanodine receptor type 3 (RyR3) impairs forms of synaptic plasticity and spatial learning. *EMBO J* 18: 5264–5273.

Balschun D, Wolfer DP, Gass P, Mantamadiotis T, Welzl H, Schutz G, Frey JU, Lipp H P (2003) Does cAMP response element-binding protein have a pivotal role in hippocampal synaptic plasticity and hippocampus-dependent memory? *J. Neurosci* 23:6304–6314.

Bannerman DM, Good MA, Butcher SP, Ramsay M, Morris RG (1995) Distinct components of spatial learning revealed by prior training and NMDA receptor blockade. *Nature* 378:182–186.

Bannerman DM, Chapman PF, Kelly PAT, Butcher SP, Morris RGM (1994) Inhibition of nitric-oxide synthase does not prevent the induction of long-term potentiation in-vivo. *J Neurosci* 14:7415–7425.

Barbour B, Szatkowski M, Ingledew N, Attwell D (1989) Arachidonic acid induces a prolonged inhibition of glutamate uptake into glial cells. *Nature* 342:918–920.

Barco A, Alancon JM, Kandel ER (2002) Expression of constitutively active CREB protein facilitates the late phase of long-term potentiation by enhancing synaptic capture. *Cell* 108:689–703.

Barnes CA (1979) Memory deficits associated with senescence: a neurophysiological and behavioral study in the rat. *J Comp Physiol Psychol* 93:74–104.

Barnes CA (1995) Involvement of LTP in memory: are we searching under the street light? *Neuron* 15:751–754.

Barnes CA, McNaughton BL, Goddard GV, Douglas RM, Adamec R (1977) Circadian rhythm of synaptic excitability in rat and monkey central nervous system. *Science* 197:91–92.

Barnes CA, McNaughton BL (1985) An age comparison of the rates of acquisition and forgetting of spatial information in relation to long-term enhancement of hippocampal synapses. *Behav Neurosci* 99:1040–1048.

Barnes CA, Jung MW, McNaughton BL, Korol DL, Andreasson K, Worley PF (1994) LTP saturation and spatial learning disruption: effects of task variables and saturation levels. *J Neurosci* 14:5793–5806.

Barnes CA, Rao G, McNaughton BL (1996) Functional integrity of NMDA-dependent LTP induction mechanisms across the life-span of F-344 rats. *Learn Mem* 3:124–137.

Barnes CA, Rao G, Houston FP (2000) LTP induction threshold change in old rats at the perforant path–granule cell synapse. *Neurobiol Aging* 21:613–620.

Barria A, Derkach V, Soderling T (1997a) Identification of the Ca^{2+}/calmodulin-dependent protein kinase II regulatory phosphorylation site in the alpha-amino-3-hydroxyl-5-methyl-4-isoxazole-propionate-type glutamate receptor. *J Biol Chem* 272:32727–32730.

Barria A, Malinow R (2005) NMDA receptor subunit composition controls synaptic plasticity by regulating binding to CaMKII. *Neuron* 48:289–301.

Barria A, Muller D, Derkach V, Griffith LC, Soderling TR (1997b) Regulatory phosphorylation of AMPA-type glutamate receptors by CaM-KII during long-term potentiation. *Science* 276:2042–2045.

Barrionuevo G, Brown T (1983) Associative long-term potentiation in hippocampal slices. *Proc Natl Acad Sci USA* 70:7347–7351.

Barrionuevo G, Shottler F, Lynch G (1980) The effects of repetitive low-frequency stimulation on control and "potentiated" synaptic responses in the hippocampus. *Life Sci* 27:2385–2391.

Barrow PA, Empson RM, Gladwell SJ, Anderson CM, Killick R, Yu X, Jefferys JG, Duff K (2000) Functional phenotype in transgenic mice expressing mutant human presenilin-1. *Neurobiol Dis* 7:119–126.

Bashir ZI (2003) On long-term depression induced by activation of G-protein coupled receptors. *Neurosci Res* 45:363–367.

Bashir ZI, Collingridge GL (1994) An investigation of depotentiation of long-term potentiation in the CA1 region of the hippocampus. *Exp Brain Res* 100:437–443.

Bashir ZI, Tam B, Collingridge GL (1990) Activation of the glycine site in the NMDA receptor is necessary for the induction of LTP. *Neurosci Lett* 108:261–6.

Bashir ZI, Alford S, Davies SN, Randall AD, Collingridge GL (1991) Long-term potentiation of NMDA receptor-mediated synaptic transmission in the hippocampus. *Nature* 349:156–158.

Bashir ZI, Bortolotto ZA, Davies CH, Berretta N, Irving AJ, Seal AJ, Henley JM, Jane DE, Watkins JC, Collingridge GL (1993) Induction of LTP in the hippocampus needs synaptic activation of glutamate metabotropic receptors. *Nature* 363:347–350.

Bast T, da Silva BM, Morris RG (2005) Distinct contributions of hippocampal NMDA and AMPA receptors to encoding and retrieval of one-trial place memory. *J Neurosci* 25:5845–5856.

Battistin T, Cherubini E (1994) Developmental shift from long-term depression to long-term potentiation at mossy fiber synapses in the rat hippocampus. *Eur J Neurosci* 6:1750–1755.

Bauer EP, LeDoux JE, Nader K (2001) Fear conditioning and LTP in the lateral amygdala are sensitive to the same stimulus contingencies. *Nat Neurosci* 4:687–688.

Bear MF (1996) A synaptic basis for memory storage in the cerebral cortex. *Proc Natl Acad Sci USA* 93:13453–13459.

Bear MF, Linden DJ (2001) The mechanisms and meaning of long-term synaptic depression in the mammalian brain. In: *Synapses* (Cowan WM, Südhof TC, Stevens CF, eds), pp 455–518. Baltimore: Johns Hopkins University Press.

Bear MF, Cooper LN, Ebner FF (1987) A physiological basis for a theory of synapse modification. *Science* 237:42–48.

Beattie EC, Carroll RC, Yu X, Morishita W, Yasuda H, von Zastrow M, Malenka RC (2000) Regulation of AMPA receptor endocytosis by a signaling mechanism shared with LTD. *Nat Neurosci* 3:1291–1300.

Beattie EC, Stellwagen D, Morishita W, Bresnahan JC, Ha BK, Von Zastrow M, Beattie MS, Malenka RC (2002) Control of synaptic strength by glial TNFalpha. *Science* 295:2282–2285.

Beck H, Goussakov IV, Lie A, Helmstaedter C, Elger CE (2000) Synaptic plasticity in the human dentate gyrus. *J Neurosci* 20:7080–7086.

Belanger A, Lavoie N, Trudeau F, Massicotte G, Gagnon S (2004) Preserved LTP and watermaze learning in hyperglycaemic-hyperinsulinemic ZDF rats. *Physiol Behav* 83:483–494.

Bellinger FP, Madamba S, Siggins GR (1993) Interleukin 1 beta inhibits synaptic strength and long-term potentiation in the rat CA1 hippocampus. *Brain Res* 628:227.

Bellinger FP, Madamba SG, Campbell IL, Siggins GR (1995) Reduced long-term potentiation in the dentate gyrus of transgenic mice with cerebral overexpression of interleukin-6. *Neurosci Lett* 198:95–98.

Benke TA, Luthi A, Isaac JT, Collingridge GL (1998) Modulation of AMPA receptor unitary conductance by synaptic activity. *Nature* 393:793–797.

Benson DL, Schnapp LM, Shapiro ML, Huntley GW (2000) Making memories stick: cell-adhesion molecules in synaptic plasticity. *Trends Cell Biol* 10:473–482.

Berberich S, Punnakkl P, Jensen V, Pawlak V, Seeburg PH, Hvalby O, Köhr G (2005) Lack of NMDA Receptor Subtype Selectivity for Hippocampal Long-Term Potentiation. *J Neurosci* 25:6907–6910.

Berger TW (1984) Long-term potentiation of hippocampal synaptic transmission affects rate of behavioral learning. *Science* 224:627–630.

Bernabeu R, Bevilaqua L, Ardenghi P, Bromberg E, Schmitz P, Bianchin M, Izquierdo I, Medina JH (1997) Involvement of hippocampal cAMP/cAMP-dependent protein kinase signaling pathways in a late memory consolidation phase of aver-sively motivated learning in rats. *Proc Natl Acad Sci USA* 94:7041–7046.

Berretta N, Berton F, Bianchi R, Brunelli M, Capogna M, Francesconi W (1991) Long-term potentiation of NMDA receptor-mediated EPSP in guinea-pig hippocampal slices. *Eur J Neurosci* 3:850–854.

Bi G-Q, Poo M-M (1998) Synaptic modifications in cultured hippocampal neurons: dependence on spike timing, synaptic strength, and postsynaptic cell type. *J Neurosci* 18:10464–10472.

Bi G-Q, Rubin J (2005) Timing in synaptic plasticity: from detection to integration. *Trends Neurosci* 28:222–228.

Bi P, Poo M-M (2001) Synaptic modification by correlated activity: Hebb's postulate revisited. *Annu Rev Neurosci* 24:139–166.

Bienenstock EL, Cooper LN, Munro PW (1982) Theory for the development of neuron selectivity: orientation specificity and binocular interaction in visual cortex. *J Neurosci* 2:32–48.

Bischofberger J, Jonas P (2002) TwoB or not twoB: differential transmission at glutamatergic mossy fiber–interneuron synapses in the hippocampus. *Trends Neurosci* 25:600–603.

Bliss T, Errington M, Fransen E, Godfraind J-M, Kauer J, Kooy RF, Maness PF, Furley AJW (2000) Long-term potentiation in mice lacking the neural cell adhesion molecule L1. *Curr Biol* 10:1607–1610.

Bliss TVP, Collingridge GL (1993) A synaptic model of memory: long-term potentiation in the hippocampus. *Nature* 361:31–39.

Bliss TVP, Dolphin AC (1984) Where is the locus of long-term potentiation in the hippocampus? In: *The neurobiology of learning and memory* (McGaugh JL, Lynch G, eds), pp 451–458. New York: Guilford Press.

Bliss TVP, Gardner-Medwin AR (1973) Long-lasting potentiation of synaptic transmission in the dentate area of the unanaesthetized rabbit following stimulation of the perforant path. *J Physiol (Lond)* 232:357–374.

Bliss TVP, Lømo T (1973) Long-lasting potentiation of synaptic transmission in the dentate area of the anaesthetized rabbit following stimulation of the perforant path. *J Physiol (Lond)* 232:331–356.

Bliss TVP, Lynch MA (1988) Long-term potentiation of synaptic transmission in the hippocampus: properties and mechanisms. In: *Long-term potentiation in the hippocampus: from biophysics to behavior* (Landfield PW, Deadwyler SA, eds), pp 3–72. New York: Alan R Liss.

Bliss TVP, Richter-Levin G (1993) Spatial-learning and the saturation of long-term potentiation. *Hippocampus* 3:123–126.

Bliss TVP, Gardner-Medwin AR, Lømo T (1973) Synaptic plasticity in the hippocampal formation. In: *Macromolecules and behavior* (Ansell GB, Bradley PB, eds), pp 193–203. Baltimore: University Park Press.

Bliss TVP, Goddard GV, Riives M (1983) Reduction of long-term potentiation in the dentate gyrus of the rat following selective depletion of monoamines. *J Physiol* 334:475–491.

Bliss TVP, Errington AL, Lynch A, Williams JH (1990) Presynaptic mechanisms in hippocampal long-term potentiation. *Cold Spring Harbor Symp Quant Biol* 55:119–129.

Bliss TVP, Collingridge GL, Morris RGM, (eds) (2003) LTP: enhancing neuroscience for 30 years. *Philos Trans R Soc B* 358:607–842.

Bliss TVP, Collingridge Gl, Laroche S (2006) From Zap to Zip: a story to forget. *Science* 313:1058–1059.

Blitzer RD, Wong T, Nouranifar R, Iyengar R, Landau EM (1995) Postsynaptic cAMP pathway gates early LTP in hippocampal CA1 region. *Neuron* 15:1403–1414.

Blitzer RD, Connor JH, Brown GP, Wong T, Shenolikar S, Iyengar G, Landau EM (1998) Gating of CaMKII by cAMP-regulated protein phosphatase activity during LTP. *Science* 280:1940–1943.

Bodensteiner KJ, Cain P, Ray AS, Hamula LA (2006) Effects of pregnancy on spatial cognition in female Hooded Long-Evan rats. *Horm Behav* 49:303–314.

Boehm J, Kang MG, Johnson RC, Esteban J, Huganir RL, Malinow R (2006) Synaptic incorporation of AMPA receptors during LTP is controlled by a PKC phosphorylation site on GluR1. *Neuron* 51:213–25.

Bohme GA, Bon C, Stutzmann JM, Doble A, Blanchard JC (1991) Possible involvement of nitric-oxide in long-term potentiation. *Eur J Pharm* 199:379–381.

Bolhuis JJ, Reid IC (1992) Effects of intraventricular infusion of the N-methyl-D-aspartate (NMDDA receptor antgonist AP5 on spatial memory of rats in a radial arm maze. *Behav Brain Res* 47:151–157.

Bolshakov V, Siegelbaum S (1994) Postsynaptic induction and presynaptic expression of hippocampal long-term depression. *Science* 264:1148–1151.

Bolshakov VY, Siegelbaum SA (1995) Regulation of hippocampal transmitter release during development and long-term potentiation. *Science* 269:1730–1734.

Bon CL, Garthwaite J (2003) On the role of nitric oxide in hippocampal long-term potentiation. *J Neurosci* 23:1941–1948.

Bortolotto ZA, Collingridge GL (1993) Characterisation of LTP induced by the activation of glutamate metabotropic receptors in area CA1 of the hippocampus. *Neuropharmacology* 32:1.

Bortolotto ZA, Collingridge GL (2000) A role for protein kinase C in a form of metaplasticity that regulates the induction of long-term potentiation at CA1 synapses of the adult rat hippocampus. *Eur J Neurosci* 12:4055–4062.

Bortolotto ZA, Bashir ZI, Davies CH, Collingridge GL (1994) A molecular switch activated by metabotropic glutamate receptors regulates induction of long-term potentiation. *Nature* 368:740–743.

Bortolotto ZA, Collingridge GL (1995) On the mechanism of long-term potentiation induced by (1S,3R)-1-aminocyclopentane-1,3-dicarboxylic acid (ACPD) in rat hippocampal slices. *Neuropharmacology* 34:1003–1014.

Bortolotto ZA, Collingridge GL (1998) Involvement of calcium/calmodulin-dependent protein kinases in the setting of a molecular switch involved in hippocampal LTP. *Neuropharmacology* 37:535–544.

Bortolotto ZA, Clarke VR, Delany CM, Parry MC, Smolders I, Vignes M, Ho KH, Miu P, Brinton BT, Fantaske R, Ogden A, Gates M, Orstein PL, Lodge D, Bleakman D, Collingridge GL (1999) Kainate receptors are involved in synaptic plasticity. *Nature* 402:297–301.

Bortolotto ZA, Anderson WW, Isaac JT, Collingridge GL (2002) Synaptic plasticity in the hippocampal slice preparation. In: *Current protocols in neuroscience* (Crawley JN, Gerfen CR, McKay R, Rogawski MA, Sibley DR, Skolnick P, eds). New York: Wiley.

Bourtchuladze R, Frenguelli B, Blendy J, Cioffi D, Schutz G, Silva AJ (1994) Deficient long-term memory in mice with a targeted mutation of the cAMP-responsive element-binding protein. *Cell* 79:59–68.

Bozdagi O, Shan W, Tanaka H, Benson DL, Huntley GW (2000) Increasing numbers of synaptic puncta during late-phase LTP: N-cadherin is synthesized, recruited to synaptic sites, and required for potentiation. *Neuron* 28:245–259.

Bradshaw KD, Emptage NJ, Bliss TVP (2003) A role for dendritic protein synthesis is hippocampal late LTP. *Eur J Neurosci* 18:3150–3152.

Bramham CR, Messaoudi E (2005) BDNF function in adult synaptic plasticity: the synaptic consolidation hypothesis. *Prog Neurobiol* 76:99–125.

Bramham CR, Srebro B (1989) Synaptic plasticity in the hippocampus is modulated by behavioral state. *Brain Res* 493:74–86.

Braunewell K-H, Manahan-Vaughan D (2001) Long-term depression: a cellular basis for learning? *Rev Neurosci* 12:121–140.

Bredt DS, Nicoll RA (2003) AMPA receptor trafficking at excitatory synapses. *Neuron* 40:361–379.

Brightwell JJ, Smith CA, Countryman RA, Neve RL, Colombo PJ (2005) Hippocampal overexpression of mutant CREB blocks long-term but not short-term memory for a socially transmitted food preference. *Learn Mem* 12:12–17.

Brown TH, McAfee DA (1982) Long-term potentiation in the superior cervical ganglion. *Science* 215:1411–1413.

Brun VH, Ytterbo K, Morris RG, Moser MB, Moser EI (2001) Retrograde amnesia for spatial memory induced by NMDA receptor-mediated long-term potentiation. *J Neurosci* 21: 356–362.

Brun VH, Otnass MK, Molden S, Steffenach HA, Witter MP, Moser MB, Moser EI (2002) Place cells and place recognition maintained by direct entorhinal-hippocampal circuitry. *Science* 296:2243–2246.

Buchs PA, Muller D (1996) Induction of long-term potentiation is associated with major ultrastructural changes of activated synapses. *Proc Natl Acad Sci USA* 93:8040–8045.

Budde T, Minta A, White JA, Kay AR (1997) Imaging free zinc in synaptic terminals in live hippocampal slices. *Neuroscience* 79:347–358.

Burgoyne RD (2004) The neuronal calcium-sensor proteins. *Biochim Biophys Acta* 1742:59–68.

Burke SN, Barnes CA (2006) Neural plasticity in the ageing brain. *Nat Rev Neurosci* 7:30–40.

Burrone J, O'Byrne M, Murthy VN (2002) Multiple forms of synaptic plasticity triggered by selective suppression of activity in individual neurons. *Nature* 420:414–418.

Bushell TJ, Sansig G, Collett VJ, van der Putten H, Collingridge GL (2002) Altered short-term synaptic plasticity in mice lacking the metabotropic glutamate receptor mGlu7. *Sci World J* 2: 730–737.

Butler MP, O'Connor JJ, Moynagh PN (2004) Dissection of tumor-necrosis factor-alpha inhibition of long-term potentiation (LTP) reveals a p38 mitogen-activated protein kinase-dependent mechanism which maps to early- but not late-phase LTP. *Neuroscience* 124:319–326.

Buzsaki G, Haas HL, Anderson EG (1987) Long-term potentiation induced by physiologically relevant stimulus patterns. *Brain Res* 435:331–333.

Caillard O, Ben-Ari Y, Gaiarsa JL (1999) Long-term potentiation of GABAergic synaptic transmission in neonatal rat hippocampus. *J Physiol (Lond)* 518:109–119.

Cain DP (1989) Long-term potentiation and kindling: how similar are the mechanisms? *Trends Neurosci* 12:6–10.

Cain DP, Hargreaves EL, Boon F, Dennison Z (1993) An examination of the relations between hippocampal long-term potentiation, kindling, afterdischarge, and place learning in the watermaze. *Hippocampus* 3:153–163.

Cain DP, Saucier D, Hall J, Hargreaves EL, Boon F (1996) Detailed behavioral analysis of watermaze acquisition under AP5 or CNQX: contribution of sensorimotor disturbances to drug-induced acquisition deficits. *Behav Neurosci* 110:86–102.

Campbell IG, Guinan MJ, Horowitz JM (2002) Sleep deprivation impairs long-term potentiation in rat hippocampal slices. *J Neurophysiol* 88:1073–1076.

Camodeca N, Breakwell NA, Rowan MJ, Anwyl R (1999) Induction of LTD by activation of group I mGluR in the dentate gyrus in vitro. *Neuropharmacology* 38:1597–1606.

Capecchi MR (1989) Altering the genome by homologous recombination. *Science* 244:1288–1292.

Caramanos Z, Shapiro ML (1994) Spatial memory and *N*-methyl-D-aspartate receptor antagonists AP5 and MK-801: memory impairments depend on familiarity with the environment, drug dose, and training duration. *Behav Neurosci* 108:30–43.

Castillo PE, Janz R, Sudhof TC, Tzounopoulos T, Malenka RC, Nicoll RA (1997a) Rab3A is essential for mossy fiber long-term potentiation in the hippocampus. *Nature* 388:590–593.

Castillo PE, Malenka RC, Nicoll RA (1997b) Kainate receptors mediate a slow postsynaptic current in hippocampal CA3 neurons. *Nature* 388:182–186.

Castillo PE, Schoch S, Schmitz F, Sudhof TC, Malenka RC (2002) RIM1alpha is required for presynaptic long-term potentiation. *Nature* 425:327–330.

Castro CA, Silbert LH, McNaughton BL, Barnes CA (1989) Recovery of spatial learning deficits after decay of electrically induced synaptic enhancement in the hippocampus. *Nature* 342: 545–548.

Cavus I, Teyler T (1996) Two forms of long-term potentiation in area CA1 activate different signal transduction cascades. *J Neurophysiol* 76:3038–3047.

Chan CS, Weeber EJ, Kurup S, Sweatt JD, Davis RL (2003) Integrin requirement for hippocampal synaptic plasticity and spatial memory. *J Neurosci* 23:7107–7116.

Chapman PF, Kairiss EW, Keenan CL, Brown TH (1990) Long-term potentiation in the amygdala. *Synapse* 6:271–278.

Chapman PF, White GL, Jones MW, Cooper-Blacketer D, Marshall VJ, Irizarry M, Younkin L, Good MA, Bliss TV, Hyman BT, Younkin SG, Hsiao KK. (1999) Impaired synaptic plasticity and learning in aged amyloid precursor protein transgenic mice. *Nat Neurosci* 2:271–276.

Chavez-Noriega LE, Bliss TVP, Halliwell JV (1989) The EPSP-spike (E-S) component of long-term potentiation in the rat hippocampal slice is modulated by GABAergic but not cholinergic mechanisms. *Neurosci Lett* 104:58–64.

Chen C, Tonegawa S (1997) Molecular genetic analysis of synaptic plasticity, activity-dependent neural development, learning, and memory in the mammalian brain. *Annu Rev Neurosci* 20: 157–184.

Chen L, Chetkovich DM, Petralia RS, Sweeney NT, Kawasaki Y, Wenthold RJ, Bredt DS, Nicoll RA (2000) Stargazin regulates synaptic targeting of AMPA receptors by two distinct mechanisms. *Nature* 408:936–943.

Chen N, Luo T, Wellington C, Metzler M, McCutcheon K, Hayden MR, Raymond LA (1999) Subtype-specific enhancement of NMDA receptor currents by mutant huntingtin. *J Neurochem* 72:1890–1898.

Chen QS, Kagan BL, Hirakura Y, Xie CW (2000) Impairment of hippocampal long-term potentiation by Alzheimer amyloid beta-peptides. *J Neurosci Res* 60:65–72.

Chen Y-L, Huang C-C, Hsu K-S (2001a) Time-dependent reversal of long-term potentiation by low-frequency stimulation at the mossy fiber-CA3 synapses. *J Neurosci* 21:2705–2714.

Chen HX, Otmakhov N, Strack S, Colbran RJ, Lisman JE (2001b) Is persistent activity of calcium/calmodulin-dependent kinase required for the maintenance of LTP? *J Neurophysiol* 85: 1368–1376.

Chetkovich DM, Gray R, Johnston D, Sweatt JD (1991) *N*-Methyl-D-aspartate receptor activation increases cAMP levels and voltage-gated Ca^{2+} channel activity in area CA1 of hippocampus. *Proc Natl Acad Sci USA* 88:6467–6471.

Chetkovich DM, Sweatt JD (1993) NMDA receptor activation increases cyclic AMP in area CA1 of the hippocampus via calcium/calmodulin stimulation of adenylyl cyclase. *J Neurochem* 61:1933–1942.

Chetkovich DM, Chen L, Stocker TJ, Nicoll RA, Bredt DS (2002) Phosphorylation of the postsynaptic density-95 (PSD-95)/discs large/zona occludens-1 binding site of stargazin regulates binding to PSD-95 and synaptic targeting of AMPA receptors. *J Neurosci* 22:5791–5796.

Chevaleyre V, Castillo PE (2002) Assessing the role of Ih channels in synaptic transmission and mossy fiber LTP. *Proc Natl Acad Sci USA* 99:9538–9543.

Chevaleyre V, Castillo PE (2003) Heterosynaptic LTD of hippocampal GABAergic synapses: a novel role of endocannabinoids in regulating excitability. *Neuron* 38:461–472.

Chevaleyre V, Castillo PE (2004) Endocannabinoid-mediated metaplasticity in the hippocampus. *Neuron* 43:871–881.

Chevaleyre V, Takahashi KA, Castillo PE (2006) Endocannabinoid-mediated synaptic plasticity in the CNS. *Annu Rev Neurosci* 29:37–76.

Cho K, Aggleton JP, Brown MW, Bashir ZI (2001) An experimental test of the role of postsynaptic calcium levels in determining synaptic strength using perirhinal cortex of rat. *J Physiol* 532: 459–466.

Cho YH, Giese KP, Tanila H, Silva AJ, Eichenbaum H (1998) Abnormal hippocampal spatial representations in alphaCaMKIIT286A and CREBalphaDelta- mice. *Science* 279:867–869.

Choi S, Klingauf J, Tsien RW (2000) Postfusional regulation of cleft glutamate concentration during LTP at 'silent synapses.' *Nat Neurosci* 3:330.

Christie BR, Abraham WC (1992) Priming of associative long-term depression in the dentate gyrus by theta frequency synaptic activity. *Neuron* 9:79–84.

Clark KA, Collingridge GL (1995) Synaptic potentiation of dual-component excitatory postsynaptic currents in the rat hippocampus. *J Physiol* 482:39–52.

Coan EJ, Saywood W, Collingridge GL (1987) Mk-801 blocks NMDA receptor-mediated synaptic transmission and long-term potentiation in rat hippocampal slices. *Neurosci Lett* 80:111–114.

Coan EJ, Irving AJ, Collingridge GL (1989) Low-frequency activation of the NMDA receptor system can prevent the induction of LTP. *Neurosci Lett* 105:205–210.

Cohen AS, Abraham WC (1996) Facilitation of long-term potentiation by prior activation of metabotropic glutamate receptors. *J Neurophysiol* 76:953–962.

Colbert CM, Levy WB (1993) Long-term potentiation of perforant path synapses in hippocampal CA1 in vitro. *Brain Res* 606:87–91.

Colbran RJ, Brown AM (2004) Calcium/calmodulin-dependent protein kinase II and synaptic plasticity. *Curr Opin Neurobiol* 14:318–327.

Cole BJ, Klewer M, Jones GH, Stephens DN (1993) Contrasting effects of the competitive NMDA antagonist CPP and non-competitive NMDA antagonist MK801 on performance of an operant delayed matching to position task in rats. *Pyschopharmacology (Berl)* 111:465–471.

Colicos MA, Collins BE, Sailor MJ, Goda Y (2001) Remodeling of synaptic actin induced by photoconductive stimulation. *Cell* 107:605–616.

Colledge M, Snyder EM, Crozier RA, Soderling JA, Jin Y, Langeberg LK, Lu H, Bear MF, Scott JD (2003) Ubiquitination regulates PSD-95 degradation and AMPA receptor surface expression. *Neuron* 40:595–607.

Collingridge GL (1985) Long term potentiation in the hippocampus: mechanisms of initiation and modulation by neurotransmitters. *Trends Pharmacol Sci* 6:407–411.

Collingridge GL, Kehl SJ, McLennan H (1983) Excitatory amino acids in synaptic transmission in the Schaffer collateral–commissural pathway of the rat hippocampus. *J Physiol* 334:33–46.

Collingridge GL, Herron CE, Lester RA (1988) Synaptic activation of N-methyl-D-aspartate receptors in the Schaffer collateral-commissural pathway of rat hippocampus. *J Physiol* 399: 283–300.

Collingridge GL, Isaac JT, Wang YT (2004) Receptor trafficking and synaptic plasticity. *Nat Rev Neurosci* 5:952–962.

Conquet F, Bashir ZI, Davies CH, Daniel H, Ferraguti F, Bordi F, Franz-Bacon K, Reggiani A, Matarese V, Conde F, et al (1994) Motor deficit and impairment of synaptic plasticity in mice lacking mGluR1. *Nature* 372:237–243.

Contractor A, Swanson G, Heinemann SF (2001) Kainate receptors are involved in short- and long-term plasticity at mossy fiber synapses in the hippocampus. *Neuron* 29:209–216.

Contractor A, Rogers C, Maron C, Henkemeyer M, Swanson GT, Heinemann SF (2002) Trans-synaptic Eph-receptor-ephrin signalling in hippocampal mossy fiber LTP. *Science* 296:1864–1869.

Cooke SF, Bliss TV (2005) Long-term potentiation and cognitive drug discovery. *Curr Opin Invest Drugs* 6:25–34.

Cooke SF, Bliss TV (2006) Plasticity in the human central nervous system. *Brain* 129:1659–1673.

Cooke SF, Wu J, Plattner F, Errington M, Rowan M, Peterson, Hirano A, Bradshaw KD, Anwyl R, Bliss TVP, Giese KP (2006) Autophosphorylation of αCaMKII is not a general requirement for NMPA receptor-dependent LTP in the adult mouse. *J Physiol* (in press).

Costa AC, Grybko MJ (2005) Deficits in hippocampal CA1 LTP induced by TBS but not HFS in the Ts65Dn mouse: a model of Down syndrome. *Neurosci Lett* 382:317–322.

Cox PR, Fowler V, Xu B, Sweatt JD, Paylor R, Zoghbi HY (2003) Mice lacking tropomodulin-2 show enhanced long-term potentiation, hyperactivity, and deficits in learning and memory. *Mol Cell Neurosci* 23:1–12.

Cremer H, Chazal G, Carleton A, Goridis C, Vincent JD, Lledo P (1998) Long-term but not short-term plasticity at mossy fiber synapses is impaired in neural cell adhesion molecule-deficient mice. *Proc Natl Acad Sci USA* 95:13242–13247.

Crépel F, Jaillard D (1991) Pairing of pre- and postsynaptic activities in cerebellar Purkinje cells induces long-term changes in synaptiic efficacy in vitro. *J Physiol* 432:123–141.

Crick F (1984) Memory and molecular turnover. *Nature* 312:101.

Cull-Candy SG, Usowicz MM (1987) Multiple-conductance channels activated by excitatory amino acids in cerebellar neurons. *Nature* 325:525–528.

Cullen WK, Wu J, Anwyl R, Rowan MJ (1996) Beta-amyloid produces a delayed NMDA receptor-dependent reduction in synaptic transmission in rat hippocampus. *Neuroreport* 8:87–92.

Cullen WK, Suh YH, Anwyl R, Rowan MJ (1997) Block of LTP in rat hippocampus in vivo by beta-amyloid precursor protein fragments. *Neuroreport* 8:3213–3217.

Cummings JA, Nicola SM, Malenka RC (1994) Induction in the rat hippocampus of long-term potentiation (LTP) and long-term depression (LTD) in the presence of a nitric oxide synthase inhibitor *Neurosci Lett* 1994 18:110–114

Cummings JA, Mulkey RM, Nicoll RA, Malenka RC (1996) Ca^{2+} signalling requirements for long-term depression in the hippocampus. *Neuron* 16:825–833.

Cunningham AJ, Murray CA, O'Neill LA, Lynch MA, O'Connor JJ (1996) Interleukin-1 beta (IL-1 beta) and tumour necrosis factor (TNF) inhibit long-term potentiation in the rat dentate gyrus in vitro. *Neurosci Lett* 203:17–20.

Curran B, O'Connor JJ (2001) The pro-inflammatory cytokine interleukin-18 impairs long-term potentiation and NMDA receptor-mediated transmission in the rat hippocampus in vitro. *Neuroscience* 108:83–90.

Curran BP, Murray HJ, O'Connor JJ (2003) A role for c-Jun N-terminal kinase in the inhibition of long-term potentiation by interleukin-1beta and long-term depression in the rat dentate gyrus in vitro. *Neuroscience* 118:347–357.

Dan Y, Poo M-M (2004) Spike timing-dependent plasticity of neural circuits. *Neuron* 44:22–30.

Dana RC, Martinez JL (1984) Effect of adrenalectomy on the circadian rhythm of LTP. *Brain Res* 308:392–395.

Danscher G, Fjerdingstad EJ, Fjerdingstad E, Fredens K (1976) Heavy metal content in subdivisions of the rat hippocampus (zinc, lead, copper). *Brain Res* 112:442–446.

Danysz W, Parsons CG, Mobius HJ, Stoffler A, Quack G (2000) Neuroprotective and symptomatological action of memantine relevant for Alzheimer's disease - a unified glutamatergic hypothesis on the mechanism of action. *Neurotox Res* 2:85–97.

Danysz W, Wroblewski JT, Costa E (1988) Learning impairment in rats by *N*-methyl-D-aspartate receptor antagonist. *Neuropharmacology* 27:653–656.

Danysz W, Zajaczkowski W, Parsons CG (1995) Modulation of learning processes by ionotropic glutamate receptor ligands. *Behav Pharmacol* 6:455–474.

Daoudal G, Hanada Y, Debanne D (2002) Bidirectional plasticity of excitatory postsynaptic potential (EPSP)-spike coupling in CA1 hippocampal pyramidal neurons. *Proc Natl Acad Sci USA* 99:14512–14517.

D'Arcangelo G, Grassi F, Ragozzino D, Santoni A, Tancredi V, Eusebi F (1991) Interferon inhibits synaptic potentiation in rat hippocampus. *Brain Res* 564:245–248.

Daumas S, Halley H, Frances B, Lassalle JM (2005) Encoding, consolidation, and retrieval of contextual memory: differential involvement of dorsal CA3 and CA1 hippocampal subregions. *Learn Mem* 12:375–382.

Davies CH, Collingridge GL (1993) The physiological regulation of synaptic inhibition by GABA$_B$ autoreceptors in rat hippocampus. *J Physiol* 472:245–265.

Davies CH, Collingridge GL (1996) Regulation of EPSPs by the synaptic activation of GABA$_B$ autoreceptors in rat hippocampus. *J Physiol* 496:451–470.

Davies SN, Collingridge GL (1989) Role of excitatory amino acid receptors in synaptic transmission in area CA1 of rat hippocampus. *Proc R Soc B* 236:373–384.

Davies CH, Davies SN, Collingridge GL (1990) Paired-pulse depression of monosynaptic GABA-mediated inhibitory postsynaptic responses in rat hippocampus. *J Physiol* 424:513–531.

Davies CH, Starkey SJ, Pozza MF, Collingridge GL (1991) GABA-B autoreceptors regulate the induction of LTP. *Nature* 349:609–611.

Davies J, Francis AA, Jones AW, Watkins JC (1981) 2-Amino-5-phosphonovalerate (2AP5), a potent and selective antagonist of amino acid-induced and synaptic excitation. *Neurosci Lett* 21:77–81.

Davies SN, Lester RA, Reymann KG, Collingridge GL (1989) Temporally distinct pre- and post-synaptic mechanisms maintain long-term potentiation. *Nature* 338:500–503.

Davis C, Harding JW, Wright JW (2003). REM sleep deprivation-induced deficits in the latency-to-peak induction and maintenance of long-term potentiation within the CA1 region of the hippocampus. *Brain Res* 973:293–297.

Davis HP, Squire LR (1984) Protein synthesis and memory: a review. *Psychol Bull* 96:518–559.

Davis S, Butcher SP, Morris RG (1992) The NMDA receptor antagonist D-2-amino-5-phosphonopentanoate (D-AP5) impairs spatial learning and LTP in vivo at intracerebral concentrations comparable to those that block LTP in vitro. *J Neurosci* 12:21–34.

Davis S, Vanhoutte P, Pages C, Caboche J, Laroche S (2000) The MAPK/ERK cascade targets both Elk-1 and cAMP response element-binding protein to control long-term potentiation-dependent gene expression in the dentate gyrus in vivo. *J Neurosci* 20:4563–4572.

Daw MI, Chittajallu R, Bortolotto ZA, Dev KK, Duprat F, Henley JM, Collingridge GL, Isaac JT (2000) PDZ proteins interacting with C-terminal GluR2/3 are involved in a PKC-dependent regulation of AMPA receptors at hippocampal synapses. *Neuron* 28:873–876.

Daw MI, Bortolotto ZA, Saulle E, Zaman S, Collingridge GL, Isaac JT (2002) Phosphatidylinositol 3 kinase regulats synapse specificity of hippocampal long-term depression. *Nat Neurosci* 5:835–836.

Day M, Good M (2005) Ovariectomy-induced disruption of long-term synaptic depression in the hippocampal CA1 region in vivo is attenuated with chronic estrogen replacement. *Neurobiol Learn Mem* 83:13–21.

Day M, Langston RF (2006) Post-training *N*-methyl-D-aspartate receptor blockade offers protection from retrograde interference but does not affect consolidation of weak or strong memory traces in the watermaze. *Neuroscience* 137:19–28.

Day M, Langston R, Morris RG (2003) Glutamate-receptor-mediated encoding and retrieval of paired-associate learning. *Nature* 424:205–209.

Dayan P, Willshaw DJ (1991) Optimising synaptic learning rules in linear associative memories. *Biol Cybern* 65:253–265.

Debanne D, Gahwiler BH, Thompson SM (1994) Asynchronous presynaptic and postsynaptic activity induces associative long-term depression in area CA1 of the rat hippocampus in vitro. *Proc Natl Acad Sci USA* 91:1148–1152.

Debanne D, Gahwiler BH, Thompson SM (1998) Long-term synaptic plasticity between pairs of individual CA3 pyramidal cells in rat hippocampal slice cultures. *J Physiol (Lond)* 507:237–247.

Debanne D, Gahwiler BH, Thompson SM (1999) Heterogeneity of synaptic plasticity at unitary CA3–CA1 and CA3–CA3 connections in rat hippocamal slice cultures. *J Neurosci* 19:10664–10671.

Deisseroth K, Bito H, Schulman H, Tsien RW (1995) A molecular mechanism of metaplasticity. *Curr Biol* 5:1334–1338.

Deisseroth K, Bito H, Tsien RW (1996) Signaling from synapse to nucleus: postsynaptic CREB phosphorylation during multiple forms of hippocampal synaptic plasticity. *Neuron* 16:89–101.

Deisseroth K, Heist EK, Tsien RW (1998) Translocation of calmodulin to the nucleus supports CREB phosphorylation in hippocampal neurons. *Nature* 392:198–202.

Derkach V, Barria A, Soderling TR (1999) Ca^{2+}/calmodulin-kinase II enhances channel conductance of alpha-amino-3-hydroxy-5-methyl-4-isoxazolepropionate type glutamate receptors. *Proc Natl Acad Sci USA* 96:3269–3274.

Derrick BE, Martinez JL (1994a) Opioid receptor activation is one factor underlying the frequency dependence of mossy fiber LTP. *J Neurosci* 14:4359–4367.

Derrick BJ, Martinez JL (1994b) Frequency-dependent associative long-term potentiation at the hippocampal mossy fiber-CA3 synapse. *Proc Natl Acad Sci USA* 91:10290–10294.

Derrick BE, Martinez JL (1996) Associative, bidirectional modifications at the hippocampal mossy fiber-CA3 synapse. *Nature* 381:429–434.

Desmond NL, Levy WB (1983) Synaptic correlates of associative potentiation/depression: an ultrastructural study in the hippocampus. *Brain Res* 265:21–30.

Desmond NL, Levy WB (1986a) Changes in the postsynaptic density with long-term potentiation in the dentate gyrus. *J Comp Neurol* 253:476–482.

Desmond NL, Levy WB (1986b) Changes in the numerical density of synaptic contacts with long-term potentiation in the hippocampal dentate gyrus. *J Comp Neurol* 253:466–475.

Desmond NL, Levy WB (1990) Morphological correlates of long-term potentiation imply the modification of existing synapses, not synaptogenesis, in the hippocampal dentate gyrus. *Synapse* 5:139–143.

DeSouza S, Fu J, States BA, Ziff EB (2002) Differential palmitoylation directs the AMPA receptor-binding protein ABP to spines or to intracellular clusters. *J Neurosci* 22:3493–3503.

Deupree DL, Turner DA, Watters CL (1991) Spatial performance correlates with in vitro potentiation in young and aged Fischer 344 rats. *Brain Res* 554:1–9.

Dev KK, Nishimune A, Henley JM, Nakanishi S (1999) The protein kinase C alpha binding protein PICK1 interacts with short but not long form alternative splice variants of AMPA receptor subunits. *Neuropharmacology* 38:635–644.

Diamond DM, Rose GM (1994) Does associative LTP underlie classicalal conditioning? *Psychobiology* 22:263–269.

Diamond DM, Bennett MC, Fleshner M, Rose GM (1992) Inverted-U relationship between the level of peripheral corticosterone and the magnitude of hippocampal primed burst potentiation. *Hippocampus* 2:421–430.

Diamond JS, Bergles DE, Jahr CE (1998) Glutamate release monitored with astrocyte transporter currents during LTP. *Neuron* 21:425–433.

Dieguez D, Jr., Barea-Rodriguez EJ (2004) Aging impairs the late phase of long-term potentiation at the medial perforant path–CA3 synapse in awake rats. *Synapse* 52:53–61.

Dineley KT, Westerman M, Bui D, Bell K, Ashe KH, Sweatt JD (2001) Beta-amyloid activates the mitogen-activated protein kinase cascade via hippocampal alpha7 nicotinic acetylcholine receptors: in vitro and in vivo mechanisms related to Alzheimer's disease. *J Neurosci* 21:4125–4133.

Dingledine R, Hynes MA, King GL (1986) Involvement of N-methyl-D-aspartate receptors in epileptiform bursting in the rat hippocampal slice. *J Physiol* 380:175–189.

Do VH, Martinez CO, Martinez JL Jr, Derrick BE (2002) Long-term potentiation in direct perforant path projections to the hippocampal CA3 region in vivo. *J Neurophysiol* 87: 669–678.

Dolphin AC, Errington ML, Bliss TV (1982) Long-term potentiation of the perforant path in vivo is associated with increased glutamate release. *Nature* 297:496–498.

Domenici MR, Berretta N, Cherubini E (1998) Two distinct forms of long-term depression coexist at the mossy fiber–CA3 synapse in the hippocampus during development. *Proc Natl Acad Sci USA* 95:8310–8315.

Dong H, O'Brien RJ, Fung ET, Lanahan AA, Worley PF, Huganir RL (1997) GRIP: a synaptic PDZ domain-containing protein that interacts with AMPA receptors. *Nature* 386:279–284.

Douglas RM, Goddard GV (1975) Long-term potentiation of the perforant path–granule cell synapse in the rat hippocampus. *Brain Res* 86:205–215.

Douglas RM, Goddard GV, Riives M (1982) Inhibitory modulation of long-term potentiation: evidence for a postsynaptic locus of control. *Brain Res* 240:259–272.

Doyère V, Laroche S (1992) Linear relationship between the maintenance of hippocampal long-term potentiation and retention of an associative memory. *Hippocampus* 2:39–48.

Doyère V, Errington ML, Laroche S, Bliss TVP (1996) Low-frequency trains of paired stimuli induce long-term depression in area CA1 but not in dentate gyrus of the intact rat. *Hippocampus* 6:52–57.

Doyère V, Srebro B, Laroche S (1997) Heterosynaptic LTD and depotentiation in the medial perforant path in the freely moving rat. *J Neurophysiol* 77:571–578.

Doyle CA, Cullen WK, Rowan MJ, Anwyl R (1997) Low-frequency stimulation induces homosynaptic depotentiation but not long-term depression of synaptic transmission in the adult anaesthetized and awake rat hippocampus in vivo. *Neuroscience* 77:75–85.

Dozmorov M, Li R, Abbas AK, Hellberg F, Farre C, Huang FS, Jilderos B, Wigstrom H (2006) Contribution of AMPA and NMDA receptors to early and late phases of LTP in hippocampal slices. *Neurosci Res* 55:182–188.

Dragoi G, Harris KD, Buzsaki G (2003) Place representation within hippocampal networks is modified by long-term potentiation. *Neuron* 39:843–853.

Dragunow M (1996) A role for immediate-early transcription factors in learning and memory. *Behav Genet* 26:293–299.

Du J-L, Poo M-M (2004) Rapid BDNF-induced retrograde modification in a developing retinotectal system. *Nature* 429:878–883.

Dudai Y, Morris RGM (2000) To consolidate or not to consolidate: what are the questions? In: *Brain, perception, memory* (Bolhuis JJ, ed), pp 149–162. Oxford: Oxford University Press.

Dudek SM, Bear MF (1992) Homosynaptic long-term depression and effects of N-methyl-D-aspartate receptor blockade. *Proc Natl Acad Sci USA* 89:4363–4367.

Dudek SM, Bear MF (1993) Bidirectional long-term modification of synaptic effectiveness in the adult and immature hippocampus. *J Neurosci* 13:2910–2918.

Dudek SM, Fields RD (2002) Somatic action potentials are sufficient for late-phase LTP-related signaling. *Proc Natl Acad Sci USA* 99:3962–3967.

Duffy SN, Craddock KJ, Abel T, Nguyen PV (2001) Environmental enrichment modifies the PKA-dependence of hippocampal LTP and improves hippocampus-dependent memory. *Learn Mem* 8:26–34.

Duffy JN, Nguyen PV (2003) Postsynaptic application of a peptide inhibitor of cAMP-dependent protein kinase blocks expression of long-lasting synaptic potentiation in hippocampal neurons. *J Neurosci* 23:1142.

Dumuis A, Sebben M, Haynes L, Pin JP, Bockaert J (1988) NMDA receptors activate the arachidonic acid cascade system in striatal neurons. *Nature* 336:68–70.

Dunwiddie T, Lynch G (1978) Long-term potentiation and depression of synaptic responses in the rat hippocampus: localization and frequency dependency. *J Physiol (Lond)* 276:353–367.

Durand GM, Kovalchuk Y, Konnerth A (1996) Long-term potentiation and functional synapse induction in developing hippocampus. *Nature* 381:71–75.

Eaton SA, Jane DE, Jones PL, Porter RH, Pook PC, Sunter DC, Udvarhelyi PM, Roberts PJ, Salt TE, Watkins JC (1993) Competitive antagonism at metabotropic glutamate receptors by (S)-4-carboxyphenylglycine and (RS)-alpha-methyl-4-carboxyphenylglycine. *Eur J Pharmacol* 244:195–197.

Eberwine J, Miyashiro K, Kacharmina JE, Job C (2001) Local translation of classes of mRNAs that are targeted to neuronal dendrites. *Proc Natl Acad Sci USA* 98:7080–7085.

Ehrlich I, Malinow R (2004) Postsynaptic density 95 controls AMPA receptor incorporation during long-term potentiation and experience-driven synaptic plasticity. *J Neurosci* 24:916–927.

Ekstrom AD, Meltzer J, McNaughton BL, Barnes CA (2001) NMDA receptor antagonism blocks experience-dependent expansion of hippocampal "place fields." *Neuron* 31:631–638.

El Husseini A, Schnell E, Dakoji S, Sweeney N, Zhou Q, Prange O, Gauthier-Campbell C, Aguilera-Moreno A, Nicoll RA, Bredt DS (2002) Synaptic strength regulated by palmitate cycling on PSD-95. *Cell* 108:849–863.

Emptage N, Bliss TV, Fine A (1999) Single synaptic events evoke NMDA receptor-mediated release of calcium from internal stores in hippocampal dendritic spines. *Neuron* 22:115–124.

Emptage NJ, Reid CA, Fine A, Bliss TVP (2003) Optical quantal analysis reveals a presynaptic component of LTP at hippocampal Schaffer-associational synapses. *Neuron* 38:797–804.

Engert F, Bonhoeffer T (1997) Synapse specificity of long-term potentiation breaks down at short distances. *Nature* 388:279–284.

Engert F, Bonhoeffer T (1999) Dendritic spine changes associated with hippocampal long-term synaptic plasticity. *Nature* 399:66–70.

English JD, Sweatt JD (1996) Activation of p42 mitogen-activated protein kinase in hippocampal long term potentiation. *J Biol Chem* 271:24329–24332.

English JD, Sweatt JD (1997) A requirement for the mitogen-activated protein kinase cascade in hippocampal long-term potentiation. J Biol Chem 272:19103–19106.

Ernfors P, Bramham CR (2003) The coupling of a trkB tyrosine residue to LTP. *Trends Neurosci* 26:171–173.

Errington ML, Lynch MA, Bliss TVP (1987) Long-term potentiation in the dentate gyrus: induction and increased glutamate release are blocked by D(-)aminophosphonovalerate. *Neuroscience* 20:279–284.

Errington ML, Bliss TVP, Richter-Levin G, Yenk K, Doyère V, Laroche S (1995) Stimulation at 1-5 Hz does not produce long-term depression or depotentiation in the hippocampus of the adult rat in-vivo. *J Neurophysiol* 74:1793–1799.

Errington ML, Bliss TVP, Morris RJ, Laroche S, Davis S (1997) Long-term potentiation in awake mutant mice. *Nature* 387:666–667.

Errington ML, Galley PT, Bliss TVP (2003). Long-term potentiation in the dentate gyrus of the anaesthetized rat is accompanied by an increase in extracellular glutamate: real-time measurements using a novel dialysis electrode. *Philos Trans R Soc B* 358:675–687.

Esteban JA, Shi SH, Wilson C, Nuriya M, Huganir RL, Malinow R (2003) PKA phosphorylation of AMPA receptor subunits controls synaptic trafficking underlying plasticity. *Nat Neurosci* 6:136–143.

Evans RH, Francis WW, Watkins JC (1977) Selective antagonism by Mg^{2+} of amino acid-induced depolarization of spinal neurones. *Experientia* 15:489–491.

Fan Y, Fricker D, Brager DH, Chen X, Lu HC, Chitwood RA, Johnston D (2005) Activity-dependent decrease of excitability in rat hippocampal neurons through increases in I(h). *Nat Neurosci* 8:1542–1551.

Fanselow MS, Kim JJ, Yipp J, De Oca B (1994) Differential effects of the *N*-methyl-D-aspartate antagonist DL-2-amino-5-phosphonovalerate on acquisition of fear of auditory and contextual cues. *Behav Neurosci* 108:235–240.

Feinmark SJ, Begum R, Tsvetkov E, Goussakov IV, Funk CD, Siegelbaum SA, Bolshakov VY (2003) 12-Lipoxygenase metabolites of arachidonic acid mediate metabotropic glutamate receptor-dependent long-term depression at hippocampal CA3–CA1 synapses. *J Neurosci* 23:11427–11435.

Feng B, Tse HW, Skifter DA, Morley R, Jane DE, Monaghan DT (2004) Structure-activity analysis of a novel NR2C/NR2D-preferring NMDA receptor antagonist: 1-(phenanthrene-2-carbonyl) piperazine-2,3-dicarboxylic acid. *Br J Pharmacol* 141:508–516.

Fifkova E, Van Harreveld A (1977) Long-lasting morphological changes in dendritic spines of dentate granular cells following stimulation of the entorhinal area. *J Neurocytol* 6:211–230.

Fischer M, Kaech S, Knutti D, Matus A (1998) Rapid actin-based plasticity in dendritic spines. *Neuron* 20:847–854.

Fitzgerald M (2005) The development of nociceptive circuits. *Nat Rev Neurosci* 6:507–520.

Fitzjohn SM, Bortolotto ZA, Palmer MJ, Doherty AJ, Ornstein PL, Schoepp DD, Kingston AE, Lodge D, Collingridge GL (1998) The potent mGlu receptor antagonist LY341495 identifies roles for both cloned and novel mGlu receptors in hippocampal synaptic plasticity. *Neuropharmacology* 37:1445–1458.

Fitzjohn SM, Morton RA, Kuenzi F, Rosahl TW, Shearman M, Lewis H, Smith D, Reynolds DS, Davies CH, Collingridge GL, Seabrook GR (2001a) Age-related impairment of synaptic transmission but normal long-term potentiation in transgenic mice that overexpress the human APP695SWE mutant form of amyloid precursor protein. *J Neurosci* 21:4691.

Fitzjohn SM, Palmer MJ, May JE, Neeson A, Morris SA, Collingridge GL (2001b) A characterization of long-term depression induced by metabotropic glutamate receptor activation in the rat hippocampus in vitro. *J Physiol* 537:421–430.

Fitzsimonds RM, Song H-J, Poo M-M (1997) Propagation of activity-dependent synaptic depression in simple neural networks. *Nature* 388:439–448.

Florian C, Roullet P (2004) Hippocampal CA3-region is crucial for acquisition and memory consolidation in Morris watermaze task in mice. *Behav Brain Res* 154:365–374.

Fonseca R, Nageri UV, Morris RGM, Bonhoeffer T (2004) Competing for memory: hippocampal LTP under regimes of reduced protein synthesis. *Neuron* 44:1011–1020.

Foy MR, Stanton ME, Levine S, Thompson RF (1987) Behavioral stress impairs long-term potentiation in rodent hippocampus. *Behav Neural Biol* 48:138–149.

Frankiewicz T, Parsons CG (1999) Memantine restores long term potentiation impaired by tonic N-methyl-D-aspartate (NMDA) receptor activation following reduction of Mg2+ in hippocampal slices. *Neuropharmacology* 38:1253–1259.

Frederickson CJ, Danscher G (1990) Zinc-containing neurons in hippocampus and related CNS structures. *Prog Brain Res* 83:71–84.

Freir DB, Holscher C, Herron CE (2001) Blockade of long-term potentiation by beta-amyloid peptides in the CA1 region of the rat hippocampus in vivo. *J Neurophysiol* 85:708–713.

French PJ, O'Connor V, Jones MW, Davis S, Errington ML, Voss K, Truchet B, Wotjak C, Stean T, Doyere V, Maroun M, Laroche S, Bliss TVP (2001) Subfield-specific immediate early gene expression associated with hippocampal long-term potentiation in vivo. *Eur J Neurosci* 13:958–976.

Frey U, Morris RGM (1997) Synaptic tagging and long-term potentiation. *Nature* 385:533–536.

Frey U, Morris RGM (1998a) Synaptic tagging: implications for late maintenance of hippocampal long-term potentiation. *TINS* 21:181–188.

Frey U, Morris RGM (1998b) Weak before strong: dissociating synaptic-tagging and plasticity-factor accounts of late-LTP. *Neuropharmacology* 37:545–552.

Frey U, Krug M, Reymann KG, Matthies H (1988) Anisomycin, an inhibitor of protein synthesis, blocks late phases of LTP phenomena in the hippocampal CA1 region in vitro. *Brain Res* 452:57–65.

Frey U, Krug M, Brodemann R, Reymann K, Matthies H (1989) Long-term potentiation induced in dendrites separated from rats CA1 pyramidal somata does not establish a late phase. *Neurosci Lett* 97:135-139.

Frey U, Schroeder H, Matthies H (1990) Dopaminergic antagonists prevent long-term maintenance of posttetanic LTP in the CA1 region of rat hippocampal slices. *Brain Res* 522:69–75.

Frey U, Huang YY, Kandel ER (1993) Effects of cAMP simulate a late stage of LTP in hippocampal CA1 neurons. *Science* 260:1661–1664.

Frey U, Schollmeier K, Reymann KG, Seidenbecher T (1995) Asymptotic hippocampal long-term potentiation in rats does not preclude additional potentiation at later phases. *Neuroscience* 67:799–807.

Frey U, Frey S, Schollmeier F, Krug M (1996) Influence of actinomycin-D, an RNA-synthesis inhibitor, on long-term potentiation in rat hippocampal neurons in vivo and in vitro. *J Physiol (Lond)* 490:703–711.

Frey S, Bergado-Rosado J, Seidenbecher T, Pape HC, Frey JU (2001) Reinforcement of early long-term potentiation (early-LTP) in dentate gyrus by stimulation of the basolateral amygdala: heterosynaptic induction mechanisms of late-LTP. *J Neurosci* 21:3697–3703.

Frick A, Magee JC, Johnston D (2004) LTP is accompanied by an enhanced local excitability of pyramidal neuron dendrites. *Nat Neurosci* 7:126–135.

Friedlander MJ, Fregnac Y, Burke JP (1993) Temporal covariance of postsynaptic membrane potential and synaptic input: role in synaptic efficacy in visual cortex. *Prog Brain Res* 95:191–205.

Froemke RC, Dan Y (2002) Spike-timing-dependent synaptic modification induced by natural spike trains. *Nature* 416:433–438.

Fujii S, Saito K, Miyakawa H, Ito K, Kato K (1991) Reversal of long-term potentiation (depotentiation) induced by tetanus stimulation of the input to CA1 neurons of guinea pig hippocampal slices. *Brain Res* 555:112–122.

Fukaya M, Kato A, Lovett C, Tonegawa S, Watanabe M (2003) Retention of NMDA receptor NR2 subunits in the lumen of endoplasmic reticulum in targeted NR1 knockout mice. *Proc Natl Acad Sci USA* 100:4855–4860.

Fukazawa Y, Saitoh Y, Ozawa F, Ohta Y, Mizuno K, Inokuchi K (2003) LTP is accompanied by enhanced F-actin content within the dendritic spine that is essential for late LTP maintenance in vivo. *Neuron* 38:447–460.

Fukunaga K, Muller D, Miyamoto E (1995) Increased phosphorylation of Ca^{2+}/calmodulin-dependent protein kinase II and its endogenous substrates in the induction of long-term potentiation. *J Biol Chem* 270:6119–6124.

Furth PA, St Onge L, Boger H, Gruss P, Gossen M, Kistner A, Bujard H, Hennighausen L (1994) Temporal control of gene expression in transgenic mice by a tetracycline-responsive promoter. *Proc Natl Acad Sci USA* 91:9302–9306.

Futatsugi A, Kato K, Ogura H, Li ST, Nagata E, Kuwajima G, Tanaka K, Itohara S, Mikoshiba K (1999) Facilitation of NMDAR-independent LTP and spatial learning in mutant mice lacking ryanodine receptor type 3. *Neuron* 24:701–713.

Gall CM, Lynch G (2004) Integrins, synaptic plasticity and epileptogenesis. *Adv Exp Med Biol* 548:12–33.

Gall CM, Hess US, Lynch G (1998) Mapping brain networks engaged by, and changed by, learning. *Neurobiol Learn Mem* 70:14–36.

Gallagher SM, Daly CA, Bear MF, Huber KM (2004) Extracellular signal-regulated protein kinase activation is required for metabotropic glutamate receptor-dependent long-term depression in hippocampal area CA1. *J Neurosci* 24:4859–4864.

Garthwaite J, Charles SL, Chess-Williams R (1988) Endothelium-derived relaxing factor release on activation of NMDA receptors suggests role as intercellular messenger in the brain. *Nature* 336:385–388.

Gasbarri A, Sulli A, Packard MG (1997) The dopaminergic mesencephalic projections to the hippocampal formation in the rat. *Prog Neuropsychopharmacol Biol Psychiatry* 21:1–22.

Ge W-P, Yang X-J, Zhang Z, Wang H-K, Shen W, Deng Q-P, Duan S (2006) Long-term potentiation of neuron-glia synapses mediated by Ca^{2+}-permeable AMPA receptors. *Science* 312:1533–1537.

Geinisman Y, de Toledo-Morrell L, Morrell F (1991) Induction of long-term potentiation is associated with an increase in the number of axospinous synapses with segmented postsynaptic densities. *Brain Res* 566:77–88.

Geinisman Y, deToledo-Morrell L, Morrell F, Heller RE, Rossi M, Parshall RF (1993) Structural synaptic correlate of long-term potentiation: formation of axospinous synapses with multiple, completely partioned transmission zones. *Hippocampus* 3:435–446.

Génin A, French P, Doyere V, Davis M, Errington ML, Maroun M, Stean T, Truchet B, Webber M, Wills T, Richter-Levin G, Sanger G, Hunt SP, Mallet J, Laroche S, Bliss TVP, O'Connor V (2003) LTP but not seizure is associated with up-regulation of AKAP-150. *Eur J Neurosci* 17:331–340.

Gerlai R (1996) Gene-targeting studies of mammalian behaviour: is it the mutation or the background genotype? *Trends Neurosci* 19:177–181.

Gerlai R, Henderson JT, Roder JC, Jia Z (1998) Multiple behavioral anomalies in GluR2 mutant mice exhibiting enhanced LTP. *Behav Brain Res* 95:37–45.

Gianotti C, Nunzi M G, Gispen W H, Corradetti R (1992) Phosphorylation of the presynaptic protein B-50 (GAP-43) is increased during electrically induced long-term potentiation. *Neuron* 8:843–848.

Gibson HE, Reim K, Brose N, Morton AJ, Jones S (2005) A similar impairment in CA3 mossy fiber LTP in the R6/2 mouse model of Huntington's disease and in the complexin II knockout mouse. *Eur J Neurosci* 22:1701–1712.

Giese KP, Fedorov NB, Filipkowski RK, Silva AJ (1998) Autophosphorylation at Thr(286) of the alpha calcium-calmodulin kinase II in LTP and learning. *Science* 279:870–873.

Goddard GV (1967) Development of epileptic seizures through brain stimulation at low intensity. *Nature* 214:1020–1021.

Goelet P, Castellucci VF, Schacher S, Kandel ER (1986) The long and the short of long-term memory—a molecular framework. *Nature* 322:419–422.

Golding NL, Staff NP, Spruston N (2003) Dendritic spikes as a mechanism for cooperative long-term potentiation. *Nature* 418:326–331.

Good M, Day M, Muir JL (1999) Cyclical changes in endogenous levels of oestrogen modulate the induction of LTD and LTP in the hippocampal CA1 region. *Eur J Neurosci* 11:4476–4480.

Gooney M, Messaoudi E, Maher CO, Bramham CR, Lynch MA (2004) BDNF-induced LTP in dentate gyrus is impaired with age: analysis of changes in cell signaling events. *Neurobiol Aging* 25:1323–1331.

Grant SG, Karl KA, Kiebler MA, Kandel ER (1995) Focal adhesion kinase in the brain: novel subcellular localization and specific regulation by Fyn tyrosine kinase in mutant mice. *Genes Dev* 9:1909–1921.

Green EJ, Greenough WT (1986) Altered synaptic transmission in dentate gyrus of rats reared in complex enviornments: evidence from hippocampal slices maintained in vitro. *J Neurophysiol* 55:739–751.

Green EJ, McNaughton BL, Barnes CA (1990) Exploration-dependent modulation of evoked responses in fascia dentata: dissociation of motor, EEG, and sensory factors and evidence for a synaptic efficacy change. *J Neurosci* 10:1455–1471.

Grosshans DR, Clayton DA, Coultrap SJ, Browning MD (2002) LTP leads to rapid surface expression of NMDA but not AMPA receptors in adult rat CA1. *Nat Neurosci* 5:27–33.

Grover LM, Teyler TJ (1990) Two components of long-term potentiation induced by different patterns of afferent activation. *Nature* 347:477–479.

Gruart A, Dolores Munoz M, Delgado-Garcia JM (2006) Involvement of the CA3-CA1 synapse in the acquisition of associative learning in behaving mice. *J Neurosci* 26:1077–1087.

Grunwald IC, Korte M, Adelmann G, Plueck A, Kullander K, Adams RH, Frotscher M, Bonhoeffer T, Klein R (2004) Hippocampal plasticity requires postsynaptic ephrinBs. *Nat Neurosci* 7:33–40.

Grutzendler J, Kasthuri N, Gan WB (2002) Long-term dendritic spine stability in the adult cortex. *Nature* 420:751–752.

Gu Y, McIlwain KL, Weeber EJ, Yamagata T, Xu B, Antalffy BA, Reyes C, Yuva-Paylor L, Armstrong D, Zoghbi H, Sweatt JD, Paylor R, Nelson DL (2002) Impaired conditioned fear and enhanced long-term potentiation in Fmr2 knock-out mice. *J Neurosci* 22:2753–2763.

Gustafsson B, Wigström H (1986) Hippocampal long lasting potentiation produced by pairing single volleys and brief conditioning tetani evoked in separate afferents. *J Neurosci* 6:1575–1582.

Gustafsson B, Wigström H, Abraham WC, Huang YY (1987) Long-term potentiation in the hippocampus using depolarizing current pulses as the conditioning stimulus to single volley synaptic potentials. *J Neurosci* 7:774–780.

Gustafsson B, Asztely F, Hanse E, Wigström H (1989) Onset characteristics of long-term potentiation in the guinea-pig hippocampal ca1 region invitro. *Eur J Neurosci* 1:382–394.

Guzowski JF, McGaugh JL (1997) Antisense oligodeoxynucleotide-mediated disruption of hippocampal cAMP response element binding protein levels impairs consolidation of memory for watermaze training. *Proc Natl Acad Sci USA* 94:2693–2698.

Guzowski JF, McNaughton BL, Barnes CA, Worley PF (1999) Environment-specific expression of the immediate-early gene Arc in hippocampal neuronal ensembles. *Nat Neurosci* 2:1120–1124.

Guzowski JF, Lyford GL, Stevenson GD, Houston FP, McGaugh JL, Worley PF, Barnes CA (2000) Inhibition of activity-dependent arc protein expression in the rat hippocampus impairs the maintenance of long-term potentiation and the consolidation of long-term memory. *J Neurosci* 20:3993–4001.

Haley JE, Schaible E, Pavlidis P, Murdock A, Madison DV (1996) Basal and apical synapses of CA1 pyramidal cells employ different LTP induction mechanisms. *Learn Mem* 3:289–295.

Haley JE, Wilcox GL, Chapman PF (1992) The role of nitric oxide in hippocampal long-term potentiation. Neuron 8:211–216.

Hanley JG, Henley JM (2005) PICK1 is a calcium-sensor for NMDA-induced AMPA receptor trafficking. *EMBO J* 24:3266–3278.

Hanse E, Gustafsson B (1992) Postsynaptic, but not presynaptic, activity controls the early time course of long-term potentiation in the dentate gyrus. *J Neurosci* 12:3226–3240.

Hardingham GE, Arnold FJ, Bading H (2001) Nuclear calcium signaling controls CREB-mediated gene expression triggered by synaptic activity. *Nat Neurosci* 4:261–267.

Harris EW, Cotman CW (1986) Long-term potentiation of guinea pig mossy fiber responses is not blocked by N-methyl-D-aspartate antagonists. *Neurosci Lett* 70:132–137.

Harris EW, Ganong AH, Cotman CW (1984) Long-term potentiation in the hippocampus involves activation of N-methyl-D-aspartate receptors. *Brain Res* 323:132–137.

Harris KM (1999) Structure, development, and plasticity of dendritic spines. *Curr Opin Neurobiol* 9:343–348.

Harris KM, Stevens JK (1989) Dendritic spines of CA1 pyramidal cells in the rat hippocampus: serial electron microscopy with reference to their biophysical characteristics. *J Neurosci* 9:2982–2997.

Harris KM, Teyler TJ (1983) Age differences in a circadian influence on hippocampal LTP. *Brain Res* 261:69–73.

Harris KM, Fiala JC, Ostroff L (2003) Structural changes at dendritic spine synapses during long-term potentiation. *Philos Trans R Soc Lond B Biol Sci* 358:745–748.

Harrison NL, Gibbons SJ (1994) Zn^{2+}: an endogenous modulator of ligand- and voltage-gated ion channels. *Neuropharmacology* 33:935–952.

Harvey J, Collingridge GL (1992) Thapsigargin blocks the induction of long-term potentiation in rat hippocampal slices. *Neurosci Lett* 139:197–200.

Harvey J, Balasubramaniam R, Collingridge GL (1993) Carbachol can potentiate N-methyl-D-aspartate responses in the rat hippocampus by a staurosporine and thapsigargin-insensitive mechanism. *Neurosci Lett* 162:165–168.

Hastings NB, Gould E (1999) Rapid extension of axons into the CA3 region by adult-generated granule cells. *J Comp Neurol* 413:146–154.

Haug FM (1967) Electron microscopical localization of the zinc in hippocampal mossy fiber synapses by a modified sulfide silver procedure. *Histochemie* 8:355–368.

Hawkins RD, Son H, Arancio O (1998) Nitric oxide as a retrograde messenger during long-term potentiation in hippocampus. *Prog Brain Res* 118:155–172.

Hayashi Y, Shi SH, Esteban JA, Piccini A, Poncer JC, Malinow R (2000) Driving AMPA receptors into synapses by LTP and CaMKII: requirement for GluR1 and PDZ domain interaction. *Science* 287:2262–2267.

Hebb DO (1949) *The organization of behavior*. New York: Wiley.

Hebbard PC, King RR, Malsbury CW, Harley CW (2003) Two organizational effects of pubertal testosterone in male rats: transient social memory and a shift away from long-term potentiation following a tetanus in hippocampal CA1. *Exp Neurol* 182:470–475.

Henderson JT, Georgiou J, Jia Z, Robertson J, Elowe S, Roder JC, Pawson T (2001) The receptor tyrosine kinase EphB2 regulates NMDA-dependent synaptic function. *Neuron* 32:1041–1056.

Hendricson AW, Miao CL, Lippmann MJ, Morrisett RA (2002) Ifenprodil and ethanol enhance NMDA receptor-dependent long-term depression. *J Pharmacol Exp Ther* 301:938–944.

Henze DA, Urban NN, Barrionuevo G (2000) The multifarious hippocampal mossy fiber pathway: a review. *Neuroscience* 98: 407–427.

Hernandez AI, Blace N, Crary JF, Serrano PA, Leitges M, Libien JM, Weinstein G, Tcherapanov A, Sacktor TC (2003) Protein kinase M zeta synthesis from a brain mRNA encoding an independent protein kinase C zeta catalytic domain. Implications for the molecular mechanism of memory. *J Biol Chem* 278: 40305–40316.

Hernandez RV, Navarro MM, Rodriquez WA, Martinez JL, LeBaron RG (2005) Differences in the magnitude of long-term potentiation produced by theta burst and high frequency stimulation protocols matched in stimulus number. *Brain Res Protocols* 15:6–13.

Herron CE, Williamson R, Collingridge GL (1985) A selective N-methyl-D-aspartate antagonist depresses epileptiform activity in rat hippocampal slices. *Neurosci Lett* 61:255–260.

Herron CE, Lester RA, Coan EJ, Collingridge GL (1986) Frequency-dependent involvement of NMDA receptors in the hippocampus: a novel synaptic mechanism. *Nature* 322:265–268.

Hessler NA, Shirke AM, Malinow R (1993) The probability of transmitter release at a mammalian central synapse. *Nature* 366: 569–572.

Hevroni D, Rattner A, Bundman M, Lederfein D, Gabarah A, Mangelus M, Silverman MA, Kedar H, Naor C, Kornuc M, Hanoch T, Seger R, Theill LE, Nedivi E, Richter-Levin G, Citri Y (1998) Hippocampal plasticity involves extensive gene induction and multiple cellular mechanisms. *J Mol Neurosci* 10:75–98.

Heynen AJ, Abraham WC, Bear MF (1996) Bidirectional modification of CA1 synapses in the adult hippocampus in vivo. *Nature* 381:163–166.

Heynen AJ, Quinlan EM, Bae DC, Bear MF (2000) Bidirectional, activity-dependent regulation of glutamate receptors in the adult hippocampus in vivo. *Neuron* 28:527–536.

Hinds HL, Tonegawa S, Malinow R (1998) CA1 long-term potentiation is diminished but present in hippocampal slices from alpha-CaMKII mutant mice. *Learn Mem* 5:344–354.

Hodgson JG, Agopyan N, Gutekunst CA, Leavitt BR, LePiane F, Singaraja R, Smith DJ, Bissada N, McCutcheon K, Nasir J, Jamot L, Li XJ, Stevens ME, Rosemond E, Roder JC, Phillips AG, Rubin EM, Hersch SM, Hayden MR (1999) A YAC mouse model for Huntington's disease with full-length mutant huntingtin, cyto-

plasmic toxicity, and selective striatal neurodegeneration. *Neuron* 23:181–192.

Holscher C, Gigg J, O'Mara SM (1999) Metabotropic glutamate receptor activation and blockade: their role in long-term potentiation, learning and neurotoxicity. *Neurosci Biobehav Rev* 23:399–410.

Hoh T, Beiko J, Boon F, Weiss S, Cain DP (1999) Complex behavioral strategy and reversal learning in the watermaze without NMDA receptor-dependent long-term potentiation. *J Neurosci* 19:RC2.

Hopkins WF, Johnston D (1988) Noradrenergic enhancement of long-term potentiation at mossy fiber synapses in the hippocampus. *J Neurophysiol* 59:667–687.

Hopper R, Lancaster B, Garthwaite J (2004) On the regulation of NMDA receptors by nitric oxide. *Eur J Neurosci* 19:1675–1682.

Horwood JM, Dufour F, Laroche S, Davis S (2006) Signalling mechanisms mediated by the phosphoinositide 3-kinase/Akt cascade in synaptic plasticity and memory in the rat. Eur J Neurosci 23:3375–3384.

Hosokawa T, Rusakov DA, Bliss TVP, Fine A (1995) Repeated confocal imaging of individual dendritic spines in the living hippocampal slice: evidence for changes in length and orientation associated with chemically-induced LTP. *J Neurosci* 15: 5560–5573.

Hou Q, Gao X, Zhang X, Kong L, Wang X, Bian W, Tu Y, Jin M, Zhao G, Li B, Jing N, Yu L (2004) SNAP-25 in hippocampal CA1 region is involved in memory consolidation. *Eur J Neurosci* 20:1593–1603.

Hou L, Klann E (2004) Activation of the phosphoinositide 3-kinase-Akt-mammalian target of rapamycin signaling pathway is required for metabotropic glutamate receptor-dependent long-term depression. *J Neurosci* 24:6352–6361.

Howell GA, Welch MG, Frederickson CJ (1984) Stimulation-induced uptake and release of zinc in hippocampal slices. *Nature* 308:736–738.

Hrabetova S, Serrano P, Blace N, Tse HW, Skifter DA, Jane DE, Monaghan DT, Sacktor TC (2000) Distinct NMDA receptor subpopulations contribute to long-term potentiation and long-term depression induction. *J Neurosci* 20:RC81, 81–86.

Hsia AY, Salin PA, Castillo PE, Aiba A, Abeliovich A, Tonegawa S, Nicoll RA (1995) Evidence against a role for metabotropic glutamate receptors in mossy fiber LTP: the use of mutant mice and pharmacological antagonists. *Neuropharmacology* 34: 1567–1572.

Hsia AY, Masliah E, McConlogue L, Yu GQ, Tatsuno G, Hu K, Kholodenko D, Malenka RC, Nicoll RA, Mucke L (1999) Plaque-independent disruption of neural circuits in Alzheimer's disease mouse models. *Proc Natl Acad Sci USA* 96:3228–3233.

Hsiao K, Chapman P, Nilsen S, Eckman C, Harigaya Y, Younkin S, Yang F, Cole G (1996) Correlative memory deficits, Ab elevation, and amyloid plaques in transgenic mice. *Science* 274: 99–102.

Hrabetova S, Serrano P, Blace N, Tse HW, Skifter DA, Jane DE, Monaghan DT, Sacktor TC (2000) Distinct NMDA receptor subpopulations contribute to long-term potentiation and long-term depression induction. *J Neurosci* 20:RC81, 81–86.

Hu GY, Hvalby O, Walaas SI, Albert KA, Skjeflo P, Andersen P, Greengard P (1987) Protein kinase C injection into hippocampal pyramidal cells elicits features of long term potentiation. *Nature* 328:426–429.

Huang CC, Hsu K-S (2001) Progress in understanding the factors regulating reversibility of long-term potentiation. *Rev Neurosci* 12:51–68.

Huang CC, Hsu KS (2006) Sustained activation of metabotropic glutamate receptor 5 and protein tyrosine phosphatases mediate the expression of (S)-3,5-dihydroxyphenylglycine-induced long-term depression in the hippocampal CA1 region. *J Neurochem* 96:179–194.

Huang CC, Luang YC, Hsu K-S (2001) Characterization of the mechanism underlying the reversal of long term potentiation by low frequency stimulation at hippocampal CA1 synapses. *J Biol Chem* 2276:48108–48117.

Huang CC, Chen Y-L, Liang Y-C, Hsu K-S (2002) Role for cAMP and protein phosphatase in the presynaptic expression of mouse hippocampal mossy fiber depotentiation. *J Physiol (Lond)* 543:767–778.

Huang CC, You JL, Wu MY, Hsu KS (2004) Rap1-induced p38 mitogen-activated protein kinase activation facilitates AMPA receptor trafficking via the GDI.Rab5 complex. Potential role in (S)-3,5-dihydroxyphenylglycene-induced long term depression. *J Biol Chem* 279:12286–12292.

Huang CS, Song-Hai S, Ule J, Ruggiu M, Barker LA, Darnell RB, Jan YN, Jan LY (2005) Common molecular pathways mediate long-term potentiation of synaptic excitation and slow synaptic inhibition. *Cell* 123:105–118.

Huang Y, Lu W, Ali DW, Pelkey KA, Pitcher GM, Lu YM, Aoto H, Roder JC, Sasaki T, Salter MW, MacDonald JF (2001b) CAKbeta/Pyk2 kinase is a signaling link for induction of long-term potentiation in CA1 hippocampus. *Neuron* 29:485–496.

Huang YY, Colino A, Selig DK, Malenka RC (1992) The influence of prior synaptic activity on the induction of long-term potentiation. *Science* 255:730–733.

Huang YY, Kandel ER (1994) Recruitment of long-lasting and protein kinase A-dependent long-term potentiation in the CA1 region of hippocampus requires repeated tetanization. *Learn Mem* 1:74–82.

Huang YY, Kandel ER (1995) D1/D5 receptor agonists induce a protein synthesis-dependent late potentiation in the CA1 region of the hippocampus. *Proc Natl Acad Sci USA* 92:2446–2450.

Huang YY, Li XC, Kandel ER (1994) cAMP contributes to mossy fiber LTP by initiating both a covalently mediated early phase and macromolecular synthesis-dependent late phase. *Cell* 79:69–79.

Hüber KM, Kayser MS, Bear MF (2000) Role for rapid dendritic protein synthesis in hippocampal mGluR-dependent long-term depression. *Science* 288:1254–1257.

Hüber KM, Roder JC, Bear MF (2001) Chemical induction of mGluR5-and protein synthesis-dependent long-term depression in hippocampal area CA1. *J Neurophysiol* 86:321–325.

Huntley GW (2002) Dynamic aspects of cadherin-mediated plasticity in synapse development and plasticity. *Biol Cell* 94:335–344.

Hvalby O, Lacaille JC, Hu GY, Andersen P (1987) Postsynaptic long-term potentiation follows coupling of dendritic glutamate application and synaptic activation. *Experientia* 43:599–601.

Hyman SE, Malenka RC (2001) Addiction and the brain: the neurobiology of compulsion and its persistence. *Nat Rev Neurosci* 2:695–703.

Ikeda H, Heinke B, Ruscheweyh R, Sandkuhler J (2003) Synaptic plasticity in spinal lamina I projection neurons that mediate hyperalgesia. *Science* 299:1237–1240.

Impey S, Obrietan K, Wong ST, Poser S, Yano S, Wayman G, Deloulme JC, Chan G, Storm DR (1998) Cross talk between ERK and PKA is required for Ca^{2+} stimulation of CREB-dependent transcription and ERK nuclear translocation. *Neuron* 21:869–883.

Isaac JT, Nicoll RA, Malenka RC (1995) Evidence for silent synapses: implications for the expression of LTP. *Neuron* 15:427–434.

Isaac JT, Luthi A, Palmer MJ, Anderson WW, Benke TA, Collingridge GL (1998) An investigation of the expression mechanism of LTP of AMPA receptor-mediated synaptic transmission at hippocampal CA1 synapses using failures analysis and dendritic recordings. *Neuropharmacology* 37:1399–1410.

Ito I, Hidaka H, Sugiyama H (1991) Effects of KN-62, a specific inhibitor of calcium/calmodulin-dependent protein kinase II, on long-term potentiation in the rat hippocampus. *Neurosci Lett* 121:119–121.

Izquierdo I, Medina JH (1997) Memory formation: the sequence of biochemical events in the hippocampus and its connection to activity in other brain structures. *Neurobiol Learn Mem* 68:285–316.

Izquierdo I, Medina JH, Bianchin M, Walz R, Zanatta MS, Da Silva RC, Bueno e Silva M, Ruschel AC, Paczko N (1993) Memory processing by the limbic system: role of specific neurotransmitter systems. *Behav Brain Res* 58:91–98.

Izquierdo I, Izquierdo LA, Barros DM, Mello e Souza T, de Souza MM, Quevedo J, Rodrigues C, Sant'Anna MK, Madruga M, Medina JH (1998) Differential involvement of cortical receptor mechanisms in working, short-term and long-term memory. *Behav Pharmacol* 9:421–427.

Izquierdo I, Schroder N, Netto CA, Medina JH (1999) Novelty causes time-dependent retrograde amnesia for one-trial avoidance in rats through NMDA receptor- and CaMKII-dependent mechanisms in the hippocampus. *Eur J Neurosci* 11:3323–3328.

Izumi Y, Zorumski CF (1999) Norepinephrine promotes long-term potentiation in the adult rat hippocampus in vitro. *Synapse* 31:196–202.

Jaffard R, Vouimba RM, Marighetto A, Garcia R (1996) Long-term potentiation and long-term depression in the lateral septum in spatial working and reference memory. *J Physiol* 90:339–341.

Jaffe D, Johnston D (1990) Induction of long-term potentiation at hippocampal mossy-fiber synapses follows a Hebbian rule. *J Neurophysiol* 64:948–961.

Jahr CE, Stevens CF (1987) Glutamate activates multiple single channel conductances in hippocampal neurons. *Nature* 325: 522–525.

Jahr CE, Stevens CF (1993) Calcium permeability of the *N*-methyl-D-aspartate receptor channel in hippocampal neurons in culture. *Proc Natl Acad Sci USA* 90:11573–11577.

Jasnow AM, Shi C, Israel JE, Davis M, Huhman KL (2005) Memory of social defeat is facilitated by cAMP response element-binding protein overexpression in the amygdala. *Behav Neurosci* 119:1125–1130.

Jeffery KJ (1997) LTP and spatial learning—where to next? *Hippocampus* 7:95–110.

Jeffery KJ, Morris RGM (1993) Cumulative long-term potentiation in the rat dentate gyrus correlates with, but does not modify, performance in the watermaze. *Hippocampus* 3:133–140.

Jeon D, Yang YM, Jeong MJ, Philipson KD, Rhim H, Shin HS (2003) Enhanced learning and memory in mice lacking Na^+/Ca^{2+} exchanger 2. *Neuron* 38:965–976.

Jester JM, Campbell LW, Sejnowski TJ (1995) Associative EPSP-spike potentiation induced by pairing orthodromic and antidromic stimulation in rat hippocampal slices. *J Physiol (Lond)* 484:589–705.

Jia Y, Jeng JM, Sensi SL, Weiss JH (2002) Zn^{2+} currents are mediated by calcium-permeable AMPA/kainate channels in cultured murine hippocampal neurones. *J Physiol* 543:35–48.

Jia Z, Agopyan N, Miu P, Xiong Z, Henderson J, Gerlai R, Taverna FA, Velumian A, MacDonald J, Carlen P, Abramow-Newerly W, Roder J (1996) Enhanced LTP in mice deficient in the AMPA receptor GluR2. *Neuron* 17:945–956.

Jia Z, Lu Y, Henderson J, Taverna F, Romano C, Abramow-Newerly W, Wojtowicz JM, Roder J (1998) Selective abolition of the NMDA component of long-term potentiation in mice lacking mGluR5. *Learn Mem* 5:331–343.

Jones MW, Errington ML, French PJ, Fine A, Bliss TVP, Garel S, Charnay P, Bozon B, Laroche S, Davis S (2001) A requirement for the immediate early gene *Zif268* in the expression of late LTP and long-term memories. *Nat Neurosci* 3:289–296.

Josselyn SA, Shi C, Carlezon WA Jr, Neve RL, Nestler EJ, Davis M (2001) Long-term memory is facilitated by cAMP response element-binding protein overexpression in the amygdala. *J Neurosci* 21:2404–2412.

Jun K, Choi G, Yang SG, Choi KY, Kim H, Chan GC, Storm DR, Albert C, Mayr GW, Lee CJ, Shin HS (1998) Enhanced hippocampal CA1 LTP but normal spatial learning in inositol 1,4,5-trisphosphate 3-kinase(A)-deficient mice. *Learn Mem* 5:317–330.

Kafitz KW, Rose CR, Thoenen H, Konnerth A (1999) Neurotrophin-evoked rapid excitation through TrkB receptors. *Nature* 401:918–921.

Kaksonen M, Pavlov I, Voikar V, Lauri SE, Hienola A, Riekki R, Lakso M, Taira T, Rauvala H (2002) Syndecan-3-deficient mice exhibit enhanced LTP and impaired hippocampus-dependent memory. *Mol Cell Neurosci* 21:158–172.

Kameyama K, Lee HK, Bear MF, Huganir RL (1998) Involvement of a postsynaptic protein kinase A substrate in the expression of homosynaptic long-term depression. *Neuron* 21:1163–1175.

Kandler K, Katz LC, Kauer JA (1998) Focal photolysis of caged glutamate produces long-term depression of hippocampal glutamate receptors. *Nat Neurosci* 1:119–123.

Kang HJ, Schuman EM (1995) Neurotrophin-induced modulation of synaptic transmission in the adult hippocampus. *J Physiol Paris* 89:11–22.

Kang H, Schuman EM (1996) A requirement for local protein synthesis in neurotrophin-induced hippocampal synaptic plasticity. *Science* 273:1402–1406.

Kapur A, Yeckel MF, Gray R, Johnston D (1998) L-Type calcium channels are required for one form of hippocampal mossy fiber LTP. *J Neurophysiol* 79:2181–2190.

Kasai H, Matsuzaki M, Noguchi K (2003) Structure-stability-function relationships of dendritic spines. *Trends Neurosci* 26:360–368.

Katagiri H, Tanaka K, Manabe T (2001) Requirement of appropriate glutamate concentrations in the synaptic cleft for hippocampal LTP induction. *Eur J Neurosci* 14:547–553.

Katsuki H, Nakai S, Hirai Y, Akaji K, Kiso Y, Satoh M (1990) Interleukin-1 beta inhibits long-term potentiation in the CA3 region of mouse hippocampal slices. *Eur J Pharmacol* 181:323–326.

Kauderer BS, Kandel ER (2000) Capture of a protein synthesis-dependent component of long-term depression. *Proc Natl Acad Sci USA* 97:13342–13347.

Kauer JA, Malenka RC, Nicoll RA (1988) A persistent postsynaptic modification mediates long-term potentiation in the hippocampus. *Neuron* 1:911–917.

Kawamura Y, Manita S, Nakamura T, Inoue M, Kudo Y, Miyakawa H

(2004) Glutamate release increases during mossy-CA3 LTP but not during Schaffer-CA1 LTP. *Eur J Neurosci* 19:1591–1600.

Kazanietz MG, Caloca MJ, Eroles P, Fujii T, Garcia-Bermejo ML, Reilly M, Wang H (2000) Pharmacology of the receptors for the phorbol ester tumor promoters: multiple receptors with different biochemical properties. *Biochem Pharmacol* 60:1417–1424.

Keith JR, Rudy JW (1990) Why NMDA-receptor-dependent long-term potentiation may not be a mechanism of learning and memory: reappraisal of the NMDA-receptor blockade strategy. *Psychobiology* 18:251–257.

Kelleher RJI, Govindarajan A, Tonegawa S (2004a) Tranlational regulatory mechanisms in persistent forms of synaptic plasticity. *Neuron* 44:59–73.

Kelleher RJI, Govindarajan A, Jung H-Y, Kang H, Tonegawa S (2004b) Translational control by MAPK signaling in long-term synaptic plasticity and memory. *Cell* 116:467–479.

Kelly A, Lynch MA (2000) Long-term potentiation in dentate gyrus of the rat is inhibited by the phosphoinositide 3-kinase inhibitor, wortmannin. *Neuropharmacology* 39:643–651.

Kelly A, Mullany PM, Lynch MA (2000) Protein synthesis in entorhinal cortex and long-term potentiation in dentate gyrus. *Hippocampus* 10:431–437.

Kelly A, Lynch A, Vereker E, Nolan Y, Queenan P, Whittaker E, O'Neill LA, Lynch MA (2001) The anti-inflammatory cytokine, interleukin (IL)-10, blocks the inhibitory effect of IL-1 beta on long term potentiation: a role for JNK. *J Biol Chem* 276:45564–45572.

Kelly A, Vereker E, Nolan Y, Brady M, Barry C, Loscher CE, Mills KH, Lynch MA (2003) Activation of p38 plays a pivotal role in the inhibitory effect of lipopolysaccharide and interleukin-1 beta on long term potentiation in rat dentate gyrus. *J Biol Chem* 278:19453–19462.

Kelso SR, Brown TH (1986) Differential conditioning of associative synaptic enhancement in hippocampal brain slices. *Science* 232:85–87.

Kelso SR, Ganong AH, Brown TH (1986) Hebbian synapses in hippocamus. *Proc Natl Acad Sci USA* 83:5326–5330.

Kemp N, Bashir ZI (2001) Long-term depression: a cascade of induction and expression mechanisms. *Prog Neurobiol* 65:339–365.

Kemp A, Manahan-Vaughan D (2004) Hippocampal long-term depression and long-term potentiation encode different aspects of novelty acquisition. *Proc Natl Acad Sci USA* 101:8192–8197.

Kemp N, McQueen J, Faulkes S, Bashir ZI (2000) Different forms of LTD in the CA1 region of the hippocampus: role of age and stimulus protocol. *Eur J Neurosci* 12:360–366.

Kentros C, Hargreaves E, Hawkins RD, Kandel ER, Shapiro M, Muller RV (1998) Abolition of long-term stability of new hippocampal place cell maps by NMDA receptor blockade. *Science* 280:2121–2126.

Kerchner GA, Wilding TJ, Huettner JE, Zhuo M (2002) Kainate receptor subunits underlying presynaptic regulation of transmitter release in the dorsal horn. *J Neurosci* 22:8010–8017.

Kerr DS, Abraham WC (1993) Associative stimulation does not facilitate long-term depression in region CA1 of the hippocampus. *Synapse* 14:305–313.

Kida S, Josselyn SA, de Ortiz SP, Kogan JH, Chevere I, Masushige S, Silva AJ (2002) CREB required for the stability of new and reactivated fear memories. *Nat Neurosci* 5:348–355.

Kim CH, Chung HJ, Lee HK, Huganir RL (2001) Interaction of the AMPA receptor subunit GluR2/3 with PDZ domains regulates hippocampal long-term depression. *Proc Natl Acad Sci USA* 98:11725–11730.

Kim CH, Takamiya K, Petralia RS, Sattler R, Yu S, Zhou W, Kalb R, Wenthold R, Huganir R (2005a) Persistent hippocampal CA1 LTP in mice lacking the C-terminal PDZ ligand of GluR1. *Nat Neurosci* 8:985–987.

Kim EY, Mahmoud GS, Grover LM (2005b) REM sleep deprivation inhibits LTP in vivo in area CA1 of the rat hippocampus. *Neurosci Lett* 388:163–167.

Kim JJ, Diamond DM (2002) The stressed hippocampus, synaptic plasticity and lost memories. *Nat Rev Neurosci* 3:453–462.

Kim JJ, Koo J-W, Lee H-J, Han J-S (2005c) Amygdalar inactivation blocks stress-induced impairments in hippocampal long-term potentiation and spatial memory. *J Neurosci* 25:1532–1539.

Kirov SA, Sorra KE, Harris KM (1999) Slices have more synapses than perfusion-fixed hippocampus from both young and mature rats. *J Neurosci* 19:2876–2886.

Kistner A, Gossen M, Zimmermann F, Jerecic J, Ullmer C, Lubbert H, Bujard H (1996) Doxycycline-mediated quantitative and tissue-specific control of gene expression in transgenic mice. *Proc Natl Acad Sci USA* 93:10933–10938.

Kitamura HW, Hamanaka H, Watanabe M, Wada K, Yamazaki C, Fujita SC, Manabe T, Nukina N (2004) Age-dependent enhancement of hippocampal long-term potentiation in knock-in mice expressing human apolipoprotein E4 instead of mouse apolipoprotein E. *Neurosci Lett* 369:173–178.

Kiyama Y, Manabe T, Sakimura K, Kawakami F, Mori H, Mishina M (1998) Increased thresholds for long-term potentiation and contextual learning in mice lacking the NMDA-type glutamate receptor epsilon1 subunit. *J Neurosci* 18:6704–6712.

Kleschevnikov AM, Sokolov MV, Kuhnt U, Dawe GS, Stephenson JD, Voronin LL (1997) Changes in paired-pulse facilitation correlate with induction of long-term potentiation in area CA1 of rat hippocampal slices. *Neuroscience* 76:829–843.

Kleschevnikov AM, Belichenko PV, Villar AJ, Epstein CJ, Malenka RC, Mobley WC (2004) Hippocampal long-term potentiation suppressed by increased inhibition in the Ts65Dn mouse, a genetic model of Down syndrome. *J Neurosci* 24:8153–8160.

Kobayashi K, Poo M-M (2004) Spike train timing-dependent associative modification of hippocampal CA3 recurrent synapses by mossy fibers. *Neuron* 41:445–454.

Kobayashi K, Manabe T, Takahashi T (1996) Presynaptic long-term depression at the hippocampal mossy fiber-CA3 synapse. *Science* 273:648–650.

Koek W, Woods JH, Winger GD (1988) MK-801, a proposed non-competitive antagonist of excitatory amino acid neurotransmission, produces phencyclidine-like behavioral effects in pigeons, rats and rhesus monkeys. *J Pharmacol Exp Ther* 245:969–974.

Kogan JH, Frankland PW, Silva AJ (2000) Long-term memory underlying hippocampus-dependent social recognition in mice. *Hippocampus* 10:47–56.

Kojima N, Wang J, Mansuy IM, Grant SG, Mayford M, Kandel ER (1997) Rescuing impairment of long-term potentiation in fyn-deficient mice by introducing Fyn transgene. *Proc Natl Acad Sci USA* 94:4761–4765.

Kojima T, Matsumoto M, Togashi H, Tachibana K, Kemmotsu O, Yoshioka M (2003) Fluvoxamine suppresses the long-term potentiation in the hippocampal CA1 field of anesthetized rats: an effect mediated via 5-HT1A receptors. *Brain Res* 959: 165–168.

Kolta A, Lynch G, Ambros-Ingerson J (1998) Effects of aniracetam after LTP induction are suggestive of interactions on the kinetics of the AMPA receptor channel. *Brain Res* 788:269–286.

Konorski J (1948) *Conditioned reflexes and neuron organization.* Cambridge, UK: Hefner.

Korol DL, Abel TW, Church LT, Barnes CA, McNaughton BL (1993) Hippocampal synaptic enhancement and spatial learning in the Morris swim task. *Hippocampus* 3:127–132.

Kombian SB, Malenka RC (1994) Simultaneous LTP of non-NMDA- and LTD of NMDA-receptor-mediated responses in the nucleus accumbens. *Nature* 368:242–246.

Korte M, Carroll P, Wolf E, Brem G, Thoenen H, Bonhoeffer T (1995) Hippocampal long-term potentiation is impaired in mice lacking brain-derived neurotrophic factor. *Proc Natl Acad Sci USA* 92:8856–8860.

Korte M, Griesbeck O, Gravel C, Carroll P, Staiger V, Thoenen H, Bonhoeffer T (1996) Virus-mediated gene transfer into hippocampal CA1 region restores long-term potentiation in brain-derived neurotrophic factor mutant mice. *Proc Natl Acad Sci USA* 93:12547–12552.

Kovalchuk Y, Eilers J, Lisman J, and Konnerth A (2000). NMDA receptor-mediated subthreshold $Ca(2+)$ signals in spines of hippocampal neurons. *J Neurosci* 20:1791–1799.

Kovalchuk Y, Hanse E, Kafitz KW, Konnerth A (2002) Postsynaptic induction of BDNF-mediated long-term potentiation. *Science* 295:1730–1734.

Krasteniakov NV, Martina M, Bergeron R (2004) Subthreshold contribution of *N*-methyl-D-aspartate receptors to long-term potentiation induced by low-frequency pairing in rat hippocampal CA1 pyramidal cells. *Neuroscience* 126:83–94.

Krucker T, Siggins GR, Halpain S (2003) Dynamic actin filaments are required for stable long-term potentiation (LTP) in area CA1 of the hippocampus. *Proc Natl Acad Sci USA* 97:6856–6861.

Krug M, Lossner B, Ott T (1984) Anisomycin blocks the late phase of long-term potentiation in the dentate gyrus of freely moving rats. *Brain Res Bull* 13:39–42.

Kuhl D, Skehel P (1998) Dendritic localization of mRNAs. *Curr Opin Neurobiol* 8:600–606.

Kulla A, Reymann KG, Manahan-Vaughan D (1999) Time-dependent induction of depotentiation in the dentate gyrus of freely moving rats: involvement of group 2 metabotropic glutamate receptors. *Eur J Neurosci* 11:3864–3872.

Kulla A, Manahan-Vaughan D (2002) Modulation of serotonin 5-HT(4) receptors of long-term potentiation and depotentiation in the dentate gyrus of freely moving rats. *Cereb Cortex* 12:150–162.

Kulla A, Reymann KG, Manahan-Vaughan D (1999) Time-dependent induction of depotentiation in the dentate gyrus of freely-moving rats: involvement of group 2 metabotropic receptors. *Eur J Neurosci* 11:3864–3872.

Kullmann DM (1994) Amplitude fluctuations of dual-component EPSCs in hippocampal pyramidal cells: implications for long-term potentiation. *Neuron* 12:1111–1120.

Kullmann DM (2003) Silent synapses: what are they telling us about long-term potentiation? *Philos Trans R Soc Lond B Biol Sci* 358:727–733.

Kullmann DM, Erdemli G, Asztely F (1996) LTP of AMPA and NMDA receptor-mediated signals: evidence for presynaptic expression and extrasynaptic glutamate spill-over. *Neuron* 17:461–474.

Kusuki T, Imahori Y, Ueda S, Inokuchi K (1997) Dopaminergic modulation of LTP induction in the dentate gyrus of the intact brain. *Neuroreport* 8:2037–2040.

Kutsuwada T, Sakimura K, Manabe T, Takayama C, Katakura N, Kushiya E, Natsume R, Watanabe M, Inoue Y, Yagi T, Aizawa S,

Arakawa M, Takahashi T, Nakamura Y, Mori H, Mishina M (1996) Impairment of suckling response, trigeminal neuronal pattern formation, and hippocampal LTD in NMDA receptor epsilon 2 subunit mutant mice. *Neuron* 16:333–344.

Kwon OB, Longart M, Vullhorst D, Hoffman DA, Buonanno A (2005) Neuregulin-1 reverses long-term potentiation at CA1 hippocampal synapses. *J Neurosci* 25:9378–9383.

Laezza F, Doherty JJ, Dingledine R (1999) Long-term depression in hippocampal interneurones: joint requirement for pre- and postsynaptic events. *Science* 285:1411–1414.

Lambert MP, Barlow AK, Chromy BA, Edwards C, Freed R, Liosatos M, Morgan TE, Rozovsky I, Trommer B, Viola KL, Wals P, Zhang C, Finch CE, Krafft GA, Klein WL (1998) Diffusible, nonfibrillar ligands derived from Abeta1-42 are potent central nervous system neurotoxins. *Proc Natl Acad Sci USA* 95:6448–6453.

Lamsa K, Heeroma JH, Kullmann DM (2005) Hebbian LTP in feedforward inhibitory interneurons and the temporal fidelity of input discrimination. *Nat Neurosci* 8:916–924.

Lanahan A, Worley P (1998) Immediate-early genes and synaptic function. *Neurobiol Learn Mem* 70:37–43.

Langdon RB, Johnson JW, Barrionuevo G (1995) Posttetanic potentiation and presynaptically induced long-term potentiation at the mossy fiber synapse in rat hippocampus. *J Neurobiol* 26:370–385.

Lapointe V, Morin F, Ratte S, Croce A, Conquet F, Lacaille JC (2003) Synapse-specific mGluR1-dependent long-term potentiation in interneurons regulates mouse hippocampal inhibition. *J Physiol (Lond)* 555:125–135.

Larkum ME, Zhu JJ, Sakmann B (1999) A new cellular mechanism for coupling inputs arriving at different cortical layers. *Nature* 398:338–341.

Laroche S, Doyere V, Bloch V (1989) Linear relation between the magnitude of long-term potentiation in the dentate gyrus and associative learning in the rat: a demonstration using commissural inhibition and local infusion of an *N*-methyl-D-aspartate receptor antagonist. *Neuroscience* 28:375–386.

Laroche S, Jay TM, Thierry AM (1990) Long-term potentiation in the prefrontal cortex following stimulation of the hippocampal CA1/subicular region. *Neurosci Lett* 114:184–190.

Larson J, Lynch G (1986) Induction of synaptic potentiation in hippocampus by patterned stimulation involves two events. *Science* 232:985–987.

Larson J, Lynch G, Games D, Seubert P (1999) Alterations in synaptic transmission and long-term potentiation in hippocampal slices from young and aged PDAPP mice. *Brain Res* 840:23–35.

Lathe R, Morris RGM (1994) Analyzing brain-function and dysfunction in transgenic animals. *Neuropathol Appl Neurobiol* 20:350–358.

Lauri SE, Bortolotto ZA, Bleakman D, Ornstein PL, Lodge D, Isaac JT, Collingridge GL (2001) A critical role of a facilitatory presynaptic kainate receptor in mossy fiber LTP. *Neuron* 32:697–709.

Lauri SE, Bortolotto ZA, Nistico R, Bleakman D, Ornstein PL, Lodge D, Isaac JT, Collingridge GL (2003) A role for Ca^{2+} stores in kainate receptor-dependent synaptic facilitation and LTP at mossy fiber synapses in the hippocampus. *Neuron* 39:327–341.

Lawrence JJ, McBain CJ (2003) Containing the detonation: feedforward inhibition in the CA3 hippocampus. *Trends Neurosci* 26:631–640.

Lebel D, Grossman Y, Barkai E (2001) Olfactory learning modifies predisposition for long-term potentiation and long-term depression induction in the rat piriform (olfactory) cortex. *Cereb Cortex* 11:485–489.

Lederer R, Radeke E, Mondadori C (1993) Facilitation of social learning by treatment with an NMDA receptor antagonist. *Behav Neural Biol* 60:220–224.

LeDoux JE (2000) Emotion circuits in the brain. Annu Rev Neurosci 23:155–184.

Lee HK, Barbarosie M, Kameyama K, Bear MF, Huganir RL (2000) Regulation of distinct AMPA receptor phosphorylation sites during bidirectional synaptic plasticity. *Nature* 405:955–959.

Lee I, Kesner RP (2002) Differential contribution of NMDA receptors in hippocampal subregions to spatial working memory. *Nat Neurosci* 5:162–168.

Lee KS, Schottler F, Oliver M, Lynch G (1980) Brief bursts of high-frequency stimulation produce two types of structural change in rat hippocampus. *J Neurophysiol* 44:247–258.

Lee PR, Cohen JE, Becker KG, Fields RD (2005) Gene expression in the conversion of early-phase to late-phase long-term potentiation. *Ann N Y Acad Sci* 1048:259–271.

Lee SH, Liu L, Wang YT, Sheng M (2002) Clathrin adaptor AP2 and NSF interact with overlapping sites of GluR2 and play distinct roles in AMPA receptor trafficking and hippocampal LTD. *Neuron* 36:661–674.

Lei S, McBain CJ (2002) Distinct NMDA receptors provide differential modes of transmission at mossy fiber-interneuron synapses. *Neuron* 33:921–933.

Lei S, Pelkey KA, Topolnik L, Congar P, Lacaille JC, McBain CJ (2003) Depolarization-induced long-term depression at hippocampal mossy fiber-CA3 pyramidal neuron synapses. *J Neurosci* 23:9786–9795.

Lein ES, Zhao X, Gage FH (2004) Defining a molecular atlas of the hippocampus using DNA microarrays and high-throughput in situ hybridization. *J Neurosci* 24:3879–3889.

Lemphrect R, Le Doux J (2004) Structural plasticity and memory. *Nat Rev Neurosci* 5:45–54.

Lengyel I, Voss K, Cammarota M, Bradshaw K, Brent V, Murphy KP, Giese KP, Rostas J, Bliss TV (2004) Autonomous activity of CaMKII is only transiently increased after the induction of long-term potentiation in the rat hippocampus. *Eur J Neurosci* 20:3063–3072.

Leonard AS, Davare MA, Horne MC, Garner CC, Hell JW (1998) SAP97 is associated with the alpha-amino-3-hydroxy-5-methylisoxazole-4-propionic acid receptor GluR1 subunit. *J Biol Chem* 1998 273:19518–19524.

Leonard BJ, McNaughton BL, Barnes CA (1987) Suppression of hippocampal synaptic plasticity during slow-wave sleep. *Brain Res* 425:174–177.

Leung LS, Shen B (2006) Hippocampal CA1 kindling but not long-term potentiation disrupts spatial memory performance. *Learn Mem* 13:18–26.

Leung LS, Shen B, Rajakumar N, Ma J (2003) Cholinergic activity enhances hippocampal long-term potentiation in CA1 during walking in rats. *J Neurosci* 23:9297-9304.

Levy WB, Steward O (1979) Synapses as associative memory elements in the hippocampal formation. *Brain Res* 175:233–245.

Levy WB, Steward O (1983) Temporal contiguity requirements for long-term associative potentiation/depression in the hippocampus. *Neuroscience* 8:791–797.

Li AJ, Katafuchi T, Oda S, Hori T, Oomura Y (1997) Interleukin-6 inhibits long-term potentiation in rat hippocampal slices. *Brain Res* 748:30–38.

Li HB, Matsumoto K, Yamamoto M, Watanabe H (1997) NMDA but not AMPA receptor antagonists impair the delay-interposed radial maze performance of rats. *Pharmacol Biochem Behav* 58:249–253.

Li L, Carter J, Gao X, Whitehead J, Tourtellotte WG (2005) The neuroplasticity-associated arc gene is a direct transcriptional target of early growth response (Egr) transcription factors. *Mol Cell Biol* 25:10286–10300.

Li S, Cullen WK, Anwyl R, Rowan MJ (2003) Dopamine-dependent facilitation of LTP induction in hippocampal CA1 by exposure to spatial novelty. *Nat Neurosci* 6:526–531.

Li Y, Hough CJ, Frederickson CJ, Sarvey JM (2001) Induction of mossy fiber (→) CA3 long-term potentiation requires translocation of synaptically released Zn^{2+}. *J Neurosci* 21: 8015–8025.

Liao D, Hessler NA, Malinow R (1995) Activation of postsynaptically silent synapses during pairing-induced LTP in CA1 region of hippocampal slice. *Nature* 375:400–404.

Linden DJ (1999) The return of the spike: postsynaptic action potentials and the induction of LTP and LTD. *Neuron* 22:661–666.

Ling DS, Benardo LS, Sacktor TC (2006) Protein kinase Mzeta enhances excitatory synaptic transmission by increasing the number of active postsynaptic AMPA receptors. *Hippocampus* 16:443–452.

Ling DS, Benardo LS, Serrano PA, Blace N, Kelly MT, Crary JF, Sacktor TC (2002) Protein kinase Mzeta is necessary and sufficient for LTP maintenance. *Nat Neurosci* 5:295–296.

Lipp HP, Wolfer DP (1998) Genetically modified mice and cognition. *Curr Opin Neurobiol* 8:272–280.

Lisman J (1989) A mechanism for the Hebb and anti-Hebb processes underlying learning and memory. *Proc Natl Acad Sci USA* 86:9574–9578.

Lisman J, Spruston N (2005) Postsynaptic depolarization requirements for LTP and LTD: a critique of spike timing-dependent plasticity. *Nat Neurosci* 8:839–841.

Lisman J, Schulman H, Cline H (2002) The molecular basis of CaMKII function in synaptic and behavioural memory. *Nat Rev Neurosci* 3:175–190.

Lisman JE (1997) Bursts as a unit of neural information: making unreliable synapses reliable. *Trends Neurosci* 20:38–43.

Lisman JE, Grace AA (2005) The hippocampal-VTA loop: controlling the entry of information into long-term memory. *Neuron* 46:703–713.

Lissin DV, Gomperts SN, Caroll RC, Christine CW, Kalman D, Kitamura M, Hardy S, Nicoll RA, Malenka RC, von Zastrow M (1998) Activity differentially regulates the surface expression of synaptic AMPA and NMDA glutamate receptors. *Proc Natl Acad Sci USA* 95:7097–7102.

Liu L, Wong TP, Pozza MF, Lingenhoehl K, Wang Y, Sheng M, Auberson YP, Wang YT (2004a) Role of NMDA receptor subtypes in governing the direction of hippocampal synaptic plasticity. *Science* 304:1021–1024.

Liu S, Ninan I, Antonova I, Battaglia F, Trinchese F, Narasanna A, Kolodilov N, Dauer W, Hawkins RD, Arancio O (2004b) Alpha-synuclein produces a long-lasting increase in neurotransmitter release. *EMBO J* 23:4506–4516.

Lledo PM, Zhang X, Sudhof TC, Malenka RC, Nicoll RA (1998) Postsynaptic membrane fusion and long-term potentiation. *Science* 279:399–403.

Lømo T (1966) Frequency potentiation of excitatory synaptic activity in the dentate area of the hippocampal formation. *Acta Physiol Scand* 68(Suppl 277):128.

Lonze B, Ginty DD (2002) Function and regulation of CREB family transcription factors in the nervous system. *Neuron* 35: 605–623.

Lopez-Garcia JC, Arancio O, Kandel ER, Baranes D (1996) A presynaptic locus for long-term potentiation of elementary synaptic transmission at mossy fiber synapses in culture system. *Proc Natl Acad Sci USA* 93:4712–4717.

Lovinger DM, Wong KL, Murakami K, Routtenberg A (1987) Protein kinase C inhibitors eliminate hippocampal long-term potentiation. *Brain Res* 436:177–183.

Lozovaya NA, Grebenyuk SE, Tsintsadze T, Feng B, Monaghan DT, Krishtal OA (2004) Extrasynaptic NR2B and NR2D subunits of NMDA receptors shape 'superslow' afterburst EPSC in rat hippocampus. *J Physiol* 558:451–463.

Lu W, Man H, Ju W, Trimble WS, MacDonald JF, Wang YT (2001) Activation of synaptic NMDA receptors induces membrane insertion of new AMPA receptors and LTP in cultured hippocampal neurons. *Neuron* 29:243–254.

Lu YM, Jia Z, Janus C, Henderson JT, Gerlai R, Wojtowicz JM, Roder JC (1997) Mice lacking metabotropic glutamate receptor 5 show impaired learning and reduced CA1 long-term potentiation (LTP) but normal CA3 LTP. *J Neurosci* 17:5196–5205.

Lu YM, Roder JC, Davidow J, Salter MW (1998) Src activation in the induction of long-term potentiation in CA1 hippocampal neurons. *Science* 279:1363–1367.

Lu YM, Mansuy IM, Kandel ER, Roder J (2000a) Calcineurin-mediated LTD of GABAergic inhibition underlies the increased excitability of CA1 neurons associated with LTP. *Neuron* 26:197–205.

Lu YM, Taverna FA, Tu R, Ackerley CA, Wang YT, Roder J (2000b) Endogenous Zn(2+) is required for the induction of long-term potentiation at rat hippocampal mossy fiber-CA3 synapses. *Synapse* 38:187–197.

Luscher C, Malenka RC, Nicoll RA (1998) Monitoring glutamate release during LTP with glial transporter currents. *Neuron* 21:435–441.

Lüscher C, Xia H, Beattie EC, Carroll RC, von Zastrow M, Malenka RC, Nicoll RA (1999) Role of AMPA receptor cycling in synaptic transmission and plasticity. *Neuron* 24:649–658.

Lüthi A, Laurent JP, Figurov A, Muller D, Schachner M (1994) Hippocampal long-term potentiation and neural cell adhesion molecules L1 and NCAM. *Nature* 372:777–779.

Lüthi A, Chittajallu R, Duprat F, Palmer M, Benke TA, Kidd FL, Henley JM, Isaac JTR (1999) Hippocampal LTD expression involves a pool of AMPARs regulated by the NSF-GluR2 interaction. *Neuron* 24:389–399.

Lüthi A, Wikström MA, Palmer MJ, Matthews P, Benke TA, Isaac JTR, Collingridge GL (2004) Bi-directional modulation of AMPA receptor unitary conductance by synaptic activity. *BMC Neurosci* 5:44.

Lyford GL, Gutnikov SA, Clark AM, Rawlins JN (1993) Determinants of non-spatial working memory deficits in rats given intraventricular infusions of the NMDA antagonist AP5. *Neuropsychologia* 31:1079–1098.

Lynch G (2006) Glutamate-based therapeutic approaches: ampakines. *Curr Opin Pharmacol* 6:82–88.

Lynch G, Baudry M (1984) The biochemistry of memory: a new and specific hypothesis. *Science* 224:1057–1063.

Lynch G, Larson J, Kelso S, Barrionuevo G, Schottler F (1983) Intracellular injections of EGTA block induction of hippocampal long-term potentiation. *Nature* 305:719–721.

Lynch GS, Dunwiddie T, Gribkoff V (1977) Heterosynaptic depres-

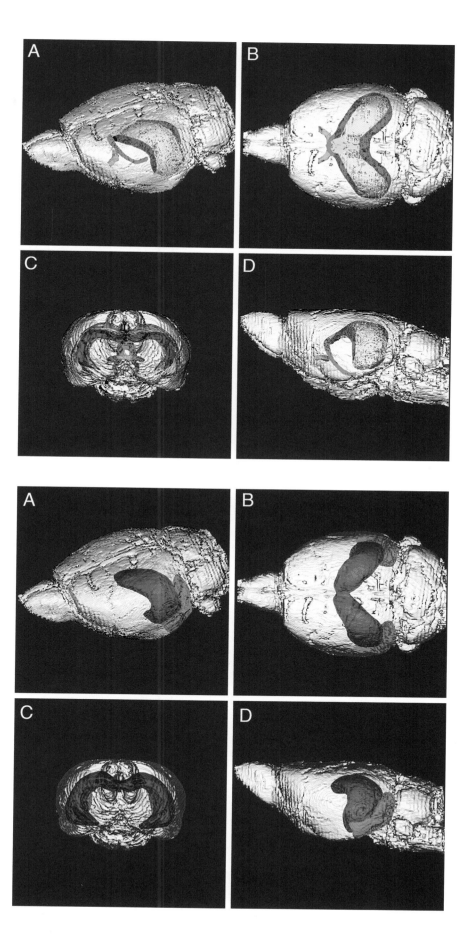

Figure 3–4. Major fiber systems of the rat hippocampal formation. Views of the rat brain are volume renderings of MRI images. The brain is seen from the left side (top left), from above (top right), from the front of the brain (bottom left), and from the ventrolateral position (bottom right). The dorsal hippocampal commissure is colored purple, the dorsal fornix is yellow, the fimbria is red. The precommissural fornix is tan colored and the ventral hippocampal commissure and the postcommissural fornix are green. (MRI images, courtesy of Dr. G. Allan Johnson, Center for In Vivo Microscopy, Duke University, NIH/NCRR National Resource [P41 05959].)

Figure 3–5. Magnetic resonance imaging of the rat brain shows the position of the hippocampus (dentate gyrus + hippocampus proper + subiculum) in red and the entorhinal cortex in green. *A.* Oblique view. *B.* dorsal view. *C.* frontal view. *D.* lateral view. (*Source*: Courtesy of Dr. G. Allan Johnson, Center for In Vivo Microscopy, Duke University.)

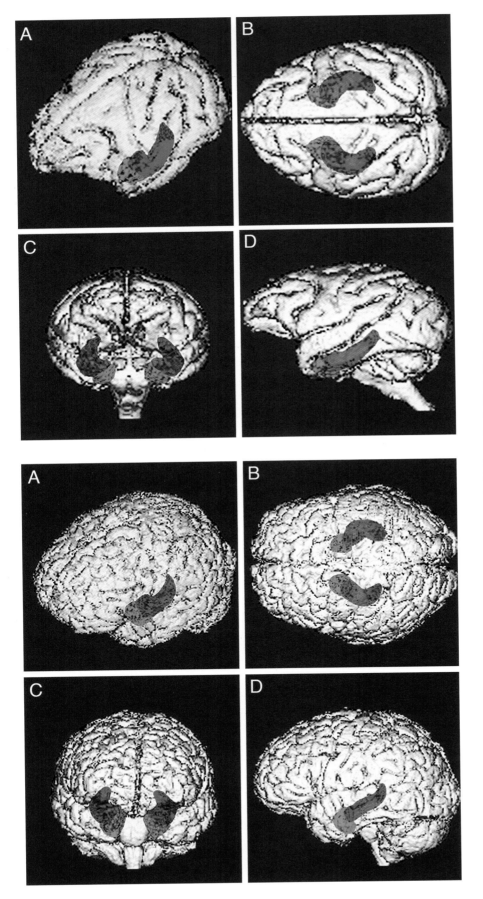

Figure 3–6. Magnetic resonance imaging of the monkey brain shows the position of the hippocampus (dentate gyrus + hippocampus proper + subiculum) in red and the entorhinal cortex in green. *A.* Oblique view. *B.* dorsal view. *C.* frontal view. *D.* lateral view.

Figure 3–7. Magnetic resonance imaging of the human brain shows the position of the hippocampus (dentate gyrus + hippocampus proper + subiculum) in red and the entorhinal cortex in green. *A.* Oblique view. *B.* dorsal view. *C.* frontal view. *D.* lateral view.

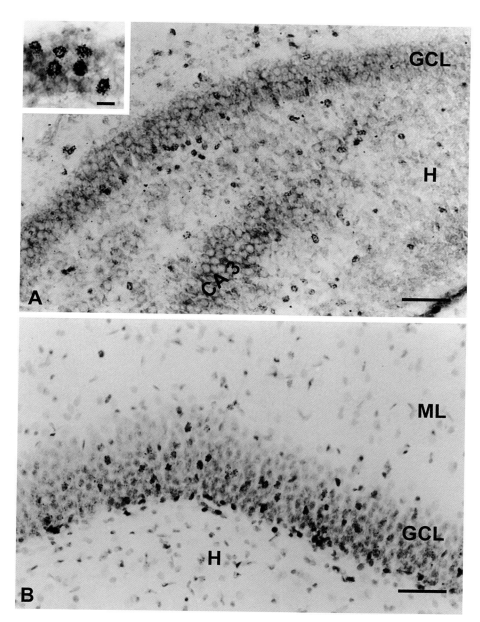

Figure 4–3. *A.* Photomicrograph showing ³H-thymidine-labeled cells (black) in the hilus (H) and granule cell layer (GCL) of the dentate gyrus of a 5-day-old rat that received a single injection of thymidine 1 hour before sacrifice. At this age, the infrapyramidal blade is still very short and hardly reaches the tip of the CA3 pyramidal layer. The large number of labeled cells above the granule cell layer suggests that glial cells are also formed at this age because the molecular layer contains only a few interneurons, which are born prenatally. Note the lack of labeling in the CA3 area of Ammon's horn where pyramidal cells are generated prenatally. *Inset.* Labeled cells in the granule cell layer of this animal at higher magnification. Section is 10 μm thick and stained with toluidine blue. *B.* BrdU-labeled cells (brown) in the suprapyramidal blade of the dentate gyrus of a 3-month-old rat that received daily injections of BrdU from P4 to P6. bars: *A, B,* 50 μm; *inset,* 10 μm.

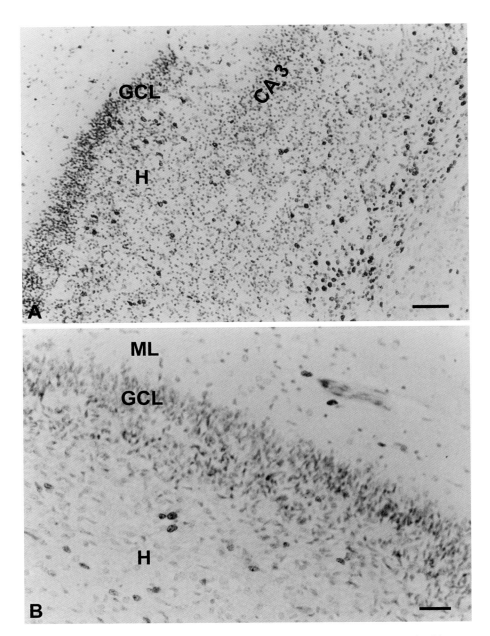

Figure 4–4. *A.* MIB-1 (Ki-67)-labeled cells (brown) in the dentate gyrus of a 16-week-old human fetus. A large number of labeled cells are seen in the hilus (H) underneath the granule cell layer (GCL). Note the absence of labeled cells in the CA3 area of Ammon's horn. In contrast, numerous labeled cells, migrating from the ventricular germinative layer along the pyramidal layer toward the hilus, are seen in the intermediate zone. *B.* MIB-1 (Ki-67)-labeled cells are still abundant in the hilus (H) of a 28-week-old fetus. The granule cell layer and molecular layer (ML) contain only a few labeled cells. Sections are 10 μm thick and are stained with cresyl violet. bars: *A,* 50 μm; *B,* 20 μm.

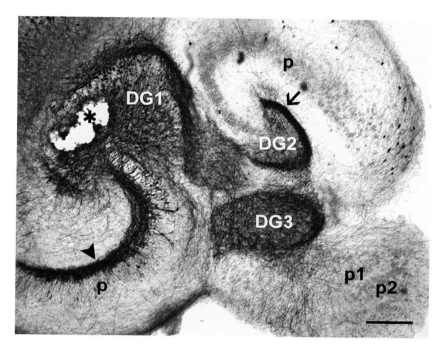

Figure 4–7. Triplet cocultures of two wild-type slices of hippocampus together with a reeler hippocampal slice. The biocytin injection site into the dentate gyrus of one of the wild-type cultures (DG1) is marked with an asterisk. Labeled commissural fibers invade the two other cultures, but only in the dentate gyrus of the second wild-type culture (DG2) do they show their characteristic compact termination in the inner molecular layer (arrow). In the reeler hippocampal culture, the commissural fibers arising from the same cells of origin have lost their laminar specificity and terminate throughout the hilar region of the dentate gyrus (DG3). Arrowhead points to the mossy fiber projection in the wild-type culture that was also labeled by the tracer injection into the hilus. p, pyramidal layer; p1, p2 two pyramidal layers in the reeler culture. Bar = 100 μm. (*Source*: Zhao et al., 2003, © 2003 by the Society for Neuroscience.)

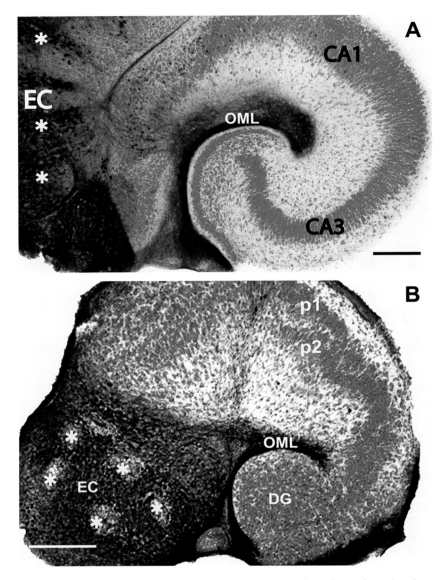

Figure 4–8. *A*. Entorhino-hippocampal projection in a complex culture of entorhinal cortex (EC) and hippocampus. Biocytin injection sites are labeled by asterisks. Note the layer-specific termination of the entorhinal fibers in the outer molecular layer (OML) of the dentate gyrus. *B*. In a slice culture of reeler hippocampus and entorhinal cortex, entorhinal fibers labeled by biocytin injection into the entorhinal cortex (asterisks) form a sharply segregated projection to the outer portion of the molecular layer of the dentate gyrus (DG) despite the malpositioned granule cells, demonstrating that the trajectory of entorhinal fibers is not influenced by the position of their target neurons. p1, p2, two pyramidal layers in the reeler hippocampus. Bar = 100 μm. (*Source*: Zhao et al., 2003; © 2003 by the Society for Neuroscience.)

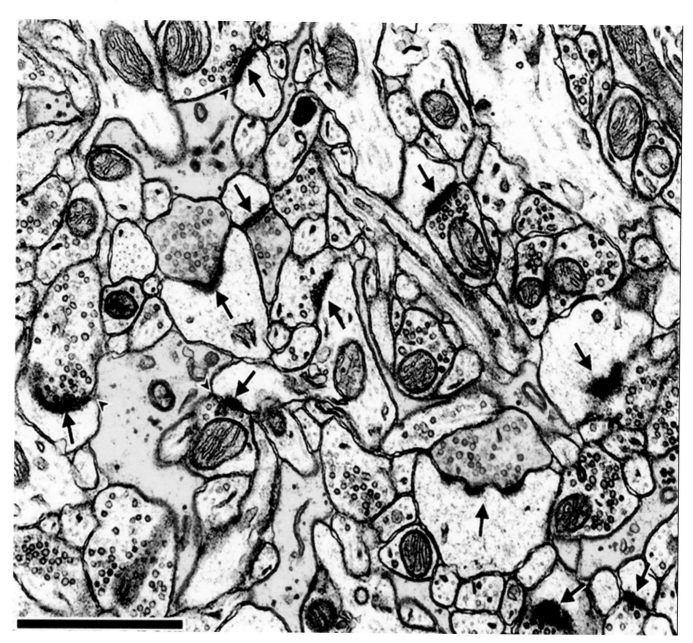

Figure 6–1. Fine structure of the hippocampal neuropil. Arrows point to individual asymmetrical (glutamatergic) synapses in a section taken from the stratum radiatum of CA1 in the rat. The presynaptic boutons contain numerous vesicles, which are frequently clustered close to membrane specializations (the active zone). A proportion of "docked" vesicles are in contact with the presynaptic membrane and are thought to be ready for exocytosis. The electron-dense area is the postsynaptic density, which distinguishes these synapses from numerically less abundant symmetrical (inhibitory) synapses (see Fig. 6–9). Three presynaptic boutons are colored green. Astrocyte profiles, colored in blue, lacking vesicles and postsynaptic densities, contact the synaptic perimeter in some cases (arrowheads). bar = 1 μm. (*Source*: Ventura and Harris, 1999, with permission.)

Figure 9–2. Most cells generated in the dentate gyrus of adults express neuronal characteristics. *A.* Photomicrograph of a BrdU-positive cell (red) in the adult rat dentate gyrus, expressing TUJ-1 (green), a marker of immature and mature neurons. *B.* Photomicrograph of a BrdU-positive cell (red) in the adult rat dentate gyrus, not expressing the astrocytic protein GFAP (green). *C.* Photomicrograph of a segment of dentate gyrus granule cell layer, triple-labeled with Hoechst, a DNA dye (blue), BrdU (red), and NeuN (green). Many but not all BrdU-positive cells express NeuN, a marker of mature neurons.

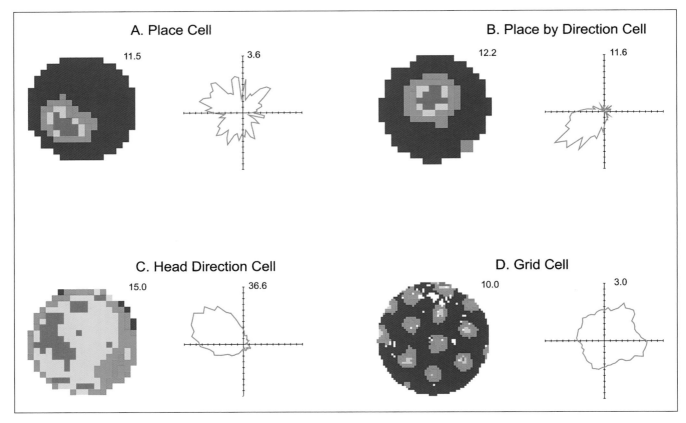

Figure 11–21. Four spatial cell types in the hippocampal formation. False color firing field maps (left) show the firing rate as a function of the animal's location in cylindrical environments irrespective of heading direction; directional polar plots (right) show the firing rate for the same cell as a function of the animal's heading direction irrespective of location. *A.* Place cell has single localized field and no directional selectivity. *B.* Place by directional cell has single localized field and strong directional selectivity. *C.* Head direction cell does not have localized firing but has strong directional selectivity. *D.* Grid cell has multiple place fields and no directional selectivity. Directional grid cells also exist. Numbers associated with the firing rate plots represent the maximum firing rate (red regions in firing rate maps and peak x and y values in polar plots). Diameter of cylinders in *A– C* is 79 cm; diameter in *D* is 2 m. (*Sources: A–C.* Courtesy of Francesca Cacucci. *D.* Courtesy of Edvard and May-Britt Moser.)

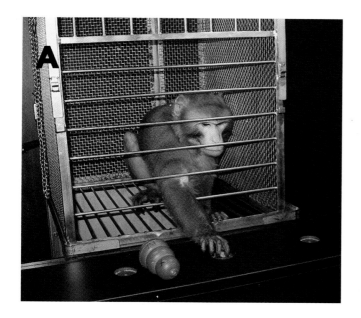

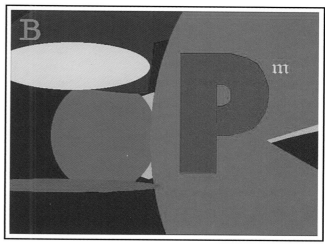

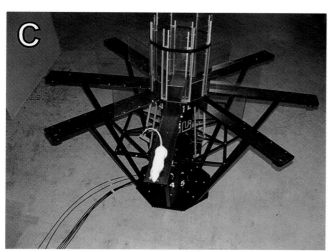

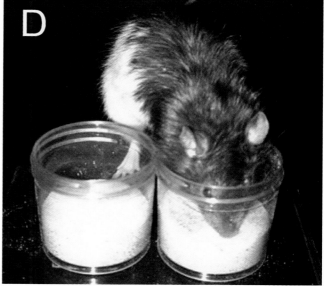

Figure 13–49. Examples of common behavioral tasks used to study hippocampal function in animals. *A.* Classic Wisconsin General Testing Apparatus for macaque monkeys. *B.* Screen shot of modern "touchscreen" display. *C.* Radial maze foraging task for rats, shown with doors. *D.* Rat making a choice in a two-pot olfactory discrimination task. Only one odor is familiar or may be cued by another odor in a paired-associate manner.

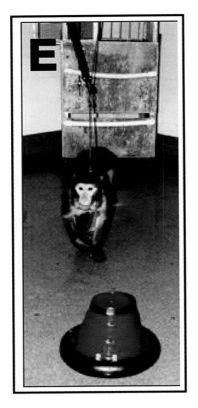

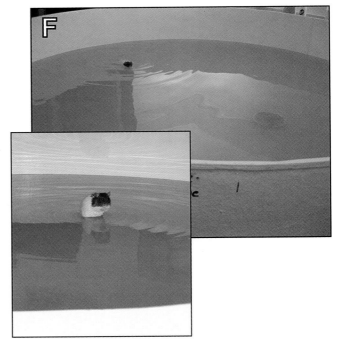

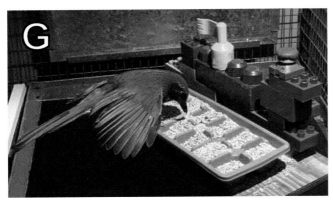

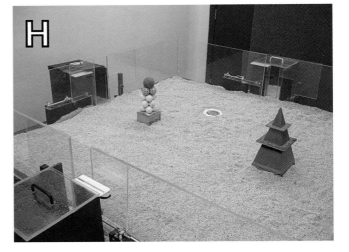

Figure 13–49. *(Continued) E.* Foraging monkey exploring objects in a laboratory. *F.* Water maze. Rat swimming in a large 2-m pool trying to find a hidden escape platform under the water surface (just visible on the right). *Inset* (below). The rat is on the platform, rearing and working out his location. *G.* Scrub-jay in an episodic-like "what-where-when" memory task in which it caches various foods in an ice-cube tray and then retrieves them selectively later. *H.* Paired-associate event arena task for rats. Different foods are found at specific locations (e.g., one shown) in the apparatus.

A

A 32 year old man presented with refractory partial epilepsy. He had a prolonged febrile seizure at the age of 18 months, and spontaneous seizures began at the age of 8 years. These seizures have continued despite trying all available antiepileptic drugs. The seizures take the form of simple partial seizures in which he perceives a sense of fear rising from his stomach, and complex partial seizures in which he has an aura as above and then loses touch with his surroundings. During the complex partial seizure he is described as making chewing movements, his right hand is postured and he fiddles with his clothes with his left hand. The seizure lasts a couple of minutes, and he is then confused and dysphasic afterwards for approximately 5 minutes.

B

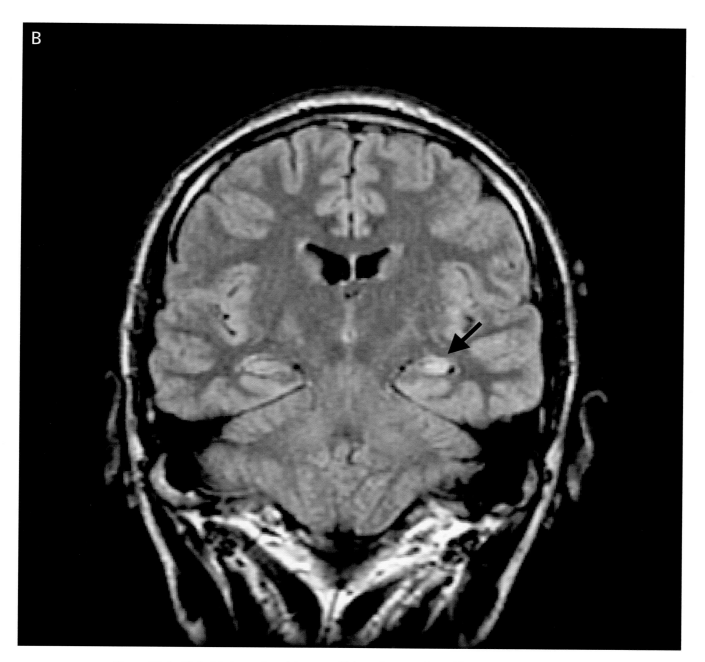

Figure 16–1. Clinical features of mesial temporal lobe epilepsy. *A*. Typical history. *B*. Magnetic resonance imaging (MRI) findings of left hippocampal sclerosis with high T2 signal in shrunken hippocampus (arrow).

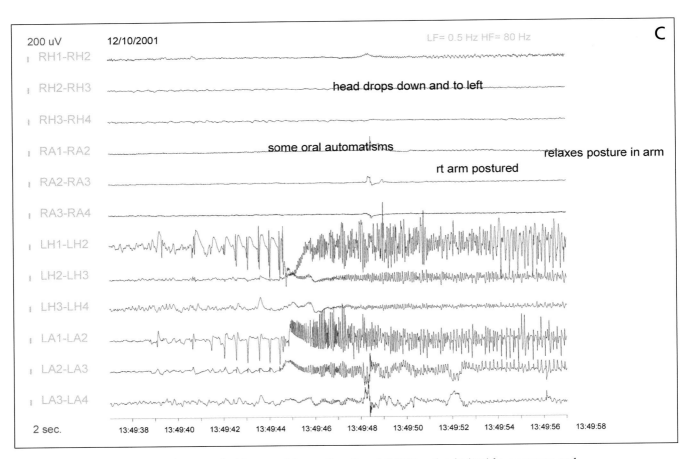

Figure 16–1. *(Continued) C.* Intracranial recordings from left (LH) and right (RH) hippocampus and left (LA) and right (RA) amydala demonstrate well localized 1- to 2-Hz spikes in left hippocampus and amygdala that evolve to low-amplitude fast activity at seizure onset.

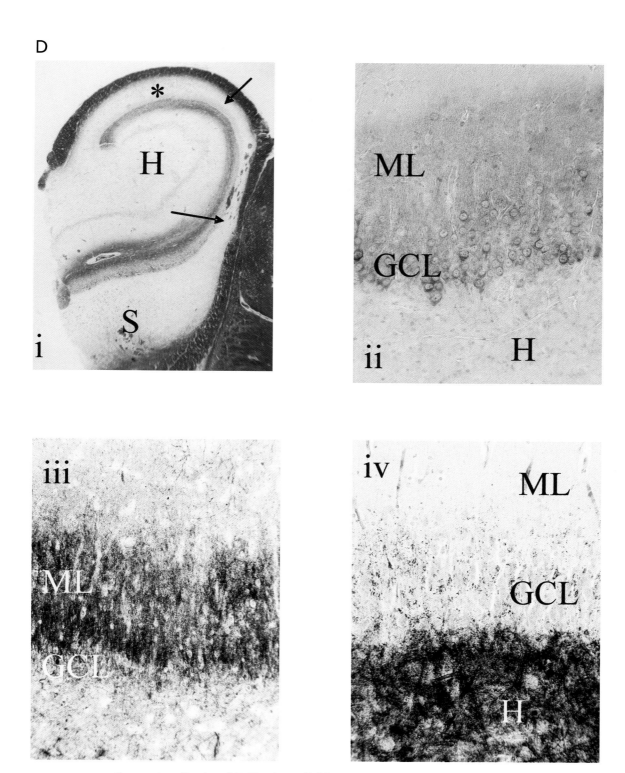

Figure 16–1. *(Continued) D.* Histology of left hippocampal sclerosis with marked cell loss in the hilus and CA1 and Timm's stain demonstrating mossy fiber sprouting.

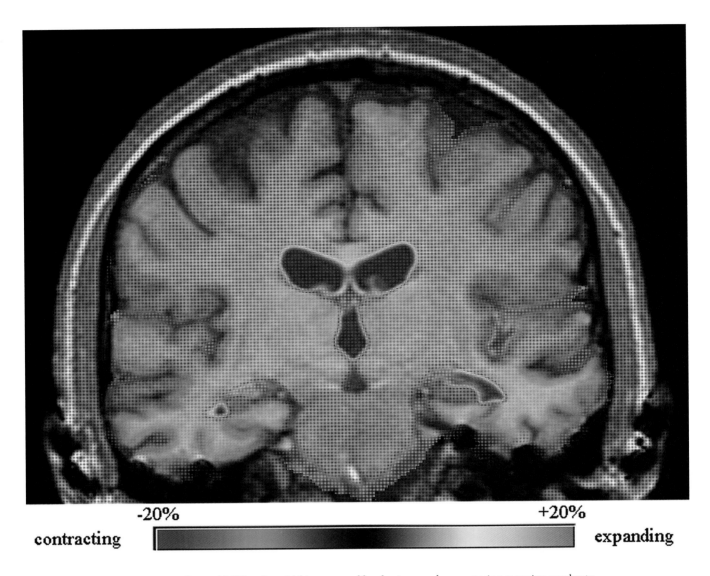

-20%   +20%

contracting   expanding

Figure 16–7. Coronal MRI at the mid-hippocampal level using voxel-compression mapping overlay to show the change in brain volume over 12 months in a patient with Alzheimer's disease (AD). Particular features to note are the marked involvement of the temporal lobes including the hippocampi, the relative symmetry of the structural changes, and the diffuse involvement of both gray and white matter.

transentorhinal stages I-II

limbic stages III-IV

neocortical stages V-VI

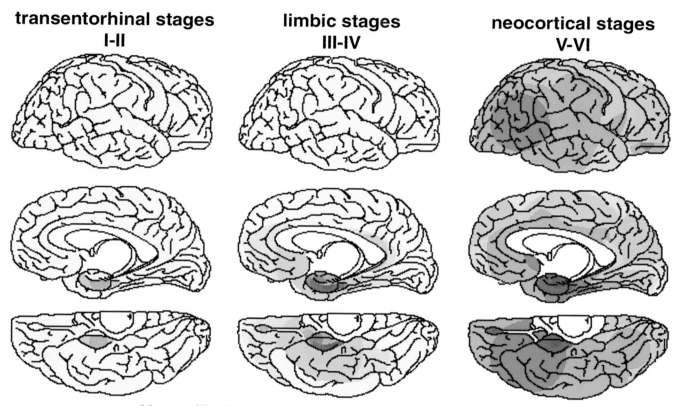

Neurofibrillary changes of the Alzheimer type

Figure 16–8. Distribution patterns of neurofibrillary changes in AD, including both neurofibrillary tangles and neuropil threads. In stages I and II the pathological changes are largely restricted to the transentorhinal region (tangles may also be found in CA1). Stages III and IV are characterized by severe involvement of the transentorhinal and entorhinal regions, with additional changes in CA1 and the subiculum. The isocortex is minimally affected. In stages V and VI the entire hippocampal formation is involved, with severe neuronal loss in CA1. The temporal lobes and cortical association areas are severely affected, but typically there is relative sparing of the primary sensory cortices. Darker colors represent more extensive tangles. (*Source*: Courtesy of Dr. Heiko Braak.)

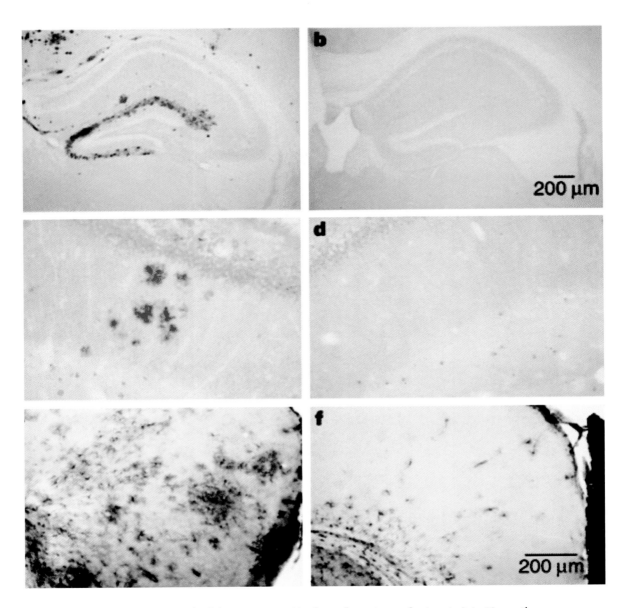

Figure 16–9. Hippocampal Aβ deposition, neuritic plaque formation, and astrocytosis in 13-month-old mice injected with phosphate-buffered saline (PBS) and Aβ$_{42}$. There is marked Aβ deposition in the outer molecular layer of the dentate gyrus of the PBS-injected mice (*a*), which contrasts with the absence of Aβ observed in the Aβ$_{42}$-injected mice. Dystrophic neurites labeled with the APP-specific monoclonal antibody 8ES were found in the hippocampal sections of the PBS-injected (*c*) but not the Aβ$_{42<}$-injected mice (*d*). Plaque-associated astrocytosis is abundant in the retrosplenial cortex of the PBS-injected (*e*) but not the Aβ$_{42}$-injected (*f*) mice. (*Source*: Schenk et al., 1999, with the permission of Dr. Dale Schenk and Nature Publishing Group.)

sion: a postsynaptic correlate of long-term potentiation. *Nature* 266:737–739.

Lynch MA (2004) Long-term potentiation and memory. *Physiol Rev* 84:87–136.

Ma L, Zablow L, Kandel ER, Siegelbaum SA (1999) Cyclic AMP induces functional presynaptic boutons in hippocampal CA3-CA1 neuronal cultures. *Nat Neurosci* 2:24–30.

Maccaferri G, McBain CJ (1996) Long-term potentiation in distinct subtypes of hippocampal nonpyramidal neurons. *J Neurosci* 16:5334–5343.

Maccaferri G, Toth K, McBain CJ (1998) Target-specific expression of presynaptic mossy fiber plasticity. *Science* 279:1368–1370.

MacDermott AB, Mayer ML, Westbrook GL, Smith SJ, Barker JL (1986) NMDA-receptor activation increases cytoplasmic calcium concentration in cultured spinal cord neurones. *Nature* 321: 519–22.

MacDonald JF, Wojtowicz JM (1980) Two conductance mechanisms activated by applications of L-glutamic, L-aspartic, DL-homocysteic, N-methyl-D-aspartic, and DL-kainic acids to cultured mammalian central neurones. *Can J Physiol Pharmacol* 58: 1393–1397.

Madani R, Hulo S, Toni N, Madani H, Steimer T, Muller D, Vassalli JD (1999) Enhanced hippocampal long-term potentiation and learning by increased neuronal expression of tissue-type plasminogen activator in transgenic mice. *EMBO J* 18: 3007–3012.

Madison DV, Schuman EM (1994) Locally distributed synaptic potentiation in the hippocampus. *Science* 263:532–536.

Magee JC, Johnston D (1997) A synaptically controlled, associative signal for Hebbian plasticity in hippocampal neurons. *Science* 275:209–213.

Magleby KL (1979) Facilitation, augmentation and potentiation of transmitter release. *Prog Brain Res* 49:175–182.

Maher FO, Nolan Y, Lynch MA (2005) Downregulation of IL-4-induced signalling in hippocampus contributes to deficits in LTP in the aged rat. *Neurobiol Aging* 26:717–728.

Mainen ZF, Jia Z, Roder J, Malinow R (1998) Use-dependent AMPA receptor block in mice lacking GluR2 suggests postsynaptic site for LTP expression. *Nat Neurosci* 1:579–586.

Malenka RC, Madison DV, Nicoll RA (1986) Potentiation of synaptic transmission in the hippocampus by phorbol esters. *Nature* 321:175–177.

Malenka RC, Kauer JA, Perkel DJ, Mauk MD, Kelly PT, Nicoll RA, Waxham MN (1989) An essential role for postsynaptic calmodulin and protein kinase activity in long-term potentiation. *Nature* 340:554–557.

Malenka RC, Lancaster B, Zucker RS (1992) Temporal limits on the rise in postsynaptic calcium required for the induction of long-term potentiation. *Neuron* 9:121–128.

Maletic-Savatic M, Malinow R, Svoboda K (1999) Rapid dendritic morphogenesis in CA1 hippocampal dendrites induced by synaptic activity. *Science* 283:1923–1927.

Malgaroli A, Ting AE, Wendland B, Bergamaschi A, Villa A, Tsien RW, Scheller RH (1995) Presynaptic component of long-term potentiation visualized at individual hippocampal synapses. *Science* 268:1624–1628.

Malinow R, Malenka RC (2002) AMPA receptor trafficking and synaptic plasticity. *Annu Rev Neurosci* 25:103–126.

Malinow R, Miller JP (1986) Postsynaptic hyperpolarization during conditioning reversibly blocks induction of long-term potentiation. *Nature* 320:529–530.

Malinow R, Tsien RW (1990) Presynaptic enhancement shown by whole-cell recordings of long-term potentiation in hippocampal slices. *Nature* 346:177–180.

Malinow R, Schulman H, Tsien RW (1989) Inhibition of postsynaptic PKC or CaMKII blocks induction but not expression of LTP. *Science* 245:862–866.

Malleret G, Haditsch U, Genoux D, Jones MW, Bliss TVP, Vanhoose AM, Weitlauf C, Kandel ER, Winder DG, Mansuy IM (2001) Inducible and reversible enhancement of learning, memory and long-term potentiation by genetic inhibitior of calcineurin. *Cell* 104:675–686.

Man HY, Wang Q, Lu WY, Ju W, Ahmadian G, Liu L, D'Souza S, Wong TP, Taghibiglou C, Lu J, Becker LE, Pei L, Liu F, Wymann MP, MacDonald JF, Wang YT (2003) Activation of PI3-kinase is required for AMPA receptor insertion during LTP of mEPSCs in cultured hippocampal neurons. *Neuron* 38:611–624.

Manabe T, Nicoll RA (1994) Long-term potentiation: evidence against an increase in transmitter release probability in the CA1 region of the hippocampus. *Science* 265:1888–1892.

Manabe T, Noda Y, Mamiya T, Katagiri H, Houtani T, Nishi M, Noda T, Takahashi T, Sugimoto T, Nabeshima T, Takeshima H (1998) Facilitation of long-term potentiation and memory in mice lacking nociceptin receptors. *Nature* 394:577–581.

Manahan-Vaughan D (1997) Group 1 and 2 metabotropic receptors play differential roles in hippocampal long-term depression and long-term potentiation in freely moving rats. *J Neurosci* 17:3303–3311.

Manahan-Vaughan D (2000) Long-term depression in freely moving rats is dependent upon strain variation, induction protocol and behavioral state. *Cereb Cortex* 10:483–487.

Manahan-Vaughan D, Braunewell KH (1999) Novelty acquisition is associated with induction of hippocampal long-term depression. *Proc Natl Acad Sci USA* 96:8739–8744.

Manahan-Vaughan D, Kulla A, Frey JU (2000) Requirement of translation but not transcription for the maintenance of long-term depression in the CA1 region of freely moving rats. *J Neurosci* 20:8572–8576.

Mansuy IM, Mayford M, Jacob B, Kandel ER, Bach ME (1998a) Restricted and regulated overexpression reveals calcineurin as a key component in the transition from short-term to long-term memory. *Cell* 92:39–49.

Mansuy IM, Winder DG, Moallem TM, Osman M, Mayford M, Hawkins RD, Kandel ER (1998b) Inducible and reversible gene expression with the rtTA system for the study of memory. *Neuron* 21:257–265.

Manzoni OJ, Weisskopf MG, Nicoll RA (1994) MCPG antagonizes metabotropic glutamate receptors but not long-term potentiation in the hippocampus. *Eur J Neurosci* 6:1050–1054.

Marder CP, Buonomano DV (2003) Differential effects of short- and long-term potentiation on cell firing in the CA1 region of the hippocampus. *J Neurosci* 23:112–121.

Marder CP, Buonomano DV (2004) Timing and balance of inhibition enhance the effect of long-term potentiation on cell firing. *J Neurosci* 24:8873–8884.

Margrie TW, Rostas JA, Sah P (1998) Long-term potentiation of synaptic transmission in the avian hippocampus. *J Neurosci* 18:1207–1216.

Markakis EA, Gage FH (1999) Adult-generated neurons in the dentate gyrus send axonal projections to field CA3 and are surrounded by synaptic vesicles. *J Comp Neurol* 406:449–460.

Markram H, Tsodyks M (1996) Redistribution of synaptic efficacy between neocortical pyramidal cells. *Nature* 382:807–810.

Markram H, Lubke J, Frotscher M, Sakmann B (1997) Regulation of synaptic efficacy by coincidence of postsynaptic APs and EPSPs. *Science* 275:213–215.

Marr D (1971) Simple memory: a theory for archicortex. *Philos Trans R Soc Lond B Biol Sci* 262:23–81.

Martin KC (2004) Local protein synthesis during axon guidance and synaptic plasticity. *Curr Opin Neurobiol* 14:305–310.

Martin KC, Kosik KS (2002) Synaptic tagging—who's it? *Nat Neurosci Rev* 3:813–820.

Martin KC, Barad M, Kandel ER (2000a) Local protein synthesis and its role in synapse-specific plasticity. *Curr Opin Neurobiol* 10:587–592.

Martin SJ (1998) Time-dependent reversal of dentate LTP by 5 Hz stimulation. *Neuroreport* 9:3775–3781.

Martin SJ, Morris RGM (1997) (R,S)-Alpha-methyl-4-car-boxyphenylglycine (MCPG) fails to block long-term potentiation under urethane anaesthesia in vivo. *Neuropharmacology* 10:1339–1354.

Martin SJ, Grimwood PD, Morris RG (2000) Synaptic plasticity and memory: an evaluation of the hypothesis. *Annu Rev Neurosci* 23:649–711.

Massey PV, Johnson BE, Moult PR, Auberson YP, Brown MW, Molnar E, Collingridge GL, Bashir ZI (2004) Differential roles of NR2A and NR2B-containing NMDA receptors in cortical long-term potentiation and long-term depression. *J Neurosci* 24:7821–7828.

Matsuda S, Mikawa S, Hirai H (1999) Phosphorylation of serine-880 in GluR2 by protein kinase C prevents its C terminus from binding with glutamate receptor-interacting protein. *J Neurochem* 73:1765–1768.

Matsuo R, Murayama A, Saitoh Y, Sakaki Y, Inokuchi K (2000) Identification and cataloging of genes induced by long-lasting long-term potentiation in awake rats. *J Neurochem* 74:2239–2249.

Matsuzaki M, Honkura N, Ellis-Davies GCR, Kasai H (2004) Structural basis of long-term potentiation in single dendritic spines. *Nature* 429:761–766.

Matthies H, Reymann KG (1993) Protein kinase A inhibitors prevent the maintenance of hippocampal long-term potentiation. *Neuroreport* 4:712–714.

Matthies H, Ruthrich H, Ott T, Matthies HK, Matthies R (1986) Low frequency perforant path stimulation as a conditioned stimulus demonstrates correlations between long-term synaptic potentiation and learning. *Physiol Behav* 36:811–821.

Matthies H, Becker A, Schroeder H, Kraus J, Hollt V, Krug M (1997) Dopamine D1-deficient mutant mice do not express the late phase of hippocampal long-term potentiation. *Neuroreport* 8:3533–3535.

Matus A (2005) Growth of dendritic spines: a continuing story. *Curr Opin Neurobiol* 15:67–72.

Matynia A, Kushner SA, Silva AJ (2002) Genetic approaches to molecular and cellular cognition: a focus on LTP and learning and memory. *Annu Rev Genet* 36:687–720.

Mauceri D, Cattabeni F, Di Luca M, Gardoni F (2004) Calcium/calmodulin-dependent protein kinase II phosphorylation drives synapse-associated protein 97 into spines. *J Biol Chem* 279:23813–23821.

Mayer ML, Westbrook GL, Guthrie PB (1984) Voltage-dependent block by Mg^{2+} of NMDA responses in spinal cord neurones. *Nature* 309:261–263.

Mayford M, Wang J, Kandel ER, O'Dell TJ (1995) CaMKII regulates the frequency-response of hippocampal synapses for the production of both LTP and LTD. *Cell* 81:891–904.

Mayford M, Bach ME, Huang Y-Y, Wang L, Hawkins R, Kandel ER (1996) Control of memory formation through regulated expression of a CaMKII transgene. *Science* 274:1678–1683.

Mayford M, Mansuy IM, Muller RU, Kandel ER (1997) Memory and behavior: a second generation of genetically modified mice. *Curr Biol* 7:R580(R589.

McBain CJ, Freund TF, Mody I (1999) Glutamatergic synapses onto hippocampal interneurons: precision timing without lasting plasticity. *Trends Neurosci* 22:228–235.

McDermott CM, LaHoste GJ, Chen C, Musto A, Bazan NG, Magee JC (2003). Sleep deprivation causes behavioral, synaptic, and membrane excitability alterations in hippocampal neurons. *J Neurosci* 23:9687–9695.

McDonald RJ, Hong NS, Craig LA, Holahan MR, Louis M, Muller RU (2005) NMDA-receptor blockade by CPP impairs post-training consolidation of a rapidly acquired spatial representation in rat hippocampus. *Eur J Neurosci* 22:1201–1213.

McEachern JC, Shaw CA (1996) An alternative to the LTP orthodoxy: a plasticity-pathology continuum model. *Brain Res Brain Res Rev* 22:51–92.

McGahon B, Holscher C, McGlinchey L, Rowan MJ, Lynch MA (1996) Training in the Morris watermaze occludes the synergism between ACPD and arachidonic acid on glutamate release in synaptosomes prepared from rat hippocampus. *Learn Mem* 3:296–304.

McGaugh JL (2000) Memory—a century of consolidation. *Science* 287:248–251.

McHugh TJ, Blum KI, Tsien JZ, Tonegawa S, Wilson MA (1996) Impaired hippocampal representation of space in CA1-specific NMDAR1 knockout mice. *Cell* 87:1339–1349.

McKernan MG, Shinnick-Gallagher P (1997) Fear conditioning induces a lasting potentiation of synaptic currents in vitro. *Nature* 390:607–611.

McKinney RA, Capogna M, Durr R, Gahwiler BH, Thompson SM (1999) Miniature synaptic events maintain dendritic spines via AMPA receptor activation. *Nat Neurosci* 2:44–49.

McMahon LL, Kauer JA (1997) Hippocampal interneurons express a novel form of synaptic plasticity. *Neuron* 18:295–305.

McNaughton BL (1980) Evidence for two physiologically distinct perforant pathways to the fascia dentata. *Brain Res* 199:1–19.

McNaughton BL (1982) Long-term synaptic enhancement and short-term potentiation in rat fascia dentata act through different mechanisms. *J Physiol* 324:249–262.

McNaughton BL (1983) Activity-dependent modulation of hippocampal synaptic efficacy: some implications for memory processes. In: *Neurobiology of the hippocampus* (Siefert W, ed), pp 233–252. London: Academic Press.

McNaughton BL, Douglas RM, Goddard GV (1978) Synaptic enhancement in fascia dentata: cooperativity among coactive afferents. *Brain Res* 157:277–293.

McNaughton BL, Barnes CA, Rao G (1984) Presynaptic versus postsynaptic control over long-term synaptic enhancement. In: *Neurobiology of learning and memory* (Lynch G, McGaugh JL and Weinberger NM, eds), pp. 466-469. New York: Guilford Press.

McNaughton BL, Barnes CA, Rao G, Baldwin J, Rasmussen M (1986) Long-term enhancement of hippocampal synaptic transmission and the acquisition of spatial information. *J Neurosci* 6:563–571.

Mehta MR, Quirk MC, Wilson MA (2000) Experience-dependent asymmetric shape of hippocampal receptive fields. *Neuron* 25:707–715.

Meiri N, Ghelardini C, Tesco G, Galeotti N, Dahl D, Tomsic D, Cavallaro S, Quattrone A, Capaccioli S, Bartolini A, Alkon DL (1997) Reversible antisense inhibition of Shaker-like Kv1.1 potassium channel expression impairs associative memory in mouse and rat. *Proc Natl Acad Sci USA* 94:4430–4434.

Meiri N, Sun MK, Segal Z, Alkon DL (1998) Memory and long-term potentiation (LTP) dissociated: normal spatial memory despite CA1 LTP elimination with Kv1.4 antisense. *Proc Natl Acad Sci USA* 95:15037–15042.

Mellor J, Nicoll RA (2001) Hippocampal mossy fiber LTP is independent of postsynaptic calcium. *Nat Neurosci* 4:125–126.

Mellor J, Nicoll RA, Schmitz D (2002) Mediation of hippocampal mossy fiber long-term potentiation by presynaptic Ih channels. *Science* 295:143–147.

Mendoza-Fernandez V, Andrew RD, Barajas-Lopez C (2000) Interferon-alpha inhibits long-term potentiation and unmasks a long-term depression in the rat hippocampus. *Brain Res* 885:14–24.

Meng Y, Zhang Y, Jia Z (2003) Synaptic transmission and plasticity in the absence of AMPA glutamate receptor GluR2 and GluR3. *Neuron* 39:163–176.

Messaoudi E, Ying SW, Kanhema T, Croll SD, Bramham CR (2002) Brain-derived neurotrophic factor triggers transcription-dependent, late phase long-term potentiation in vivo. *J Neurosci* 22:7453–7461.

Micheau J, Riedel G (1999) Protein kinases: which one is the memory molecule? *Cell Mol Life Sci* 55:534–548.

Micheva KD, Buchanan J, Holz RW, Smith SJ (2003) Retrograde regulation of synaptic vesicle endocytosis and recycling. *Nat Neurosci* 6:925–932.

Migaud M, Charlesworth P, Dempster M, Webster LC, Watabe AM, Makhinson M, He Y, Ramsay MF, Morris RG, Morrison JH, O'Dell TJ, Grant SG (1998) Enhanced long-term potentiation and impaired learning in mice with mutant postsynaptic density-95 protein. *Nature* 396:433–439.

Miller B, Sarantis M, Traynelis SF, Attwell D (1992) Potentiation of NMDA receptor currents by arachidonic acid. *Nature* 235:722–725.

Miller SG, Kennedy MB (1986) Regulation of brain type II Ca^{2+}/calmodulin-dependent protein kinase by autophosphorylation: a Ca^{2+}-triggered molecular switch. *Cell* 44:861–870.

Minogue AM, Schmid AW, Fogarty MP, Moore AC, Campbell VA, Herron CE, Lynch MA (2003) Activation of the c-Jun N-terminal kinase signaling cascade mediates the effect of amyloid-beta on long term potentiation and cell death in hippocampus: a role for interleukin-1beta? *J Biol Chem* 278:27971–27980.

Mizuno T, Kanazawa I, Sakurai M (2001) Differential induction of LTP and LTD is not determined solely by instantaneous calcium concentration: an essential involvement of a temporal factor. *Eur J Neurosci* 14:701–708.

Mockett B, Coussens C, Abraham WC (2002) NMDA receptor-mediated metaplasticity during the induction of long-term depression by low-frequency stimulation. *Eur J Neurosci* 15:1819–1826.

Mockett BG, Brooks WM, Tate WP, Abraham WC (2004) Dopamine D1/D5 receptor activation fails to initiate an activity-independent late-phase LTP in rat hippocampus. *Brain Res Rev* 1021:92–100.

Monaghan DT, Cotman CW (1885) Distribution of N-methyl-D-aspartate-sensitive L-[^{3}H]-binding sites in rat brain. *J Neurosci* 5:2909–2919.

Mondadori C, Weiskrantz L (1991) Memory facilitation by NMDA receptor blockade. In: *Long-term potentiation: a debate of current issues* (Baudry M, Davis J, eds), pp 259–266. Cambridge, MA: MIT Press.

Mondadori C, Weiskrantz L (1993) NMDA receptor blockers facilitate and impair learning via different mechanisms. *Behav Neural Biol* 60:205–210.

Mondadori C, Weiskrantz L, Buerki H, Petschke F, Fagg GE (1989) NMDA receptor antagonists can enhance or impair learning performance in animals. *Exp Brain Res* 75:449–456.

Mondadori C, Borkowski J, Gentsch C (1996) The memory-facilitating effects of the competitive NMDA-receptor antagonist CGP 37849 are steroid-sensitive, whereas its memory-impairing effects are not. *Psychopharmacology (Berl)* 124:380–383.

Moechars D, Dewachter I, Lorent K, Reverse D, Baekelandt V, Naidu A, Tesseur I, Spittaels K, Haute CV, Checler F, Godaux E, Cordell B, Van Leuven F (1999) Early phenotypic changes in transgenic mice that overexpress different mutants of amyloid precursor protein in brain. *J Biol Chem* 274:6483–6492.

Monfils MH, Teskey GC (2004) Skilled-learning-induced potentiation in rat sensorimotor cortex: a transient form of behavioural long-term potentiation. *Neuroscience* 125:329–336.

Montgomery JM, Madison DV (2002) State-dependent heterogeneity in synaptic depression between pyramidal cell pairs. *Neuron* 33:765–777.

Montgomery JM, Pavlidis P, Madison DV (2001) Pair recordings reveal all-silent synaptic connections and the postsynaptic expression of long-term potentiation. *Neuron* 29:691–701.

Moore CI, Browning MD, Rose GM (1993) Hippocampal plasticity induced by primed burst, but not long-term potentiation, stimulation is impaired in area CA1 of aged Fischer 344 rats. *Hippocampus* 3:57–66.

Moosmang S, Haider N, Klugbauer N, Adelsberger H, Langwieser N, Muller J, Stiess M, Marais E, Schulla V, Lacinova L, Goebbels S, Naye K-L, Storm DR, Hofmann F, Kleppisch T (2005) Role of hippocampal $Ca_V1.2$ Ca^{2+} channels in NMDA receptor-independent synaptic plasticity and spatial memory. *J Neurosci* 25:9883–9892.

More JC, Nistico R, Dolman NP, Clarke VR, Alt AJ, Ogden AM, Buelens FP, Troop HM, Kelland EE, Pilato F, Bleakman D, Bortolotto ZA, Collingridge GL, Jane DE (2004) Characterisation of UBP296: a novel, potent and selective kainate receptor antagonist. *Neuropharmacology* 47:46–64.

Morris R, Anderson E, Lynch GS, Baudry M (1986) Selective impairment of learning and blockade of long-term potentiation by an N-methyl-D-aspartate receptor antagonist, AP5. *Nature* 319:774–776.

Morris RG (1989) Synaptic plasticity and learning: selective impairment of learning rats and blockade of long-term potentiation in vivo by the N-methyl-D-aspartate receptor antagonist AP5. *J Neurosci* 9:3040–3057.

Morris RG, Halliwell RF, Bowery N (1989) Synaptic plasticity and learning. II. Do different kinds of plasticity underlie different kinds of learning? *Neuropsychologia* 27:41–59.

Morris RGM, Davis S, Butcher SP (1990) Hippocampal synatic plasticity and NMDA receptors: a role in information storage? *Philos Trans R Soc Lond* 329:187–204.

Morton RA, Kuenzi FM, Fitzjohn SM, Rosahl TW, Smith D, Zheng H, Shearman M, Collingridge GL, Seabrook GR (2002) Impairment in hippocampal long-term potentiation in mice under-expressing the Alzheimer's disease related gene presenilin-1. *Neurosci Lett* 319:37–40.

Moser E, Moser M-B (1999) Is learning blocked by saturation of synaptic weights in the hippocampus? *Neurosci Biobehav Rev* 23:661–672.

Moser E, Mathiesen I, Andersen P (1993a) Association between brain temperature and dentate field potentials in exploring and swimming rats. *Science* 259:1324–1326.

Moser E, Moser M-B, Andersen P (1993b) Synaptic potentiation in the rat dentate gyrus during exploratory learning. *Neuroreport* 5:317–320.

Moser MB, Trommald M, Andersen P (1994) An increase in dendritic spine density on hippocampal CA1 pyramidal cells following spatial learning in adult rats suggests the formation of new synapses. *Proc Natl Acad Sci USA* 91:12673–12675.

Moser EI, Krobert KA, Moser MB, Morris RG (1998) Impaired spatial learning after saturation of long-term potentiation. *Science* 281:2038–2042.

Moult PR, Schnabel R, Kilpatrick IC, Bashir ZI, Collingridge GL (2002) Tyrosine dephosphorylation underlies DHPG-induced LTD. *Neuropharmacology* 43:175–180.

Moult PR, Gladding CM, Sanderson TM, Fitzjohn SM, Bashir ZI, Molnar E, Collingridge GL (2006) Tyrosine phosphatases regulate AMPA receptor trafficking during metabotropic glutamate receptor-mediated long-term depression. *J Neurosci* 26:2544–2554.

Mouly AM, Fort A, Ben-Boutayab N, Gervais R (2001) Olfactory learning induces differential long-lasting changes in rat central olfactory pathways. *Neuroscience* 102:11–21.

Moyer JRJ, Thompson LT, Disterhoft JF (1996) Trace eyeblink conditioning increases CA1 excitability in a transient and learning-specific manner. *J Neurosci* 16:5536–5546.

Mulkey RM, Malenka RC (1992) Mechanisms underlying induction of homosynaptic long-term depression in area CA1 of the hippocampus. *Neuron* 9:967–975.

Mulkey RM, Herron CE, Malenka RC (1993) An essential role for protein phosphatases in hippocampal long-term depression. *Science* 261:1051–1055.

Mulkey RM, Endo S, Shenolikar S, Malenka RC (1994) Involvement of a calcineurin/inhibitor-1 phosphatase cascade in hippocampal long-term depression. *Nature* 369:486–488.

Muller D, Joly M, Lynch G (1988) Contributions of quisqualate and NMDA receptors to the induction and expression of LTP. *Science* 242:1694–1697.

Muller D, Bittar P, Boddeke H (1992) Induction of stable long-term potentiation in the presence of the protein kinase C antagonist staurosporine. *Neurosci Lett* 135:18–22.

Muller D, Hefft S, Figurov A (1995) Heterosynaptic interactions between LTP and LTD in CA1 hippocampal slices. *Neuron* 14:599–605.

Muller D, Wang D, Skibo G, Toni N, Cremer H, Calaora V, Rougon G, Kiss JZ (1996) PSA-NCAM is required for activity-induced synaptic plasticity. *Neuron* 17:413–422.

Munro CAM, Walling SG, Evans JH, Harley CW (2001) β-Adrenergic blockade in the dentate gyrus in vivo prevents high frequency-induced long-term potentiation of EPSP slope, but not long-term potentiaion of population spike amplitude. *Hippocampus* 11:329–336.

Murai KK, Pasquale EB (2004) Eph receptors, ephrins, and synaptic function. *Neuroscientist* 10:304–414.

Murai KK, Nguyen LN, Irie F, Yamaguchi Y, Pasquale EB (2003) Control of hippocampal dendritic spine morphology through ephrin-A3/EphA4 signaling. *Nat Neurosci* 6: 153–160.

Murase S, Schuman EM (1999) The role of cell adhesion molecules in synaptic plasticity and memory. *Curr Opin Cell Biol* 11: 549–553.

Murase S, Mosser E, Schuman EM (2002) Depolarization drives beta-catenin into neuronal spines promoting changes in synaptic structure and function. *Neuron* 35:91–105.

Murphy KP, Carter RJ, Lione LA, Mangiarini L, Mahal A, Bates GP, Dunnett SB, Morton AJ (2000) Abnormal synaptic plasticity and impaired spatial cognition in mice transgenic for exon 1 of the human Huntington's disease mutation. *J Neurosci* 20: 5115–5123.

Murphy KPSJ, Williams JH, Bettache N, Bliss TVP (1994) Photolytic release of nitric-oxide modulates NMDA receptor-mediated transmission but does not induce long-term potentiation at hippocampal synapses. *Neuropharmacology* 33: 1375–1385.

Murray CA, Lynch MA (1998) Evidence that increased hippocampal expression of the cytokine interleukin-1 beta is a common trigger for age- and stress-induced impairments in long-term potentiation. *J Neurosci* 18:2974–2981.

Nagappan G, Lu B (2005) Activity-dependent modulation of the BDNF receptor TrKB: mechanisms and implications. *Trends Neurosci* 28:464–471.

Nagase T, Ito K-I, Kato K, Kaneko K, Kohda K, Hoshino A, Matsumoto M, Inoue T, Fujii S, Kato A, Mikoshiba K (2003) Long-term potentiation and long-term depression in hippocampal CA1 neurons of mice lacking the IP3 type 1 receptor. *Neuroscience* 117:821–830.

Nakagawa T, Futai K, Lashuel HA, Lo I, Okamoto K, Walz T, Hiyashi Y, Sheng M (2004) Quarternary structure, protein dynamics, and synaptic function of SAP97 controlled by L27 domain interactions. Neuron 44:453–467.

Nakamura K, Manabe T, Watanabe M, Mamiya T, Ichikawa R, Kiyama Y, Sanbo M, Yagi T, Inoue Y, Nabeshima T, Mori H, Mishina M (2001) Enhancement of hippocampal LTP, reference memory and sensorimotor gating in mutant mice lacking a telencephalon-specific cell adhesion molecule. *Eur J Neurosci* 13:179–189.

Nakanishi K, Saito H, Abe K (2001) The supramammillary nucleus contributes to associative EPSP-spike potentiation in the rat dentate gyrus in vivo. *Eur J Neurosci* 13:793–800.

Nakazawa K, Quirk MC, Chitwood RA, Watanabe M, Yeckel MF, Sun LD, Kato A, Carr CA, Johnston D, Wilson MA, Tonegawa S (2002) Requirement for hippocampal CA3 NMDA receptors in associative memory recall. *Science* 297:211–218.

Nakazawa K, Sun LD, Quirk MC, Rondi-Reig L, Wilson MA, Tonegawa S (2003) Hippocampal CA3 NMDA receptors are crucial for memory acquisition of one-time experience. *Neuron* 38:305–315.

Nalbantoglu J, Tirado-Santiago G, Lahsaini A, Poirier J, Goncalves O, Verge G, Momoli F, Welner SA, Massicotte G, Julien JP, Shapiro ML (1997) Impaired learning and LTP in mice expressing the carboxy terminus of the Alzheimer amyloid precursor protein. *Nature* 387:500–505.

Navakkode S, Sakijumar S, Frey JU (2004) The type IV-specific phosphodiesterase inhibitor rolipram and its effects on hippocampal long-term potentiation and synaptic tagging. *J Neurosci* 24: 7740–7744.

Nayak A, Zastrow DJ, Lickteig R, Zahniser NR, Browning MD (1998) Maintenance of late-phase LTP is accompanied by PKA-dependent increase in AMPA receptor synthesis. *Nature* 394:680–683.

Ngezahayo A, Schachner M, Artola A (2000) Synaptic activity modulates the induction of bidirectional synaptic changes in adult mouse hippocampus. *J Neurosci* 20:2451–2458.

Nguyen PV, Abel T, Kandel ER (1994) Requirement for a critical period of transcription for induction of a late phase of LTP. *Science* 265:1104–1107.

Nguyen PV, Woo NH (2003) Regulation of hippocampal synaptic plasticity by cyclic AMP-dependent protein kinases. *Prog Neurobiol* 71:401–437.

Nguyen PV, Duffy SN, Young JZ (2000) Differential maintenance and frequency-dependent tuning of LTP at hippocampal synapses of specific strains of inbred mice. *J Neurophysiol* 84:2484–2493.

Nicholls JG, Martin AR, Wallace BG, Fuchs PA (2001) *From neuron to brain: celluar approach to the function of the nervous system*, 4th ed. Sunderland, MA: Sinauer.

Nicoll RA, Schmitz D (2005) Synaptic plasticity at hippocampal mossy fiber synapses. *Nat Rev Neurosci* 6:863–876.

Nimchinsky EA, Sabatini BL, Svoboda K (2002) Structure and function of dendritic spines. *Annu Rev Physiol* 64:313–353.

Nishimune A, Isaac JT, Molnar E, Noel J, Nash SR, Tagaya M, Collingridge GL, Nakanishi S, Henley JM (1998) NSF binding to GluR2 regulates synaptic transmission. *Neuron* 21:87–97.

Nishiyama M, Hong K, Mikoshiba K, Poo M-M, Kato K (2000) Calcium stores regulate the polarity and input specificity of synaptic modification. *Nature* 408:584–588.

Noel J, Ralph GS, Pickard L, Williams J, Molnar E, Uney JB, Collingridge GL, Henley JM (1999) Surface expression of AMPA receptors in hippocampal neurons is regulated by an NSF-dependent mechanism. *Neuron* 23:365–376.

Norris CM, Korol DL, Foster TC (1996) Increased susceptibility to induction of long-term depression and long-term potentiation reversal during aging. *J Neurosci* 16:5382–5392.

Nosten-Bertrand M, Errington ML, Murphy KP, Tokugawa Y, Barboni E, Kozlova E, Michalovich D, Morris RG, Silver J, Stewart CL, Bliss TV, Morris RJ (1996) Normal spatial learning despite regional inhibition of LTP in mice lacking Thy-1. *Nature* 379:826–829.

Nowak L, Bregestovski P, Ascher P, Herbet A, Prochiantz A (1984) Magnesium gates glutamate-activated channels in mouse central neurones. *Nature* 307:462–465.

Obenaus A, Mody I, Baimbridge KG (1989) Dantrolene-Na (Dantrium) blocks induction of long-term potentiation in hippocampal slices. *Neurosci Lett* 98:172–178.

O'Connor JJ, Rowan MJ, Anwyl R (1994) Long-lasting enhancement of NMDA receptor-mediated synaptic transmission by metabotropic glutamate receptor activation. *Nature* 367: 557–559.

O'Connor JJ, Rowan MJ, Anwyl R (1995) Tetanically induced LTP involves a similar increase in the AMPA and NMDA receptor components of the excitatory postsynaptic current: investigations of the involvement of mGlu receptors. J Neurosci 15:2013–2020.

O'Dell TJ, Kandel ER (1994) Low-frequency stimulation erases LTP through an NMDA receptor-mediated activation of protein phosphatases. *Learn Mem* 1:129–139.

O'Dell TJ, Kandel ER, Grant SG (1991) Long-term potentiation in the hippocampus is blocked by tyrosine kinase inhibitors. *Nature* 353:558–560.

O'Dell TJ, Hawkins RD, Kandel ER, Arancio O (1991b) Tests of the roles of two diffusible substances in long-term potentiation: evidence for nitric oxide as a possible early retrograde messenger. *Proc Natl Acad Sci USA* 88:11285–11289.

O'Doherty A, Ruf S, Mulligan C, Hildreth V, Errington ML, Cooke S, Sesay A, Modino S, Vanes L, Hernandez D, Linehan JM, Sharpe PT, Brandner S, Bliss TV, Henderson DJ, Nizetic D, Tybulewicz VL, Fisher EM (2005) An aneuploid mouse strain carrying human chromosome 21 with Down syndrome phenotypes. *Science* 309:2033–2037.

Oh MC, Derkach VA, Guire ES, Soderling TR (2006) Extrasynaptic membrane trafficking regulated by GluR1 serine 845 phosphorylation primes AMPA receptors for long-term potentiation. *J Biol Chem* 281:752–758

Oh MM, Kuo AG, Wu WW, Sametsky EA, Disterhoft JF (2003) Watermaze learning enhances excitability of CA1 pyramidal neurons. *J Neurophysiol* 90:2171–2179.

Ohno M, Frankland PW, Chen AP, Costa RM, Silva AJ (2001) Inducible, pharmacogenetic approaches to the study of learning and memory. *Nat Neurosci* 4:1238–1243.

Ohno M, Frankland PW, Silva AJ (2002) A pharmacogenetic inducible approach to the study of NMDA/alphaCaMKII signaling in synaptic plasticity. *Curr Biol* 12:654–656.

Okada T, Yamada N, Tsuzuki K, Horikawa HP, Tanaka K, Ozawa S (2003) Long-term potentiation in the hippocampal CA1 area and dentate gyrus plays different roles in spatial learning. *Eur J Neurosci* 17:341–349.

Okamoto K-I, Nagai T, Miyawaki A, Hayashi Y (2004) Rapid and persistent modulation of actin dynamics regulates postsynaptic reorganisation underlying bidirectional plasticity. *Nat Neurosci* 7:1104–1112.

Okumoto S, Looger LL, Micheva KD, Reimer RJ, Smith SJ, Frommer WB (2005) Detection of glutamate release from neurons by genetically encoded surface-displayed FRET nanosensors. *Proc Natl Acad Sci USA* 102:8740–8745.

Oliet SHR, Malenka RC, Nicoll RA (1997) Two distinct forms of long-term depression co-exist in CA1 hippocampal pyramidal cells. *Neuron* 18:969–982.

O'Mara SM, Commins S, Anderson M (2000) Synaptic plasticity in the hippocampal area CA1-subiculum projection: implications for theories of memory. *Hippocampus* 10:447–456.

Opazo P, Watabe AM, Grant SG, O'Dell TJ (2003) Phosphatidylinositol 3-kinase regulates the induction of long-term potentiation through extracellular signal-related kinase-independent mechanisms. *J Neurosci* 3679:3679–3688.

Osten P, Srivastava S, Inman GJ, Vilim FS, Khatri L, Lee LM, States BA, Einheber S, Milner TA, Hanson PI, Ziff EB (1998) The AMPA receptor GluR2 C terminus can mediate a reversible, ATP-dependent interaction with NSF and alpha- and beta-SNAPs. *Neuron* 21:99–110.

Osten P, Khatri L, Perez JL, Kohr G, Giese G, Daly C, Schulz TW, Wensky A, Lee LM, Ziff EB (2000) Mutagenesis reveals a role for ABP/GRIP binding to GluR2 in synaptic surface accumulation of the AMPA receptor. *Neuron* 27:313–325.

Ostroff LE, Fiala JC, Allwardt B, Harris KM (2002) Polyribosomes redistribute from dendritic shafts into spines with enlarged synapses during LTP in developing rat hippocampal slices. *Neuron* 35:535–545.

Otani S, Abraham WC (1989) Inhibition of protein synthesis in the dentate gyrus, but not the entorhinal cortex, blocks maintenance of long-term potentiation in rats. *Neurosci Lett* 106:175–180.

Otani S, Marshall CJ, Tate WP, Goddard GV, Abraham WC (1989) Maintenance of long-term potentiation in rat dentate gyrus requires protein synthesis but not messenger RNA synthesis immediately post-tetanization. *Neuroscience* 28:519–526.

Otmakhova NA, Lisman JE (1996) D1/D5 dopamine receptor activation increases the magnitude of early long-term potentiation at CA1 hippocampal synapses. *J Neurosci* 16:7478–7486.

Otmakhova NA, Otmakhov N, Mortenson LH, Lisman JE (2000) Inhibition of the cAMP pathway decreases early long-term potentiation at CA1 hippocampal synapses. *J Neurosci* 20:4446–4451.

Otnaess MK, Brun VH, Moser MB, Moser EI (1999) Pretraining prevents spatial learning impairment after saturation of hippocampal long-term potentiation. *J Neurosci* 19:RC49.

Packard MG, Teather LA (1997) Posttraining injections of MK-801 produce a time-dependent impairment of memory in two watermaze tasks. *Neurobiol Learn Mem* 68:42–50.

Palmer CL, Lim W, Hastie PG, Toward M, Korolchuk VI, Burbidge SA, Banting G, Collingridge GL, Isaac JT, Henley JM (2005) Hippocalcin functions as a calcium sensor in hippocampal LTD. *Neuron* 47:487–494.

Palmer MJ, Irving AJ, Seabrook GR, Jane DE, Collingridge GL (1997) The group I mGlu receptor agonist DHPG induces a novel form of LTD in the CA1 region of the hippocampus. *Neuropharmacology* 36:1517–532.

Palmer MJ, Isaac JT, Collingridge GL (2004) Multiple, developmentally regulated expression mechanisms of long-term potentiation at CA1 synapses. *J Neurosci* 24:4903–4911.

Parent A, Linden DJ, Sisodia SS, Borchelt DR (1999) Synaptic transmission and hippocampal long-term potentiation in transgenic mice expressing FAD-linked presenilin 1. *Neurobiol Dis* 6:56–62.

Parsons CG, Danysz W, Quack G (1999) Memantine is a clinically well tolerated *N*-methyl-D-aspartate (NMDA) receptor antagonist—a review of preclinical data. *Neuropharmacology* 38:735–767.

Parsons CG, Gruner R, Rozental J, Millar J, Lodge D (1993) Patch clamp studies on the kinetics and selectivity of N-methyl-D-aspartate receptor antagonism by memantine (1-amino-3,5-dimethyladamantan). *Neuropharmacology* 32:1337–1350.

Passafaro M, Piech V, Sheng M (2001) Subunit-specific temporal and spatial patterns of AMPA receptor exocytosis in hippocampal neurons. *Nat Neurosci* 4:917–926.

Pastalkova E, Serrano P, Pinkhasova D, Wallace E, Fenton AA, Sacktor TC (2006) Storage of spatial information by the maintenance mechanism of LTP. *Science*, 313:1141–1144.

Patterson SL, Abel T, Deuel TA, Martin KC, Rose JC, Kandel ER (1996) Recombinant BDNF rescues deficits in basal synaptic transmission and hippocampal LTP in BDNF knockout mice. *Neuron* 16:1137–1145.

Paulsen O, Li Y-G, Hvalby O, Andersen P, Bliss TVP (1993) Failure to induce long-term depression by an anti-correlation procedure in area CA1 of the rat hippocampal slice. *Eur J Neurosci* 5:1241–1246.

Pelkey KA, Lavezzari G, Racca C, Roche KW, McBain CJ (2005) mGluR7 is a metaplastic switch controlling bidirectional plasticity of feedforward inhibition. *Neuron* 46:89–102.

Perez Y, Morin F, Lacaille JC (2001) A Hebbian form of long-term potentiation dependent on mGluR1a in hippocampal inhibitory interneurones. *Proc Natl Acad Sci USA* 98:9401–9406.

Petersen CCH, Malenka RC, Nicoll RA, Hopfield JJ (1998) All-or-none potentiation at CA3-CA1 synapses. *Proc Natl Acad Sci USA* 95:4732–4737.

Pettit DL, Perlman S, Malinow R (1994) Potentiated transmission and prevention of further LTP by increased CaMKII activity in postsynaptic hippocampal slice neurons. *Science* 266:1881–1885.

Philpot BD, Esinosa JS, Bear MF (2003) Evidence for enhanced NMDA receptor function as a basis for metaplasticity in visual cortex. *J Neurosci* 23:5583–5588.

Pickard L, Noel J, Duckworth JK, Fitzjohn SM, Henley JM, Collingridge GL, Molnar E (2001) Transient synaptic activation of NMDA receptors leads to the insertion of native AMPA receptors at hippocampal neuronal plasma membranes. *Neuropharmacology* 41:700–713.

Pike FG, Meredith RM, Olding AW, Pauslen O (1999) Postsynaptic bursting is essential for 'Hebbian' induction of associative long-term potentiation at excitatory synapses in rat hippocampus. *J Phyiol (Lond)* 518:571–576.

Pineda VV, Athos JI, Wang H, Celver J, Ippolito D, Boulay G, Birnbaumer L, Storm DR (2004) Removal of G(ialpha1) constraints on adenylyl cyclase in the hippocampus enhances LTP and impairs memory formation. *Neuron* 41: 153–163.

Piomelli D, Volterra A, Dale N, Siegelbaum SA, Kandel ER, Schwartz JH, Berladetti F (1987) Lipoxygenase metabolites of arachidonic acid are second messengers for presynaptic inhibition of *Aplysia* sensory cells. *Nature* 328:38–43.

Pittenger C, Huang YY, Paletzki RF, Bourtchouladze R, Scanlin H, Vronskaya S, Kandel ER (2002) Reversible inhibition of CREB/ATF transcription factors in region CA1 of the dorsal hippocampus disrupts hippocampus-dependent spatial memory. *Neuron* 34:447–462.

Plant K, Pelkey KA, Bortolotto ZA, Morita D, Terashima A, McBain CJ, Collingridge GL, Isaac JT (2006) Transient incorporation of native GluR2-lacking AMPA receptors during hippocampal long-term potentiation. *Nat Neurosci* 9:602–4.

Pokorska A, Vanhoutte P, Arnold FJL, Silvagno F, Hardingham GE, Bading H (2003) Synaptic activity induces signalling to CREB without increasing global levels of cAMP in hippocampal neurons. *J Neurochem* 84:447–452.

Poncer JC, Esteban JA, Malinow R (2002) Multiple mechanisms for the potentiation of AMPA receptor-mediated transmission by alpha-Ca^{2+}/calmodulin-dependent protein kinase II. *J Neurosci* 22:4406–4411.

Popov VI, Davies HA, Rogachevsky VV, Patrushev IV, Errington ML, Gabbott PLA, Bliss TVP, Stewart MG (2004) Remodelling of synaptic morphology but unchanged synaptic density during late phase LTP: a serial section electron micrographic study of the dentate gyrus in the anesthetized rat. *Neuroscience* 128:251–262.

Purcell AL, Carew TJ (2003) Tyrosine kinases, synaptic plasticity and memory: insights from vertebrates and invertebrates. *Trends Neurosci* 26:625–630.

Quinta-Ferreira ME, Matias CM (2004) Hippocampal mossy fiber calcium transients are maintained during long-term potentiation and are inhibited by endogenous zinc. *Brain Res* 1004: 52–60.

Racine RJ, Milgram NW, Hafner S (1983) Long-term potentiation phenomena in the rat limbic forebrain. *Brain Res* 260: 217–231.

Rae MG, Martin DJ, Collingridge GL, Irving AJ (2000) Role of Ca^{2+} stores in metabotropic L-glutamate receptor-mediated supralinear Ca^{2+} signaling in rat hippocampal neurons. *J Neurosci* 20:8628–8636.

Rajji T, Chapman D, Eichenbaum H, Greene R (2006) The role of CA3 hippocampal NMDA receptors in paired associate learning. *J Neurosci* 26:908–915.

Rammes G, Zeilhofer HU, Collingridge GL, Parsons CG, Swandulla D (1999) Expression of early hippocampal CA1 LTP does not lead to changes in AMPA-EPSC kinetics or sensitivity to cyclothiazide. *Pflugers Arch* 437:191–196.

Rammes G, Palmer M, Eder M, Dodt H-U, Zieglgansberger W, Collingridge GL (2003) Activation of mGlu receptors induces LTD without affecting postsynaptic sensitivity of CA1 neurons in rat hippocampal slices. *J Physiol* 546:455–460.

Raymond CR, Redman SJ (2006) Spatial segregation of neuronal calcium signals encodes different forms of LTP in rat hippocampus. *J Physiol (Lond)* 570:97–111.

Raymond CR, Redman SJ, Crouch MF (2002) The phosphoinositide 3-kinase and p70 S6 kinase regulate long-term potentiation in hippocampal neurons. *Neuroscience* 109:531–536.

Reid CA, Dixon D, Takahashi M, Bliss TVP, Fine A (2004) Optical quantal analysis indicates LTP at single hippocampal mossy fiber synapses is expressed through increased release probability, recruitment of new release sites and activation of silent synapses. *J Neurosci* 24:3618–3626.

Reid IC, Stewart CA (1997) Seizures, memory and synaptic plasticity. *Seizure* 6:351–359.

Reisel D, Bannerman DM, Schmitt WB, Deacon RM, Flint J, Borchardt T, Seeburg PH, Rawlins JN (2002) Spatial memory dissociations in mice lacking GluR1. *Nat Neurosci* 5:868–873.

Ribeiro S, Mello CV, Velho T, Gardner TJ, Jarvis ED, Pavlides C (2002) Induction of hippocampal long-term potentiation during waking leads to increased extrahippocampal zif-268 expression during ensuing rapid-eye-movement sleep. *J Neurosci* 22:10914–10923.

Richter-Levin G, Akirav I (2003) Emotional tagging of memory formation—in the search for neural mechanisms. *Brain Res Brain Res Rev* 43:247–256.

Richter-Levin G, Errington ML, Maegawa H, Bliss TV (1994) Activation of metabotropic glutamate receptors is necessary for long-term potentiation in the dentate gyrus and for spatial learning. *Neuropharmacology* 33:853–857.

Richter-Levin G, Canevari L, Bliss TV (1995) Long-term potentiation and glutamate release in the dentate gyrus: links to spatial learning. *Behav Brain Res* 66:37–40.

Richter-Levin G, Canevari L, Bliss TVP (1997) Spatial training and high-frequency stimulation engage a common pathway to enhance glutamate release in the hippocampus. *Learn Mem* 4:445–450.

Riedel G, Reymann K (1993) An antagonist of the metabotropic glutamate receptor prevents LTP in the dentate gyrus of freely moving rats. *Neuropharmacology* 32:929–931.

Riedel G, Platt B, Micheau J (2003) Glutamate receptor function in learning and memory. *Behav Brain Res* 140:1-47.

Rioult-Pedotti MS, Friedman D, Hess G, Donoghue JP (1998) Strengthening of horizontal cortical connections following skill learning. *Nat Neurosci* 1:230–234.

Rioult-Pedotti M-S, Friedman D, Donoghue JP (2000) Learning-induced LTP in neocortex. *Science* 290:533–536.

Roberson ED, English JD, Adams JP, Selcher JC, Kondratick C, Sweatt JD (1999) The mitogen-activated protein kinase cascade couples PKA and PKC to cAMP response element binding protein phosphorylation in area CA1 of hippocampus. *J Neurosci* 19:4337–4348.

Roberts L, Greene JR (2003) Post-weaning social isolation of rats leads to a diminution of LTP in the CA1 to subiculum pathway. *Brain Res* 991:271–273.

Roberts M, Shapiro M (2002) NMDA receptor antagonists impair memory for nonspatial, socially transmitted food preference. *Behav Neurosci* 116:1059–1069.

Rogan MT, Staubli UV, LeDoux JE (1997) Fear conditioning induces associative long-term potentiation in the amygdala. *Nature* 390:604–607.

Roman FS, Truchet B, Chaillan FA, Marchetti E, Soumireu-Mourat B (2004) Olfactory associative discrimination: a model for studying modifications of synaptic efficacy in neuronal networks supporting long-term memory. *Rev Neurosci* 15:1–17.

Romcy-Pereira R, Pavlides C (2004) Distinct modulatory effects of sleep on the maintenance of hippocampal and medial prefrontal cortex LTP. *Eur J Neurosci* 20:3453–3462.

Rose GM, Dunwiddie TV (1986) Induction of hippocampal long-term potentiation using physiologically patterned stimulation. *Neurosci Lett* 69:244–248.

Rosenblum K, Dudai Y, Richter-Levin G (1996) Long-term potentiation increases tyrosine phosphorylation of the *N*-methyl-D-aspartate receptor subunit 2B in rat dentate gyrus in vivo. *Proc Natl Acad Sci USA* 93:10457–10460.

Rosenmund C, Clements JD, Westbrook GL (1993) Nonuniform probability of glutamate release at a hippocampal synapse. *Science* 262:754–757.

Rosenzweig ES, Rao G, McNaughton BL, Barnes CA (1997) Role of temporal summation in age-related long-term potentiation-induction deficits. *Hippocampus* 7:549–558.

Rosenzweig ES, Barnes CA, McNaughton BL (2002) Making room for new memories. *Nat Neurosci* 5:6–8.

Ross FM, Allan SM, Rothwell NJ, Verkhratsky A (2003) A dual role for interleukin-1 in LTP in mouse hippocampal slices. *J Neuroimmunol* 144:61–67.

Ross ST, Soltesz I (2001) Long-term plasticity in interneurons in the dentate gyrus. *Proc Natl Acad Sci USA* 98:8874–8879.

Rostas JA, Brent VA, Voss K, Errington ML, Bliss TV, Gurd JW (1996) Enhanced tyrosine phosphorylation of the 2B subunit of the *N*-methyl-D-aspartate receptor in long-term potentiation. *Proc Natl Acad Sci USA* 93:10452–10456.

Rotenberg A, Mayford M, Hawkins RD, Kandel ER, Muller RU (1996) Mice expressing activated CaMKII lack low frequency LTP and do not form stable place cells in the CA1 region of the hippocampus. *Cell* 87:1351–1361.

Rouach N, Byrd K, Petralia RS, Elias GM, Adesnik H, Tomita S, Karimzadegan S, Kealey C, Bredt DS, Nicoll RA (2005) TARP gamma-8 controls hippocampal AMPA receptor number, distribution and synaptic plasticity. *Nat Neurosci* 8:1525–1533.

Routtenberg A, Rekart JL (2005) Post-translational protein modification as the substrate for long-term memory. *Trends Neurosci* 28:12–19.

Routtenberg A, Lovinger D (1985) Selective increase in phosphorylation of a 47 kDA protein (F1) directly related to long-term potentiation. *Behav Neural Biol* 43:3–11.

Routtenberg A, Cantallops I, Zaffuto S, Serrano P, Namgung U (2000) Enhanced learning after genetic overexpression of a brain growth protein. *Proc Natl Acad Sci USA* 97:7657–7662.

Rowan MJ, Klyubin I, Cullen WK, Anwyl R (2003) Synaptic plasticity in animal models of early Alzheimer's disease. *Philos Trans R Soc Lond B Biol Sci* 358:821–828.

Rozov A, Burnashev N (1999) Polyamine-dependent facilitation of postsynaptic AMPA receptors counteracts paired-pulse depression. *Nature* 401:594–598.

Rumbaugh G, Sia GM, Garner CC, Huganir RL (2003) Synapse-associated protein-97 isoform-specific regulation of surface AMPA receptors and synaptic function in cultured neurons. *J Neurosci* 23:4567–4576.

Rumelhart DE, Hinton GE, Williams RJ (1986) Learning representations by back-propagation errors. *Nature* 323:533–536.

Rumpel S, LeDoux J, Zador A, Malinow R (2005) Postsynaptic receptor trafficking underlying a form of associative learning. *Science* 308:83–88.

Rush AM, Wu J, Rowan MJ, Anwyl R (2002) Group I metabotropic glutamate receptor (mGluR)-dependent long-term depression mediated via p38 mitogen-activated protein kinase is inhibited by previous high-frequency stimulation and activation of mGluRs and protein kinase C in the rat dentate gyrus in vitro. *J Neurosci* 22:6121–6128.

Sabatini BL, Oertner TG, Svoboda K (2002) The life cycle of Ca(2+) ions in dendritic spines. *Neuron* 33:439–52.

Sacchetti B, Lorenzini CA, Baldi E, Bucherelli C, Roberto M, Tassoni G, Brunelli M (2001) Long-lasting hippocampal potentiation and contextual memory consolidation. *Eur J Neurosci* 13:2291–2298.

Sacchetti B, Lorenzini CA, Baldi E, Bucherelli C, Roberto M, Tassoni G, Brunelli M (2002) Time-dependent inhibition of hippocampal LTP in vitro following contextual fear conditioning in the rat. *Eur J Neurosci* 15:143–150.

Sacchetti B, Scelfo B, Tempia F, Strata P (2004) Long-term synaptic changes induced in the cerebellar cortex by fear conditioning. *Neuron* 42:973–982.

Sacktor TC, Osten P, Valsamis H, Jiang X, Naik MU, Sublette E (1993) Persistent activation of the zeta isoform of protein kinase C in the maintenance of long-term potentiation. *Proc Natl Acad Sci U S A* 90:8342–8346.

Sajikumar S, Frey JU (2004a) Resetting of 'synaptic tags' is time- and activity dependent in rat hippocampal CA1 in vitro. *Neuroscience* 129:503–507.

Sajikumar S, Frey JU (2004b) Late-associativity, synaptic tagging, and the role of dopamine during LTP and LTD. *Neurobiol Learn Mem* 82:12–25.

Sajikumar S, Navakkode S, Sacktor TC, Frey JU (2005) Synaptic tagging and cross-tagging: the role of protein kinase Mzeta in maintaining long-term potentiation but not long-term depression. *J Neurosci* 25:5750–5756.

Sakamoto T, Porter LL, Asanuma H (1987) Long-lasting potentiation of s ynaptic potentials in the motor cortex produced by stimulation of the sensory cortex in the cat: a basis of motor learning. *Brain Res* 413:360–364.

Sakimura K, Kutsuwada T, Ito I, Manabe T, Takayama C, Kushiya E, Yagi T, Aizawa S, Inoue Y, Sugiyama H, et al. (1995) Reduced hippocampal LTP and spatial learning in mice lacking NMDA receptor epsilon 1 subunit. Nature 373:151–155.

Salin PA, Weisskopf MG, Nicoll RA (1995) A comparison of the role of dynorphin in the hippocampal mossy fiber pathway in guinea-pig and rat. *J Neurosci* 15:6939–6945.

Salin PA, Scanziani M, Malenka RC, Nicoll RA (1996) Distinct short-term plasticity at two excitatory synapses in the hippocampus. *Proc Natl Acad Sci USA* 93:13304–13309.

Salt TE (1986) Mediation of thalamic sensory input by both NMDA receptors and non-NMDA receptors. *Nature* 322:263–265.

Salt TE, Eaton SA (1989) Function of non-NMDA receptors and NMDA receptors in synaptic responses to natural somatosensory stimulation in the ventrobasal thalamus. *Exp Brain Res* 77:646–652.

Sanes JR, Lichtman JW (1999) Can molecules explain long-term potentiation? *Nat Neurosci* 2:597–604.

Sanna PP, Cammalleri M, Berton F, Simpson C, Lutjens R, Bloom FE, Francesconi W (2002) Phosphatidylinositol 3-kinase is required for the expression but not for the induction or the maintenance of long-term potentiation in the hippocampal CA1 region. *J Neurosci* 22:3359–3365.

Sastry BR, Goh JW, Auyeung A (1986) Associative induction of post-tetanic and long-term potentiation in CA1 neurons of rat hippocampus. *Science* 232:988–990.

Saucier D, Cain DP (1995) Spatial learning without NMDA receptor-dependent long-term potentiation. *Nature* 378:186–189.

Saucier D, Hargreaves EL, Boon F, Vanderwolf CH, Cain DP (1996) Detailed behavioral analysis of watermaze acquisition under systemic NMDA or muscarinic antagonism: nonspatial pretraining eliminates spatial learning deficits. *Behav Neurosci* 110: 103–116.

Scammell TE, Arrigoni E, Thompson MA, Ronan PJ, Saper CB, Greene RW (2003) Focal deletion of the adenosine A1 receptor in adult mice using an adeno-associated viral vector. *J Neurosci* 23:5762–5770.

Scanziani M, Malenka RC, Nicoll RA (1996) Role of intercellular interactions in heterosynaptic long-term depression. *Nature* 380:446–450.

Scattton B, Simon H, Le Moal M, Bischoff S (1980) Origin of dopaminergic innervation of the rat hippocampal formation. *Neurosci Lett* 18:125–131.

Schinder AF, Gage FH (2004) A hypothesis about the role of adult neurogenesis in hippocampal function. *Physiology (Bethesda)* 19:253–261.

Schinder AF, Poo M-M (2000) The neurotrophin hypothesis for synaptic plasticity. *Trends Neurosci* 23:639–645.

Schmidt-Hieber C, Jonas P, Bischofberger J (2004) Enhanced synaptic plasticity in newly generated granule cells of the adult hippocampus. *Nature* 429:184–187.

Schmitt WB, Sprengel R, Mack V, Draft RW, Seeburg PH, Deacon RM, Rawlins JN, Bannerman DM (2005) Restoration of spatial working memory by genetic rescue of GluR-A-deficient mice. *Nat Neurosci* 8:270–272.

Schmitz D, Mellor J, Nicoll RA (2001) Presynaptic kainate receptor mediation of frequency facilitation at hippocampal mossy fiber synapses. *Science* 291:1972–1976.

Schmitz D, Mellor J, Breustedt J, Nicoll RA (2003) Presynaptic kainate receptors impart an associative property to hippocampal mossy fiber long-term potentiation. *Nat Neurosci* 6: 1058–1063.

Schnabel R, Kilpatrick IC, Collingridge GL (1999) An investigation into signal transduction mechanisms involved in DHPG-induced LTD in the CA1 region of the hippocampus. *Neuropharmacology* 38:1585–1596.

Schnabel R, Kilpatrick IC, Collingridge GL (2001) Protein phosphatase inhibitors facilitate DHPG-induced LTD in the CA1 region of the hippocampus. *Br J Pharmacol* 132:1095–1101.

Schneider I, Reverse D, Dewachter I, Ris L, Caluwaerts N, Kuiperi C, Gilis M, Geerts H, Kretzschmar H, Godaux E, Moechars D, Van Leuven F, Herms J (2001) Mutant presenilins disturb neuronal calcium homeostasis in the brain of transgenic mice, decreasing the threshold for excitotoxicity and facilitating long-term potentiation. *J Biol Chem* 276:11539–11544.

Schroeder BW, Shinnick-Gallagher P (2005) Fear learning induces persistent facilitation of amygdala synaptic transmission. *Eur J Neurosci* 22:1775–1783.

Schubert M, Siegmund H, Pape HC, Albrecht D (2005) Kindling-induced changes in plasticity of the rat amygdala and hippocampus. *Learn Mem* 12:520–526.

Schulz PE, Cook EP, Johnston D (1994) Changes in paired-pulse facilitation suggest presynaptic involvement in long-term potentiation. *J Neurosci* 14:5325–5337.

Schuman EM, Madison DV (1991) A requirement of the intercellular messenger nitric oxide in long-term potentiation. *Science* 254:1503–1506.

Schwartzkroin PA, Wester K (1975) Long-lasting facilitation of a synaptic potential following tetanization in the in vitro hippocampal slice. *Brain Res* 89:107–119.

Seabrook GR, Smith DW, Bowery BJ, Easter A, Reynolds T, Fitzjohn SM, Morton RA, Zheng H, Dawson GR, Sirinathsinghji DJ, Davies CH, Collingridge GL, Hill RG (1999) Mechanisms contributing to the deficits in hippocampal synaptic plasticity in mice lacking amyloid precursor protein. *Neuropharmacology* 38:349–359.

Segal M, Auerbach JM (1997) Muscarinic receptors involved in hippocampal plasticity. *Life Sci* 13/14:1085–1091.

Seidenbecher T, Balschun D, Reymann KG (1995) Drinking after water deprivation prolongs unsaturated LTP in the dentate gyrus of rats. *Physiol Behav* 57:1001–1004.

Sejnowski TJ (1977) Storing covariance with nonlinearly interacting neurons. *J Math Biol* 4:303–321.

Selig DK, Hjelmstad GO, Herron C, Nicoll RA, Malenka RC (1995a) Independent mechanisms for long-term depression of AMPA and NMDA responses. *Neuron* 15:417–426.

Selig DK, Lee HK, Bear MF, Malenka RC (1995b) Reexamination of the effects of MCPG on hippocampal LTP, LTD, and depotentiation. *J Neurophysiol* 74:1075–1082.

Selig DK, Nicoll RA, Malenka RC (1999) Hippocampal long-term potentiation preserves the fidelity of postsynaptic responses to presynaptic bursts. *J Neurosci* 19:1236–1246.

Sergueeva OA, Fedorov NB, Reymann KG (1993) An antagonist of glutamate metabotropic receptors, (RS)-alpha-methyl-4-arboxyphenylglycine, prevents the LTP-related increase in postsynaptic AMPA sensitivity in hippocampal slices. *Neuropharmacology* 32:933–935.

Serrano P, Yao Y, Sacktor TC (2005) Persistent phosphorylation by protein kinase Mzeta maintains late-phase long-term potentiation. *J Neurosci* 25:1979–1984.

Sevelinges Y, Gervais R, Messaoudi B, Granjon L, Mouly AM (2004) Olfactory fear conditioning induces field potential potentiation in rat olfactory cortex and amygdala. *Learn Mem* 11:761–769.

Sharp PE, McNaughton BL, Barnes CA (1989) Exploration-ependent modulation of evoked response in fascia dentata: fundamental observations and time-course. *Psychobiology* 17:257–269.

Shew T, Yip S, Sastry BR (2000) Mechanisms involved in tetanus-induced potentiation of fast IPSCs in rat hippocampal CA1 neurons. *J Neurophysiol* 83:3388–3401.

Shi S, Hayashi Y, Esteban JA, Malinow R (2001) Subunit-specific rules governing AMPA receptor trafficking to synapses in hippocampal pyramidal neurons. *Cell* 105:331–343.

Shi SH, Hayashi Y, Petralia RS, Zaman SH, Wenthold RJ, Svoboda K, Malinow R (1999) Rapid spine delivery and redistribution of AMPA receptors after synaptic NMDA receptor activation. *Science* 284:1811–1816.

Shimizu E, Tang YP, Rampon C, Tsien JZ (2000) NMDA receptor-dependent synaptic reinforcement as a crucial process for memory consolidation. *Science* 290:1170–1174.

Shors TJ, Matzel LD (1997) Long-term potentiation: what's learning got to do with it? *Behav Brain Sciences* 20:597–655.

Shors TJ, Seib TB, Levine S, Thompson RF (1989) Inescapable versus escapable shock modulates long-term potentiation in the rat hippocampus. *Science* 244:224–226.

Shors TJ, Miesegaes G, Beylin A, Zhao M, Rydel T, Gould E (2001) Neurogenesis in the adult is involved in the formation of trace memories. *Nature* 410:372–376.

Shors TJ, Townsend DA, Zhao M, Kozorovitskiy Y, Gould E (2002) Neurogenesis may relate to some but not all types of hippocampal-dependent learning. *Hippocampus* 12:578–584.

Shouval HZ, Bear MF, Cooper LN (2002) A unified model of NMDA receptor-dependent bidirectional synaptic plasticity. *Proc Natl Acad Sci USA* 99:10831–10836.

Si K, Lindquist S, Kandel ER (2003) A neuronal isoform of the aplysia CPEB has prion-like properties. *Cell* 115:879–891.

Siarey RJ, Stoll J, Rapoport SI, Galdzicki Z (1997) Altered long-term potentiation in the young and old Ts65Dn mouse, a model for Down syndrome. *Neuropharmacology* 36:1549–1554.

Siarey RJ, Carlson EJ, Epstein CJ, Balbo A, Rapoport SI, Galdzicki Z (1999) Increased synaptic depression in the Ts65Dn mouse, a model for mental retardation in Down syndrome. *Neuropharmacology* 38:1917–1920.

Siarey RJ, Villar AJ, Epstein CJ, Galdzicki Z (2005) Abnormal synaptic plasticity in the Ts1Cje segmental trisomy 16 mouse model of Down syndrome. *Neuropharmacology* 49:122–128.

Sillito AM (1985) Inhibitory circuits and orientation selectivity in the visual cortex. In: *Models of the visual cortex* (Dobson DRaVG, ed), pp 396–407. New York: Wiley.

Silva AJ, Paylor R, Wehner JM, Tonegawa S (1992a) Impaired spatial learning in alpha-calcium calmodulin kinase II mutant mice. *Science* 257:206–211.

Silva AJ, Stevens CF, Tonegawa S, Wang Y (1992b) Deficient hippocampal long-term potentiation in alpha-calcium-calmodulin kinase II mutant mice. *Science* 257:201–206.

Simonyi A, Schachtman TR, Christoffersen GR (2005) The role of metabotropic glutamate receptor 5 in learning and memory processes. *Drug News Perspect* 18:353–361.

Singer W (1990) The formation of cooperative cell assemblies in the visual cortex. *J Exp Biol* 153:177–197.

Skrede KKR, Westgaard RH (1971) The transverse hippocampal slice: a well-defined cortical structure maintained in vitro. *Brain Res* 35:589–593.

Snyder EM, Philpot BD, Huber KM, Dong X, Fallon JR, Bear MF (2001) Internalization of ionotropic glutamate receptors in response to mGluR activation. *Nat Neurosci* 4: 1079–1085.

Soderling TR, Derkach VA (2000) Postsynaptic protein phosphorylation and LTP. *Trends Neurosci* 23:75–80.

Sokolov MV, Rossokhin AV, Kasyanov A, Gasparini S, Berretta N, Cherubini E, Voronin L (2003) Associative mossy fiber LTP induced by pairing presynaptic stimulation with postsynaptic hyperpolarization of CA3 neurons in rat hippocampal slice. *Eur J Neurosci* 17:1425–1437.

Son H, Hawkins RD, Martin K, Kiebler M, Huang PL, Fishman MC, Kandel ER (1996) Long-term potentiation is reduced in mice that are doubly mutant in endothelial and neuronal nitric oxide synthase. *Cell* 87:1015–1023.

Song H, Stevens CF, Gage FH (2002) Neural stem cells from adult hippocampus develop essential properties of functional CNS neurons. *Nat Neurosci* 5:438–445.

Song I, Kamboj S, Xia J, Dong H, Liao D, Huganir RL (1998) Interaction of the *N*-ethylmaleimide-sensitive factor with AMPA receptors. *Neuron* 21:393–400.

Song S, Miller KD, Abbott LF (2000) Competitive Hebbian learning through spike-timing-dependent synaptic plasticity. *Nat Neurosci* 3:919–926.

Sorra KE, Harris KM (1998) Stability in synapse number and size at 2 hr after long-term potentiation in the hippocampus. *J Neurosci* 18:658–671.

Sourdet V, Russier M, Daoudal G, Ankri N, Debanne D (2003) Long-term enhancement of neuronal excitability and temporal fidelity mediated by metabotropic glutamate receptor subtype 5. *J Neurosci* 23:10238–10248.

Spangenberger H, Nikmanesh FG, Igelmund P (1995) Long-term potentiation at low temperature is stronger in hippocampal slices from hibernating Turkish hamsters compared to warm-acclimated hamsters and rats. *Neurosci Lett* 194:127–129.

Sprengel R, Suchanek B, Amico C, Brusa R, Burnashev N, Rozov A, Hvalby O, Jensen V, Paulsen O, Andersen P, Kim JJ, Thompson RF, Sun W, Webster LC, Grant SG, Eilers J, Konnerth A, Li J, McNamara JO, Seeburg PH (1998) Importance of the intracellular domain of NR2 subunits for NMDA receptor function in vivo. *Cell* 92:279–289.

Squire LR, Barondes SH (1972) Variable decay of memory and its recovery in cycloheximide-treated mice. *Proc Natl Acad Sci USA* 69:1416–1420.

Srivastava S, Ziff EB (1999) ABP: a novel AMPA receptor binding protein. *Ann NY Acad Sci* 868:561–564.

Staff NP, Spruston N (2003) Intracellular correlate of EPSP-spike potentiation in CA1 pyramidal neurons is controlled by GABAergic modulation. *Hippocampus* 13:801–805.

Stanton PK, Sejnowski TJ (1989) Associative long-term depression in the hippocampus induced by Hebbian covariance. *Nature* 339:215–218.

Stanton PK, Sarvey JM (1985) Depletion of norepinephrine, but not serotonin, reduces long-term potentiation in the dentate gyrus of rat hippocampal slices. *J Neurosci* 5:2169–2176.

Stanton PK, Heinemann U, Muller W (2001) FM1-43 imaging reveals cGMP-dependent long-term depression of presynaptic transmitter release. *J Neurosci* 21:RC167.

Stanton PK, Winterer J, Bailey CP, Kyrozis A, Raginor I, Laube G, Veh RW, Nguyen CP, Muller W (2003) Long-term depression of presynaptic release from the readily releasable vesicle pool induced by NMDA receptor-dependent retrograde nitric oxide. J Neurosci 23:5935–5944.

Stanton PK, Winterer J, Zhang XL, Muller W (2005) Imaging LTP of presynaptic release of FM1-43 from the rapidly recycling vesicle pool of Schaffer collateral-CA1 synapses in rat hippocampal slices. *Eur J Neurosci* 22:2451–2461.

Staubli U, Chun D (1996) Factors regulating the reversibility of long-term potentiation. *J Neurosci* 16:853–860.

Staubli U, Lynch G (1987) Stable hippocampal long-term potentiation elicited by theta-pattern stimulation. *Brain Res* 435:227–234.

Staubli U, Lynch G (1990) Stable depression of potentiated synaptic responses in the hippocampus with 1-5 Hz stimulation. *Brain Res* 513:113–118.

Staubli U, Xu FB (1995) Effects of 5-HT3 receptor antagonism on hippocampal theta rythm, memory and LTP induction in the freely moving rat. *J Neurosci Methods* 15:2445–2452.

Staubli U, Ivy G, Lynch G (1984) Hippocampal denervation causes rapid forgetting of olfactory information in rats. *Proc Natl Acad Sci USA* 81:5885–5887.

Staubli U, Thibault O, DiLorenzo M, Lynch G (1989) Antagonism of NMDA receptors impairs acquisition but not retention of olfactory memory. *Behav Neurosci* 103:54–60.

Staubli U, Perez Y, Xu FB, Rogers G, Ingvar M, Stone Elander S, Lynch G (1994) Centrally active modulators of glutamate receptors facilitate the induction of long-term potentiation in vivo. *Proc Nat Acad of Sci USA* 91:11158–11162.

Staubli U, Chun D, Lynch G (1998) Time-dependent reversal of long-term potentiation by an integrin antagonist. *J Neurosci* 18:3460–3469.

Steele RJ, Morris RG (1999) Delay-dependent impairment of a matching-to-place task with chronic and intrahippocampal infusion of the NMDA-antagonist D-AP5. *Hippocampus* 9:118–136.

Stein V, House DR, Bredt DS, Nicoll RA (2003) Postsynaptic density-95 mimics and occludes hippocampal long-term potentiation and enhances long-term depression. *J Neurosci* 23:5503–5506.

Stellwagen D, Malenka RC (2006) Synaptic scaling mediated by glial TNF-alpha. *Nature* 440:1054–1059.

Stent GS (1973) A physiological mechanism for Hebb's postulate of learning. *Proc Natl Acad Sci USA* 70:997–1001.

Stephan A, Laroche S, Davis S (2001) Generation of aggregated beta-amyloid in the rat hippocampus impairs synaptic transmission and plasticity and causes memory deficits. *J Neurosci* 21:5703-5714.

Stevens CF (1998) A million dollar question: does LTP = memory? *Neuron* 20:1–2.

Stevens CF, Wang Y (1993) Reversal of long-term potentiation by inhibitors of haem oxygenase. *Nature* 364:147–149.

Stevens CF, Wang Y (1994) Changes in reliability of synaptic function as a mechanism for plasticity. *Nature* 371:704–707.

Steward O (1983) Alterations in polyribosomes associated with dendritic spines during the reinnervation of the dentate gyrus of the adult rat. *J Neurosci* 3:177–188.

Steward O, Schuman E (2001) Protein synthesis at synaptic sites on dendrites. *Annu Rev Neurosci* 24:299–235.

Steward O, Schuman EM (2003) Compartmentalized synthesis and degradation of proteins in neurons. *Neuron* 40:347–359.

Straube T, Frey JU (2003) Time-dependent depotentiation in the dentate gyrus of freely moving rats by repeated brief 7 Hz stimulation. *Neurosci Lett* 339:82–84.

Straube T, Korz V, Balschun D, Frey JU (2003) Requirement of beta-adrenergic receptor activation and protein synthesis for LTP-reinforcement by novelty in rat dentate gyrus. *J Phyiol (Lond)* 552:953–960.

Stringer JL, Greenfield LJ, Hackett JT, Guyenet PG (1983) Blockade of long-term potentiation by phencyclidine and sigma opiates in the hippocampus in vivo and in vitro. *Brain Res* 280:127–138.

Stuart GJ, Sakmann B (1994) Active propagation of somatic action potentials into neocortical pyramidal cell dendrites. *Nature* 367:69–72.

Sun MK, Alkon DL (2002) Impairment of hippocampal CA1 heterosynaptic transformation and spatial memory by beta-amyloid(25-35). *J Neurophysiol* 87:2441–2449.

Sun MK, Alkon DL (2005) Protein kinase C isozymes: memory therapeutic potential. *Curr Drug Targets CNS Neurol Disord* 4:541–552.

Sutherland RJ, Dringenberg HC, Hoesing JM (1993) Induction of long-term potentiation at perforant path dentate synapses does not affect place learning or memory. *Hippocampus* 3:141–147.

Sweatt JD (2001a) Protooncogenes subserve memory formation in the adult CNS. *Neuron* 31:671–674.

Sweatt JD (2001b) The neuronal MAP kinase cascade: a biochemical signal integration system subserving synaptic plasticity and memory. *J Neurochem* 76:1–10.

Sweatt JD (2004) Mitogen-activated protein kinases in synaptic plasticity and memory. *Curr Opin Neurobiol* 14:311–317.

Talwar SK, Gerstein GL (2001) Reorganization in awake rat auditory cortex by local microstimulation and its effect on frequency-discrimination behavior. *J Neurophysiol* 86:1555–1572.

Tanaka H, Shan W, Phillips GR, Arndt K, Bozdaghi O, Shapiro L, Huntley GW, Benson DL, Colman DR (2000) Molecular modification of N-cadherin in response to synaptic activity. *Neuron* 25:93–107.

Tancredi V, Zona C, Velotti F, Eusebi F, Santoni A (1990) Interleukin-2 suppresses established long-term potentiation and inhibits its induction in the rat hippocampus. *Brain Res* 525:149–151.

Tancredi V, D'Arcangelo G, Grassi F, Tarroni P, Palmieri G, Santoni A, Eusebi F (1992) Tumor necrosis factor alters synaptic transmission in rat hippocampal slices. *Neurosci Lett* 146:176–178.

Tang J, Wotjak CT, Wagner S, Williams G, Schachner M, Dityatev A (2001) Potentiated amygdaloid auditory-evoked potentials and freezing behavior after fear conditioning in mice. *Brain Res* 919:232–241.

Tang J, Wagner S, Schachner M, Dityatev A, Wotjak CT (2003) Potentiation of amygdaloid and hippocampal auditory evoked potentials in a discriminatory fear-conditioning task in mice as a function of tone pattern and context. *Eur J Neurosci* 18:639–650.

Tang L, Hung CP, Schuman EM (1998) A role for the cadherin family of cell adhesion molecules in hippocampal long-term potentiation. *Neuron* 20:1165–1175.

Tang YG, Zucker RS (1997) Mitochondrial involvement in post-tetanic potentiation of synaptic transmission. *Neuron* 18:483–491.

Tang Y-P, Shimizu E, Dube GR, Rampon C, Kerchner GA, Zhuo M, Liu G, Tsien JZ (1999) Genetic enhancement of learning and memory in mice. *Nature* 401:63–69.

Tao H, Zhang LI, Bi G, Poo M-M (2000) Selective presynaptic propagation of long-term potentiation in defined neural networks. *J Neurosci* 20:3233–3243.

Tardin C, Cognet L, Bats C, Lounis B, Choquet D (2003) Direct imaging of lateral movements of AMPA receptors inside synapses. *EMBO J* 22:4656–4665.

Tashiro A, Yuste R (2003) Structure and molecular organization of dendritic spines. *Histol Histopathol* 18:617–634.

Terashima A, Cotton L, Dev KK, Meyer G, Zaman S, Duprat F, Henley JM, Collingridge GL, Isaac JT (2004) Regulation of synaptic strength and AMPA receptor subunit composition by PICK1. *J Neurosci* 24:5381–5390.

Thiels E, Barrionuevo G, Berger T (1994) Excitatory stimulation during postsynaptic inhibition induces long-term depression in hippocampus in vivo. *J Neurophysiol* 72:3009–3116.

Thiels E, Norman ED, Barrionuevo G, Klann E (1998) Transient and persistent increases in protein phosphatase activity during long-term depression in the adult hippocampus in vivo. *Neuroscience* 86:1023–1029.

Thiels E, Kanterewicz BI, Norman ED, Trzaskos JM, Klann E (2002) Long-term depression in the adult hippocampus in vivo involves activation of extracellular signal-regulated kinase and phosphorylation of Elk-1. *J Neurosci* 22:2054–2062.

Thomas GM, Huganir RL (2004) MAPK cascade signalling and synaptic plasticity. *Nat Rev Neurosci* 5:173–183.

Thomas KL, Laroche S, Errington ML, Bliss TV, Hunt SP (1994) Spatial and temporal changes in signal transduction pathways during LTP. *Neuron* 13:737–745.

Thomas MJ, O'Dell TJ (1995) The molecular switch hypothesis fails to explain the inconsistent effects of the metabotropic glutamate receptor antagonist MCPG on long-term potentiation. *Brain Res* 695:45–52.

Thomas MJ, Watabe AM, Moody TD, Makhinson M, O'Dell TJ (1998) Postsynaptic complex spike bursting enables the induction of theta frequency synaptic stimulation. *J Neurosci* 18:7118–7126.

Tiedtke PI, Bischoff C, Schmidt WJ (1990) MK-801-induced stereotypy and its antagonism by neuroleptic drugs. *J Neural Transm Gen Sect* 81:173–182.

Togashi H, Abe K, Mizoguchi A, Takaoka K, Chisaka O, Takeichi M (2002) Cadherin regulates dendritic spine morphogenesis. *Neuron* 35:77–89.

Tombaugh GC, Rowe WB, Chow AR, Michael TH, Rose GM (2002) Theta-frequency synaptic potentiation in CA1 in vitro distinguishes cognitively impaired from unimpaired aged Fischer 344 rats. *J Neurosci* 22:9932–9940.

Tomita S, Adesnik H, Sekiguchi M, Zhang W, Wada K, Howe JR, Nicoll RA, Bredt DS (2005) Stargazin modulates AMPA receptor gating and trafficking by distinct domains. *Nature* 435:1052–1058.

Tomita S, Fukata M, Nicoll RA, Bredt DS (2004) Dynamic interaction of stargazin-like TARPs with cycling AMPA receptors at synapses. *Science* 303:1508–1511.

Tong G, Malenka RC, Nicoll RA (1996) Long-term potentiation in cultures of single hippocampal granule cells: a presynaptic form of plasticity. *Neuron* 16:1147–1157.

Tong L, Thornton PL, Balazs R, Cotman CW (2001) Beta -amyloid-(1-42) impairs activity-dependent cAMP-response element-binding protein signaling in neurons at concentrations in which cell survival Is not compromised. *J Biol Chem* 276:17301–17306.

Toni N, Buchs PA, Nikonenko I, Bron CR, Muller D (1999) LTP promotes formation of multiple spine synapses between a single axon terminal and a dendrite. *Nature* 402:421–425.

Tonkiss J, Rawlins JNP (1991) The competitive NMDA antagonist AP5, but not the noncompetitive antagonist MK801, induces a delay-related impairment in spatial working memory in rats. *Exp Brain Res* 85:349–358.

Tonkiss J, Morris RGM, Rawlins JNP (1988) Intra-ventricular infusion of the NMDA antagonist AP5 impairs performance on a non-spatial operant DRL task in the rat. *Exp Brain Res* 73:181–188.

Trachtenberg JT, Chen BE, Knott GW, Feng G, Sanes JR, Welker E, Svoboda K (2002) Long-term in vivo imaging of experience-dependent synaptic plasticity in adult cortex. *Nature* 420:788–794.

Tricklebank MD, Singh L, Oles RJ, Preston C, Iversen SD (1989) The behavioural effects of MK-801: a comparison with antagonists acting non-competitively and competitively at the NMDA receptor. *Eur J Pharmacol* 167:127–135.

Trommald M, Hulleberg G, Andersen P (1996) Long-term potentiation is associated with new excitatory spine synapses on rat dentate granule cells. *Learn Mem* 3:218–228.

Trommer BL, Shah C, Yun SH, Gamkrelidze G, Pasternak ES, Ye GL, Sotak M, Sullivan PM, Pasternak JF, LaDu MJ (2004) ApoE isoform affects LTP in human targeted replacement mice. *Neuroreport* 15:2655–2658.

Tsien JZ, Chen DF, Gerber D, Tom C, Mercer EH, Anderson DJ, Mayford M, Kandel ER, Tonegawa S (1996a) Subregion-and cell type-restricted gene knockout in mouse brain. *Cell* 87:1317–1326.

Tsvetkov E, Carlezon WA, Benes FM, Kandel ER, Bolshakov VY (2002) Fear conditioning occludes LTP-induced presynaptic enhancement of synaptic transmission in the cortical pathway to the lateral amygdala. *Neuron* 34:289–300.

Turrigiano GG, Nelson SB (2004) Homeostatic plasticity in the developing nervous system. *Nat Rev Neurosci* 5:97–107.

Turski L, Klockgether T, Turski WA, Schwarz M, Sontag KH (1990) Blockade of excitatory neurotransmission in the globus pallidus induces rigidity and akinesia in the rat: implications for excitatory neurotransmission in pathogenesis of Parkinson's diseases. *Brain Res* 512:125–131.

Tzounopoulos T, Janz R, Sudhof TC, Nicoll RA, Malenka RC (1998) A role for cAMP in long-term depression at hippocampal mossy fiber synapses. *Neuron* 21:837–845.

Ueno S, Tsukamoto M, Hirano T, Kikuchi K, Yamada MK, Nishiyama N, Nagano T, Matsuki N, Ikegaya Y (2002) Mossy fiber Zn^{2+} spillover modulates heterosynaptic N-methyl-D-aspartate receptor activity in hippocampal CA3 circuits. *J Cell Biol* 158:215–220.

Uetani N, Kato K, Ogura H, Mizuno K, Kawano K, Mikoshiba K, Yakura H, Asano M, Iwakura Y (2000) Impaired learning with enhanced hippocampal long-term potentiation in PTPdelta-deficient mice. *EMBO J* 19:2775–2785.

Urban NN, Barrionuevo G (1996) Induction of Hebbian and non-Hebbian mossy fiber long-term potentiation by distinct patterns of high-frequency stimulation. *J Neurosci* 16:4293–4299.

Urban NN, Henze DA, Lewis DA, Barrionuevo G (1996) Properties of LTP induction in the CA3 region of the primate hippocampus. *Learn Mem* 3:86–95.

Usdin MT, Shelbourne PF, Myers RM, Madison DV (1999) Impaired synaptic plasticity in mice carrying the Huntington's disease mutation. *Hum Mol Genet* 8:839–846.

Vaillend C, Billard JM, Laroche S (2004) Impaired long-term spatial and recognition memory and enhanced CA1 hippocampal LTP in the dystrophin-deficient Dmd(mdx) mouse. *Neurobiol Dis* 17:10–20.

Valastro B, Ghribi O, Poirier J, Krzywkowski P, Massicotte G (2001) AMPA receptor regulation and LTP in the hippocampus of young and aged apolipoprotein E-deficient mice. *Neurobiol Aging* 22:9–15.

Valastro B, Cossette J, Lavoie N, Gagnon S, Trudeau F, Massicotte G (2002) Up-regulation of glutamate receptors is associated with LTP defects in the early stages of diabetes mellitus. *Diabetologia* 45:642–650.

Van Harreveld A, Fifkova E (1975) Swelling of dendritic spines in the fascia dentata after stimulation of the perforant fibers as a mechanism of post-tetanic potentiation. *Exp Neurol* 49: 736–749.

Van Praag H, Christie BR, Sejnowski TJ, Gage FH (1999) Running enhances neurogenesis, learning and long-term potentiation in mice. *Proc Natl Acad Sci USA* 96:13427–13431.

Vereker E, Campbell V, Roche E, McEntee E, Lynch MA (2000a) Lipopolysaccharide inhibits long term potentiation in the rat dentate gyrus by activating caspase-1. *J Biol Chem* 275: 26252–26258.

Vereker E, O'Donnell E, Lynch MA (2000b) The inhibitory effect of interleukin-1beta on long-term potentiation is coupled with increased activity of stress-activated protein kinases. *J Neurosci* 20:6811–6819.

Vereker E, O'Donnell E, Lynch A, Kelly A, Nolan Y, Lynch MA (2001) Evidence that interleukin-1beta and reactive oxygen species production play a pivotal role in stress-induced impairment of LTP in the rat dentate gyrus. *Eur J Neurosci* 14:1809–1819.

Vickers CA, Dickson KS, Wyllie DJ (2005) Induction and maintenance of late-phase long-term potentiation in isolated dendrites of rat hippocampal CA1 pyramidal neurones. *J Physiol (Lond)* 568:803–813.

Vignes M, Collingridge GL (1997) The synaptic activation of kainate receptors. *Nature* 388:179–182.

Villani F, Johnston D (1993) Serotonin inhibits induction of long-term potentiation at commissural synapses in hippocampus. *Brain Res* 606:304–308.

Villarreal DM, Do V, Haddad E, Derrick BE (2001) NMDA receptor antagonists sustain LTP and spatial memory: active processes mediate LTP decay. *Nat Neurosci* 5:48–52.

Volianskis A, Jensen MS (2003) Transient and sustained types of long-term potentiation in the CA1 area of the rat hippocampus. *J Physiol (Lond)* 550:459–492.

Walling SG, Harley CW (2004) Locus ceruleus activation initiates delayed synaptic potentiation of perforant path input to the dentate gyrus in awake rats: a novel beta-adrenergic- and protein synthesis-dependent mammalian plasticity mechanism. *J Neurosci* 24:598–604.

Walsh DM, Klyubin I, Fadeeva JV, Cullen WK, Anwyl R, Wolfe MS, Rowan MJ, Selkoe DJ (2002) Naturally secreted oligomers of amyloid beta protein potently inhibit hippocampal long-term potentiation in vivo. *Nature* 416:535–539.

Wang HW, Pasternak JF, Kuo H, Ristic H, Lambert MP, Chromy B, Viola KL, Klein WL, Stine WB, Krafft GA, Trommer BL (2002) Soluble oligomers of beta amyloid (1-42) inhibit long-term potentiation but not long-term depression in rat dentate gyrus. *Brain Res* 924:133–140.

Wang JH, Alger BE (1995) GABAergic and developmental influences on homosynaptic LTD and depotentiation in rat hippocampus. *J Neurosci* 15:1577–1586.

Wang Z, Xu N-I, Wu C-P, Duan S, Poo M-M (2003) Bidirectional changes in spatial dendritic integration accompany long-term synaptic modifications. *Neuron* 37:463–472.

Warren SG, Humphreys AG, Juraska JM, Greenough WT (1995) LTP varies across the estrous cycle: enhanced synaptic plasticity in proestrus rats. *Brain Res* 703:26–30.

Wasling P, Hanse E, Gustafsson B (2002) Long-term depression in the developing hippocampus: low induction threshold and synapse nonspecificity. *J Neurosci* 22:1823–1830.

Watabe AM, Carlisle HJ, O'Dell TJ (2002) Postsynaptic induction and presynaptic expression of group 1 mGlurR-dependent LTD in the hippocampal CA1 region. *J Neurophysiol* 87:1395–1403.

Wathey JC, Lytton WW, Jester JM, Sejnowski TJ (1992) Computer simulations of EPSP-spike (E-s) potentiation in hippocampal CA1 pyramidal cells. *J Neurosci* 12:607–618.

Weinberger NM (2004) Specific long-term memory traces in primary auditory cortex. *Nat Rev Neurosci* 5:279–290.

Weiss JH, Koh JY, Christine CW, Choi DW (1989) Zinc and LTP. *Nature* 338:212.

Weisskopf MG, Nicoll RA (1995) Presynaptic changes during mossy fiber LTP revealed by NMDA receptor-mediated synaptic responses. *Nature* 376:256–259.

Weisskopf MG, Zalutsky RA, Nicoll RA (1993) The opioid peptide dynorphin mediates heterosynaptic depression of hippocampal mossy fiber synapses and modulates long-term potentiation. *Nature* 362:423–427.

Weisskopf MG, Castillo PE, Zalutsky RA, Nicoll RA (1994) Mediation of hippocampal mossy fiber long-term potentiation by cyclic AMP. *Science* 265:1878–1882.

Weisz DJ, Clark GA, Thompson RF (1984) Increased responsivity of dentate granule cells during nictitating membrane response conditioning in rabbit. *Behav Brain Res* 12:145–154.

West AE, Griffith EC, Greenberg ME (2002) Regulation of transcription factors by neuronal activity. *Nat Rev Neurosci* 3: 921–931.

Whitlock, J.R., Heynen, A.J., Shuler MG, Bear MF (2006) Learning induces LTP in the hippocampus. *Science* 313:1093–1097.

Wibrand K, Messaoudi E, Havik B, Steenslid V, Lovlie R, Steen VM, Bramham CR (2006) Identification of genes co-upregulated with Arc during BDNF-induced long-term potentiation in adult rat dentate gyrus in vivo. *Eur J Neurosci* 23:1501–1511.

Wigström H, Gustafsson B (1983) Facilitated induction of hippocampal long-lasting potentiation during blockade of inhibition. *Nature* 301:603–604.

Wigström H, Gustafsson B (1985) On long-lasting potentiation in the hippocampus—a proposed mechanism for its dependence on coincident presynaptic and postsynaptic activity. *Acta Physiol Scand* 123:519–522.

Wigström H, Gustafsson B, Huang C-C, Abraham WC (1986) Hippocampal long-term potentiation is induced by pairing single afferent volleys with intracellularly injected depolarizing current pulses. *Acta Physiol Scand* 126:317–319.

Wikström MA, Matthews P, Roberts D, Collingridge GL, Bortolotto ZA (2003) Parallel kinase cascades are involved in the induction of LTP at hippocampal CA1 synapses. *Neuropharmacology* 45:828–836.

Wilkinson DG (2001) Multiple roles of Eph receptors and ephrins inneural development. *Nat Rev Neurosci* 2:155–164.

Williams CE, Guevremont D, Kennard JT, Mason-Parker SE, Tate WP, Abraham WC (2003) Long-term regulation of *N*-methyl-D-aspartate receptor subunits and associated synaptic proteins following hippocampal synaptic plasticity. *Neuroscience* 118: 1003–1013.

Williams JH, Bliss TVP (1988) Induction but not maintenance of calcium-induced long-term potentiation in dentate gyrus and area CA1 of the hippocampal slice is blocked by nordihydroguaiaretic acid. *Neurosci Lett* 88:81–85.

Williams JH, Errington ML, Lynch MA, Bliss TVP (1989) Arachidonic acid induces a long-term activity-dependent enhancement of synaptic transmission in the hippocampus. *Nature* 341: 739–742.

Williams S, Johnston D (1989) Long-term potentiation of hippocampal mossy fiber synapses is blocked by postsynaptic injection of calcium chelators. *Neuron* 3:583–588.

Williams JH, Li YG, Nayak A, Errington ML, Murphy KP, Bliss TV (1993) The suppression of long-term potentiation in rat hippocampus by inhibitors of nitric oxide synthase is temperature and age dependent. *Neuron* 11:877–884.

Willshaw D, Dayan P (1990) Optimal plasticity from matrix memories: what goes up must come down. *Neural Comput* 2: 85–93.

Wilson RI, Nicoll RA (2001) Endogenous cannabinoids mediate retrograde signalling at hippocampal synapses. *Nature* 410: 588–592.

Winder DG, Mansuy IM, Osman M, Moallem TM, Kandel ER (1998) Genetic and pharmacological evidence for a novel, intermediate phase of long-term potentiation suppressed by calcineurin. *Cell* 92:25–37.

Wisden W, Errington ML, Williams S, Dunnett SB, Waters C, Hitchcock D, Evan G, Bliss TV, Hunt SP (1990) Differential expression of immediate early genes in the hippocampus and spinal cord. *Neuron* 4:603–614.

Wolfer DP, Stagljar-Bozicevic M, Errington ML, Lipp HP (1998) Spatial memory and learning in transgenic mice: fact or artifact? *News Physiol Sci* 13:118–123.

Woo NH, Nguyen PV (2003) Protein synthesis is required for synaptic immunity to depotentiation. *J Neurosci* 23:1125–1132.

Woo NH, Teng HK, Siao CJ, Chiaruttini C, Pang PT, Milner TA, Hempstead BL, Lu B (2005) Activation of p75NTR by proBDNF facilitates hippocampal long-term depression. *Nat Neurosci* 8:1069–1077.

Wood MA, Kaplan MP, Park A, Blanchard EJ, Oliveira AM, Lombardi TL, Abel T (2005) Transgenic mice expressing a truncated form of CREB-binding protein (CBP) exhibit deficits in hippocampal synaptic plasticity and memory storage. *Learn Mem* 12:111–119

Woodin MA, Ganguly K, Poo M-M (2003) Coincident pre- and postsynaptic activity modifies GABAergic synapses by postsynaptic changes in Cl⁻ transporter. *Neuron* 39:807–820.

Woolley DE, Gould E, Frankfurt M, McEwen BS (1990) Naturally occurring fluctuations in dendritic spine density on adult hippocampal pyramidal neurons. *J Neurosci* 10:4035–4039.

Wu H, Nash JE, Zamorano P, Garner CC (2002) Interaction of SAP97 with minus-end-directed actin motor myosin. VI. Implications for AMPA receptor trafficking. *J Biol Chem* 277: 30928–30934.

Wu J, Anwyl R, Rowan MJ (1995a) Beta-amyloid-(1-40) increases long-term potentiation in rat hippocampus in vitro. *Eur J Pharmacol* 284:R1–R3.

Wu J, Anwyl R, Rowan MJ (1995b) Beta-amyloid selectively augments NMDA receptor-mediated synaptic transmission in rat hippocampus. *Neuroreport* 6:2409–2413.

Wu J, Rush A, Rowan MJ, Anwyl R (2001) NMDA receptor- and metabotropic glutamate receptor-dependent synaptic plasticity induced by high frequency stimulation in the rat dentate gyrus in vitro. *J Physiol* 533:745–755.

Wu L, Saggau P (1994) Presynaptic calcium is increased during normal synaptic transmission and paired-pulse facilitation, but not in long-term potentiation in area CA1 of hippocampus. *J Neurosci* 14:645–654.

Wu J, Rowan MJ, Anwyl R (2006) Long-term potentiation is mediated by multiple kinase cascades involving αCaMKII or either PKA or p42/44 MAPK in the adult rat dentate gyrus in vitro. *J Neurophysiol* 95:3519–27.

Wu Z-L, Thomas SA, Villacres EC, Xia Z, Simmons ML, Chavkin C, Palmiter RD, Storm DR (1995) Altered behavior and long-term potentiation in type I adenyl cyclase mutant mice. *Proc Natl Acad Sci USA* 92:220–224.

Wyllie DJ, Nicoll RA (1994) A role for protein kinases and phosphatases in the Ca(2+)-induced enhancement of hippocampal

AMPA receptor-mediated synaptic responses. *Neuron* 13: 635–643.

Xia J, Zhang X, Staudinger J, Huganir RL (1999) Clustering of AMPA receptors by the synaptic PDZ domain-containing protein PICK1. *Neuron* 22:179–187

Xiang Z, Greenwood AC, Kairiss EW, Brown TW (1994) Quantal mechanism of long-term potentiation in hippocampal mossy-fiber synapses. *J Neurophysiol* 71:2552–2556.

Xiao MY, Karpefors M, Gustafsson B, Wigström H (1995) On the linkage between AMPA and NMDA receptor-mediated EPSPs in homosynaptic long-term depression in the hippocampal CA1 region of young rats. *J Neurosci* 15:4496–4506.

Xiao MY, Wasling P, Hanse E, Gustafsson B (2004) Creation of AMPA-silent synapses in the neonatal hippocampus. *Nat Neurosci* 7:236–243.

Xie X, Smart TG (1994) Modulation of long-term potentiation in rat hippocampal pyramidal neurons by zinc. *Pflugers Arch* 427: 481–486.

Xiong H, Boyle J, Winkelbauer M, Gorantla S, Zheng J, Ghorpade A, Persidsky Y, Carlson KA, Gendelman HE (2003) Inhibition of long-term potentiation by interleukin-8: implications for human immunodeficiency virus-1-associated dementia. *J Neurosci Res* 71:600–607.

Xu L, Anwyl R, Rowan MJ (1997) Behavioural stress facilitates the induction of long-term depression in the hippocampus. *Nature* 387:497–500.

Xu L, Anwyl R, Rowan MJ (1998) Spatial exploration induces a persistent reversal of long-term potentiation in rat hippocampus. *Nature* 394:891–894.

Yamagata M, Sanes JR, Weiner JA (2003) Synaptic adhesion molecules. *Curr Opin Cell Biol* 15:621–632.

Yamamoto C, Sawada S, Kamiya H (1992) Enhancement of postsynaptic responsiveness during long-term potentiation of mossy fiber synapses in guinea-pig hippocampus. *Neurosci Lett* 138:111–114.

Yamazaki M, Fukaya M, Abe M, Ikeno K, Kakizaki T, Watanabe M, Sakimura K (2001) Differential palmitoylation of two mouse glutamate receptor interacting protein 1 forms with different N-terminal sequences. *Neurosci Lett* 304:81–84.

Yang CH, Huang CC, Hsu KS (2004) Behavioral stress modifies hippocampal synaptic plasticity through corticosterone-induced sustained extracellular signal-regulated/mitogen-activated proein kinase activation. *J Neurosci* 24:11029–11034.

Yang CH, Huang CC, Hsu KS (2005) Behavioral stress enhances hippocampal CA1 long-term depression through the blockade of the glutamate uptake. *J Neurosci* 25:4288–4293.

Yang SN, Tang YG, Zucker RS (1999) Selective induction of LTP and LTD by postsynaptic [Ca^{2+}]$_i$ elevation. *J Neurophysiol* 81: 781–787.

Yang XD, Connor J, Faber D (1994) Weak excitation and simultaneous inhibition induce long-term depression in hippocampal CA1 neurons. *J Neurophysiol* 71:1586–1590.

Yasuda H, Barth AL, Stellwagen D, Malenka RC (2003) A developmental switch in the signaling cascades for LTP induction. *Nat Neurosci* 6:15–16.

Ye B, Liao D, Zhang X, Zhang P, Dong H, Huganir RL (2000) GRASP-1: a neuronal RasGEF associated with the AMPA receptor/GRIP complex. *Neuron* 26:603–617.

Yeckel MF, Kapur A, Johnston D (1999) Multiple forms of LTP in hippocampal CA3 neurons use a common postsynaptic mechanism. *Nat Neurosci* 2:625–633.

Ying SW, Futter M, Rosenblum K, Webber MJ, Hunt SP, Bliss TVP, Bramham CR (2002) Brain-derived neurotrophic factor induces long-term potentiation in intact adult hippocampus: requirement for ERK activation coupled to CREB and upregulation of Arc synthesis. *J Neurosci* 22:1532–1540.

Yokoi M, Kobayashi K, Manabe T, Takahashi T, Sakaguchi I, Katsuura G, Shigemoto R, Ohishi H, Nomora S, Nakamura K, Nakao K, Katsuki M, Nakanishi S (1996) Impairment of hippocampal mossy fiber LTD in mice lacking mGluR2. *Science* 273: 645–647.

Yu H, Saura CA, Choi SY, Sun LD, Yang X, Handler M, Kawarabayashi T, Younkin L, Fedeles B, Wilson MA, Younkin S, Kandel ER, Kirkwood A, Shen J (2001) APP processing and synaptic plasticity in presenilin-1 conditional knockout mice. *Neuron* 31:713–726

Yuan LL, Adams JP, Swank M, Sweatt JD, Johnston D (2002) Protein kinase modulation of dendritic K$^+$ channels in hippocampus involves a mitogen-activated protein kinase pathway. *J Neurosci* 22:4860–4868.

Yuste R, Bonhoeffer T (2001) Morphological changes in dendritic spines associated with long-term plasticity. *Annu Rev Neurosci* 24:1071–1089.

Yuste R, Denk W (1995). Dendritic spines as basic functional units of neuronal integration. *Nature* 375: 682–684.

Zakharenko SS, Patterson SL, Dragatsis I, Zeitlin SO, Siegelbaum SA, Kandel ER, Morozov A (2003) Presynaptic BDNF required for a presynaptic but not postsynaptic component of LTP at hippocampal CA1–CA3 synapses. *Neuron* 39:975–990.

Zalutsky RA, Nicoll RA (1990) Comparison of two forms of long-term potentiation in single hippocampal neurons. *Science* 248:1619–1624.

Zalutsky RA, Nicoll RA (1992) Mossy fiber long-term potentiation shows specificity but no apparent cooperativity. *Neurosci Lett* 138:193–197.

Zaman SH, Parent A, Laskey A, Lee MK, Borchelt DR, Sisodia SS, Malinow R (2000) Enhanced synaptic potentiation in transgenic mice expressing presenilin 1 familial Alzheimer's disease mutation is normalized with a benzodiazepine. *Neurobiol Dis* 7:54–63.

Zamanillo D, Sprengel R, Hvalby O, Jensen V, Burnashev N, Rozov A, Kaiser KM, Koster HJ, Borchardt T, Worley P, Lubke J, Frotscher M, Kelly PH, Sommer B, Andersen P, Seeburg PH, Sakmann B (1999) Importance of AMPA receptors for hippocampal synaptic plasticity but not for spatial learning. *Science* 284:1805–1811.

Zeng H, Chattarji S, Barbarosle M, Rondi-Reig L, Philpot BD, Miyakawa T, Bear MF, Tonegawa S (2001) Forebrain-specific calcineurin knockout selectively impairs bidirectional synaptic plasticity and working/episodic-like memory. *Cell* 107:617–629.

Zhang W, Linden DJ (2003) The other side of the engram: experience-driven changes in neuronal intrinsic excitability. *Nat Rev Neurosci* 4:885–900.

Zhu JJ, Qin Y, Zhao M, Van Aelst L, Malinow R (2002a) Ras and Rap control AMPA receptor trafficking during synaptic plasticity. *Cell* 110:443–455.

Zhuo M, Zhang W, Son H, Mansuy I, Sobel RA, Seidman J, Kandel ER (1999) A selective role of calcineurin Aa in synaptic depotentiation in hippocampus. *Proc Natl Acad Sci USA* 96: 4650–4655.

Zucker RS, Regehr WG (2002) Short-term synaptic plasticity. *Annu Rev Physiol* 64:355–405.

11

John O'Keefe

Hippocampal Neurophysiology in the Behaving Animal

11.1 Overview

This chapter addresses a central question in the study of the hippocampus: What information is represented in hippocampal electrical activity? When asking this question, we are immediately confronted with one of the central problems in neuroscience, the nature of how information is coded in the nervous system. Historically, there have been two answers to this question: On the one hand is the view that the nervous system is composed of a large set of individual computing elements, the neurons, and that these neurons interact with each other by passing discrete bundles of information along their axons. An alternative view is that the system is organized on more holistic principles, with large numbers of cells acting in concert perhaps reflected in synchronous neuronal firing or in rhythmical electroencephalographic (EEG) activity.

The general position taken in this chapter is that the hippocampus uses both strategies. There is ample evidence that individual hippocampal pyramidal cells code for specific locations in an environment by a marked increase in firing rate; but, equally, that part of the code for location involves the timing of cell firing relative to a clock wave, represented by the EEG theta wave and associated interneurons, and that groups of pyramidal cells can act cooperatively in an ensemble fashion. On this view, each pyramidal cell acts as an oscillator, and a sophisticated set of mechanisms exists for producing these oscillations. Each cell has the biophysical machinery to oscillate in isolation from other cells or external inputs. These individual oscillators are stabilized and synchronized by a set of inhibitory feedback circuits primarily involving inhibitory interneurons. Neurons in the septum and brain stem provide the neuromodulatory inputs necessary for hippocampal pyramidal cells to enter the oscillatory state and may also provide a driving signal that sets the overall frequency of the oscillations.

One powerful approach to the study of the functions of a brain region is to correlate the electrical activity of its neurons with some aspect of observed behavior or inferred cognition. This approach reveals what information is available to that part of the brain and when it is available. Furthermore, it is sometimes possible to record both the inputs and the outputs of an area, and under these conditions it may be possible to compute what transfer function is being performed.

Several patterns of electrical activity have been recorded from the hippocampus, and they have been correlated with behavioral or psychological states. During the mid-1960s, Vanderwolf placed a relatively large electrode into the hippocampus of the freely moving rat and recorded the EEG activity during a wide range of behaviors (Vanderwolf, 1969). He identified three distinct states: the rhythmical theta state, the large irregular amplitude activity (LIA) state, and the small irregular amplitude activity (SIA) state. Theta, in turn, could be classified into two subtypes on the basis of behavioral correlate and pharmacological sensitivity. In this chapter, these two types are called a-theta (for arousal/attention theta), which is sensitive to anticholinergic drugs such as atropine, and t-theta (for translation movement theta), which may be serotoninergic and glutamatergic.

The behavioral/psychological correlates of the two types of theta activity have been characterized best in rats: In this animal, the atropine-resistant component or t-theta occurs during a class of movements that may be loosely characterized as those that normally change the spatial relation between the animal's head and the environment. The correlates of the atropine-sensitive theta, or a-theta, are less well defined and are best summed up as psychological states such as arousal, attention, or intention to move. The behavioral correlates of LIA are those that do not change the animal's location in the environment: quiet sitting, eating, drinking, and grooming in the absence of postural shifts. The SIA state occurs during behavioral transitions, often when the animal awakens from slow-wave or rapid-eye-movement (REM) sleep or when it abruptly stops running. It has not received much attention, and its behavioral correlates and physiological function are less well understood.

The rhythmical theta state reflects the synchronous membrane oscillations of large numbers of pyramidal cells in the CA1 field and dentate gyrus that are locked into synchrony by the inhibitory interneuronal network. One of its functions is to provide a clock signal against which the action potentials of the individual pyramidal cells can be timed. Another function might be to set up the optimal circumstances for the induction of long-term potentiation (LTP) (see Chapter 10). The nonrhythmical LIA state has a more random, broader spectrum especially in the lower-frequency range and may represent an inactive, relaxed state of the same network when it is not being driven. Alternatively, it may be an active state in its own right in which memories previously encoded in the hippocampus are strengthened and/or transferred to other regions of the brain. LIA is characterized by sharp waves of about 100 ms duration that occur randomly, with an average interval of 1 second. Associated with them are higher-frequency "ripple" oscillations of 100 to 200 Hz, which also may reflect the operation of the inhibitory network. In addition to oscillations in the theta and ripple bands, oscillations at intermediate frequencies (beta: 12–30 Hz; gamma: 30–100 Hz) have been recorded in association with various aspects of olfactory behavior.

Placing a microelectrode rather than a gross electrode into the CA1 hippocampal cell layer reveals a much richer and surprising set of behavioral correlates correlations between physiology and behavior. On the basis of the EEG recordings one might expect to see cell-firing patterns that are correlated with the animal's movements, and indeed this is observed. However, it is not the whole story. Ranck (1973) placed microelectrodes into the pyramidal cell layers of CA3 and CA1 and found two classes of cellular response. One type, which he called the theta cell, fired at frequencies ranging from 10 Hz (when the animal sat quietly or engaged in other "LIA" behaviors) to as high as 100 Hz (as it ran around the environment or engaged in other "theta" behaviors). Furthermore, they burst at the same frequency and showed consistent correlations with different phases of the various EEG waves. Here, at the level of the single cell, was one clear correlate of the EEG patterns, banishing forever any lingering skepticism about their functional significance. The second class of cell, the complex spike cell, had a much lower baseline firing rate, and many were effectively "silent" for long periods of time. Their defining characteristic is the occasional short burst of action potentials with successively decreasing amplitudes. Their major behavioral correlate was first identified by O'Keefe and Dostrovsky (1971) as the animal's location. They reported that these place cells were typically silent as the rat moved around the environment until it entered a small patch of the environment when the cell began to fire (the place field). It is now recognized that, within the place field, these cells also fire

in a rhythmical bursting pattern during the EEG theta state. Unlike the theta cells, however, the frequency of bursts is slightly higher than the gross EEG theta, causing each successive burst to precess to earlier phases of the theta cycle as the animal moves through the place field. This temporal code works together with the overall rate code to identify the animal's location. In addition, variations in firing rate can signal aspects of behavior that occur in the place field or the presence (or absence) of objects encountered there. The same cells often fire in different environments, but the preferred locations are unrelated if the environments are sufficiently dissimilar to each other. One notable feature of these place cells is that in unconstrained open fields—environments in which the animal is free to move in all directions—the cells fire in the place field irrespective of the direction in which the animal is facing. In environments that constrain the animal's behavior, the cells become directionally sensitive and may be said to represent the successive locations along a path. In addition to the animal's location, some pyramidal cells signal the presence or absence of particular objects within the place field or the performance of particular behaviors there.

In addition to *representing* locations and features of the environment, the place cells have been shown to *learn* about new environments or changes in a familiar environment. For example, place cells initially treat similar environments as identical but can learn to differentiate between them with repeated exposure.

Place cells are typically recorded from the hippocampus proper but have also been recorded from other parts of the hippocampal formation, namely the subiculum, presubiculum, parasubiculum, and entorhinal cortex as well as the hippocampus. The properties of cells in these various regions vary, and it is still not clear how this diverse population of place cells is organized into a functional network or which functions are performed by each region.

Two other major classes of spatial cell have been found in the hippocampal formation: the head direction (HD) cell and the grid cell. The HD cell is sensitive to the orientation of the rat's head with respect to the environmental frame, irrespective of the animal's location in that environment. These cells have been found in several regions, most notably the anterior thalamus and dorsal presubiculum. Different cells have different preferred directional orientations. The animal's orientation is given partly by environmental cues and partly by interoceptive cues derived from vestibular and/or proprioceptive inputs. In addition to directly controlling behavior based on environmental directions, these cells may provide directional information to the place cells. The third major class of spatial cell, the grid cell, provides a metric for marking off distances in the environment. These cells have been found in layers 2/3 of the medial entorhinal cortex, which sends a major projection to the hippocampus proper, and in the lower layers, which receive inputs from the hippocampus. Each of these cells lays a grid-like pattern of firing on top of every environment the animal encounters. The orientation and spacing of the grid varies in a systematic fashion from cell to cell and appears to depend on information generated by the animal's self motion.

Place cells have also been described in primates including humans, as have a variety of other spatial cells: HD cells and spatial view cells, which respond when the animal looks at a particular location.

Nonspatial behavioral correlates of hippocampal complex spike cells have also been reported in rodents and primates. Simple sensory stimuli, such as tones or somatosensory stimuli, appear to be relatively ineffective in the untrained animal, although there are several reports that pyramidal cells respond to these stimuli following classic conditioning or discrimination learning tasks. Furthermore, increased firing in complex-spike cells has been reported to correlate with different aspects of behavior in approach tasks, such as whether the animal is approaching an area containing cues to be recognized or discriminated or containing a reward. Some authors have argued that these findings support the idea that the hippocampus is involved in many types of relational processing in addition to those in the spatial domain. As we shall see, it is sometimes difficult to decide whether the firing of a hippocampal cell in a particular task is spatial or nonspatial. Whether these nonspatial correlates can eventually be explained within a spatial framework or alternatively, signal the need for an extension of the functions attributed to the hippocampus into nonspatial domains is discussed.

11.2 Hippocampal Electroencephalogram Can Be Classified into Distinct Patterns, with Each Providing Information About an Aspect of Hippocampal Function

If an electrode is placed in the hippocampus and electrical activity in the frequency range 1 to 200 Hz is recorded as the animal goes about its daily business, distinct patterns of electrical activity are seen that vary as a function of state of alertness, sensory stimulation, behavior, and anatomical location. These patterns of electrical activity are known collectively as the "electroencephalogram," or EEG. The EEG reflects the activity of large numbers of neurons and probably includes contributions from action potentials in disparate cell types, excitatory and inhibitory synaptic potentials, and dendritic and glial slow potentials. As such, it can provide a measure of information about the overall function of a brain region but not at the same level of precision as the activity of single units. It is probably most useful for signaling when large numbers of neurons are acting together synchronously. Because this is an important mode of operation of cortical areas such as the hippocampus, it follows that different EEG patterns can serve as a bridge between behavior on the one hand and single or multiple unit activity on the other. As we shall see in this chapter, there are several types of hippocampal EEG pattern, and each type provides information about a different aspect of hip-

pocampal function, although none tells the whole story on its own. Theta and LIA have been studied most and so receive the most attention here.

11.2.1 Hippocampal EEG Can Be Classified into Four Types of Rhythmical and Two Types of Nonrhythmical Activity

In the hippocampus of the freely moving rat, six prominent EEG patterns have been identified: four rhythmical and two nonrhythmical. Rhythmical patterns (and their frequency ranges) include theta (6–12 Hz), beta (12–30 Hz), gamma (30–100 Hz), and ripple (100–200 Hz) waves. Nonrhythmical patterns include LIA and SIA. Figure 11–1 shows examples of each. Some patterns can co-occur (e.g., LIA with ripples, theta with gamma), whereas others appear to be mutually exclusive (e.g., theta, LIA, and SIA). The latter three waveforms appear to correspond to mutually exclusive states of hippocampal functioning.

Theta consists of rhythmical, often sinusoidal oscillations that vary in frequency from 6 to 12 Hz in the rat but can be as low as 4 Hz in the rabbit and cat (Fig. 11–1A, traces 1–4). The frequency power spectrum is narrow (Fig. 11–1B, walking), with a sharp peak around 7 to 10 Hz and often associated with higher harmonics (second peak around 16 Hz in Fig. 11–1B, walking). The LIA pattern looks much more random and is often characterized by sharp waves that resemble the spike and wave of epileptiform tissue (see Fig. 11–1A, traces 6, 7). The LIA power spectrum is flatter, with fewer peaks than are seen in theta and more power in the lower (1–5 Hz) frequencies (Figs. 11–1B, still and 11–2G). High-frequency 200-Hz ripples occur on the LIA sharp waves (Fig. 11–1C). SIA is a low-amplitude pattern that contains a broad spectrum of high frequencies and occurs only occasionally (Figs. 11–1A, 7, pencil tap and 11–2C). Beta waves occupy the frequency range 12 to 20 Hz (Fig. 11–1D) and gamma waves the frequency range 20 to 100 Hz (Fig. 11–1E). Either can occur alone or in combination with theta, LIA, or SIA.

11.2.2 Each EEG Pattern Has Distinct Behavioral Correlates

The simplest behavioral correlates of the various EEG patterns occur in the rat, and here we follow Vanderwolf's general description (Whishaw and Vanderwolf, 1973; Vanderwolf, 2001). It should be noted, however, that theta, in particular, has slightly different behavioral correlates in different species. In the awake rat, theta occurs primarily during movements that can loosely be described as "translational"—those that change the location of the animal's head with respect to the environment: walking, running, swimming, jumping, exploratory head movements, struggling (see examples in Fig. 11–1A, 1–4). Theta also occurs during REM sleep and occasionally during immobile attention or arousal. In the rabbit and guinea pig, this immobile attention-related theta

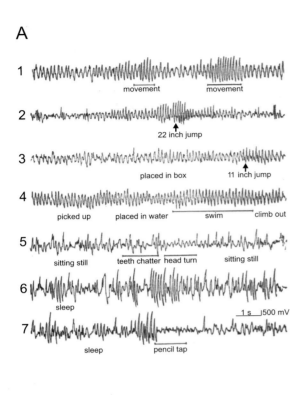

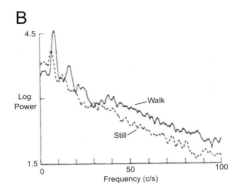

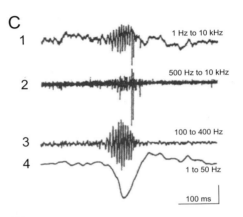

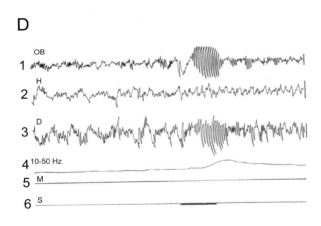

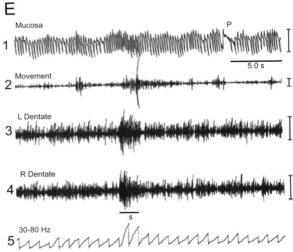

Figure 11–1. Hippocampal electroencephalography (EEG) patterns. *A.* Theta during rapid-eye-movement (REM) sleep (trace 1), jumping (2, 3), and swimming (4). Large irregular amplitude activity (LIA) during quiet sitting (5) and slow-wave sleep (6, 7). Note the large amplitude sharp waves especially prominent during slow-wave sleep. Small irregular amplitude activity (SIA) during brief arousal from slow-wave sleep after a pencil tap (7). (*Source*: Whishaw and Vanderwolf, 1973.) *B.* Frequency power spectrum during walking and standing still. Note the peaks around 8 and 16 Hz and the generally higher amplitude in the beta and gamma bands during walking. (*Source*: Leung, 1992.) *C.* LIA ripples and sharp waves in broad-band (trace 1) and filtered (2–4) recordings. Ripples (3) and sharp waves (4) are accompanied by bursts of action potentials (2) in hippocampal interneurons (small spikes) and principal cells (large spikes). (*Source*: Buzsaki et al., 1992.) *D.* Beta activity in the olfactory bulb (OB) and dentate gyrus (D) during sniffing toluene (thickening of s in trace 6). Note the absence of beta in the hippocampus (2, H) and the absence of gross movement (5, M). *E.* Gamma activity (3, 4) in the dentate during sniffing (s). Trace 5 shows the increase in breathing recorded during sniffing. (*Source*: Vanderwolf, 2001.)

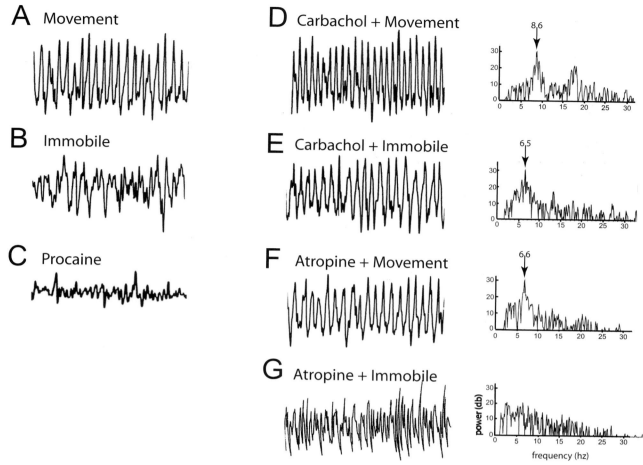

Figure 11–2. EEG patterns and frequency power spectra during movement and immobility in the rat. *A.* Theta during spontaneous movement. *B.* LIA during quiet immobility. *C.* All theta is abolished by a procaine injection into the medial septum. *D.*Theta during movement following intraseptal injection of the cholinomimetic carbachol. *E.* a-Theta during immobility following intraseptal injection of the cholinomimetic carbachol has a lower frequency than in *D.* *F.* t-Theta during movement is not blocked by an intraseptal injection of the anticholinergic atropine. *G.* LIA during immobility following intraseptal atropine. All EEG traces are 3 s long except *C,* which is 2 seconds. Arrows in *D, E,* and *F* indicate peak theta frequency in hertz. (*Source*: After Lawson and Bland, 1993, with permission.)

occurs more often. In the cat, it is related to active exploratory eye movements.

LIA occurs during behaviors that do not change the animal's location, such as sitting quietly, eating, drinking, grooming, and during slow wave sleep (SWS) (Fig. 11–1A, 5–7). SIA is seen infrequently: in the awake rat when ongoing movement is abruptly halted after a long train of theta, during sudden, motionless transitions from rest/sleep to alertness (Fig. 11–1A, 7, pencil tap), and during periods of SWS after REM episodes. Much less is known about the full range of behavioral correlates of beta and gamma, but they both have been shown to be associated with different types of olfactory input. Gamma occurs when the animal sniffs at a wide range of odors (Fig. 11–1E), whereas beta waves have been observed only during the sniffing of odors associated with predators (Fig. 11–1D).

11.3 Hippocampal Theta Activity

11.3.1 Hippocampal Theta Activity: Historical Overview

Theta activity and its behavioral correlates have been studied extensively ever since its discovery in the rabbit hippocampus by Jung and Kornmuller in 1938 (Jung and Kornmuller, 1938). The initial skepticism about the possibility that such regular large amplitude waves could be generated in the brain was overcome when Green and Arduini (1954) repeated the observations during the 1950s and showed that the theta pattern correlated inversely with neocortical desynchronization, suggesting that it represented the hippocampal arousal pattern. Later, attempts were made to correlate the theta rhythm with aspects of learning: Adey et al. (1960) in the United States reported frequency shifts during simple discrimination learning, and Grastyan et al. (1959) in Hungary found high-frequency theta during orienting behavior early in auditory-reward conditioning but a desynchronized SIA pattern later, after the animal had learned to approach the reward. Studies by Gray (1971) in Britain suggested that particular frequencies of hippocampal theta activity (ca. 7.7 Hz) in the rat may also occur in association with reactions to nonreward.

These differences of opinion from different laboratories led to speculation that the behavioral correlate of theta varied from species to species and perhaps from task to task. Some measure of order was brought to the field by Vanderwolf's careful observations of the strictly behavioral correlates of hippocampal EEG patterns (Vanderwolf, 1969). He made the important point that changes of the kind seen by Adey and Grastyan that appeared to be correlated with different phases of learning were also correlated with specific changes in behavior at the same time. The changes in theta frequency seen by Adey, for example, tended to be correlated with changes in motor behavior during the course of learning. Vanderwolf argued that it was the strictly behavioral correlate of these EEG patterns that was primary. In various rodent species, he and his colleagues observed that theta activity was associated with what he termed "voluntary movements," whereas LIA occurred during stereotyped "fixed-action patterns." His subsequent observation that there were two types of theta, each with different behavioral correlates, clarified matters further (Kramis et al., 1975). One type is associated with arousal or attention, whether in association with movement or immobility, and the other with a class of movement alone. These two types are expressed to different degrees in different species and depend on different neuromodulatory inputs. The changes in hippocampal EEG during classic conditioning in the rabbit are examined in more detail in the section on nonspatial learning and memory (see Section 11.11).

11.3.2 Hippocampal Theta Activity Is Comprised of Two Components, a-Theta and t-Theta, Which Can Be Distinguished on the Basis of Behavioral Correlates and Pharmacology

In addition to differences in their behavioral correlates, the two components of theta recorded in freely moving animals also differ in their pharmacology. One is affected by drugs that act at cholinergic synapses, such as the antagonists atropine and scopolamine, the agonist carbachol, and the anticholinesterase, eserine. Vanderwolf and colleagues (Kramis et al., 1975) called this component atropine-sensitive theta, but we refer to it here by the more psychological name, arousal- or attentional-theta (*a-theta* for short). The second component of theta is correlated with translational movements and is unaffected by cholinergic drugs. There is some evidence that it is dependent on the transmitters serotonin and glutamate. It is called translation-movement theta (*t-theta* for short).

Theta is not uniformly distributed in the hippocampal formation but varies in both phase and amplitude in different parts. Whereas synchronous, large-amplitude theta waves are prominent in the dentate gyrus and CA1 areas of the hippocampus, most mapping studies report the absence of theta in area CA3. Despite this, CA3 cells can show good phase correlates to the EEG recorded elsewhere (e.g., in CA1 or the dentate gyrus). The implication is that the presence or absence of theta waves in the EEG is not a simple function of the underlying single-cell activity. The presence of theta must depend, at least in part, on other factors, such as the anatomical arrangement of the cells and the phase relations of their activity (see Buzsaki, 2002 for a recent review of the cellular basis of theta).

11.3.3 Both Types of Theta Activity Are Dependent on the Medial Septal/DBB but Only t-Theta Is Dependent on the Entorhinal Cortex

As discussed in Chapter 3, the major cholinergic input to the hippocampal formation arises from the medial septal nucleus and the nucleus of the diagonal band of Broca. The relative contributions of the medial septal nucleus and entorhinal cortex to the overall hippocampal theta pattern have been dissected using a combination of lesions and pharmacological manipulations (Bland and Oddie, 2001; Buzsaki, 2002). Lesions of the medial septal nucleus and associated diagonal band eliminate both types of theta activity. Injection of various drugs into the septum reveals differences in the pharmacological basis of a- and t-theta (Lawson and Bland, 1993). Inactivation by intraseptal injections of the local anesthetic procaine or the γ-aminobutyric acid (GABA)ergic drug muscimol eliminates all theta from the hippocampus (Fig. 11–2 C). Intraseptal injection of cholinergic antagonists (such as atropine) also block both thetas if the animal sits quietly (Fig. 11–2G) but leave movement-related t-theta intact (Fig. 11–2F). Conversely, injections of cholinergic agonists such as carbachol produce a state of continuous theta in the hippocampus regardless of whether the animal is moving (Fig. 11–2D) or sitting quietly (Fig. 11–2E). The frequency of the a-theta that occurs during immobility is about 2 Hz lower than when the animal is moving (compare power spectra in Fig. 11–2, D and E).

Lesions of the entorhinal cortex, in contrast, eliminate t-theta but leave a-theta intact (Kramis et al., 1975). Following such lesions, injections of atropine eliminate the remaining theta. Chronic injections of para-chlorophenylalanine (PCPA) or reserpine, both of which reduce the levels of serotonin in the brain, appear to eliminate t-theta. Because the *N*-methyl-D-aspartate (NMDA) receptor blocker ketamine also eliminates t-theta and results in a depth profile similar to urethane, it is likely that the glutamatergic afferents from the entorhinal cortex to the distal dendrites of CA1 and CA3 are responsible for this subcomponent of theta (Buzsaki, 2002).

The simplest explanation of these findings is that t-theta depends on fibers that pass through, or synapse in, the medial septum on their way to the entorhinal cortex with onward connection to the hippocampus. On the other hand, a-theta requires the integrity of the direct cholinergic projection from the medial septal-diagonal band of Broca to the hippocampus perhaps through the activation of networks of inhibitory interneurons (see Chapter 8).

11.3.4 t-Theta Occurs During Movement Through Space

Following Vanderwolf's observational studies, the tight coupling between t-theta and certain types of movement was strengthened by the results of "theta-conditioning" experiments by Black (1975). The idea was to reward animals for producing short trains of theta activity under two training conditions: In one they were allowed to move, but in the other they were forced to hold still. Training to produce theta with frequencies greater than 7 Hz (t- theta) was successful only when movement was allowed. Thus, movement is necessary for t-theta, but what aspect of such movement is being signaled by theta activity?

Vanderwolf's original suggestion that theta was correlated with some aspect of voluntary behavior is not operational enough because it is not clear whether, in the case of animals, a movement can ever be said to be truly volitional. Considering the movements during which theta occurs most readily—walking, running, swimming, jumping—the likely common factor is translation through space. The fact that small head movements during exploratory sniffing are also accompanied by theta suggests that the crucial factor is the translation of the *head* through space or, more specifically, the generation of motor outputs that would normally result in translation of the head through space. Changes in the frequency of theta activity are correlated with either the animal's speed of movement through the environment (Rivas et al., 1996; Slawinska and Kasicki, 1998) or the rapidity with which a movement is initiated. The latter has been shown in experiments in which rats have been trained to jump up onto a ledge or to initiate running in a runway (Whishaw and Vanderwolf, 1973).

The behavioral correlate of theta amplitude is less clear. Although Vanderwolf and colleagues failed to find a positive correlation between amplitude and speed, Rivas et al. (1996) reported a positive correlation between both the frequency and the amplitude of theta and the speed of movement in the guinea pig when movements are initiated in simple runways. On the other hand, there is no correlation in jumping experiments between amplitude and speed of movement. It seems that there are many factors contributing to the amplitude of theta, such that a consistent correlate of amplitude is not always seen.

11.3.5 a-Theta Occurs During Arousal and/or Attention as well as Movement

a-Theta may correlate with psychological states such as arousal or attention. It rarely occurs in isolation in the rat but is much more common in rabbits, guinea pigs, and cats. In rats, it occurs naturally only when the animal freezes following a noxious stimulus, in response to an aversive conditioned stimulus, or when the animal is immobile but preparing to move (such as just before a jump). It also co-occurs with t-theta during movement. In rabbits and guinea pigs, it is readily produced in immobile animals by innocuous visual, auditory, or tactile stimuli. Repeated stimulation, however, leads to habituation of this response. Sainsbury and colleagues (1987a,b) have shown that the ability of a stimulus to elicit hippocampal a-theta is dependent on the preexisting level of arousal. A relatively neutral stimulus such as a tone, which ordinarily has little effect, readily elicits a-theta if the animal has previously been "sensitized" with an arousing stimulus such as the sound of an owl or the sight of a predator. One possibility is that a-theta represents a subthreshold activation of the motor system. Experiments in support of this idea have been carried out by Sinnamon and his colleagues (Sinnamon, 2000; Sinnamon et al., 2000). They recorded theta activity in urethane-anesthetized rats before, during, and after hind-limb stepping movements elicited by electrical stimulation of the hypothalamus or pharmacological block of the midbrain raphe nucleus. Both manipulations elicited low-frequency premovement (presumptive a- type) theta activity as well as the higher-frequency (presumptive t- type) theta, which accompanied the hind-limb stepping movements. It might be that a- theta reflects the activation of movement programs in the absence of the movement itself. Alternatively or in addition, it might reflect the organization of sensory inputs as reflected in the correlation of single-unit activity in different sensory nuclei with hippocampal theta (see Section 11.3.7).

11.3.6 Theta and Sleep

Theta occurs during the REM phase of sleep; LIA and SIA occur during slow-wave sleep; and SIA bursts frequently come at the termination of an REM episode. Pharmacological studies have shown that the theta recorded during the actual eye movements of the REM phase of sleep is unaffected by cholinergic drugs and therefore resembles t-theta, and that outside of these episodes is a-theta.

11.3.7 Theta Activity in Nonhippocampal Areas

In the rat, the theta system is centred on the hippocampal formation, taken here to include the septum, subicular area, and entorhinal cortex (Alonso and Garcia-Austt, 1987a,b; Brankack et al., 1993). However there are also reports of EEG and cellular activity phase-locked to theta in the cingulate cortex (Leung and Borst, 1987), prefrontal cortex (Hyman et al., 2005; Jones and Wilson, 2005; Siapas et al., 2005), perirhinal cortex (Muir and Bilkey, 1998), posterior hypothalamus including the mammillary bodies (Kirk and McNaughton, 1991; Bland et al., 1995; Slawinska and Kasicki, 1995; Kocsis and Vertes, 1997), brain stem reticular formation (Nunez et al., 1991), amygdala (Paré and Gaudreau, 1996; Seidenbecher et al., 2003), and superior (Natsume et al., 1999) and inferior (Pedemonte et al., 1996) colliculi. Some of these areas, such as the posterior hypothalamus and the brain stem reticular formation, are involved in the circuitry that generates the hippocampal theta rhythm and might be expected to show activity synchronized with theta, whereas others are part of the sensory systems (the colliculi) or the limbic system (amygdala and cingulate cortex). These latter correlations must represent a fairly widespread function for theta, such as the synchronization or binding together of neurons in many sensory, motor, and emotional/motivational centers as well as those involved in spatial perception and memory.

11.3.8 Does the Hippocampal EEG in Monkeys and Humans Have a Theta Mode?

Although theta patterns are readily observed in cats, dogs, and rodents, it has been difficult to establish whether a clear rhythmic theta pattern can been recorded from either monkey or human hippocampus. There have been hints over the years that it might exist. For example, Stewart and Fox (1991) reported a theta-like pattern (7–9 Hz) in the hippocampal EEG of urethane-anesthetized monkeys. In an earlier study, Watanabe and Niki (1985) reported the existence of the rhythmical theta-like firing patterns in monkey hippocampal cells. Similarly, rare experiments using depth electrodes in the human hippocampus have observed activity at theta frequencies, although their behavioral correlates were not clear (Halgren et al., 1978; Arnolds et al., 1980). This paucity of data has led some authors to suggest that theta may not exist in monkeys and primates or may not have the same behavioral correlates as in other mammals. Some reasons for the failure to record prominent theta patterns in the primate EEG are examined in the next section.

First, the existence of an oscillatory theta pattern in the EEG depends not only on the rhythmical firing of cells but also on the correct cytoarchitectonic orientation of pyramidal cells to create the appropriate electrical dipole. As was seen in the section on theta activity in field CA3, cells can burst with a theta pattern in the absence of pronounced theta waves in the EEG. Different neuroarchitecture could account for a theta system in primates in the absence of rodent-like theta patterns in the gross EEG.

A second problem is that most monkey and human recording is done while the subject is immobile, a condition that is not conducive to recording t-theta. Thirdly, most recordings in humans have been from the scalp, and it is possible that the skull and scalp are acting as filters, effectively screening out the theta patterns. Some evidence to support the last two possibilities comes from recent findings (Kahana et al., 1999) that theta patterns could be recorded from electrodes placed on the surface of the human neocortex while subjects navigated through a virtual reality maze. Theta activity was recorded from several cortical regions, but temporal lobe theta showed the best correlation with maze difficulty. More theta activity was seen during traverses through more difficult 12-choice mazes than through simpler 6-choice mazes. The same group has used depth as well as subdural electrodes in humans performing a virtual taxi driver task (Caplan et al., 2003) to show

that theta oscillations in humans are found during virtual movement, exploratory search, and goal-seeking. One difference from the rat is that human theta bursts tend to be of shorter duration. These kinds of studies confirm the suspicion that the difficulty recording primate theta has more to do with inappropriate behavioral paradigms and recording techniques than with the absence of a theta system per se.

There has also been recent interest in the related field of frequency analysis of EEGs recorded from scalp electrodes. For example, increases in the power present in the EEG at theta frequencies have been shown to be related to the successful encoding of new information (for a review see Klimesch, 1999). However, these studies typically do not demonstrate the peak in the power spectrum at theta frequencies or the long continuous records of trains of theta activity shown by Kahana and colleagues in their virtual reality study. Localizing the source of theta in scalp-recorded EEGs is even more problematical than with subdural electrodes; one experiment where it was attempted implicated the anterior cingulate rather than the hippocampus (in a task showing increased theta with increased working memory load) (Gevins et al., 1997). Spectral peaks at theta frequencies have been found in experiments using magnetoencephalography and have been interpreted as consistent with a generator near the hippocampus (Tesche and Karhu, 2000), although this technique also suffers from problems of accurate source localization. Nevertheless, these findings, and particularly the subdural recordings of Kahana et al., clearly show that theta activity exists in the human brain and tempt one to speculate that it might be related to the hippocampal system. There is a more extensive discussion of recording of the EEG and evoked potentials from the human brain in Chapter 12.

11.3.9 Functions of Theta

Work on the rat hippocampus suggests three possible functions for theta. First, it acts as a global synchronizing mechanism, essentially locking the entire hippocampal formation into one global processing mode and organizing the activity in each hippocampal region with respect to the others. Simultaneous recordings of the EEG in different hippocampal locations have shown that theta activity at comparable locations (e.g., in the CA1 pyramidal layer) is in synchrony and coherent across large areas of the hippocampal formation (Mitchell and Ranck, 1980; Fox et al., 1986; Bullock et al., 1990). This means that if two cells have firing patterns that are systematically related to the local theta cycle, they have systematic temporal relations to each other, even if they are located far apart in the hippocampus. Although the theta rhythm is centered on the hippocampal formation, sensory and motivational areas are also brought under its sway. We begin to see here evidence for a widespread system of oscillations that organizes the activity of many disparate brain areas.

A second function of the theta oscillations is to provide a periodic clocking system for the timing of hippocampal spikes. As set out in greater detail in Section 11.7.9, the phase relation of each pyramidal cell measured against the concurrent theta activity is not constant but can vary from one cycle to the next (O'Keefe and Recce, 1993; Skaggs et al., 1996). As a rat runs through the firing field of a spatially coded pyramidal cell (the place field), the cell fires bursts of spikes at an interburst frequency slightly higher than that of the concomitant EEG theta. This leads to a precession of the phase of firing to earlier points on each successive cycle. Over the course of the five to seven theta cycles that comprise the typical place field, the phase of the EEG at which the cell fires may precess through a full 360°, although smaller amounts of precession are also seen. Furthermore, the phase of firing is highly correlated with the animal's location within the place field (more so than with the duration spent in the field). Thus, temporal variation in spike firing conveys information about the animal's spatial location. An analysis of this phenomenon (Jensen and Lisman, 2000) shows that the temporal information provided by the phase precession can improve localization of the animal's position by more than 40% compared to that obtained by the use of firing rates alone.

A third function for theta is to provide temporal control over long-term potentiation (LTP) induction and, by inference, the storage and retrieval of information from the hippocampus. As noted in Chapter 10, theta-burst electrical stimulation of hippocampal afferents is an effective way to induce LTP. Furthermore, there is some evidence that volleys arriving at different phases of the ongoing theta are differentially effective (Pavlides et al., 1988; Huerta and Lisman, 1995; Holscher et al., 1997; Hyman et al., 2003). Inputs arriving at the positive phase of CA1 theta result in synaptic potentiation, whereas those arriving at the negative phase yield depotentiation or depression. On the basis of this and other evidence, Hasselmo (2005) proposed that the various phases of theta oscillation represent different modes of operation. Specifically, the peak of the CA1 theta is the period during which encoding of new information entering the hippocampus from the entorhinal cortex takes place, and the trough is the period during which retrieval of information from the hippocampus to the entorhinal cortex occurs.

11.4 Non-theta EEG Patterns in the Hippocampal EEG: LIA, SIA, Ripples, Beta, and Gamma

11.4.1 Sharp Waves, Ripples, and Single Units During Large Irregular Activity

During LIA, large sharp waves occur in the hippocampal EEG (Fig. 11–1A, traces 5–7 and Fig.11–1C, trace 4). In CA1, the sharp waves occur most frequently during slow wave sleep and quiet sitting, less frequently during eating and drinking, and least frequently during grooming. They appear to occur during periods of low arousal and are often, but not always, inhibited by arousing stimuli. They may represent a resting state of the hippocampus as a whole or the absence of some aspect of hippocampal function such as the theta state; functionally, it has been suggested that they represent a neural correlate of memory consolidation. Each sharp wave lasts 50 to 100 ms and has a maximum amplitude in the stratum radiatum that can be as large as 1 mV or more. Their resemblance to the interictal spike and wave complex of epileptogenic cortex may give some clues to the peculiar susceptibility of the hippocampus to seizure activity (Bragin, 1999; Draguhn et al., 2000; Buzaki and Draguhn, 2004). They occur more or less synchronously over large areas of the CA1 field of the dorsal hippocampus: Recordings at different points along the septo-temporal axis of the hippocampus have shown that they are in phase over the entire extent (Buzsaki et al., 1992; Chrobak and Buzsaki, 1996). They reverse polarity in the pyramidal cell layer and reach their maximum amplitude several hundred microns into the stratum radiatum (O'Keefe and Nadel, 1978, pp. 150–153). Buzsaki and colleagues have suggested that sharp waves originate in the CA3 field and that the sharp waves recorded in CA1 are the summated extracellular excitatory postsynaptic potentials (EPSPs) of the Schaffer collaterals that result from synchronous firing of the CA3 pyramidal cells (Csicsvari et al., 2000). Direct stimulation of these fibres results in evoked potentials with similar shape and depth profiles.

Around the time of the negative peak of the sharp wave, there is a high-frequency oscillation of between 120 and 200 Hz whose peak amplitude occurs in the CA1 pyramidal cell layer (O'Keefe and Nadel, 1978, pp. 150–153; Buzsaki et al., 1992) (Fig. 11–1C). During these "ripples" there are synchronous bursts in almost all theta interneurons and in about 1 in 10 of the complex-spike pyramidal cells. Intracellular recordings from the soma of pyramidal cells during ripples reveals intracellular oscillations that mirror the extracellular pattern. Hyperpolarization results in a reduction of ripple amplitude at −70 mV, with a reversal at more negative potentials. This sequence of events suggests that the sharp wave itself reflects the synchronous barrage of afferent activity from CA3 cells onto the apical dendrites of CA1 cells. The rapid activation of inhibitory interneurons causes synchronized hyperpolarizing inhibitory postsynaptic potentials (IPSPs) in the somata of pyramidal cells.

Are sharp waves and ripples confined to the hippocampus proper, or do they spread to other structures? Recordings in the subiculum and the deep layers of the entorhinal cortex show that sharp waves also occur in these structures at about the same time as those in hippocampus. The sharp wave in layers V and VI of the entorhinal cortex, which receive inputs from the hippocampus, followed those in the hippocampus by 5 to 30 ms (Chrobak and Buzsaki, 1996). In contrast, the presence of hippocampal sharp waves is not reflected in the activity of the upper layers (II and III) of the entorhinal cortex, which project to the dentate gyrus, hippocampus, and subiculum. Recordings from the dentate gyrus show that the granule cells are also influenced by the sharp-wave activity of CA3. The anatomical basis for this retrograde effect is not entirely clear.

There are projections from CA3 into the polymorph layer, and these fibers may be ending on mossy cells, which in turn project to the dentate granule cells. In the ventral tip of the hippocampus, there appear to be some CA3 pyramidal cells that project directly into the molecular layer of the dentate gyrus.

11.4.2 Dentate EEG Spikes During LIA

Sharp-wave activity during LIA also occurs in the granule cell layers of the dentate gyrus. It is also associated with a high-frequency ripple, although the frequency is not as high as that of the CA1 ripple. Most granule cells do not fire during dentate sharp waves, but intracellular recordings have shown that they are nevertheless depolarized at this time. Surprisingly, the overall effect of dentate spikes on CA3 cells is inhibitory. This presumably reflects the heavy innervation of interneurons by the mossy fibers (Acsady et al., 1998) (see Chapter 5, Section 5.7).

11.4.3 Pharmacology of LIA

Little is known about the pharmacology of LIA, the sharp waves, or the ripples. Ripples are eliminated under halothane anesthesia, and their frequency is reduced under urethane and ketamine to around 100 Hz (Ylinen et al., 1995). In the mouse, sharp waves and ripples can be elicited by application of KCl to the dendrites of pyramidal cells following pharmacological block of $GABA_A$ receptors, making it unlikely that they are due to activity in networks of the inhibitory interneurons (Nimmrich et al., 2005). Synchronization between ripples appears to depend on gap junctions. Consistent with the idea that the LIA state is a passive absence of theta, procaine or muscimol suppression of the medial septum, which inhibits theta activity, has only a small effect on the power of hippocampal LIA (Bland et al., 1996). Recordings of medial septal and diagonal band cells during LIA show that the firing rates of most of these cells are reduced relative to theta, strengthening this suggestion. On the other hand, cholinergic activation of the septum completely suppresses hippocampal LIA, replacing it with low-frequency theta even in the immobile animal (Fig. 11–2E). Theta appears to be the active state driven from the medial septum, and LIA is the passive state that occurs in its absence.

11.4.4 Behavioral Correlates and Functions of LIA

In their discussion of hippocampal sharp waves and ripples during LIA, O'Keefe and Nadel (1978, pp. 150–153) suggested that one way to think about this EEG state was as an absence of the theta state—it is the hippocampus in a non-theta idling mode. This suggestion was based partly on the observation that there was always a period of at least a few seconds between the onset of an LIA-associated pattern of behavior (such as immobility) and the onset of the sharp wave and ripples. They also argued that the nearly synchronous bursts in a

sizable percentage of the pyramidal cells, when compared with their highly differentiated patterns of activity during the theta state as the animal moved around an environment, would be unlikely to convey much information. Perhaps most tellingly, it was found that lesions of the fornix decreased neither the frequency nor the amplitude of ripples and sharp waves; if anything, they increased them—again suggesting release of the hippocampus from an activated theta state. In this view, the LIA state is the passive activity of a system with extensive positive and negative feedback loops and other oscillatory mechanisms.

An alternative hypothesis is that LIA is an active, rather than an idling, state of the hippocampus whose function is to strengthen synaptic modifications that have occurred during the immediately prior periods (Buzsaki, 1989). Pointing to the similarity between the synchronous volleys of afferent activity impinging on the dendrites of CA1 dendrites during LIA and the type of tetanic stimulation known to cause LTP, Buzsaki suggested that synaptic potentiation occurs naturally during LIA. He went on to propose that this potentiation acts as a boost to synapses that had been only weakly modified during the previous theta behaviors and perhaps plays a role in a memory consolidation process. Evidence in support of this idea comes from experiments by Skaggs and McNaughton (1996). They looked at pairs of CA1 pyramidal cells with overlapping place fields in freely moving rats that were running around a small triangular runway. When identified cells were recorded before and after the animal had run around for extended periods, they observed during LIA an increase in the cross-correlation between cells that had been simultaneously active during the previous period. That is, cells with firing fields that were close together in the environment were more likely to fire close together in time during an ensuing period of slow-wave sleep than cells with more distant fields. The small number of collateral fibers between CA1 pyramidal cells suggests that this effect might be due to an increase in the efficacy of the common input from CA3 or the entorhinal cortex onto these cells, rather than to the direct connections between them. In the consolidation view of LIA, the uncoupling of the hippocampus from the septum during LIA is merely a necessary condition for hippocampal consolidation to occur.

A related idea is that LIA is a period involving transfer of information from hippocampus to neocortex. Support for this view comes from experiments (Siapas and Wilson, 1998) that showed a correlation between hippocampal sharp waves and neocortical spindle waves during slow-wave sleep. The hypothesis that information might be transferred from the hippocampus to the neocortex as a result of LIA-associated sharp waves is consonant with evidence from behavioral experiments addressing the question of long-term storage of memory "traces" in or outside of the hippocampus. Chapter 12 presents evidence that lesions to the hippocampus in animals and humans can sometimes cause temporally graded amnesia. One interpretation of such a gradient is that memory traces are stored only in the hippocampus for a short period before being sent to the neocortex for permanent storage (see Chapter 13, Section 13.3 for a more extensive discussion of consolidation). After this period, damage to the hippocampus would no longer result in memory loss. Although the sharp waves may be part of such a mechanism, there is some evidence against this general idea. For example, Leonard and colleagues (1987) have shown that LTP cannot be induced in the hippocampus during slow-wave sleep. If this finding can be generalized to other parts of the brain, it would greatly reduce the attractiveness of the hypothesis that sharp waves could serve as a basis for consolidation because no new LTP-based learning could take place. There is clearly much more to understand about ripple/sharp-wave states. A possible role in memory formation may not be restricted within the confines of the currently dominant theory of intrahippocampal consolidation or hippocampo-neocortical trace transfer during sleep. For example, ripple/sharp-wave events may have a purely intrahippocampal *housekeeping* function. To take just one possibility, synaptic renormalization or overall gain control processes might occur during LIA.

11.4.5 Small Irregular Activity

Small irregular activity (SIA) is characterized by low-amplitude irregular activity in the hippocampus and desynchronization in the neocortical EEG. In 1967, Pickenhain and Klingberg reported low-amplitude irregular activity in the hippocampus of rats during transitions to alertness where no orienting movements were made, such as when a click awakened them from sleep. Vanderwolf and Whishaw (Whishaw and Vanderwolf, 1971) noted a similar pattern during transitions to alertness but added the observation that SIA, as they called it, occurred when rats abruptly halt voluntary movement.

Jarosiewicz and colleagues (2002) have extended the characterization of SIA to include periods during sleep. Sleep SIA bursts occur repeatedly during all periods of slow-wave sleep and after nearly every REM episode. Each burst typically lasts a few seconds, with a range from 200 ms to many seconds. A brief tone presented in sleep routinely elicited an increase in electromyographic (EMG) and neocortical arousal accompanied by hippocampal SIA, suggesting that it is a state intermediary between LIA and theta (Jarosiewicz and Skaggs, 2004b). Sleep SIA is characterized by the cessation of firing in most pyramidal cells. The 3% to 5% that continue to fire do so actively and repeatedly over successive bursts. These place cells are probably continuing to represent the location where the rat fell asleep because rotating the platform and the sleeping rat away from a given cell's place field location relative to the testing laboratory did not have an effect on SIA firing (Jarosiewicz and Skaggs, 2004a).

11.4.6 Beta/Gamma Activity in the Hippocampus

In addition to the low-frequency EEG activity seen during theta and LIA, and the higher frequency ripple activity characteristic of sharp waves and dentate spikes, intermediate frequency 10- to 100-Hz waves have also been described. This band is further divided into beta (10–20 Hz) (Leung, 1992) (Fig. 11–1D) and gamma (20–100 Hz) (Fig. 11–1E) activity. Gamma waves were first described in the cat amygdala by Lesse in 1955 and have since been reported in widespread brain regions of animals and humans (Singer and Gray, 1995). It has been suggested that gamma synchrony between various regions of the neocortex binds together the simple elements of a complex representation. In the hippocampal formation, they occur most clearly in the entorhinal cortex and dentate but have also been reported in the CA fields (Csicsvari et al., 2003). They may be related to 40-Hz oscillations that have been reported in the olfactory (Freeman, 1975) and visual (Singer and Gray, 1995) systems.

Gamma activity is slightly depressed in the rat by both septal lesions and cholinergic antagonists (Leung, 1985). In rabbits, drugs that stimulate a-theta during immobility (e.g., physostigmine) increase the amount of this intermediate frequency. However, this increase does not seem to occur in immobile rats. Seizures cause a dramatic increase in the amount of beta/gamma activity, an effect blocked by cholinergic antagonists and unaffected by the animal's ongoing behavior (Leung, 1992). The extent to which this beta/gamma activity is a reflection of the underlying behavior of neural elements (principal cells or interneurons) is unclear, although it may be a correlate of the activity of hilar theta cells.

11.4.7 Olfactory Stimulation Can Elicit Hippocampal Gamma and Beta Waves

In the rat hippocampal formation, both beta and gamma waves occur preferentially during olfaction. The dentate gamma waves appear to occur during the sniffing of odors in general but do not occur during odorless sniffing or other sensory stimulation (Vanderwolf, 2001) (Fig. 11–1E). The behavioral correlates of the CA1/CA3 gamma have not been established. In general, gamma and theta occur independently, but under some (undefined) circumstances they become synchronized, with the gamma occurring preferentially at the positive peak of the dentate theta waves. The dentate, but not the CA1, gamma is dependent on the perforant path input from the entorhinal cortex, as lesions of the entorhinal cortex abolish the dentate gyrus gamma but enhance the CA1/CA3 gamma (Bragin et al., 1995). Dentate gamma waves may be part of the mechanism for synchronizing the olfactory inputs arriving via the entorhinal cortex with the hippocampal theta. Beta waves have a more restricted olfactory correlate than gamma waves. They occur in the dentate gyrus in response to olfactory inputs that signal, or mimic those that signal, the presence of predators (Fig. 11–1D) (Vanderwolf, 2001): compounds found in the anal scent gland secretions of weasels and foxes, most organic solvents including toluene and xylene, and phytochemicals derived from plants such as eucalyptol and salicylaldehyde. In general, these odors also elicit a fear response and behavioral avoidance. Other strong smells, such as ammonia, cadaverine, or putrescine, which are either approached or not avoided, do not elicit dentate beta waves. Vanderwolf has argued that these olfactory correlates of gamma and beta waves in the hippocampus suggest a primary olfactory function for this structure, but it is more likely that, like the theta waves, they represent one aspect of a more complex overall function, such as cognitive mapping or associative memory formation.

11.5 Single-cell Recording in the Hippocampal Formation Reveals Two Major Classes of Units: Principal Cells and Theta Cells

Although EEG recordings provide some information about the circumstances under which large numbers of neurons in a brain region become synchronously active, it is generally accepted that a complete understanding of function can be gained only by looking at the behavioral correlates of single units. One reason for this is that although neighboring neurons often share common functional properties they may not always respond to the same specific stimulus or behavior. As we shall see, this is particularly true of the hippocampus, where neighboring pyramidal cells share the property of representing places in an environment. However, because different cells become active in different parts of an environment, this property is not revealed in the hippocampal EEG.

The recording of individual neuronal responses in the hippocampus of the awake freely moving rat began during the early 1970s with the work of Ranck (1973) and O'Keefe (O'Keefe and Dostrovsky, 1971). They both encouraged their animals to move around the environment, engaging in every-

day tasks such as eating, drinking, sleeping, and searching for food and water. This emphasis on naturalistic behavioral correlates led to several important discoveries. The first was that they noticed that there were two major classes of cells that could be distinguished by differences in their anatomical and physiological properties (e.g., firing rates, action potential width, and relative locations in the hippocampus). Ranck termed these two classes complex-spike and theta cells, and these terms are still in general usage. We describe their properties in a subsequent section. Perhaps more importantly, they discovered that the firing patterns of the two cell types had repeatable behavioral correlates. Ranck had trained his animals to approach one location to obtain food and another to get water, and emphasized the relation of the complex-spike cell firing pattern to the behavioral approach to reward. O'Keefe was more impressed by the spatial correlate and named the cells *place* cells. It is now widely accepted that the location of the animal in a familiar environment is the major determinant of when such cells fire.

The second class of neurons, the *theta* cells, has less specific behavioral correlates. As the name implies, their behavioral correlates are closely related to those of the gross EEG waves and in particular theta. They tend to change rate during hippocampal EEG theta, and many display strong phase locking to the individual theta waves.

Extracellular recordings in the freely moving rat enable complex-spike and theta cells to be distinguished on the basis of differences in their wave shapes, firing rates, and other properties (Fig. 11–3). Complex-spike place cells have a much broader action potential than theta cells (Fig. 11–3B–D), often display a complex-spike burst pattern in which the later spikes in a burst are smaller in amplitude and of longer duration than the first (Fig. 11–3A), and have a lower spontaneous

Figure 11–3. Complex-spike cells and theta cells have different physiological properties. *A.* Theta cells have a steady firing rate and constant size amplitude spikes, whereas C-S cells sometimes emit a complex-spike burst in which the later action potentials in the burst are lower in amplitude and broader. *B–D.* Action potentials of C-S cells (pyr) are broader and have a larger initial hump than those of

theta cells (int). *E.* C-S cells have a narrower range of interspike intervals (ISI) *F.* Three-dimensional plot of firing rate against mean ISI and spike asymmetry (a-b in *D*) separates the overall population into two clusters. (*Source: A,B.* After Christian and Deadwyler, 1986; *C–F.* After Csicsvari et al., 1998 with permission.)

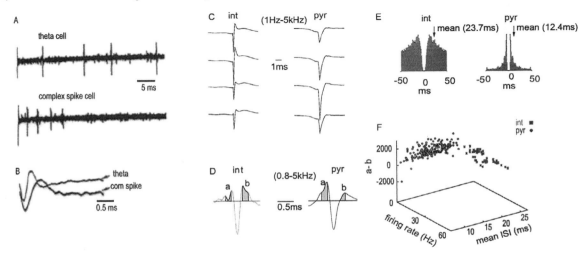

background firing rate (generally about 1 Hz) (Fig. 11–3F). In contrast, theta cells have a much higher firing rate (10–100 Hz) (Fig. 11–3F) with all action potentials being of the same amplitude (Fig. 11–3A) and of shorter duration (Fig. 11–3B-D). An important caveat is that in the rabbit this separation of spikes into two nonoverlapping classes is less clear as there appears to be a large subclass of complex-spike cells with spontaneous firing rates as high as 6 Hz.

It is highly likely that in the rat the complex spike cells are pyramidal cells and the theta cells are one or more types of interneuron. Intracellular staining of neurons that display complex spikes in brain slices reveals they have the morphology of pyramidal cells, whereas those without complex spikes are interneurons. Sometimes it is possible to activate complex spike cells antidromically from electrodes placed in hippocampal outflow pathways, but the theta cells can only be driven orthodromically (Berger and Thompson, 1978; Fox and Ranck, 1981; Christian and Deadwyler, 1986). Another strong piece of evidence in support of the idea that complex-spike cells are pyramidal cells and theta cells are interneurons comes from the temporal relation between their firing patterns. Most pyramidal cells innervate neighboring interneurons via an axon collateral, which should give rise to an increased probability of firing in the theta cell shortly after an action potential in the pyramidal cell. Just such a relation

has been reported. Some theta cells tend to fire a few milliseconds after a complex-spike cell recorded on the same tetrode (see Box 11–1), and this is reflected in a short latency cross-correlation between their spike trains (Csicsvari et al., 1998) (Fig. 11–4B-D and Box 11–2).

The same generalizations can be made for rabbits. However, there appears to be an additional group of intermediate cells that exhibit complex spikes and that can be antidromically activated by stimulation of projection pathways; but they have a resting firing rate that is intermediate between the theta and complex-spike cell firing rates shown in rats (Berger et al., 1983).

11.5.1 Distinctive Spatial Cells—Complex-spike Place Cells, Head-direction Cells, and Grid Cells—Are Found in Various Regions of the Hippocampal Formation

Discovery of the place cells led to the development of the *cognitive map theory* of hippocampal function by O'Keefe and Nadel (1978), which has guided much of the subsequent research and theorizing on hippocampal function (see Chapter 13, Section 13.4). Equally important for our understanding of the spatial functions of the hippocampal formation was the discovery of two other classes of spatial cell: In

---

Box 11–1
Microelectrode Recording Technique

Microelectrodes placed in the extracellular space in the vicinity of a neuron detect the current flow associated with action potentials. Experience has shown that relatively large electrodes with flat tips are preferable for recording in chronic animals because they do not puncture the cells and therefore do less damage during small movements of the electrode relative to the brain. One problem with the use of single electrodes in a structure such as the hippocampus is that it is difficult to isolate single units on the basis of action potential amplitude and shape. This is because of the close packing of the identically sized and shaped cells. Action potentials from all cells on a sphere with the electrode at the center are identical. There is a danger that all such spikes are considered to have come from one neuron. Template-matching algorithms, which are so useful when different cell types are in close proximity, offer no way out of this ambiguity and also have difficulty coping with the fact that a single pyramidal cell sometimes fires simple spikes and sometimes complex spike bursts in which the later action potentials in the burst have reduced amplitude and broader waveforms than the initial spike (Fig. 11–3A). One solution, introduced by McNaughton et al. (1983b), is to use multiple electrodes whose tips are close enough to sense the action potentials from a group of neurons but, being spaced a short distance apart, cannot both be at the center of a notional sphere. Each electrode tip is a slightly different distance from a given cell and, consequently, records its action potential with a slightly different amplitude and shape. These sometimes subtle differences can be used to distinguish a multiunit recording from several electrodes into spikes emanating from different cells. The principle is analogous to a "stereophonic" recording in which two or more microphones are used to capture the sound of an orchestra; hence, the earliest electrodes of this type used two wires and were called "stereotrodes." In general, $n + 1$ electrodes are necessary to identify uniquely the action potential from a neuron in n-space. In the hippocampus, "triotrodes" with three tips oriented in the plane of the quasi-two-dimensional pyramidal cell layer would probably suffice; but in practice, "tetrodes" are commonly used to ensure adequate isolation (O'Keefe and Recce, 1993; Wilson and McNaughton, 1993). Figure 11–4A shows the profile of action potentials of complex-spike and theta cells on the four electrodes of a tetrode.

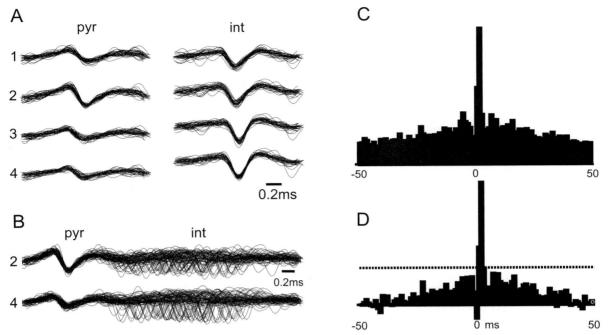

Figure 11–4. Hippocampal interneurons sometimes fire a few milliseconds after neighboring pyramidal cells. *A.* Waveforms of a pyramidal (pyr) and an interneuron (int) recorded on the same tetrode (traces 1–4). *B.* Multiple sweeps triggered on the pyramidal cell show that the interneuron often fired at a short but variable latency shortly after, suggesting a monosynaptic coupling between the two. *C.* Cross-correlogram between the firing trains of the two cells in *B* shows the interneuron fires at a peak latency of 2 ms following the spike in the pyramidal cell. *D.* Controlling for the repetitive rhythmical pattern of firing within each of the spike trains does not eliminate the short-term causal relation between the two. Horizontal line in *D* indicates a significance level above which the correlation is highly significant. (*Source*: After Csicsvari et al., 1998, with permission.)

Box 11–2
Auto-correlation and Cross-correlation Functions

Correlation techniques are used to investigate the temporal relations of spike occurrences to themselves (auto-correlation) (Fig. 11–3 E), to the occurrence of spikes in other neurons (cross-correlation) (Fig. 11–4C,D), and to other brain events (e.g., theta waves) (Fig. 11–5) or to sensory and motor events in the environment (e.g., peristimulus event histogram) (see Fig. 11–17, later). The auto-correlation function is useful for revealing repetitive or rhythmical patterns of firing. A graph is constructed in which the x-axis represents time intervals before and after each spike event, and the y-axis represents the probability that the cell will fire during each interval before or after that spike event. A period of 50 ms is a useful period of time for looking at the complex spike properties of principal cells in which the cell fires repetitively within 10 ms (Fig. 11–3A,E); 500 ms is a useful length of time for demonstrating the rhythmical pattern of theta cell firing. The cross-correlation function reveals the tendency of two cells to fire with a particular temporal relation to each other. Here one cell is chosen as the target, and its spikes fix the zero point on the time axis. The probability of the other cell firing at times earlier and later is calculated and displayed as a histogram. This type of analysis is useful for identifying potential synaptic relations between cells or the existence of common inputs to the cells. The cross-correlogram between a complex-spike cell and a theta cell is shown in Figure 11–4C,D. The peak at 2 ms suggests that there is a short-latency excitatory synaptic connection from the pyramidal cell to the theta cell. The probability associated with this peak gives some indication of the strength of this connection. The correlation between hippocampal units and the phase of the global EEG theta signal is useful for showing the temporal relations of different types of unit to the EEG and to each other (Fig. 11–5). A final use of correlation techniques is to look for a relation of spike firing to a sensory event or motor action in the external world or to another brain event. Illustrated in Figures 11–17 to 11–19 are peristimulus histograms of hippocampal unit responses to auditory stimuli as a result of conditioning experiments and in Figure 11–20 (see later) the increase in activity during different aspects of the behavioral learning paradigm.

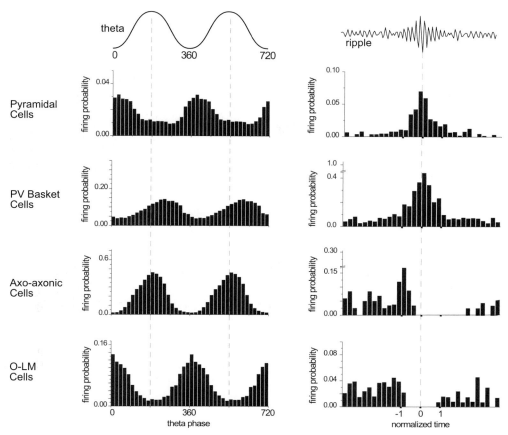

Figure 11–5. Phase relations of pyramidal cells and various classes of interneurons for theta (*top left*) and sharp-wave ripples (*top right*). Note that the various interneurons have phase relations different from those of theta activity. Note also that pyramidal cells and basket cells fire during the ripples, axo-axonic cells fire slightly before, and both they and the O-LM cells are silent during the ripples. (*Source:* After Klausberger et al., 2003.)

1984, Ranck described the *head direction* units, and in 2005 Hafting and colleagues discovered the *entorhinal grid* cells. The availability of directional and distance information to the mapping system was a prediction of the theory, and the discovery of these cell types in the hippocampal formation provides strong support for it.

Head direction cells were first discovered in the dorsal presubiculum (or postsubiculum) (Ranck, 1984; Taube et al., 1990a). The activity of these cells complements that of the place cells: They do not take into account the animal's location but signal the direction in which it is pointing relative to the environmental frame. They are rarely found in the hippocampus proper but mainly in another part of the hippocampal formation, the dorsal presubiculum, which has strong anatomical connections to the hippocampus via its projections to the entorhinal cortex, perhaps to the grid cells located there. The best estimate is that about 25% of the cells in this area are sensitive to head direction, whereas other cells there have angular head velocity, running speed, locational, and both directional and locational correlates (Sharp, 1996; Cacucci et al., 2004). They are discussed in Section 11.9.

The grid cells are found in the medial entorhinal cortex. Their firing maps lay down a regular pattern of locations across all environments the animal encounters. They are well suited to provide the self-motion or idiothetic information for the construction of place cells, as well as the distances and directions between them. They are considered in greater detail in Section 11.7.7.

Not everyone who has recorded from principal cells in the hippocampus agrees with this spatially conditioned way of looking at the data. For example, there have been reports of temporal correlates between pyramidal cell firing with eyelid responses during nictitating membrane conditioning and sensory, motor, and task-related correlates during olfactory learning and memory tasks. These reports have suggested a function for the hippocampus broader than spatial memory and navigation, perhaps as a storage device for nonspatial as well as spatial relations. Several authors, most notably Eichenbaum and Cohen (Cohen and Eichenbaum, 1993; Eichenbaum and Cohen, 2001), have returned to the original Ranck description of these cells as having behavioral approach as well as spatial and relational correlates. The next sections focus on the extensive literature on place cells, theta cells, and on other spatially related cells in particular, head-direction cells, and grid cells. Work on nonspatial correlates is described in later sections (see Section 11.11).

11.6 Theta Cells

The second major class of cells in the rodent hippocampal formation is the theta cell. These cells are distinguishable from the complex-spike cells by having a briefer action potential, a higher firing rate, and a different anatomical location (Fig. 11–3). They also have a different relation to the hippocampal EEG. Given the predominance of theta EEG activity during certain behaviors, it is not surprising to find that many cells in the hippocampus have a rhythmical pattern of firing that is related to theta. Theta cells were originally defined by their strong, consistent phase correlation to the EEG theta pattern and by their increased firing rate during theta, irrespective of the animal's location. Subsequently, the class was broadened to include cells that decrease their firing rates during theta. In contrast, the timing of complex-spike action potentials relative to the theta waves is more complex and changes as the animal moves through the place field (see Section 11.7.9). In the rest of this section, the relation of theta cells to the EEG, their pharmacology, and their correlation with behavior are described.

11.6.1 Theta Cells Fire with a Consistent Phase Relation to EEG Theta

The defining feature of theta cells is their close relation to the hippocampal EEG. Bland and his colleagues (Colom and Bland, 1987) have identified four classes of theta cell, theta-on and theta-off cells, each of which is subdivided into phasic and tonic subtypes. Theta-on cells increase their firing rates during theta activity, whereas theta-off cells decrease their activity. Phasic cells have strong constant phase relations to theta; tonic ones do not. The theta-off cells are found much less frequently than theta-on cells and are particularly rare in the freely moving rat.

In the urethane-anesthetized rat, both CA1 and dentate theta cells fire close to the negative peak of the dentate theta. In contrast, in the awake animal, maximal firing is found much closer to the positive peak of the dentate theta (Fox et al., 1986). In addition, there is a broad range of preferred phases in the various cells pointing to a heterogeneous population of theta cells. It is likely that more than one class of interneuron is involved, corresponding to the different classes of hippocampal interneuron identified in Chapter 8. Different types of interneuron have different phase correlates to theta and the LIA sharp waves. For example, Klausberger (2003) reported that the basket cells, which have their cell body in the pyramidal cell layer and inhibit the perisomatic region of the pyramidal cells, preferentially fire on the positive/negative part of the theta wave and on each wave of the sharp-wave rip-

ple oscillation; oriens/lacunosum-moleculare cells, with their somata in the stratum oriens and their axons targeted on the distal dendrites of the pyramidal cells, fire on the negative phase of the theta wave and are silent during sharp waves; axo-axonic cells, which target the axon hillock of the pyramidal cells, fire on the positive theta wave and are also silent on the sharp waves (Fig. 11–5).

In the rabbit, the same cells take part in both a-theta and t-theta. Typically, the firing rate during a-theta is lower than during t-theta even for the same frequency of theta. Within each type of theta, the firing rates of the theta cells vary as a function of the frequency of theta. In Section 11.7.9, we discuss in greater detail the temporal relation between the complex-spike and theta cells and the EEG theta.

11.6.2 Pharmacology of Theta Cells

As we have seen in Chapters 3 and 8, interneurons in the hippocampus receive both GABAergic and cholinergic inputs from the septal nuclei, GABAergic and endorphin peptidergic inputs from other inhibitory interneurons, and glutamatergic inputs from the pyramidal cells. Finally, they receive catecholaminergic inputs from the brain stem and might be expected to respond to transmitters such as noradrenaline (norepinephrine). Firing rates of theta cells recorded in the urethane-anesthetized rat decreased by up to 75% following iontophoretic application of atropine or scopolamine (Stewart et al., 1992). There was, however, no change in the phase relation between the remaining spikes and the EEG theta. This is markedly different from the effect of the same drugs on complex-spike cells, which did not change their rate of firing but altered their patterns of firing from the usual complex-spike burst pattern to more continuous firing. This suggests that the cholinergic input to the hippocampus from the medial septal nucleus makes direct contact with the theta cells and increases their firing rate but has no influence on their theta burst mode of firing. It further suggests that the pattern of activity in complex spike cells, in contrast to the rate, has only a modest influence on the pattern of firing of the theta cell interneurons. Opiates have a different effect: They directly inhibit the interneurons and indirectly disinhibit the pyramidal cells, increasing their discharge rate firing (Pang and Rose, 1989). Finally norepinephrine has an effect that is broadly opposite to that of the opiates, exciting interneurons and inhibiting the principal cells in both the CA1 field (Pang and Rose, 1987) and the dentate gyrus (Rose and Pang, 1989).

11.6.3 Hippocampal Theta Cells Have Behavioral Correlates Similar to Those of the Hippocampal EEG

In the rat, theta-on cells increase their firing rates during the EEG theta and begin to fire in a bursting pattern in phase with the theta rhythm. This normally occurs during behaviors such as walking and swimming, which change the animal's location in an environment. During LIA behaviors (e.g., slow-wave sleep, quiet sitting, eating, drinking, grooming), theta cell firing is lower in frequency and more random in pattern. Interestingly, low-frequency theta mode firing occurs during the postural shifts of grooming, such as changes from face-washing to flank-grooming.

Theta-off cells have the opposite behavioral correlates, increasing their firing rate during LIA and decreasing their rates during theta. There are differences between the behavioral correlates of theta in the rat and rabbit (see above), and similar differences are found in the correlates of theta cells in these two animals. For example, a-theta in the rabbit occurs much more readily in response to arousing stimuli in the absence of movement. It is no surprise, then, that the theta cells also fire during arousing stimuli as well as during movements such as walking and hopping. As we shall see in the section on conditioned responses in single hippocampal units (11.11.5), this a-theta related firing may help explain the involvement of the hippocampus in the timing of such responses to the (arousing) conditioned stimulus.

An important pointer to one function of the theta cells comes from an interesting observation by Nitz and McNaughton (2004). They found that a large number of CA1 theta cells turn off during the first exposure to a novel environment, whereas the dentate interneurons increased firing rates. Perhaps the CA1 interneurons are part of a mechanism for identifying familiar and novel environments and for controlling the processes of learning that occur in CA1 pyramidal cells when the animal is confronted with environmental novelty.

11.7 Complex-spike Cells and Spatial Processing

The primary correlate of hippocampal complex-spike cell firing is the animal's location in an environment. For this reason they have been called *place* cells (Fig. 11–21A, see color insert). This section begins with a description of the properties of place cells, followed by the factors that control the location, size, and shape of place fields. Both exteroceptive sensory cues and internal proprioceptive/vestibular cues play a role in determining place field structure and location. The frame of reference for the spatial coordinates of place fields can vary depending on the environment. It is known that the spatial code is conveyed by the temporal firing pattern of the complex-spike cells as well as by their absolute rate of firing. The animal's location in an environment is not given by the activity of a single place cell but by the pattern of firing across a large number of such cells. It follows, therefore, that it is important to look at the network properties of place cells. Place cells have been found in areas outside of the hippocampus, in particular in the subiculum and entorhinal cortex; and the properties of these cells and how they differ from those in hippocampus are discussed. The final section examines the data suggesting that place cell firing is controlled by activity in

brain regions outside the hippocampal formation and in particular by cells in the septal region and in the thalamus.

11.7.1 Place Cells Signal the Animal's Location in an Environment

Place cells were discovered by O'Keefe and Dostrovsky in 1971 (O'Keefe and Dostrovsky, 1971). After recording from rat CA1 complex-spike cells during various behavioral tasks and in response to various types of sensory stimulation, they noticed that the activity of some cells was more closely related to the animal's location than to any aspect of the task in which it was engaged. O'Keefe (1976) confirmed and extended these observations by recording from rats as they ran between the arms of a three-arm maze to obtain different rewards. He christened these cells *place cells* and called the location where each cell fired its *place field*. There were several aspects of the firing patterns of these cells that suggested they were signaling the abstract concept of place rather than acting as simple sensory cells. First, it was not possible to identify any single sensory stimulus that reliably controlled the cell's activity. Second, after the rat had some experience with running on the maze in the dark as well as in the light, many of the complex-spike cells continued to fire in the appropriate location with the lights out. Third, on the broad-armed maze used by O'Keefe, many cells fired equally well as the animal faced in any direction. Finally, place field firing did not seem to depend on the animal's motivation or incentive for visiting a location. For example, interchanging the food and water rewards at the ends of the different arms of the maze had no effect on place cell firing. Thus, complex-spike cells did not appear to be tuned to specific sensory stimuli, they tolerated radical changes in lighting, and they were omnidirectional and uninfluenced by reward. The notion that something more abstract was being signaled—such as location—seemed an appropriate conclusion.

Some skepticism greeted the first qualitative reports of the properties of these cells. However, the introduction of photographic methods and, later, the development of computational methods of obtaining objective data gradually convinced the most ardent skeptics (Box 11–3 and Fig. 11–6). Over the years, improvements in single-cell isolation (see Box 11–2), coupled to ever more sophisticated behavioral procedures and unusual bits of apparatus (e.g., "morph" boxes with walls that can be reconfigured), have helped unravel many of the properties and determinants of place cells.

O'Keefe (1976) noted that although many complex-spike cells could be classified as simple place cells, others had more complex properties. For these cells, the firing rate was dependent on factors in addition to location. For example, some cells increased their firing rates if the animal experienced an object in their place field or engaged in a particular type of behavior there (e.g., running or sniffing). The clearest example of this type of cell was one that fired maximally when the animal went to a specific location on the maze and either failed to find something that had been there often before or found something new. These complex spatial cells were called *mis-*

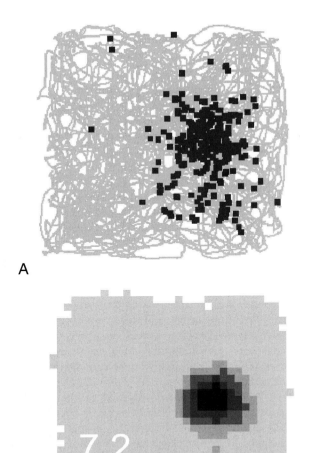

A

B

7.2

Figure 11–6. Firing field of a CA1 place cell. *A*. Raw data from a rat foraging for food in a square box for 10 minutes. Gray line traces the animal's path through the environment; black boxes show firing of place cell. *B*. Place firing field as a grayscale map where darker colors represent higher firing rates. Inset number in white gives the peak firing rate. (*Source*: After Wills et al., 2005, with permission.)

Box 11–3
Quantitative Recording of Place Fields

An objective description of the firing field of a place cell is achieved by constructing a map of firing frequencies across the surface of an environment (see Fig. 11–6). The location of a small light fixed to the animal's head is monitored by an overhead television camera, and the animal's position is recorded throughout the trial. The environment is broken up into a set of squares, and two independent measures are computed for each square: the amount of time the animal spent there and the number of times the cell fired while the animal occupied that square. A firing rate per square can be calculated by dividing the number of spikes in each square by the amount of time the animal spent there. Spatial firing rates are often portrayed as false color or grayscale maps in which different colors or shades of gray represent different firing rates. In some laboratories, the data are spatially averaged and smoothed before this step. The colors or grayscales allocated to the different firing rates are usually adjusted relative to each cell's peak firing rate (auto-scaling) to give comparable field pictures from high- and low-firing cells. When fields are created for the same cell across different conditions, it is often useful to fix all of the color map levels to the first one to facilitate comparisons. In some experiments, two differently colored lights or infrared lights of different intensities are fixed at different positions on the animal's head so the computer monitoring the animal's movements can compute the instantaneous heading direction as well as location. The best estimates of spatial firing are achieved during tasks in which the animal visits each section of the environment for an equal amount of time.

---

place cells. Whether the firing of these misplace cells was due to the absence of the expected object or reward or to the myostatial (exploratory) sniffing elicited by the mismatch was not clear. Ranck (1973) noted similar behavioral correlates of hippocampal complex-spike cells but did not identify their spatial properties. He labeled one class "approach-consummate" cells because they fired as the animal ran toward the food or the water reward. Another class he called "approach-consummate mismatch" cells because they fired maximally when the animal sniffed around the reward location when the reward was withheld. It now seems likely that many and perhaps all of Ranck's first class of cells are synonymous with O'Keefe's category of place cells and his second class synonymous with the misplace cells. Eichenbaum and his colleagues have recorded cells during odor discrimination tasks with properties similar to those described by Ranck and

questioned whether all of these cells are best described as having spatial fields. This work is described in more detail later (see Section 11.11).

11.7.2 Basic Properties of Place Fields

The size and shape of place fields vary with the shape and perhaps also the size of the testing enclosure as well as with the part of the hippocampus from which the recordings are taken. In the dorsal hippocampus, fields on small, open platforms have a tendency to be located along the edges or just off them (seen when the animal peers over the edge), whereas those in closed cylinders or rectangular boxes tend to be equally distributed around the environment (Muller et al., 1987) (Fig. 11–7). On mazes, fields may be located anywhere, with no tendency for them to cluster in particular arms or in particular parts of the maze such as at choice points (O'Keefe, 1976; Olton et al., 1978; McNaughton et al., 1983a; O'Keefe and Speakman, 1987). There are, however, occasional reports that provide exceptions to this generalization: Hetherington and Shapiro (1997) reported that fields tended to cluster closer to walls than in the center of rectangular boxes, and Hollup et al. (2001) found a greater representation of fields in the region of the goal in an annular-shaped swimming pool.

Place fields of 32 simultaneously recorded complex-spike cells

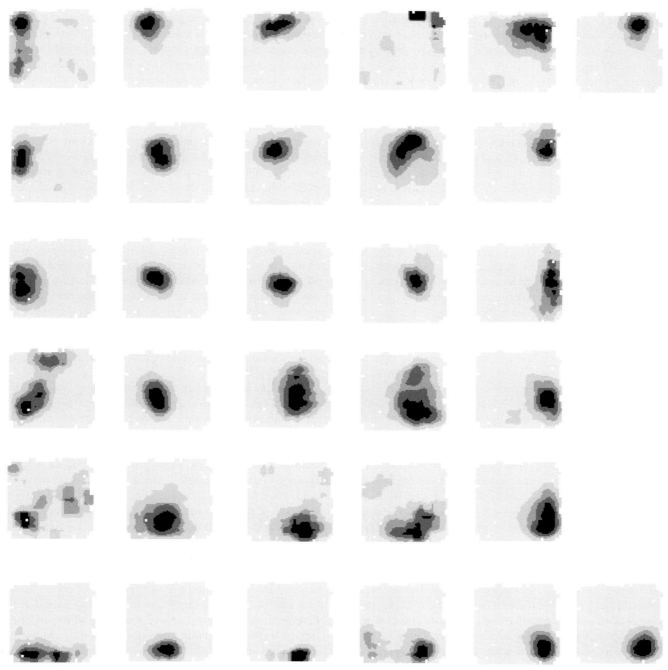

Figure 11–7. Firing fields of 32 place cells simultaneously recorded while a rat foraged for food in a 62-cm² box. The place field maps are arranged topographically so fields in the northwest of the box are located at the upper left, fields in the southwest are located at the lower left, and so on. In reality there is no topographical relation between the location of cells in the hippocampus and the location of their fields in an environment. (*Source*: After Lever et al., 2002, with permission.)

One distinctive feature of the representation of any particular environment by the hippocampal place cells is the absence of topographical mapping of function onto anatomy, such as is seen in the neocortex. That is, place cells located next to each other in the hippocampus are no more likely to have fields located next to each other than those far away (O'Keefe et al., 1998). In contrast, there have been some reports that neighboring cells have fields closer than expected by chance (Eichenbaum et al., 1989) or that cells in the hippocampus are functionally organized in bands separated by 300 to 400 μm along the long axis (Hampson et al., 1999). A definitive resolution of the question seems to have been given by Redish and colleagues (2001). Using tetrodes to ensure adequate spike isolation, they collected a large number of recordings of pairs of complex-spike cells during tasks in which the animals ran along circular or linear tracks. They compared the place fields of cells recorded from the same tetrode (see Box 11–2) and therefore anatomically neighboring each other, with those of cells from different tetrodes and therefore more distant from each other. They found no tendency for the place fields of neighboring cells to be closer to each other than would be expected for cells located at any two points in the hippocampus. They also recorded the activation of the immediate early gene *Arc*, which identifies active cells, as the animal explored two different environments. In neither case did they find any evidence for clustering of cells with similar spatial or temporal correlates. One is tempted to speculate that there must exist some mechanism for preventing neighboring cells with their overlapping inputs from adopting similar place fields in any environment. Perhaps one function of the inhibitory interneuronal networks is to allow some pyramidal cells to capture a territory in an environment and to exclude their neighbors from firing in that region.

Place cells rarely have more than one field in a single environment (typical testing environments are less than 1 m²). The best current estimate is that cells with double fields comprise no more than about 5% to 10% of the total. The sizes of place fields in the dorsal hippocampus vary considerably. To some extent, field size is a function of the threshold used for separating signal from noise and the location of the recording site along the dorsal septo-temporal axis of the hippocampus. Using a 1-Hz threshold as the minimum rate within a place field, field sizes in a cylinder of 76 cm radius ranged from a minimum of 4% of the surface area to a maximum of 62%, with a median size of 18% (Muller et al., 1987). (These data were obtained with single-electrode recording techniques; it is likely that the actual place field sizes are even smaller.) As can be seen from Figure 11–7, there appears to be a slight tendency for the fields in the center of the environment to be larger than those toward the periphery, but this has not been quantified.

The average size of the place field varies with location along the long axis of the hippocampus. As the recording electrode is moved to more ventral portions of the hippocampus, the size of place fields expands. Fields in the middle region of the hippocampus are almost twice as large as those in the septal hippocampus (Jung et al., 1994). The most ventral regions

of the hippocampus were not extensively explored in these studies, but a small number of cells recorded there (Maurer et al., 2005) appear to have fields twice the size of those in the middle region. It seems reasonable to assume, therefore, that field sizes increase as one goes from the dorsal to the ventral hippocampus; and some fields in the most ventral hippocampus might be very large, covering areas the size of the usual laboratory testing enclosures or even larger. This wide range of field sizes has important implications for analysis of the sensory correlates of hippocampal cells and for analysis of the differences in behavioral functions of the dorsal versus ventral hippocampus. Some authors have claimed that hippocampal complex-spike cells respond to specific sensory inputs (e.g., an odor) in the absence of a spatial correlate because the cells did not fire at higher rates in one part of the testing apparatus than in any other (e.g., Wood et al., 1999). Clearly, however, if some spatial firing fields can be as large as or even larger than the size of the apparatus, this conclusion is not warranted. At the very least, it is necessary to test sensory responses in two enclosures located in different laboratories. Similarly, when trying to discern the differences in function between the dorsal and ventral hippocampi, it is important to take this average field size difference into account. Fields that cover an entire testing enclosure might be described as spatial context neurons and in conditioning paradigms, for example, might have the primary function of distinguishing between two testing boxes rather than identifying different locations within the same testing box.

How quickly are place fields formed, and how do they develop? The answers to these questions can provide some indication of whether some or all of the representation of an environment is prefigured and what rules govern the plasticity involved in the initial development of the spatial representation. Several studies have provided reasonably good answers. On a small sample of 15 place cells, Hill (1978) found that 11 had fully fledged fields on the first entry into the relevant part of the environment. On a larger sample of cells and using tetrode recordings, Wilson and McNaughton (1993) allowed their rats to explore one-half of an open field box until it was familiar; they then removed a partition wall of the box, giving access to the whole. They reported that all place fields had stabilized within 10 to 15 minutes of entry into this new part of the enclosure. Frank et al. (2004) looked at the development of fields on a three-arm maze when one of the usual arms was closed and a new one with a different angular orientation was opened. They found that about one-quarter of the new fields on the novel arm developed rapidly within the first 2 minutes and that most fields had stabilized after 5 to 6 minutes of experience with this arm. Interestingly, cells that had less than 4 minutes of novel experience on the first day showed considerable plasticity on the second day, whereas those with more than 4 minutes' experience were much more stable. The firing in some fields strengthened in the initial location, that of others weakened, and some shifted to a new location altogether. Still others were initially silent on the arm, but after several minutes of exposure to the new arm turned on from this zero baseline and began to fire. The authors pointed out that the latter phenomenon is incompatible with a role for postsynaptic spike timing-dependent plasticity in the recorded cells as the mechanism underlying place field development. This mechanism suggests that presynaptic activity coincident with postsynaptic spiking strengthens the active synapses, and the absence of postsynaptic cell firing prior to the development of the full-blown place field rules it out. Of course, it could be that the changes are taking place in an earlier part of the circuit with postsynaptic cells that are initially active. Our own studies (Lever, Cacucci, Burton, O'Keefe, unpublished) have examined CA1 place field dynamics during the first exposure to an entirely novel environment: a 60-cm sided square box located in a curtained environment of which the animal had no prior experience. In agreement with Frank and colleagues, we found that place field establishment was rapid and could occur within 2 to 3 minutes. Most of the CA1 cells that developed fields during the first exposure to an environment maintained these fields, but some stopped firing or changed field location. This is reminiscent of the process of place field development upon exposure to a new part of a familiar environment, described above. Setting up a representation of a new environment or part of an otherwise familiar environment seems to involve a competitive competition among a group of neighboring cells perhaps mediated by the inhibitory interneuronal networks. Initially, a small number of seed cells have place fields from the moment the animal enters the environment, although the field firing rate may increase or decrease with continued experience. These cells prevent neighbors from firing in their territories through activation of inhibitory interneurons. Other cells gradually fill in the unclaimed territory until the entire space is represented, at which point no other cells are allowed to develop place fields in that environment and the representation stabilizes. Both Wilson and McNaughton (1993) and Frank and colleagues (2004) noted that some theta cells showed a marked

reduction in firing rate during the first entry into the novel environment, although according to Frank et al. this lasted only for the first minute of exploration. In a subsequent section, evidence is presented in support of O'Keefe's (O'Keefe, 1976) original idea that place cells could be activated in the place field by sensory cues experienced there or by path integration signals that compute the distance and direction from other locations. McNaughton et al. (1996) has speculated that when an animal first enters a novel environment the firing of place cells is driven by the path integration inputs and that only subsequently are the environmental stimuli experienced in each location associated with these place fields. A plausible alternative is that the small number of seed cells are driven by the appropriate combination of environmental cues from the first exposure (perhaps including the animal's own urine), and the rest of the cells are subsequently co-opted by the path integration system as the animal moves around the environment relative to these known locations. Further experimentation is needed to distinguish between these alternatives.

11.7.3 Place Fields are Nondirectional in Unrestricted Open-field Environments but Directional When Behavior Is Restricted to Routes

Place field firing sometimes depends on the direction in which the animal faces and sometimes it does not. In open-field environments, the place fields are nondirectional (Muller et al., 1994) (Figs. 11–8A; see Fig. 11–21A, color insert); on radial arm mazes (McNaughton et al., 1983a; Muller et al., 1994; Markus et al., 1995) and narrow linear tracks (O'Keefe and Recce, 1993; Gothard et al., 1996a), they are highly directional (Fig. 11–8B). Whereas in the first situation each cell may be said to represent a location, in the second it might more properly be described as representing a serial position along a path.

Figure 11–8. Place fields are nondirectional in open-field environments but directional on linear tracks. *A.* Central panel shows the firing field of a place cell in a 78 cm diameter cylinder regardless of the direction in which the rat is facing. The four outer panels show the field when the animal is facing in the four cardinal directions: northward at the top, eastward to the right, and so on. (Peak rates are shown in black: 12 center, 10 north, 12 east, 9 south, 9 west.) *B.*

Firing fields of three cells recorded simultaneously as the rat runs back and forth on a 1.5-m linear track for food reward at each end. Cells 1 and 2 fired as the animal ran from left to right but not in the opposite direction; cell 3 fired during right to left runs. (Peak rates shown in black: 9 top, 10 middle, 7 bottom.) (*Source*: Courtesy of O'Keefe.)

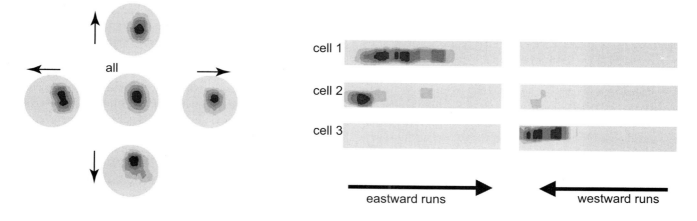

The difference between the two situations appears to be due, in part, to the constraints that the shape of the testing apparatus places on the animal's behavior. It is not a matter of sampling from two cell populations because the same cells can have directional or nondirectional fields in different testing apparatuses or under different behavioral constraints (Muller et al., 1994; Markus et al., 1995). The most important variables appear to be whether the animal can turn around in any given location and if it approaches the same location from many directions. If it can, cells are relatively nondirectional. However, if the animal always runs through the same location along the same one or two paths, place cells tend to be directional. Note that one can induce narrow and stereotypical pathtaking in open fields by reward shaping. Markus et al. (1995) originally trained rats to perform random foraging in an open cylinder and then retrained them to take direct paths in the same cylinder among four reward locations in either clockwise or anticlockwise sequences. The proportion of place fields defined as directional doubled from about 20% in the random foraging condition to 40% in the direct path condition. An important study has reexamined directionality in CA1 cells (Battaglia et al., 2004). These authors trained rats to run on narrow linear and circular tracks of the kind that would normally induce a high proportion of unidirectional place fields. Their finding across experiments was that placing various proximal multimodal cues along the tracks significantly increased the proportion of bidirectional place fields. This is puzzling because there are usually no distinctive local cues in open fields where the cells are typically nondirectional. The dynamics of (non)directionality need further study; there are no published reports examining directionality on first exposures in linear tracks. Does omnidirectionality appear as soon as a place field develops, or do the fields start out with a directional bias and only lose this directionality with further experience of the environment (Kali and Dayan, 2000)?

The existence of both directional and nondirectional modes of spatial representation raises the question of whether the hippocampus is providing fundamentally different types of information in these two situations. Specifically, does the spatial localization system, of which the place cells are a part, "know" that the rat is in the same location when, say, traveling east as when traveling west? Perhaps it is only acting to its fullest capacity when the cells are omnidirectional and is showing limited functionality when they are unidirectional. Against this is the recent demonstration (Rosenzweig et al., 2003) of a good correlation between the degree to which place cells recorded on a linear track used a particular reference frame and the animal's ability to localize an unmarked location defined within that framework. Place cells were recording on a linear track where locations could be identified in one of two conflicting frameworks: in the framework of (1) a goal box that changed location along the track from trial to trial or (2) stable room cues. The target location remained fixed relative to the stable room cues but moved from trial to trial relative to the moving goal box. The authors showed that the higher the percentage of place cells that related to the framework of the stable room cues in each rat's hippocampus, the more likely the animal was to be successful at the task. The relation of place fields to different environmental reference frames is considered at greater length in a subsequent section.

One major difference between directional and nondirectional field firing is the influence on the firing rate within the field of the overall trajectory of the path in the former but not, so far as is known, in the latter. During behavioral tasks that promote directional firing and require the rat to traverse the same part of the apparatus as part of two different paths, place cells fire differently in the place field on the two paths (Frank et al., 2000; Wood et al., 2000; Ferbinteanu and Shapiro, 2003). For example, Wood and colleagues (2000) trained animals on a continuous alternation task in a T maze that had been fitted with return tracks from each goal to the start of the stem so the animal could run in a continuous figure-of-eight path by turning left or right alternatively at the choice point of the T junction. Activity in two-thirds of the place fields in the stem of the T varied markedly depending on whether the animal entered the stem following a return from the left-hand or right-hand goal. In the Wood et al. study, it was not possible to distinguish between firing owing to the previous part of the path (retrospective coding) and the future part of the path (prospective coding). Two of the three studies (Frank et al., 2000; Ferbinteanu and Shapiro, 2003), however, did allow for this distinction and reported that, in addition to the retrospective effect of the previous path on place cell firing, the subsequent path (i.e., the upcoming turn to be made at the T junction) also had an effect on firing in the stem (a prospective effect), although the effect was seen in only a few hippocampal cells in the Frank et al. study and was much more prominent in cells in the entorhinal cortex.

These effects appear to be due to the animal repeatedly running in a continuous trajectory in the same direction through the entire path and thus activating a fixed sequence of place cells. These prospective and retrospective effects have not been reported in nondirectional fields in open-field environments, suggesting they have something to do with the stereotyped ballistic nature of the paths taken on linear tracks. In the one study in which the effect was not seen, the animals were trained to alternate on a Y maze with broad arms (Lenck-Santini et al., 2001a). They had to return to the start arm following each visit to a goal arm, resulting in a start arm → left goal → start arm → right goal → start arm, etc. alternation pattern. This behavioral pattern would activate the same cells in a different order on successive runs, and the wide arms would allow the rat to take slightly differing paths on each run. Interestingly, one observation in the Ferbineatu and Shapiro study suggests that the effect is not due solely to the activation of the immediately prior place cell in the sequence or the execution of the immediately preceding turn. On error trials in which the animal first visited an incorrect arm before entering the correct goal arm for that trial, about one-half of the cells with place fields in the goal arm continued to fire correctly. This shows that small deviations from the standard path through the environment do not disrupt the effect. The authors suggested that it is the overall journey from one place to another that is important, not the actual sequence of locations traversed. Buzsaki (2005) has speculated that the firing of any given place cell may be influenced by place cells from early stages in the path and not just by the immediately preceding cell in the sequence. At this stage, it is not clear how much these effects are due to the beginning and end points of the path and how much to particular motor behaviors, such as body turns made during the path. One possibility is that the firing of many cells on these tracks is driven by the path integration system (see Section 11.7.7), and activation of the motor, proprioceptive, and vestibular systems at the turn into the stem of the T maze marks an important location on the path and is carried over to the rest of the path. This would explain some of the retrospective effects but would not explain the prospective effects unless there is activation of the turning machinery some period of time prior to reaching the turn itself.

These studies have been interpreted by their authors as pointing to a place cell basis for the episodic functions of the hippocampus (see Chapter 13, Section 13.4). O'Keefe and Nadel (1978, 1979) originally suggested that the spatial functions of the rat hippocampus could be elaborated into a spatiotemporal episodic memory in humans by adding a temporal time-stamp signal, which would allow each set of events occurring in the same location to be distinguished from each other on the basis of their time of occurrence. The present results, however, do not provide evidence for this unique time-stamp signal, which would enable different runs to be identified as independent episodes. Rather, it seems to be more appropriately interpreted as evidence of the organization of place cells into integrated, ordered sequences, as might be expected for the representation of paths.

To conclude this section, it is clear that the place cells can be directional or nondirectional depending on the specific circumstances in which they are recorded. It is important to emphasize that the nondirectional mode of place cell activity rules out the possibility that they are simply responding to a particular configuration of distal sensory cues. They cannot be responsive just to a particular view or scene in front of the animal (sometimes called the "local view"), as this would change radically as a function of the heading direction. Moreover, as these experiments routinely control for local sensory inputs such as intramaze smells and textures, nondirectionality is evidence in favor of the idea that these cells can signal something quite abstract.

11.7.4 What Proportion of Complex-spike Cells Are Place Cells?

To estimate the proportion of complex-spike cells that are place cells, it is necessary to record from the same cells in several environments. This is because most place cells do not have a place field in every environment. For example, early studies (O'Keefe and Conway, 1978; Kubie and Ranck, 1983) reported that whereas some complex-spike cells had fields in two or more recording environments others had fields in one but not the other. A second problem is that many complex-spike cells

are silent most of the time, making it difficult to estimate the population number. Thompson and Best (1989) tried to get an accurate estimate of the population by recording during slow-wave sleep or while the rat was under light barbiturate anesthesia. Both procedures are known to enhance the spontaneous firing rates of complex-spike cells and may therefore provide a better estimate of the total population under the recording electrode than can be obtained during the active, awake state. They also recorded complex spikes in three environments: an elevated eight-arm radial maze, an enclosed cylinder, and an enclosed rectangular environment. They concluded that slightly more than a third of the cells that could be identified under barbiturate anesthesia had place fields in at least one of the three environments. Almost all of the other cells recorded had very low spontaneous rates in all environments (and were thus termed "silent cells"), with many firing no spikes for the entire period of testing. Only 14% of cells had fields in two environments, and only 1% had fields in all three environments. That is, many cells with fields in one environment acted like silent cells in the other environments. On the basis of the physiological similarities between the place cells and the silent cells, and the distribution of fields across the three boxes, Thompson and Best suggested that if enough environments were tested every complex-spike cell would have a field in at least one of them. In several studies, McNaughton and his colleagues (Wilson and McNaughton, 1993a; Gothard et al., 1996a) have sampled large groups of complex-spike cells and find that 30% to 70% have place fields in a given environment. Their group (Guzowski et al., 1999) has used the immediate early gene *Arc* to label all of the CA1 cells active in two groups of animals, each exploring a different environment. In one group 44% of CA1 cells were active and in the other group 45%—in broad agreement with the results from single-unit recordings. In animals that were allowed to explore both boxes and in which double staining was carried out, 22% of the cells were active in one environment, 23% in the other, and 16% in both. These studies make it clear that a large proportion of complex-spike cells have a place field in some environments, consistent with the view that spatial representation is one of the primary functions of the hippocampus.

Is there any relation between the size or shape of the place fields that a cell displays in one environment and those obtained in another? The answer depends on the similarity between the environments and the amount of experience the animal has had with them. When the environments are sufficiently different, such as the eight-arm radial maze without walls and a small enclosed rectangular box used in the study of Thompson and Best (1989), and the animal has had considerable experience in both, the fields are very different. In contrast, when both environments have walls and the animal is inexperienced, most fields are initially similar in shape and location despite differences of shape or color between boxes. With experience, the place cells begin to differentiate between the two environments, and after a period of time most cells fire differently in the two boxes (Bostock et al., 1991; Lever et al., 2002; Wills et al., 2005). This phenomenon is called remapping and is a good example of a type of learning that is reflected in hippocampal cell firing. Most of the remapping that occurred between square and circular environments involves the cessation of firing in one of the two environments; more rarely, there is a shift in field location between the two (Lever et al., 2002). One important factor influencing whether a complex-spike cell has a place field in any given environment might be the overall level of inhibition experienced by that cell in that environment. Thompson and Best found higher background rates in environments in which the cell had a place field than in environments in which it did not. A reasonable speculation, therefore, is that silent cells are potential place cells whose level of inhibition is high in the "silent" environment perhaps due to enhanced excitatory inputs to its inhibitory interneurons from place cells with maintained fields in that environment.

11.7.5 Frame of Reference of Place Fields

If place cells identify an animal's location, they must do so ultimately on the basis of sensory information. In this section, this issue is addressed from the perspective of frames of reference. In the next, the role of specific sensory modalities is examined. The framework to which place fields are referenced might be egocentric or allocentric. An egocentric framework is one that is anchored to the animal's body (or some part of it, such as the trunk, head, or eye) and that travels with the animal as it moves through the environment. An allocentric framework, on the other hand, is one that is fixed to some part of the environment. It is therefore a framework in which the animal's position changes as it traverses the environment. The fact that complex-spike cells recorded in an open field environment fire in their place field irrespective of the direction in which the animal is facing appears to rule out a purely egocentric reference framework. On the other hand, the fact that complex-spike cells can sometimes be directional (e.g., on linear tracks) shows that under some circumstances they can be egocentric or that the inputs to these cells may be coded in egocentric frameworks.

In open fields, where place cells appear to be anchored within an allocentric reference frame, it has been shown that this frame can be a reference to the room, the testing box, or the maze in which the animal has been placed. When recording takes place on symmetrical elevated mazes or open fields with low side-walls, the room generally provides the overall framework. This is readily revealed by rotating the testing apparatus. The usual result is that place fields follow cues located outside the apparatus (O'Keefe, 1976; Olton et al., 1978) (see Fig. 11–12B, later). This is not to say that the intra-apparatus, or what are commonly referred to as "intramaze," cues are without influence. They ordinarily may contribute to place field size or location but be overshadowed in importance by more distal, or "extramaze," cues when the two types are put in opposition. Maze rotation, however, sometimes gives rise to locational ambiguity. A cell may develop two place fields immediately after the rotation, but they quickly resolve into one field with repeated experience of the new configuration (O'Keefe, 1976; Thompson and Best, 1989).

In boxes with high walls and limited views of the room, place cells often use the box itself as the frame of reference. Rotation of the box or rotation of a "cue-card" suspended prominently on the interior wall of the box, generally causes equal rotation of the place fields (Kubie and Ranck, 1983; Muller and Kubie, 1987). On multi-arm mazes with high walls, the fields sometimes take their reference from specific arms and not from the entire maze. Under these circumstances, interchanging arms can result in the fields following a specific arm of the maze irrespective of its allocentric location (Shapiro et al., 1997). In this situation, the cells do not fire all over the surface of the arm but maintain a localized firing field relative to the "frame of the arm" and can thus still be said to be spatially coded. It should not be thought, however, that there is a sharp distinction between extramaze and intramaze cues and frameworks or that any given cell is forced to choose between them. In an experiment described in more detail later, O'Keefe and Burgess (1996) found that although most place fields were controlled by either the animal's location relative to the walls of the testing box or relative to the laboratory frame, some were responsive to combinations of one wall of the testing box and an extramaze cue, such as the wall of the testing room. Bures and colleagues (Rossier et al., 2000) developed an elegant behavioral paradigm for dissociating intramaze from extramaze frames of reference. Rats are trained to avoid a prohibited area of a static circular platform with a good view of the surrounding laboratory. Under these circumstances, the prohibited area can be defined with reference to the extramaze laboratory reference frame or the intramaze frame of the platform itself. Recording from place cells with the platform rotating slowly showed that the firing fields of some are fixed to the extramaze room cues, whereas those of others remain with the rotating intramaze cues. Turning off the lights increased the number of intramaze fields. A large proportion of place fields disintegrated when the two frames of reference were dissociated, suggesting that information from both was required.

In a subsequent experiment, Zinyuk et al. (2000) demonstrated that the proportion of cells related to the extramaze frame, the intramaze frame, or both depended on whether the animal was trained to navigate within the environment. The animals in the navigation group were trained to use the extramaze environmental cues to go to an unmarked location in the static open-field box to receive food pellets. Each entry into this target zone triggered the release of a food reward into a random location for which the rats had to forage. When the intra- and extramaze frames of reference were dissociated by rotating the box at 1 rpm, 38% of the place fields stayed with the extramaze framework, 9% with the rotating intramaze framework, and 31% with the conjunction of both. Cells in this last category fired only at that point of the cycle when the two frameworks coincided. The firing fields of only one-fifth of the cells were disrupted during rotation. In contrast, when another group of animals carried out a random foraging task in the same environment without the navigational component, almost three-fifths of the cells were disrupted by rotating the platform. Of the small number of intact fields, 21%

stayed with the extramaze environment framework, 14% with the rotating intramaze framework, and 7% with both. This study makes several important points. First, it confirms that place cells can be anchored by the extramaze environmental cues, the intramaze box cues, or both, in agreement with previous findings. Second, it shows that training the animals to pay attention to the extramaze cues increases the proportion of place cells that use these cues, alone or in combination, from less than one-third to more than two- thirds. Third, somewhat surprisingly, training to attend to the extramaze cues markedly increases the proportion of cells responsive to the conjunction of the relevant extramaze cues and the irrelevant intramaze framework. It appears that in the absence of explicit training to attend to the spatial aspects of the environment many place cells take their inputs from combinations of a small number of weak distal and local intra-maze cues which are easily disrupted by the rotation. In animals trained to attend to the distal cues the cells incorporate much more robust information especially about the extra-maze cues and are less easily disrupted when these cues are placed into conflict. Support for this interpretation comes from experiments in the same testing paradigm using blockade of one hippocampus by injection of tetrodotoxin. This has no effect on the ability of rats to avoid a place successfully on the basis of either extramaze or intramaze cues alone but blocks their ability to avoid a place on the basis of extramaze cues *in the face of* conflicting intramaze cues (Wesierska et al., 2005). The effects of unilateral blockade are probably due to the disruptive effect of the procedure on the other intact hippocampus (Olypher et al., 2006). These results should serve as a warning that some of the conclusions drawn from studies on animals foraging in the open fields in the absence of an explicit requirement to encode the spatial aspects of the environment might not be providing an accurate picture of the full range of the spatial capacities of the hippocampus.

Interestingly, this group has also shown that training rats to use room-based but not arena-based cues to navigate increases the amount of total variance in place cell firing that is accounted for by position (Olypher et al., 2002). Accordingly, they speculated that some of the variance in place cell firing not accounted for by position (Fenton and Muller, 1998) is attributable to attentional switches between alternative spatial reference frames. Their analysis may provide an interesting window into ostensibly unstable coding of place by hippocampal cells in some experiments.

11.7.6 Place Fields Can Be Controlled by Exteroceptive Sensory Cues

What sensory information does a place cell use to determine where it fires? O'Keefe (1976) suggested that two sources of information were available.

Each place cell receives two different inputs, one conveying information about the large number of environmental stimuli or events, and the other from a

navigational system which calculates where an animal is in an environment independently of the stimuli impinging on it at that moment. The input from the navigational system gates the environmental input, allowing only those stimuli occurring when the animal is in a particular place to excite a particular cell. One possible basis for the navigational system relies on the fact that information about changes in position and direction in space could be calculated from the animal's movement. When the animal had located itself in an environment (using environmental stimuli), the hippocampus could calculate subsequent positions in that environment on the basis of how far, and in what direction the animal had moved in the interim. . . . In addition to information about distance traversed, a navigational system would need to know about changes in direction of movement either relative to some environmental landmark or within the animal's own egocentric space. . . . (O'Keefe, 1976, pp. 107–108)

Both hypotheses have received experimental support: Place fields can be controlled by exteroceptive information from the environment or by movement-generated proprioceptive and vestibular stimuli. This section looks at the external sensory information arising from the environment and asks: Are some sensory modalities privileged over others? Which cues determine the angular orientation of a field in a symmetrically shaped environment, and do these differ from those that control its distance from the borders of the environment? The following section examines the role of internal cues generated by the animal's own behavior in providing estimates of distance and direction traveled.

We begin by asking: Are some sensory modalities privileged over others? There are two ways to identify the role of sensory inputs in controlling place fields. The first follows the pioneering methods of Honzik (1936) in his study of the sensory control of maze learning. Here, a specific sensory modality is eliminated by lesion or occlusion and the consequences examined. The second approach is to construct artificial environments in which there are a few controlled cues that can be experimentally manipulated. Various manipulations have been explored: Cues have been rotated; the distance between them changed; the geometry of the environment altered; associative value or cue meaning taken into account. The results show that many place cells receive information from more than one sensory input; they can use subsets of this total input to identify correctly the preferred place; and geometrical information about distance to features of the environment is particularly important.

A simple manipulation to test the role of vision is to turn out the room lights (O'Keefe, 1976; Quirk et al., 1990; Markus et al., 1994). Some cells are unaffected, but others show a more interesting response. For example, the field may disappear on the first visit to the preferred area but return on the second or third visit. In a cylindrical open-field apparatus, place fields tend to remain intact if the animal is in the environment when the lights are extinguished. However, if the animal is removed from the environment and then put back into it in the dark, about half of the fields change (Quirk et al., 1990). New fields may appear, and they are maintained even if the lights are now turned on. In contrast, there are many fewer cells that retain similar fields in the light and the dark on the radial arm maze. Furthermore, of the cells firing in both light and dark, the firing in the light was more reliable. Such observations offer yet another indication that place cells act in distinct ways in differing environments. It appears that, in a cylindrical arena or rectangle, once a pattern of place fields is set up for a particular environment it is relatively stable to alterations of exteroceptive cues—unless the animal is removed from the environment. In contrast, place cells are more sensory-bound on radial arm mazes and in other situations that restrict an animal's movements to a linear path.

Eliminating sensory modalities by occlusion or using lesions indicates that there are still place cells after the elimination of olfactory, visual, or both visual and auditory inputs. Save and colleagues (1998) found that rats blind from birth have completely normal place fields when tested as adults. The only discernible difference was a decreased firing rate of place cells compared to controls. Hill and Best's study (1981) of animals deprived of both vision and audition during adulthood revealed they also had apparently normal place fields. However, rotating the arms of the maze showed that, on average, these animals were much more "bound" to the local cues of an arm. Further experiments on the small group of cells that had fields anchored to the allocentric room frame of reference showed that rapid rotation of the animal for 20 to 30 seconds prior to running on the maze caused their fields also to come under the control of the intramaze cues. On the assumption that the rotation primarily affected the vestibular system, these results suggest that, in the absence of distal visual and auditory cues, the angular orientation of place cells can be controlled by olfactory/tactile cues on the maze and by vestibular cues. The latter may be mediated by inputs from the head direction system (see Sections 11.9 and 11.10).

Several studies have attacked the problem of cue control by constructing environments in which the distal stimuli were explicitly identified and controlled. O'Keefe and Conway (1978) trained animals on a T maze located within a set of curtains that excluded visual cues from the rest of the laboratory. Four objects were hung around the periphery of a T maze inside the curtains, and the animal was taught to choose an arm of the maze. The four cues were rotated from trial to trial. Place fields always rotated with the cues (see Fig. 11–12B, later, for a similar result). Removal of one or more cues on each trial showed that a few fields depended on one specific cue, but most were maintained so long as any two of the four cues were present. Muller and colleagues (Muller and Kubie, 1987) showed similar cue dependence of place fields recorded from rats foraging for food in cylinders or rectangular boxes. A single white cue-card fixed to the wall exerted control over the angular location of the field but not its distance from the wall. Rotation of the card rotated the fields by the same

amount. Neither the shape of the field nor its distance from the walls of the box was affected, but there was a slight loss of place specificity.

The location of the controlling cues within the environment can be important. Cressant et al. (1997) found that three objects placed in a triangular configuration in the center of a cylinder did not control the orientation of place fields, but they did do so when these same objects were moved to the periphery. This result was interpreted as suggesting that distal peripheral landmarks are more important for fixing the orientation of the place fields, perhaps because the animal's movement relative to centrally placed local cues causes constant reordering of their positions relative to each other within the egocentric frameworks of the distal sensory modalities, whereas movements relative to distal cues do not. Central object A is sometimes seen to the left of central object B and sometimes to its right.

If the angular orientation of a place field in a symmetrical environment is controlled by distal cues, what determines its shape and size and its radial distance from the walls of the environment? The first clue came from an experiment (Muller and Kubie, 1987) that showed that doubling the dimensions of a cylinder or a rectangular box had two effects: In many cells, the fields remapped to unpredictable shapes and locations; in about one-third of the place cells, however, field size increased to about twice the original size without significant effect on field shape. This is less than the fourfold increase that would have represented an exact proportion to the increased area of the recording chamber. Factors other than simple scaling seemed to be at work. A related experiment (Wilson and McNaughton, 1993b) looked at field changes after a partition was removed, converting a square box to a rectangular box whose long dimension was twice that of its short one. Here cells with fields in the square were maintained, whereas other cells began to fire in the new section of the box. It appears, then, that under some circumstances the field sizes are influenced by the size of the testing environment, but under others they are not. The factors controlling this difference are still unclear, but they may relate to whether the animal is, or is not, in the box when the change is made. If in it, the animal is better placed to see the change happening in front of him, which triggers exploration. Under these circumstances the existing fields are maintained intact and new ones created to represent the new part of the environment. However, when the animal is removed from a recording chamber with which it is familiar and placed in a dilated version of it, the system may be tricked into treating this as the "same" environment with the resulting alteration of existing fields.

O'Keefe and Burgess (1996) employed the second procedure to look at the effect of changing box size and shape on established place fields. Combining features of the preceding studies, the same cell was studied while the rat foraged for food in four differently shaped boxes: two squares, one with double the dimensions of the others; and two rectangles, each with its small side taken from the dimensions of the small square and its large side from the large square (Fig. 11–9). One

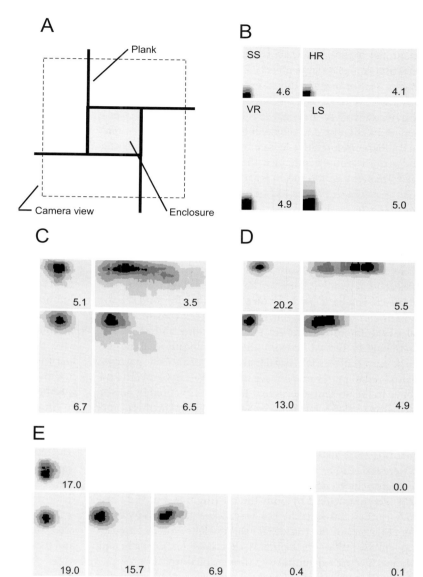

Figure 11–9. Place fields in four rectilinear enclosures reveal that each field is comprised of several subcomponents. *A*. Layout of the testing area shows how the small square (61 cm²) is constructed from four wooden planks set on their edges. The same set of planks can be joined in different configurations to make rectangular (61 by 122 cm) and large square (122 by 122 cm) enclosures. *B*. Place field with strong inputs from the left and bottom walls does not change its relative location in the various boxes. *C*. A different place field with strong inputs from the top, left, and right walls is elongated in the horizontal rectangle. *D*. A field similar to that shown in *C* breaks into two components in the horizontal rectangle. *E*. A cell with fields in the small square and vertical rectangle (two left-hand panels) shows steadily diminishing firing rates in the boxes intermediate to the vertical rectangle and the large square. Numbers in each panel represent the peak field firing rate (shown in black). (*Source*: After O'Keefe and Burgess, 1996, with permission.)

rectangle was oriented with its long side parallel to the long dimension of the testing laboratory and the other with its long side perpendicular to this dimension. The same construction materials were used, and the floor covering was interchanged frequently, eliminating local olfactory and tactile cues as determinants of field shape and location. The important finding was that for most cells the field location and shape was determined by the distance to two or more walls usually of the box but, more rarely, of the room itself. Some cells were controlled by the distance to two box walls in orthogonal directions (e.g., the south and west walls) (Fig. 11–9B); others were sensitive to the distance to three or four walls (e.g., Fig. 11–9C,D). The expansion of field width along one dimension sometimes resulted in double peaks or even the apparent splitting of a field into two (Fig. 11–9D). Some cells (e.g., Fig. 11–9E) that had a field in one box (vertical rectangle) but were silent in an adjacent box (big square) could be shown to

reduce their rates in an incremental way in boxes intermediate to these two. A small number of cells had one of their field dimensions determined by the distance to the room walls and the other by a wall of the box. One important observation was that no cells used the framework of the shape of the box itself. If this had been the case, one would expect to see cells with fields that rotated by 90° in the two rectangular configurations or that fired only in the small and large squares. These patterns were never observed. The experiment shows that in environments in which the animal has sufficient distal information to fix its directional orientation it is not the geometry of the testing box that is being captured by the place field but the intersection of distances to two or more elongated features of the environment (see Chapter 13 for a further discussion of the geometry of the spatial representation and Chapter 14 for a discussion of a computational model that accounts for these findings).

Gothard and her colleagues obtained similar results (Gothard et al., 1996b). Place cells were recorded while the rat attempted to find a reward hidden at a fixed distance and direction from two large objects. Each trial began with the rat leaving a small box and ended when it returned to it where it was also rewarded. The location of the box, like that of the objects, was moved around the room from trial to trial. Cells were found that fired as the rat entered or exited the start/goal box; others fired relative to one or other of the goal objects; and a third group maintained their field location relative to the framework of the room, regardless of the location of the goal or start box. This study complemented that of Burgess and O'Keefe in showing that relative location to objects or walls is important. It also reinforced the notion that different place cells recorded at the same time may use two or more frames of reference in a single environment.

In another study, Gothard et al. (1996a) examined the "frame of reference" issue further by recording cells in rats trained to run back and forth on a linear track for food reward at each end. The goal at one end of the track remained fixed relative to the room, whereas that at the other end was a box that could be moved between one of five locations along the track from trial to trial. Recall that on linear tracks or narrow-armed radial mazes many place cells tend to have directional fields. In the present experiment just over 42% fired in one of the two directions, another 45% in the opposite direction, and just over 12% in both directions and these usually did not bear a close spatial relation to each other. Place fields closer to the goal box were tied to it and moved with it, whereas those closer to the other end of the track tended to stay fixed with respect to the room and the fixed goal location. A number of cells were influenced by both the moving box and the fixed goal. In these cases, as the box was moved farther away from the other end of the track there was evidence for the stretching and splitting of the fields described by O'Keefe and Burgess in their expanding two-dimensional world.

Two interpretations of these results are possible. Gothard and her colleagues suggest that there are two representations or charts of the space on the track: one related to the framework of the box and the other to the room. As the animal runs along the track, it switches from one map or chart of the environment to the other. The animal was, in some sense, treating this single runway as two separate environments: a world in which it was located relative to the goal box while it was in its vicinity and a world in which it was located in the room frame as it got farther from the moving box. These authors further interpreted the constant distance of the box- related fields from the box as evidence for a path integration mechanism.

O'Keefe and Burgess favor the alternative view: that under the conditions of these experiments, the normal map-like omnidirectionality and connectedness between place cells has been lost, and they are essentially acting as isolated individuals. Each individual cell is influenced by the box and the fixed goal in proportion to the distance of its field from each. Cells close to the box are almost entirely controlled by a box, whereas those far from it are controlled by the fixed room

cues. The distance from each set of cues could be computed on the basis of sensory inputs from that cue or from path integration signals (see Chapter 14, Section 14.3 for a more detailed discussion of this model).

Fenton et al. (2000a,b) investigated the problem of cue-control of place fields in a different experimental paradigm. They recorded while rats foraged for food pellets in cylinders with two distinct cue cards on the wall and varied the angle between the cards by small amounts. Removal of either card had no effect on place fields, and rotation of the remaining card caused equal rotation of the place fields, demonstrating independent control over the fields by each card. In contrast, changing the angle between the cards from 135° to either 160° or 110° caused subtle changes in the location and shape of the fields. In general, fields shifted and transformed in the direction of card movement. Fields closer to the cards were more influenced than those farther away. An interesting finding was that the peak firing rate was highest for the original card configuration and decreased as the cards were brought closer together or placed farther apart. Although carried out under different experimental circumstances and interpreted somewhat differently by the authors, these results are broadly in line with those of O'Keefe and Burgess and of Gothard et al. in showing that place fields are determined by distances from specific environmental features.

An overview of all the experiments reviewed in this section suggests that there are at least two independent exteroceptive determinants of place fields. The directional orientation of a place field in a symmetrical enclosure is controlled by polarizing distal cues in the room or at the periphery of the testing box. On the other hand, the location and shape of the field is determined by the distance of the animal from two or more walls or by other features of the environment. In addition, it is clear that interoceptive cues can influence place field shape and location, which we discuss in the next section.

11.7.7 Idiothetic Cues Can Control Place Fields

Place fields can also be located on the basis of idiothetic cues generated by an animal's own movements, which consist of interoceptive stimuli such as head, neck and limb proprioceptors, vestibular signals, and motor reafference signals from intended movements together with exteroceptive stimuli derived from optic flow and whisker-detected airflow. We noted earlier that rats blind from birth have completely normal place fields when tested as adults (Save et al., 1998). Detailed analysis of the behavior of these animals suggested that they used olfactory and tactile information to recognize objects in the recording environment and then "updated" the locations of place fields on the basis of interoceptive cues associated with their own movements. Whereas some 80% of place cells in the sighted control rats in this study fired in the appropriate location before the animal had made contact with any of the objects, none of the place cells in the blind rats did so. However, after contact with one of the objects, 60% of cells fired appropriately in a single place, and 75% did so after

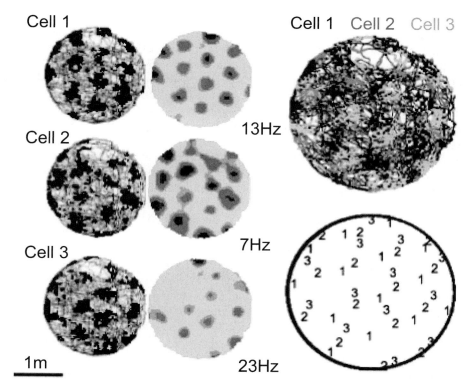

Figure 11–10. Entorhinal cortex grid cells. Raw data (left) and firing fields (right) for three grid cells. Note the regularity of the firing, which forms a triangular grid pattern in each cell. Numbers indicate the peak rate. Peaks of the three cells (top in grayscale, bottom as numbers 1–3) are slightly offset from each other so when superimposed they tend to tesselate the space. (*Source*: After Hafting et al., 2005, by permission.)

exploring two objects. Completely normal firing patterns were seen after contact with all three objects.

Maintaining spatial specificity in this way represents a form of "memory." It is presumably an "active" or "working" memory that is maintained by some form of inertial navigation or path-integration mechanism. Once an animal had identified its location in an environment on the basis of exteroceptive cues, a path integration mechanism could continuously update its position by calculating the changes in distance and direction from the original position resulting from the animal's movements. This type of mechanism might explain the short-term memory properties of place cells, which are discussed in greater detail in Section 11.8.

Further evidence for idiothetic influences on place fields comes from experiments in which animals have been passively rotated. As we saw in the experiment of Hill and Best, rotating animals deprived of vision and audition before placing them on a radial arm maze results in the rotation of place fields. Several groups (Sharp et al., 1995; Wiener et al., 1995; Bures et al., 1997; Jeffery et al., 1997) have studied the effect of rotating the testing enclosure, or parts of it, with the animal inside it. Sharp et al. (1995) rotated the cylinder walls or floor separately at a fast or slow speed and in the light or dark. It was assumed that the slow rotations were below the speed detectable by the vestibular system and would not be compensated for: The fields rotated with the rotating enclosure relative to the laboratory frame. Both visual and vestibular signals influenced the angular location of place fields to about the same extent. Slow rotation of the rat in a separate chamber outside of the testing enclosure also led to rotated place

fields when the rat was replaced into the enclosure (Jeffery et al., 1997). In both experiments the rotations were brief, and their effects were subsequently assessed in a stationary environment. Similar findings with head direction cells (Blair and Sharp, 1996) raise the possibility of a coupling between the spatial localization and head direction system. The interactions between the two are discussed in Section 11.10.

A movement-generated estimate of distance and direction would explain the instances of place cell stability in the shift from light to dark in memory tasks and following lesions that limit access to exteroceptive cues. The source of this "path-integration" signal is either input from interoceptive cues or "collateral discharges" arising from motor structures actively generating movements. This information arrives at the hippocampus via several routes. Information about the animal's heading direction is carried by the head direction cells and enters the hippocampal system through the presubiculum projection to the medial entorhinal cortex. We discuss the properties of the head direction cells in greater detail in Section 11.9 and their interaction with the place cells in Section 11.10. When it arrives to the medial entorhinal cortex, head direction information is combined with distance information in a set of grid cells (Hafting et al., 2005). One of the functions of the grid cells is to convey information about distances in specific environmental directions. Each grid cell fires in several locations in an environment, with the locations forming a regular pattern as though they were nodes on a triangular grid (Fig. 11–10; see also Fig. 11–21D, color centerfold). Different cells recorded at the same location have the same grid spacing and orientation relative to the environment. They differ, however, in the location of the nodes such that the firing peaks of one cell are slightly shifted from those of its neighbor. The multiple interdigitated fields of several such cells together cover the environment (Fig. 11–10, right). For each cell, the size of the grid appears to be independent of the size or shape of the environment. The orientation of the grid relative to the environment, however, is dependent on the location of a polarizing visual cue on the wall of the enclosure in much same way as are the postsubicular head direction (Taube et al., 1990b) and the hippocampal place cells (Muller and Kubie, 1987). It seems likely, then, that the orientation of each grid is controlled by the head direction cells of the presubiculum. Cells located at increasing depths from the postrhinal border form grids whose nodes have fields of increasing size and spacing. In summary, the grid cells probably do not form a map of a given environment by themselves but provide the Euclidean distance and direction metric postulated by the cognitive map theory of hippocampal function (O'Keefe and Nadel, 1978). This idiothetic information is combined with sensory information about each environment to create the specific map of that environment in the hippocampus.

To maintain the appropriate distance between grid points as the animal moves around the environment, the grid cells must take its speed into account. Information about speed may arise in posterior hypothalamic areas that are known to provide theta-related inputs to the hippocampus and where electrical stimulation produces running or jumping, with the speed of the movement increasing as a function of the stimulation intensity (Bland and Vanderwolf, 1972). Integration of a speed signal over time as the animal ran in a constant direction would give a measure of distance traveled during that time. There is direct evidence that information about an animal's speed of movement is available to the hippocampus. A small number of nonprincipal "speed" cells have been recorded in the hippocampus. The firing rates of these cells directly correlates with the animal's speed of running regardless of direction or location (O'Keefe et al., 1998). Second, higher running speeds tend to increase place cell firing rates (McNaughton et al., 1983a; Wiener et al., 1989; Zhang et al., 1998). Furthermore, the firing frequencies of many place cells from a stationary animal running in a wheel located in the place field were positively correlated with the speed of running (Czurko et al., 1999; Hirase et al., 1999). Some cells asymptoted within the range of speeds reached in the wheel. Cells that wholly or partially code for speed have also been found in the presubiculum (Sharp, 1996), which projects to the hippocampus via the medial entorhinal cortex. In all, we can conclude that information about both an animal's heading direction and its speed of movement through the environment is available to the hippocampal formation, and this information most likely is combined in the medial entorhinal grid cells.

The path integration system suffers from the fact that errors accumulate rapidly as the animal's heading direction and distance from the original location are continuously updated. On the basis of data from several studies in which attempts were made to remove exteroceptive information after initial localization or make it irrrelevant, it has been estimated that place fields can be maintained for only 1 to 2 minutes on the basis of path integration information alone (Save et al., 2000).

11.7.8 Are Place Cells Influenced by Goals, Rewards, or Punishments?

If place cells are part of a navigational system that can guide an animal to locations containing desirable objects such as food and water or to avoid dangerous places, one might expect to find goal cells whose activity was sensitive to goal location or navigation to a goal or, more generally, a change in place cell firing following a shift in the valence of parts or all of an environment. These "goal" or "valence" cells might exhibit any of several characteristics: The location of their place fields might alter when the valence of the environment changes, and it might happen in a way that reflects the goal location in an environment; there might be a disproportionate number of place cells with fields located at reward sites; or there might be nonlocational cells whose firing rate depended on which goal was being sought or navigated toward. Several experiments have searched for the first type by shifting goal locations: Some reported no effect (O'Keefe, 1976; Speakman and O'Keefe, 1990; Zinyuk et al., 2000), while others found concomitant place field shifts (Breese et al., 1989; Kobayashi et al., 1997; Hollup et al., 2001). Here we need to bear in mind that rewards have both sensory and incentive properties, and field shifts might be due to the former rather than the latter. Three recent studies employed experimental paradigms in which the goal was not marked by any physical stimulus. The rats in the Hollup et al (Hollup et al., 2001) experiment searched for a hidden platform in a modified annular watermaze and the fields of some cells shifted when the goal location was changed. Kobayashi used rewarding brain stimulation of the hypothalamus in order to designate particular locations as goals and reported that six of 31 place cells either developed additional new fields in the rewarded location or shifted their place field to that location {Kobayashi et al., 1997}. Finally, Zinyuk et al. (2000) used a paradigm similar to that of Kobayashi et al. but rewarded the animals with random food pellets rather than electrical brain stimulation; they found no changes in place fields when the reward location was moved. Because there was no physical reward at the goal locations in these experiments, the explanation of the discrepancies cannot rely solely on the perceptibility of the goal or its role as a sensory cue. We note that many of the cells that shifted fields in the Kobayashi et al. experiment had very low (< 1 Hz) place field rates, below those normally accepted in these types of experiment. These considerations, however, do not apply to the Hollup findings (Hollup et al., 2001).

Moita et al. (2004) used aversive electrical stimulation of the orbit of the eye to condition rats to an auditory conditioned stimulus (CS) or to the background context. They found that as a result of training some place fields were altered. More place cells changed their firing fields in the context than in the cue-conditioned group and more in the conditioning box than in a different control box. Furthermore, they found that following cue conditioning the place cells began to fire with a short latency response to the auditory cue but only if the animal was in the place field of that cell when the CS was delivered (Moita et al., 2003). This result is discussed further in Section 11.11.3.

Evidence for the second type of goal representation comes from Hollup et al. (2001), who found twice as many cells representing the unmarked goal in their annular watermaze than would be expected by chance. The third type of active goal cell was reported in a study of temporal and frontal cells recorded in human epileptic patients while they played a taxicab game in which they searched for passengers in a small virtual reality town and took them to their destinations in the form of specific storefronts (Ekstrom et al., 2003). About one-fifth of the cells recorded were sensitive to the goal being sought, almost three-fourths of which responded while searching for a specific location. An additional 7% were involved as the subject searched for more than one store and 22% while searching for passengers. A small number of cells showed a place by goal interaction, firing in a particular location if the subject crossed it en route to a particular goal. These goal cells were located throughout the temporal and frontal lobes and not concentrated in the hippocampus or parahippocampal gyrus as were the place and spatial-view cells (see below) recorded in the same study.

It seems clear, then, that changing the valence of an environment or regions within that environment can cause the firing fields of some place cells to shift. The functional significance of this is not clear, unless it turns out that the cells that changed had fields where the animal was located during the occurrence of the rewarding or punishing event. At present, it is not clear exactly how goals are represented or whether goal location is stored in the hippocampus or outside of it. When no distal sensory information is available, the sensory qualities of rewards may be used to locate place fields. In a "richer" environment, food and water may be "categorized" as objects that are potentially unstable over time. Food sources become depleted and new ones become available, and this happens over a time scale quite different from that of other cues such as trees or bushes. Nonetheless, the locations of reward have to be stored somewhere. However, on balance, the experimental results, although not conclusive, suggest that the information about goal location is probably not stored in any simple fashion in the CA3 or CA1 areas of the hippocampus itself. Regions such as the lateral septum subiculum, nucleus accumbens, or prefrontal cortex, which receive inputs from the hippocampal formation, might be the site of such place-reward cells. In support of this hypothesis is a recent study strongly suggesting that one type of goal cell can be found in the prelimbic/infralimbic areas situated in the rat's medial prefrontal cortex (Hok et al., 2005). Rats were trained in a cylinder to spend a short period of time in a localized but unmarked region to receive a pellet of food elsewhere. The pellets dropped from an overhead dispenser into a localized zone but then bounced elsewhere, ending up all over the enclosure. There were thus two localized but unmarked zones, a goal zone, which upon entry triggered the reward, and a landing zone, where the pellets initially dropped. Most pellets, however, were retrieved and eaten elsewhere. One-fourth of the cells in the prelimbic/infralimbic areas had place fields and these were about three to four times larger than those found in the hippocampus. The centers of a large percentage of these fields were concentrated in the trigger (36%) and landing (42%) zones. Rotating the cue card on the wall of the enclosure rotated the animal's representation of the trigger zone location, as judged by its behavior, but had no effect on the landing zone place fields. Conversely, changing the location of the pellet dispenser and thus the location of the landing zone caused a shift in the landing zone fields to the new area but had no effect on the behavioral approach to the trigger zone. The large size of the prefrontal place fields and the concentration of their centers at goal regions to which the animal navigated make them much better potential candidates for goal cells than hippocampal neurons. They bear some resemblance to the goal cells postulated in the models of spatial navigation of Burgess and colleagues (Burgess et al., 1994; Burgess and O'Keefe, 1996) (see Chapter 14, Section 14.4).

11.7.9 Temporal Patterns of Place Cell Firing

Complex-spike cells do not fire in a continuous pattern when the rat runs through a place field but burst with a frequency close to that of the EEG theta rhythm. In several studies (Fox and Ranck, 1975; Buzsaki et al., 1983) recordings were made while the rats were running on a treadmill. Unfortunately, pyramidal cells do not fire at their maximal rate in such a situation unless the animal is in that part of the environment that the cell represents (its place field). On a treadmill, CA1 complex-spike cells often fire at a low rate and display a preference for the positive peak of the dentate gyrus theta. Phase correlates have also been studied on narrow tracks as the rat runs through a cell's place field (O'Keefe and Recce, 1993; Skaggs et al., 1996; Harris et al., 2002; Mehta et al., 2002; Yamaguchi et al., 2002; Huxter et al., 2003), and a different, more interesting pattern has emerged. O'Keefe and Recce first noted that instead of remaining correlated to a constant phase of the EEG theta cycle, as on treadmills, the phase of firing changed in a systematic way. When the rat entered the cell's place field, the cell began firing at a particular phase of theta. However, as the animal progressed through the field, the bursts of unit firing occurred on an earlier phase of each successive theta cycle (Fig. 11–11C). The phase of firing correlates with the animal's location in the place field (Fig. 11–11B,D), and this correlation is higher than for time after entry into the field (Fig. 11–11E) or instantaneous firing rate (Fig. 11–11F). This *phase precession* phenomenon is partly explained by cells firing rhythmically at a frequency higher than that of theta. Dentate granule cells also phase shift but by a lesser amount, and the onset of firing is at an earlier phase of the theta cycle than that seen in the CA1 cells (Skaggs et al., 1996).

Is there information in the phase correlate of place cell firing beyond that contained in the firing rate? If there is, does it add greater precision to the locational information contained in the rate, or are the two coding for independent variables

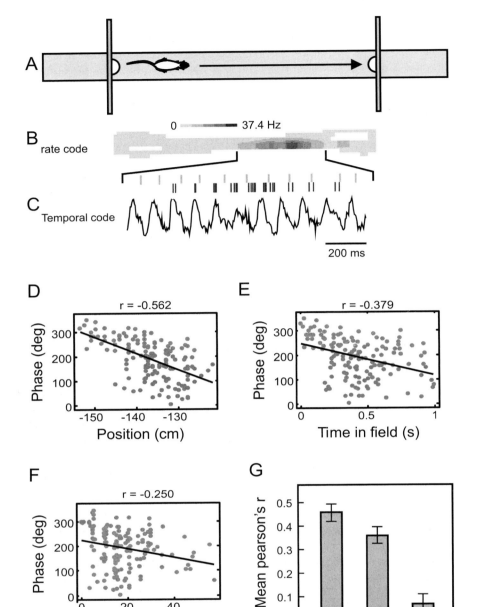

Figure 11–11. Temporal coding of location in hippocampal pyramidal cells. *A.* Rat shuttled from left to right and then back again to receive a food reward at each end wall of a linear track. *B.* Firing rate field map of the cell based on multiple runs. *C.* Spikes on a single run through the field show phase precession, moving to earlier phases of the EEG theta cycle with each successive wave. Spikes are shown in black; lighter tick marks above identify the zero crossing point of the EEG. *D.* Plot of theta phase versus the position for multiple runs through the field of an example cell. The correlation between phase and position (*D*) is higher than the correlation with the time in field (*E*) or the instantaneous firing rate (*F*) for an average cell. *G.* Correlation of phase with position, time, and instantaneous firing rate across a population of 94 place fields. Best correlation is with position. (*Source*: After Huxter et al., 2003, by permission.)

(O'Keefe, 1991)? Jensen and Lisman (2000) have used data collected by Skaggs et al. (1996) and shown that, with certain assumptions, the accuracy of locating an animal's position on a narrow track can be increased by more than 40% when phase is taken into account in addition to rate. In this view, phase acts like a vernier, permitting finer-grain location of the animal within the place field. Evidence for the dual coding hypothesis comes from a linear track study showing that phase and rate could vary independently (Huxter et al., 2003). The rate within the field varied as a function of the animal's running speed, and phase coded for the proportion of the place field the animal had traversed. Changing the size of the field by changing the distance between the walls at the ends of the track increased the rate of phase precession to maintain

the correlation between phase and a fixed proportion of the total field size. Whether phase and rate can represent variables other than location and speed is an open question. It has been known for some time that the firing rate in the place field can vary considerably from one traverse to the next (see above), and there is some evidence that different odors located in a place can be coded by different rates (Wiebe and Staubli, 1999; Wood et al., 1999a). Some evidence in support of the idea that phase can represent a nonspatial as well as a spatial variable comes from the running wheel experiments of Hirase et al. (1999) and Harris et al. (2002). They found that whereas the rate of firing of the place cells was a function of the animal's speed of running, the phase with respect to theta was relatively constant at low firing rates but occasionally changed at higher rates in the absence of changed location. One variable that caused a change in phase in some cells was the directional orientation of the wheel, and thus the animal, to the room.

One important consequence of the phase precession effect is that the spatial overlap between the firing fields of two place cells is represented within each theta cycle by the amount of time the bursting pattern in the cell of the first field entered precedes that of the second field. This temporal difference can be demonstrated in the cross correlation between the firing patterns of the two cells (Skaggs et al., 1996). The farther apart the field borders, the larger is the temporal gap between firing peaks within each theta cycle.

Part of the phase precession effect might be explained by a coupling between the amount of cellular depolarization and the time of firing of the cell (Harris et al., 2002; Mehta et al., 2002). As the animal advances farther toward the center of the field, the cell would be more depolarized, fire more spikes on each cycle, and begin firing at an earlier phase of the cycle. This cannot be the whole story, however, as the phase continues to precess in the latter part of the field when the firing rate (and presumably the level of depolarization) is falling. An alternative explanation for phase precession invokes a mechanism based on the interaction of two theta-like waves (O'Keefe and Recce, 1993; Lengyel et al., 2003). These waves would normally be of the same frequency but 180° phase-reversed so that, when added together, they cancel each other. A slight increase in the frequency of one of these oscillators relative to the other would result in an interference pattern when the two waves are added together. If it is assumed that the extracellular EEG represents the lower frequency of the two oscillators, and that place cells fire on the peaks of the interference pattern, the precession phenomenon would be seen. The dual oscillator model predicts that the size of the place field is dependent on the difference between the frequencies of the two oscillators. The closer the two frequencies are together, the larger is the field. An article by Maurer et al. (2005) provides experimental evidence in support of this predicted relation between field size and the oscillatory frequency of the pyramidal cell. They showed that the average sizes of place fields are not uniform along the long (septo-temporal) axis of the hippocampus but increase in the temporal direction. In parallel with this field expansion, place cells in the dorsal hippocampus have a higher (intrinsic) frequency of oscillation than those located more ventrally despite no differences in the frequency of the EEG theta or the theta cells in the two regions. The dual oscillator interference model suggests there is a causal link between these two phenomena, with the dorsoventral gradient in intrinsic frequency (higher in the dorsal hippocampus) leading to the gradient in the spatial extent of the firing fields (smaller fields in the dorsal hippocampus).

The origin of the two separate but interacting theta rhythms and the site of their interaction are unknown. The latter may be in the hippocampus proper. One may be internal to CA3 and CA1 pyramidal cells, which can oscillate under the cholinergic influence of the septal nuclei. The other theta rhythm might arise from the direct projection from the entorhinal cortex to the CA3 and CA1 areas. Kamondi et al.

(1998) studied the oscillations inside the dendrites of CA1 cells during theta and showed that they are 180° phase-shifted with respect to those in the soma, as predicted by the wave interference hypothesis. They also found that depolarization of the dendrites causes an increase in the frequency of these oscillations. This and other models of the phase shift are considered in greater detail in Chapter 14.

Alternatively, the site of phase shift generation may ultimately be found in areas outside of the hippocampus but projecting to it, such as the entorhinal cortex. A study by Zugaro and colleagues (2005) lends strong support to the idea of an extrahippocampal origin. They trained rats to shuttle between two ends of a linear track and recorded the phase precession in hippocampal place cells. During some runs through the place field, a single 0.1 ms duration electric shock was delivered to the fibers of the ventral hippocampal commissure. This had the effect of resetting the phase of the hippocampal theta and inhibiting all recorded cells for approximately 200 to 250 ms. They found that when the cells recovered and began firing again they did so at the correct phase of the (reset) theta to code correctly for the animal's location at that point. This finding appears to argue against a primary role for the hippocampus itself in the phase precession and points in the direction of structures afferent to the hippocampus that might not have been affected by the brief intervention. The most likely source of this preserved positional information is the entorhinal cortex, which has direct projections to the CA3 and CA1 pyramidal cells as well as to the dentate granule cells and which was probably not affected by the electrical shock to the ventral hippocampal commissure. Evidence that it escaped comes from an observation by Zugaro et al. They looked for but did not see a rebound evoked potential in the hippocampus in response to the shock, suggesting that the entorhinal-hippocampal pathways were not greatly affected via the CA1-to-entorhinal return pathway. As we have seen, the medial entorhinal cortex contains grid cells that are theta-modulated and might be able to identify changes in the animal's location in the environment independent of the hippocampus.

11.7.10 Place Fields in Young and Aged Animals

In altricial animals, which depend on their mother after birth (such as the rat), the brain and in particular the hippocampus continues to develop for considerable periods of time after birth. For example, the dentate gyrus continues to generate large numbers of new granule cells for several weeks after birth and at a lesser rate throughout life (see Chapter 9), and inhibitory processes do not reach their full adult level of functioning until postnatal age 28 days (P28). Tests of spatial memory and navigation suggest that the hippocampus is not fully functioning until P40. Schenk (1985) trained rats of different ages on two versions of the Morris watermaze: the standard version in which the platform was hidden and the animal had to use distant spatial cues throughout learning and a version in which the platform was hidden but its location was marked by a visible proximal cue. This meant the task could be learned by a hippocampal or a nonhippocampal strategy. Which of these methods was used was probed by trials in which the proximal cue was removed. Schenk found that animals aged P28 took longer to learn a new platform task than did adults and reached adult levels of performance only at ages greater than 40 days. Animals at age P35 could perform the version of the task with the proximal visual cue; but when the cue was removed, they failed to show transfer to the distal cues. This finding suggests that they had developed all of the abilities necessary to solve the watermaze task except formation of the distal cue-based spatial representation needed to navigate to the goal in the absence of the visible proximal cue. A longitudinal study in which rats were originally trained on the hidden platform version of the watermaze at age 21 and then given daily trials for 69 days put the development of spatial navigation ability somewhat earlier (Clark et al., 2005). They found that the performance of the animals rose above chance level after the second day of training and steadily increased over the next 10 days to asymptote at adult levels at approximately P35. It is reasonable to conclude that the ability to form allocentric spatial memories and to perform spatial navigation does not fully develop until around 35 to 40 days of age in rats.

In the only study of the development of place cells in young animals, Martin and Berthoz (2002) recorded complex-spike cells from animals at ages P27, P29, P34, P40, and P52 and above while they were searching for random food pellets on an open field platform. They found that the place fields of younger animals were larger and more diffuse than those of adults and became more compact with age, finally reaching adult values at about P52. Furthermore, the place fields recorded on successive 10-minute trials were unstable in younger animals, shifting location from one trial to the next, and reached adult levels of stability only at age P52. In contrast, a small number of head direction cells, which signal the orientation of the animal's head relative to environmental cues (see Section 11.9), were recorded from the cingulum at P30 and appeared to be indistinguishable from those reported in the adult. Previous work on the development of hippocampal theta had suggested that theta waves could be recorded on the hippocampal EEG as early as P10, developing to adult levels over the next 2 weeks (Leblanc and Bland, 1979). It seems reasonable to conclude from both the behavioral and the electrophysiological data that the rat hippocampus continues to develop over the first month of life and reaches the mature adult level of functioning only at ages 40 to 50 days after birth. The head direction and the theta systems, on the other hand, appeared to be functioning at earlier ages, reaching maturity by P30.

At the other end of the life cycle, when animals get older, their spatial learning abilities decrease (for a review see Rosenzweig and Barnes, 2003) and their hippocampal place cells appear to undergo changes. There seems to be little overall agreement as to whether place fields get larger or become less reliable as animals age. In the first study that compared the sizes of place fields in adult and aged animals, it was reported

that the older animals had larger firing fields (Barnes et al., 1983). Subsequent studies, however, have not been able to replicate this change but have found that the field sizes of the aged animals were normal or, under some circumstances, even more compact than those of the adult controls (Mizumori et al., 1996; Tanila et al., 1997a). There is also disagreement as to whether the place fields in aged animals are more or less reliable than in younger animals. Whereas Barnes and colleagues (1983, 1997) found that the CA1 place fields in aged animals are less reliable, Tanila et al. (1997a) found that, if anything, they were more reliable. Mizumori et al. (1996) found that they were more reliable in the CA1 pyramidal cells but less reliable in the hilar cells. Barnes et al. (1997) has suggested a reconciliation of these apparently conflicting results. They also found no difference in field size between groups but found that older animals spontaneously remapped between trials in the absence of any environmental changes. In the earlier Barnes et al. study, data were averaged across trials. If spontaneous remapping occurred between trials, it might lead to the impression that the firing fields were more dispersed and less reliable. The cause of the spontaneous remapping is not clear but may signal weakening of control of the head direction system over the hippocampal place fields with age. Spatial behavior in the watermaze also appears to reflect a decrease in the consistency of the spatial representation in older animals in that they sometimes head directly for the hidden platform and on some trials take much longer to get there, resulting in a bimodal distribution of scores (Barnes et al., 1997).

Tanila and colleagues (1997a) looked at whether cue control over place fields changed with aging. Aged animals were divided into spatial memory-impaired and spatial memory-unimpaired groups following testing in the Morris watermaze. They were then trained on the four-arm radial maze, with both distal visual cues and local visual, tactile, and olfactory cues available on the arms of the maze. Their place cells were then recorded. Probe trials in which either set of cues was rotated or scrambled were also conducted to determine which set of cues was controlling the fields. About two-fifths of the fields of young animals remapped when the distal and local cues were rotated by 90° in opposite directions, and approximately another third followed the distal cues. A smaller percentage (about one-fifth) followed the local cues. In contrast, more than three-fourths of the place fields in the aged animals with memory deficits followed the distal cues with fewer than one-fifth remapping. Scrambling the distal cues caused the latter group of place cells to become responsive to the local cues, showing that the predominant influence of the distal cues in the double rotation probes was not due to a sensory deficit. It appears as though the cells of the younger animals were relying on all of the cue information, whereas those of the memory-impaired aged animals were selectively attending to the distal visual cues. It is not clear why this shift should occur with age or how to explain it. It is especially puzzling because the aged animals were selected on the basis of their deficits in the Morris watermaze, which requires attention to distal cues for its solution. The authors noted that all of the animals had adopted a strategy of entering adjacent arms of the maze to solve the task and therefore may not have been using a spatial strategy. Whether forcing them to use a spatial strategy would have made a difference is not clear.

Rosenzweig and colleagues (2003) looked at environmental control of place fields in a different way and compared it with the animal's performance in a spatial task. They trained animals in a task where they (and their place fields) could locate themselves within one of two frameworks (Gothard et al., 1996a). The goal at one end of a linear track was fixed relative to the room cues, whereas the goal at the other end was located inside a box that moved along the track from one run to the next. Place fields located close to the moving box tended to move with the box, whereas those distant from it stayed fixed relative to the room framework. As the animal ran from the box to the fixed end of the track, the population of cells could be said to switch frameworks. Rosenzweig et al. trained the rats to slow down at an unmarked location on the track to receive positively rewarding electrical brain stimulation. This goal location stayed fixed relative to the room cues and thus would be better located after the population response of the cells had switched into the room frame of reference. They found that the adult animals learned the task better than the aged animals and that as a group the adult animals switched from the box framework to the room framework earlier on the track than the aged animals. Furthermore, on an animal-by-animal basis there was a good correlation between the point at which the ensemble of place cells recorded switched and the ability of the animal to distinguish between the goal location and a control location. Although it was not formally tested, it seems reasonable to conclude that the ability to switch into the fixed room framework was at least in part dependent on the ability of room cues to influence the place fields and that this was deficient in the aged animals.

11.7.11 Hippocampal Place Cell Firing Is Influenced by Other Areas of the Brain

Lesions of the septal or entorhinal projections to the hippocampus have been reported to cause a decrease in the number of place cells that are found and, in the case of entorhinal lesions, to a shift in the stimulus control of place field firing (Miller and Best, 1980). Following entorhinal cortex lesions, the fields rotated with the maze, unlike the fields of normal animals, which remain anchored to extramaze cues. These findings are consistent with the idea that CA1 and CA3 cells have access to distal sensory input via the entorhinal cortex. The importance of direct entorhinal–CA1 connections has been highlighted by Brun et al. (2002), who removed the input from CA3 (and thus the dentate gyrus as well) onto CA1 cells and showed that CA1 place cells could still form well defined, stable place fields in repeated exposures to a familiar environment.

The influence of the medial septal nucleus is somewhat different from that of the entorhinal cortex. Recall that it

provides powerful cholinergic and GABAergic inputs to the hippocampal formation and has a major influence on hippocampal theta activity. As we shall see in Section 11.12.6, many medial septal cells are theta cells that have a good phase relation with the hippocampal theta. Its role in the control of place field firing has been studied by Mizumori et al., 1989). They trained rats in an eight-arm radial maze and recorded from place cells in CA1 and CA3 during performance of the task. Surprisingly, blocking the medial septum with the anesthetic procaine left place fields intact despite disrupting maze performance. Subsequent experiments have suggested that firing in the subiculum is disrupted and that this area of the hippocampal formation thus contributes to the control of behavior in this task. Leutgeb and Mizumori (1999) replicated this observation but found a difference between the place cells in the lesioned animals and controls when the animals were placed in a new environment or faced with altered spatial cues. Interestingly the place fields of the lesioned animals showed less transfer from light to dark and slightly greater transfer between rooms.

Lesions or temporary inactivation of other regions have been shown to affect place fields in different ways. Lesions of the perirhinal cortex, which projects to the entorhinal cortex and therefore might be providing sensory information to the hippocampal place cells, have no effect on basic field parameters but reduce the consistency of locational firing (Muir and Bilkey, 2001): In contrast to the stability of field locations in the control animals, field centers in the lesioned rats frequently moved from one exposure to the testing box to the next. A similar effect on the stability of hippocampal place fields was found after lesions of the prefrontal cortex (Kyd and Bilkey, 2005), and this may have been mediated by frontal projections to the entorhinal/perirhinal cortex.

Temporary inactivation of the retrosplenial cortex (Cooper and Mizumori, 2001) disrupt an animal's performance on the radial arm maze in the dark and during the initial learning phase in the light. During inactivation, the location of place fields shift on the maze. There are head direction (HD) cells and more complex HD, location, and movement cells in retrosplenial cortex (Chen et al., 1994; Cho and Sharp, 2001). This suggests that the retrosplenial cortex is more involved in nonvisual (perhaps path integration) control of place cells and spatial behavior. On the other hand, the role of objects placed at the periphery of the environment in controlling the orientation of place fields in a symmetrical environment seems to be mediated, at least in part, by the visual and the parietal cortices. After lesions of the visual cortex, 70% of place fields did not rotate in step with the rotation of the landmarks. In comparison, 100% of place fields in the controls did so (Paz-Villagran et al., 2002) (see Section 11.7.6 regarding how place fields can be controlled by exteroceptive sensory cues). When the objects were removed, the fields in both lesioned and control animals remained in the standard position fixed relative to the room. The parietal cortex also seems to be involved in the control of place cell orientation relative to the landmark objects but in a different way (Save et al., 2005). Following lesions to the parietal cortex, most cells (78%) still rotated with the objects but, unlike in control animals, did not maintain this rotated location when the objects were subsequently removed. This type of short-term memory for the visual location of landmarks is discussed in greater detail in Section 11.8 and appears to be dependent on the integrity of the parietal cortex.

11.7.12 Primate Hippocampal Units also Exhibit Spatial Responses

The spatial properties of single units in the hippocampus of primates including humans have been studied. This is important because it establishes the generality of the spatial nature of the hippocampus and shows that the findings in rodents are not unique. However, if there is broadening of the function of the human hippocampus to include episodic memory as well as spatial memory, it might be expected that the cells in humans and, more generally, primates might have a broader spectrum of response properties than those found in rodents. Furthermore, the standard approach to recording single units in primates is markedly different from that found in the freely moving rat. Primates are usually restrained with their heads fixed, and stimuli are often presented in ways that make it difficult to identify a spatial correlate or to dissociate the different frames of reference that might be used for the localization. It is also known that restraining rats severely depresses the locational correlate of the hippocampal complex-spike cells (Foster et al., 1989). These constraints have been partially overcome in a few studies by giving the animals increased mobility either in movable chairs or carts or by allowing them to move freely around a large cage. We should not be surprised, then, if there are differences between the unit/behavioral correlates found in primates and those in rodents. The spatial responses are described in this section; the nonspatial responses are described separately in Sections 11.11. 1 and 8.

Several types of spatial response have been found in primate hippocampal units. Responses to the location of the stimulus on a VDU screen, spatial-view cells that respond to the location at which the animal is looking, and place cells similar to those in the rodent have all been described. When the response of hippocampal units to the identity of a stimulus is compared to its spatial location, considerably higher percentages of units are found to the latter variable. Rolls and his colleagues (1993) tested monkeys on object recognition tasks and compared unit responses to object familiarity with those to object location. They reported that about 9% of cells in the hippocampal region responded differentially to the location of the stimulus on a display screen. In contrast, only a small percentage (2%) of cells responded to familiar objects (see Section 11.11.8). Colombo et al. (1998) recorded units in the primate hippocampus during a similar delayed matching to sample task in which either the spatial location or the object identity of the sample stimulus had to be remembered. They found 41 neurons that responded during the delay period, and of these 15(37%) were related exclusively to spatial position

and 5 (12%) to object identity. The remaining 21 responded to both. Most of the responses were inhibitory. Interestingly, the spatial neurons were more heavily concentrated in the posterior hippocampus, which is the analogue of the dorsal hippocampus in rodents. Ringo and colleagues (Ringo et al., 1994; Sobotka et al., 1997; Nowicka and Ringo, 2000) investigated the role of eye movements in hippocampal single unit responses. Monkeys were trained to look to one of five locations in the light or in the dark to receive rewards. In an early study, about one-third of the units changed their rate during saccades; in a subsequent study, 13% of the cells were shown to be sensitive to position and another 17% were shown to be sensitive to direction. Because the animal's head was fixed in these experiments, it is not possible to say whether the effective saccades were to locations in the laboratory or in a head-centered framework. Remembering the location of a stimulus on a computer screen might not be the same type of spatial task as locating oneself in an environment and might more easily be solved using egocentric spatial strategies dependent on parietal than hippocampal cortex (Burgess et al., 1999). Wirth et al. (2003) studied the responses of hippocampal neurons during a task that required the monkeys to learn the association between specific scenes and specific locations. Novel pictures of scenes were presented on a VDU screen, and the animal's task was to learn to move its eyes to one of four locations on the screen at the end of the presentation to obtain a reward. Each scene was presented for 0.5 second followed by a 700-ms delay during which the screen was blank before the animal was allowed to move its eyes to the required location. In all, 61% of the hippocampal cells recorded had firing rates that were significantly altered during the presentation of one of the scenes, during the delay that followed it, or both. Furthermore, there was a good correlation between the altered firing during the trial and the learning of the behavioral response. Changes in firing rate preceded the behavioral learning by a small number of trials for 14 cells, occurred at the same time in 4 cells, and followed learning in 19 cells. This suggests that although the firing rate of some cells may have been related to the learning of the scene-location association it may have been involved in learning other aspects of the scene in others. Control trials involved the presentation of familiar scenes that required the same eye movement as the novel scene. This rules out the possibility that the hippocampal firing was related to a particular eye movement or to a specific location on the screen. Although it is possible to describe this task as learning an arbitrary association between a scene and an eye movement to a location defined relative to the VDU screen, it is also possible that the animals were learning to attend to a particular location in each new scene, to remember the scene and the location during the delay, and to look at the location when allowed to do so after the delay. On this view, these cells would be closely related to the spatial-view cells, which respond when an animal looks at a location rather than goes there (Rolls et al., 1997) (see next paragraph).

Several groups have also looked for spatially coded cells in the hippocampus of monkeys free to move around the environment. Rolls and colleagues (1997) have found a type of spatial cell not described in the rodent: the spatial-view cell. Spatial-view cells respond selectively when the animal looks at particular locations in the testing room irrespective of where the animal is situated in the room when it looks at that location. For example, one cell increased its firing rate markedly when the animal looked at a particular corner of the room regardless of where it was located in the room itself and regardless of the orientation of gaze required to look there. Some of these cells continued to respond when the target location is screened off by curtains, suggesting that the cells are not responding to particular sensory features in that location. This group has also reported the existence of whole body motion cells (O'Mara et al., 1994), which may be related to the speed cells in the rat described above. In contrast, this group has looked for but not found place cells comparable to those seen in rats. The existence of spatial-view cells might be an indication that primates have developed the ability to identify places and their contents without physically visiting those places, an important step in the evolution of the spatial mapping system.

Ono and his colleagues (1993) found place-coded neurons in the hippocampal formation of monkeys that could visit different locations in an environment while performing different tasks. The monkeys were trained to sit in an enclosed cart and to move it to nine different locations in the testing environment by pressing a lever. About 13% of the cells fired more when the animal was at one location than when it was in other locations. In a subsequent task, the animals were required to perform an object-in-place discrimination. The cart was moved to a particular location and the view window was opened, allowing the animal a sight of an object at that location. About one-fourth of cells responded when objects were shown to the animal in this task. A subset of these cells (5% of the total) were object-in-place cells that responded differentially when the animal was shown an object in a particular location and not in other locations. These cells were also not interested in a different object in the preferred location. They appear to have properties similar to those of the place and object-in-place cells described in the rat. Further evidence that the cells are appropriately described as place cells comes from an experiment by Nishijo et al. (1997) in the same laboratory. Here the animal in the cart was moved backward as well as forward through the environment, and the cells continued to fire at the same location. This manipulation reverses the cues in egocentric space but leaves allocentric cues unchanged. This group has also used virtual reality environments to provide testing environments more related to the open field tasks used with rodents (Hori et al., 2005). Monkeys were trained to use a joystick to move between five reward locations in a large 100 m virtual diameter space containing a 20 m diameter arena surrounded by landmarks such as a tree, a house, and the building. Almost one-third of the hippocampal units displayed spatial fields. When the distal cues were rearranged, two-thirds of the cells tested remapped by either ceasing to fire or by changing the spatial pattern of firing. The

monkeys were also trained in a two-dimensional screen-based task in which they had to move a pointer to different parts of the screen. A subset of cells were recorded in both the virtual reality task and the screen-based task. Of the cells with spatial responses in either or both tasks, about one-third had spatial activity in both, one-half in the virtual reality task alone, and only 15% in the screen-based task. It appears that large-scale allocentric spatial tasks are better for activating primate hippocampal neurons than are screen-based egocentric tasks.

If we are to compare hippocampal physiology in rodents and primates appropriately, more recordings are needed from primates whose heads are unrestrained and who are free to locomote around a complex environment (see Section 11.2). There has been some interesting progress along these lines. In the first study in completely freely moving monkeys, rodent-like place cells with high signal-to-noise ratios in the hippocampus proper were found in squirrel monkeys performing a spatial memory task in three dimensions (Ludvig et al., 2004). Interestingly, many of these cells had fields that involved the walls of the wire-mesh testing cage, areas that would not have been sampled in the floor-bound experiments of Rolls and Ono.

Another approach has been to record units from human epilepsy patients (awaiting determination of seizure foci). In early studies the responses to faces, objects, and scenes were studied (see Section 11.11.9). Of relevance here is a study of unit activity during virtual locomotion in a taxi-driver game (Ekstrom et al., 2003). This study recorded units from the temporal lobe and frontal cortex and looked for evidence of cell activity responsive to the variables of place, view, and goal-seeking and of conjuctions between these variables. Place responses clustered in the hippocampus to a greater extent than in the parahippocampus (24% of hippocampal cells being "pure" place cells versus 8% in the parahippocampus), and "pure" location-independent spatial-view cells clustered in the parahippocampus (17% vs. 5% in the hippocampus). The goal cells were distributed evenly throughout the temporal and frontal cortices (see above). The place-responsive cells were found to be nondirectional, as would be predicted from the rodent literature, given that the subjects were free to move through areas in the virtual town from different directions. In an important control, Eckstrom et al. looked for unit responses to isolated landmarks before the patients learned to use them to navigate in a virtual reality environment; they failed to find any.

11.8 Place Cells Are Memory Cells

A role for the hippocampal formation in memory is suggested by activity-dependent synaptic plasticity, such as long-term potentiation (LTP) and long-term depression (LTD) (see Chapter 10) and the profound amnesia associated with damage to the medial temporal lobe (see Chapters 12 and 13). Is this mnemonic capability also reflected by place cells? This chapter presents evidence that these cells can maintain their firing fields over a period of a few minutes in a working memory task, that place field characteristics can change with experience over the course of a day, that sensory control of place cell firing can become more differentiated with experience over days and weeks or can shift from exteroceptive to interoceptive cues when the animal learns that the former are unstable, that place cell activity during sleep reflects experience in the prior waking period and may be involved in consolidation of recently acquired spatial memories, and finally that several properties of normal place cell behavior in familiar and novel environments, such as place field stability, are based on memory and depend on the NMDA receptor implicated in LTP.

11.8.1 Hippocampal Place Cells "Remember" the Animal's Location for Several Minutes During a Spatial Working Memory Task

When discussing the properties of place cells, we saw that they displayed "memory" properties such as continuing to fire in appropriate places when the lights have been turned off. The cells use environmental cues to set up their firing pattern, but once established the pattern is sometimes surprisingly free of environmental influences. The clearest demonstration of this "memory" phenomenon was in experiments in which the environmental cues controlling place fields have been identified; and it was shown that place fields were maintained following the removal of these cues (Muller and Kubie, 1987; O'Keefe and Speakman, 1987; Save et al., 2005). We concentrate here on the O'Keefe and Speakman experiment in which place cell firing pattern was shown to be correlated with the animal's behavior.

O'Keefe and Speakman (1987) recorded cells during a spatial memory task in a cue-controlled environment (Fig. 11–12). Rats were first trained on a plus shaped elevated maze to go to a goal defined by a set of cues within the curtained environment (Fig. 11–12A). Rotation of the cues and goal between trials ensured that the rats learned to use these cues. Place fields rotated in step with the cue rotations (Fig. 11–12B). On some trials, the cues were removed while the rat was still in the start arm before it was allowed to choose. Tests on normal rats had established that well trained animals could remember the location of the goal for periods as long as 30 minutes after the cues were removed. Of 30 cells with fields on the maze, 27 maintained these fields following removal of the cues (Fig. 11–12C). Cells with fields on the nonstart arms for a particular trial also fired in the correct place, demonstrating that place cell "memory" is more than the continuous persistence of a trace set up during the registration period; the system can, in addition, compute the correct location on the maze of place fields for cells that are inactive in the start arm. One explanation for this memory phenomenon points to a role for the distal cues at the periphery of an environment in orienting the head direction system. Once this has been set by the orientation of the control cues on a given trial, exterocep-

tive and interoceptive cues other than these might be capable of maintaining it (see Section 11.9). As we saw in Section 11.7.11, a role for the parietal cortex in this short-term spatial memory has been demonstrated (Save et al., 2005).

A final observation on these cells was made during control trials in which the animal was not placed in the start arm until after the controlled cues had been removed, preventing the animal from knowing which arm contained the reward. Under these circumstances, choice performance falls to chance levels, but the pattern of place cell firing still stayed appropriate for the animal's choice of goal (Fig. 11–12D). This constitutes strong evidence that these cells are not firing to the actual environmental location but to where the animal "thinks" it is. Other studies have also found a good relation between place field activity and behavioral choices (Zinyuk et al., 2000; Lenck-Santini et al., 2001a, 2002; Rosenzweig et al., 2003) but there has also been failure to find this (Jeffery et al., 2003). In the latter experiment, rats continued to perform a hippocampus-dependent spatial task, albeit at a reduced level, following a change in the testing box that caused remapping of most of the CA1 place fields. Here, it is plausible to assume that place cells in other areas of the hippocampal formation did not remap and continued to support the behavior.

11.8.2 Place Field Plasticity During Unidirectional Locomotion

One interesting line of investigation has involved changes in place field characteristics over time as rats run along a track. When animals are run on narrow tracks, many of the fields are directional, firing in one direction of movement but not the other. The experiments described in this section test models describing the effects of temporally asymmetrical LTP and the encoding of sequence-related information (see discussion in Chapter 14; see also Section 11.7.3). Mehta and colleagues (1997, 2000) have shown that over the course of a few dozen traverses in the same direction along a track, CA1 place fields shift backward relative to that direction of motion and become larger. They also found that an experience-dependent skewness develops in the place fields; that is, on the animal's first runs of the day a given cell's place field is symmetrical, but with continued exposure the place cell tends to fire at a higher rate when the animal leaves the place field than as it enters it. However, this increased skewness in CA1 place fields has not been found by others (Huxter et al., 2003). The development of place field expansion and backward shift has been shown to depend on NMDA receptors (Ekstrom et al., 2001). An intriguing aspect of the phenomenon in CA1 is that the effect resets overnight, as if the cells do not remember the previous day's experience on the track (Mehta et al., 2000). Evidence from Lee et al. (2004) confirms and extends this finding but in addition shows a difference betweeen the CA3 and CA1 fields: CA3 fields develop skewness and shift backward immediately on exposure to a newly altered track and maintain these changes on subsequent days, whereas CA1 fields shift back-

A   Plus maze with 6 distal cues

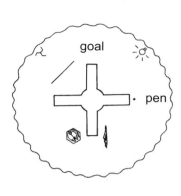

B   Place fields rotate with distal cues

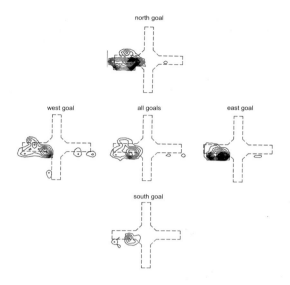

C   Place cells remember locations

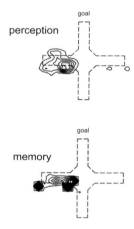

D   Place cells predict spatial choice

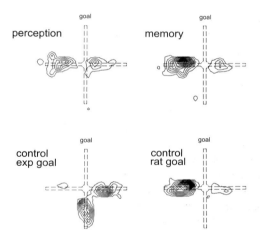

Figure 11–12. Place cell activity during a spatial working memory task. *A.* Layout of the testing environment showing an elevated plus-shaped maze surrounded by six cues and a set of curtains. *B.* Place cell with a field on the arm 90° counterclockwise to the goal (−90°, inner panel). The firing field remains constant with respect to the distal cues and goal as they are rotated by multiples of 90° relative to the laboratory frame (outside panels). Trials have been rotated so the goal is always shown at the top. More contours indicate a higher firing rate. *C.* Same cell as in *B* maintains its field dur-

ing the perceptual (top) and memory (bottom) phases of the experiment. *D.* A different place cell fires strongly in the −90° arm and weakly in the +90° arm on both perceptual and memory trials (upper left and right). During control trials, it fails to fire with correct relation to the (unknown) goal (lower left) but fires with correct relation to the animal's choice of goal arm at the end of the trial (lower right). In *B* and *C*, each contour = 0.7 spikes s⁻¹; in *D*, each contour = 1.5 spikes s⁻¹. (*Source*: After O'Keefe and Speakman, 1987, with permission.)

ward only from the second day of testing and do *not* maintain the changes. Lee et al. interpreted these findings as suggesting that the CA3, but not the CA1, network can store sequence information in the long term, and that CA1 is more involved in novelty detection. Note that CA1 cells can show long-term plasticity in other paradigms (see Section 11.8.3).

11.8.3 Cue Control over Hippocampal Place Cells Can Change as a Function of Experience

Experience with an environment can change which features of that environment control place fields. Such features include the color of a polarizing cue and the geometrical shape of the environment. Bostock et al. (1991) studied place fields in two recording chambers that were identical except for a white or black polarizing card at the periphery. They found that when the black card was first substituted for the white card most of the place fields remained the same. However, as the rat continued to experience the white and black card environments, the place cells began to distinguish between them. The remapped fields fell into three classes: (1) the field in the black card environment was a rotation of that in the white card environment, or (2) the cell ceased to fire in the black card environment, or (3) the fields in the two environments were completely different in location and shape. The second and third classes were described as "complex remapping" and were found to be all-or-none: If one place cell showed complex remapping, so did another simultaneously recorded cell. Learned remapping can also occur between environments of different geometrical shapes (Muller and Kubie, 1987).

Lever et al. (2002) and Wills et al. (2005) studied the development of shape remapping in CA1 place cells in detail. Both experiments studied remapping between square and circular enclosures. In the Lever et al experiment, the enclosures differed only in shape and were identical in color, texture, and odor; in the Wills experiment they differed across all four dimensions. The activity of several hippocampal place cells was recorded on each day of the experiment; often they were different cells, but in some cases recordings were taken from the same cells over many consecutive days. Remapping was rapid and coherent in the latter experiment but slow and individualistic in the former. As in the Bostock et al. experiment described above, Lever found that on first exposure to a circular and a square environment most place fields were identical in the two shapes. With continued exposure, however, the cells began to differentiate between the environments. Unlike Bostock et al., they found that different cells differentiated between the environments at different rates, so after a few days some of the place fields were still similar in the two environments whereas others had clearly remapped. After 1 to 3 weeks of exposure to both environments, most of the cells had different fields in the two. Recording from individual cells through their remapping transition period showed that it took one of three forms. The most common form involved a gradual reduction of firing rate in one of the two shapes until it reached zero. Other forms of remapping involved the development of a new field in one of the shapes in tandem with the decline of the original field in that shape or, more rarely, a shift of the field in one shape to a new location. Once the cells had learned to differentiate between the two different-shaped boxes, rats were placed back in their home cages for delay periods of up to 39 days without any exposure to the shapes; upon reexposure, most of the cells continued to discriminate the two shaped boxes. CA1 place cells thus demonstrated long-term memory for this learned discrimination. Note that in both this and the Bostock et al. study the rats were not trained to discriminate the environments but were equally rewarded in both. Thus, the learning is *incremental* (see also

Tanila et al., 1997b), *latent* because it does not necessarily manifest in behavior, and *incidental* because it takes place in the absence of explicit reward.

In the Wills et al. study (2005a), the boxes were more different from each other to begin with, differing not only in shape but also in the color, odor, and texture of the walls. Original training took place in a white wooden circle and a brown morph square. Under these circumstances, the remapping took place over a period of minutes, and most of the cells had differentiated between the two environments by the end of the first few exposures. Furthermore, the remapped cells act in a unitary ensemble fashion, as was revealed by challenging them with shapes intermediate between the circle and the square. After several days' experience with the original training enclosures the animals were transferred to circles and squares constructed from the same brown morph box. It was then possible to probe the basis for each cell's differentiation between circle and square by recording in a series of octagons that vary systematically from the circle-like (regular octagon, adjacent side ratio 4:4) to the square-like (adjacent side ratio 7:1) (Fig. 11–13). Most of the remapped cells shifted abruptly from a square to circle firing pattern (for example, by treating the 6:2 octagon as a square and the 5:3 octagon as a circle). Furthermore, in all animals tested on this probe, all of the simultaneously recorded cells show the abrupt shift at exactly the same point in the sequence of octagons. This suggests that there are two mechanisms at work: pattern separation and pattern association (see Chapter 14). The first would permit the abrupt switch from the circle to square pattern despite a very small change in the geometry of the boxes. The second would be based on some type of cooperation among the active subset of place cells, perhaps revealing the operation of an attractor network and would account for the coherent behavior of the network.

11.8.4 Control of the Angular Orientation of Place Cells in a Symmetrical Environment Can Be Altered by the Animal's Experience of Cue Instability

In a symmetrically shaped environment such as a cylinder, an animal's sense of direction can be controlled by distal polarizing cues, such as a card on the wall of the environment, or by internal path integration cues, such as the amount it has turned around. Commonly, the visual information provided by a distal cue overshadows the internal cues, and rotating the cue causes an equal rotation of the fields (see Section 11.7.6). Jeffery and colleagues (Jeffery et al 1997; Jeffery 1998) showed that given certain experiences the animal could learn to give priority to internal path integration signals over the external cue. They tested the effectiveness of the cue card by rotating it when the animal was out of the enclosure and the effectiveness of the internal path integration system by slow rotations (subvestibular threshold) of the animal relative to the framework of the enclosure. As expected, they found that, initially, the visual cue card controlled place field orientation.

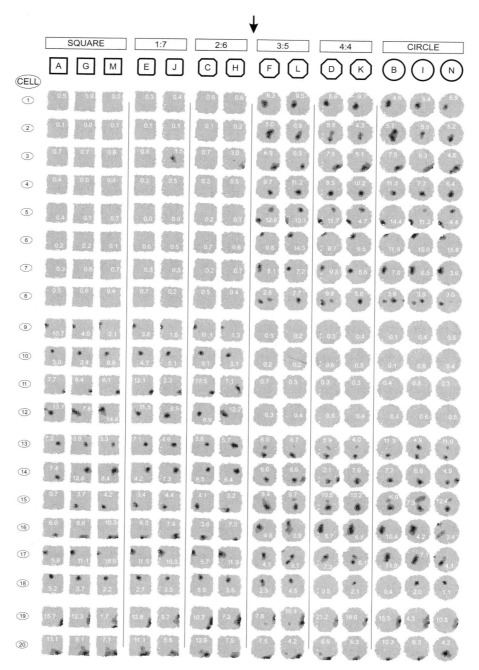

Figure 11–13. Abrupt coherent switch from square-like pattern to circle-like pattern in an incrementally changing series of octagons. Fields of 20 simultaneously recorded place cells following fast remapping training. Cells 1–17 met the criterion for remapping, and all switched abruptly from the square-like to circle-like

pattern at the same point in the series between the 2:6 and 3:5 octagon (arrow at top). The order in which the octagons were experienced is indicated by the letters A to N in the second row. Numbers in panels are peak rates. (*Source*: After Wills et al., 2005, with permission.)

However, following experience in which the rat could see the cue card move relative to the background environment and therefore was not a stable landmark, control of place field orientation passed from this visual cue to the interoceptive path integration system. Now the fields were no longer controlled by rotations of the visual cue but could be shifted by slow rotations of the animal relative to the framework of

the enclosure, demonstrating that they were under the control of the vestibular system. Rotations of the cue when the animal could not see it move did not produce the shift away from cue control. It seems likely that the site for this cue-instability learning is in the head-direction system itself (see Sections 11.9 and 11.10), perhaps in the presubiculum. This is suggested by two key features of the data. First, all the cells behave as a map-like ensemble, following *either* exteroceptive cues *or* interoceptive cues. Second, once the path integration system surplants the visual cue card in the control of orientation, it generalizes to novel situations. Following remapping induced by changing the color of the environment's walls, the newly remapped population of CA1 cells immediately follows the interoceptive rather than the visual cues, without needing to relearn the cue instability (Chakraborty et al., 2004).

11.8.5 Complex-spike Cell Firing and Connectivity During Sleep Is Modulated by Prior Spatial Learning Experiences

It has been suggested that consolidation of memories might take place during sleep and, in particular, during REM sleep (Maquet, 2001; Stickgold et al., 2001). Therefore, one might expect neuronal firing patterns to reflect this consolidation activity. Furthermore, if consolidation involves the transfer of information from hippocampus to neocortex (an idea developed further in Chapters 12 and 13), one might expect there to be increased interaction between cells in these brain areas during and after sleep. Experiments have suggested that the cell activity during ripples and sharp waves, or that related to the theta waves of REM sleep, could be the neural signature of this information transfer/consolidation process.

Pavlides and Winson (1989) recorded pairs of place cells in rats during sleep sessions that followed experience on a radial arm maze. The rats were allowed to visit the place field of one of the two cells prior to each sleep session but not the other. Remarkably, there was a selective increase in firing during both the slow-wave sleep and REM sleep periods of the cell that had been allowed to be active in its place field prior to sleep. The other cell showed no change in firing rate. In another study following place cell activation on a runaway during waking, the theta phase at which these cells fired during subsequent REM sleep shifted to the positive peak (Poe et al., 2000). Because LTP is more likely to occur at this phase, this finding might be an indication that recently experienced cells are more susceptible to plastic modification. Evidence for such changes comes from studies on changes in cell connectivity. Wilson and McNaughton (1994) examined the effects of spatial experience on changes in functional connectivity between CA1 cells. Using cross-correlation techniques (see Box 11–2), they found an increase in the correlation between pairs of cells with overlapping place fields in slow-wave sleep *after*, compared to before, the environmental experience; these correlations were more pronounced during ripples (see also Kudrimoti et al., 1999). There was evidence from another study (Qin et al., 1997) that some of this increased connectivity takes place between cells that were already connected prior to the environmental experience. Skaggs and McNaughton (1996) ran rats in one direction on a narrow triangular track and found that the temporal ordering of firing between cells with partially overlapping fields was replicated in a compressed form during slow wave

sleep. Firing sequence replay has been replicated by Wilson's group for slow-wave sleep (Lee and Wilson, 2002) and for REM sleep (Louie and Wilson, 2001). It should be emphasized that the replay time scales relative to the waking spatial experience differ markedly for these types of sleep, involving about 20-fold compression during slow-wave sleep and basically no compression during REM sleep. Second, it seems that slow-wave sleep replays sequences immediately after they were experienced, whereas REM sleep replays experience at least a day old. Finally, cross-correlational analysis showed that increased correlations were found between pairs of neocortical cells as well as pairs of hippocampal cells and, most intriguingly, between pairs of hippocampal and neocortical cells (Qin et al., 1997; Siapas and Wilson, 1998). The latter finding may be taken as evidence for increases in the "functional connectivity" between, as well as within, structures.

In all, these results indicate selective, orderly reactivation of cells that have recently taken part in a spatial experience. They also suggest that co-activation of place cells during the waking experience might lead to increased connectivity and further consolidation during sleep states. These studies have involved CA1 cells. A future goal is to compare CA3 and CA1 cells and relate these findings to the experience-dependent place field changes during unidirectional track running described above in this section. The mechanisms that immediately produce sequence replay during sleep in CA1 appear to reset (Lee and Wilson, 2002), like the CA1 place field changes such as skewness and backward shift. Given that these are maintained on subsequent days in CA3 cells (Lee et al., 2004), one might predict that experience-dependent changes in CA3–CA3 connectivity in sleep would also be less transient.

What is needed to take these results forward and demonstrate a causal relation between the sleep phenomenon and subsequent memory capacity is a physiological or pharmacological technique for selectively disrupting postexperience LIA or REM theta activity or, even better, altering the patterning of place cell activity during these periods.

11.8.6 NMDA Receptor Confers Mnemonic Properties on Place Cell Firing

Several studies have pointed to a role for the NMDA receptor (NMDAR) in conferring mnemonic properties on place cell function (reviewed by Nakazawa et al., 2004). McHugh et al. (1996) studied the place cells of mice in which the NMDA receptor subunit NR1 had been knocked out only in CA1 pyramidal cells. Deletion of this subunit renders the receptor inoperable. Rotenberg et al. (1996) looked at the fields of place cells in animals that transgenically expressed a mutated calcium-independent form of CAMKII, part of the intracellular signaling pathway that mediates the effects of the NMDA receptor. Both groups of animals had deficits in LTP and spatial memory (Rotenberg et al., 1996; Tsien et al., 1996). In both experiments fewer place cells were found in the mutants and the quality of the mutant place fields was degraded, a result that has also been seen in other mutant mice with disrupted

NMDAR-dependent plasticity (Cho et al 1998). In a different mutant. Rotenberg et al found that place fields were less stable over repeated exposures to the environment (Rotenberg et al., 2000). In the McHugh et al. experiment, the place cells showed an interesting loss of the usual temporal relation between the firing patterns of cells with overlapping place fields. As we saw in Section 11.7.9, place cells fire with a theta-like bursting pattern as the animal runs through the firing field, which is revealed by strong periodicity in the cross-correlogram of the two spike trains (see Box 11–2). The absence of this periodicity in the McHugh et al. experiment suggests a fundamental breakdown in the temporal firing pattern of the place cells or the temporal relations between cells lacking a functional NMDA receptor.

The global role of the NMDA receptor in the long-term stability of place fields was studied by Kentros et al. (1998). They showed that systemic administration of the competitive NMDA channel blocker CPP had no effect on established place fields in an environment long familiar to the rats or on the formation of newly "remapped" place fields in a novel environment, nor on the short-term stability of these new, remapped place fields, as measured over a couple of hours. However, on the second day of exposure to the novel environment, the previous day's place fields had been "forgotten": Again the cells remapped the new environment, but the new patterns of firing bore no relation to those of the previous day. This finding suggests that the NMDA receptor is more important for the stability of place fields in the long term than it is in their initial establishment or their short-term maintenance.

Highly informative studies have used conditional CA3-restricted NMDA receptor knockout mice to explore the contribution of long-term CA3 plasticity to CA1 place cell firing and spatial behavior (Nakazawa et al., 2002, 2003). These studies suggest two important roles for CA3 plasticity: pattern completion (see Chapter 14), whereby only a subset of cues are sufficient to reinstate a pattern of firing originally associated with the full cue set; and rapid, single-exposure, learning. Pattern completion is suggested by the finding that although CA1 cells in the mutants showed normal firing in full-cue reexposures to an environment they showed significantly reduced levels of firing (albeit in the appropriate locations) in partial-cue reexposures. Impaired behavior was also seen in probe trials during the watermaze task under partial-cue conditions. A CA3 plasticity-dependent role in rapid environmental learning is suggested by the poorer quality of the mutants' CA1 place fields in novel environments and by impaired performance in the delayed match-to-place version of the watermaze (see Chapter 13).

11.8.7 Summary of Place Cell Plasticity

The evidence summarized in this section indicates that place cells show several forms of plasticity, some of which can be correlated with the animal's behavior in spatial memory tasks. These various forms of plasticity last for markedly different periods of time, ranging from a few minutes to longer than a month. Some of them are activity-dependent and temporary, lasting only the length of a single trial in a working memory task or a session on a maze, whereas others appear to be permanent, such as the differentiation between two boxes following slow remapping. Some of these changes clearly depend on the integrity of the NMDA receptor in different parts of the hippocampus, but others may not. Indeed, for many of these changes it has not yet been firmly established that the underlying synaptic plasticity takes place in the hippocampus itself rather than in structures afferent to the hippocampus and is merely being passively reflected by the cells there. Finally, there is substantial evidence that some type of consolidation process takes place during sleep following an experience, and it is reflected in place cell firing. Whether this involves intrahippocampal processes, such as the strengthening of synapses between cells with overlapping fields, or involves the transfer of information from hippocampal stores to neocortical ones, must await further experimentation. It is clear that there are sufficient examples of plasticity reflected in place cell firing to make them one of the more fruitful targets in the study of the neural basis of memory. In a subsequent section (see Section 11.11), we examine the evidence for changes in hippocampal cell activity during nonspatial learning and memory tasks.

11.9 Head Direction Cells

Another well characterized class of spatial cells recorded in the hippocampal formation of freely moving awake animals is the head-direction (HD) cells, found in the dorsal presubiculum and regions connected with the presubiculum, such as the anterior thalamus (Ranck, 1984; Taube et al., 1990a; Taube, 1995a, 1998). As already noted, HD cells fire whenever the rat's head points in a specific direction relative to the environment, irrespective of its location or whether it is moving or still (see Fig. 11–21C, color centerfold). The primary correlate is the azimuthal orientation of the head in the horizontal plane. Pitch and roll appear to be relatively unimportant, as is the orientation of the rest of the body. Figure 11–14A shows the firing rate for three of these HD units plotted as a function of the direction of heading. Each cell has a single preferred direction, and firing falls off rapidly, symmetrically, and almost linearly as the head direction rotates away from the preferred direction. We refer to these directions in terms of compass headings but do not imply that these cells are sensitive to geomagnetism. The portion of the 360° circle covered by a given cell ranges from about 60° to 140°, with the average being about 90° (Fig. 11–14A). An impressively Euclidean property of HD cells is that the preferred direction is remarkably independent of position (Taube et al., 1990a; Burgess et al., 2005); the preferred direction vectors in the various parts of an environment appear *not* to converge (e.g., upon a salient distal cue, as one might have expected) but are parallel. The distribution of peak firing directions across the population of cells is uniform, with no direction preferred over any other.

A   3 Head Direction Cells Firing Fields

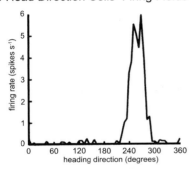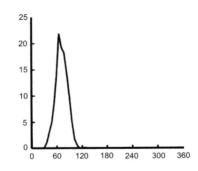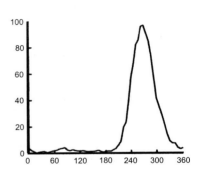

B   Fields rotate with cue card

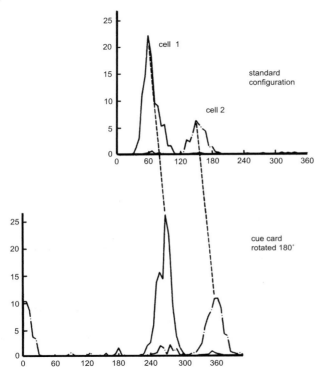

C   Fields shift after cue card removal

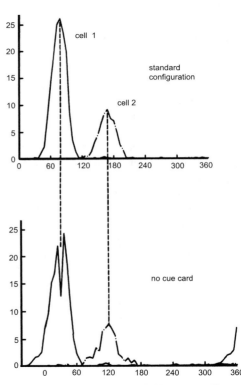

Figure 11–14. Head direction cells in the dorsal presubiculum. *A.* Firing fields of three cells as a function of the animal's heading direction. Note that each firing field subtends an angle of about 90° but that the firing rates differ. (*Source:* After Taube et al., 1990a.) *B.* Rotation of a cue card on the wall of the cylindrical enclosure by 180° rotates the angular orientation of two simultaneously recorded fields by a similar amount. Note that the relative angle between the two fields tends to remain the same, as shown by the dashed parallel lines. *C.* Removal of the cue card shifts firing fields of two cells recorded at the same time. Again, both fields shift by approximately 40° and maintain a constant difference in their preferred heading directions. The x axes in the bottom figures of *B* and *C* have been extended beyond 360°, and part of the field is duplicated to show the entire shape of the firing fields around 0/360°. (*Source: B, C.* Afer Taube et al., 1990b, both with permission.)

Similarly, there does not appear to be any topography to the directions represented by neighboring neurons, an arrangement reminiscent of the lack of environmental topography in the layout of place cells. Importantly, unlike hippocampal place cells, which signal location in some locations but are silent in others, HD cells fire in all environments tested.

11.9.1 Head Direction Cells are Controlled by Distal Sensory Cues

Taube et al. (1990a) found that rotations of a cue card fixed to the apparatus wall by multiples of 90° produced almost commensurate rotations of the directional firing field (Fig.

11–14B). Slight deviations from perfect rotation, however, suggested that in the experimental setup used the card was not the only environmental cue exerting stimulus control over the preferred direction. This was confirmed in tests in which the card was removed altogether. Card removal revealed two interesting properties of these cells (Fig. 11–14C). First, the width of the directional firing field remained the same, as did the peak firing rate. This suggests that these properties depend on factors intrinsic to the cell itself or to the network in which it is embedded, not on environmental inputs. Second, the preferred direction shifted to a new unpredictable compass point in almost two-thirds of the cells. Shifts ranged from 108° in the clockwise direction to 66° in the counterclockwise direction. The preferred direction appeared to remain approximately the same in the remaining one-third of cells. Zugaro et al. (2001) tested the relative influence of distal and proximal cues in determining the orientation of HD cells. As Cressant et al. (1997) had shown with place field orientation, Zugaro found that the rotation of three distinct objects at the periphery of a platform, bounded by a cylindrical enclosure, caused an equal rotation in the preferred directions of all anterior thalamus HD cells tested. The cylinder prevented the rats from seeing more distal background cues, such as geometrically configured black curtains along the walls of the room. When the same object-set rotation was performed in the absence of the cylinder, the preferred directions of all the HD cells were essentially unaltered. Although the cylinder-absent, background-visible condition was always performed second, the consistency of the responses provides further evidence that the orientation system is preferentially controlled by the most distal cues available.

In addition to cue card shifts, Taube and colleagues (1990b) found that changing the shape of the testing enclosure from a cylinder to a square or rectangle also caused changes in the preferred direction. In both right-angled boxes, the polarizing cue card occupied the same location relative to the environment as it had in the cylinder. When tested in the rectangular enclosure, most cells (8/10) shifted directions by large amounts; but on subsequent testing of these cells in the square enclosure, fewer than half (3/8) had preferred directions shifted relative to those they had displayed in the cylinder. As with card removal, the peak firing and angular width remained constant. Golob and Taube (1997) found that only 2 of 11 cells changed their preferred direction by more than 18° from the standard cylinder to a square box. As previously, more radical shape changes (i.e., from the cylinder to triangular or rectangular enclosures) caused large shifts in directional preference; all 17 cells tested shifting by at least 36°. (One minor caveat: This study tested HD cell activity in hippocampal-lesioned animals only.)

Goodridge et al. (1998) looked at the role of sensory modalities other than vision on the firing of head direction cells. Whereas a simple auditory cue, such as a localized series of clicks or bursts of noise, was ineffective, a localized smell did exert a small but significant control over the preferred direction. Rotation of the walls and floor of the testing chamber in blindfolded rats also had a small effect that subsequent tests revealed was mostly attributable to the floor. There was also some evidence that the preferred direction in blindfolded rats was less stable.

11.9.2 Angular Distance Between any Given Pair of Head Direction Cells Always Remains Constant

An important property of HD cells is "obligatory coupling"— the angular distance between the preferred directions of pairs of HD cells is remarkably resistant to alteration (Fig. 11–14B,C). Regardless of the cue-control manipulation, both cells of a simultaneously pair are always found to rotate by the same amount. Figure 11–14C illustrates this nicely: Following cue removal, the preferred head direction of cell 1 rotates by approximately 40° accompanied by a similar rotation in cell 2. The important implication of this coupling of preferred directions between cells is that there must be some kind of "hard-wiring" of the network of HD cells such that the population of cells firing at any one time gives an accurate and, above all, unambiguous representation of heading direction. The maintenance of a constant angular distance between HD cell pairs in the face of environmental change is well modeled by attractor networks (e.g., Redish and Touretzky, 1996; Zhang, 1996) (see Chapter 14).

11.9.3 Head Direction Cells Can also Be Controlled by Idiothetic Cues

In a fashion similar to the place cells, some HD cells maintain their preferred direction following removal of the cue card. One interpretation of this finding is that the sense of direction is continually updated in the absence of environmental cues on the basis of idiothetic or inertial navigation cues including those from the vestibular and proprioceptive systems. Consistent with this possibility is the finding that vestibular lesions cause cells to lose their preferred direction (Stackman and Taube, 1997). It must be stressed, however, that idiothetic cues *alone* are almost certainly insufficient to maintain a constant preferred direction over a long period of nonstereotyped locomotion. For instance, in darkness, olfactory signals from the cylinder and/or floor are probably required in tandem with idiothetic cues for stable orientation, as suggested by the place cell results of Save et al. (2000) (Section 11.7.7).

Additional evidence for the role of vestibular cues on preferred heading direction comes from experiments in which the floor (and therefore the rat) and the black-and-white striped walls of the recording chamber were rotated together in tandem or independently (Blair and Sharp, 1996). There were two rates of rotation, one above and the other below that assumed to be detectable by the vestibular system. These manipulations were carried out both in the light and in the dark in an attempt to dissociate visual motion cues from vestibular effects. In the light, slow rotation of the wall and floor together resulted in the comparable rotation of the preferred heading direction in all cells tested. In contrast, rapid rotation of the wall or floor individually or together was ignored by most cells, which maintained their preferred direction relative to the laboratory frame. A few cells did show partial or complete rotations under these conditions, revealing some influence of idiothetic cues. The picture was different in the dark. Now both fast and slow rotations changed the preferred heading direction for many but not all of the cells. This pattern of results suggests that the preferred direction is controlled by several factors, which include visual information from the laboratory itself and visual motion and vestibular information derived from the animal's movements. The latter become more effective in the absence of the distal visual cues.

Disorientating or disruptive rotations of the animal carried out before it is placed in the environment have also been examined. If these are carried out on a routine daily basis for several weeks prior to recording, HD cells have a less stable relation to the frame of the laboratory both within and across recording sessions. They are also less well controlled by explicit visual cues (Knierim et al., 1995). Even in animals that had not been disorientated in this way and that displayed strong stable control by visual cues, subsequent introduction of the disorienting procedure prior to each daily recording session caused the HD cells to become progressively uncoupled from strong visual control. Knierim and colleagues suggested that this is evidence that path integration navigation cues predominate when an animal first enters a new environment and that environmental cues gain control over the head direction system only after a period in which they maintain a stable relation to the path integration system. Stability, it is thought, initially derives from the path integration system. On this argument, the association of the head direction system to environmental cues would provide corrections for the inevitable accumulation of errors to which the path integration system is subject. This requires that the system, which originally used the path integration system as the basis for assigning stability (or a direction) to the visual cue, would then be able to use that cue to correct the drift in the system. This boot-strap operation appears to require rapid association of specific cues (e.g., those provided by a cue card) to an otherwise stable but preexisting framework. The amount of exposure time for a visual cue card to gain control over preferred orientation was studied in passing in earlier studies. Goodridge et al. (1998), for instance, found that 8 minutes was sufficient for all cells tested, but that as little as 1 minute sufficed for some cells. Zugaro et al. (2000) found that preferred directions shifted to a new, fairly stable orientation within 15 seconds of a cue card rotation. More recently, an interesting study designed specifically to examine this issue (Zugaro et al., 2003) has shown that reorientation induced by 90° rotation of a peripheral cue card in the dark can occur with a latency on the order of 100 ms after the cue-card shift becomes visually apparent. The authors reasonably concluded that such latencies are more compatible with an abrupt jump from one preferred direction to another than with a gradual

rotation through intermediate directions. In familiar environments, control of the head direction system by visual stimuli can be rapid indeed. Perhaps the slower figures are due to the time it takes for the animal to notice the changed position of the cue card.

11.9.4 Head Direction Cells Are Found in Different Anatomically Connected Brain Areas

Head-direction cells have been recorded in areas of the brain in addition to the dorsal presubiculum, where they were first discovered. These areas include the anterior dorsal thalamic nucleus (Taube, 1995a), lateral mammillary nucleus (Stackman and Taube, 1998), lateral dorsal thalamic nuclei (Mizumori and Williams, 1993), retrosplenial cortex (Chen et al., 1994; Cho and Sharp, 2001), and striatum (Wiener, 1993). Apart from the striatum, these areas are all strongly interconnected. The HD cells in the lateral mammillary nucleus, anterior thalamus, and dorsal presubiculum have been most studied, and this section concentrates on the differences in their properties. Do they tell us anything about the way in which the head direction signal is constructed? What is the contribution of each part of the circuit? In addition to the characterization of the properties of the HD cells in each area, two additional approaches to these questions have been used. The first looks at the relative timing of the signal in the various areas, and the second asks what the effect of a lesion in one area is on the activity in another. With the first approach, the best temporal correlation between the HD cell firing and the animal's heading direction is computed. The idea is to see whether cell firing is better related to the animal's current heading or to its heading in the immediate past or future. The assumption is that if the best correlated cell firing precedes the current heading direction, it is more likely to reflect some aspect of neural activity in the motor system that is producing the head movements; conversely, if the best correlated cell firing lags behind the behavior, it is more likely to reflect sensory feedback generated by the movement. The latter assumption is not infallible, however, because it is equally possible that lagged cell firing represents aspects of the neural control of movement shifted by a time delay.

The second use of time shift correlation analyses is to compare the temporal relations between the areas in which HD cells are found. If the cells in one area show a firing pattern that is earlier relative to the current heading direction than those of a second area, it is reasonable to suppose that the first brain area makes computations that come "earlier" in the circuit than the second. In a modular system with strictly serial connections between the modules, the relative latencies with respect to an external event may be taken as an indication of the functional and perhaps causal connectivity between brain areas.

There is a clear consensus that, on average, the firing of HD cells in the dorsal presubiculum is approximately in synchrony with the current direction of heading. HD cells in the lateral mammillary nucleus lead those of the anterior dorsal thalamus (by about 60–70 ms), and the anterior dorsal thalamus leads the dorsal presubiculum (by about 20–30 ms) (Blair et al., 1997; Stackman and Taube, 1998; Taube and Muller, 1998). Although it is clear that there are average time shifts between the areas, there is also a wide distribution of shifts within any area, resulting in an overlap of shifts between areas. The pattern of temporal correlations suggests a functional pathway that originates in the lateral mammillary nucleus, passes information to the anterior dorsal thalamic nucleus, and thence to the dorsal presubiculum. Remarkably, this is part of the classic Papez circuit originally believed to provide the neural substrate for emotions (see Chapter 2), and there is abundant evidence of its anatomical basis from numerous tract tracing studies (see Chapter 3). It is important to remember, however, that there are also substantial connections in the opposite direction and, as we shall see in the next section, good reason to be cautious when putting forward any simple serial theory of the elements of the head direction system in rodents.

A similar story emerges from lesion experiments. Lesions of the anterior dorsal thalamic nucleus abolish the head direction signal in the dorsal presubiculum (Goodridge and Taube, 1997). In contrast, lesions in the dorsal presubiculum do not abolish the anterior dorsal thalamic nucleus signal but have more subtle effects on it. The clearest of these is an increase in the amount of time by which anterior dorsal thalamic nucleus HD cell firing anticipates the animal's heading direction. This suggests that a contribution of the feedback from the dorsal presubiculum to the anterior dorsal thalamic nucleus is to reduce the anticipatory interval expressed in the anterior dorsal thalamic nucleus leg of the system. A second effect of dorsal presubiculum lesions is to abolish the control of a cue card over the preferred heading direction of anterior dorsal thalamic nucleus cells (Goodridge and Taube, 1997) and to reduce the consistency and stability of the preferred heading direction between recording sessions.

Blair and colleagues (1999) investigated the effects of bilateral or unilateral lesions of the lateral mammillary nuclei on the properties of HD cells in the anterior thalamus. Following unilateral lesions, thalamic cells still had preferred directions, but they sometimes differed from prelesion ones, the peak firing rates were often reduced, and the turning curves were broader. In general, the HD cell firing properties shifted to resemble those in the mammillary bodies. Following bilateral lesions, no directional cells could be found in the anterior thalamus.

The overall pattern of changes following lesions of various nuclei support the notion that directional signals travel from the hypothalamus through the thalamus to the cortex. Furthermore, they are consistent with the idea that the dorsal presubiculum is the site at which visual sensory information gains access to the HD system, and the lateral mammillary nucleus/anterior dorsal thalamic nucleus pathway is the source of path integration control based on vestibular information.

11.9.5 Dorsal Tegmental Nucleus of Gudden Provides Information About the Direction and Angular Velocity of the Animal's Head Rotation

The midbrain nucleus called the dorsal tegmental nucleus of Gudden (DTN) is reciprocally connected to the lateral mammillary nucleus and contains cells whose firing rate correlates with the angular velocity of the head (Bassett and Taube, 2001; Sharp et al., 2001). Integration of the angular velocity over time would produce a signal proportional to the change in angular direction, which could be used to update the current heading direction. There appear to be several types of angular velocity cell in the DTN: Many show strong correlations with velocity of movement regardless of the direction of the movement, increasing their firing rates in both directions, whereas others are asymmetrical, increasing their firing rates in one direction and decreasing them or firing at a constant rate in the other. In addition to these angular velocity cells, the DTN contains a small number of HD cells, and there is evidence that some of the angular velocity cells also show head direction or head pitch correlates.

11.10 Interactions Between Hippocampal Place Cells and Head Direction Cells

What is the relation between place cells and HD cells? In the original formulation of the cognitive map theory, O'Keefe and Nadel suggested that the map of an environment consisted of a set of place representations bound together by information about the direction and distance between them (O'Keefe, 1976; O'Keefe and Nadel, 1978) (see Section 11.7). In this view a place representation could be activated either by direct sensory information impinging on the animal when it occupied that place or by activation of a different place representation together with the appropriate distance and direction inputs between that place and the target place. The theory was extended in 1991 (O'Keefe, 1991a,b) by the suggestion that place cells were dependent on the input from two or more HD cells for directional information and that rotation of the HD system relative to the environmental frame would produce the rotation of place fields seen in these experiments. McNaughton and colleagues (1996) suggested that the place cell firing field was determined by the distance to a single object in a specific direction and that this directional signal was provided by the HD system. Evidence in favor of the idea that the place system is dependent on the HD system comes from the following.

Both place and HD cells respond similarly to rotation and removal of polarizing cues, such as the cue card in the standard cylinder (Muller and Kubie, 1987; Taube et al., 1990b; Cressant et al., 1997; Zugaro et al., 2001). Vestibular lesions abolish anterior thalamic directional firing and location-specific firing in hippocampal place cells (Stackman and

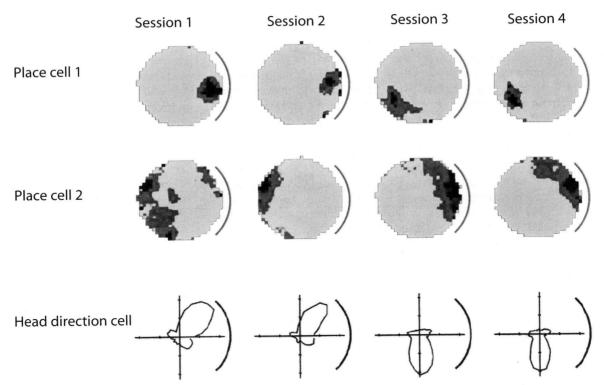

Figure 11–15. Place and head direction cells recorded simultaneously maintain the same angular orientation despite both rotating relative to the environment. Top two rows show the place fields of two cells that rotate by about 135° following disorientation of the animal by gentle spinning between sessions two and three. Bottom row shows the field of a head-direction (HD) cell recorded at the same time, which also rotates. Both place fields and preferred direction of the HD cell are stable before (sessions one and two) and after (sessions three and four) the intervention. Note that the fields of both place cells and the HD cell maintain a constant angular relation to each other. (*Source*: After Knierim et al., 1995, with permission.)

Taube, 1997; Stackman et al., 2002; Russell et al., 2003). In the one experiment (Knierim et al., 1995) in which HD cells and place cells were recorded simultaneously, they stayed in register even under circumstances where the control by environmental stimuli was lost: Rotating the animal prior to the recording session often led to unpredictable rotation of both the preferred heading direction of the HD cell and the angular orientation of the place cell, but they maintained their fixed relation to each other (Fig. 11–15).

Lesions to the anterior thalamus or the dorsal presubiculum significantly increased the directionality of place fields recorded in the cylinder in comparison with control animals (Calton et al., 2003). Recall that in normal rats the place fields are essentially nondirectional in this testing apparatus (Muller et al., 1994) (see Section 11.7). Such lesions also reduce the spatial coherence of the place fields. The relation between the standard cue card and the place fields depends on the lesion locus. Note that in intact animals, as discussed above, rotation of the card causes the preferred direction of most HD cells to reorient rapidly so as to maintain a fixed relation to the card. Calton et al. (2003) found that in animals with lesions of the dorsal presubiculum the angular locations of hippocampal place fields were not controlled by the cue card but shifted unpredictably from trial to trial. Although intertrial variability was also reliably seen in anterior thalamus-lesioned animals, the effect was mild in these cases. Similarly, removing the cue card caused large shifts in the place fields' angular location in the dorsal presubicular animals but minor shifts in the anterior thalamic lesioned animals.

In contrast to the large effect that dorsal presubicular lesions have on hippocampal place cells, there is little evidence that hippocampal lesions have a major effect on the basic firing characteristics of HD cells. Golob and Taube (1997) reported that about the usual number of HD cells were recorded in the anterior thalamic nuclei and dorsal presubiculum following hippocampal lesions, and that they were under control of the visual cue card to the same extent. Furthermore, changes in the preferred firing direction in novel enclosures of different shapes were broadly similar to previous studies of nonlesioned animals. In a follow-up experiment, the effect of combined lesions of the hippocampus and overlying neocortex on the control of the HD cells by idiothetic path integration signals was examined (Golob and Taube, 1999). The preferred head direction was monitored as the animals moved from a familiar environment to an unfamiliar one. In normal animals, the self-movement cues provided sufficient information to maintain the heading direction in the new environment consonant with that in the old familiar one, consistent with previous work (Taube and Burton, 1995). HD cells in lesioned animals, however, were not able to do this and, furthermore, took up to 4 minutes to reach a stable preferred orientation in the new environment. On the other hand, a cue card in the new environment was capable of establishing control over the HD preferred orientation, showing that there was no deficit in this part of the system. The primary influence of the hippocampus on the head direction system appears to be to maintain a consistent preferred direction in the HD cells as an animal moves between different enclosures in the same laboratory, presumably on the basis of path integration signals or context information about the laboratory. The only caveat here is that lesions of the overlying neocortex resulted in effects that were similar but of lesser magnitude, and it is not possible therefore to rule out a role for the neocortex or a more general, nonspecific effect of the lesions.

As we shall see in Chapter 13, there is evidence that hippocampus-lesioned rats can learn an allocentric spatial memory task in which they are required to go to a location defined by its distance from a single object in a specific environmental direction. This capability appears to depend on the HD system but not, because it depends on a single vector, on the hippocampal system.

In summary, the evidence strongly suggests that the place system relies on the HD system to provide it with the directional basis of a fixed framework, which acts as the scaffolding for the representation of an environment. Two HD cell characteristics are crucial to this: First, the angular distance between HD cells remains constant; and second, the vectors created by the signaling of each HD cell firing in different portions of an environment are parallel. Whereas environmental changes can cause the distance between different place fields to shift relative to each other, the HD cells appear to be rigidly fixed relative to each other, and it is only the relation between the total constellation of cells and the environment that can be altered. Rotation of the HD system rotates the entire place system. The most likely route for the influence of the HD system on the hippocampal place cells is via the medial entorhinal cortical grid cells whose orientation relative to the environment is also controlled by distal cues (see Section 11.7.7). The contribution of the hippocampal place system to the HD system is less clear. It may be the origin of information about the wider context that allows the animal to maintain a constant heading direction relative to distant cues as it moves from a familiar part of a territory to an unfamiliar one.

11.11 Hippocampal Complex-spike Cells Have Been Implicated in Nonspatial Perception and Learning

In addition to the widely reported spatial and movement correlates of hippocampal cells, there have been reports of other correlates from several laboratories. They have suggested to some that the functions of the hippocampus are more general

than the processing and storage of specifically *spatial* information. We return to this question in Chapter 13 on lesion results, as a successful theory must account for the data from several experimental domains. Suffice it to mention here that nonspatial responses in hippocampal units do not per se argue against a spatial function for the hippocampus. A spatial system would need to incorporate information about the locations of objects, rewards, and dangers as well as using nonspatial information in the construction of place representations.

The data on nonspatial unit responses fall into two primary classes: those suggesting a role in nonspatial sensory processing and those showing a correlation with some aspect of a nonspatial learning process. They are discussed in separate sections.

11.11.1 Hippocampal Cells Have Been Implicated in the Processing of Nonspatial Sensory Information

Studies by McLean, Ranck, and O'Keefe during the 1960s and early 1970s looked for, but could not find, selective sensory inputs to the hippocampal complex-spike cells. On the other hand, Vinogradova (1977) and colleagues reported a nonspecific effect of sensory stimulation in the awake rabbit; however, it appears likely from the firing rates of her cells, the absence of complex spikes, and subsequent work on the correlates of theta cells in the rabbit (Sinclair et al., 1982) that many of her cells were theta cells. As pointed out above, theta cells in the rabbit increase their firing during theta EEG episodes, and in the rabbit these episodes occur during nonmovement arousal as well as during movement.

Ranck (1973) and O'Keefe (1976) studied the role of sensory inputs in the freely moving rat and, aside from a few olfactory responses reported by O'Keefe, neither found much evidence for these inputs. However, some of the unit responses to the cues used in more recent learning experiments could be interpreted as unlearned responses to the stimuli themselves. For example, Wood et al. (1999a) reported that 8% of cells in the rat hippocampus responded to the olfactory cues in an olfactory recognition task. Likewise, Tamura et al. (1992) reported that 10% of units in the hippocampus and surrounding regions of the monkey responded to specific objects. Creutzfeldt and colleagues (Vidyasagar et al., 1991; Salzmann et al., 1993) found that as many as 38% of hippocampal and parahippocampal units in the monkey changed activity in response to arousing stimuli such as the presentation of a raisin or the sight of the experimenter. It is not clear whether these are perceptual, learned, or general arousal responses. These studies are examined in more detail in the section on nonspatial learning, below.

Perceptual responses to stimuli have also been reported in studies on the human hippocampal formation. In one experiment (Kreiman et al., 2000b), subjects viewed a series of pictures drawn from nine classes: household objects, unknown faces portraying different emotions, famous faces, spatial layouts including the facades of houses and natural scenes, animals, drawings of famous people or cartoon characters, cars, food items, and abstract drawings. Overall, 14% of units from medial temporal lobe sites showed a visual response to one or more stimuli. Interestingly, of the 32 hippocampal units responsive to visual stimuli, 29% responded selectively to spatial layouts, 12% to famous faces, and less than 10% to stimuli drawn from the other categories. Therefore, although hippocampal cells responded to famous faces and other stimuli, pictures portraying the layout of environments or buildings were by far the most effective of these visual stimuli. The human hippocampus, like that of the rodent and nonhuman primate, appears to prefer information about spaces over faces and objects.

11.11.2 Hippocampal Unit Activity May Show Correlations with Different Aspects of Nonspatial Learning Tasks

In pioneering studies conducted during the 1960s, Jim Olds and Menahem Segal recorded unit activity in the hippocampus during classical conditioning to a tone. They saw an increase in firing to the tone following conditioning. These studies were the first of a number that have looked at the responses of hippocampal neurons during or after nonspatial learning, primarily using conditioning paradigms or discrimination learning. Some of these studies were carried out using multiunit recording techniques, which, like EEG, register only the collective properties of a group of neurons. As we have seen, the spatial coding of environmental features in complex-spike cells is carried out at the single-cell level, and group recordings would not reveal this spatial code. We therefore concentrate primarily on studies that have recorded single-unit activity and refer to the multiunit studies only when they add something different.

Two types of behavioral paradigm have often been used to look at nonspatial learning: (1) classical conditioning in which the animal's response has no effect on the stimulus-reward contingencies and (2) signaled operant conditioning in which it does. A good example of the former are experiments on classical conditioning of the rabbit nictitating membrane (NM) response; a good example of the latter would be a nose poke, go/no-go instrumental task taught to a rat. In the sections that follow, we turn first to classical conditioning experiments in the rat and rabbit and then examine the somewhat more extensive literature on operant conditioning in rats and monkeys.

11.11.3 Hippocampal Unit Activity During Aversive Classical Conditioning

Hippocampal unit activity has been recorded during aversive classical conditioning: a single conditioned stimulus (CS) followed after a short period by an unconditioned stimulus (US) consisting of a shock or other noxious stimulus. After sufficient pairings, the CS comes to elicit a conditioned response

(CR) such as an eyeblink or suppressed heart rate. In a more complicated differential conditioning paradigm, two stimuli (CS$^+$ and CS$^-$) are interspersed randomly, one followed by the US and the other not. In this latter paradigm, the animal learns to discriminate between the stimuli, coming eventually to respond to the first but not the second. Typically, during the early stages of learning, both stimuli elicit responses and only subsequently does the animal learn to inhibit its response to the CS$^-$. In addition, there is a learned arousal response that is not specific to the hippocampus but can be reflected in the activity of hippocampal cells.

Delacour (1984) trained rats on an aversive differential conditioning paradigm. During slow-wave sleep two different tones served as the conditioning stimuli and mild electric shock to the neck as the unconditioned stimulus. He recorded increased neck muscle tone as the conditioned response (CR) and the cortical EEG as an independent measure of arousal. During the early stages of training, both the CS$^+$ and CS$^-$ elicited a muscle activation CR that was associated with cortical arousal; during the later stages, there was a decrease in the cortical arousal to both stimuli as well as the development of a differential neck muscle response, with the response to the CS$^+$ remaining high and that to the CS$^-$ steadily declined to baseline (Fig. 11–16A). The initial increase in the EMG activation to both stimuli was thought to reflect general arousal, whereas the later differentiation between them reflected movement to the CS$^+$. Unit responses to the CSs of single hippocampal complex-spike cells, hippocampal theta cells, and dentate granule cells were monitored. During the early phase of training, all cell types increased activity to both stimuli in parallel with EMG activation, the complex-spike cells somewhat faster than the theta cells. During the latter phases, however, they acted differently: The hippocampal complex-spike cells ceased firing to both positive and negative conditioning stimuli, paralleling the decrease in cortical arousal. Like the cortical arousal, at no time during training did they differentiate between the two CSs (Fig. 11–16B). In contrast, the responses of the hippocampal theta and dentate granule cells followed the pattern of the EMG response and began to differentiate between the stimuli as the behavioral differentiation developed (Fig. 11–16C). As a control for the specificity of these responses, Delacour recorded from thalamic cells as well and found that they also divided into two classes: Those in the centre median acted similar to the complex spike cells, whereas those recorded in the dorsomedial nucleus resembled the theta cells. On the basis of these results, Delacour argued rather convincingly that the response of the complex-spike cells was a reflection of general arousal, whereas the pattern of activity of the theta/granule cells was a reflection of the learned differential increase in neck muscle activation to the two conditioned stimuli. The latter response may reflect the movement correlates of the hippocampal theta cells. He further argued that these were not specific responses but were representative of more general responses in arousal and movement systems that could be recorded elsewhere in the brain as well. Laroche and Bloch (Bloch and Laroche, 1981; Laroche et

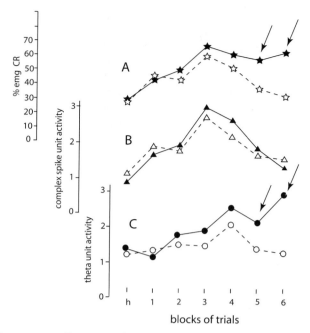

Figure 11–16. Two types of response in hippocampal unit activity during classic conditioning of the arousal response to positive and negative tones. *A.* Neck electromyography (EMG) increases during the early trials and then begins to differentiate between the CS+ (black stars) and CS– (open stars) by the last two blocks of trials (arrows). *B.* Principal hippocampal neurons increase their firing rate during the early part of the trial in parallel with the EMG response but then fall off to both stimuli. *C.* Hippocampal theta cells and dentate granule cells also show an initial increase but then differentiate between the CSs in a manner that parallels the EMG activity. Solid symbols are CS+ responses, and open symbols are CS– responses in all panels. h, habituation trials. (*Source*: Delacour, 1984.)

al., 1983) found a similar increase to a CS in the dentate multiple unit response after conditioning.

Moita and colleagues (2003, 2004) have carried out an important classical conditioning experiment in the rat that may throw further light on the role of hippocampal cells in these tasks. They recorded the responsiveness of complex-spike and theta cells to an auditory stimulus before and after delay classical conditioning in which the stimulus was paired with a brief electric shock to the eyelid. No complex-spike cells responded with a short latency to the tone prior to conditioning, but many did so after conditioning. However, they did so only if the animal was located in the place field of the cell during CS presentation (Fig. 11–17). As Figure 11–17 shows, the same cell might give a strong, brisk response to the auditory stimulus when the animal was in the place field but respond little or not at all to the same stimulus when the animal was outside the field. The animal's location in the place field appeared to gate the response to the CS rather than simply summate with it. Moita and colleagues (2004) also found that place cells can develop a place field or can shift field location in the conditioning box following conditioning, and this

effect was greater following conditioning to the context of the box than when there was an explicit auditory stimulus. These results may give some insight into the role of the hippocampus in this behavioral paradigm, at least in the rat. It is possible that, in addition to the conditioning of arousal responses, some conditioned responses in hippocampal units in immobile animals reflect the fact that during conditioning some cells shift their place fields to the animal's location and begin to respond to the CS in that location. Against this interpretation is the fact that restraining the rat abolishes the firing in the place field (Foster et al., 1989). However the possibility remains that restraint may not abolish the gating function on conditioned stimuli. We return to this possibility following a discussion of unit activity during the nictitating conditioning paradigm.

11.11.4 Nictitating Membrane Conditioning in the Rabbit: Role of Theta

Conditioning of the rabbit nictitating membrane (NM) has been used successfully as a model system for studying the neural bases of learning and memory since it was introduced by Richard Thompson in 1976 (Thompson, 1976). In this paradigm, the CS (e.g., a 6 KHz tone) is paired with a US, which can be a puff of air to the eye or a small electric shock to the orbit. By varying the temporal relation between the CS and US, one can investigate various types of classical conditioning. In delay conditioning, the US overlaps the last portion of the CS, so both terminate together. In trace conditioning, the CS ends before the US begins, and there is a temporal gap between the two. As we saw with classical conditioning in the rat (Delacour, 1984), there is an important role for arousal in this form of learning. There is clear evidence that theta activity gets conditioned to various aspects of the task during classical conditioning experiments in the rabbit. Powell and Joseph (1974) conditioned the corneoretinal potential in the rabbit using a mild electric shock to the eye as the US. This was preceded by a CS. A second stimulus was not followed by the US and served as a CS–. During the early stages of learning, before differential responses to these two stimuli had been established, there was a high incidence of theta to both CSs; after differential conditioning, when the CS+ but not the CS– consistently elicited the US, a considerably higher amount of theta occurred to the CS+. During this second phase of conditioning there was a differential response of the neck EMG to the CS+. This pattern of responses is similar to that seen in the rat (see above) and indicates that the early theta activity was related to general arousal, and the later theta activity was related, at least in part, to the motor response. Experiments that manipulate the animal's arousal have shown that it has a strong effect on learning rates and that this effect may be mediated in part via its effect on the baseline rate of theta activity. Berry and colleagues (Berry, 1989) showed that the pretraining background amount of hippocampal theta was a good predictor of NM conditioning rates and that this variable was strongly influenced by the level of arousal. Following

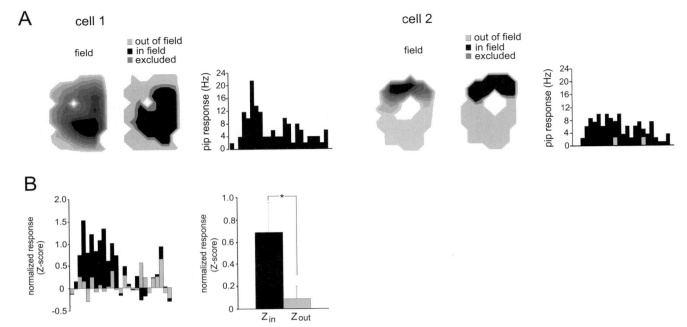

Figure 11–17. Response of hippocampal complex spike cells to auditory CS following classic eyeblink conditioning. The cells respond only when the animal is in the place field. *A.* Responses in two individual cells. On the left of each panel, place fields are shown with the higher firing rates in the darker colors; on the right of each panel are histograms of the unit responses while the animal is inside the place field (black color) and outside the field (light color). The middle panels show the portion of the environment included as part of the field, the portion considered to be outside the field, and an immediate zone not considered as part of either. Both cells showed a strong response to the stimulus inside the field and no (cell 1) or few (cell 2) spikes outside the field. *B.* Population response histograms to stimulus presented inside (dark shading) and outside (light shading) the field of each cell. Across the population there is a significant difference between the in-the-field and out-of-field responses (histogram, right). The x-axes in the unit response histograms are 250 ms in total, which was the period of CS presentation. (*Source:* Moita et al., 2003.)

mild water deprivation, there was a faster rate of learning. A similar pattern was found with trace conditioning (Kim et al., 1995).

11.11.5 Single-unit Recording in the Hippocampus During Nictitating Membrane Conditioning of Rabbits

Several laboratories have recorded the activity of single units and multiple units from the hippocampus of rabbits during classical conditioning of the NM response. Berger and colleagues (1983) recorded single units in the rabbit hippocampus during simple delay NM conditioning. Pyramidal cells were identified by their antidromic activation from fornix stimulation. They comprised the largest proportion of cells recorded; and following conditioning, many increased their firing rates during the CS period (Fig. 11–18A–C). They typically emitted one or more bursts of spikes during each trial, some showing a pattern of activity that closely modeled the NM response (Fig. 11–18A) whereas others were more selective, firing during different time epochs of the trial (Fig. 11–18B,C). One type of theta cell increased its overall level of activity during the trial (Fig. 11–18D,E), whereas another type showed an overall decrease in activity (Fig. 11–18F,G). Theta cells were typically activated by the CS to fire a series of theta-like bursts, which often continued throughout the trial and in some cases continued beyond the termination of the trial. Berger and colleagues also reported a third category of cells, "silent" cells, which constituted 11% of the neurons recorded; they had exceptionally low spontaneous firing rates (< 0.2/second), were not activated by fornix stimulation, and did not participate in the conditioned response. As we shall see below, this estimate of the percentage of cells in this category may be low.

Weiss et al. (1996) recorded single units from rabbit hippocampus during trace conditioning of the NM, a version of the conditioning task that is sensitive to hippocampal lesions: Either the CR is abolished, or its timing is altered (see Chapter 12). They also reported the existence of the same three classes of cells reported by Berger and colleagues in their delay conditioning experiments; but in other respects the results differed markedly. Weiss et al. found a much larger percentage of cells that did not participate in the conditioning (40% in contrast to Berger's 11%) and relatively few units that were significantly excited (in contrast to inhibited) during the CS or trace period in the conditioned animals in comparison with unpaired controls. Thus, in CA1, 14% of pyramidal cells were excited during the CS period in contrast to 9% of the unpaired

Pyramidal cells

Theta cells

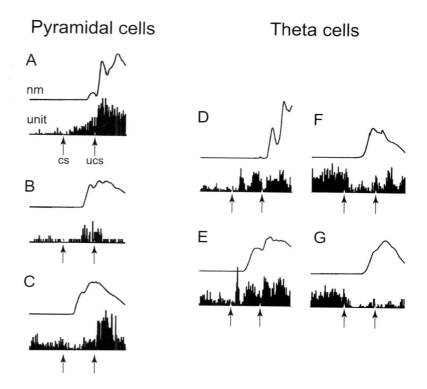

Figure 11–18. Firing patterns of hippocampal units following nictitating membrane conditioning in the rabbit. *A–C.* Pyramidal cells. *D, E.* Excited theta cells. *F, G.* Inhibited theta cells. Top trace in each panel is the nictitating membrane record; bottom trace is the histogram of the average unit response. The first arrow indicates CS onset and the second arrow UCS onset, an interval of 250 ms. Note the theta bursting at approximately 8 Hz following the CS onset in the theta cells. (*Source*: Berger et al., 1983.)

controls; and 11% were excited during the trace period in contrast to 9% of the controls. In contrast to the findings of Berger and colleagues, the increase in inhibitory responses relative to the controls was twice as large as the increase in excitatory responses. McEchron and Disterhoft (1997) obtained similar results in animals conditioned in a trace paradigm when recordings were taken after asymptotic performance had been reached. In addition, they recorded from some animals during the earlier stages of learning. They found that the maximal activation in complex spike units occurred on the trials just *prior* to the onset of learning; as behavioral conditioning proceeded and the conditioned responses appeared more frequently, these unit responses actually diminished. Finally, when looked at on a trial-by-trial basis, there was no correlation between the unit activity and the occurrence of the conditioned response. This pattern suggests that the hippocampus may not be involved directly in the generation or timing of the motor response. Rather, it may be involved only indirectly, perhaps playing a role in the creation of a temporary behavioral state that precedes the motor learning but is a necessary condition for it to occur. Lesions of the hippocampus do not generally affect delay conditioning but do affect trace conditioning, changing the timing of the conditioned response in the trace version of the task (for a review see O'Keefe, 1999). Thus, if we compare the effects of hippocampal lesions on the NM conditioning with the results of single-unit recording experiments, we are left with a paradox. Delay conditioning, in which there are a sizable number of pyramidal cells whose temporal activation profile precedes and models the CR, does not require the hippocampus,

whereas trace conditioning, during which few such unit responses are found, does require an intact hippocampus.

How might the hippocampus be involved in trace but not delay conditioning? There are three distinct but related possibilities. The first suggests that the hippocampus provides the information that the animal is in a frightening place, the second that the animal is in a place where frightening events happen, and the third that it provides information about the timing of the unpleasant event. The first two make clear links to the spatial functions of the hippocampus, whereas the third does not necessarily do so. We deal with these in turn.

Our first two mechanisms relate to ones suggested by Nadel and colleagues (1985). According to them, the spatial functions of the hippocampus might lead to its being involved in conditioning in two ways: as the substrate for a direct association between the background cues and the US or less directly as the basis for an association between the CS–US event and the overall context. Evidence for a hippocampal role in conditioning to the background cues (the fearful context hypothesis) comes from experiments showing that animals with hippocampal lesions do not condition to the context (Phillips and LeDoux, 1994; Kim et al., 1995). This could come about either because there is an association of fear with the entire testing box or with specific locations in it. Recall that the ventral hippocampus contains place cells with large fields that may extend to an entire testing environment, and they could provide the basis for context conditioning. An alternative is that the more localized place fields in the dorsal hippocampus could shift following context conditioning so the overall pattern of place cell firing was different, perhaps signifying a dangerous environment (Moita et al., 2004).

The second possibility is that the cells showing conditioned responses are place cells whose fields coincide with the location of the testing box, and the responses to the CS are signaling the occurrence of an event in that place. As we have seen above in the experiments of Moita and colleagues (2003), complex-spike cells in the rat, which are normally not responsive to auditory stimuli, begin to respond to the CS following delay conditioning but only if the animal occupies the firing field of that cell. If the same changes are occurring in the rabbit, this might explain the increased responsiveness of cells with fields in the conditioning location; moreover, the fields of some cells might shift to that location following conditioning. With this interpretation, the increased responsiveness might reflect the fact that the hippocampus is now signaling that the animal is in a dangerous location and, furthermore, that the auditory cue predicts the onset of danger in that place. More evidence for a role for the hippocampus in contextual gating of CS–US events comes from a context shift experiment. Although lesions of the hippocampu have no obvious effect on simple delay conditioning, they do affect the role the background cues (i.e., the room in which conditioning takes place) play in that conditioning. Penick and Solomon (1991) showed that simple delay conditioning was disrupted in normal rabbits when the animal was moved into a new room after conditioning was completed but hippocampal-lesioned animals were not affected. This result fits nicely with the idea that the hippocampus provides spatial contextual information that gates the conditioning of fear to the CS. This information might not be necessary for simple delay conditioning, but it might be essential for trace conditioning.

The third possibility is that the hippocampus provides information about the timing of the US. The interpretation of the altered timing response in trace conditioning following dorsal hippocampal lesions is unclear. Why, for that matter, does the conditioned unit response occur just prior to the unconditioned stimulus in normals? The original rationale of the NM learning paradigm was to rule out any instrumental contribution to the learning and in particular the possibility that the conditioned response would protect the eye from the US or otherwise attenuate its impact (Thompson, 1976). If, on the other hand, one accepts that the conditioned response in these conditioning paradigms is a reflection of the prediction of the US, the timing of the CS is important; and the lesion results suggest that the hippocampus is involved in setting up the conditions under which the short-term prediction of stimuli can occur. Both Rawlins (1985) and Wallenstein and colleagues (1998) have suggested that the hippocampus is needed to bridge a temporal gap between two stimuli to be associated. This role would be particularly important in paradigms such as trace conditioning, where there is a CS–US interval and normal animals generate a CR just prior to the US. What might the underlying mechanism be? One possibility is that hippocampal a-theta is being used as a timing mechanism to allow a short-term signal to bridge the CS–US

gap. Theta oscillations, with their relatively constant period, could act as a clock over short intervals. During conditioning of the rabbit NM response, this clock signal can be reset by the CS and could therefore be used to predict the occurrence of the US. Even here there might be a secondary role for the spatial functions of the hippocampus. Recall that a-theta in the rabbit can be driven by arousing stimuli (e.g., the CS) much more easily than in the rat (see Section 11.3). That required level of arousal might be based on conditioning to the apparatus and other nonspatial cues, but it might also be driven by hippocampus-mediated fear conditioning to the background context as well. Under circumstances where the arousal level is appropriate, pyramidal cells may be able to count theta cycles and use this clock signal to predict the timing of the US. This timing signal would then be available to brain stem regions to control the occurrence of the CR. In the absence of this signal (e.g., following hippocampal damage), conditioning would still occur but the timing of the CR would be controlled by other factors. Some support for this view comes from an experiment on trace conditioning of the heart rate in rabbits (McEchron et al., 2003). Pairing a CS with an aversive US results in slowing of the heart rate in anticipation of the US; this can be conditioned with trace intervals as long as 20 seconds. McEchron and colleagues used trace intervals of 10 and 20 seconds in two groups of animals and found that one-fourth of complex-spike cells showed a burst of activity timed to coincide with the end of the trace interval. The effect was weak on any given trial; but when summed over trials there was a discernible response. The problem for the theta-counting hypothesis is that 10 seconds is a long time to count theta cycles. For further discussion of the contributions that contexts make to learning, see Chapter 13.

11.11.6 Hippocampal Unit Recording During Operant Tasks

During operant conditioning tasks, the animal must emit a response to gain a reward or avoid punishment. Often the availability of reinforcement is signaled by a sensory stimulus such as a tone. Christian and Deadwyler (1986) recorded from complex-spike and theta cells during an appetitive operant conditioning task. They trained thirsty rats to poke their noses into a small antechamber in the wall of a box to receive a water reward. For some animals, the availability of reward was signaled by a tone, and no sensory discrimination was required; for others, a differential CS⁺/CS⁻ procedure was used. Following successful conditioning to the single tone stimulus (Fig. 11–19A), theta cells showed a consistent increase in firing rate during the 200 ms following tone onset (Fig. 11–19A, theta). In contrast, no change from the background rate was seen in the complex spike cells (Fig. 11–19A, complex spike). During two-tone differential conditioning, the theta cells showed an increase to both stimuli with a greater increase to the CS⁺ (Fig. 11–19B, theta). In contrast, the pyramidal cells registered a marginal but nonsignificant change to the CS⁺ (Fig. 11–19B, complex-spike). Recordings

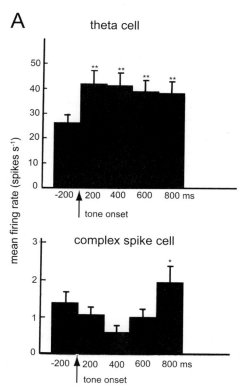

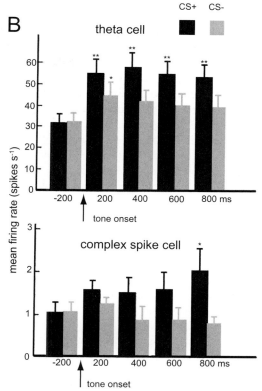

Figure 11–19. Theta and complex spike cell responses following nose-poke conditioning to tones. Theta cells (top) show increased firing above the pre-tone background rate in response to the tone in both simple (*A*) and compound (*B*) conditioning paradigms. In the latter, the unit response to the CS$^+$ is more marked than to the CS$^-$. Complex spike cells (bottom) do not respond in either the simple conditioning paradigm (*A*) or the complex compound conditioning paradigm (*B*). Single asterisks indicate a significant difference from pre-tone firing rates at the 0.05 level of significance and double asterisks at the 0.01 level of significance. The apparent increase in firing rate in the complex spike cells 800 ms following the tone in both *A* and *B* is an artifact from the reward dispenser. (*Source:* Christian and Deadwyler, 1986.)

taken from animals while they acquired the task showed that the changes in theta cell firing occurred in parallel to acquisition of the conditioned EMG response and disappeared with subsequent extinction. Again no changes were seen in complex-spike cells during the course of acquisition.

In a subsequent experiment from the same laboratory, Foster and colleagues (1987) did find a small but significant increase in firing in their population of complex-spike cells to both conditioned stimuli but still no differential activity to the CS$^+$. A more detailed look at the differential response that did occur in the theta cell group revealed that the difference in response to the two stimuli was due to an initial increase in firing to both stimuli, which peaked at about 80 to 100 ms after tone onset and was then maintained throughout the 1-second tone period to the CS$^+$ but fell back to baseline in response to the CS$^-$.

The simplest explanation for the pattern of results observed in these studies is that there are two independent factors operating during conditioning: arousal and preparation for the motor response. Both contribute to the firing of theta cells, but only one of them, arousal, influences the

pyramidal cells. The initial short-latency response of hippocampal interneurons and granule cells to either a CS$^+$ or a CS$^-$ is presumably activation reflecting an arousal input from the brain stem; at about the same time, a small percentage of pyramidal cells, in some studies, also show an arousal response. Depending on the stage and type of training, this can either be an inhibitory or a weak excitatory response. The later phase (> 200 ms after CS onset) of the unit activity is related to the behavioral response. For the theta and granule cells there is prolonged activation continuing throughout the CS$^+$ period but no such response to the CS$^-$. The pyramidal cells do not participate in this second longer-latency phase.

Eichenbaum and his colleagues have studied the behavioral correlates of hippocampal cells in various olfactory recognition and discrimination tasks. They recorded two major behavioral correlates: Some cells fired when the animal sniffed at the odor cues, whereas others changed their firing rates during various stages of the approach to the cues or to the goal. In a successive go/no-go discrimination task (Eichenbaum et al., 1987), the rat was presented with one odor of a pair and had to poke its nose into the single-odor port in response to the CS⁺ but not to the CS⁻. Water reward was available on the other side of the testing box, requiring the animal to shuttle continuously between opposite sides of the box. Three behavioral correlates of unit response were identified: cells that fired when the animal was sniffing at the odor ("cue sampling" 15%); cells that fired when the animal approached the sniff port or ran from the sniff port to the water cup at the other end of the box ("reward/port approach" 60%) (Fig. 11–20A); and theta cells (10%). Many of the cue sampling units had firing patterns that were maximally synchronized to the onset of cue sniffing. No evidence was found for cells that preferred one odor over others. Almost all cue sampling cells fired more to the positive stimulus that signaled the availability of water reward in another part of the environment. In addition, there was evidence that in the trials that followed a CS⁻ trial the cells gave a larger response than in those that followed a CS⁺. A follow-up study (Otto and Eichenbaum, 1992) looked at complex-spike cell firing during a continuous recognition olfactory memory task in which any one of 32 odors could be presented, and the availability of

water nearby was signaled by a mismatch between the current and previous stimulus. Again, cells that had peak firing rates at different points in the task were found, including 12% that peaked during the cue sampling period. Somewhat disappointingly however, only eight cells (3%) had firing patterns that could be unambiguously classified as signaling a mismatch between successive stimuli. As we shall see below in the section on primate studies of delayed nonmatch to sample, there are also very few cells in these studies that responded selectively to the familiarity or unfamiliarity of a stimulus.

In a forced-choice discrimination trial, Wiener and colleagues (1989) used simultaneous rather than successive odor discrimination. Both the CS⁺ and CS⁻ were presented at the same time from two adjacent odor ports. In total, 22% of complex-spike cells had increased activity during cue sampling (Fig. 11–20A, center panel). However, closer examination of these data showed that only 13% of cue-sampling cells discriminated between odors irrespective of location, and 44% took the stimulus location into account. Figure 11–20B

Figure 11–20. Hippocampal cell firing correlates with various aspects of an odor discrimination task. *A.* Firing rate histograms of cells that fired best when the animal approached the odor sampling port (top trace), sniffed at the odors (middle trace), and approached the reward cup (bottom trace). Arrows in the top two traces indicate initiation of the behavior; arrow in the bottom trace indicates a nose-poke into the reward cup. *B.* Firing pattern of an odor/spatial

cell that responded maximally when the animal sniffed at a particular odor (odor 1) on the left side of the odor sampling port and a second (different) odor (odor 2) on the right side. Top trace: best response to odor 1 on the left and odor 2 on the right; second trace: same odors from the opposite ports gives a lower response; third and fourth traces: different odors are also less effective. Dotted line marks initiation of the trials. (*Source:* Wiener et al., 1989.)

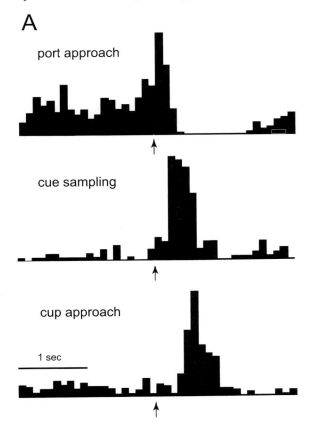

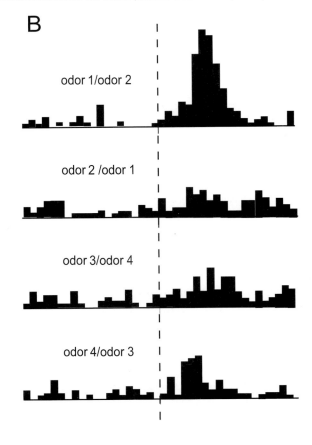

shows an example of a cell that had a strong spatial component. It fired best to a particular odor pair when one was presented on the left and the other on the right. Somewhat more surprising, 44% of cup-approach cells signaling approach to the reward cup on the opposite side of the box also had responses that depended on the position of the prior nose poke or the odor/position interaction. It is difficult to interpret these data, but one possibility is that the rats may have been turning in different directions away from the odor port as they headed toward the reward. If this is true, the cup approach response in this ostensibly nonspatial task may depend on whether the animal turns toward the left or right on its exit from the sniff port and thus passes through a place field on one side of the sniff port as it turns in one direction but not in the other. Alternatively, this may be an example of the dependence of some place cells firing on the prior turn taken by the animal before entry to the place field (see Section 11.7.3). One can conclude that a small number of complex-spike cells respond to the CS$^+$ in a differential go/no-go discrimination but that, in general, few hippocampal cells code for the specific odor quality, and that many cells take the location of the odor into account.

On the basis of these and other results (see Chapter 13), Eichenbaum and his colleagues proposed that the hippocampus stores information about a wide range of relations, both nonspatial and spatial. Unit responses to odors and approaches to the odor port or reward dispenser might be taken as evidence of nonspatial representations and unit responses signaling the identity between two successive stimuli as evidence of one type of nonspatial relationship: the identity relation between two stimuli experienced at different times.

As described earlier in the chapter (see Section 11.7.1), many place cells fire more when the animal sniffs at a location when the stimulus in that location has been altered in some way, and these results from odor discrimination paradigms may provide additional information about the conditions under which this mismatch response occurs. To identify cell responses as being due to the odor cue independently of its location, it is necessary to present the same odor in two or more locations. The demonstration that place fields can be rather large, encompassing a large part of the testing box (see Section 11.7.2), means that it may be necessary to test the same odors in two different laboratories as well as in two testing boxes in the same laboratory before concluding that hippocampal cells do not have a spatial correlate. Similarly, the cells that fire selectively during port approach and cup approach have much in common with place cells recorded on linear tracks. Recall that under conditions that constrain the animal to move along narrow pathways, the place cells are unidirectional. To distinguish a goal-oriented response from a motivationally neutral place response, it is necessary to have two identical goals in the environment or two different goals that can be interchanged. O'Keefe (1976) reported that interchanging the water and food at the end of a three-arm maze did not change the location of complex-spike firing fields on

the maze. O'Keefe and Recce (1993) used a linear track with identical food reward at both ends and found that some cells fire in one direction and other cells fired in the opposite direction. Even if one were tempted to describe these cells as goal approach cells, it is not the approach to the food or the food container per se that is being signaled but their locations at different ends of the track. It does not seem warranted to describe the cells reported in the experiments of Eichenbaum and colleagues as cue-sampling or goal-approach cells in the absence of similiar manipulations.

Two experiments have provided evidence about the efficacy of cues and goals in isolation from their location (Wiebe and Staubli, 1999; Wood et al., 1999). Wood et al. recorded from hippocampal cells during a variant of a continuous olfactory recognition task in which they tried to dissociate location, odor, and the match/mismatch aspects of the task. Rats were trained on an open platform to approach a small cup containing sand scented with one of nine odors. In each trial the cup was placed in one of nine locations. If a cup had an odor different from that of the previous one, it contained food for which the animal could dig (nonmatch); if the odor was the same, there was no food (match), and digging went unrewarded. Cells were recorded during the 1 second prior to arrival at each cup. An analysis of variance showed that of the total 127 cells, 8% responded to odor in the absence of any other correlate, 11% solely to location, and 10% solely to the match/mismatch aspect of the task. The remainder of the responsive cells took interactions between these variables into account. In all, 20% of cells had nonspatial correlates, and 32% took location into account. (Another 20% changed their firing rate as the animal approached any of the cups. The latter may simply be movement- or speed-related—because this was not measured, it is not discussed further.) These results are notable as a higher percentage of cells with a match/mismatch correlate irrespective of location was found than in the previous reports from the same laboratory (see above). Furthermore, there are fewer purely spatially coded cells than are usually found. This may be because the experimental design required the animal to approach each cup from a different angle during different trials and therefore via different locations; this might lead to a significant underestimation of the number of place cells. Approaching a cup from the north would not force the animal to cross the same region of space as approaching the same cups from the south. It is also not clear how much of the difference between cellular match and nonmatch responses can be attributed to the different behaviors of digging and turning away from the cup that were used as the response measures, rather than the relational judgment itself. Nevertheless, taken at face value, these results provide evidence for the more general relational theory. Significantly, this task has been shown by the authors of the Wood et al. study themselves (Dudchenko et al., 2000) not to be disrupted by selective hippocampal damage.

Wiebe and Straubli (1999) used a Y maze task that forced the animal to traverse the same locations on the approaches to the goals and came to a conclusion different from that of

Wood and colleagues. Animals were trained on a delayed non-match-to-sample odor task with each trial comprised of three discrete periods: a sampling period during which the animal sniffed one of two odors in the start arm, a delay period during which it was confined to the start arm and had to remember the recently smelled odor, and a test period during which it was required to choose one of the other two arms containing the odor it had not recently experienced. During the first two periods, everything happened within the same arm, and cellular activity could be correlated only with the odor presented on that trial and with subsequent correct or incorrect performance on the choice part of the trial. During the third (test) period the animal could enter one of two goal arms, and therefore a correlation with location as well as odor and performance could be sought. Overall, most of the 1101 cells recorded from the dentate gyrus, CA3, and CA1 had significant correlations with one or more aspects of the task. Some of the results are shown in Table 11–1. Several conclusions can be drawn from these results. First, during the sample phase, which always took place in the same arm and therefore did not allow the contribution of location to be examined, a small percentage of cells had significant changes in firing rate to the specific odor presented (5%), to whether the subsequent choice would be correct or incorrect (2%), or to the interaction between two (4%). None of these firing rate changes, however, carried over into the delay phase of the trial (Table 11–1, delay) suggesting that the hippocampus does not maintain an active trace of the correct odor choice, as it does of location in a comparable spatial memory task (O'Keefe and Speakman, 1987). Second, in marked contrast to what was seen in the sample phase, during the test phase only a tiny percentage of cells fired to the odor, to the correctness of the choice, or to the interaction between them (all < 1%). This represents a large discrepancy with the odor and performance correlates found in the sample arm. Third, in contrast to the

weak representation of odor or performance in the test arms, there was a strong representation of the animal's location. Of the 571 cells with behavioral correlates in the test arms either alone or as an interaction with another correlate, 70% had a spatial correlate, whereas only 27% had an odor correlate and 21% a performance correlate. More significantly, 37% of the cells with spatial correlates were pure place cells with no other correlates, whereas most of the cells with olfactory and performance correlates also had spatial correlates (92% and 93%, respectively). It is difficult to escape the conclusion that when the testing situation allows them to be identified spatial responses predominate either as pure place responses or as place combined with some other aspect of the task, even in tasks where the spatial component is irrelevant to the solution.

A potential criticism of the Wiebe and Straubli experiment is that they only used two odors, but there might be more than one location in each of the test arms. This points up an important methodological problem in these studies. To equate two tasks on the number of odors and locations, it is important to have an accurate measure of these items. It might be thought, for example, that the number of place fields in each arm of the maze is greater than the number of odors, but the odors used in the tasks are typically compounds and may be distinguished on the basis of many different elemental aspects of the compound. In the absence of more information about the elemental components of locations and smells in any given task, the best one can do is try to vary each variable systematically to see what effect it has on the results.

11.11.7 Comparison of Hippocampal Cells During Operant Conditioning and Place Tasks in Rats

Are the neurons that show place responses the same as those that take part in nonspatial learning tasks conditioning, or are there two separate populations of cells? Several studies have compared the response of the same hippocampal neurons during place tasks and conditioning tasks. Three studies have asked whether complex-spike cells might be specifically involved in the place task and the theta cells might be specifically involved in the conditioning tasks. Christian and Deadwyler (1986) used antidromical stimulation of projection pathways to identify complex-spike cells as pyramidal cells. They found a clear double dissociation of the cells involved in the two tasks. In total, 81% of complex-spike cells had place fields in the place task in comparison with none of the theta cells. Conversely, 81% of the theta cells participated in the conditioning task whereas none of the complex-spike cells did. In two experiments, Eichenbaum and his colleagues (Eichenbaum et al., 1987; Wiener et al., 1989) asked whether cells that were related to events in their olfactory discrimination task also had place fields in the same or different tasks. In the first study, they found that 43% of cells with correlates in the odor discrimination task had place fields in the same

Table 11–1.
Percentages of Total Number of Recorded Cells with Significant Correlates to Various Aspects of an Olfactory Delayed Nonmatch-to-Sample Task

Parameter	Sample phase (%)	Delay phase (%)	Test phase phase (%)
Odor	4.8	0	0.9
Performance	2.1	0	0.6
Odor × performance	4.3	0	0.2
Position	–		26.8
Position × odor	–		8.4
Position × performance	–		5.6
Position × odor × performance	–		4.5
Position exclusively	–		13.5
Odor exclusively	2.4		0.8
Performance exclusively	2.1		0.4

After Wiebe & Staubli, 1999.

environment; in the second study, they recorded some complex-spike cells in a spatial task, some in the odor discrimination task, and a third group in both tasks. They found 75% of the complex-spike cells had place fields in the spatial task compared to 58% with correlations in the odor discrimination task. Of cells collected in both tasks, 85% had place fields in contrast to 54% that had correlates in the odor task.

We can conclude that in conditioning tasks involving rats that were not required to move around the environment to any great extent, most or all hippocampal cells taking part in the conditioning response were theta cells. Complex-spike cells, by contrast, either did not take part or showed slight inhibition of their resting firing rate. In discrimination conditioning tasks in which the animal is required to move, the complex-spike cells also become engaged. The clearest example of cells that may not have a spatial correlate are the cue-sampling cells reported in the Eichenbaum studies. However, even some of these responses may be covert place responses, as clearly suggested by the Wiebe and Straubli experiments.

11.11.8 Hippocampal Units During Nonspatial Learning in Nonhuman Primates

Tamura et al. (1991) reported that 10% of cells in the hippocampal formation responded differentially to the presentation of three-dimensional objects, some of which had been conditioned to rewarding (3%) or aversive (2%) stimuli. In a follow-up study (Tamura et al., 1992), they showed that 61% of object-responsive cells tested in the same apparatus varied their response as a function of the location of the stimulus in egocentric or allocentric space. The latter study indicates that apparently perceptual responses in the hippocampus may be spatially modulated. Such responses may underlie object-in-place associativity, which like odor-place associativity, is often shown to be hippocampus-dependent, unlike odor-object associativity, which is hippocampus-independent (Gilbert and Kesner, 2002).

Hippocampal units have been recorded from primates while they performed in one of the paradigmatic relational tasks: delayed match or non-match-to-sample. On these tasks, the animal must signal whether two successive stimuli separated by an interval are the same or different. It is now widely accepted that these tasks can be solved in two ways. The animal can either assess the strength of the familiarity of the two stimuli presented during the test phase and choose the least familiar, or it can remember which stimulus was previously presented in the present situation or context and choose the one it has not experienced there before. The second strategy is clearly both spatial and relational, but it could be argued that the first strategy is also relational although clearly nonspatial. To judge a stimulus as familiar or novel, it is necessary to compare it to the representation of a previous stimulus and to decide whether the relation between the two is one of equality. Recognition tasks of this sort were originally thought to depend on the integrity of the hippocampus but are now known to depend on the perirhinal/parahippocampal cortices and only minimally (Alvarez et al., 1995) or not at all (Murray and Mishkin, 1998) on the hippocampus itself (see Chapter 13) (Aggleton and Brown, 1999). In keeping with the lesion results, it has been found that only a small number of cells show a differential response to the familiarity of the stimuli (0%–2.3% in various studies (Riches et al., 1991; Tamura et al., 1992; Rolls et al., 1993; Salzmann et al., 1993; Brown and Xiang, 1998). In contrast, Wilson et al. (1990) found that 40% of their hippocampal cells in this task correlated with the response, signaling whether the animal was reaching to the left or right position during their task. Salzmann and Creutzfeldt (Salzmann et al., 1993) reported that 28% of hippocampal and 33% of parahippocampal neurons responded to both presentations of the visual stimuli in a delayed match-to-sample task but that even more cells (38% in each area) fired when the animal was presented with a raisin. Vidyasagar and Creutzfeldt (Vidyasagar et al., 1991) reported similar results but that arousing events such as the cage door being opened or closed or the experimenter entering or leaving the room also produced a response in these cells. On the basis of these findings, they attributed hippocampal single-unit activity to the animal's behavioral state rather than to any specific memory. These studies provide no evidence for the representation of stimulus familiarity in the hippocampus.

In contrast and in keeping with the lesion results, there is evidence that cells in the rhinal cortex are involved in familiarity judgments. Brown and colleagues (Brown and Xiang, 1998) reported that about one-fourth of cells in the rhinal cortex and area TE showed a decreased response to the second presentation of the stimulus in a delayed match-to-sample task.

Rolls and his colleagues (Rolls et al., 1993) have tested monkeys on object recognition tasks and compared unit responses to object familiarity with those to object location. Only a small percentage (2%) of cells responded to familiar objects (see above). In contrast, they reported that about 9% of cells in the hippocampal region responded differentially to the location of the stimulus on a display screen. As part of a study of the place properties of primate hippocampal neurons, Ono and his colleagues (1993) found that 17% of cells responded to objects such as a moving experimenter or apple when presented in a particular part of the visual field. Just over half of these were object-in-place cells, which responded differentially when the animal was shown the object in a particular location and not in other locations. They appear to have properties similar to those of the misplace cells described in the rat (O'Keefe, 1976).

11.11.9 Hippocampal Units During Nonspatial Learning in Humans

Single units have been recorded from medial temporal lobe regions in patients with intractable epilepsy during both recognition and recall memory tasks (Heit et al., 1988; Fried et al., 1997, 2002; Cameron et al., 2001) as well as during the perceptual categorization tasks described in Section 11.11.1. In general, a sizable percentage of hippocampal units was found to participate in both types of memory task. In a recognition memory task, Fried and colleagues (2002) presented a set of male and female faces portraying various emotions; and after an interval of 1 to 12 hours they showed the same faces again together with an equal number of foils. A significant number of hippocampal neurons responded to faces during encoding (25%) and a somewhat larger percentage during the recognition phase (41%). Perhaps surprisingly, a large proportion of the hippocampal responses (62%) consisted of firing rate decreases. Almost one-half the hippocampal neurons with an excitatory response but only one-sixth of those with an inhibitory response showed some selectivity for gender or emotion. Similar findings were reported by Heit and colleagues (1988), who used lists of words to be remembered and found most hippocampal units selective for one of the words on the list. When tested with a second list of different words, slightly less than half of these cells (13/30) were also selective for a word in that list. As the authors remarked, this suggests that rather than being preordained to respond to specific stimuli the cells were tuning into the current context and selecting one aspect of it (such as position along a list?). The result is reminiscent of the way in which a given pyramidal cell in the rat hippocampus may have unrelated place fields in two or more environments. Hippocampal units have also been recorded during a paired-associate recall task (Cameron et al., 2001). A series of word pairs were presented, and after 1 to 2 minutes the subject had to respond with the second of the pair when prompted with the first: 29% of hippocampal units responded during stimulus encoding and 44% during recall. These percentages are similar to those found in the entorhinal cortex and amygdala in the same study and in the face recognition study of Fried et al. (2002) but significantly higher than the response to faces and other nonspatial visual stimuli in the perceptual classification study of Kreiman et al., 2000a), suggesting a specific role for learning. An interesting aspect of the study was that one-fifth of the hippocampal cells showed a differential firing rate during encoding between word pairs that were subsequently remembered correctly and those that were forgotten. Most intriguingly, most of these cells showed a *smaller* increase in firing rate to the word pairs that were subsequently remembered than to the ones that were forgotten. Whatever the role being played by the hippocampus in these tasks, it cannot simply be that increased firing in hippocampal neurons during encoding leads to a stronger memory trace and therefore to better recall.

Although one must be cautious when comparing across studies, even from the same laboratory, the results can be summarized as follows. (1) The percentage of cells responding to faces and words is higher when they are part of a memory task than when they are simply perceived; (2) these stimuli are equally well represented in both recognition and recall memory tasks; and finally (3) the response of hippocampal units to a stimulus during the encoding phase of a recall test correlates with subsequent recall of that stimulus but in a counterintuitive fashion. The cells increase firing to both remembered and forgotten stimuli but the increase is smaller to the subsequently remembered stimuli than to those forgotten.

11.11.10 Conclusions

In all species tested, a small percentage of hippocampal cells have been reported to fire to nonspatial stimuli. The data are clearest in humans, where about 12% of cells responded to the sight of famous faces, but this fell well below the proportion (29%) that responded to spatial stimuli such as pictures of houses or interiors. Hippocampal unit responses to stimuli used as discriminanda in learning experiments have been reported in all species tested: rats, rabbits, monkeys, and humans. There is some suggestion that the responses in the rat may be due to a place-gated mechanism because the one study that tested this carefully found that the conditioned stimuli only elicited a pyramidal cell response after conditioning if it was presented while the animal was in the place field of the cell (Moita et al., 2003). Theta cells are much less sensitive to location and may account for a large percentage of the responses reported in the early studies, which did not distinguish between cell types. In general, monkey experiments reported few cells responding to objects per se but more to location or object-in-places. In keeping with the lesion results (see Chapter 13), units responding to objects and their familiarity were more plentiful in the rhinal cortex than in the hippocampus.

There are clearly cells in the human medial temporal lobe that respond to words as well as faces and other stimuli in both recognition and recall paradigms. Furthermore, in one study of verbal paired associate learning, hippocampal unit responses during encoding of a pair predicted the success of subsequent recall (Cameron et al., 2001). Somewhat surprisingly, there was only a hint of lateralization of these responses to the left hemisphere, as might be expected from the lesion data. It is clear that the human hippocampus is involved in the storage of verbal as well as nonverbal material.

In general then, there is evidence that nonspatial information is represented in the hippocampus but that the number of cells involved is considerably smaller than those involved in spatial information and often the nonspatial responses are secondary to a primary spatial correlate. The larger percentage of responses to nonspatial stimuli reported in humans is consonant with the wider function attributed to the human hippocampus in narrative and episodic memory (O'Keefe and Nadel, 1978; O'Keefe, 1996, 2001; Burgess et al., 2002).

11.12 Other Distinctive Cells in the Hippocampal Formation and Related Areas

As we have seen, the hippocampal formation is part of a widespread system of anatomically related regions involved in memory and navigation. In addition to the CA fields and the dentate gyrus, the hippocampal formation contains two anatomically distinct regions: the subicular complex and the parahippocampal cortex. Response properties of cells in some of these other regions have been touched on at different points in this chapter where appropriate. For example in Sections 11.9 and 11.10, we summarized the properties of head-direction (HD) cells found in the presubiculum and, in addition, regions of the Papez circuit, which forms the inputs to these cells. In this section, we briefly summarize the properties of cells in some of these other related brain regions and touch upon the question of whether these cells are afferent to the hippocampal formation, providing spatial information, or alternately should be thought of as efferent output structures, receiving spatial and memory information from the hippocampal formation.

There are three ways this question might be approached. The first is to look at the effects of lesions elsewhere in the circuit on hippocampal place cell firing (Brun et al., 2002; Calton et al., 2003) and presubicular HD cell firing (Golob and Taube, 1997) as described in Sections 11.7.4 and 11.9/11.10, respectively. The second examines the relative latency of the neurons in each area to respond to the stimulus or behavior under study. This approach depends on the assumption that neurons in a region that projects to a second region in a serial fashion, on average, fire earlier in response to the appropriate stimulus or during the relevant behavior than the neurons in that second region. On the assumption that many cells in the hippocampal formation and related areas have spatial aspects of behavior as their primary correlate, it is possible to compare the temporal correlation of cells in different hippocampal regions in response to manipulations of these spatial variables to estimate the temporal relation between cells in different regions indirectly. For example, one might study the latency to onset of firing of HD cells with the same preferred orientation in different parts of the Papez circuit. Ideally, this ought to be done with simultaneous recording from the two (or more) regions in question to control for variations between rats in behavior and location of the tracking lights on the head. The third method is based on a comparison of the place correlates of the neurons in the two areas. If one has a serial model of place field construction, it might be possible to attribute some neuronal responses to earlier stages in that process than others. For example, Barnes and colleagues (1990) compared the field sizes of place cells in different regions of the hippocampal formation and subiculum. As we shall see, some generalizations arise from this third type of analysis. The locational code in the CA fields of the hippocampus is more environment-specific than in other regions. Hippocampal place cells often fire in distinct patterns in different environments ("remapping"); indeed, many hippocampal cells are or become silent in a given environment (see Section 11.7.4). By contrast, the locational region(s) signaled by nonhippocampal cells are much more likely to be in similar places across dissimilar environments. Moreover, in other regions, such as the subiculum and superficial entorhinal cortex, principal cells are never silent.

Taking the results of all three methods into account, it is difficult but not impossible to make suggestions about the functional circuit diagram of the interconnections between these regions of the hippocampal formation that underlies spatial behavior and memory.

11.12.1 Subicular Region Has Fewer Place Cells than the Hippocampus Proper, and Their Properties Differ

Place cells and theta cells have been recorded from several subdivisions of the subicular region. We consider the similarities and differences between cells in the next sections. The subiculum contains both place cells and theta cells (Sharp and Green, 1994; Sharp, 1997). The percentage of theta cells is approximately the same as found in the hippocampus proper (10%), and most of the remaining cells have strong spatial signals. There are no complex-spike cells, but one group (29% of total) shows a bursting pattern with a peak interspike interval of 2 to 4 ms. These cells do not seem to differ in any other respect from the nonbursting types except that they have a stronger theta modulation. The field sizes and average firing rates of the subicular place cells are much larger when compared to those in the hippocampus. A typical subicular cell fires over the entire environment with an average rate of 5 to 15 Hz (in contrast to 0.5–2.5 Hz in the hippocampus) and has one or more areas of increased firing. Like the place cells of the hippocampus, subicular place cells recorded in a cylinder are under the influence of a cue card on the wall and rotate in step with it. It has been claimed that the subicular cells have a stronger directional component than the hippocampal cells, but this claim must be treated with caution. The amount of variance in subicular firing rate that is explained by direction is actually very small (Sharp and Green, 1994).

One important difference from hippocampal place cells is that subicular cells are far less likely to remap across environments that differ in shape (Sharp and Green, 1994), shape and visual markings (Sharp, 1997), or size (Sharp, 1999b). For instance, whereas many of the hippocampal cells displayed markedly different fields in a cyclinder and a rectangle, the subicular fields were similar in the two environments. This is reminiscent of what is found in the spatially coded cells in the superficial layers of the entorhinal cortex (see below) and to hippocampal place cells during the animal's initial experiences of the two (see Section 11.8.3). A study of the timing of subicular cell firing relative to the animal's location suggests that subicular cells fire slightly earlier on average than CA1 cells (70 vs. 40 ms), perhaps indicating that they come earlier in the computational chain (Sharp, 1999a). This result may seem paradoxical in light of the strong connections from CA1 to the subiculum, but it is consistent with the data showing that subicular cells do not remap the environments that CA1 cells do.

In conclusion, various approaches to the functional relation between the subiculum and the hippocampus proper suggest that the subicular place cells cannot receive their spatial properties solely by virtue of their inputs from the hippocampus proper. They may be more dependent on direct inputs from the entorhinal cortex and/or they themselves may provide a source of spatial inputs to the entorhinal cells.

11.12.2 Presubiculum Contains Several Classes of Spatial Cell

The dorsal presubiculum (or postsubiculum in some authors' terminology) contains other types of spatial cell in addition to the HD cells described above (see Section 11.9). A survey study (Sharp, 1996) of presubicular cells in the standard cylinder also reported cells with correlates for angular velocity, running speed (see also Lever et al., 2003), location and direction, and location. The nature of these correlates suggests an important role for the presubiculum in navigation and spatial memory. One class of these cells, called theta-modulated place-by-direction (TPD) cells, has been examined in detail (Cacucci et al., 2004) (Fig. 11–21B, see color insert). TPD cells generally have a strong tendency to fire at or just before the trough of the local theta oscillation. Their depth of theta modulation is high and comparable to that of cells in the medial septum/diagonal band of Broca (King et al., 1998). The quantitative analyses of Cacucci et al. indicate that both loca-

tional and directional signals are stable and robust in TPD cells, with the directional signal carrying more information. The directional and locational signals are dissociable in different environments. The preferred direction of a given TPD cell appears to be environment-invariant, being similar across different locations in the testing room (like the HD cells) and across different enclosures in the same location (cylinder versus an open circular platform). In contrast, the locational fields tend to differ more between environments; notably, TPD cells generally have different locational fields in the cylinder and open circular platform. TPD cell firing represents an integration of location-related and direction-related information. It is possible that directional information may have to be incorporated into and distributed in theta wave packets to be used by the navigation system. Neither anterodorsal thalamic nor presubicular HD cells show theta modulation. Cacucci et al. provided evidence that a robust orientation signal operating in theta mode exists in the hippocampal formation.

There have been no published reports of cells recorded from the ventral portions of either the presubiculum or the parasubiculum. By analogy with the differences between dor-

Figure 11–21. Four spatial cell types in the hippocampal formation. False color firing field maps (left) show the firing rate as a function of the animal's location in cylindrical environments irrespective of heading direction; directional polar plots (right) show the firing rate for the same cell as a function of the animal's heading direction irrespective of location. *A.* Place cell has single localized field and no directional selectivity. *B.* Place by directional cell has single localized field and strong directional selectivity. *C.* Head direction cell does not have localized firing but has strong directional selectivity. (*Source: A–C.* Courtesy of Francesca Cacucci.) *D.* Grid cell has multiple place fields and no directional selectivity. Directional grid cells also exist. Numbers associated with the firing rate plots represent the maximum firing rate (red regions in firing rate maps and peak x and y values in polar plots). Diameter of cylinders in *A–C* is 79 cm; diameter in *D* is 2 m. (*Source:* Edvard and May-Britt Moser.)

A. Place Cell

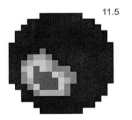 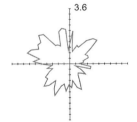

B. Place by Direction Cell

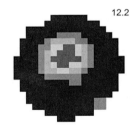 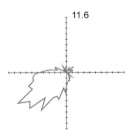

C. Head Direction Cell

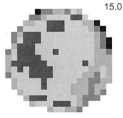 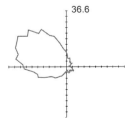

D. Grid Cell

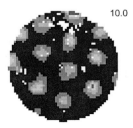 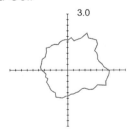

sal and ventral hippocampus (Jung et al., 1994), these ventral regions might be expected to contain lower levels of spatial signaling and/or larger spatial fields.

11.12.3 Parasubiculum

The parasubiculum contains location-specific neurons, although in much lower percentages (ca. 10%) than are found in the hippocampus proper or the subiculum (Taube, 1995b). In contrast, it contains a much higher percentage of theta cells (41%). No complex-spike cells have been found there. In comparison with the hippocampus, the firing fields of the parasubicular place cells are significantly larger and have less spatial information content. In common with all place and HD cells recorded thus far, their place fields rotate in step with the rotation of the cue card on the wall of the environment. Analysis of the temporal relations of the firing fields of these cells to the animal's location showed a variety of relations, but on average the cell firing preceded the animal's location by about 60 ms. This is less than the average of about 120 ms for hippocampal cells, suggesting that the parasubicular neurons may be later in the circuit than the hippocampal cells.

11.12.4 Spatial Cells in the Entorhinal Cortex

Quirk and colleagues (1992) recorded from cells in layers 2 and 3 of the medial entorhinal cortex under conditions similar to those in which hippocampal place cells have been recorded (Muller et al., 1987). They found both place-coded and theta cells. Two properties of the spatial cells were different from those displayed by the hippocampal place cells but similar to those found in the subiculum. The entorhinal cortex (EC) fields were larger and less spatially compact; and unlike the hippocampal cells but like the subicular cells, they showed less sensitivity to the shape of the enclosure. Whereas many of the hipppocampal place cells displayed markedly different fields in the cylinder and the square, the EC cell fields were similar in the two environments. Unlike the hippocampus, where this similarity between fields in the two boxes occurs only during the initial experience of the environments, the EC cells appear not to learn to discriminate. As we saw earlier (Mizumori et al., 1992; Jeffery et al., 1995), the theta cells in the EC are dependent on the integrity of the medial septum in the same way as the hippocampal theta cells.

As discussed in Section 11.7, work by Fynn, Hafting, and colleagues (Fyhn et al., 2004; Hafting et al., 2005) suggests that at least one class of cells in the superficial layers of the medial entorhinal cortex lays a grid-like structure on every environment the animal visits. Each grid cell fires in several locations in each environment, with the locations forming a regular pattern as though they were nodes on a triangular grid (see Figs 11–10 and 11–21D, see color insert). Different cells recorded at the same location have the same grid spacing and orientation relative to the environment but differ in the location of the nodes, such that the firing peaks of one cell are slightly shifted from those of its neighbor. The result is that the overall set of fields of several such cells covers the entire environment. For each cell, the size of the grid appears to be independent of the size or shape of the environment. As one goes more ventral in the medial entorhinal cortex, the size of the grid gets larger. This grid system appears to be based on path integration inputs generated by the animal's own movements and may provide the hippocampal mapping system with distance and directional information on which to construct maps of individual environments.

Frank and colleagues (2000) recorded from neurons in the hippocampus proper and in the superficial and deep layers of the entorhinal cortex while rats ran along single or double U-shaped tracks (the latter termed W-shaped tracks). On the single U-shaped track, the animal shuttled back and forth between the two prongs of the U to receive rewards at each end; on the W track it shuttled first between the left-hand and middle prongs and then between the middle and right-hand ones and vice-versa. Similar to the findings of Quirk et al. (see above), they found that: (1) EC cells fire at rates about five times those of CA1 cells; (2) the locational fields of cells in both the superficial and deep layers of the entorhinal cortex were larger (by about three times) and contained less locational information than those in CA1. Deep EC cells contained more locational information than superficial EC cells. Some cells in all three regions were sensitive to the place from which the animals had recently come (retrospective coding) or to which they were intending to go (prospective coding) (cf. Section 11.7.3 for a discusssion of retrospective and prospective coding in hippocampal cells). However, the deep entorhinal cortex contained a significantly higher proportion of prospectively coding cells than the CA1 or the superficial entorhinal cortex. Cells in the deep entorhinal layers were also more likely to reflect environment-invariant aspects of the paths taken along these tracks. For instance, one deep EC cell fired on both the U and W tracks as the animal ran away from a prong and turned left into the adjacent arm. These findings suggest that the deeper layers of the entorhinal cortex, which receive strong inputs from the CA1 field and the subiculum, may be using spatial information provided by these regions to construct routes between known locations. Alternatively, the results may be related to the regular field structure of grid cells reported by Hafting and colleagues (see above).

11.12.5 Cells in the Perirhinal Cortex Code for the Familiarity of Stimuli

Cells in the perirhinal cortex of the monkey and rat (Brown et al., 1987) are sensitive to the familiarity of the stimulus. The amplitude of the cell's response to the second and subsequent repetitions of an object is smaller than that to the first presentation, and this decreased response recovers as a function of the time and number of intervening items since the previous exposure to that stimulus. This fits with the suggestion that the deficit in delayed non-match-to-sample in the monkey or human following large lesions in the mesial temporal lobes is due primarily to the involvement of these rhinal structures

(Brown and Aggleton, 2001) (see Section 11.11.8 and Chapter 13 for further discussion).

11.12.6 Cells in the Medial Septum Are Theta Cells

Cholinergic and GABAergic cells in the medial septum and diagonal band of Broca (DBB) supply the driving inputs that set the frequency of hippocampal theta. As we saw in Section 11.3.3, lesions of this region abolish hippocampal theta. Ranck (1973) recorded from cells in the medial septum of freely moving rats and confirmed earlier reports by Petsche and Stumpf that cells there had a rhythmical bursting pattern that was phase-locked to hippocampal theta. About 50% of the septal cells showed this pattern. Attempts have been made to classify septal cells into those likely to be cholinergic or GABAergic on the basis of their waveform (Matthews and Lee, 1991; King et al., 1998). Cells have also been classified on the basis of the strength of their correlation to the hippocampus theta. In one study (King et al., 1998) , 47% showed a strong phase relation to the hippocampal theta with strong peaks in the auto-correlation at the theta period. Each cell had its own individual preferred phase, which was constant over days. The rest of the septal cells show weaker relations to theta. There is, however, only a slight preference for a particular phase across the whole population with all phases represented. Putative cholinergic cells (on the basis of wave shape) tended to be concentrated in the less rhythmical class than putative GABAergic cells. On the other hand, GABAergic medial septal neurons, which selectively target hippocampal interneurons, appear to form two distinct populations tightly coupled either to the trough (178°) or the peak (330°) of hippocampal theta waves (Borhegyi et al., 2004).

As we saw in Section 11.3.4 on the theta rhythms and the EEG, there is some evidence that the frequency of theta is correlated with the speed with which an animal moves in an environment. A similar correlation was found in the rhythmical theta cells of the septum (King et al., 1998). Rhythmical cells showed a burst frequency that was correlated with the speed of movement on a linear track. The slope of the regression linear curve was about 0.9 Hz/m/s with an intercept at 8.4 Hz. A small number of rhythmical septal cells had an interesting directional response. They fired with a strong rhythmicity when the animal ran in one direction but lost their rhythmicity when it ran in other directions.

11.12.7 Summary of Extrahippocampal Place Field Properties

The firing of extrahippocampal cells tends to be more environment-invariant than hippocampal place cell firing, generalizing across the various environments explored and routes taken. Thus, cells in the subiculum and entorhinal cortex may signal broadly equivalent locations, or similar points along a route, in different environments. Whereas extrahippocampal cells generalize, hippocampal place cells basically discriminate (especially after experience). This is revealed at the population level: In any single environment, half or more of the cells in the hippocampus proper are silent. Outside the hippocampus proper, principal cells are generally not silent and indeed tend to fire at higher rates than hippocampal place cells. Further study is required to disentangle the particular role played by each of the regions in the hippocampal formation.

Relative to hippocampal place cells, cells in some neighboring extrahippocampal regions tend to, have larger fields, and are less sensitive to environmental changes such as alterations in the shape of the enclosure. It seems reasonable to suggest that the presubicular HD cells are afferent to the medial EC grid cells, which in turn are afferent to the hippocampal place cells; and the anatomical connections between these regions are consonant with this functional relation. Less clear is the relation between the subiculum and the hippocampus. The greater susceptibility of hippocampal place cells to environmental change and the latency data suggest that the subiculum provides environmental inputs to the hippocampus perhaps in the form of the distance to one or more boundaries; on the other hand, the anatomy suggests a strong projection from the CA1 field to the subiculum that is not reciprocated. The perirhinal and lateral entorhinal cells most likely provide information about environmental landmarks and other objects to the hippocampus where it is integrated with the place information to support behavior based on object-in-place knowledge. The deeper layers and the lateral septum are the major efferent targets of the CA1 and CA3 pyramids, respectively. Little is known about the behavioral correlates of deep layers of the entorhinal cortex and the prefrontal cortex, but they may be the first stages in the transformation of the hippocampal signal into environmentally specific route information or where it is used to program the approach to goal locations. The hippocampal projection to the EC may stabilize the grid cell location relative to a given environment.

11.13 Overall Conclusions

This chapter has focused on the neural correlates of hippocampal EEG and single-unit activity. We found that the EEG could be categorized into several frequency bands: theta, beta, gamma, and the high-frequency ripples. Each of these has a different behavioral correlate and is reflected by different firing patterns in hippocampal interneurons. In rodents, the beta and gamma oscillations relate primarily to olfactory stimuli, but theta and the ripples have much broader correlates. There are two types of theta, which are differentially sensitive to cholinergic drugs: a-Theta is activated during periods of arousal or attention, and t-theta is related to movements (e.g., walking, swimming, jumping) that translate the animal's position relative to the environment. Hippocampal interneurons fire in synchrony with the concurrent theta; and various types of interneuron, targeting different parts of the pyramidal cell, preferentially fire on different phases of theta. One function of theta activity is to coordinate and perhaps bind together neural activity in different parts of the nervous system. Theta-related firing patterns have been found in cells in such disparate regions of the nervous system as the prefrontal cortex, amygdala, and inferior colliculus. Theta also organizes the temporal relation between the firing of cells in the hippocampus such that inputs to a cell at one phase of theta produce larger synaptic modifications (LTP) than at other phases. Finally, each theta cycle acts as a timing cycle against which the phase of hippocampal pyramidal cell firing can be measured. This phase coding complements the locational signal carried in the gross firing rate and allows rate modulations above the baseline to code for variables such as the speed of running in addition to location (see below). Dual phase and firing rate coding may be a general strategy for binding together the representations of different aspects of the world in the train of action potentials of a single cell. The high-frequency ripples occur in conjunction with the large irregular activity (LIA) state of the hippocampal EEG, which occurs during nontranslational activities such as sleeping, quiet resting, grooming, drinking, and eating. Theta and LIA/ripples appear to be mutually exclusive states of the hippocampus, never occurring at the same time. It has been suggested that the synchronized bursts of activity that occur in hippocampal neurons during the ripples may reflect the transfer of information from the hippocampus to the neocortex as part of a memory consolidation process.

Three classes of cells with spatial correlates have been reported in the hippocampal formation: the place cells in the hippocampus itself (Fig. 11–21A, see color insert); the head direction (HD) cells in the dorsal presubiculum (Fig. 11–21C, see color insert); and the grid cells in the medial entorhinal cortex (Fig. 11–21D, see color insert). In addition, there are cells that combine two types of information, such as the "place by direction" cells found in the presubiculum (Fig. 11–21B, see color insert). Place cells signal the animal's location, HD cells signal the animal's direction of heading, and grid cells provide information about distances moved in particular directions. It seems reasonable to assume that the place cell firing patterns are constructed from combinations of grid cell inputs, which in turn get their directional orientation from the head direction input. Together these three cell types provide the information required to construct a mapping system that identifies the animal's location in an environment and relates these locations to each other on the basis of the distance and direction from one to the other. It should also allow the animal to move from one location in that environment to another along any available path, supporting flexible navigation. As we mentioned above, hippocampal pyramidal cells also code for events or stimuli that occur in particular places, laying the basis for the more general episodic memory system seen in the human hippocampus. A true episodic memory system would incorporate the time of occurrence of events as well as their location.

Encoding of events as well as locations in hippocampal pyramidal cells is made possible by a dual coding strategy: Location is conveyed by a combination of increased firing rate above a low-level baseline and the phase of firing relative to the ongoing hippocampal EEG theta activity; events and stimuli occurring in that location are signaled by variations in the firing rate above the baseline. The existence of temporal coding strategies in the nervous system means that one must be cautious when interpreting the results of recording techniques that reflect only relative rates of neural activity in contrast to the timing of action potentials. This is especially true when the representation is distributed across a population of cells with some cells increasing and others decreasing their firing rates in addition to shifting phases.

Several types of learning have been demonstrated in hippocampal pyramidal cells: short-term changes in the orientation of place fields relative to the environment lasting for the duration of the trial; longer changes in the shape of the place field lasting for the duration of the testing session; and long-term discrimination between similar environments that appears to be permanent. One type of environmental discrimination appears to involve the collective behavior of pyramidal cells, perhaps operating as a discrete attractor in which the behavior of neighboring pyramidal cells, in addition to environmental inputs, is taken into account in the final representation.

The location of place fields depends on factors in addition to the animal's physical location in an environment. Under certain circumstances, fields may depend on the animal's previous behavior, such as the turn that it has just made at a choice point or one that it intends to make. Training on aversive tasks such as eyeblink conditioning in the rat has also been shown to shift the location of fields. Whether this means that the animal conceives of these environments as different is not clear at present.

It has also been reported that pyramidal cells respond to nonspatial stimuli such as the odors used in a running recognition task or the auditory cues in a nictitating membrane conditioning task. The existence of such responses together with deficits in some types of conditioning tasks (e.g., trace conditioning following hippocampal lesions) has suggested a broader function for the hippocampus than purely spatial. On the other hand, several studies have suggested that when the locations in which these stimuli occur are varied, these "nonspatial" responses are gated by the animal's location. In a rat eyeblink conditioning experiment, the auditory conditioned stimulus only elicited short latency response in hippocampal cells when the animal was in the place field of that cell. In an olfactory delayed match-to-sample task, cells appeared to respond to the olfactory cues alone when position was not varied in the start arm of a Y maze; in contrast, only olfactory responses gated by position were seen in the two goal arms where position was available as a factor. To rule out position as a contribution to hippocampal unit responses, it is important to provide the stimulus in more than one location.

Studies of single-unit activity in monkey hippocampus suggest that although place responses also dominate there is evidence of nonspatial inputs as well. As primate research moves in the direction of the use of freely moving monkeys, and especially when the animal can explore the walls as well as the floor of the environment, we will begin to get a better picture of the relation between these nonspatial and spatial inputs. There are also a small number of studies of hippocampal unit activity in humans. Units responding to pictures of faces and household objects have been reported, but the percentage of cells responding to pictures of houses and locations in the same studies has been higher. Responses to words have been reported frequently, especially when they are presented in a learning paradigm. This may be an indication that the function of the human hippocampus is broader than purely spatial. This is in line with the original suggestion of the cognitive map theory that the incorporation of verbal and temporal inputs into its original spatial functions would result in employment of the hippocampus as an episodic and narrative memory system as well a spatial one.

ACKNOWLEDGMENTS

I am grateful to my co-editors for extensive and helpful comments on earlier drafts of the chapter. I also thank Dr. Colin Lever (Leeds University) who made extensive comments and suggestions on an earlier version. Support for the research from my own laboratory cited in this chapter came from the Medical Research Council UK, Wellcome Trust, and the BBSRC.

REFERENCES

Acsady L, Kamondi A, Sik A, Freund T, Buzsaki G (1998) GABAergic cells are the major postsynaptic targets of mossy fibers in the rat hippocampus. *J Neurosci* 18:3386–3403.

Adey WR, Dunlop CW, Hendrix CE (1960) Hippocampal slow waves: distribution and phase relations in the course of approach learning. *Arch Neurol* 3:74–90.

Aggleton JP, Brown MW (1999) Episodic memory, amnesia, and the hippocampal-anterior thalamic axis. *Behav Brain Sci* 22: 425–490.

Alonso A, Garcia-Austt E (1987a) Neuronal sources of theta rhythm in the entorhinal cortex of the rat. I. Laminar distribution of theta field potentials. *Exp Brain Res* 67:493–501.

Alonso A, Garcia-Austt E (1987b) Neuronal sources of theta rhythm in the entorhinal cortex of the rat. II. Phase relations between unit discharges and theta field potentials. *Exp Brain Res* 67: 502–509.

Alvarez P, Zola-Morgan S, Squire LR (1995) Damage limited to the hippocampal region produces long-lasting memory impairment in monkeys. *J Neurosci* 15:3796–3807.

Arnolds DE, Lopes da Silva FH, Aitink JW, Kamp A, Boeijinga P (1980) The spectral properties of hippocampal EEG related to behavior in man. *Electroencephalogr Clin Neurophysiol* 50: 324–328.

Barnes CA, McNaughton BL, O'Keefe J (1983) Loss of place specificity in hippocampal complex spike cells of senescent rat. *Neurobiol Aging* 4:113–119.

Barnes CA, McNaughton BL, Mizumori SJ, Leonard BW, Lin LH (1990) Comparison of spatial and temporal characteristics of neuronal activity in sequential stages of hippocampal processing. *Prog Brain* Res 83:287–300.

Barnes CA, Suster MS, Shen J, McNaughton BL (1997) Multistability of cognitive maps in the hippocampus of old rats. *Nature* 388:272–275.

Bassett JP, Taube JS (2001) Neural correlates for angular head velocity in the rat dorsal tegmental nucleus. *J Neurosci* 21:5740–5751.

Battaglia FP, Sutherland GR, McNaughton BL (2004) Local sensory cues and place cell directionality: additional evidence of prospective coding in the hippocampus. *J Neurosci* 24: 4541–4550.

Berger TW, Thompson RF (1978) Identification of pyramidal cells as the critical elements in hippocampal neuronal plasticity during learning. *Proc Natl Acad Sci USA* 75:1572–1576.

Berger TW, Rinaldi PC, Weisz DJ, Thompson RF (1983) Single-unit analysis of different hippocampal cell types during classical conditioning of rabbit nictitating membrane response. *J Neurophysiol* 50:1197–1219.

Berry SD, Swain RA (1989) Water deprivation optimizes hippocampal activity and facilitates nictitating membrane conditioning. *Behav Neurosci* 103:71–76.

Black A (1975) Hippocampal electrical activity and behavior. In: *The hippocampus: a comprehensive treatise* (Isaacson RL, Pribram KH, eds), pp 129–167. New York: Plenum Press.

Blair HT, Sharp PE (1996) Visual and vestibular influences on head-direction cells in the anterior thalamus of the rat. *Behav Neurosci* 110:643–660.

Blair HT, Lipscomb BW, Sharp PE (1997) Anticipatory time intervals of head-direction cells in the anterior thalamus of the rat: implications for path integration in the head-direction circuit. *J Neurophysiol* 78:145–159.

Blair HT, Cho J, Sharp PE (1999) The anterior thalamic head-direction signal is abolished by bilateral but not unilateral lesions of the lateral mammillary nucleus. *J Neurosci* 19:6673–6683.

Bland BH, Oddie SD (2001) Theta band oscillation and synchrony in the hippocampal formation and associated structures: the case for its role in sensorimotor integration. *Behav Brain Res* 127:119–136.

Bland BH, Vanderwolf CH (1972) Diencephalic and hippocampal mechanisms of motor activity in the rat: effects of posterior hypothalamic stimulation on behavior and hippocampal slow wave activity. *Brain Res* 43:67–88.

Bland BH, Konopacki J, Kirk IJ, Oddie SD, Dickson CT (1995) Discharge patterns of hippocampal theta-related cells in the caudal diencephalon of the urethane-anesthetized rat. *J Neurophysiol* 74:322–333.

Bland BH, Trepel C, Oddie SD, Kirk IJ (1996) Intraseptal microinfusion of muscimol: effects on hippocampal formation theta field activity and phasic theta-on cell discharges. *Exp Neurol* 138:286–297.

Bloch V, Laroche S (1981) Conditioning of hippocampal cells: its acceleration and long-term facilitation by post-trial reticular stimulation. *Behav Brain Res* 3:23–42.

Borhegyi Z, Varga V, Szilagyi N, Fabo D, Freund TF (2004) Phase segregation of medial septal GABAergic neurons during hippocampal theta activity. *J Neurosci* 24:8470–8479.

Bostock E, Muller RU, Kubie JL (1991) Experience-dependent modifications of hippocampal place cell firing. *Hippocampus* 1:193–205.

Bragin A, Engel J Jr, Wilson CL, Fried I, Buzsaki, G (1999) High-frequency oscillation in human brain. *Hippocampus* 9: 137–142.

Bragin A, Jando G, Nadasdy Z, Hetke J, Wise K, Buzsaki G (1995) Gamma (40–100 Hz) oscillation in the hippocampus of the behaving rat. *J Neurosci* 15:47–60.

Brankack J, Stewart M, Fox SE (1993) Current source density analysis of the hippocampal theta rhythm: associated sustained potentials and candidate synaptic generators. *Brain Res* 615:310–327.

Breese CR, Hampson RE, Deadwyler SA (1989) Hippocampal place cells: stereotypy and plasticity. *J Neurosci* 9:1097–1111.

Brown MW, Aggleton JP (2001) Recognition memory: what are the roles of the perirhinal cortex and hippocampus? *Nat Rev Neurosci* 2:51–61.

Brown MW, Xiang JZ (1998) Recognition memory: neuronal substrates of the judgement of prior occurrence. *Prog Neurobiol* 55:149–189.

Brown MW, Wilson FA, Riches IP (1987) Neuronal evidence that inferomedial temporal cortex is more important than hippocampus in certain processes underlying recognition memory. *Brain Res* 409:158–162.

Brun VH, Otnass MK, Molden S, Steffenach HA, Witter MP, Moser MB, Moser EI (2002) Place cells and place recognition maintained by direct entorhinal-hippocampal circuitry. *Science* 296:2243–2246.

Bullock TH, Buzsaki G, McClune MC (1990) Coherence of compound field potentials reveals discontinuities in the CA1-subiculum of the hippocampus in freely-moving rats. *Neuroscience* 38:609–619.

Bures J, Fenton AA, Kaminsky Y, Rossier J, Sacchetti B, Zinyuk L (1997) Dissociation of exteroceptive and idiothetic orientation cues: effect on hippocampal place cells and place navigation. *Philos Trans R Soc Lond B Biol Sci* 352:1515–1524.

Burgess N, O'Keefe J (1996) Neuronal computations underlying the firing of place cells and their role in navigation. *Hippocampus* 6:749–762.

Burgess N, Recce M, O'Keefe J (1994) A model of hippocampal function. *Neural Networks* 7:1065–1081.

Burgess N, Jeffery KJ, O'Keefe J (1999) Intergrating hippocampal and parietal functions: a spatial point of view. In: *The hippocampal and parietal foundations of spatial cognition* (Burgess N, Jeffery KJ, O'Keefe J, eds), pp 3–29. Oxford, UK: Oxford University Press.

Burgess N, Maguire EA, O'Keefe J (2002) The human hippocampus and spatial and episodic memory. *Neuron* 35:625–641.

Burgess N, Cacucci F, Lever C, O'Keefe J (2005) Characterizing multiple independent behavioral correlates of cell firing in freely moving animals. *Hippocampus* 15:149–153.

Buzsaki G (1989) Two-stage model of memory trace formation: a role for "noisy" brain states. *Neuroscience* 31:551–570.

Buzsaki G (2002) Theta oscillations in the hippocampus. *Neuron* 33:325–340.

Buzsaki G (2005) Theta rhythm of navigation: link between path integration and landmark navigation, episodic and semantic memory. *Hippocampus* 15:827–840.

Buzsaki G, Draguhn A (2004) Neuronal oscillations in cortical networks. *Science* 304: 1926–1929.

Buzsaki G, Leung LW, Vanderwolf CH (1983) Cellular bases of hippocampal EEG in the behaving rat. *Brain Res* 287:139–171.

Buzsaki G, Horvath Z, Urioste R, Hetke J, Wise K (1992) High-frequency network oscillation in the hippocampus. *Science* 256:1025–1027.

Cacucci F, Lever C, Wills TJ, Burgess N, O'Keefe J (2004) Theta-modulated place-by-direction cells in the hippocampal formation in the rat. *J Neurosci* 24:8265–8277.

Calton JL, Stackman RW, Goodridge JP, Archey WB, Dudchenko PA, Taube JS (2003) Hippocampal place cell instability after lesions of the head direction cell network. *J Neurosci* 23:9719–9731.

Cameron KA, Yashar S, Wilson CL, Fried I (2001) Human hippocampal neurons predict how well word pairs will be remembered. *Neuron* 30:289–298.

Caplan JB, Madsen JR, Schulze-Bonhage A, Aschenbrenner-Scheibe R, Newman EL, Kahana MJ (2003) Human theta oscillations related to sensorimotor integration and spatial learning. *J Neurosci* 23:4726–4736.

Chakraborty S, Anderson MI, Chaudhry AM, Mumford JC, Jeffery KL (2004) Context-independent directional cue learning by hippocampal place cells. *Eur J Neurosci* 20: 281–292.

Chen LL, Lin LH, Green EJ, Barnes CA, McNaughton BL (1994) Head-direction cells in the rat posterior cortex. I. Anatomical distribution and behavioral modulation. *Exp Brain Res* 101:8–23.

Cho J, Sharp PE (2001) Head direction, place, and movement correlates for cells in the rat retrosplenial cortex. *Behav Neurosci* 115:3–25.

Cho YH, Giese KP, Tanila H, Silva AJ, Eichenbaum H (1998) Abnormal hippocampal spatial representations in alphaCaMKIIT286A and CREBalphaDelta mice. Science 279:867–869.

Christian EP, Deadwyler SA (1986) Behavioral functions and hippocampal cell types: evidence for two nonoverlapping populations in the rat. *J Neurophysiol* 55:331–348.

Chrobak JJ, Buzsaki G (1996) High-frequency oscillations in the output networks of the hippocampal- entorhinal axis of the freely behaving rat. *J Neurosci* 16:3056–3066.

Clark RE, Broadbent, Squire LR (2005) Imparied remote spatial memory after hippocampal lesions despite extensive training beginning early in life. *Hippocampus* 15:340–346.

Cohen NJ, Eichenbaum H (1993) *Memory, amnesisa and the hippocampal system*. Cambridge, MA: MIT Press.

Colom LV, Bland BH (1987) State-dependent spike train dynamics of hippocampal formation neurons: evidence for theta-on and theta-off cells. *Brain Res* 422:277–286.

Colombo M, Fernandez T, Nakamura K, Gross CG (1998) Functional differentiation along the anterior-posterior axis of the hippocampus in monkeys. *J Neurophysiol* 80:1002–1005.

Cooper BG, Mizumori SJ (2001) Temporary inactivation of the retrosplenial cortex causes a transient reorganization of spatial coding in the hippocampus. *J Neurosci* 21:3986–4001.

Cressant A, Muller RU, Poucet B (1997) Failure of centrally placed objects to control the firing fields of hippocampal place cells. *J Neurosci* 17:2531–2542.

Csicsvari J, Hirase H, Czurko A, Buzsaki G (1998) Reliability and state dependence of pyramidal cell-interneuron synapses in the hippocampus: an ensemble approach in the behaving rat. *Neuron* 21:179–189.

Csicsvari J, Hirase H, Mamiya A, Buzsaki G (2000) Ensemble patterns of hippocampal CA3-CA1 neurons during sharp wave-associated population events. *Neuron* 28:585–594.

Csicsvari J, Jamieson B, Wise KD, Buzsaki G (2003) Mechanisms of gamma oscillations in the hippocampus of the behaving rat. *Neuron* 37:311–322.

Czurko A, Hirase H, Csicsvari J, Buzsaki G (1999) Sustained activation of hippocampal pyramidal cells by 'space clamping' in a running wheel. *Eur J Neurosci* 11:344–352.

Delacour J (1984) Two neuronal systems are involved in a classical conditioning in the rat. *Neuroscience* 13:705–15.

Draguhn A, Traub RD, Bibbig A, Schmitz (2000) Ripple (approximately 200-Hz) oscillations in temporal structures. *J Clin Neurophysiol* 17:361–376.

Dudchenko PA, Wood ER, Eichenbaum H (2000) Neurotoxic hippocampal lesions have no effect on odor span and little effect on odor recognition memory but produce significant impairments on spatial span, recognition, and alternation. *J Neurosci* 20:2964–2977.

Eichenbaum H, Cohen N (2001) *From conditioning to conscious recollection*. Oxford, UK: Oxford University Press.

Eichenbaum H, Kuperstein M, Fagan A, Nagode J (1987) Cuesampling and goal-approach correlates of hippocampal unit activity in rats performing an odor-discrimination task. *J Neurosci* 7:716–732.

Eichenbaum H, Wiener SI, Shapiro ML, Cohen NJ (1989) The organization of spatial coding in the hippocampus: a study of neural ensemble activity. *J Neurosci* 9:2764–2775.

Ekstrom AD, Meltzer J, McNaughton BL, Barnes CA (2001) NMDA receptor antagonism blocks experience-dependent expansion of hippocampal "place fields." *Neuron* 31:631–638.

Ekstrom AD, Kahana MJ, Caplan JB, Fields TA, Isham EA, Newman EL, Fried I (2003) Cellular networks underlying human spatial navigation. *Nature* 425:184–188.

Fenton AA, Muller RU (1998) Place cell discharge is extremely variable during individual passes of the rat through the firing field. *Proc Natl Acad Sci USA* 95:3182–3187.

Fenton AA, Csizmadia G, Muller RU (2000a) Conjoint control of hippocampal place cell firing by two visual stimuli. I. The effects of moving the stimuli on firing field positions. *J Gen Physiol* 116:191–209.

Fenton AA, Csizmadia G, Muller RU (2000b) Conjoint control of hippocampal place cell firing by two visual stimuli. I. A vector-field theory that predicts modifications of the representation of the environment. *J Gen Physiol* 116:211–221.

Ferbinteanu J, Shapiro ML (2003) Prospective and retrospective memory coding in the hippocampus. *Neuron* 40:1227–1239.

Foster TC, Christian EP, Hampson RE, Campbell KA, Deadwyler SA (1987) Sequential dependencies regulate sensory evoked responses of single units in the rat hippocampus. *Brain Res* 408:86–96.

Foster TC, Castro CA, McNaughton BL (1989) Spatial selectivity of rat hippocampal neurons: dependence on preparedness for movement. *Science* 244:1580–1582.

Fox SE, Ranck JB Jr (1975) Localization and anatomical identification of theta and complex spike cells in dorsal hippocampal formation of rats. *Exp Neurol* 49:299–313.

Fox SE, Ranck JB Jr (1981) Electrophysiological characteristics of hippocampal complex-spike cells and theta cells. *Exp Brain Res* 41:399–410.

Fox SE, Wolfson S, Ranck JB Jr (1986) Hippocampal theta rhythm and the firing of neurons in walking and urethane anesthetized rats. *Exp Brain Res* 62:495–508.

Frank LM, Brown EN, Wilson M (2000) Trajectory encoding in the hippocampus and entorhinal cortex. *Neuron* 27:169–178.

Frank LM, Stanley GB, Brown EN (2004) Hippocampal plasticity across multiple days of exposure to novel environments. *J Neurosci* 24:7681–7689.

Freeman WJ (1975) *Mass action in the nervous system*. San Diego: Academic Press.

Fried I, MacDonald KA, Wilson CL (1997) Single neuron activity in human hippocampus and amygdala during recognition of faces and objects. *Neuron* 18:753–765.

Fried I, Cameron KA, Yashar S, Fong R, Morrow JW (2002) Inhibitory and excitatory responses of single neurons in the human medial temporal lobe during recognition of faces and objects. *Cereb Cortex* 12:575–584.

Fyhn M, Molden S, Witter MP, Moser EI, Moser MB (2004) Spatial representation in the entorhinal cortex. *Science* 305:1258–1264.

Gevins A, Smith ME, McEvoy L, Yu D (1997) High-resolution EEG mapping of cortical activation related to working memory: effects of task difficulty, type of processing, and practice. *Cereb Cortex* 7:374–385.

Gilbert PE, Kesner RP (2002) Role of the rodent hippocampus in paired-associate learning involving associations between a stimulus and a spatial location. *Behav Neurosci* 116:63–71.

Golob EJ, Taube JS (1997) Head direction cells and episodic spatial information in rats without a hippocampus. *Proc Natl Acad Sci USA* 94:7645–7650.

Golob EJ, Taube JS (1999) Head direction cells in rats with hippocampal or overlying neocortical lesions: evidence for impaired angular path integration. *J Neurosci* 19:7198–7211.

Goodridge JP, Taube JS (1997) Interaction between the postsubiculum and anterior thalamus in the generation of head direction cell activity. *J Neurosci* 17:9315–9330.

Goodridge JP, Dudchenko PA, Worboys KA, Golob EJ, Taube JS (1998) Cue control and head direction cells. *Behav Neurosci* 112:749–761.

Gothard KM, Skaggs WE, McNaughton BL (1996a) Dynamics of mismatch correction in the hippocampal ensemble code for space: interaction between path integration and environmental cues. *J Neurosci* 16:8027–8040.

Gothard KM, Skaggs WE, Moore KM, McNaughton BL (1996b) Binding of hippocampal CA1 neural activity to multiple reference frames in a landmark-based navigation task. *J Neurosci* 16:823–835.

Grastyan, E., Lissak, K., Madarasz, I, Donhoffer, H. (1959) Hippocampal electrical activity during the development of conditioned reflexes. *Electroencephalogr Clin Neurophysiol* 11:409–430.

Gray JA (1971) Medial septal lesions, hippocampal theta rhythm and the control of vibrissal movement in the freelymoving rat. *Electroencephalogr Clin Neurophysiol* 30:189–197.

Green JD, Arduini AA (1954) Hippocampal electrical activity in arousal. *J Neurophysiol* 17:533–557.

Guzowski JF, McNaughton BL, Barnes CA, Worley PF (1999) Environment-specific expression of the immediate-early gene Arc in hippocampal neuronal ensembles. *Nat Neurosci* 2:1120–1124.

Hafting T, Fyhn M, Molden S, Moser MB, Moser EI (2005) Microstructure of a spatial map in the entorhinal cortex. *Nature* 436:801–806.

Halgren E, Babb TL, Crandall PH (1978) Human hippocampal formation EEG desynchronizes during attentiveness and movement. *Electroencephalogr Clin Neurophysiol* 44:778–781.

Hampson RE, Simeral JD, Deadwyler SA (1999) Distribution of spatial and nonspatial information in dorsal hippocampus. *Nature* 402:610–614.

Harris KD, Henze DA, Hirase H, Leinekugel X, Dragoi G, Czurko A, Buzsaki G (2002) Spike train dynamics predicts theta-related phase precession in hippocampal pyramidal cells. *Nature* 417:738–741.

Hasselmo ME (2005) What is the function of hippocampal theta rhythm? Linking behavioral data to phasic properties of field potential and unit recording data. *Hippocampus* 15:936–949.

Heit G, Smith ME, Halgren E (1988) Neural encoding of individual words and faces by the human hippocampus and amygdala. *Nature* 333:773–775.

Hetherington PA, Shapiro ML (1997) Hippocampal place fields are altered by the removal of single visual cues in a distance-dependent manner. *Behav Neurosci* 111:20–34.

Hill AJ (1978) First occurrence of hippocampal spatial firing in a new environment. *Exp Neurol* 62:282–297.

Hill AJ, Best PJ (1981) Effects of deafness and blindness on the spatial correlates of hippocampal unit activity in the rat. *Exp Neurol* 74:204–217.

Hirase H, Czurko HH, Csicsvari J, Buzsaki G (1999) Firing rate and theta-phase coding by hippocampal pyramidal neurons during 'space clamping.' *Eur J Neurosci* 11:4373–4380.

Hok V, Save E, Lenck-Santini PP, Poucet B (2005) Coding for spatial goals in the prelimbic/infralimbic area of the rat frontal cortex. *Proc Natl Acad Sci USA* 102:4602–4607.

Hollup SA, Molden S, Donnett JG, Moser MB, Moser EI (2001) Accumulation of hippocampal place fields at the goal location in an annular watermaze task. *J Neurosci* 21:1635–1644.

Holscher C, Anwyl R, Rowan MJ (1997) Stimulation on the positive phase of hippocampal theta rhythm induces long-term potentiation that can be depotentiated by stimulation on the negative phase in area CA1 in vivo. *J Neurosci* 17:6470–6477.

Honzik CH (1936) The sensory basis of maze learning in rats. *Comp Psychol Monogr* 13:1–113.

Hori E, Nishio Y, Kazui K, Umeno K, Tabuchi E, Sasaki K, Endo S, Ono T, Nishijo H (2005) Place-related neural responses in the monkey hippocampal formation in a virtual space. *Hippocampus* 15:991–996.

Huerta PT, Lisman JE (1995) Bidirectional synaptic plasticity induced by a single burst during cholinergic theta oscillation in CA1 in vitro. *Neuron* 15:1053–1063.

Huxter J, Burgess N, O'Keefe J (2003) Independent rate and temporal coding in hippocampal pyramidal cells. *Nature* 425:828–832.

Hyman JM, Wyble BP, Goyal V, Rossi CA, Hasselmo ME (2003) Stimulation in hippocampal region CA1 in behaving rats yields long-term potentiation when delivered to the peak of theta and long-term depression when delivered to the trough. *J Neurosci* 23:11725–11731.

Hyman JM, Zilli EA, Paley AM, Hasselmo ME (2005) Medial prefrontal cortex cells show dynamic modulation with the hippocampal theta rhythm dependent on behavior. *Hippocampus* 15:739–749.

Jarosiewicz B, Skaggs WE (2004a) Hippocampal place cells are not controlled by visual input during the small irregular activity state in the rat. *J Neurosci* 24:5070–5077.

Jarosiewicz B, Skaggs WE (2004b) Level of arousal during the small irregular activity state in the rat hippocampal EEG. *J Neurophysiol* 91:2649–2657.

Jarosiewicz B, McNaughton BL, Skaggs WE (2002) Hippocampal population activity during the small-amplitude irregular activity state in the rat. *J Neurosci* 22:1373–1384.

Jeffery KJ (1998) Learning of landmark stability and instability by hippocampal place cells. *Neuropharmacology* 37:677–687.

Jeffery KJ, Donnett JG, O'Keefe J (1995) Medial septal control of theta-correlated unit firing in the entorhinal cortex of awake rats. *Neuroreport* 6:2166–2170.

Jeffery KJ, Donnett JG, Burgess N, O'Keefe JM (1997) Direc-

tional control of hippocampal place fields. *Exp Brain Res* 117:131–142.

Jeffery KJ, Gilbert A, Burton S, Strudwick A (2003) Preserved performance in a hippocampal-dependent spatial task despite complete place cell remapping. *Hippocampus* 13:175–189.

Jensen O, Lisman JE (2000) Position reconstruction from an ensemble of hippocampal place cells: contribution of theta phase coding. *J Neurophysiol* 83:2602–2609.

Jones MW, Wilson MA (2005) Theta rhythms coordinate hippocampal-prefrontal interactions in a spatial memory task. *PLoS Biol* 3:e402.

Jung MW, Wiener SI, McNaughton BL (1994) Comparison of spatial firing characteristics of units in dorsal and ventral hippocampus of the rat. *J Neurosci* 14:7347–7356.

Jung R, Kornmuller AE (1938) Eine methodik der ableitung lokalisierter Potentialschwankungen aus subcorticalen Hirngebieten. *Arch Psychiatry* 109:1–30.

Kahana MJ, Sekuler R, Caplan JB, Kirschen M, Madsen JR (1999) Human theta oscillations exhibit task dependence during virtual maze navigation. *Nature* 399:781–784.

Kali S, Dayan P (2000) The involvement of recurrent connections in area CA3 in establishing the properties of place fields: a model. *J Neurosci* 20:7463–7477.

Kamondi A, Acsady L, Wang XJ, Buzsaki G (1998) Theta oscillations in somata and dendrites of hippocampal pyramidal cells in vivo: activity-dependent phase-precession of action potentials. *Hippocampus* 8:244–261.

Kentros C, Hargreaves E, Hawkins RD, Kandel ER, Shapiro M, Muller RV (1998) Abolition of long-term stability of new hippocampal place cell maps by NMDA receptor blockade. *Science* 280:2121–2126.

Kim JJ, Clark RE, Thompson RF (1995) Hippocampectomy impairs the memory of recently, but not remotely, acquired trace eyeblink conditioned responses. *Behav Neurosci* 109:195–203.

King C, Recce M, O'Keefe J (1998) The rhythmicity of cells of the medial septum/diagonal band of Broca in the awake freely moving rat: relationships with behavior and hippocampal theta. *Eur J Neurosci* 10:464–477.

Kirk IJ, McNaughton N (1991) Supramammillary cell firing and hippocampal rhythmical slow activity. *Neuroreport* 2:723–725.

Klausberger T, Magill PJ, Marton LF, Roberts JD, Cobden PM, Buzsaki G, Somogyi P (2003) Brain-state- and cell-type-specific firing of hippocampal interneurons in vivo. *Nature* 421:844–848.

Klimesch W (1999) EEG alpha and theta oscillations reflect cognitive and memory performance: a review and analysis. *Brain Res Brain Res Rev* 29:169–195.

Knierim JJ, Kudrimoti HS, McNaughton BL (1995) Place cells, head direction cells, and the learning of landmark stability. *J Neurosci* 15:1648–1659.

Kobayashi T, Nishijo H, Fukuda M, Bures J, Ono T (1997) Task-dependent representations in rat hippocampal place neurons. *J Neurophysiol* 78:597–613.

Kocsis B, Vertes RP (1997) Phase relations of rhythmic neuronal firing in the supramammillary nucleus and mammillary body to the hippocampal theta activity in urethane anesthetized rats. *Hippocampus* 7:204–214.

Kramis R, Vanderwolf CH, Bland BH (1975) Two types of hippocampal rhythmical slow activity in both the rabbit and the rat: relations to behavior and effects of atropine, diethyl ether, urethane, and pentobarbital. *Exp Neurol* 49:58–85.

Kreiman G, Koch C, Fried I (2000a) Category-specific visual responses of single neurons in the human medial temporal lobe. *Nat Neurosci* 3:946–953.

Kubie JL, Ranck JB Jr (1983) Sensory-behavioral correlates of individual hippocampal neurons in three situations: space and context. In: *Neurobiology of the hippocampus* (Siefert W, ed), pp 433–447, New York: Academic Press.

Kudrimoti HS, Barnes CA, McNaughton BL (1999) Reactivation of hippocampal cell assemblies: effects of behavioral state, experience, and EEG dynamics. *J Neurosci* 19:4090–4101.

Kyd RJ, Bilkey DK (2005) Hippocampal place cells show increased sensitivity to changes in the local environment following prefrontal cortex lesions. *Cereb Cortex* 15:720–731.

Laroche S, Falcou R, Bloch V (1983) Post-trial reticular facilitation of associative changes in multiunit activity; comparison between dentate gyrus and entorhinal cortex. *Behav Brain Res* 9:381–387.

Lawson VH, Bland BH (1993) The role of the septohippocampal pathway in the regulation of hippocampal field activity and behavior: analysis by the intraseptal microinfusion of carbachol, atropine, and procaine. *Exp Neurol* 120:132–144.

Leblanc MO, Bland BH (1979) Developmental aspects of hippocampal electrical activity and motor behavior in the rat *Exp Neurol* 66:220–237.

Lee AK, Wilson MA (2002) Memory of sequential experience in the hippocampus during slow wave sleep. *Neuron* 36:1183–1194.

Lee I, Rao G, Knierim JJ (2004) A double dissociation between hippocampal subfields: differential time course of CA3 and CA1 place cells for processing changed environments. *Neuron* 42:803–815.

Lenck-Santini PP, Save E, Poucet B (2001a) Evidence for a relationship between place-cell spatial firing and spatial memory performance. *Hippocampus* 11:377–390.

Lenck-Santini PP, Save E, Poucet B (2001b) Place-cell firing does not depend on the direction of turn in a Y-maze alternation task. *Eur J Neurosci* 13:1055–1058.

Lenck-Santini PP, Muller RU, Save E, Poucet B (2002) Relationships between place cell firing fields and navigational decisions by rats. *J Neurosci* 22:9035–9047.

Lengyel M, Szatmary Z, Erdi P. (2003) Dynamically detuned oscillators account for the coupled rate and temporal code of place cell firing. *Hippocampus* 13:700–714.

Leonard BJ, McNaughton BL, Barnes CA (1987) Suppression of hippocampal synaptic plasticity during slow-wave sleep. *Brain Res* 425:174–177.

Leung LW (1985) Spectral analysis of hippocampal EEG in the freely moving rat: effects of centrally active drugs and relations to evoked potentials. *Electroencephalogr Clin Neurophysiol* 60:65–77.

Leung LS (1992) Fast (beta) rhythms in the hippocampus: a review. *Hippocampus* 2:93–98.

Leung LW, Borst JG (1987) Electrical activity of the cingulate cortex. I. Generating mechanisms and relations to behavior. *Brain Res* 407:68–80.

Leutgeb S, Mizumori SJ (1999) Excitotoxic septal lesions result in spatial memory deficits and altered flexibility of hippocampal single-unit representations. *J Neurosci* 19:6661–6672.

Lever C, Cacucci F, Wills TJ, Burton S, McClelland, Burgess N, O'Keefe J (2003) Spatial coding in the hippocampal formation: input, information type, plasticity, and behavior. In: *The neurobiology of spatial behavior* (Jeffrey KJ, ed), pp 199–225. Oxford, UK: Oxford University Press.

Lever C, Wills T, Cacucci F, Burgess N, O'Keefe J (2002) Long-term plasticity in hippocampal place-cell representation of environmental geometry. *Nature* 416:90–94.

Louie K, Wilson MA (2001) Temporally structured replay of awake hippocampal ensemble activity during rapid eye movement sleep. *Neuron* 29:145–156.

Ludvig N, Tang HM, Gohil BC, Botero JM (2004) Detecting location-specific neuronal firing rate increases in the hippocampus of freely-moving monkeys. *Brain Res* 1014:97–109.

Maquet P (2001) The role of sleep in learning and memory. *Science* 294:1048–1052.

Markus EJ, Barnes CA, McNaughton BL, Gladden VL, Skaggs WE (1994) Spatial information content and reliability of hippocampal CA1 neurons: effects of visual input. *Hippocampus* 4:410–421.

Markus EJ, Qin YL, Leonard B, Skaggs WE, McNaughton BL, Barnes CA (1995) Interactions between location and task affect the spatial and directional firing of hippocampal neurons. *J Neurosci* 15:7079–7094.

Martin PD, Berthoz A (2002) Development of spatial firing in the hippocampus of young rats. *Hippocampus* 12:465–480.

Matthews RT, Lee WL (1991) A comparison of extracellular and intracellular recordings from medial septum/diagonal band neurons in vitro. *Neuroscience* 42:451–462.

Maurer AP, Vanrhoads SR, Sutherland GR, Lipa P, McNaughton BL (2005) Self-motion and the origin of differential spatial scaling along the septo-temporal axis of the hippocampus. *Hippocampus* 15:841–852.

McEchron MD, Disterhoft JF (1997) Sequence of single neuron changes in CA1 hippocampus of rabbits during acquisition of trace eyeblink conditioned responses. *J Neurophysiol* 78:1030–1044.

McEchron MD, Tseng W, Disterhoft JF (2003) Single neurons in CA1 hippocampus encode trace interval duration during trace heart rate (fear) conditioning in rabbit. *J Neurosci* 23:1535–1547.

McHugh TJ, Blum KI, Tsien JZ, Tonegawa S, Wilson MA (1996) Impaired hippocampal representation of space in CA1-specific NMDAR1 knockout mice. *Cell* 87:1339–1349.

McNaughton BL, Barnes CA, O'Keefe J (1983a) The contributions of position, direction, and velocity to single unit activity in the hippocampus of freely-moving rats. *Exp Brain Res* 52:41–49.

McNaughton BL, O'Keefe J, Barnes CA (1983b) The stereotrode: a new technique for simultaneous isolation of several single units in the central nervous system from multiple unit records. *J Neurosci Methods* 8:391–397.

McNaughton BL, Barnes CA, Gerrard JL, Gothard K, Jung MW, Knierim JJ, Kudrimoti H, Qin Y, Skaggs WE, Suster M, Weaver KL (1996) Deciphering the hippocampal polyglot: the hippocampus as a path integration system. *J Exp Biol* 199(Pt 1):173–185.

Mehta MR, Barnes CA, McNaughton BL (1997) Experience-dependent, asymmetric expansion of hippocampal place fields. *Proc Natl Acad Sci USA* 94:8918–8921.

Mehta MR, Quirk MC, Wilson MA (2000) Experience-dependent asymmetric shape of hippocampal receptive fields. *Neuron* 25:707–715.

Mehta MR, Lee AK, Wilson MA (2002) Role of experience and oscillations in transforming a rate code into a temporal code. *Nature* 417:741–746.

Miller VM, Best PJ (1980) Spatial correlates of hippocampal unit activity are altered by lesions of the fornix and endorhinal cortex. *Brain Res* 194:311–323.

Mitchell SJ, Ranck JB Jr (1980) Generation of theta rhythm in medial entorhinal cortex of freely moving rats. *Brain Res* 189:49–66.

Mizumori SJ, Williams JD (1993) Directionally selective mnemonic properties of neurons in the lateral dorsal nucleus of the thalamus of rats. *J Neurosci* 13:4015–4028.

Mizumori SJ, Barnes CA, McNaughton BL (1989) Reversible inactivation of the medial septum: selective effects on the spontaneous unit activity of different hippocampal cell types. *Brain Res* 500:99–106.

Mizumori SJ, Ward KE, Lavoie AM (1992) Medial septal modulation of entorhinal single unit activity in anesthetized and freely moving rats. *Brain Res* 570:188–197.

Mizumori SJ, Lavoie AM, Kalyani A (1996) Redistribution of spatial representation in the hippocampus of aged rats performing a spatial memory task. *Behav Neurosci* 110:1006–1016.

Moita MA, Rosis S, Zhou Y, LeDoux JE, Blair HT (2003) Hippocampal place cells acquire location-specific responses to the conditioned stimulus during auditory fear conditioning. *Neuron* 37:485–497.

Moita MA, Rosis S, Zhou Y, LeDoux JE, Blair HT (2004) Putting fear in its place: remapping of hippocampal place cells during fear conditioning. *J Neurosci* 24:7015–7023.

Muir GM, Bilkey DK (1998) Synchronous modulation of perirhinal cortex neuronal activity during cholinergically mediated (type II) hippocampal theta. *Hippocampus* 8:526–532.

Muir GM, Bilkey DK (2001) Instability in the place field location of hippocampal place cells after lesions centered on the perirhinal cortex. *J Neurosci* 21:4016–4025.

Muller RU, Kubie JL (1987) The effects of changes in the environment on the spatial firing of hippocampal complex-spike cells. *J Neurosci* 7:1951–1968.

Muller RU, Kubie JL, Ranck JB Jr (1987) Spatial firing patterns of hippocampal complex-spike cells in a fixed environment. *J Neurosci* 7:1935–1950.

Muller RU, Bostock E, Taube JS, Kubie JL (1994) On the directional firing properties of hippocampal place cells. J Neurosci 14:7235–7251.

Murray EA, Mishkin M (1998) Object recognition and location memory in monkeys with excitotoxic lesions of the amygdala and hippocampus. J Neurosci 18:6568–6582.

Nadel L, Willner J, Kurz E (1985) Cognitive maps and environmental contex. In: *Context and learning* (Balsam P, Tomie A, eds), pp 385–406. Hillside, NJ: Erlbaum.

Nakazawa K, Quirk MC, Chitwood RA, Watanabe M, Yeckel MF, Sun LD, Kato A, Carr CA, Johnston D, Wilson MA, Tonegawa S (2002) Requirement for hippocampal CA3 NMDA receptors in associative memory recall. *Science* 297:211–218.

Nakazawa K, Sun LD, Quirk MC, Rondi-Reig L, Wilson MA, Tonegawa S (2003) Hippocampal CA3 NMDA receptors are crucial for memory acquisition of one-time experience. *Neuron* 38:305–315.

Nakazawa K, McHugh TJ, Wilson MA, Tonegawa S (2004) NMDA receptors, place cells and hippocampal spatial memory. *Nat Rev Neurosci* 5:361–372.

Natsume K, Hallworth NE, Szgatti TL, Bland BH (1999) Hippocampal theta-related cellular activity in the superior colliculus of the urethane-anesthetized rat. *Hippocampus* 9:500–509.

Nimmrich V, Maier N, Schmitz D, Draguhn A (2005) Induced sharp wave-ripple complexes in the absence of synaptic inhibition. *J Physiol* 563(Pt 3):663–670.

Nishijo H, Ono T, Eifuku S, Tamura R (1997) The relationship between monkey hippocampus place-related neural activity and action in space. *Neurosci Lett* 226:57–60.

Nitz D, McNaughton B (2004) Differential modulation of CA1 and dentate gyrus interneurons during exploration of novel environments. *J Neurophysiol* 91:863–872.

Nowicka A, Ringo JL (2000) Eye position-sensitive units in hippocampal formation and in inferotemporal cortex of the macaque monkey. *Eur J Neurosci* 12:751–759.

Nunez A, de Andres, I, Garcia-Austt E (1991) Relationships of nucleus reticularis pontis oralis neuronal discharge with sensory and carbachol evoked hippocampal theta rhythm. *Exp Brain Res* 87:303–308.

O'Keefe J (1976) Place units in the hippocampus of the freely moving rat. *Exp Neurol* 51:78–109.

O'Keefe J (1991a) The hippocampal cognitive map and navigational strategies. In: *Brain and space* (Paillard J, ed), pp 273–295. Oxford, UK: Oxford University Press.

O'Keefe J (1991b) An allocentric spatial model for the hippocampal cognitive map. *Hippocampus* 1:230–235.

O'Keefe J (1996) The spatial prepositions in English, vector grammar and the cognitive map theory. In: *Language and space* (Bloom P, Peterson M, Nadel L, Garrett M, eds), pp 277–316. Cambridge, MA: MIT Press.

O'Keefe J (1999) Do hippocampal pyramidal cells signal non-spatial as well as spatial information? *Hippocampus* 9:352–364.

O'Keefe J (2001) Vector grammar, places, and the functional role of the spatial prepositions in English. In: *Axes and vectors in language and space* (van der Zee E, Slack J, eds). Oxford, UK: Oxford University Press.

O'Keefe J, Burgess N (1996) Geometric determinants of the place fields of hippocampal neurons. *Nature* 381:425–428.

O'Keefe J, Conway DH (1978) Hippocampal place units in the freely moving rat: why they fire where they fire. *Exp Brain Res* 31:573–590.

O'Keefe J, Dostrovsky J (1971) The hippocampus as a spatial map: preliminary evidence from unit activity in the freely-moving rat. *Brain Res* 34:171–175.

O'Keefe J, Nadel L (1978) *The hippocampus as a cognitive map.* Oxford, UK: Oxford University Press.

O'Keefe J, Nadel L (1979) Precis of O'Keefe and Nadel's The Hippocampus as a Cognitive Map. Behav Brain Sci 2:487–533.

O'Keefe J, Recce ML (1993) Phase relationship between hippocampal place units and the EEG theta rhythm. *Hippocampus* 3:317–330.

O'Keefe J, Speakman A (1987) Single unit activity in the rat hippocampus during a spatial memory task. *Exp Brain Res* 68:1–27.

O'Keefe J, Burgess N, Donnett JG, Jeffery KJ, Maguire EA (1998) Place cells, navigational accuracy, and the human hippocampus. *Philos Trans R Soc Lond B Biol Sci* 353:1333–1340.

O'Mara SM, Rolls ET, Berthoz A, Kesner RP (1994) Neurons responding to whole-body motion in the primate hippocampus. *J Neurosci* 14:6511–6523.

Olton DS, Branch M, Best PJ (1978) Spatial correlates of hippocampal unit activity. *Exp Neurol* 58:387–409.

Olypher AV, Lansky P, Fenton AA (2002) Properties of the extrapositional signal in hippocampal place cell discharge derived from the overdispersion in location-specific firing. *Neuroscience* 111:553–566.

Olypher AV, Klement D, Fenton AA (2006) Cognitive disorganization in hippocampus: a physiological model of the disorganization in psychosis. *J Neurosci* 26:158–168.

Ono T, Nakamura K, Nishijo H, Eifuku S (1993) Monkey hippocampal neurons related to spatial and nonspatial functions. *J Neurophysiol* 70:1516–1529.

Otto T, Eichenbaum H (1992) Neuronal activity in the hippocampus during delayed non-match to sample performance in rats: evidence for hippocampal processing in recognition memory. *Hippocampus* 2:323–334.

Pang K, Rose GM (1987) Differential effects of norepinephrine on hippocampal complex-spike and theta-neurons. *Brain Res* 425:146–158.

Pang K, Rose GM (1989a) Differential effects of methionine5-enkephalin on hippocampal pyramidal cells and interneurons. *Neuropharmacology* 28:1175–1181.

Paré D, Gaudreau H (1996) Projection cells and interneurons of the lateral and basolateral amygdala: distinct firing patterns and differential relation to theta and delta rhythms in conscious cats. *J Neurosci* 16:3334–3350.

Pavlides C, Winson J (1989) Influences of hippocampal place cell firing in the awake state on the activity of these cells during subsequent sleep episodes. *J Neurosci* 9:2907–2918.

Pavlides C, Greenstein YJ, Grudman M, Winson J (1988) Long-term potentiation in the dentate gyrus is induced preferentially on the positive phase of theta-rhythm. *Brain Res* 439:383–387.

Paz-Villagran V, Lenck-Santini PP, Save E, Poucet B (2002) Properties of place cell firing after damage to the visual cortex. *Eur J Neurosci* 16:771–776.

Pedemonte M, Pena JL, Velluti RA (1996) Firing of inferior colliculus auditory neurons is phase-locked to the hippocampus theta rhythm during paradoxical sleep and waking. *Exp Brain Res* 112:41–46.

Penick S, Solomon PR (1991) Hippocampus, context, and conditioning. *Behav Neurosci* 105:611–617.

Phillips RG, LeDoux JE (1994) Lesions of the dorsal hippocampal formation interfere with background but not foreground contextual fear conditioning. *Learn Mem* 1:34–44.

Pickenhain, L., and Klingberg, F. (1967) Hippocampal slow wave activity as a correlate of basic behavioural mechanisms in the rat. In *Progress in brain research*, Vol. 27 (Adley WR, Tokizane T, eds), pp 218–27. Elsevier, Amsterdam.

Poe GR, Nitz DA, McNaughton BL, Barnes CA (2000) Experience-dependent phase-reversal of hippocampal neuron firing during REM sleep. *Brain Res* 855:176–180.

Powell DA, Joseph JA (1974) Autonomic-somatic interaction and hippocampal theta activity. *J Comp Physiol Psychol* 87:978–986.

Qin YL, McNaughton BL, Skaggs WE, Barnes CA (1997) Memory reprocessing in corticocortical and hippocampocortical neuronal ensembles. *Philos Trans R Soc Lond B Biol Sci* 352:1525–1533.

Quirk GJ, Muller RU, Kubie JL (1990) The firing of hippocampal place cells in the dark depends on the rat's recent experience. *J Neurosci* 10:2008–2017.

Quirk GJ, Muller RU, Kubie JL, Ranck JB Jr (1992) The positional firing properties of medial entorhinal neurons: description and comparison with hippocampal place cells. *J Neurosci* 12:1945–1963.

Ranck JB (1973) Studies on single neurons in dorsal hippocampal formation and septum in unrestrained rats. I. Behavioral correlates and firing repertoires. *Exp Neurol* 41:461–531.

Ranck JB (1984) Head-direction cells in the deep cell layers of the dorsal presubiculum in freely moving rats. *Soc Neurosci Abstr* 10:599.

Rawlins JNP (1985) Associations across time: the hippocampus as a temporary memory store. *Brain Behav Sci* 8:479–496.

Redish AD, Touretzky DS (1996) Modeling interactions of the rat's place and head direction systems. In: *Neural information processing systems 8* (Touretzky DS, Mozer MC, Hasselmo ME, eds), pp 61–67. Cambridge, MA: MIT Press.

Redish AD, Battaglia FP, Chawla MK, Ekstrom AD, Gerrard JL, Lipa P, Rosenzweig ES, Worley PF, Guzowski JF, McNaughton BL, Barnes CA (2001) Independence of firing correlates of anatomically proximate hippocampal pyramidal cells. *J Neurosci* 21:RC134.

Riches IP, Wilson FA, Brown MW (1991) The effects of visual stimulation and memory on neurons of the hippocampal formation and the neighboring parahippocampal gyrus and inferior temporal cortex of the primate. *J Neurosci* 11:1763–1779.

Ringo JL, Sobotka S, Diltz MD, Bunce CM (1994) Eye movements modulate activity in hippocampal, parahippocampal, and inferotemporal neurons. *J Neurophysiol* 71:1285–1288.

Rivas J, Gaztelu JM, Garcia-Austt E (1996) Changes in hippocampal cell discharge patterns and theta rhythm spectral properties as a function of walking velocity in the guinea pig. *Exp Brain Res* 108:113–118.

Rolls ET, Cahusac PM, Feigenbaum JD, Miyashita Y (1993) Responses of single neurons in the hippocampus of the macaque related to recognition memory. *Exp Brain Res* 93:299–306.

Rolls ET, Robertson RG, Georges-Francois P (1997) Spatial view cells in the primate hippocampus. *Eur J Neurosci* 9:1789–1794.

Rose GM, Pang KC (1989) Differential effect of norepinephrine upon granule cells and interneurons in the dentate gyrus. *Brain Res* 488:353–356.

Rosenzweig ES, Barnes CA (2003) Impact of aging on hippocampal function: plasticity, network dynamics, and cognition. *Prog Neurobiol* 69:143–179.

Rosenzweig ES, Redish AD, McNaughton BL, Barnes CA (2003) Hippocampal map realignment and spatial learning. *Nat Neurosci* 6:609–615.

Rossier J, Kaminsky Y, Schenk F, Bures J (2000) The place preference task: a new tool for studying the relation between behavior and place cell activity in rats. *Behav Neurosci* 114:273–284.

Rotenberg A, Mayford M, Hawkins RD, Kandel ER, Muller RU (1996) Mice expressing activated CaMKII lack low frequency LTP and do not form stable place cells in the CA1 region of the hippocampus. *Cell* 87:1351–1361.

Rotenberg A, Abel T, Hawkins RD, Kandel ER, Muller RU (2000) Parallel instabilities of long-term potentiation, place cells, and learning caused by decreased protein kinase A activity. *J Neurosci* 20:8096–8102.

Russell NA, Horii A, Smith PF, Darlington CL, Bilkey DK (2003) Long-term effects of permanent vestibular lesions on hippocampal spatial firing. *J Neurosci* 23:6490–6498.

Sainsbury RS, Harris JL, Rowland GL (1987a) Sensitization and hippocampal type 2 theta in the rat. *Physiol Behav* 41:489–493.

Sainsbury RS, Heynen A, Montoya CP (1987b) Behavioral correlates of hippocampal type 2 theta in the rat. *Physiol Behav* 39:513–519.

Salzmann E, Vidyasagar TR, Creutzfeldt OD (1993) Functional comparison of neuronal properties in the primate posterior hippocampus and parahippocampus (area TF/TH) during different behavioral paradigms involving memory and selective attention. *Behav Brain Res* 53:133–149.

Save E, Cressant A, Thinus-Blanc C, Poucet B (1998) Spatial firing of hippocampal place cells in blind rats. *J Neurosci* 18: 1818–1826.

Save E, Nerad L, Poucet B (2000) Contribution of multiple sensory information to place field stability in hippocampal place cells. *Hippocampus* 10:64–76.

Save E, Paz-Villagran V, Alexinsky T, Poucet B (2005) Functional interaction between the associative parietal cortex and hippocampal place cell firing in the rat. *Eur J Neurosci* 21:522–530.

Schenk F (1985) Development of place navigation in rats from weaning to puberty. *Behav Neural Biol* 43:69–85.

Seidenbecher T, Laxmi TR, Stork O, Pape HC (2003) Amygdalar and hippocampal theta rhythm synchronization during fear memory retrieval. *Science* 301:846–850.

Shapiro ML, Tanila H, Eichenbaum H (1997) Cues that hippocampal place cells encode: dynamic and hierarchical representation of local and distal stimuli. *Hippocampus* 7:624–642.

Sharp PE (1996) Multiple spatial/behavioral correlates for cells in the rat postsubiculum: multiple regression analysis and comparison to other hippocampal areas. *Cereb Cortex* 6:238–259.

Sharp PE (1997) Subicular cells generate similar spatial firing patterns in two geometrically and visually distinctive environments: comparison with hippocampal place cells. *Behav Brain Res* 85:71–92.

Sharp PE (1999a) Comparison of the timing of hippocampal and subicular spatial signals: implications for path integration. *Hippocampus* 9:158–172.

Sharp PE (1999b) Subicular place cells expand or contract their spatial firing pattern to fit the size of the environment in an open field but not in the presence of barriers: comparison with hippocampal place cells. *Behav Neurosci* 113:643–662.

Sharp PE, Green C (1994) Spatial correlates of firing patterns of single cells in the subiculum of the freely moving rat. *J Neurosci* 14:2339–2356.

Sharp PE, Blair HT, Etkin D, Tzanetos DB (1995) Influences of vestibular and visual motion information on the spatial firing patterns of hippocampal place cells. *J Neurosci* 15:173–189.

Sharp PE, Tinkelman A, Cho J (2001) Angular velocity and head direction signals recorded from the dorsal tegmental nucleus of gudden in the rat: implications for path integration in the head direction cell circuit. *Behav Neurosci* 115:571–588.

Siapas AG, Wilson MA (1998) Coordinated interactions between hippocampal ripples and cortical spindles during slow-wave sleep. *Neuron* 21:1123–1128.

Siapas AG, Lubenov EV, Wilson MA (2005) Prefrontal phase locking to hippocampal theta oscillations. *Neuron* 46:141–151.

Sinclair BR, Seto MG, Bland BH (1982) Theta-cells in CA1 and dentate layers of hippocampal formation: relations to slow-wave activity and motor behavior in the freely moving rabbit. *J Neurophysiol* 48:1214–1225.

Singer W, Gray CM (1995) Visual feature integration and the temporal correlation hypothesis. *Annu Rev Neurosci* 18:555–586.

Sinnamon HM (2000) Priming pattern determines the correlation between hippocampal theta activity and locomotor stepping elicited by stimulation in anesthetized rats. *Neuroscience* 98:459–470.

Sinnamon HM, Jassen AK, Ilch C (2000) Hippocampal theta activity and facilitated locomotor stepping produced by GABA injections in the midbrain raphe region. *Behav Brain Res* 107:93–103.

Skaggs WE, McNaughton BL (1996) Replay of neuronal firing sequences in rat hippocampus during sleep following spatial experience. *Science* 271:1870–1873.

Skaggs WE, McNaughton BL, Wilson MA, Barnes CA (1996) Theta phase precession in hippocampal neuronal populations and the compression of temporal sequences. *Hippocampus* 6: 149–172.

Slawinska U, Kasicki S (1995) Theta-like rhythm in depth EEG activity of hypothalamic areas during spontaneous or electrically induced locomotion in the rat. *Brain Res* 678:117–126.

Slawinska U, Kasicki S (1998) The frequency of rat's hippocampal theta rhythm is related to the speed of locomotion. *Brain Res* 796:327–331.

Sobotka S, Nowicka A, Ringo JL (1997) Activity linked to externally cued saccades in single units recorded from hippocampal, parahippocampal, and inferotemporal areas of macaques. *J Neurophysiol* 78:2156–2163.

Speakman A, O'Keefe J (1990) Hippocampal complex spike cells do not change their place fields if the goal is moved within a cue controlled environment. *Eur J Neurosci* 7:544–555.

Stackman RW, Taube JS (1997) Firing properties of head direction cells in the rat anterior thalamic nucleus: dependence on vestibular input. *J Neurosci* 17:4349–4358.

Stackman RW, Taube JS (1998) Firing properties of rat lateral mammillary single units: head direction, head pitch, and angular head velocity. *J Neurosci* 18:9020–9037.

Stackman RW, Clark AS, Taube JS (2002) Hippocampal spatial representations require vestibular input. *Hippocampus* 12: 291–303.

Stewart M, Fox SE (1991) Hippocampal theta activity in monkeys. *Brain Res* 538:59–63.

Stewart M, Luo Y, Fox SE (1992) Effects of atropine on hippocampal theta cells and complex-spike cells. *Brain Res* 591:122–128.

Stickgold R, Hobson JA, Fosse R, Fosse M (2001) Sleep, learning, and dreams: off-line memory reprocessing. *Science* 294: 1052–1057.

Tamura R, Ono T, Fukuda M, Nishijo H (1991) Role of monkey hippocampus in recognition of food and nonfood. *Brain Res Bull* 27:457–461.

Tamura R, Ono T, Fukuda M, Nakamura K (1992) Spatial responsiveness of monkey hippocampal neurons to various visual and auditory stimuli. *Hippocampus* 2:307–322.

Tanila H, Shapiro M, Gallagher M, Eichenbaum H (1997a) Brain aging: changes in the nature of information coding by the hippocampus. *J Neurosci* 17:5155–5166.

Tanila H, Shapiro ML, Eichenbaum H (1997b) Discordance of spatial representation in ensembles of hippocampal place cells. *Hippocampus* 7:613–623.

Taube JS (1995a) Head direction cells recorded in the anterior thalamic nuclei of freely moving rats. *J Neurosci* 15:70–86.

Taube JS (1995b) Place cells recorded in the parasubiculum of freely moving rats. *Hippocampus* 5:569–583.

Taube JS (1998) Head direction cells and the neuropsychological basis for a sense of direction. *Prog Neurobiol* 55:225–256.

Taube JS, Burton HL (1995) Head direction cell activity monitored in a novel environment and during a cue conflict situation. *J Neurophysiol* 74:1953–1971.

Taube JS, Muller RU (1998) Comparisons of head direction cell activity in the postsubiculum and anterior thalamus of freely moving rats. *Hippocampus* 8:87–108.

Taube JS, Muller RU, Ranck JB Jr (1990a) Head-direction cells recorded from the postsubiculum in freely moving rats.

I. Description and quantitative analysis. *J Neurosci* 10: 420–435.

Taube JS, Muller RU, Ranck JB Jr (1990b) Head-direction cells recorded from the postsubiculum in freely moving rats. II. Effects of environmental manipulations. *J Neurosci* 10: 436–447.

Tesche CD, Karhu J (2000) Theta oscillations index human hippocampal activation during a working memory task. *Proc Natl Acad Sci USA* 97:919–924.

Thompson LT, Best PJ (1989) Place cells and silent cells in the hippocampus of freely-behaving rats. *J Neurosci* 9:2382–2390.

Thompson RF (1976) The search for the engram. *Am Psychol* 31:209–227.

Tsien JZ, Huerta PT, Tonegawa S (1996) The essential role of hippocampal CA1 NMDA receptor-dependent synaptic plasticity in spatial memory. *Cell* 87:1327–1338.

Vanderwolf CH (1969) Hippocampal electrical activity and voluntary movement in the rat. *Electroencephalogr Clin Neurophysiol* 26:407–418.

Vanderwolf CH (2001) The hippocampus as an olfacto-motor mechanism: were the classical anatomists right after all? *Behav Brain Res* 127:25–47.

Vidyasagar TR, Salzmann E, Creutzfeldt OD (1991) Unit activity in the hippocampus and the parahippocampal temporobasal association cortex related to memory and complex behavior in the awake monkey. *Brain Res* 544:269–278.

Vinogradova OS, Brazhnik ES (1977) Neuronal aspects of septo-hippocampal relations *Ciba Found Symp* 145–177.

Wallenstein GV, Eichenbaum H, Hasselmo ME (1998) The hippocampus as an associator of discontiguous events. *Trends Neurosci* 21:317–323.

Watanabe T, Niki H (1985) Hippocampal unit activity and delayed response in the monkey. *Brain Res* 325:241–254.

Weiss C, Kronforst-Collins MA, Disterhoft JF (1996) Activity of hippocampal pyramidal neurons during trace eyeblink conditioning. *Hippocampus* 6:192–209.

Wesierska M, Dockery C, Fenton AA (2005) Beyond memory, navigation, and inhibition: behavioral evidence for hippocampus-dependent cognitive coordination in the rat. *J Neurosci* 25:2413–2419.

Whishaw IQ, Vanderwolf CH (1971) Hippocampal EEG and behavior: effects of variation in body temperature and relation of EEG to vibrissae movement, swimming and shivering. *Physiol Behav* 6:391–397.

Whishaw IQ, Vanderwolf CH (1973) Hippocampal EEG and behavior: changes in amplitude and frequency of RSA (theta rhythm) associated with spontaneous and learned movement patterns in rats and cats. *Behav Biol* 8:461–484.

Wiebe SP, Staubli UV (1999) Dynamic filtering of recognition memory codes in the hippocampus. *J Neurosci* 19:10562–10574.

Wiener SI (1993) Spatial and behavioral correlates of striatal neurons in rats performing a self-initiated navigation task. *J Neurosci* 13:3802–3817.

Wiener SI, Paul CA, Eichenbaum H (1989) Spatial and behavioral correlates of hippocampal neuronal activity. *J Neurosci* 9:2737–2763.

Wiener SI, Korshunov VA, Garcia R, Berthoz A (1995) Inertial, substratal and landmark cue control of hippocampal CA1 place cell activity. *Eur J Neurosci* 7:2206–2219.

Wills TJ, Lever C, Cacucci F, Burgess N, O'Keefe J (2005) Attractor dynamics in the hippocampal representation of the local environment. *Science* 308:873–876.

Wilson FA, Riches IP, Brown MW (1990) Hippocampus and medial temporal cortex: neuronal activity related to behavioral responses during the performance of memory tasks by primates. *Behav Brain Res* 40:7–28.

Wilson MA, McNaughton BL (1993) Dynamics of the hippocampal ensemble code for space. *Science* 261:1055–1058.

Wilson MA, McNaughton BL (1994) Reactivation of hippocampal ensemble memories during sleep. *Science* 265:676–679.

Wirth S, Yanike M, Frank LM, Smith AC, Brown EN, Suzuki WA (2003) Single neurons in the monkey hippocampus and learning of new associations. *Science* 300:1578–1581.

Wood ER, Dudchenko PA, Eichenbaum H (1999) The global record of memory in hippocampal neuronal activity. *Nature* 397:613–616.

Wood ER, Dudchenko PA, Robitsek RJ, Eichenbaum H (2000) Hippocampal neurons encode information about different types of memory episodes occurring in the same location. *Neuron* 27:623–633.

Yamaguchi Y, Aota Y, McNaughton BL, Lipa P (2002) Bimodality of theta phase precession in hippocampal place cells in freely running rats. *J Neurophysiol* 87:2629–2642.

Ylinen A, Bragin A, Nadasdy Z, Jando G, Szabo I, Sik A, Buzsaki G (1995) Sharp wave-associated high-frequency oscillation (200 Hz) in the intact hippocampus: network and intracellular mechanisms. *J Neurosci* 15:30–46.

Zhang K (1996) Representation of spatial orientation by the intrinsic dynamics of the head-direction cell ensemble: a theory. *J Neurosci* 16:2112–2126.

Zhang K, Ginzburg I, McNaughton BL, Sejnowski TJ (1998) Interpreting neuronal population activity by reconstruction: unified framework with application to hippocampal place cells. *J Neurophysiol* 79:1017–1044.

Zinyuk L, Kubik S, Kaminsky Y, Fenton AA, Bures J (2000) Understanding hippocampal activity by using purposeful behavior: place navigation induces place cell discharge in both task-relevant and task- irrelevant spatial reference frames. *Proc Natl Acad Sci USA* 97:3771–3776.

Zugaro MB, Tabuchi E, Wiener SI (2000) Influence of conflicting visual, inertial and substratal cues on head direction cell activity. *Exp Brain Res* 133:198–208.

Zugaro MB, Berthoz A, Wiener SI (2001) Background, but not foreground, spatial cues are taken as references for head direction responses by rat anterodorsal thalamus neurons. *J Neurosci* 21:RC154.

Zugaro MB, Arleo A, Berthoz A, Wiener SI (2003) Rapid spatial reorientation and head direction cells. *J Neurosci* 23:3478–3482.

Zugaro MB, Monconduit L, Buzsaki G (2005) Spike phase precession persists after transient intrahippocampal perturbation. *Nat Neurosci* 8:67–71.

12 · Craig Stark

Functional Role of the Human Hippocampus

12.1 Overview

This chapter examines data from human amnesic patients, data from electrophysiological recordings in humans, and data from functional neuroimaging studies that attempt to shed light on the question, *What does the human hippocampus do?* In broad terms, we have learned a great deal about the kinds of memory in which the hippocampus is and is not involved. The hippocampus is part of a system that plays a critical role in the encoding and retrieval of long-term memory for facts and events. As a whole, the system is vital for this "declarative" or "explicit" form of memory but is not involved in other forms of long term memory, in nonmnemonic aspects of cognition, or in immediate (or "working") memory. Furthermore, its involvement in declarative memory is not permanent but is time-limited in nature (the bases for each of these conclusions are laid out later in the chapter).

We therefore know a great deal about the role of this system in human memory. Our understanding of the roles played by the individual components of the system is much less complete. In the human, the system is often described as consisting of two major sets of structures. One set of structures, often defined as the "hippocampal region," consists of the CA fields of the hippocampus itself, the dentate gyrus, and the subiculum. For obvious reasons, most of the studies in humans do not contain histological analyses. Unfortunately, without histological analyses, it is quite difficult to isolate these components from each other (see Sections 12.3.3 and 12.3.5), so most studies that report data from the "hippocampus" include data from the more extended hippocampal region. The second set of structures consist of the adjacent cortical structures that lie along the parahippocampal gyrus. This set consists of the entorhinal, perirhinal (occasionally divided into temporopolar and posterior regions), and parahippocampal cortices.

As is discussed here and in Chapter 13, there have been a number of attempts to arrive at a description of hippocampal function. One class of theories proposes a functional distinction that qualitatively sets the hippocampal region apart from the adjacent structures in the medial temporal lobe, defining what it is that the hippocampal region specifically does that other structures do not and vice versa. Such theories have linked the function of the hippocampal region to conjunctive (e.g., Sutherland and Rudy, 1989; O'Reilly and Rudy, 2000), relational (e.g., Cohen et al., 1997), and/or episodic, recollective, or associative (e.g., Brown and Aggleton, 2001) forms of memory. A second theory (the declarative memory hypothesis—see Chapter 13) is more quantitative in nature in suggesting that the hippocampal region "combines and extends" the processing of the adjacent cortical structures that together form the medial temporal lobe memory system (Squire and Zola-Morgan, 1991).

The conclusion on this question is that the data from human studies do not unambiguously support any of the existing theories. In particular, the data suggest differentiation of function within the medial temporal lobe but not along versions of any of the binary dissociations proposed. The differentiation of function is likely to be a complex and graded one that is most consistent with the second theory—that the hippocampal region combines and extends the processing of the adjacent cortical structures. However, this theory is still underspecified, as we do not have the data at hand to understand the precise nature of the way in which the hippocampus combines and extends adjacent processing or of the dynamic interplay among the structures. Thus, although we have certainly learned a great deal about the human hippocampus and its role in memory, but it would be a mistake to believe that we have a full and satisfactory answer to the fundamental question: What does the human hippocampus do?

12.2 Patient H.M.

It would be almost impossible to begin a discussion of the role of the hippocampal region in human memory without considering the patient H.M. In a successful attempt to relieve otherwise intractable epilepsy, H.M. underwent bilateral resection of the medial portions of the temporal lobe (Fig. 12–1). Although scattered hints in the literature prior to this suggested that damage to the hippocampal region might affect memory, the detailed study of H.M. had an influence on both the study of memory and on neurosurgical practice that was unprecedented. Following a brief initial report (Scoville, 1954) describing the profound memory loss that resulted from the surgery, Scoville and Milner (1957) presented a detailed neuropsychological assessment of H.M. and nine

other patients with varying degrees and locations of resection. This seminal work concluded with the following text.

> Bilateral medial temporal lobe resection in man results in a persistent impairment of recent memory whenever the removal is carried far enough posteriorly to damage portions of the anterior hippocampus and hippocampal gyrus. ... In two cases in which bilateral resection was carried to a distance of 8 cm posterior to the temporal tips the loss was particularly severe. ... The memory loss in these cases of medial temporal lobe excision involved both anterograde and some retrograde amnesia, but left early memories and technical skills intact. There was no deterioration in personality or general intelligence, and no complex perceptual disturbance such as is seen after a more complete bilateral temporal lobectomy. It is concluded that the anterior hippocampus and [para]hippocampal gyrus, either separately or together, are critically concerned in the retention of current experience. It is not known

Figure 12–1. *Top*. Extent of H.M.'s lesion is shown by comparing the coronal magnetic resonance imaging (MRI) scan of H.M. (*left*) with that of a matched healthy volunteer (*right*). The hippocampus (H), amygdala (A), collateral sulcus (CS), perirhinal cortex (PR), entorhinal cortex (EC), and medial mammillary nucleus (MMN) are identified, and all show signs of damage in H.M. *Bottom*. Summary of the extent of the lesion. Both hemispheres are damaged, with one shown intact for comparison only. (*Source*: Corkin et al., 1997, with permission. © 1997 Society for Neuroscience.)

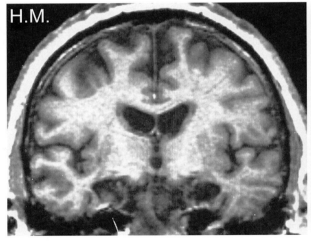
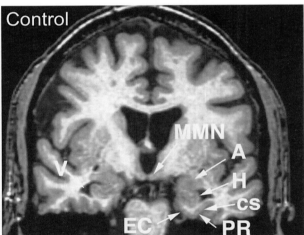

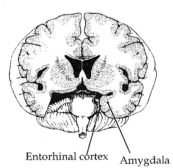
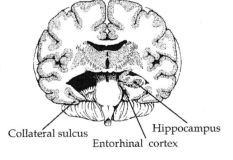
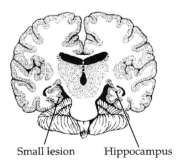

whether the amygdala plays any part in this mechanism, since the hippocampal complex has not been removed alone, but always together with uncus and amygdala. (Scoville and Milner, 1957, p. 21)

Subsequent testing of H.M. was able to reveal not only the breadth and severity of H.M.'s memory impairment but, critically, it also showed a vast array of cognitive and mnemonic function that was unaffected by his large bilateral lesion. The pattern of data allowed Milner (Milner et al., 1968; Milner, 1972) to make several conclusions that expanded on those noted above and helped lay the foundation for subsequent investigation into the amnesic syndrome.

First, Milner noted that damage to the medial portions of the temporal lobe results in profound inability to acquire long-term memory for new facts or events (anterograde amnesia) although memories from early life appear to be intact. Conversely, there was some clear loss of memory of information acquired for some time prior to the operation (retrograde amnesia). Together, these observations indicated that the medial temporal lobe might not be a permanent repository for memory but that it plays a time-limited, albeit critical, role in memory. Second, she noted that there was no loss in general intellect or perceptual ability, indicating clear dissociation between memory and other aspects of cog-

nition. Third, she noted that short-term memory remained intact, indicating clear dissociation between immediate, or "working," memory and permanent, long-term memory. Finally, she noted that damage to the medial portions of the temporal lobe did not abolish all forms of long-term learning and memory, indicating that the medial temporal lobes were not required for at least some forms of long-term memory (Fig. 12–2).

Overall, subsequent data from severely amnesic patients such as H.M. and data from animal models of amnesia (see Chapter 13) have supported Milner's basic conclusions rather well (although there is still no consensus as to whether each claim is entirely or only largely true). In a more recent extension of these conclusions, Squire and Zola-Morgan (1991) identified what they referred to as a medial temporal lobe memory system (MTL), consisting of the hippocampal region (defined as the CA fields of the hippocampus proper, the dentate gyrus, and the subiculum) and the adjacent entorhinal, perirhinal, and parahippocampal cortices (which together form the parahippocampal gyrus—see Chapter 3). Together, this system is posited to be critically involved in the acquisition of new fact ("semantic") and event ("episodic") memory. Notably, this system is not the permanent storage site for this "declarative" or "explicit" memory, nor is it the locus of other cognitive functions or other forms of memory. For example, it

Figure 12–2. Patient H.M.'s performance on the Rey-Osterreith figure-drawing task (*top*). With the original drawing in front of him, his direct copy is accurate, demonstrating intact perceptual abilities and a range of intact cognitive abilities. After an hour delay, H.M. was unable to produce any drawing and did not remember having previously seen and copied the figure. (Data provided by Suzanne Corkin, personal communication, March 6, 2005.) In contrast, H.M. showed learning that lasted over multiple days in the mirror-drawing task (*bottom*). A typical stimulus is shown on the left. Participants view the shape in a mirror and attempt to trace the shape while staying inside the lines (gray line shows the author's first attempt). H.M.'s performance improved steadily both within testing sessions and across 3 days of testing (right), despite having no conscious memory of having performed the task on previous days. (Source: Adapted from Milner et al., 1998, with permission. © 1998 Elsevier.)

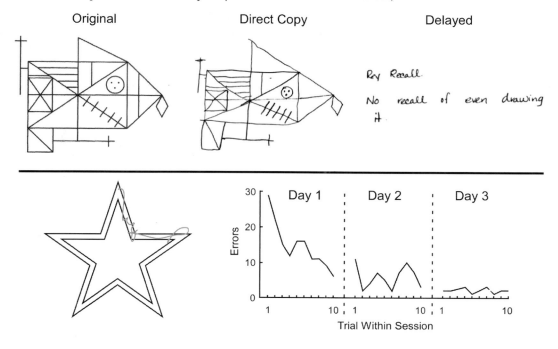

is not involved in immediate (or "working") memory, and it is not involved in a wide range of "nondeclarative" (or "implicit") long-term memory tasks (e.g., delay conditioning, perceptual repetition priming, habit learning). These ideas amplify and develop Milner's suppositions in several ways.

As a component of this interconnected system, the hippocampal region participates in declarative memory in some way. However, the exact nature or particular memory functions in which it participates cannot be unambiguously determined from patients such as H.M. or other severely amnesic patients with extensive damage to the medial temporal lobes or from animal models with analogous lesions. Thus, knowing that H.M. is impaired regarding tasks of recognition memory (e.g., Milner et al., 1968) or that a similar patient (E.P.) is entirely at chance during tests of recognition memory (Hamann and Squire, 1997; Stark and Squire, 2000b; Stefanacci et al., 2000) does not definitively implicate the hippocampal region in recognition memory (or any other individual MTL region, as the entire MTL is extensively damaged). Indeed, many researchers have proposed functional dissociations within the MTL such that extrahippocampal structures (e.g., perirhinal cortex) support recognition memory (or at least one form of recognition memory) and that the hippocampal region is not involved in recognition memory tasks (see Section 12.4.5). Of course, the study of what is not impaired in patients with more extensive damage (e.g., H.M. or E.P.) can be informative as well in letting us determine what forms of memory do not require the hippocampal region (see Section 12.4.1).

To move beyond an understanding of what is and what is not impaired overall in the amnesia that follows damage to the medial temporal lobe to an understanding of the specific contributions of the components of the MTL (e.g., the hippocampus), we must shift our focus. We must turn our study to patients (and animals) with lesions to specific structures of the medial temporal lobe and to recording or imaging techniques that allow us to measure signals confidently from these structures. Three sources of such data exist for studying the human hippocampus. First, anoxia or ischemia can lead to fairly selective bilateral damage to the hippocampal region. Although this damage is incomplete and although anoxia is by no means certain to damage only the hippocampus (see Section 12.3.3), when it does the study of the memory impairments in such patients can inform our understanding of the role of the hippocampus itself. Second, advances in diagnostic techniques for localization of epileptic seizure foci have led to several cases in which depth electrodes have been placed into the hippocampal region and recordings made during various memory tasks. The study of such patients provides a clear bridge between electrophysiology in animal models (e.g., rats or nonhuman primates) and studies of the human hippocampus. Finally, recent advances in noninvasive neuroimaging techniques have led to several methods by which correlates of neural activity can be localized with sufficient precision to differentiate signals from the components of the MTL. In particular, positron emission tomography (PET) and functional magnetic resonance imaging (fMRI) have become popular tools for noninvasive monitoring of neural activity (in the form of local blood flow or oxygenation) throughout the brain. When data analysis techniques are applied that respect and account for the morphological variability of MTL structures across individuals, fMRI data in particular can provide highly valuable data for understanding normal human hippocampal function (see Section 12.3.5).

What follows is first an overview of these methods, with particular attention to their strengths and limitations for the study of the human hippocampus. This serves as the background for the rest of the chapter, which focuses on the function of the human hippocampus. Particular attention is paid to the role of the hippocampus in declarative memory and how it might be functionally dissociated from the adjacent cortical structures of the parahippocampal gyrus.

12.3 Methods for Studying Human Hippocampal Function

Each of the three sources of data discussed in the following sections (hippocampal lesions, electrophysiology via depth electrodes, functional neuroimaging) has its own particular strengths and limitations in providing data to help us understand the function of the human hippocampus. Moreover, none of them can produce meaningful insight into understanding hippocampal function without an understanding of the behavioral tasks used to assess memory performance. As such, the cognitive and behavioral tasks used to assess memory in humans are discussed first. In addition, none of the three methods alone is sufficiently free of limitations to be able to answer the fundamental questions surrounding the hippocampus. In Chapter 13, general theoretical concerns from these lines of data are discussed (e.g., the interpretation of correlational datasets—see also Henson, 2005), but several specific concerns exist for each. These strengths and weaknesses are discussed below (see Sections 12.3.3–12.3.5).

12.3.1 Behavioral Tasks and Terms

Unlike assessing memory in nonverbal animals, assessing memory performance in humans (or at least adult humans) can be exceptionally straightforward. If we want to know whether a participant remembers a previously seen list of items, we can simply ask him or her to recall as many items as possible. The simplicity of this *free recall* task and the fact that it is an obvious test of human memory but not of animal memory should not be overlooked. No training on the task is required, as it is perhaps the archetypal everyday memory task. Despite the prevalence of free recall, or its cousin *cued recall* (in which some portion of the to-be-remembered item is provided) in everyday life, neither task is easily captured in animal studies of memory.

A second style of memory task, called a *recognition memory* task, is more easily captured in animal models. Like tests of recall, recognition memory tasks begin with a study phase that can either be *intentional* (participants are explicitly instructed to learn the item for a later test) or *incidental* (no instructions are given to learn the items and no mention is made of a later test, often using an entirely unrelated task to serve as a disguise). During the test phase, unlike recall tasks, entire items from the study list (*target* or *old* items) and entire items that were not on the study list (*foil* or *new* items) are presented. In the simplest version of a recognition memory task, *yes/no recognition*, single items (either targets or foils) are presented to the participant with the instructions to indicate whether each item was on the study list. In a second typical version, *two-alternative forced-choice recognition*, a target item and a foil item are presented, and the participant is instructed to indicate which of the two items was on the study list.

In making their responses to recognition memory probes, participants are thought to use two types of memory or sources of information: *recollection* and *familiarity* (for review see Yonelinas, 2002). Recollection provides information about a specific prior event or episode and gives one the sense of being placed back in that moment in time. Certainly, if this is the reaction one has to an item presented during a recognition memory task, the item is endorsed as having been on the study list. In contrast, one can still have a strong sense that the item is familiar without having a recollective experience. Such a feeling that the item is familiar, albeit with no specific information about the study episode, can still lead to endorsing the item in a recognition memory test. Thus, two sources of information can be used when endorsing an item at time of recognition. A variant on the yes/no recognition memory task, known as the *Remember/Know* task (Tulving, 1985), asks participants to split their endorsements into recollective ("Remember") and familiarity-based ("Know") responses in an attempt to isolate the two sources of information.

A key question that arises when discussing recollection and familiarity is whether these two types of information represent the operation of two separate neural systems. If they do, a second question that arises is whether this functional dissociation maps onto a division of labor in the medial temporal lobe: for example, that the hippocampus is particularly involved in recollective-based memory and the structures of the adjacent parahippocampal gyrus are particularly involved in familiarity-based memory. This possibility is discussed in Section 12.4.5.

Many variations on these basic tasks exist, each designed to assess different kinds of memory. For example, for a *paired-associates* task two stimuli are presented and the participant is instructed to learn the association between the two items. For the test, a single item can be presented and the participant asked to recall the target member of the pair (cued recall) or to pick out the target item from a list of choices that include one or more foil items (forced-choice recognition). Furthermore, pairs of items can be presented at the test that are either intact or recombined versions of the studied pairs. As such, each trial presents only familiar components, and performance must be governed by memory for the associations between the individual items. Finally, just as the study phase can be conducted in an incidental way, the test phase can be an incidental test of memory. For example, participants may be asked to complete the word-beginning *win____* with the first word that comes to mind (*stem-completion task*), making no reference to the prior study episode. Such *implicit*, or *non-declarative*, tests of memory are forms of long-term memory that do not appear to rely upon the MTL (see Section 12.4.1).

12.3.2 Behavioral Measures

In any of these tasks, performance can be quantified in several ways. The most straightforward is to calculate an overall percent correct—simply the percentage of correct trials out of the total number of trials. In a yes/no recognition task with 20 target items and 20 foil items, 16 correct "yes" responses to the targets and 16 correct "no" responses to foil items would result in 80% correct (Table 12–1). Although quite straightforward and intuitive, percent correct has significant difficulty in accurately capturing the underlying strength of the memory when participants exhibit a strong bias toward one response. An uneven distribution of "yes" and "no" responses can arise quite easily from either natural individual participant biases or task instruction and result in an underestimation of the true

Table 12–1.
Comparison of Various Measures of Recognition Memory Performance

Memory capability	Hits (rate)	False alarms (rate)	% Correct	Pr	Br	d'
Normal	16 (0.8)	4 (0.2)	80	0.6	0.5	1.7
Normal, "no" bias	10 (0.5)	1 (0.05)	72	0.45	0.1	1.6
Normal, "yes" bias	19 (0.95)	10 (0.5)	72	0.45	0.9	1.6
Moderate	14 (0.7)	6 (0.3)	70	0.4	0.5	1.0
Chance	10 (0.5)	10 (0.5)	50	0	0.5	0
Chance, "yes" bias	16 (0.8)	16 (0.8)	50	0	0.5	0

Typical behavioral measures—hit rate, false alarm rate, percent correct, "corrected rejection" (Pr), "bias" (Br), and "discriminability" (d')—are shown for three levels of underlying memory capability (Normal, unimpaired memory; Moderate, mildly impaired memory; Chance, no actual memory); and under conditions of response biases.

strength of the memory. For example, if one were to reward participants with a small sum of money for each correct "yes" response but administer a strong shock for each incorrect "yes" response, participants would be generally less likely to respond "yes" and do so only when they are quite confident they are accurate. In our above example, this might reduce the correct "yes" responses to 10 and increase the correct "no" responses to 19, with a resulting percent correct of 72%. There is good reason to believe, however, that the actual memory is the same in these two cases, and this change in response rates is the result of a shift in the participant's response bias.

Several measures are commonly used to measure or remove the detrimental effect of response biases. Response biases can be easily seen by dividing the recognition responses into four categories: (1) *hits*, defined as correct "yes" responses to studied target items; (2) *misses*, defined as incorrect "no" responses to studied target items; (3) *correct rejections*, defined as correct "no" responses to unstudied foil items; and (4) *false alarms*, defined as incorrect "yes" responses to unstudied foil items. Comparing the hit rate and correct rejection rate is one method for determining whether a bias is present. A second method uses the "corrected recognition" score, often denoted *Pr*. *Pr* is simply the probability of a correct "yes" response (a "hit") minus the probability of an incorrect "yes" response (a "false alarm"). *Pr* scores are in a range between 0 and 1, with 0 indicating chance performance. By themselves, *Pr* scores do not fully remove the effects of response biases; however, a complementary measure of bias, *Br*, accurately estimates any response bias that exists.

$$Br = \text{false alarm rate} \div (1 - Pr)$$

The most common method to correct for any bias that exists is to calculate d', the discriminability measure from the signal detection theory (Green and Swets, 1966). Here, it is assumed that there are two normal distributions of stimuli (a distribution of targets and a distribution of foils) that differ along a single parameter (e.g., some representation of perceived memory strength or familiarity at time of retrieval). It is further assumed that participants set a threshold or criterion value for this single parameter and respond "yes" if the stimulus presented for recognition exceeds this threshold and "no" if the stimulus does not exceed this threshold. Thus, there are four categories of responses corresponding to the hits, misses, correct rejections, and false alarms defined above.

With respect to memory tasks, the amount of memory present is viewed as the distance between the target and the foil distributions along this axis of familiarity (e.g., Morrell et al., 2002). That is, the effect of studying the target stimuli is to shift the distribution away from the unstudied distribution. The amount it has been shifted corresponds to the amount of memory the participant has for the studied items. If the distribution has been shifted a lot, it is easy to discriminate the target from the foil distributions, whereas if the distribution has been shifted very little, it is more difficult to discriminate whether a given item presented at test was drawn from the target or foil distribution. The measure d' is the distance between the two distributions and, as such, does not depend on where the participant decides to set the criterion threshold. Values of zero represent no memory, and positive values represent accurate memory (negative values indicate a propensity to say "yes" to foil items and "no" to target items and, when reliable, indicate reliably below-chance performance). Different thresholds result in different biases (different propensities to respond "yes" or "no") but merely represent different values of this single parameter that are used to threshold both distributions. As such, d' can index memory in a manner that is independent of individual response biases.

Finally, one more means of quantification must be discussed because simply knowing the overall percent correct or d' in a memory task only tells a part of the story. For example, if we measured recognition memory performance in a task and obtained an average of 85% correct for a group of healthy control participants and 75% correct for a patient with damage to the hippocampus, it is still unclear whether this patient's performance is impaired. If the control participants' scores ranged from 80% to 90%, the patient is likely to be truly impaired, but if the control scores ranged from 60% to 100%, the participant is likely to be performing at a normal level.

In addition to the ubiquitous *t*-tests and analyses of variance (ANOVAs) used throughout behavioral testing, analysis by *z-scores* is prevalent in the memory literature and in particular in the analysis of small numbers of memory-impaired patients covered in Section 12.4. A z-score is simply the number of standard deviations away from the mean a given observation lies. As such, it gives a way to determine how aberrant a single observation is (e.g., a single amnesic patient's recognition memory score). Critically, this analysis relies on an accurate estimate of both the average performance of the control population and an accurate estimate of the variance in control performance. A z-score of 0 represents performance equal to the mean of the control population. A z-score of ± 1.0 corresponds to a likelihood that the patient's score was, in fact, drawn from the normal population (alpha level, two-tailed) of 0.32. A z-score of ± 1.96 has this probability drop to the traditional threshold of significance (0.05).

12.3.3 Anoxia and Bilateral Hippocampal Lesions

Neuropsychology—study of the relation between brain and behavior—has a long history of studying the cognitive and behavioral results of brain lesions and using this information to help understand the function of specific brain regions. Many common etiologies, and even many etiologies that produce memory impairments, do not provide data that cleanly isolate hippocampal function. For example, although a common and valuable source of neuropsychological data, patients who have suffered damage due to stroke are not common sources of restricted bilateral hippocampal damage, as the vasculature does not provide a mechanism for selective bilateral hippocampal damage. For example, although rupture or blockage of the posterior communicating artery often results

Direct Copy

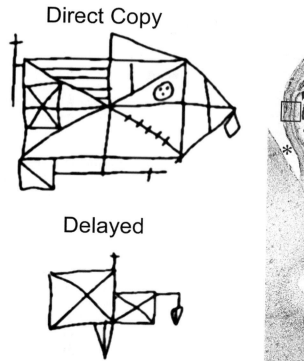

Delayed

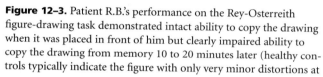

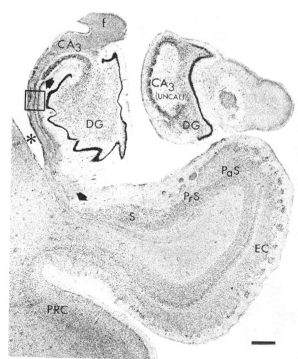

Figure 12–3. Patient R.B.'s performance on the Rey-Osterreith figure-drawing task demonstrated intact ability to copy the drawing when it was placed in front of him but clearly impaired ability to copy the drawing from memory 10 to 20 minutes later (healthy controls typically indicate the figure with only very minor distortions at this delay). Postmortem histological analyses revealed his anoxic episode resulted in severe cell loss limited to the CA1 fields of the left and right hippocampus (left shown). Location and extent of damage are indicated by the asterisk and arrows. (Source: Zola-Morgan et al., 1986, with permission. © 1986 by the Society for Neuroscience.)

in MTL damage (and amnesia), the damage is not restricted to the hippocampus and is unilateral. Thus, although stroke or aneurysm can lead to memory impairment, it does not give us the most powerful means of assessing hippocampal function.

Similarly, although physical infarct can lead to amnesia (e.g., the case of N.A. who suffered mammillary body damage following an accident involving a miniature fencing foil), it is hard to imagine how a physical infarct would selectively lesion the hippocampus bilaterally given the physical location of the hippocampus buried within the MTL. Alzheimer's disease does result in bilateral damage to the hippocampus, but it also results in damage to the entorhinal cortex and damage outside the MTL (particularly as it progresses). The thiamine deficiency associated with chronic alcohol abuse and Korsakoff's disease results in diencephalic damage and amnesia. Many highly informative and influential studies of amnesia have been conducted with patients suffering from Korsakoff's disease (e.g., the seminal work of Warrington and Weiskrantz, 1968). However, as with patient N.A., it is clear that the damage suffered in such patients does not allow us to isolate the function of the hippocampus itself.

In contrast, anoxia (reduction in oxygen) and ischemia (reduction in blood flow) have the potential to damage the hippocampal region selectively and bilaterally. Such cases, even if quite rare, can prove to be highly informative. Several patients have been reported to show quantifiable bilateral damage to the hippocampal region, little or no damage outside the hippocampal region, and behavior consistent with the amnesic syndrome after anoxic or ischemic episodes (Cummings et al., 1984; Zola-Morgan et al., 1986; Rempel-Clower et al., 1996; Spiers et al., 2001; Hopkins et al., 2004). In one such case, that of R.B. (Zola-Morgan et al., 1986) (Fig. 12–3), postmortem histological analysis confirmed that the damage was almost entirely limited to the CA1 field of the hippocampus with only minor damage observed elsewhere (and located outside the MTL).

The presence of these cases does not indicate that anoxia or ischemia necessarily result in selective damage to the hippocampus. Although histological analyses such as R.B.'s are rarely available (and only postmortem), even relatively basic MRI techniques have been shown to correlate with postmortem analyses of hippocampal damage, albeit at a coarser resolution and potentially with less sensitivity (Rempel-Clower et al., 1996). Using current quantitative MRI techniques, a study of anoxia resulting from carbon monoxide poisoning and obstructive sleep apnea (Gale and Hopkins, 2004) reported that only 30% to 36% of the patients were observed to have hippocampal damage. Cortical atrophy (in the form of the ventricle/brain ratio) was present in 35% of the patients with damage resulting from carbon monoxide poisoning. Furthermore, in a review of 43 patients with damage following anoxia (Caine and Watson, 2000), 32 showed evidence of cortical damage and 31 showed evidence of damage to the pallidum or striatum. The hippocampal region was only the third most common site of damage (30 cases). Damage was also reported commonly in the basal ganglia and the thalamus. Most strikingly, in only 18% of these anoxic cases (8/43) was the damage present in and limited to the hippocampal region.

Thus, it should be quite clear that the study of patients with damage resulting from anoxia or ischemia does not necessarily imply the study of selective hippocampal damage or even hippocampal damage at all. To use anoxic patients as a route to studying the consequences of hippocampal damage, detailed structural neuroimaging assessment of the damage (whenever possible) and detailed neuropsychological assessment of their behavior is certainly required. Improved techniques for quantifying damage and for addressing the possibility of "covert" damage not resolved by current techniques are certainly warranted as well. In particular, detailed comparison of postmortem histological analyses and premorbid neuroimaging analyses are required to improve and further validate the neuroimaging analyses. However, even if current neuroimaging techniques do not provide a definitive assessment of the damage, they are infinitely better than assessing damage merely by etiology, as the above review has shown. Unfortunately, although assessments to the best of current standards have been done for some of studies of memory, they have certainly not been done for all.

12.3.4 Depth Electrode Recordings

Implanting electrodes and recording from neurons in the hippocampal region and adjacent cortical structures has been a common technique for studying rodents and nonhuman primates (see Chapter 13), but electrophysiology has not been used extensively to study the human hippocampal region for obvious reasons. There have been a number of cases, however, in which depth electrodes have been placed in the human MTL to help identify the topography of epileptic seizures when other techniques for neurosurgical planning have not proved sufficient. In a limited number of these cases, single-unit recordings from the depth electrodes have been made during various explicit memory tasks (Heit et al., 1988, 1990; Fried et al., 1997, 2002; Fernandez et al., 1999b, 2002; Kreiman et al., 2000; Cameron et al., 2001; Paller and McCarthy, 2002; Fell et al., 2003) (Fig. 12–4).

Such data are certainly highly important, but they are also scarce. Unfortunately, the scarcity of the data extends not only to the small number of studies but to the small number of recordings per participant in these studies. In electrophysiological studies of the monkey hippocampus, one can expect to see data collected from 50 to 100 hippocampal neurons in each monkey (e.g., Wirth et al., 2003). In depth electrode recordings on humans, one may see data from this same number of neurons (e.g., Fried et al., 2002), but they are spread across a large number of participants, yielding single-digit numbers per participant. This is a limitation of the methodology, not of the experimenters, as multiple electrode drops and

Figure 12–4. Electrophysiological data in the human. *Left panel.* Trajectory of a depth electrode with microwires placed in the hippocampus (arrow indicates where wires protrude from electrode). Both peri-event spike-train histograms (middle) and field potentials (right) can be collected from such electrodes. *Middle panel.* A hippocampal neuron recorded from the electrode indicated on the left demonstrates an increase in activity at retrieval upon presentation of

the cue item in a paired-associate task. (*Source*: Left and middle panels: Cameron et al., 2001, with permission. © 2001 Elsevier. Right panel: Paller and McCarthy, 2002, with permission. © 2002 Wiley-Liss, a subsidiary of John Wiley & Sons.) *Right panel.* Field potentials from electrodes in the posterior portion of the hippocampus are shown for three patients demonstrating differences in activity for the sample and match phases of a delayed match-to-sample task.

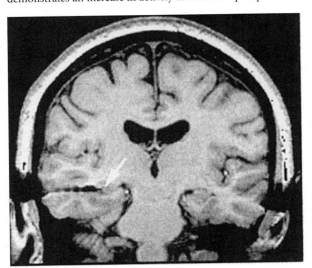

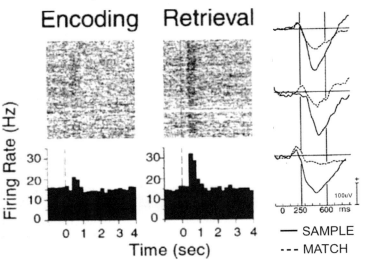

continual adjustment of the electrode location or even initial placement of the electrode to isolate as many hippocampal neurons as possible is not an option. The electrode placement must be motivated by the neurosurgical planning of which these data are a by-product.

Furthermore, we must remember that the recordings are coming from brains that are decidedly not normal. The recordings are being made from patients with epilepsy severe enough to warrant neurosurgical intervention that is most likely going to target the medial temporal lobes. Whether and how this affects the data cannot be known at present. To address this concern, data are often analyzed only from sites in the unoperated hemisphere or otherwise distant from the epileptic foci.

12.3.5 Neuroimaging

The initial set of neuroimaging studies exploring memory and the medial temporal lobe using either PET or fMRI presented a mixed set of results. There were a number of initial PET studies with positive reports of MTL activity during memory tasks (e.g., Squire et al., 1992; Grasby et al., 1993; Nyberg et al., 1995; Schacter et al., 1995). However, at the time there were also a sizable number of studies that observed memory-related activity outside the MTL but no memory-related activity in the MTL itself (e.g., Kapur et al., 1994; Shallice et al., 1994; Tulving et al., 1994; Buckner et al., 1995). For example, Shallice et al. (1994) contrasted activity during word-pair encoding and cued recall with activity during a low-level baseline control task (e.g., hearing the pair "one thousand, two thousand" repeatedly). Although the contrasts revealed numerous regions of brain activity (e.g., prefrontal cortex), no MTL activity was present. As both contrast activity during what are clearly mnemonic tasks that are impaired in amnesic patients with activity during tasks that have no mnemonic demands and that are not impaired in amnesic patients, the negative results were unsettling. Many hypotheses for the unreliability of findings were put forth, such as the idea that the MTL might always be active (thus reducing the contrast between states) or that MTL signals may be too weak to resolve (resulting from either poor imaging signals from the MTL or inherently weak activity). It was even suggested that the MTL might not be involved in long-term memory after all.

Developments in neuroimaging techniques and further studies have now led to many positive results, supporting the former two hypotheses (and several new ones as well) but not the latter. In fact, as of this writing, more than 1300 articles indexed by PubMed during the last 5 years contained the key words "fMRI" and "hippocampus" or "medial temporal lobe." The numbers would certainly be significantly higher if other neuroimaging techniques were included. The popularity of neuroimaging attests to the fact that it can provide useful data to further our understanding of the neural mechanisms that underlie memory.

However, although useful and compelling data can be obtained using neuroimaging techniques, these techniques have constraints and challenges that place limits on what one can conclude from their results. If the challenges are well met and experiments designed and interpreted with the constraints clearly kept in mind, neuroimaging studies can be highly informative (Henson, 2005). If they are not, they can present a confusing or conflicting state of affairs (much as was present at the time of the early studies).

The first constraint is that, on the whole, neuroimaging and electrical recording techniques provide correlational data and cannot provide evidence as to the necessity (or even actual use of) a structure in a particular function. For example, although single-unit recording shows strong hippocampal activity during delay eyeblink conditioning in the rabbit (e.g., Berger et al., 1980) and activity has similarly been observed in humans using PET (e.g., Blaxton et al., 1996), complete bilateral lesions of the hippocampus do not impair acquisition or expression of the response (e.g., Mauk and Thompson, 1987; Clark and Squire, 1998). Therefore, the activity observed in a region may be incidental to the task at hand or may be the result of processing in another region that has projections into the observed area. Whereas the use of parametric designs or other clever experimental manipulations that attempt to link imaging data to specific components of behavior (e.g., the recent attempts to link MTL activity to aspects of implicit tasks reported by Rose et al., 2002 and Schendan et al., 2003) can provide stronger evidence for a causal link than the use of simpler designs, neuroimaging data cannot be resolute in this regard.

A second problem faced by neuroimaging techniques is the lack of a baseline. Although particularly problematic for BOLD (blood oxygenation level-dependent) fMRI (Fig. 12–5), which has a signal with an arbitrary offset and arbitrary units of measurement, the lack of a clearly defined level of activity associated with a region not being involved in a task is endemic to all neuroimaging techniques. (How many spikes per second constitute "no activity" in the neuron, and what is an animal actually doing when this is assessed?) Neuroimaging techniques are contrastive in nature. Our data take the form of a higher BOLD fMRI signal, greater regional cerebral blood flow (rCBF), more spikes per second, a steeper excitatory postsynaptic potential (EPSP) slope, or a sharper tuning function during task A than during task B. These numbers can often be quantified and varied parametrically, but it is frequently difficult to interpret a result "zero activity." This contrasts with behavioral data. For example, in two alternative forced choice recognition, scores necessarily vary between chance and 100%; and for free recall, performance necessarily varies between 0% and 100%. Where there may be floor and ceiling effects to consider, one can, in principle, identify both perfect memory and absent memory.

As noted, this lack of a standard of comparison may be especially problematic for BOLD fMRI with its arbitrary units and its complete lack of an estimate of what measurement "zero activity" in a region should be. For example, Stark and Squire (2001b) have shown that when randomly interspersed 3-second periods of rest were used as a baseline to assess "zero

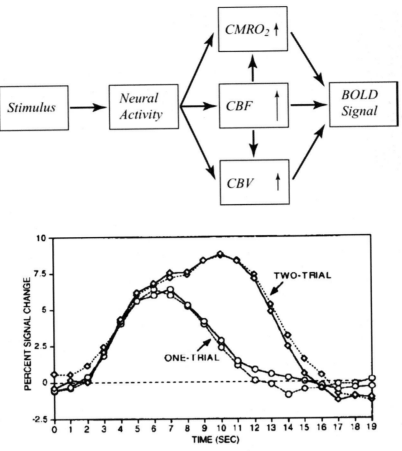

Figure 12–5. *Left.* A current model of the chain of events that leads to the blood oxygenation level-dependent (BOLD) effect measured on functional MRI (fMRI). Underlying neural activity results in local increases in the cerebral metabolic rate of oxygen extraction ($CMRO_2$), cerebral blood flow (CBF), and cerebral blood volume (CBF). Local increases in CBF affect the other two, and all combine to change the ratio of oxygenated relative to deoxygenated hemoglobin in a local area that is measured on fMRI. This signal is called the BOLD effect. *Right.* Typical BOLD effects. Here, visual activity was recorded in response to either a single 1-second visual stimulus (flickering checkerboard) or to two 1-second trials, spaced 5 seconds apart. In both cases, the percent change from a baseline of signals during no visual stimulation is plotted. Note how the BOLD effect is a temporally low-pass filtered response of the underlying neural activity. One second of neural activity was recorded as a protracted response that peaked approximately 6 seconds after onset and did not return to baseline until approximately 12 seconds after offset of the stimulus. Note also, though, that the response to two trials is a roughly linear summation of the response to two individual trials. (*Sources*: Left: Buxton, 2001, p. 419, with permission of Cambridge University Press. Right: Dale and Buckner, 1997, with permission. © 2002, Wiley-Liss, a subsidiary of John Wiley & Sons.)

activity," viewing novel or familiar pictures failed to elicit any apparent activity in the hippocampal region. However, when an active but menial task was used as a baseline (deciding whether digits were odd or even), robust activity was observed.

Similarly, Law et al. (2005) collected fMRI images as participants learned a concurrent set of arbitrarily paired associates gradually over multiple trials (Fig. 12–6). Each trial contained both encoding and cued-recall components as participants learned through trial and error which abstract geometric shapes were associated with which response options. Notably, a number of MTL regions exhibited activity that increased in conjunction with the strength of the participant's memory for a particular region. Equally notable, however, was

the observation that the choice of baseline task determined whether activity during the mnemonic trials was above or below "zero." When a trivially easy nonmnemonic perceptual task was used, activity increased with memory strength but was all "negative." When a more difficult version of the same task was used as the baseline, activity again increased with memory strength but was now all "positive." Contrasting the two baseline tasks revealed substantially greater activity in the MTL for the easy task than for the difficult task, presumably the result of participants' minds wandering during the trivially easy trials. Such mind wandering is likely to include incidental encoding and retrieval of information, the hallmark of MTL function. This result draws into sharp focus the difficulty of not having an estimate of zero activity in a region.

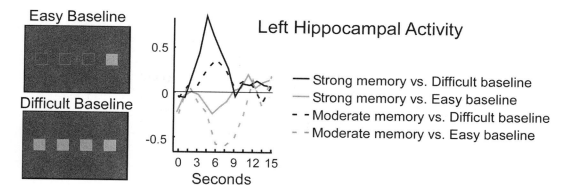

Figure 12–6. Activity in a region of the left hippocampus during a paired associate task is shown for both strong, highly accurate memories and for memories that are above chance levels of performance but still only moderately accurate. Two perceptual tasks were used to estimate "zero" activity, neither of which was overtly mnemonic. In both, the task was to identify the brightest square. The task was trivial in the Easy condition (98% correct) and challenging in the Difficult condition (54% correct). When the Easy condition was used as an estimate of "zero," strong memories yielded small "negative" activity, and moderate strength memories yielded large "negative" activity. When the Difficult condition was used as an estimate of zero, the same exact memory task trials yielded large and small "positive" activities, respectively.

These data demonstrate the effect of activity during the baseline task. Substantial activity in the hippocampus during the Easy baseline task (presumably resulting from incidental encoding and retrieval unrelated to this rather boring task) served to deflect activity during the memory task "below zero." Note, however, that the relative differences between the curves are maintained, irrespective of baseline choice. fMRI has no baseline, and all data must be interpreted in a relative manner. All we actually know from these data is that Difficult baseline > Strong memories > Moderate memories > Easy baseline. This property is often ignored yet is a clear source of several failures to observe activity. (*Source*: Data are from Law et al., 2005, with permission. © Society for Neuroscience.)

fMRI (and most other imaging techniques) yield purely relative measures, and no claims can be made about a region's absolute level of activity in any task. The only measures available are relative measures between tasks or conditions. Furthermore, simply because a task does not require a cognitive component (memory, in this case) does not mean the component is not actually being used and that the region is not active during the task.

Finally, if one considers BOLD fMRI, the most popular neuroimaging technique used in humans, we still have limited temporal (~ 1 second) and spatial (~ 3 mm³ or ~10,000 neurons) resolution; and we still do not have a complete understanding of the relation between neural events and the BOLD fMRI signal (or the measured by PET). Progress along these dimensions is being made, with some evidence from experiments that BOLD is more closely linked to synaptic activity than to spiking activity (Logothetis et al., 2001). One consequence of this is that inhibitory inputs may paradoxically serve to increase the BOLD effect rather than decrease it. Strong inhibition in a region results in substantial synaptic activity (and metabolic activity), even if spiking is reduced. Direct tests of this hypothesis in the rat have yielded increases in the CBF, a precursor of the BOLD effect (Caesar et al., 2003), indicating that inhibition would result in an increase rather than a decrease in BOLD. Thus, our current understanding of how to relate electrophysiological findings to neuroimaging findings is certainly incomplete, although it does appear that BOLD fMRI measures offer a relatively linear assessment of neural activity (Boynton et al., 1996; Rees et al., 2000; Logothetis et al., 2001).

12.3.6 Technical Challenge: Alignment of MTL Regions Across Participants

Even if the above challenges are met and the constraints respected, one significant challenge remains if neuroimaging techniques are to be able to help answer questions concerning the functional role played by the various structures in the MTL. For neuroimaging to do so, it must be possible to localize signals of the specific subregions of the MTL. Therefore, the data must be of sufficient resolution to allow confidence in localization; and if group analyses are desired, it must be possible to transform the data from multiple participants in such a way that cross-participant tests respect anatomical divisions in the MTL. Techniques such as PET and magnetoencephalography (MEG) have clear strengths. PET can directly quantify CBF and can be used to tag specific chemicals (e.g., neurotransmitters) in ways no other technique can; and MEG has millisecond temporal resolution. The spatial resolution and localization accuracy of both techniques have improved over recent years, but they still cannot approach the resolution possible with fMRI. The resolution in typical fMRI studies is typically 3 to 4 mm³ but can be pushed into the cubic millimeter range (Hyde et al., 2001; Kirwan et al., in press), making fMRI a leading candidate for imaging the small structures of the MTL.

However, even if the spatial resolution is theoretically sufficient to have some confidence in localization, it is still vital that any cross-participant analyses respect the structural boundaries in the MTL. It would be pointless to attempt to discern what factors affect activity in the perirhinal cortex if

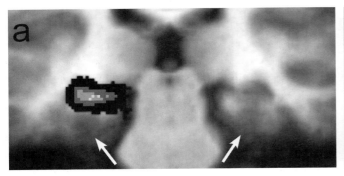 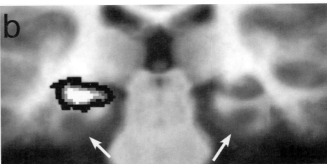

Figure 12–7. Coronal structural MRI sections through the hippocampus of 20 participants, averaged following Talairach alignment (*a*) and region of interest alignment (ROI-AL) (*b*). White arrows indicate the location of the collateral sulcus used to identify the parahippocampal gyrus. Overlay on the left hippocampus indicates the amount of cross-participant overlap of manual segmentations of each participant's left hippocampus when brains were aligned using each technique. The left hippocampus of each partici-

pant was initially manually segmented and then transformed along with the structural image using both techniques. In this group overlay, white is ideal (no voxels in *a* and 23 voxels in *b*) and indicates that all 20 participants' aligned segmentations identified the voxel as part of the left hippocampus. Black indicates 1 to 10 aligned segmentations identified the voxel as part of the left hippocampus. Light, medium, and dark gray indicate that 19, 18, and 16 segmentations overlap, respectively.

our alignment techniques normalized brains in such a way that a given voxel in a group analysis was located in the perirhinal cortex of one participant, the entorhinal cortex of another, the hippocampal region of a third, and outside, in the ambient cistern, of a fourth. Unfortunately, human brains are sufficiently dissimilar from each other that alignment with popular techniques (e.g., alignment to the atlas of Talairach and Tournoux, 1988) often leaves us in this situation.

An example of this problem is shown in Figure 12–7a. Here, 20 structural MRI scans were first individually aligned to the Talairach atlas before an average of the 20 scans was created (shown as a coronal image cropped around the MTL). The white arrows indicate where the collateral sulcus (a defining structure for the parahippocampal gyrus) is most likely to be. As one can see, it is far from clearly defined, indicating that the averaging across participants blurred this feature (which is plainly visible in each individual scan) into an undifferentiated mass. This poor level of cross-participant alignment arises from both global variability across participants (overall shifts in the location, orientation, and size of structures) and from differences in the shape of structures (Preuessner et al., 2002).

In addition to averaging the structural MRI images, Figure 12–7a shows the result of averaging segmentations of the left hippocampal region. Each participant's left hippocampal region was manually segmented, and the same Talairach transformation was applied to each segmentation prior to averaging the segmentations across participants. The result of this averaging is a grayscale overlay that indicates how well the Talairach transformation was able to align all 20 hippocampi. In this slice, there are no voxels in which there was overlap across all 20 manual segmentations of the left hippocampal region, and there are only three voxels in which 19 of the 20 segmentations overlap. Even if our only goal is to assess activity in the hippocampal region overall (not in subregions of the hippocampus), this level of alignment is insufficient as signals

from one hippocampal region are combined with another participant's entorhinal cortex and a third participant's ventricle. If one extends this analysis to segmentations of all subregions of the MTL, the picture is worse still. Between any two participant's MTLs, only about half of the voxels are typically identified as belonging to the same structure in both participants (Stark and Okado, 2003; Kirwan et al., in press).

Imperfect cross-participant alignment results in a blur of the data that has two detrimental effects. First, the blur reduces the localization accuracy for any observed activity, as signals from multiple regions may be combined. Second, the blur reduces statistical power. If separate regions (or subregions) are behaving differently, the spatial blur smears activity across regions, introducing noise that prevents a consistent pattern of activity from being observed. For example, the main result of a study by Stark and Okado (2003) demonstrating activity associated with encoding during a retrieval task was not observed when the data were aligned with traditional Talairach techniques but was observed when the data were aligned using more sophisticated techniques.

Recently, there have been three approaches taken to address this issue: simple anatomical region of interest (ROI) analyses, cortical unfolding applied to the MTL, and ROI-AL (region of interest alignment). All three approaches can address the issue of improving cross-participant alignment and, in so doing, open up the possibility of using fMRI to help differentiate the role of individual structures in the MTL. Figure 12–7b shows the result of aligning the medial temporal lobe structures from the same 20 participants from Figure 12–7a but using one of these approaches (the ROI-AL method of Stark and Okado, 2003). Here, one can clearly resolve the collateral sulcus (white arrow) and differentiate it from the hippocampal region immediately above. The 20 segmentations aligned with this technique have perfect overlap in 23 voxels; and if one extends this to near-perfect (19/20) levels, the count rises to 34 voxels (versus 0 and 3 in the case of Talairach alignment). These three approaches give us hope that fMRI may be able to isolate hippocampal function from that of adjacent regions and perhaps even differentiate contributions of hippocampal subfields.

With the most straightforward technique, several articles have collapsed activity across all voxels within a set of anatomically defined ROIs (e.g., Stark and Squire, 2000a; Small et al., 2001; Reber et al., 2002, 2003). Thus, there may be a single measure that represents activity for each participant's anterior left hippocampal region in a given condition. Although this technique has the potential for perfect alignment across participants, it suffers from two drawbacks. First, by combining all voxels in an anatomically defined region into a single measure (a single, large, irregularly shaped voxel), any functional variability in that region is lost. For example, if all data from the right hippocampal region were treated as if it were one large voxel, and if two opposing patterns of activity were present in different subregions of the right hippocampal region, this functional variability would be lost. A second, related drawback is that if only a small subregion in the anatomically defined ROI is active, noise from other included voxels distort the observed activity.

A second approach has been to adapt cortical unfolding techniques to the problem of unfolding the cortical MTL structures and the spiral structure of the hippocampal region (Zeineh et al., 2000, 2003). With this approach, anatomically localized boundaries are defined and used to map the three-dimensional data onto a common two-dimensional "flat map" and to align individual participant's flat maps. Unlike collapsing all voxels in the anatomically defined ROIs, this technique has the advantage of preserving the topography in each region. In addition, because of the requirement for very high resolution of the functional data ($1.6 \times 1.6 \times 4$ mm) and the technique's ability potentially to unfold the spiral structure of the hippocampal region, this technique holds the promise of differentiating signal from regions in the hippocampus itself. However, the unwarping process is not entirely invertible, as functional voxels that lie within a fold can be associated with two different regions of the unfolded map.

A third approach has been to use anatomically defined ROIs to guide alignment directly (Stark and Squire, 2001a; Stark and Okado, 2003; Miller et al., 2005; Kirwan et al., in press). This technique (dubbed "ROI-AL" by Stark and Okado, 2003) shares with the unfolding technique the advantage of preserving topography in regions with the unfolding technique but does not require very high-resolution functional voxels. ROI-AL takes a direct approach to aligning regions across participants. Instead of using structural MRI to align gray matter, white matter, and cerebrospinal fluid (CSF) across participants, ROI-AL attempts to align anatomically defined regions of interest based on rough segmentations of the regions. Furthermore, instead of attempting to arrive at the best fitting alignment across the entire brain, ROI-AL focuses only on alignment of a particular structure (or set of structures). Thus, all of the transformation parameters used

to align two brains with typical techniques (e.g., rotation, translation, scaling, shearing) are focused on aligning a single region (e.g., left hippocampal region). The net result is vastly improved cross-participant alignment, bringing with it improved statistical power. Furthermore, by using anatomically defined regions, ROI-AL (and unfolding) can localize results from cross-participant analyses to specific anatomically defined regions of interest (e.g., perirhinal versus parahippocampal cortices). The exact location of any region of activity in a group analysis can be compared with the segmentations from each participant (or with a composite anatomical model based on the individual participants' anatomically defined regions of interest). Thus, one can project backward from the group result to the individual participants' anatomy and determine with some precision where a signal was generated.

12.4 Dissociating Hippocampal Function

In the following sections, five aspects or potential divisions in long-term memory are discussed with particular attention paid to isolating the function of the hippocampus. For each of these aspects, the relevant data from patients with bilateral damage limited to the hippocampal region, from depth electrode recordings, and from neuroimaging studies are discussed.

12.4.1 Explicit Versus Implicit

Perhaps the clearest example of functional dissociation in long-term memory is that between *explicit*, or *declarative*, memory and *implicit*, or *nondeclarative*, memory. Explicit memory refers to "intentional or conscious recollection of prior experiences, as assessed in the laboratory by traditional tests of recall or recognition," whereas implicit memory refers to "changes in performance or behavior, produced by prior experiences, on tests that do not require any intentional or conscious recollection of those experiences" (Schacter, 1999, p. 233). These descriptive terms relate to specific task demands rather than distinctions between memory systems or specific brain structures. Yet, a wealth of data shown has shown that this descriptive distinction is strongly correlated with hippocampal function. The terms declarative and nondeclarative are defined in similar terms when applied to the human. The declarative/nondeclarative distinction goes a bit further, however, to embrace the apparent functional dissociation between multiple memory systems. Declarative memory "identifies a biologically real category of memory abilities" (Squire, 1992, p. 232) that require structures in the medial temporal lobes, whereas nondeclarative memory identifies a heterogeneous collection of memory systems that bear resemblance to each other behaviorally (all are observed with implicit memory tasks) but appear to rely on many brain structures.

Despite obvious memory impairments, it may come as a surprise to some that patients with damage limited to the hippocampal region and those with extensive damage to the medial temporal lobes demonstrate normal levels of performance on a wide range of long-term memory tasks. In an early report (Milner, 1962), H.M. was found to acquire a perceptual motor skill (learning to trace the outline of a shape when viewed in a mirror) over several days at normal rates despite not remembering the prior day's training (see Fig. 12–2). Subsequent studies have shown that even severely amnesic patients exhibit normal rates of delay eyeblink conditioning (e.g., Weiskrantz and Warrington, 1979; Clark and Squire, 1998). Furthermore, the phenomenon of categorization appears to be intact. In one task, a random dot pattern (resembling an imaginary constellation of stars) is created, and numerous distorted versions of this "prototype" are created as well by moving the dots by random amounts (Posner and Keele, 1968). After studying only highly distorted versions, even severely amnesic patients such as E.P. incidentally learn to abstract features of the prototype (or the category) so they can later correctly classify new patterns as either members or nonmembers of the studied category (e.g., Knowlton and Squire, 1993; Squire and Knowlton, 1995). They do so, however, without any knowledge that they have ever performed the task and without any ability consciously to recognize any of the previously studied dot patterns (even if the study phase consisted of seeing the same dot pattern 40 times). Thus, there appears to be a dissociation between the ability to learn in these implicit tasks gradually and the ability to remember the study episodes or contents of those episodes consciously or explicitly.

The term "priming" refers to another class of implicit memory tasks that are not affected by MTL damage. In perceptual priming tasks, exposure to a word or a picture (often incidentally, with no instruction to study the item) improves the ability to perceive the item later, usually taking the form of increased accuracy or decreased reaction time during degraded presentation. There is a long history in cognitive psychology dissociating perceptual priming and recognition memory in healthy individuals (for review see Schacter, 1994). This behavioral dissociation is relevant here in that long-term memory for an item in the form of a repetition priming effect is normal following hippocampal damage, whereas explicit memory for the same item is clearly impaired.

Warrington and Weiskrantz (1968, 1974) were the first to show that despite poor recognition memory after studying lists of words or pictures, amnesic patients had an intact form of perceptual memory for these items. When tested with a fragmented or degraded version of either type of stimulus and asked to complete this partial cue, studied items were completed more accurately or at greater levels of degradation than nonstudied items. This perceptual priming effect was normal in the amnesic patients. Likewise, if words are presented rapidly at a test so correct identification is below ceiling levels, previously studied words are identified more accurately than nonstudied words (e.g., Jacoby and Dallas, 1981). This per-

ceptual identification priming is normal even in the case of E.P., who performs at chance when given a recognition memory test under similar circumstances (Hamann and Squire, 1997).

In perhaps the most extreme example of this dissociation between intact priming and impaired recognition (Stark and Squire, 2000b), E.P. studied a list of words (e.g., "window") and after a 10-minute delay was presented with a test of repetition priming ("What is the first word that comes to mind that begins *win____*") and a test of recognition memory ("Which word did you see on the list 10 minutes ago: *window* or *winter*?") on each trial. E.P. showed a normal priming effect in the form of a 26% increased likelihood of generating the studied word (relative to baseline completion rates of generating this word). However, his recognition memory performance was at chance, averaging 48% correct. Therefore, within seconds of each other, E.P. showed intact implicit memory for a word (in the form of stem completion priming) and no detectible explicit memory for that same word. Given E.P.'s complete hippocampal loss (Stefanacci et al., 2000), it is clear that the hippocampus cannot be vital for this form of implicit memory.

We should note that when comparing an amnesic patient's level of performance on repetition priming tasks (or indeed on many implicit memory tasks) relative to healthy controls, there is always the possibility that the amnesic patient's performance may be impaired relative to that of the healthy controls because the latter group may make use of covert explicit memory. Although not the case in the above-mentioned studies overall, the repetition priming task is susceptible to "explicit contamination"—the use of explicit memory on an implicit memory task. For example, if at this point in the chapter the reader were asked to complete the word stem *win____* with the first word that comes to mind, you might follow these instructions faithfully and respond with the first word that simply pops into your mind. However, you might also realize that in the preceding paragraph the word *window* was used as a sample study item (especially if this were done in the context of not one implicit probe but an entire list of them). Therefore, you might respond with "window" not because it was the first word that freely popped into your mind, but because you tried to remember what study word began with the letters *win____*. Thus, despite the task instructions, participants may treat an implicit task as a thinly disguised explicit task and show enhanced levels of performance. For example, in the above-mentioned study with E.P. that combined a repetition priming task with a forced-choice recognition memory task during each trial (Stark and Squire, 2000b, experiment 4), all but one of the controls had priming effects ranging from 0.21 to 0.29. The other control had a priming effect of 0.53, approximately 8 standard deviations (SD) away from the mean priming effect. Although we do not know for certain that this particular control adopted an explicit strategy, it almost perfectly matches the mean hit rate in the recognition task, leaving this as the most reasonable hypothesis. Therefore, simply knowing

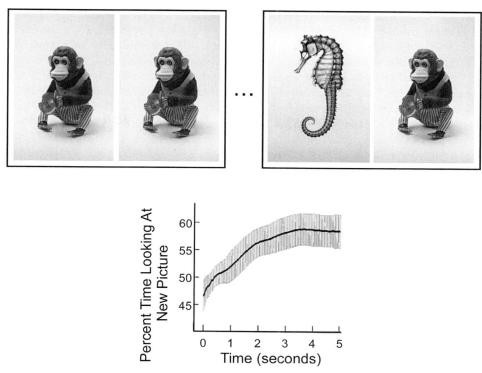

Figure 12–8. Visual-paired comparison task. Participants view two copies of the same image and after a variable delay are shown a new image and the old image. A bias exists to spend more time looking at the new image. This is an implicit memory task, yet the bias to look at the novel picture is dependent on the medial temporal lobes. (*Source*: Data are from Manns et al., 2000.)

that the task requires no more than implicit memory does not guarantee that the participants will treat it as an implicit task when there are multiple routes to solve the problem. Where implicit tasks or any other tasks are impaired in persons with amnesia, this possibility must certainly be considered.

A second form of priming, known as conceptual priming, is also apparently intact in amnesia. Here, the test presents an item or a category that is semantically or conceptually related to the studied item. For example, if the word *peach* had been presented at study (again, the study task is often incidental), participants might be asked to generate exemplars of a category (e.g., generate examples of fruits), verify category membership (e.g., how long it takes to verify that *peach* is a fruit), or perform a free-association task (e.g., free-associate to the word *pear*). In each of these, amnesic patients with damage including but not limited to the hippocampus have shown normal levels of conceptual priming (Graf et al., 1984; Shimamura and Squire, 1984; Vaidya et al., 1995; Keane et al., 1997; Levy et al., 2004) while being impaired in explicit tests for the same type of information.

A task called visual-paired comparison appears to be the one exception to the rule that implicit memory tasks are nondeclarative in nature and are not impaired by damage to the hippocampal region. In this task, two copies of an object or a scene are presented to the participant for several seconds (Fig.

12–8). During this time, the participant is free to examine either copy of the object at will, and no task instructions are given. After some delay (in which intervening items may be presented), a copy of the previously exposed object or scene is presented along with a novel object or scene; and again the participant is free to examine either stimulus at will. The task, is quite implicit in instruction and behavior. Participants have a tendency to spend a greater amount of time looking at the novel stimulus than the familiar stimulus. A small bias or change is made in behavior as a result of experience on a task that makes no reference to the prior study episode—hallmarks of implicit memory tasks. In fact, the task is commonly used to assess memory in infants who would certainly not understand any explicit instructions even if given (Fagan, 1970). Yet, the task is dependent on the hippocampus in that no such bias is seen following hippocampal damage in humans (McKee and Squire, 1993; Manns et al., 2000; Pascalis et al., 2004), the monkey (Bachevalier et al., 1993; Pascalis and Bachevalier, 1999; Zola et al., 2000), or the rat (Clark et al., 2000). Furthermore, the degree of bias shown in the visual paired comparison task is predictive of subsequent recognition memory for the items shown, whereas the amount of repetition priming exhibited is not (Manns et al., 2000). Thus, even though the task requirements are implicit in nature (no reference is made to the study episode) and even though the memory is observed in the form of a change in a behavioral bias, the task relies on the same underlying mechanisms that are responsible for declarative memory.

One final task deserves consideration when discussing the role of the hippocampus in relation to explicit and implicit memory. Chun and Phelps (1999) embedded an implicit memory task within a visual search task (locate a rotated T among numerous rotated L distractors). Although the displays appeared to be random, a set of 12 displays were repeatedly intermixed with random displays throughout the experiment. As one might expect, the reaction time to locate the target item in the random displays gradually decreased over the course of the task. This basic practice effect or increased skill in performing the task was similar in a control group and an amnesic group (two anoxic patients and two patients with encephalitic damage that included, but extended beyond, the hippocampal region), consistent with other implicit or nondeclarative tasks. Furthermore, although approximately half of the healthy controls reported noticing repetition of several displays when later asked, not even they could identify which they were (54% correct). Critically, however, the controls' reaction times to the repeated items were faster than their reaction times to the random items in the later epochs of training. Although they lacked explicit knowledge of the repeated items, they had implicit knowledge of this repetition, evidenced by their reaction time. In marked contrast, the amnesic patients did not show this effect. The amnesic patients exhibited identical reductions in reaction time for repeated and random displays.

Thus, a second task exists in which the task demands and memory are implicit in nature, yet performance requires structures in the medial temporal lobes. This said, performance may not require the hippocampus itself. A follow-up study by Manns and Squire (2001) solidly replicated the basic findings of Chun and Phelps (1999). Here, however, the amnesic patient group was large enough to separate into two groups based on size and extent of the lesion. Five patients had damage limited to the hippocampal region or only mildly extending into the parahippocampal gyrus. A separate group of three were encephalitic patients who had extensive, near-complete damage to the MTL and mild damage that extended into the lateral temporal cortex (consistent with this etiology). Notably, the only group that did not show reduced reaction times specific to repeated displays was the group with extensive MTL damage. These patients performed similarly to the mixed etiology group in Chun and Phelps' (1999) study. In contrast, the patients with damage more restricted to the hippocampal region performed much like the healthy control volunteers in both studies, demonstrating improved reaction times for repeated displays. Therefore, our best understanding of this task is that implicit memory for the repeated displays is not derived from the hippocampal region itself but, rather, is derived from some other temporal lobe structure.

In summary, we can conclude that although the hippocampus plays a role in explicit or declarative memory tasks, it does not play a role in implicit or nondeclarative memory tasks (at least when the task is solved in an implicit way). The visual-paired comparison task is the one apparent exception to this rule, highlighting the importance of extending or refining the descriptive distinctions created to understand human behavior (e.g., implicit/explicit) to more fully encompass data from other sources. The simple description of the task requirements does an admirable job of dissociating two classes of tasks, yet there is clearly something about the visual-paired comparison task that, despite its "implicit" nature, makes it dependent on the hippocampal region and the adjacent medial temporal lobe cortices.

12.4.2 Encoding Versus Retrieval

Whereas studies of patients with damage to the hippocampal region have been able to demonstrate a dissociation between declarative memory tasks that involve the hippocampus and nondeclarative memory tasks that do not, studies of patients are not particularly well suited to isolating the role of the hippocampus in encoding (or storage) versus retrieval processes. The inability to make accurate judgments in a recognition memory task or to recall items from a study list could be the result of failure to encode the items initially or failure to retrieve a well encoded item. The observation that amnesic patients can retrieve fact or event-type memory that was learned well prior to the onset of their amnesia (see Section 12.4.3) can be taken as evidence that the hippocampus is not continually required for declarative memory retrieval; however, it still leaves open the possibility that when anterograde and retrograde amnesia are observed the central impairment is one of retrieval rather than encoding or storage (e.g., Warrington and Weiskrantz, 1970).

Thus, in humans, determining whether the hippocampus plays a differential role in encoding or retrieval relies heavily on electrophysiological and neuroimaging data. Complementing this, studies of animals offer the opportunity of employing reversible lesions, blockade of long-term potentiation (LTP), and other manipulations (discussed in Chapters 8 and 13). One of the challenges that faces all such attempts is the observation that during memory retrieval tasks participants unwittingly encode the test items and can often accurately remember whether an item was present during the test (for review see Glover, 1989). fMRI activity associated with this incidental encoding has been observed in numerous frontal and parietal regions (Buckner et al., 2001) and bilaterally in the hippocampal region, perirhinal cortex, and parahippocampal cortex (Stark and Okado, 2003).

This challenge aside, hippocampal activity has been observed relating to both encoding and retrieval success. A number of fMRI studies (Small et al., 2001; Davachi and Wagner, 2002; Reber et al., 2002; Strange et al., 2002; Davachi et al., 2003; Stark and Okado, 2003; Kirwan and Stark, 2004) have observed hippocampal activity correlated with encoding success. In this so-called *Dm* (differences due to memory) effect (Paller and Wagner, 2002), there is greater activity during the successful encoding of items that are later remembered than during the unsuccessful encoding of items that are later not remembered. Similar *Dm* effects have been observed in several studies employing recording from the hippocampal region using depth electrodes as well (Fernandez et al., 1999b; Cameron et al., 2001; Fernandez et al., 2002; Fell et al., 2003). We should note that these *Dm* effects have been frequently observed in the parahippocampal cortex (e.g., Brewer et al., 1998; Wagner et al., 1998; Fernandez et al., 1999b; Otten et al., 2001; Davachi and Wagner, 2002; Fernandez et al., 2002; Strange et al., 2002; Davachi et al., 2003) and the entorhinal or perirhinal cortices (Fernandez et al., 1999b; Cameron et al., 2001; Davachi and Wagner, 2002; Fernandez et al., 2002; Strange et al., 2002; Davachi et al., 2003; Fell et al., 2003; Kirwan and Stark, 2004) as well.

Similarly, a number of fMRI studies have demonstrated activity in the hippocampal region related to retrieval success (e.g., Gabrieli et al., 1997; Eldridge et al., 2000; Stark and Squire, 2000a, 2000c, 2001a; Stark and Okado, 2003; Kirwan and Stark, 2004). Here, successful retrieval (e.g., responding "old" to previously studied targets) usually elicits greater activity than unsuccessful retrieval (e.g., responding "new" to unstudied foil items). Similar effects have been observed using depth electrode recordings (Paller and McCarthy, 2002) and magnetic source imaging (Papanicolaou et al., 2002).

Although apparently engaged in both successful encoding and retrieval processes, a dissociation between the two is still possible; and several studies have observed differences in the hippocampal region between memory encoding processes and retrieval processes. For example, Zeineh et al. (2003) used the above-mentioned unfolding techniques to isolate encoding and retrieval-related activity for face–name pairs. They reported above-baseline (visual fixation on a cross) activity during encoding but not retrieval in CA2, CA3, and the dentate gyrus, with this activity decreasing across repeated presentations (evidence of encoding-related activity was seen in the parahippocampal cortex as well). In contrast, retrieval (and to some degree encoding) was associated with activity in the subiculum, also showing a decrease in activity with repeated presentations. Thus, some differentiation between encoding and retrieval was observed in components of the hippocampus.

In addition to differentiating encoding from retrieval across these subregions (see Chapter 3), several attempts have been made to differentiate activity along the anterior-posterior (or longitudinal) axis (Gabrieli et al., 1997; LePage et al., 1998; Fernandez et al., 1999a). However, it appears as if the initial support for this hypothesis has not been confirmed in the further analysis of these and subsequent studies (Schacter and Wagner, 1999). For example Small et al. (2001) used an anatomical ROI analysis to examine encoding- and retrieval-related activity along the longitudinal axis of the hippocampal region (eight ROIs for each participant along this axis). Here, they observed activity in different locations along the longitudinal axis for encoding faces and for encoding names. They

also observed a combination of these locations (and several others) during the encoding of face–name pairs. At retrieval, when participants were cued with a face and asked to recall the name, the pattern of activity in the hippocampal region was quite similar to the pattern of activity observed when encoding the face–name pair. Similarly, using an anatomical ROI analysis, Reber et al. (2002) observed encoding effects for both words and pictures throughout the longitudinal axis of the hippocampal region and the adjacent cortical structures (differences were observed between picture and word encoding, however).

Furthermore, in a study that attempted to reduce the effects of incidental encoding during retrieval (Stark and Okado, 2003), encoding and retrieval each resulted in activity in the hippocampal region and in the perirhinal and parahippocampal cortices. It should be noted, however, that in this study the exact voxels associated with intentional encoding, incidental encoding, and retrieval were not always the same. Likewise, Pihlajamaki et al. (2003) found evidence for greater activity during retrieval than encoding and greater activity during encoding than retrieval in areas of the perirhinal and parahippocampal cortices and the hippocampal region. Thus, it is apparent that although there may be differentiation between encoding- and retrieval-related functions on a fine scale, encoding and retrieval processes appear to be present throughout the MTL.

12.4.3 Time-limited Role in Declarative Memory

At the beginning of the chapter, we noted Milner's observation that patient H.M.'s remote memory appeared to be intact in the face of both his profoundly impaired ability to learn new information and a profound loss of information that he had been exposed to for some amount of time prior to his operation. Given his intact childhood memories, she concluded that the medial temporal lobes were not the ultimate storage site for what we now refer to as declarative memory. Therefore, some form of systems-level "consolidation" occurs by which memories that initially rely on structures in the medial temporal lobe become independent of the medial temporal lobe over time. (This is not to be confused with an alternative use of the term "consolidation" to refer to the fixation of a memory over the course of seconds to hours.) This phenomenon, termed "temporally graded retrograde amnesia," has been observed frequently in amnesic patients since first being described by Ribot more than 100 years ago (Ribot, 1887).

This observation has been frequent but not entirely consistent. Although some have described it as temporally graded (e.g., Squire and Alvarez, 1995), others have described it as constant (e.g., Warrington and McCarthy, 1988). Some have found evidence that memory for both facts (semantic memory) and events (episodic memory) acquired before the onset of amnesia are similarly impaired (e.g., Verfaellie et al., 1995; Reed and Squire, 1998), whereas others have found more selective (and constant) impairment in episodic memory (e.g., Nadel and Moscovitch, 1997). One potential source of variability in the data stems from the fact that all studies of retrograde memory in human amnesic patients are retrospective and quasi-experimental in nature. When testing a patient's memory for knowledge acquired before the experiment (and potentially years or decades before the experiment), we cannot know how well the information had been learned prior to the onset of amnesia or even if it had been learned at all. Furthermore, we cannot know whether the information had been retrieved, and therefore reencoded, at some time following the initial learning. Such retrieval-induced encoding could easily affect the presence or absence of a temporal gradient. Likewise, it is a matter of debate whether such retrospective tests should employ information that shows a forgetting gradient in healthy controls or they should employ information that can be retrieved at a constant level of performance across the supposed delay.

Additionally, the exact location and extent of the hippocampal lesion is often not known nor whether it extends beyond the medial temporal lobes. There are a relatively small number of cases in which damage appears to be limited to the hippocampal region and retrograde amnesia has been assessed (Zola-Morgan et al., 1986; Reed and Squire, 1998; Kapur and Brooks, 1999; Holdstock et al., 2002a). In all but one patient (Y.R. in Holdstock et al., 2002a), a temporally graded retrograde amnesia spanning several years was observed for both episodic and semantic memory. In the case of Y.R., no retrograde amnesia was detected at all in this study. However, follow-up testing on Y.R. has revealed evidence for at least some retrograde amnesia. Its precise nature with respect to temporal gradients and with respect to selectivity for any kind of information or task is currently not known, however (unpublished data, Andrew Mayes, personal communication, February 22, 2005).

Using neuroimaging to study the time-limited nature of hippocampal function is also associated with a number of challenges. One clear challenge is the problem of activity associated with incidental encoding. It is quite plausible, for example, that if memories have been consolidated and no longer require structures in the MTL the retrieval of such a memory (e.g., a childhood memory that has not been thought about for some time) induces encoding in the MTL. If participants can tell you what memories they had retrieved while inside the scanner, activity associated with this incidental encoding could mask (or even reverse) any retrograde gradient (Stark and Okado, 2003).

A second challenge that perhaps faces studies of consolidation more strongly than most is the difficulty posed by the choice of baseline tasks. Several studies have shown that there is significant activity throughout the brain (including the MTL) during rest or other baseline tasks that do not actively engage the participant (Binder et al., 1999; Gusnard et al., 2001; Gusnard and Raichle, 2001; Newman et al., 2001; Stark and Squire, 2001b). One explanation for such activity is that during rest and other low-level baseline tasks participants are

actually engaged in an undetermined and uncontrolled task (e.g., reflecting upon the experiment). When activity during episodic recollection (e.g., "Reflect upon your visit to Paris as a child") is contrasted with rest, it is quite plausible that this reflection is carried into the rest periods. Such activity during rest could reduce the magnitude of an effect such that it might not be observed or, if the amount of reflection during rest or the actual "task" performed during rest varied with condition (e.g., participants might be more likely to reminisce or attempt to further elaborate a memory following retrieval of a very old than a recent memory), one could create or even invert a gradient purely as an artifact (Stark and Squire, unpublished data).

Given these challenges, it is not entirely surprising that in neuroimaging studies of consolidation the results have been mixed. For example, Ryan et al. (2001) asked participants to generate very remote ($>$ 20 years) and relatively recent ($<$ 4 years) episodic memories while outside the scanner. Inside the scanner, they were asked to recall these memories for 20 seconds. In bilateral hippocampal regions that showed an overall difference in activity between recollection and rest, there was no difference in activity between activity for very remote and relatively recent memories (an alternate baseline of sentence completion was also used and did not differ from rest, but as this task required one sentence completion in 5 seconds it may be open to the same difficulties as explicit rest). Furthermore, no significant activity was observed in any of the subjects in a remote-versus-recent contrast.

Similarly, Maguire et al. (2001) collected data as participants performed a verification task on both public event information and autobiographical information from periods ranging from several weeks to more than 20 years prior to scanning (e.g., "Yes or no: You were at Tim's wedding in London"). Although hippocampal activity during both tasks was greater than baseline (listening to a set of function words), and it was greater for autobiographical than public-event verification, it did not vary parametrically with memory age. However, the participant's knowledge of this information had been assessed several weeks prior to scanning, raising the possibility that they were retrieving the information from the recent reencoded episode.

Finally, Stark and Squire (2000a) attempted a prospective study of consolidation by having participants study pictures of nameable objects at varying delays prior to scanning. At test, the names of the objects were presented. In so doing, much of the incidental encoding-related activity appears to be confined to the left hemisphere, leaving retrieval-related activity for the nameable objects relatively uncontaminated in the right hemisphere (Stark and Squire, 2001a). Activity in anatomically defined ROIs in the MTL did not differ as a function of study-test interval. It should be noted, however, that the delays employed were all relatively short, ranging from an hour to a week.

In contrast to these negative findings, there have been several studies that have shown gradients in MTL activity as a function of memory age. In the first such study, Haist et al.

(2001) used the "famous faces" task (Marslen-Wilson and Teuber, 1975) in which participants were presented with photographs of faces from various decades (of both famous and nonfamous people) and attempted to recall the names of each. An analysis identifying regions whose activity varied linearly by decade (activity determined by a contrast between famous faces from each decade and rest) isolated activity in a region that appeared to be the right entorhinal cortex. Here, activity was greatest when participants attempted to recall names from the 1990s and 1980s and lowest when participants attempted to recall names from the 1940s. No other region showed this linear trend.

In a second study, Niki and Luo (2002) used a version of the episodic reflection task in which participants attempted mentally to revisit places they had visited either recently or more than 7 years prior to scanning. In the direct comparison between recent and remote memories, activity in the left parahippocampal gyrus was observed, with greater activity for recent than remote memories. Although a number of other regions throughout the brain also showed this pattern, a substantial number showed the reverse, with greater activity for remote than recent memories.

Finally, Maguire and Frith (2003) again examined autobiographical and public event knowledge as a function of remoteness using a task similar to that in their previous work, described above (Maguire et al., 2001). Although they again observed greater hippocampal activity for autobiographical than public event memory, they did observe a gradient in right hippocampal activity as a function of remoteness of the autobiographical memory (no gradient was observed in the left hippocampal region).

Thus, with respect to the expectation that a time-limited role of the MTL in declarative memories produces a gradient in the BOLD fMRI signal, the current state of affairs is mixed. There are several null results in which no gradient was observed. There are, however, several positive results as well. None of the studies has been able to address fully the issue of incidental encoding (and how it might vary with remoteness), and many suffer from the difficulty that it is unclear whether participants are recalling events from several decades ago or from their retrieval during prescreening sessions. Furthermore, all studies have ignored the possibility that over the course of decades the representation of the memory may change in such a way that the BOLD fMRI signal is affected without altering the functional role of a particular region (e.g., recently consolidated memories may have qualitatively different representations in the tens of thousands of neurons in a typical fMRI voxel than very long-standing memories). One might consider this a clear criticism of the current studies, and the solution to these problems is not clear; nor is it clear how this question can be better approached with neuroimaging. The study of retrograde memory in humans has always been exceedingly difficult with most tasks being retrospective rather than prospective in nature. When combined with the above-mentioned difficulties presented by the limitations of current neuroimaging techniques, it seems obvious

that our best evidence for any time-limited role of MTL structures will be gained from animal models of amnesia. Controlled prospective studies have been conducted in that arena that, by and large, reveal temporal gradients following hippocampal damage (for review see Squire et al., 2001).

12.4.4 Spatial Memory

The notion of a hippocampal "place cell" whose activity codes for the current location in a spatial environment is covered extensively in Chapter 11. The hypothesis that the hippocampus is primarily or even uniquely involved in spatial processing and spatial storage is laid out there, drawing extensively on electrophysiological data from the rat. This hypothesis is considered again in Chapter 13, where a wide array of data from rats, monkeys, and humans are considered. Before this more comprehensive treatment, the data concerning the role of the human hippocampus in spatial memory and spatial processing are considered. In so doing, the principal question is not whether damage to the hippocampus impairs performance on spatial memory tasks or whether place cells are observed in the human hippocampus. In fact, neuropsychological (e.g., Holdstock et al., 2000) and electrophysiological data (Ekstrom et al., 2003) have demonstrated both, implicating the human hippocampus in spatial memory tasks.

For example, Ekstrom et al. (2003) recorded data from depth electrodes implanted in the hippocampal region, parahippocampal gyrus, amygdala, and several frontal sites as participants navigated in a virtual town. Their task was to pretend to be a taxi driver, picking up and dropping off passengers. Several codes were observed in the data. In particular, 11% of the cells (31/279) could be confidently classified as place cells, with their distribution skewed toward being found in the hippocampal region. Approximately 24% of hippocampal neurons could be confidently classified as place cells, whereas significantly fewer neurons in the parahippocampal gyrus, approximately 8% of those sampled, could be confidently classified as place cells. A second code was observed primarily in the parahippocampal gyrus. These cells, termed "location-independent view cells," were observed to code for particular objects or landmarks irrespective of their location. A total of 14 of the 279 neurons (5%) were classified as such and were observed largely in the parahippocampal gyrus. Approximately 15% of neurons in the parahippocampal gyrus were location-independent view cells (7 total) whereas only 1 of 55 neurons in the hippocampal region coded for this information. Although this dissociation was observed, one should note that the numbers of cells and their proportion to the total number sampled is quite small. For example, of the 55 hippocampal cells recorded, 43 (78%) showed main effects of factors other than place or coded for combinations of several factors.

Thus, the question at hand is not whether the hippocampus plays a role in spatial memory. Rather, the question is whether the function of the human hippocampus can be tied strongly to spatial processing or the human hippocampus is better viewed as playing a mnemonic role, with spatial memory being only one example of hippocampal function.

One approach to this question that has been explored extensively in the rodent (see Chapter 11) (Eichenbaum et al., 1999) is to ask whether damage limited to the hippocampal region impairs memory on nonspatial tasks. If such impairment exists and if spatial contributions to the task can be eliminated, one could posit a role for the human hippocampus outside of spatial memory or processing. Although there are many reports of such impairment (see Spiers et al., 2001 for review), it is almost impossible to rule out the option that healthy human control participants engage in a spatial strategy on such nonspatial tasks. For example, even on tests of verbal recognition memory, control participants might imagine the stimuli, imagine relations between stimuli, or use other mnemonic techniques such as the method of loci to improve their performance. Were such spatial strategies not available to patients with hippocampal lesions, their performance might be impaired for spatial, rather than mnemonic, reasons. As tests of recognition memory in humans have not aimed to address the spatial hypothesis directly, they have not controlled for these potential spatial aspects of the tests as carefully as in much of the work in the rodent literature.

An alternative approach to addressing the question is to assess the spatial abilities of patients who have lesions that include the entirety of the hippocampus bilaterally. If spatial processing appears normal despite a complete hippocampal lesion, it would be difficult to conclude that the hippocampus is required for spatial processing in humans. The case of patient E.P. has provided compelling evidence that spatial memory and processing may be intact despite hippocampal loss (Teng and Squire, 1999). Unlike patient H.M., patient E.P. has what is most likely complete loss of the hippocampal region bilaterally (Stefanacci et al., 2000), with only a small "tag" of tissue (~ 10% of the volume) remaining. With the complete lack of entorhinal cortex in E.P., it is doubtful (even if this tissue contains healthy neurons, which it may well not) that it would be functional in any way. Yet, despite this complete loss of the hippocampal region, E.P. can perform a number of complex spatial tasks at normal levels. When asked to navigate in the town in which he grew up, E.P. not only can mentally navigate along familiar routes (from his childhood house to other local landmarks), he can mentally navigate along novel routes (paths between randomly chosen landmarks) and along novel routes with key paths blocked (e.g., imagine that a main road is closed). He also can perform a dead reckoning task (imagine being at one landmark and point in the direction of another landmark) at a level indistinguishable from that of healthy control volunteers who grew up with E.P. and who also left during their young adulthood (Teng and Squire, 1999). The matched control volunteers had an easier time mentally navigating in their current environments, scoring at the ceiling (100% correct). E.P., however, emphatically did not have an easier time navigating in the area he had moved into 6 years prior to testing (and 1 year after he became amnesic). His performance dropped from 83% correct in his childhood environment to 0% correct in his current environment on the navigation tasks. Despite living on a hill that overlooks the Pacific Ocean a mere 2 miles away, E.P. was not even able to point in its direction. Thus, E.P. can retrieve spatial information and navigate in a spatial environment learned long before the onset of his amnesia but apparently has not learned any spatial information about his environment after the onset of his amnesia. With complete hippocampal loss, spatial *processing* therefore appears normal despite complete inability to acquire new spatial *information*.

Neuroimaging studies have also begun to provide useful data on the role of MTL structures in spatial processing and, consistent with lesion evidence (e.g., Epstein et al., 2001), have clearly implicated the posterior portions of the parahippocampal gyrus in topographical memory tasks. For example, in an early study, Aguirre et al. (1996) observed MTL activity that was confined to the posterior parahippocampal gyrus (likely parahippocampal cortex) as participants learned to navigate in a three-dimensional maze viewed from a first-person perspective (activity relative to a low-level control task). Using a similar task, Maguire et al. (1998) also reported parahippocampal gyrus activity associated with exploring and learning the topography of a virtual three-dimensional environment (at least when the environment contained objects that could serve as landmarks). Whether the activity is specifically related to topographical processing or is representative of more general mnemonic function cannot be determined from these data. However, it is of interest that they implicate the posterior portions of the parahippocampal gyrus and not the hippocampal region in these topographical learning tasks.

Consistent with these findings, Shelton and Gabrieli (2002) also observed activity in the posterior parahippocampal gyrus (with this region of activity extending into the posterior hippocampal region) as participants encoded a virtual three-dimensional environment when viewed from a first-person, or "route," perspective. Of interest, the pattern clearly differed when participants encoded environments from an aerial, or "survey," perspective. Despite similar subsequent memory for environments learned from the two perspectives, activity in the posterior parahippocampal gyrus was greater when participants encoded the environment from a route perspective than from a survey perspective. The authors suggest that this difference may be the result of qualitatively different mnemonic demands placed on participants in the two conditions. For route encoding, participants must continually bind together a representation of their present position to their past and future positions to create a layout of the entire environment. Although still spatial in nature, encoding the environment from a survey perspective did not place this same sort of demand on participants. In a subsequent task that asked participants to draw maps of the environment, the sequential order of presentation was preserved following route learning and was not preserved following survey learning, further suggesting a difference in the way the two environments were encoded that may have led to the observed difference in activity in the parahippocampal gyrus.

Hartley et al. (2003) contrasted activity associated with navigating in a large-scale virtual environment either by way-finding (via route-based spatial knowledge gained by free exploration) or by route-following (traversing the same route that had been well learned during study). Unlike the simple route-following task, which required only recapitulation of a well learned route, the way-finding task required knowledge of the global spatial relations in the environment and navigation along a novel path. Within the MTL, Hartley et al. (2003) reported greater activity in the posterior parahippocampal gyrus overall during the way-finding task than during the route-following task. Perhaps of more interest, with the way-finding condition, activity in the hippocampal region was correlated with accuracy of performance (ceiling effects made this test impossible with the route-following task). Furthermore, in an individual differences analysis that examined correlations between the participant's overall performance in way-finding and neural activity differences between way-finding and route-finding, Hartley et al. (2003) reported a significant positive correlation in what is likely the perirhinal cortex and a significant negative correlation in the head of the right caudate. A positive correlation in the hippocampal region fell just short of significance. Thus, participants who were better at navigation showed greater MTL recruitment during the way-finding task relative to the route-finding task than participants who performed more poorly. Conversely, these same good navigators showed greater caudate recruitment during the route-finding task relative to the way-finding task than participants who performed more poorly.

One logical interpretation of these data (although not the only one, given the contrastive, or relative, nature of fMRI) is that the better navigators recruited structures in the MTL more for the way-finding task and that they recruited the caudate more for the route-finding task. Furthermore, these results make the tantalizing suggestion that this differential recruitment might be causally related to their better performance. Hartley et al. (2003) interpreted their results as being supportive of a role of the hippocampus in the use of a cognitive map, but McNamara and Shelton (2003) suggested that the correlations observed in the hippocampal region are also consistent with the view that the hippocampus processes memory in a way that allows for its flexible use in guiding behavior (e.g., Eichenbaum, 2000). Moreover, in the study of Hartley et al. (2003), the most reliable positive correlation in the individual differences analysis was observed in the perirhinal cortex, not the hippocampal region. (One reliable correlation was observed in the left hippocampal region, but this was using a mnemonically laden contrast.) That the contrast between way-finding and route-finding in the perirhinal cortex would strongly correlate with navigation skill provides a novel datapoint to help us understand the differentiation of function across structures in the MTL.

Thus, the evidence from humans suggests that the hippocampus is involved in spatial memory tasks but that its function is more generally mnemonic and not limited to spatial memory. In humans, spatial memory is an excellent example of complex, declarative memory.

12.4.5 Associations, Recollections, Episodes, or Sources

A large amount of the research on the human hippocampus has been aimed at functionally dissociating the role of the hippocampus from the role of adjacent cortical structures. As noted at the beginning of the chapter, a popular idea draws on the anatomy to suggest that the hippocampus integrates information from and combines the processing of the adjacent cortical structures that feed into the hippocampus. Two fundamental hypotheses that share this basic idea and that are both driven by data from human and nonhuman studies have been proposed and explored. One hypothesis states that there is a clear dissociation of function between the hippocampus and the adjacent structures. For example, the hippocampus has been described as being involved in memory that is associational, multi-item, spatial, episodic, and recollective, whereas the perirhinal cortex (and by extension at times the parahippocampal cortex) is involved in memory that is automatic, noneffortful, single-item, and familiarity, or recency-based (in contrast to recollective), with this distinction being qualitative rather than quantitative (Brown and Aggleton, 2001).

The other hypothesis states that the dissociation of function is more quantitative than qualitative in nature and that the hippocampus and the adjacent structures in the parahippocampal gyrus are all broadly involved in declarative memory. This is not to say that the medial temporal lobe is equipotential in nature. By virtue of being farther up in the hierarchical structure of the medial temporal lobe (see Chapter 3), the hippocampus is proposed to "combine and extend" the processing carried out by the entorhinal, perirhinal, and parahippocampal cortices (Squire and Zola-Morgan, 1991). By virtue of receiving input from both perirhinal and parahippocampal cortices (via the entorhinal cortex), the hippocampus is in a position to be able to integrate information across these structures and sources of information. Thus, "associative," or "conjunctive," processing can be attributed to the hippocampus. However, the structures in the parahippocampal gyrus also receive input from a wide range of sources, putting them in a position to perform "associative" or "conjunctive" processing as well. As the input to the hippocampus consists of more refined and further processed information (its major input arrives from the entorhinal cortex, which receives approximately two-thirds of its input from the perirhinal and parahippocampal cortices), the hippocampus is in a position to perform different, potentially more abstract or complex associative or conjunctive processing. This is not to say, however, that there is binary dissociation of function between the hippocampus and the adjacent cortical structures according to associative or conjunctive versus single-item, episodic versus semantic, recollection versus familiarity, and so on.

The hypothesis that the hippocampus combines and extends the processing of the adjacent cortex is underspecified, as the current theories that take this view do not detail how this process takes place (nor, often, do the theories that propose a more binary dissociation). Data from amnesic patients with damage limited to the hippocampus and data from neuroimaging studies are presented in the following two sections. Overall, the data are not consistent with a clean, binary division of labor between the hippocampus and the cortical components of the medial temporal lobes. They are more consistent with either the graded division of labor implied by the concept of "combine and extend" or with a division of labor along lines that have yet to be explored significantly using these two techniques.

Amnesic Patients

The data available from amnesic patients with bilateral damage thought to be limited to the hippocampal region are far from allowing consensus in support of either hypothesis. For example, Yonelinas et al. (2002) reported data from 56 hypoxic patients with presumed (although not confirmed—see Section 12.3.3) bilateral damage to the hippocampal region. When compared to a similar-sized group of healthy controls, the patients were impaired on both recall and recognition memory tasks. When transformed into z-scores (so the patients' performance is expressed relative to the mean and standard deviation of the controls' performance—see Section 12.3.2), the impairment in recall was larger than the impairment in recognition. Thus, if recall tasks place greater demands on episodic or recollective processing than recognition memory tasks, these data point to a differential role for the hippocampus in this kind of memory.

In the same study, four of the hypoxic patients were tested using the Remember-Know procedure to assess recollective and familiarity components of recognition (Tulving, 1985). In this task, participants indicate at the time of retrieval whether their memory is best described as recollective, containing episodic components and clear knowledge of the source of the memory (a "Remember" response), or best described as a feeling of familiarity (a "Know" response). Whereas patients with MTL damage known to extend beyond the hippocampal region were impaired in both recollective and familiarity components, the hypoxic patients were significantly impaired only in the recollective component. Thus, barring any concern about the lesion locations in the hypoxic patients, these data appear to support the conclusion that the hippocampus plays a key role in recall and in recollective processing, and that these processes may not be able to be supported by the adjacent cortex. Conversely, if the lack of familiarity impairment is true (in the four participants the 23% impairment was unreliable, but this may be the result of insufficient statistical power), the hippocampal region may not provide any familiarity signal to be used during recognition. Thus, we would have clear functional dissociation between the hippocampal region and the adjacent cortex.

The difficulty is that this pattern is not consistently observed. For example, Manns et al. (2003) tested a group of seven patients with bilateral damage limited to the hippocampal region (as determined by MRI) using the same tasks employed by Yonelinas et al. (2002). Consistent with the results of Yonelinas et al. (2002), the patients were impaired on both tests of recognition and recall. However, there was no evidence of disproportional impairment. When recall performance was measured against recognition performance, the patients' recall score was in the 30.5th percentile of their recognition distribution and the controls' recall score was in the 30.6th percentile of their recognition distribution. When the same z-score analysis was performed, the amnesics' recognition performance was *worse* than their recall performance, indicating greater impairment in recognition than recall. Furthermore, the amnesics' performance on the Remember-Know task showed similar impairments for both Remember (60% reduction) and Know (60–71% reduction, depending on the scoring method) responses. Thus, although a null result, the data of Manns et al. (2003) leave little room to support a clear functional dissociation between the hippocampal region and the adjacent MTL structures with respect to recollective processes.

Unfortunately, neither finding is entirely atypical of the results found in the literature. With regard to a specialized role for the hippocampus in this form of memory, the results are decidedly mixed, indicating a critical gap in our theories of hippocampal function or a critical methodological problem (such as the often-suggested possibility that our assessment of the damage in these patients is incomplete—see Section 12.3.3). In the particular case of these two studies, there is a potential solution to the disparity in the findings in the methodology. The potential solution serves to highlight how difficult this research can be and how tenuous the observations of differential impairments often are.

In a detailed reanalysis of the individual participant data from both data sets, Wixted and Squire (2004) noted that a single control participant of the 55 tested in the Yonelinas et al. (2002) study had a recognition score that was a marked outlier in the distribution of scores. The effect of this data-point was sufficient to skew the z-score analysis (see Section 12.3.2) and mask the apparent recognition memory impairment.

Results such as these led to a confused state of affairs in the literature, as it was often unclear what to make of the conflicting data and what factors have influenced the differing results. Looking at the effects on recall versus recognition, recollection versus familiarity, associations versus single-items, or episodic versus semantic memory, conflicting results abound. For example, Jon, a developmental-amnesic patient (neonatal hypoxia) with damage limited to the hippocampal region (as assessed by MRI), has been shown to exhibit clearly impaired episodic memory but has done relatively well in school and obtained a solid vocabulary despite his amnesia (Vargha-Khadem et al., 1997). Jon has also been shown to demonstrate relatively normal levels of recognition memory (except on cross-modal tasks), relatively intact familiarity, and impaired recollection (Baddeley et al., 2001; Vargha-Khadem et al., 2001). Although Jon's amnesia was neonatal, it appears that this is not the source of the dissociation. While examining early-onset (perinatal to 3 months) versus late-onset (6–14 years) amnesia in children with MRI-confirmed hippocampal damage, Vargha-Khadem et al. (2003) noted substantial impairments on several standardized tests of episodic memory in both groups. In contrast, semantic memory, as assessed by measures of vocabulary acquired outside the laboratory, was in the low-average range in both groups, perhaps indicating only mild impairment (unfortunately, it is difficult to know if the amount of vocabulary training in the school or at home was similar to that of normals in these patients. (See Vargha-Khadem et al., 2001 for a similar finding.)

Furthermore, Y.R., an adult-onset amnesic patient (Holdstock et al., 2002a,b; Mayes et al., 2002) showed a similar impairment pattern. Across a series of 34 recall tests, Y.R. was substantially impaired relative to a group of healthy controls, obtaining an average z-score of –3.6. However, across a series of 43 recognition memory tests, Y.R. was only mildly impaired, averaging a z-score of –0.5 (Mayes et al., 2002). (Interestingly, by not showing a bias to view the novel item, Y.R. exhibits impaired performance in the visual paired comparison task at 5- to 10-second delays). Thus, even in a case of adult-onset amnesia, selective impairment in recall relative to recognition has been observed following hippocampal damage.

In contrast with the reports on Y.R. and the developmental amnesic patients, several studies other than that of Manns et al. (2003) have shown substantial impairments in item-recognition memory tasks in patients with hippocampal damage (Hopkins et al., 1995; Reed and Squire, 1997; Stark and Squire, 2000b, 2003; Stark et al., 2002). Thus, in some patients, hippocampal damage leads to substantial recognition memory impairments that are similar to their recall impairments. Furthermore, in two of these studies (Stark et al., 2002; Stark and Squire, 2003), single-item recognition (e.g., "Did you see this object before"?) was compared with associative recognition (e.g., "You've seen both these objects before, but were they paired together?") in patients with damage limited to the hippocampal region. In both, single-item and associative recognition patients with hippocampal damage were impaired—and to the same degree (e.g., 15% impairment in single-item recognition and 13% impairment in associative recognition in Stark et al., 2002, experiment 1).

Thus, we have a number of studies that report a dissociation showing selective impairment in recall, recollection, or associative memory following hippocampal damage and a number of studies that clearly show no such dissociation. Currently, there is no clear means of explaining the varying patterns of results. Whether this is due to differences in undetected extrahippocampal damage, damage in the hippocampal region (location or extent), the stimuli, the tasks, or the manner in which the patients approach the tasks is currently unknown. Perhaps most critically, the disparate results could arise from attempting to find evidence for the wrong dissociation. If the functional role of the hippocampus is correlated with episodic, recollective, and recall aspects of declarative memory, but in fact none of these aspects best describes its role, we could be left with a pattern of positive and negative results such as we currently face. For each positive result, some aspect of the task or stimuli correlated better with the unknown true functional role of the hippocampus than for each negative result.

Neuroimaging

A significant number of recent neuroimaging studies have sought to complement the amnesic patient data on the functional dissociation between the hippocampal region and the adjacent cortical structures with respect to the associative, recollective, or source components of declarative memory. Although several patterns are beginning to emerge, the recent neuroimaging data also do not support a clean distinction between the role of the hippocampal region and the role of the adjacent cortical structures along these lines. Clearly, most studies to date have observed activity in the hippocampal region associated with associative, recollective, or source components of memory. However, in almost all of these studies, activity in the (presumed) parahippocampal cortex mirrors that in the hippocampal region. Furthermore, several have reported associative, recollective, or source components in (presumed) perirhinal or entorhinal cortices. In contrast, activity correlated with single-item memory or familiarity may not be limited to the parahippocampal gyrus, or even the perirhinal cortex specifically (see Section 12.4.5). For example, Henson and colleagues (2003) reported activity associated with familiarity in several studies within anterior portions of the MTL that appear to include entorhinal/perirhinal cortices and the hippocampal region as well. Thus, the conclusion best drawn from the following review is that the existing data are certainly not supportive of a clean functional distinction between the hippocampal region and the adjacent structures according to the recollective, associative, or source components of declarative memory.

Several studies (e.g., Henson et al., 1999; Eldridge et al., 2000) have examined the dissociation between recollection and familiarity using the Remember-Know (Tulving, 1985) task. In this task, Remember responses are used to index recollective memory, and Know responses are used to index recognition based on familiarity. Thus, a contrast between the two might be used to assess whether a region such as the hippocampus is particularly involved in recollective forms of memory retrieval. Henson and colleagues (1999) reported little differentiation between Remember and Know responses in the MTL, with no differences observed at the time of the test and only a small region in the parahippocampal gyrus showing less activity for subsequent Remember responses than Know responses at the time of the study (significant differences were observed in frontal and parietal regions).

In contrast, Eldridge and colleagues (2000) observed greater activity for Remember judgments than Know judgments, correct rejections, and misses in the hippocampal region. These data are consistent with a greater role for the hippocampal region in Remember responses than in Know responses. However, there are some limitations to the Remember-Know task. First, it is difficult to perform in the fMRI scanner because it requires two steps to avoid becoming a simple confidence rating (Hicks and Marsh, 1999). If two steps are used (as was done in Eldridge et al., 2000), two cognitive processes are being engaged (first deciding yes/no recognition and then classifying the retrieval as Remember or Know), and it is impossible in fMRI data to separate activity from two events that always immediately follow each other (see Section 12.3.5). Additionally, it is difficult to ascribe the enhanced activity for Remember responses entirely to a functional dissociation favoring the recollective component of recognition. It is quite plausible that any more detail-rich retrieval would result in more activity than a detail-poor retrieval. As such, Remember responses might yield more activity than Know responses in a region not particularly involved in the recollective component itself. Finally, even if one reasonably assumes that some portion of the enhanced activity for Remember responses over Know responses can be attributed to recollective or associative aspects of processing, Eldridge et al. (2000) observed greater activity for Remember than Know responses not only in the hippocampal region but also in the parahippocampal gyrus (likely to be in the parahippocampal cortex). Thus, this recollective signal was not limited to the hippocampal region.

Activity tied to familiarity must be considered as well. Henson and colleagues (2003) reported activity associated with familiarity in several studies in anterior portions of the MTL that appear to include entorhinal/perirhinal cortices and the hippocampal region as well. Likewise, Stark and Squire (2000c, 2001a) reported activity in the hippocampal region during simple recognition memory tasks that can rely purely on familiarity, with no apparent increase in activity when the task became more associative or recollective (Stark and Squire, 2001a). Thus, the data do not support a clean functional dissociation between recollective processing in the hippocampal region and familiarity processing in the structures of the parahippocampal gyrus.

Several other studies have examined activity during the formation or retrieval of paired associates that may be used to determine whether the hippocampal region might be more involved in associative components of declarative memory than in nonassociative or single-item components. In one case (Sperling et al., 2001), associative encoding-related activity was observed in the hippocampal formation (defined as the hippocampus proper, subiculum, and entorhinal cortex) without observing significant activity elsewhere in the parahippocampal gyrus, supporting the notion that the hippocampus is particularly involved in associative aspects of memory. However, in a similarly designed study, but one that

restricted its analysis to the hippocampal region (Small et al., 2001), activity was observed not only for the encoding and retrieval of face–name associations but also for the encoding and retrieval of individual faces and names (although hippocampal activity for face–name associations was more widespread than the combination of activity for faces and activity for names alone). In both, a blocked design was used to contrast activity associated with viewing novel face–name pairs with activity associated with viewing repeated face–name pairs. Unfortunately, the blocked nature of the design impeded the ability to isolate individual encoding trials based on the quality or amount of information subsequently retrieved. Thus, in this study, it is difficult to know whether the greater activity associated with viewing novel face–name pairs was the result of encoding the face, the name, or the association or whether the activity resulted from a novelty detection (e.g., Strange et al., 1999).

Other studies contrasting associative and nonassociative memory have observed more widespread activity. For example Henke and colleagues (1997) used PET to measure activity during the encoding and retrieval of face–house pairs. More recently, Henke et al. (1999) used fMRI to measure activity during the encoding of semantic associations between words. In both studies, greater activity for associative relative to nonassociative memory was observed in both the hippocampal region and the parahippocampal gyrus. Similarly, in an fMRI study of recognition memory, Yonelinas et al. (2001) reported greater activity during associative than nonassociative recognition in both the hippocampal region and the posterior parahippocampal gyrus. Likewise, Pihlajamaki et al. (2003) observed their most consistent activity during the encoding of picture pairs not in the hippocampal region itself (where there was some evidence) but in the perirhinal cortex; and Sperling et al. (2003) reported activity associated with high-confidence encoding of face–name pairs in anterior portions of the MTL that covered the hippocampal region and the parahippocampal gyrus bilaterally (but whose most active voxels were in the hippocampal region bilaterally and in the right entorhinal cortex).

In addition to studying arbitrary associations, a number of attempts have been made to examine the automatic associations that are formed between memory for an item itself and the "source memory" or episodic knowledge of when and where that item was encountered (e.g., Did you see this item? If so, which study task was it in?). In an elegant example that looked at encoding activity that predicted subsequent memory for an item along with the source relative to encoding activity that predicted memory for the item alone, Davachi et al. (2003) reported a functional dissociation. Activity predicting subsequent source memory was somewhat widespread, with this associative activity observed bilaterally in the hippocampal region and in the left parahippocampal cortex. In contrast, item-only activity was observed solely in the left perirhinal cortex. Here, activity at encoding predicted subsequent memory in general (using as contrast greater activity at the time of encoding for items subsequently remembered relative to items subsequently forgotten), but the activity did not differ as a function of whether the source aspect was subsequently remembered. Thus, the hippocampal region and the parahippocampal cortex appeared to play a role in encoding the source component, whereas the perirhinal cortex appeared to play a role only in encoding the item component of the memory (see Ranganath et al., 2003 for a similar finding).

In a related study, Kirwan and Stark (2004) examined activity during both the encoding and the retrieval of face–name pairs. Like Davachi et al. (2003), greater activity during the successful encoding of associations relative to their unsuccessful encoding (an "associative" pattern) was observed in the hippocampal region and the parahippocampal cortex (right unilateral in this case). Also like Davachi et al. (2003), a portion of perirhinal cortex showed a general subsequent memory effect that did not vary with the associative component (a "single item" pattern). Thus, associative signals were observed in the hippocampal region and the parahippocampal cortex whereas single-item signals were observed in the perirhinal cortex.

However, unlike Davachi et al. (2003), reliable signals that ran counter to this simple dissociation were observed as well. First, the associative pattern was observed in one portion of the right parahippocampal cortex during encoding, whereas the single-item signal was observed in a different portion of the right parahippocampal cortex. Thus, at the time of encoding, there was no clear differentiation observed between an associative hippocampal region and parahippocampal cortex and a nonassociative perirhinal cortex (nor, of course, was there clear differentiation between the hippocampal region and the parahippocampal gyrus as a whole). Furthermore, when examining activity during recognition memory testing, the left perirhinal cortex, right entorhinal cortex, right hippocampal region, and right parahippocampal cortex all showed an associative pattern of activity (greater activity during retrieval of the face(name pair and their association relative to the retrieval of the face and name without their association). Thus, at time of retrieval, greater activity in the associative than in the nonassociative condition was observed throughout the regions of the MTL, with similar amounts of associative activity (contrast between associative and nonassociative retrieval) across MTL structures.

Dobbins et al. (2002) reported a similar dissociation during retrieval of source information (what task was performed at the study?) and recency information (which word appeared more recently on the study list?). When examining activity in the source retrieval task, activity in the hippocampal region, the posterior parahippocampal gyrus (likely the parahippocampal cortex), and activity in the entorhinal/perirhinal cortex all were associated with greater activity during correct source retrieval than incorrect source retrieval. In the hippocampal region and the posterior parahippocampal gyrus, an overall task effect was observed, with both regions showing greater overall activity during source than recencyjudgments. In contrast, although activity in the entorhinal/perirhinal cortex indexed accuracy in the source retrieval task (it was affected by accuracy of source judgments), its activity was similar for source and recency judgments overall. Therefore,

whereas the hippocampal and posterior parahippocampal gyrus activity could be easily explained as indexing source retrieval, the entorhinal/perirhinal activity was a more complex combination of source and recency-related activity.

Thus, the current neuroimaging evidence has clearly implicated both the hippocampal region (Henke et al., 1997, 1999; Eldridge et al., 2000; Small et al., 2001; Sperling et al., 2001, 2003; Stark and Squire, 2001a; Yonelinas et al., 2001; Dobbins et al., 2002; Davachi et al., 2003; Ranganath et al., 2003; Kirwan and Stark, 2004) and the parahippocampal cortex (Henke et al., 1997, 1999; Eldridge et al., 2000; Yonelinas et al., 2001; Dobbins et al., 2002; Davachi et al., 2003; Ranganath et al., 2003; Kirwan and Stark, 2004) in recollective and associative memory encoding and retrieval. Furthermore, there has been some support for the perirhinal cortex and the entorhinal cortex in this regard as well (Dobbins et al., 2002; Pihlajamaki et al., 2003; Sperling et al., 2003; Kirwan and Stark, 2004) (see also the discussion of Hartley et al., 2003, in Section 12.4.4). Thus, it would be an oversimplification of the data to conclude that the fMRI data support a specific or unique role for the hippocampal region in associative or recollective aspects of declarative memory, as the same patterns of activity clearly extend into the adjacent cortical structures (most often the parahippocampal cortex). Likewise, it would be an oversimplification to conclude that the fMRI data support a specific or unique role for any of the adjacent cortical structures in nonassociative forms of declarative memory. Although there is evidence for nonassociative or familiarity-based activity in the entorhinal and perirhinal cortices (Dobbins et al., 2002; Davachi et al., 2003; Henson et al., 2003; Ranganath et al., 2003; Kirwan and Stark, 2004), there is evidence for such activity in the parahippocampal cortex (Kirwan and Stark, 2004) and in the hippocampal region (Stark and Squire, 2000c; Small et al., 2001; Stark and Squire, 2001a; Henson et al., 2003). In addition, each of these structures has been shown to respond according to the associative or recollective nature of the task as well. Accordingly, although these neuroimaging data cannot be resolute with respect to function (all are correlational data sets), they certainly do not support clean dissociation of function in the MTL according to recollective, associative, or source components of declarative memory.

12.5 Conclusions

We began this chapter by asking the question, *What does the human hippocampus do?* The significant amount of research that has followed Milner's initial hypotheses has allowed us to reach a number of clear conclusions. First, along with the adjacent cortical structures in the parahippocampal gyrus, the human hippocampal region is critically involved in memory for facts and events (explicit or declarative memory). Second, this involvement is time-limited. Third, the hippocampal region and the adjacent cortex are not involved in immediate or working memory process and are not involved in a wide range of implicit or nondeclarative long-term memory process (although they may be used in working memory or implicit tasks that evoke declarative processes). Fourth, the hippocampal region is not involved in nonmnemonic aspects of cognition including spatial processing (although spatial memory is a clear example of its time-limited mnemonic role).

However, despite these strides, the differentiation of function between the hippocampal region and the adjacent cortical structures of the parahippocampal gyrus is not currently apparent. That the hippocampus is involved in associative, recollective, or source components of declarative memory is quite clear. Lesions to the hippocampal region yield deficits on tasks that assess these forms of memory, and neuroimaging studies have observed activity correlated with them as well. However, it is equally clear that the hippocampus can be involved in single-item, nonassociative, and familiarity-based components of declarative memory as well. Hippocampal lesions have resulted in deficits on these tasks, and hippocampal activity has been observed during them. Furthermore, the adjacent cortical structures (most notably the parahippocampal cortex) may also serve to support associative, recollective, or source components of declarative memory. Thus, the available data do not support a clean division of labor along any of the lines proposed.

Some differentiation exists. Not only does the anatomy suggest functional differentiation, the research to date has often yielded solid evidence of functional dissociations. However, pushing our interpretations of these dissociations and the theories that fall out of them has often led to clear disconnects between the theoretical predictions and additional data.

There is a difficulty faced when one tries to assign function to a region based on the impairment observed following damage or based on a set of signals recorded from the region. If a hippocampal lesion impairs task X, does it mean that the hippocampus *does* task X? Difficulties with dissociations aside (which are also discussed in Chapter 13), even if we are certain that the ability to perform task X critically depends on processing that occurs in the hippocampus, it is still a large leap to the conclusion that the purpose of the hippocampus is to give us the processing required by task X. Yet, this is the kind of conclusion the dissociation approach can easily encourage unless one is extremely cautious about the interpretation of the data.

A more concrete example might make this problem clear. Suppose there is a task that requires one-trial learning of associative, complex, cross-modal, relational, novel, arbitrary information. Further suppose that a complete bilateral lesion to the hippocampus entirely removes the ability to perform this task at above-chance levels. One might conclude quite reasonably that the hippocampus allows us to, or is necessary to, perform one-trial learning of associative, complex, cross-modal, relational, novel, and arbitrary information. However, it would not be reasonable to conclude that this is the only thing the hippocampus does. The hippocampus might well be involved in one-trial associative, complex, cross-modal, and relational memories between pieces of information that are

not entirely novel or arbitrary. If it were not, we'd have a hippocampus that is rarely doing anything at all, as few experiences would satisfy the extreme end points of the dimensions laid out here.

Furthermore, it might well be that if one or more of these constraints were dropped or weakened, adjacent cortical regions might be able to perform the task to some degree. With the bias toward visual information found in perirhinal cortex, perhaps associative, complex, relational, novel, and arbitrary information could be learned to at least some degree if it were not heavily multimodal and if the test were not all-or-none but sensitive to somewhat more gradual learning. By still being somewhat multimodal, perirhinal cortex may support learning of multimodal information but only when other constraints are weakened.

In this situation (which parallels the data at least in spirit), what would we claim to be the function of the hippocampus? Are there tasks that only the hippocampus can perform? Yes, but, is that all that the hippocampus does? No. Is there a single feature of a task that allows us to determine that the hippocampus and only the hippocampus can perform the task? Not really. There is a combination of features, each of which points toward strengths of the hippocampus that, when taken together, isolate it as the only structure capable of performing the required task. By virtue of the anatomy, the hippocampus receives the most highly processed, multimodal information and is well designed to learn new arbitrary information rapidly. Structures such as the perirhinal cortex receive less processed, more modal-specific information and are less well designed to learn new arbitrary information rapidly.

Therefore, despite finding what might be a task clearly to isolate the hippocampus, we may very well be right back in the opposite class of theory. Even with a task that dissociates the hippocampus from the rest of the brain, the hippocampus may be combining and extending the processing of the adjacent cortex in the medial temporal lobe. It is not that the hippocampus is doing anything all that different from the adjacent cortex, it is merely that it has access to more complete, more refined information and can learn a bit more rapidly. Thus, what initially appears as a clear qualitative dissociation may, in truth, be far more quantitative in nature.

This is not meant to discourage the quest for dissociations. By finding such dissociations, we get to know in what tasks the hippocampus (or any other structure) plays a critical role. In so doing, and when looking across data sets, we can attempt to discern just what aspects make a task fully dependent on the hippocampus and what aspects make a task partially dependent on the hippocampus; we therefore can then define just what the hippocampus may be doing for us. What this is meant to argue against is the simple extension from dissociation to functional interpretation. The shorthand of labeling a structure such as the hippocampus as "performing task X memory" or "being responsible for" a particular kind of memory implies that it does not perform task Y memory, and other structures cannot be responsible for this kind of memory. It is not the dissociation in the data that is problematical but its interpretation as a binary functional dissociation that does injustice to the data and oversimplifies the operation of a complex, highly interconnected and dynamic system.

What we are then currently left with is incomplete understanding of the medial temporal lobe and the role the hippocampus plays in its function. As several have suggested, the division of labor is likely to be graded rather than absolute (e.g., Lavenex and Amaral, 2000; Suzuki and Eichenbaum, 2000; Stark et al., 2002; Norman and O'Reilly, 2003). Although it may best be thought of currently in terms of combining and extending the processing of the adjacent cortex, this is still an unsatisfying definition of the role of the hippocampus. We still do not know the exact nature of this division of labor, what exactly can be combined and extended, how it is done, and how the collection of structures interact to perform this mnemonic function. We also do not know the role of the perirhinal, entorhinal, and parahippocampal cortices; and we do not know how they all interact as a dynamic system. These issues represent currently active areas of experimentation and theoretical development, and all can benefit from the recent methodological advances laid out earlier in the chapter. In short, although our present understanding of human hippocampal function is far from complete, we have certainly made great strides. This is an exciting time for human hippocampal research.

In conclusion, one final point needs to be addressed. Throughout this chapter, the hippocampus and the rest of the medial temporal lobes have been discussed as providing a critical role in declarative or explicit long-term memory. The reader should not take this to mean that the structures of the medial temporal lobe are the only ones responsible for long-term memory performance. Their role is essential, as they appear to act as a repository for this kind of information or at least for some compressed version of this information (i.e., a "pointer") for some period of time. However, encoding and retrieval tasks engage structures well beyond the medial temporal lobes. For example, in cued recall, the cue must be assembled in some format suitable for probing memory's contents, and the results of the retrieval must be interpreted and evaluated. Quite likely, the results of the initial retrieval attempt leads to an extended or revised cue that is again used in a retrieval attempt. Much of this appears to be the purview of structures outside the medial temporal lobe (of frontal structures in particular), making memory, and even long-term declarative memory, the operation of a large system of structures. The medial temporal lobe and the hippocampus in particular are but one component, albeit a vital component, of this larger system.

ACKNOWLEDGMENTS

The author thanks Shauna Stark, Brock Kirwan, Yoko Okado, Marci Flanery, and Richard Morris for their comments on drafts of the chapter; Susan Corkin for providing previously unpublished data on H.M.; and the National Science Foundation for support.

REFERENCES

Aguirre G, Detre J, Alsop D, D'Esposito MD (1996) The parahippocampus subserves topographical learning in man. *Cereb Cortex* 6:823–829.

Bachevalier J, Brickson M, Hagger C (1993) Limbic-dependent recognition memory in monkeys develops early in infancy. *Learn Mem* 4:77–80.

Baddeley A, Vargha-Khadem F, Mishkin M (2001) Preserved recognition in a case of developmental amnesia: implications for the acquisition of semantic memory? *J Cogn Neurosci* 13:357–369.

Berger T, Laham R, Thompson R (1980) Hippocampal unit-behavior correlations during classical conditioning. *Brain Res* 193: 229–248.

Binder J, Frost J, Hammeke T, Bellgowan P, Rao S, Cox RW (1999) Conceptual processing during the conscious resting state: a functional MRI study. *J Cogn Neurosci* 11:80–93.

Blaxton T, Zeffiro T, Gabrieli JD, Bookheimer SY, Carrillo M, Theodore W, Disterhoft J (1996) Functional mapping of human learning: a positron emission tomography activation study of eyeblink conditioning. *J Neurosci* 16:4032–4040.

Boynton G, Engel SA, Glover GH, Heeger D (1996) Linear systems analysis of functional magnetic resonance imaging in human V1. *J Neurosci* 16:4207–42212.

Brewer JB, Zhao Z, Desmond JE, Glover GH, Gabrieli JD (1998) Making memories: brain activity that predicts how well visual experience will be remembered. *Science* 281:1185–1187.

Brown MW, Aggleton JP (2001) Recognition memory: what are the roles of the perirhinal cortex and hippocampus? *Nat Rev Neurosci* 2:51–61.

Buckner RL, Petersen SE, Ojemann JG, Miezin FM, Squire LR, Raichle ME (1995) Functional anatomical studies of explicit and implicit memory retrieval tasks. *J Neurosci* 15:12–29.

Buckner RL, Wheeler ME, Sheridan MA (2001) Encoding processes during retrieval tasks. *J Cogn Neurosci* 13:406–415.

Buxton RB (2001) *Introduction to functional magnetic resonance imaging: principles and techniques* (translated). Cambridge: Cambridge University Press.

Caesar K, Gold L, Lauritzen M (2003) Context sensitivity of activity-dependent increases in cerebral blood flow. *Proc Natl Acad Sci USA* 100:4239–4244.

Caine D, Watson J (2000) Neuropsychological and neuropathological sequelae of cerebral anoxia: a critical review. *J Int Neuropsychol Soc* 6:86–99.

Cameron K, Yashar S, Wilson C, Fried I (2001) Human hippocampal neurons predict how well word pairs will be remembered. *Neuron* 30:289–298.

Chun MM, Phelps EA (1999) Memory deficits for implicit contextual information in amnesic subjects with hippocampal damage. *Nat Neurosci* 2:844–847.

Clark RE, Squire LR (1998) Classical conditioning and brain systems: the role of awareness. *Science* 280:77–81.

Clark RE, Zola SM, Squire LR (2000) Impaired recognition memory in rats after damage to the hippocampus. *J Neurosci* 20: 8853–8860.

Cohen NJ, Poldrack RA, Eichenbaum H (1997) Memory for items and memory for relations in the procedural/declarative memory framework. *Memory* 5:131–178.

Corkin S, Amaral DG, Gonzalez RG, Johnson KA, Hyman BT (1997) H.M.'s medial temporal lobe lesion: findings from magnetic resonance imaging. *J Neurosci* 17:3964–3979.

Cummings JL, Tomiyasu U, Read S, Benson DF (1984) Amnesia with hippocampal lesions after cardiopulmonary arrest. *Neurology* 34:679–681.

Dale AM, Buckner RL (1997) Selective averaging of rapidly presented individual trials using fMRI. *Hum Brain Mapp* 5:329–340.

Davachi L, Wagner AD (2002) Hippocampal contributions to episodic encoding: insights from relational and item-based learning. *J Neurophysiol* 88:982–990.

Davachi L, Mitchell J, Wagner AD (2003) Multiple routes to memory: distinct medial temporal lobe processes build up item and source memories. Proc Natl Acad Sci USA 100:2157–2162.

Dobbins IG, Rice HJ, Wagner AD, Schacter DL (2002) Memory orientation and success: separable neurocognitive components underlying episodic recognition. *Neuropsychologia* 41:318–333.

Eichenbaum H (2000) A cortical-hippocampal system for declarative memory. *Nat Rev Neurosci* 1:41–50.

Eichenbaum H, Dudchenko P, Wood E, Shapiro M, Tanila H (1999) The hippocampus, place cells, and memory: is it spatial memory or a memory space? *Neuron* 23:209–226.

Ekstrom A, Kahana M, Caplan J, Fields T, Isham E, Newman E, Fried I (2003) Cellular networks underlying human spatial navigation. *Nature* 425:184–187.

Eldridge LL, Knowlton BJ, Furmanski CS, Bookheimer SY, Engel SA (2000) Remembering episodes: a selective role for the hippocampus during retrieval. *Nat Neurosci* 3:1149–1152.

Epstein R, DeYoe E, Press D, Rosen A, Kanwisher N (2001) Neuropsychological evidence for a topographical learning mechanism in parahippocampal cortex. *Cogn Neuropsychol* 18:481–508.

Fagan J (1970) Memory in the infant. *J Exp Child Psychol* 9:217–226.

Fell J, Klaver P, Elfadil H, Schaller C, Elger C, Fernandez G (2003) Rhinal-hippocampal theta coherence during declarative memory formation: interaction with gamma synchronization? *Eur J Neurosci* 17:1082–1088.

Fernandez G, Brewer JB, Zhao Z, Glover GH, Gabrieli JD (1999a) Level of sustained entorhinal activity at study correlates with subsequent cued-recall performance: a functional magnetic resonance imaging study with high acquisition rate. *Hippocampus* 9:35–44.

Fernandez G, Effern A, Grunwald T, Pezer N, Lehnertz K, Dumpelmann M, Van Roost D, Elger CE (1999b) Real-time tracking of memory formation in the human rhinal cortex and hippocampus. *Science* 285:1582–1585.

Fernandez G, Klaver P, Fell J, Grunwald T, Elger CE (2002) Human declarative memory formation: segregating rhinal and hippocampal contributions. *Hippocampus* 12:514–519.

Fried I, MacDonald K, Wilson C (1997) Single neuron activity in human hippocampus and amygdala during recognition of faces and objects. *Neuron* 18:753–765.

Fried I, Cameron K, Yashar S, Fong R, Morrow J (2002) Inhibitory and excitatory responses of single neurons in the human medial temporal lobe during recognition of faces and objects. *Cereb Cortex* 12:575–584.

Gabrieli JD, Brewer JB, Desmond JE, Glover GH (1997) Separate neural bases of two fundamental memory processes in the human medial temporal lobe. *Science* 276:264–266.

Gale S, Hopkins R (2004) Effects of hypoxia on the brain: neuroimaging and neuropsychological findings following carbon monoxide poisoning and obstructive sleep apnea. *J Int Neuropsychol Soc* 10:60–71.

Glover JA (1989) The "testing" phenomenon: not gone, but nearly forgotten. *J Educ Psychol* 81:392–399.

Graf P, Squire LR, Mandler G (1984) The information that amnesic patients do not forget. *J Exp Psychol Learn Mem Cogn* 10:164–178.

Grasby P, Frith C, Friston K, Bench C, Frackowiak R, Dolan RJ (1993) Functional mapping of brain areas implicated in auditory-verbal memory function. *Brain* 116:1–20.

Green D, Swets J (1966) *Signal detection theory and psychophysics* (translated). New York: Wiley.

Gusnard D, Raichle ME (2001) Searching for a baseline: functional imaging and the resting human brain. *Nat Rev Neurosci* 2:685–694.

Gusnard D, Akbudak E, Shulman G, Raichle ME (2001) Medial prefrontal cortex and self-referential mental activity: relation to a default mode of brain activation. *Proc Natl Acad Sci USA* 98:4259–4264.

Haist F, Gore J, Mao H (2001) Consolidation of human memory over decades revealed by functional magnetic resonance imaging. *Nat Neurosci* 4:1139–1145.

Hamann SB, Squire LR (1997) Intact perceptual memory in the absence of conscious memory. *Behav Neurosci* 111:850–854.

Hartley T, Maguire E, Spiers H, Burgess N (2003) The well-worn route and the path less traveled: distinct neural bases of route following and wayfinding in humans. *Neuron* 2003.

Heit G, Smith M, Halgren E (1988) Neural encoding of individual words and faces by the human hippocampus and amygdala. *Nature* 333:773–775.

Heit G, Smith M, Halgren E (1990) Neuronal activity in the human medial temporal lobe during recognition memory. *Brain* 113:1093–1112.

Henke K, Buck A, Weber B, Wieser HG (1997) Human hippocampus establishes associations in memory. *Hippocampus* 7:249–256.

Henke K, Weber B, Kneifel S, Wieser HG, Buck A (1999) Human hippocampus associates information in memory. *Proc Natl Acad Sci USA* 96:5884–5889.

Henson R (2005) What can functional neuroimaging tell the experimental psychologist? *Q J Exp Physiol* 58:193–233.

Henson RNA, Rugg MD, Shallice T, Josephs O, Dolan RJ (1999) Recollection and familiarity in recognition memory: an event-related functional magnetic resonance imaging study. *J Neurosci* 19:3962–972.

Henson RNA, Cansino S, Herron J, Robb W, Rugg MD (2003) A familiarity signal in human anterior medial temporal cortex? *Hippocampus* 13:301–304.

Hicks JL, Marsh RL (1999) Remember-know judgments can depend on how memory is tested. *Psychonom Bull Rev* 6:117–122.

Holdstock JS, Mayes AR, Cezayirli E, Isaac C, Aggleton JP, Roberts N (2000) A comparison of egocentric and allocentric spatial memory in a patient with selective hippocampal damage. *Neuropsychologia* 38:410–425.

Holdstock JS, Mayes AR, Isaac C, Gong Q, Roberts N (2002a) Differential involvement of the hippocampus and temporal lobe cortices in rapid and slow learning of new semantic information. *Neuropsychologia* 40:748–768.

Holdstock JS, Mayes AR, Roberts N, Cezayirli E, Isaac C, O'Reilly RC, Norman KA (2002b) How recall and recognition are affected by focal damage to the human hippocampus. *Hippocampus* 12:341–351.

Hopkins R, Kesner R, Goldstein M (1995) Item and order recognition memory in subjects with hypoxic brain injury. *Brain Cogn* 27:180–201.

Hopkins R, Myers C, Shohamy D, Grossman S, Gluck MA (2004) Impaired probabilistic category learning in hypoxic subjects with hippocampal damage. *Neuropsychologia* 42.

Hyde JS, Biswal B, Jesmanowicz A (2001) High-resolution fMRI using multislice partial k-space GR-EPI with cubic voxels. *Magn Reson Med* 46:114–125.

Jacoby LL, Dallas M (1981) On the relationship between autobiographical memory and perceptual learning. *J Exp Psychol Gen* 110:306–240.

Kapur N, Brooks D (1999) Temporally-specific retrograde amnesia in two cases of discrete bilateral hippocampal pathology. *Hippocampus* 9:247–254.

Kapur N, Craik FIM, Tulving E, Wilson A, Houle S, Brown G (1994) Neuroanatomical correlates of encoding in episodic memory: levels of processing effect. *Proc Natl Acad Sci USA* 91:2008–2011.

Keane M, Gabrieli JD, Monti L, Fleischman DA, Cantor J, Noland J (1997) Intact and impaired conceptual memory processes in amnesia. Neuropsychology 11:59–69.

Kirwan C, Stark CEL (2004) Medial temporal lobe activation during encoding and retrieval of novel face-name pairs. *Hippocampus* 14:910–930.

Kirwan CB, Jones C, Miller MI (in press) High-resolution *f*MRI investigation of the medial temporal lobe. *Hum Brain Mapp*.

Knowlton BJ, Squire LR (1993) The learning of categories: parallel brain systems for item memory and category knowledge. *Science* 262:1747–1749.

Kreiman G, Koch C, Fried I (2000) Category-specific visual responses of single neurons in the human medial temporal lobe. *Nat Neurosci* 3:946–953.

Lavenex P, Amaral DG (2000) Hippocampal-neocortical interaction: a heirarchy of associativity. *Hippocampus* 10:420–430.

Law JR, Flanery MA, Wirth S, Yanike M, Smith AC, Frank LM, Suzuki WA, Brown EN, Stark CEL (2005) fMRI activity during the gradual acquisition and expression of paired-associate memory. *J Neurosci* 25:5720–5729.

LePage M, Habib R, Tulving E (1998) Hippocampal PET activation of memory encoding and retrieval: the HIPER model. *Hippocampus* 8:313–322.

Levy D, Stark CEL, Squire LR (2004) Intact conceptual priming in the absence of declarative memory. *Psychol Sci* 15:680–686.

Logothetis N, Pauls J, Augath M, Trinath T, Oeltermann A (2001) Neurophysiological investigation of the basis of the fMRI signal. *Nature* 412:150–157.

Maguire E, Frith CD (2003) Lateral asymmetry in the hippocampal response to the remoteness of autobiographical memories. *J Neurosci* 23:5302–5307.

Maguire E, Frith CD, Burgess N, Donnett J, O'Keefe J (1998) Knowing where things are: parahippocampal involvement in encoding objection locations in a virtual large-scale space. *J Cogn Neurosci* 10:61–76.

Maguire E, Henson RNA, Mummery C, Frith CD (2001) Activity in prefrontal cortex, not hippocampus, varies parametrically with the increasing remoteness of memories. *Neuroreport* 12:441–444.

Manns JR, Squire LR (2001) Perceptual learning, awareness, and the hippocampus. *Hippocampus* 11:776–782.

Manns J, Stark C, Squire L (2000) The visual paired-comparison task as a measure of declarative memory. *Proc Natl Acad Sci USA* 97:12375–12379.

Manns JR, Hopkins R, Reed JM, Kitchener EG, Squire LR (2003) Recognition memory and the human hippocampus. *Neuron* 37:171–180.

Marslen-Wilson W, Teuber H (1975) Memory for remote events in anterograde amnesia: Recognition of public figures from news photographs. *Neuropsychologia* 13:353–364.

Mauk M, Thompson R (1987) Retention of classically conditioned eyelid responses following acute decerebration. *Brain Res* 403:89–95.

Mayes AR, Holdstock JS, Isaac C, Hunkin N, Roberts N (2002) Relative sparing of item recognition memory in a patient with adult-onset damage limited to the hippocampus. *Hippocampus* 12:325–340.

McKee R, Squire LR (1993) On the development of declarative memory. *J Exp Psychol Learn Mem Cogn* 19:397–404.

McNamara T, Shelton A (2003) Cognititve maps and the hippocampus. *Trends Cogn Sci* 7:333–335.

Miller MB, Beg M, Ceritogulu C, Stark CEL (2005) Improving statistical power and fMRI data localization using large deformation metric mapping. *Proc Natl Acad Sci USA* 102:9685–9690.

Milner B (1962) Les troubles de la mémoire accompagnant des lésions hippocampiques bilatérales. In: *Physiologie de l'hippocampe*, pp 257–272. Paris: Centre National de la Recherche Scientifique.

Milner B (1972) Disorders of learning and memory after temporal-lobe lesions in man. *Clin Neurosurg* 19:421–446.

Milner B, Corkin S, Teuber H (1968) Further analysis of the hippocampal amnesic syndrome: 14-year follow-up study of H.M. *Neuropsychologia* 6:215–234.

Milner B, Squire LR, Kandel ER (1998) The cognitive neuroscience of memory. *Neuron* 20:445–468.

Morrell H, Gitman S, Wixted J (2002) On the nature of the decision axis in signal-detection-based models of recognition memory. *J Exp Psychol Learn Mem Cogn* 28:1095–1110.

Nadel L, Moscovitch M (1997) Memory consolidation, retrograde amnesia, and the hippocampal complex. *Curr Opin Neurobiol* 7:217–227.

Newman S, Tweig D, Carpenter P (2001) Baseline conditions and subtractive logic in neuroimaging. *Hum Brain Mapp* 14: 228–235.

Niki K, Luo J (2002) An fMRI study on the time-limited role of the medial temporal lobe in long-term topographical autiobiographic memory. *J Cogn Neurosci* 14:500–507.

Norman KA, O'Reilly RC (2003) Modeling hippocampal and neocortical contributions to recognition memory: a complementary learning systems approach. *Psychol Rev* 110:611–646.

Nyberg L, Tulving E, Habib R, Nilsson L, Kapur S, Houle S, Cabeza R, McIntosh A (1995) Functional brain maps of retrieval mode and recovery of episodic information. *Neuroreport* 7:249–252.

O'Reilly RC, Rudy JW (2000) Computational principles of learning in the neocortex and hippocampus. *Hippocampus* 10:389–397.

Otten LJ, Henson RNA, Rugg MD (2001) Depth of processing effects on neural correlates of memory encoding: relationship between findings across- and within-task comparisons. *Brain* 124: 399–412.

Paller KA, McCarthy G (2002) Field potentials in the human hippocampus during the encoding and recognition of visual stimuli. *Hippocampus* 12:415–420.

Paller KA, Wagner AD (2002) Observing the transformation of experience into memory. *Trends Cogn Sci* 6:93–102.

Papanicolaou AC, Panagiotis GS, Castillo EM, Breier JI, Katz JS, Wright AA (2002) The hippocampus and memory of verbal and pictorial material. *Learn Mem* 9:99–104.

Pascalis O, Bachevalier J (1999) Neonatal aspiration lesions of the hippocampal-formation impair visual recognition memory when assessed by the paired-comparison task but not by delayed nonmatching-to-sample task. *Hippocampus* 9:609–616.

Pascalis O, Hunkin N, Holdstock JS, Isaac C, Mayes AR (2004) Visual paired comparison performance is impaired in a patient with selective hippocampal lesions and relatively intact item recognition. *Neuropsychologia* 24:1293–1300.

Pihlajamaki M, Tanila H, Hanninen T, Kononen M, Mikkonen M, Jalkanen V, Partanen K, Aronen H, Soininen H (2003) Encoding of novel picture pairs activates the perirhinal cortex: an fMRI study. *Hippocampus* 13:67–80.

Posner MI, Keele SW (1968) On the genesis of abstract ideas. *J Exp Psychol* 77:353–363.

Preuessner J, Kohler S, Crane J, Pruessner M, Lord C, Byrne A, Kabani N, Collins DL, Evans AC (2002) Volumetry of temporopolar, perirhinal, entorhinal, and parahippocampal cortex from high-resolution MR images: considering the variability of the collateral sulcus. *Cereb Cortex* 12:1342–1353.

Ranganath C, Yonelinas AP, Cohen MX, Dy CJ, Tom SM, D'Esposito MD (2003) Dissociable correlates of recollection and familiarity within the medial temporal lobes. *Neuropsychologia* 42:2–13.

Reber PJ, Wong EC, Buxton RB (2002) Encoding activity in the medial temporal lobe examined with anatomically constrainted fMRI analysis. *Hippocampus* 12:363–376.

Reber PJ, Gitelman D, Parrish T, Mesulam M (2003) Dissociating explicit and implicit category knowledge with fMRI. *J Cogn Neurosci* 15:574–583.

Reed JM, Squire LR (1997) Impaired recognition memory in patients with lesions limited to the hippocampal formation. *Behav Neurosci* 111:667–675.

Reed JM, Squire LR (1998) Retrograde amnesia for facts and events: findings from four new cases. *J Neurosci* 18:3943–3954.

Rees G, Friston K, Koch C (2000) A direct quantitative relationship between the functional properties of human and macaque V5. *Nat Neurosci* 3:716–723.

Rempel-Clower NL, Zola SM, Squire LR, Amaral DG (1996) Three cases of enduring memory impairment after bilateral damage limited to the hippocampal formation. *J Neurosci* 16:5233–5255.

Ribot T (1887) *Diseases of memory: an essay in the positive psychology* (Smith WH, translator). New York: Appleton.

Rose M, Haider H, Weiller C, Buchel C (2002) The role of medial temporal lobe structures in implicit learning: an event-related fMRI study. *Neuron* 36:1221–1231.

Ryan L, Nadel L, Keil K, Putnam K, Schnyer D, Trouard T, Moscovitch M (2001) Hippocampal complex and retrieval of recent and very remote autobiographical memories: evidence from functional magnetic resonance imaging in neurologically intact people. *Hippocampus* 11:707–714.

Schacter DL (1994) Priming and multiple memory systems: perceptual mechanisms of implicit memory. In: *Memory systems 1994* (Schacter DL, Tulving E, eds), pp 233–268. Cambridge, MA: MIT Press.

Schacter DL (1999) The seven sins of memory. *Am Psychol* 54:182–203.

Schacter DL, Wagner AD (1999) Medial temporal lobe activations in fMRI and PET studies of episodic encoding and retrieval. *Hippocampus* 9:7–24.

Schacter DL, Reiman E, Uecker A, Polster M, Yun LS, Cooper L (1995) Brain regions associated with retrieval of structurally coherent visual information. *Nature* 376:587–590.

Schendan H, Searl M, Melrose R, Stern CE (2003) An fMRI study off the role of the medial temporal lobe in implicit and explicit sequence learning. *Neuron* 37:1013–1025.

Scoville WB (1954) The limbic lobe in man. *J Neurosurg* 11:64–66.

Scoville WB, Milner B (1957) Loss of recent memory after bilateral hippocampal lesions. *J Neurol Neurosurg Psychiatry* 20:11–21.

Shallice T, Fletcher PC, Frith CD, Grasby P, Frackowiak R, Dolan RJ (1994) Brain regions associated with acquisition and retrieval of verbal episodic memory. *Nature* 368:633–635.

Shelton A, Gabrieli JD (2002) Neural correlates of encoding space from route and survey perspectives. *J Neurosci* 22:2711–2717.

Shimamura AP, Squire LR (1984) Paired-associate learning and priming effects in amnesia: a neuropsychological study. *J Exp Psychol Gen* 113:556–570.

Small S, Arun A, Perera G, De La Paz R, Mayeaux R, Stern Y (2001) Circuit mechanisms underlying memory encoding and retrieval in the long axis of the hippocampal formation. *Nat Neurosci* 4:442–449.

Sperling RA, Bates JF, Cocchiarella AJ, Schacter DL, Rosen BR, Albert MS (2001) Encoding novel face-name associations: a functional MRI study. *Hum Brain Mapp* 14:129–139.

Sperling R, Chua E, Cocchiarella A, Rand-Giovannetti E, Poldrack RA, Schacter DL, Albert M (2003) Putting names to faces: successful encoding of associative memories activates the anterior hippocampal formation. *Neuroimage* 20:1400–1410.

Spiers H, Maguire E, Burgess N (2001) Hippocampal amensia. *Neurocase* 7:357–382.

Squire LR (1992) Declarative and nondeclarative memory: multiple brain systems supporting learning and memory. *J Cogn Neurosci* 4:232–243.

Squire LR, Alvarez P (1995) Retrograde amnesia and memory consolidation: a neurobiological perspective. *Curr Opin Neurobiol* 5:169–177.

Squire LR, Knowlton BJ (1995) Learning about categories in the absence of memory. *Proc Natl Acad Sci USA* 92:12470–12474.

Squire LR, Zola-Morgan S (1991) The medial temporal lobe memory system. *Science* 253:1380–1386.

Squire LR, Ojemann JG, Miezin FM, Petersen SE, Videen TO, Raichle ME (1992) Activation of the hippocampus in normal humans: a functional anatomical study of memory. *Proc Natl Acad Sci USA* 89:1837–1841.

Squire LR, Clark RE, Knowlton BJ (2001) Retrograde amnesia. *Hippocampus* 11:50–55.

Stark CEL, Okado Y (2003) Making memories without trying: medial temporal lobe activity associated with incidental memory formation during recognition. *J Neurosci* 23:6748–6753.

Stark CEL, Squire LR (2000a) fMRI activity in the medial temporal lobe during recognition memory as a function of study-test interval. *Hippocampus* 10:329–337.

Stark CEL, Squire LR (2000b) Recognition memory and familiarity judgments in severe amnesia: no evidence for a contribution of repetition priming. *Behav Neurosci* 114:459–467.

Stark CEL, Squire LR (2000c) Functional magnetic resonance imaging (fMRI) activity in the hippocampal region during recognition memory. *J Neurosci* 20:7776–7781.

Stark CEL, Squire LR (2001a) Simple and associative recognition memory in the hippocampal region. *Learn Mem* 8:190–197.

Stark CEL, Squire LR (2001b) When zero is not zero: the problem of ambiguous baseline conditions in fMRI. *Proc Natl Acad Sci USA* 98:12760–12766.

Stark CEL, Squire LR (2003) Hippocampal damage equally impairs memory for single-items and memory for conjunctions. *Hippocampus* 13:281–292.

Stark CEL, Bayley PJ, Squire LR (2002) Recognition memory for single items and for associations is similarly impaired following damage limited to the hippocampal region. *Learn Mem* 9:238–242.

Stefanacci L, Buffalo EA, Schmolck H, Squire LR (2000) Profound amnesia after damage to the medial temporal lobe: a neuroanatomical and neuropsychological profile of patient E.P. *J Neurosci* 20:7024–7036.

Strange BA, Fletcher PC, Henson RNA, Friston KJ, Dolan RJ (1999) Segregating the functions of human hippocampus. *Proc Natl Acad Sci USA* 96:4034–4039.

Strange BA, Otten LJ, Josephs O, Rugg MD, Dolan RJ (2002) Dissociable human perirhinal, hippocampal, and parahippocampal roles during verbal encoding. *J Neurosci* 22:523–528.

Sutherland RJ, Rudy JW (1989) Configural association theory: the role of the hippocampal formation in learning, memory, and amnesia. *Psychobiology* 17:129–144.

Suzuki WA, Eichenbaum H (2000) The neurophysiology of memory. *Ann N Y Acad Sci* 911:175–191.

Talairach J, Tournoux P (1988) *A co-planar stereotaxic atlas of the human brain* (translated). New York: Thieme Medical.

Teng E, Squire LR (1999) Memory for places learned long ago is intact after hippocampal damage. *Nature* 400:675–677.

Tulving E (1985) Memory and consciousness. *Can J Psychol* 26:1–12.

Tulving E, Kapur N, Markowitsch H, Craik FIM, Habib R, Houle S (1994) Neuroanatomical correlates of retrieval in episoidc memory: auditory sentence recognition. *Proc Natl Acad Sci USA* 91:2012–2015.

Vaidya C, Gabrieli JD, Keane M, Monti L (1995) Perceptual and conceptual memory processes in global amnesia. *Neuropsychology* 9:580–591.

Vargha-Khadem F, Gadian DG, Watkins KE, Connelly A, Van Praesschen W, Mishkin M (1997) Differential effects of early hippocampal pathology on episodic and semantic memory. *Science* 277:376–380.

Vargha-Khadem F, Gadian DG, Mishkin M (2001) Dissociaitons in cognitive memory: the syndrome of developmental amnesia. *Philos Trans R Soc Lond B Biol Sci* 356:1435–1440.

Vargha-Khadem F, Salamond C, Watkins KE, Friston K, Gadian DG, Mishkin M (2003) Developmental amnesia: effect of age at injury. *Proc Natl Acad Sci USA* 100:10055–10060.

Verfaellie M, Reiss A, Roth H (1995) Knowledge of new English vocabulary in amnesia: an examination of premorbidly acquired semantic memory. *J Int Neuropsychol Soc* 1:443–452.

Wagner AD, Schacter DL, Rotte M, Koutstaal W, Maril A, Dale AM, Rosen BR, Buckner RL (1998) Building memories: remembering and forgetting of verbal experiences as predicted by brain activity. *Science* 281:1188–1191.

Warrington E, McCarthy G (1988) The fractionation of retrograde amnesia. *Brain Cogn* 7:184–200.

Warrington E, Weiskrantz L (1968) New method of testing long-term retention with special reference to amnesic patients. *Nature* 217:972–974.

Warrington E, Weiskrantz L (1970) The amnesic syndrome: consolidation or retrieval? *Nature* 228:628–630.

Warrington E, Weiskrantz L (1974) The effect of prior learning on subsequent retention in amensic patients. *Neuropsychologia* 12419–428.

Weiskrantz L, Warrington E (1979) Conditioning in amnesic patients. *Neuropsychologia* 17:187–194.

Wirth S, Yanike M, Frank L, Smith A, Brown E, Suzuki WA (2003) Single neurons in the monkey hippocampus and learning of new associations. *Science* 300:1578–1581.

Wixted J, Squire LR (2004) Recall and recognition are equally impaired in patients with selective hippocampal damage. *Cogn Affect Behav Neurosci* 4:58–66.

Yonelinas AP (2002) The nature of recollection and familiarity: a review of 30 years of research. *J Mem Lang* 46:441–517.

Yonelinas A, Hopfinger J, Buonocore M, Kroll N, Baynes K (2001) Hippocampal, parahippocampal and occipital-temporal contributions to associative and item recognition memory: an fMRI study. *Neuroreport* 12:359–363.

Yonelinas AP, Kroll NEA, Quamme J, Lazzara MM, Suave M, Widaman K, Knight RT (2002) Effects of extensive temporal lobe damage or mild hypoxia on recollection and familiarity. *Nat Neurosci* 5:1236–1241.

Zeineh MM, Engel SA, Bookheimer SY (2000) Application of cortical unfolding techniques to functional MRI of the human hippocampal region. *Neuroimage* 11:668–683.

Zeineh MM, Engel SA, Thompson PM, Bookheimer SY (2003) Dynamics of the hippocampus during encoding and retrieval of face-name pairs. *Science* 299:577–580.

Zola SM, Squire LR, Teng E, Stefanacci L, Buffalo EA, Clark RE (2000) Impaired recognition memory in monkeys after damage limited to the hippocampal region. *J Neurosci* 20:451–463.

Zola-Morgan S, Squire LR, Amaral DG (1986) Human amnesia and the medial temporal lobe region: enduring memory impairment following a bilateral lesion limited to field CA1 of the hippocampus. *J Neurosci* 6:2950–2967.

13 ▦ Richard Morris

Theories of Hippocampal Function

13.1 Overview

What does the hippocampal formation do? Does it have one function or many? Can we understand its functions in isolation from that of other areas of the brain? The theories we review in this chapter all focus on the idea that it is a special kind of "memory machine." The link between the hippocampus and memory is an old idea, having its roots in clinical and experimental observations on patients who sustained brain damage that included the hippocampus but all too often extended into other areas of the medial temporal lobe or midbrain (see Chapter 2). Careful study of the small number of patients with more selective damage (see Chapter 12) and that of animals given experimental lesions or other interventions (see later in this chapter) has provided further grounds for believing that the integrity of the hippocampal formation is causally involved in implementing some but not all types of memory. Given that multiple "types" of memory have now been proposed—such as declarative, spatial, and episodic memory—the focus of this chapter is on identifying which of these or other putative types of memory are mediated by the hippocampal formation. Success in this task requires that we recognize that the hippocampus operates in conjunction with other networks and brain structures, including neuromodulatory afferent systems emanating from the midbrain and diverse regions of the neocortex. Any claim that the integrity of the hippocampus is required for one or another type of memory does not, therefore, mean that other brain areas are not involved as well. Discussion of types of memory and their anatomical substrate carries us forward to consider the logically distinct issue of the various "phases" of memory processing in which the hippocampus may be engaged—the encoding of information into memory, the storage of memory traces as biochemical and structural changes in the nervous system, the consolidation processes responsible for their stability over time, and the subsequent retrieval and reactivation of hippocampus-dependent memories during recall. Newer research techniques, such as functional magnetic resonance imaging (fMRI) in humans and invasive techniques with animals such as ensemble single-cell recording and selective neuropharmacological perturbations, all point to a role for specific aspects of hippocampal neural activity in successive phases of memory processing.

Two theories have dominated research on hippocampal function over the past quarter century. The first, discussed in Section 13.3, is that it is involved in the formation of memories for everyday facts and events that can be consciously recalled—collectively called *declarative memory* (Squire, 1992; Squire et al., 2004). Complementing the human studies of the preceding chapter, a particular focus has been the development of a primate model of amnesia built largely on studies of recognition memory. Other behavioral tasks have also been examined, but they have been secondary to testing a key issue: whether the hippocampus is involved in recognizing stimuli that have been presented before. The other major theory (see Section 13.4), emerging from observations first made during the recording of single-cell activity in freely moving rodents (see Chapter 11), is the idea that it is involved in *spatial memory* and, more specifically, the formation of cognitive maps and their use in navigation through space (O'Keefe and Nadel, 1978; Burgess et al., 2002). This theory makes testable predictions about the cell activity that occurs during spatial navigation and the impact of hippocampal dysfunction on spatial memory. Although enormously influential, and often at loggerheads with each other, it will become clear that neither of these two major theories offers a fully satisfactory account of the available data.

Section 13.5 discusses a range of alternative theories, particularly those built around how memory systems handle ambiguity, associative-relations, and context. In 1984, Schmajuk identified more than 20 psychological theories of hippocampal function (Schmajuk, 1984). There have been yet others since. Here we focus on certain particularly influential ideas of the past 25 years, namely that the hippocampus implements a learning process involving the formation of *stimulus configurations* (Sutherland and Rudy, 1989a; O'Reilly and Rudy, 2001), that it is involved in *the relational processing* of stimuli in a manner that enables flexible retrieval (Cohen and Eichenbaum, 1993; Eichenbaum and Cohen, 2001), or that it provides the substrate for encoding and retrieval of information in relation to the *spatiotemporal context* in which that information occurs. Contexts, relations, and configurations may each help disambiguate conflicting associative relations in which a specific stimulus occurs (Hirsh, 1974; Good and Honey, 1991). Although perhaps less prominent than the two major theories, these ideas have been important in expanding our concepts of what memory is all about and its mediation by diverse structures in the brain.

The present focus on memory is, arguably, too exclusive. The hippocampus has also been implicated in a range of other brain functions, including behavioural inhibition and anxiety (Kimble, 1968; Gray, 1982; Davidson and Jarrard, 2004), sensorimotor function (Vanderwolf and Cain, 1994), and acting as a comparator to detect novelty (Gray, 2000). The presence in the hippocampus of a high density of receptors for adrenocortical hormones such as cortisol and corticosterone has also implicated the hippocampus in the cognitive regulation of stress and the hypothalamic-pituitary axis (Sapolsky, 1985; McEwen and Sapolsky, 1995; de Kloet et al., 1999). For clarity, these issues are considered separately in Chapter 15.

Certain concepts relevant to identifying hippocampal function in relation to memory are excluded from detailed discussion in this chapter because it seemed most appropriate to outline them elsewhere. They include the widely discussed idea that activity-dependent synaptic plasticity, such as long-term potentiation (LTP) and long-term depression (LTD), might play a role in learning and memory (Martin et al., 2000; Bliss et al., 2004). This important topic is discussed at the end of Chapter 10. Hebb's concepts of the "cell assembly" and "phase sequence" (Hebb, 1949) and Marr's proposal that distributed associative memories could be implemented by hippocampal local circuitry (Marr, 1971) were both touched on in our historical overview (see Chapter 2) and are developed more fully in Chapter 14. Neural network modeling is a field in its own right that has matured to a level of conceptual and mathematical precision that is beyond the scope of this chapter (Willshaw and Buckingham, 1990; O'Reilly, 1998; Rolls and Treves, 1998; Lisman and Zhabotinsky, 2001; O'Reilly and Norman, 2002).

The chapter concludes by zeroing in on the idea that neural activity in the hippocampal formation contributes to episodic memory (Tulving, 1983; Aggleton and Brown, 1999; Redish, 1999). This contribution has been variously characterized as remembering the "scenes" in which events take place (Gaffan, 1994a), or as processing the "automatic" components of recording and recalling experience that are downstream of neocortical attentional systems (Morris and Frey, 1997). In animals, where the phenomenological aspects of memory are

so difficult to capture (Hampton and Schwartz, 2004), this is now often referred to as "episodic-like" memory (Clayton and Dickinson, 1998). Although also applied elsewhere, it is in this section that we see the greatest implementation of new research technologies, such as novel behavioral tasks, reversible pharmacological manipulations, and region-specific gene targeting. This new way of thinking about hippocampal function also draws more explicitly on the anatomical, physiological, and cell biological ideas discussed in earlier chapters of this book.

In each section, the main concepts of each theory are outlined followed by an examination of exemplar experimental work that supports or conflicts with it and then a general critique. Given the scale of the literature, no attempt has been made to be definitively inclusive, and the choice of studies cited is inevitably subjective. When possible, an attempt is made to refer to ideas about hippocampal function that have emerged from the principles discussed in earlier chapters. Understanding the hippocampal memory machine is an ambitious exercise that requires integrating "top-down" psychological concepts about the distinct types and processing phases of memory with "bottom-up" physiological and cell biological ideas about the local networks, cells, and signal transduction pathways that constitute this beautiful brain structure.

13.2 Cognitive and Behavioral Neuroscience, Interventional Techniques, and the Hippocampus

13.2.1 Value of Interventional Studies to Identify Function

If you want to learn how a machine works, it is a good idea to watch it working. An appropriate next step is to look at selective interventions that disrupt one part of the machine or another and study the various changes in the machine's operation that then occur. In the case of a modular organ such as the brain, it is essential to complement studies that involve its cells being cut up, put under microscopes, poked with electrodes, or bathed in drugs (see Chapters 3–11) with studies of selective interventions that may affect its behavior. This is part of what cognitive and behavioral neuroscientists do to try to understand the functions of the distinct but interacting regions of the brain. Lesion studies in animals, on which we largely focus in this chapter, have been the classic "interventionist" technique for testing theories of function. They have their methodological and interpretative problems, as do pharmacological and genetic techniques. Intervention is, however, the only way to secure definitive information about whether the integrity of a particular anatomical region of the brain or specific physiological and cell biological processes in it is *necessary* for a particular function.

In humans, damage to the brain may arise because of a tumor, a stroke, or a viral infection, or it may be incurred through neurosurgery undertaken to prevent further brain damage (e.g., the surgical management of epilepsy). A few striking and analytically valuable exceptions aside, lesions that arise from these causes are rarely restricted to anatomically circumscribed areas of the brain; nor when they are is the damage incurred ever complete (see Chapter 12). In animal studies, in contrast, specific brain regions can be subject to selective lesions to evaluate whether one or more functions can still be carried out normally. Postmortem histological techniques complement the behavioral observations, providing a vital, relatively immediate check on an experimentalist's intentions with respect to the site and size of the lesion. It is also now possible to use histologically calibrated structural MRI techniques in vivo to establish the accuracy and extent of damage before extensive behavioral testing is undertaken (Malkova et al., 2001).

The lesion method is, of course, used widely in biology, the modern variants of it being pharmacological techniques directed at specific receptors or targeted molecular engineering to investigate gene function ("gene knockouts"). The common analytical principle underlying such approaches is that the study of dysfunction offers insights into normal function. Creating dysfunction does not necessarily require invasive interventions—the study of visual illusions being a case in point—but the neurological approach, as twentieth century neurologist Sir Henry Head put it so well, is one in which "it should not be the injury that captures our attention but how, through injury or disease, normal function is laid bare."

There are, however, problems strewn along the path of laying things bare. In some cases it is the pitfalls of the approach that lead an investigator astray. First, a brain reacts to permanent damage with repair mechanisms—cerebrovascular, neural, glial—that collectively result in dynamic changes from the moment the damage occurs. It may be some while before brain function restabilizes after surgically induced diaschisis (Stein et al., 1983; Finger et al., 2004). Second, even when it does restabilize, we should not assume that adjacent undamaged brain areas necessarily function normally, as the neural activity carried on input pathways may have been affected by the nearby damage. Lesions can also induce structural changes, such as axonal growth and synaptogenesis (see Chapter 9). This "sprouting" can be compensatory and thus homeostatic, or it may give rise to abnormal circuitry not usually seen in the normal brain (Lynch et al., 1973; Steward et al., 1974). Third, even if postlesion reorganization achieves relatively little in the way of compensation for lost tissue, the person or animal may still alter his behavior in a manner that enables him to compensate for lost function through the use of undamaged systems. Behavioral compensation can help mask a neurological deficit. With respect to damage to the medial temporal lobe and the ensuing amnesia, for example, the use of memory aids such as electronic devices to remind people to do things is one example of such "compensatory" behavior (Wilson, 1999). Desirable as these aids are therapeutically, the possibility that behavioral compensation occurs naturally over the course of time adds difficulties

to the neuroscientist's efforts to interpret lesion effects in relation to the functional theories they are intended to test. Notwithstanding these obstacles along the path, interventional techniques can be used successfully, provided a number of conceptual issues are also considered.

13.2.2 Lesions, Functional Hypotheses, and Behavioral Tasks

Dissociations, Double Dissociations, and Hypotheses

Experimental lesions are widely used to establish functional dissociations between tasks that are thought to depend on distinct forms of information processing. Thus, if behavior A is *impaired* by a lesion made in area X and, simultaneously, behavior B is *unaffected* by lesion X, there are grounds for suspecting that behaviors A and B may, at least in part, depend on different brain circuits. The confidence in such assertions grows when a so-called double dissociation is obtained— when a different lesion Y impairs behavior B but not behavior A (Teuber, 1955). However, discovering a list of behaviors that are affected or unaffected by a particular set of lesions (or other intervention) is only the first step toward such a theory.

An essential parallel step is the development of hypotheses about information processing in the brain (Shallice, 1988). Numerous hypotheses have been developed by cognitive neuroscientists to account for the cerebral organization of perceptual processes, attention, language processing, executive function. and memory (Shallice, 1988; McCarthy and Warrington, 1990; Gazzaniga, 2002). With respect to the hippocampal formation, numerous hypotheses have been developed and are discussed in this chapter. As we saw in the overview, these theories differ in their claims about the character and timing of the information processing that is taking place in the hippocampal formation during learning and memory.

Learning, Performance, and Hippocampus-dependent Learning and Memory Tasks

One important theme in studies of learning and memory is the distinction between *learning* and *performance*. In a behaving animal, performance is what we can see and measure, whereas learning reflects a variety of covert processes that we presume are taking place in the brain. It is these covert processes that are responsible for the acquisition of knowledge. Performance is the expression of this knowledge. Of course, performance may also itself be learned, as occurs with sensorimotor skills, but it is often a reflection of learning rather than being a participant in such a process. Obstructing performance in some way (e.g., by putting a barrier in a maze that an animal has been trained to run through) may prevent the usual expression of learned performance, but it does not affect what the animal "knows." The animal generally tries to find an alternative way in which to express this knowledge, such as its memory of where some desired food is located (Tolman, 1948).

The concept of learning itself must also be fractionated as the brain has evolved to have a number of qualitatively distinct forms of learning. Most theories of hippocampal function are statements about the type (or types) of learning and memory in which this group of structures is engaged. There is passionate debate about how to characterize them. Over the years, a range of learning tasks have been developed that are now widely used in studies with rodents, primates, and birds to try to identify which of them involve hippocampus-dependent processes. Widely used tasks for rats and mice include alternation protocols in T mazes and cross mazes, foraging for food in radial mazes, and other spatial tasks such as finding the way home in an open arena or swimming to safety in a watermaze. Recognition memory can be studied by presenting novel and familiar objects or by taking advantage of rats' superb olfactory sense and then "asking" which object or smell is familiar. One widely used protocol is the conditioning of fear to the context where testing takes place, and another examines the social transmission of food preferences. Certain protocols of some of these tasks seem to be "hippocampus-dependent" (i.e., affected by hippocampal lesions), whereas others are not. The community that conducts research on temporal lobe function in primates has its family of tried and trusted tasks for investigating memory ranging from manual protocols with three-dimensional objects to automated touch-screen technology, some of which has now seen application as neuropsychological tests for humans (Robbins et al., 1994). Birds are also used extensively, with due consideration to their natural behavioral ecology. Innovation has gone into the design and development of rigorous laboratory-based tasks such as food caching and recovery (Suzuki and Clayton, 2000). In using this range of tasks, there is ongoing debate about the relative value of standardization on a subset of tasks that are then used in a common way within and across laboratories and of innovation with respect to procedure in the search for better ways of characterizing hippocampus-dependent learning and memory.

One complication is that there is rarely, if ever, a simple one-to-one mapping between a specific task and a single putative type of learning. All of them rely on effective sensory/perceptual processing in "upstream" brain structures and on effective motor processing "downstream." Researchers have then to be careful that any alteration in task performance caused by interventions is really due to an interruption of a neural process mediated by the hippocampus or to some secondary effect on upstream or downstream processes. The conceptual boundary between input, cognition, and output is hazy, particularly as it becomes ever more apparent that "bottom-up" processes can be modulated by "top-down" mechanisms. Indeed some researchers of a behaviorist persuasion even question whether the conceptual boundary between learning and performance exists, in part because an animal may appear to be unable to learn when, in practice, a treatment has been given that has affected only its ability to sense afferent stimuli or to move around effectively (Vanderwolf and Cain, 1994).

What, How, and When: Different Aspects of Hippocampus-dependent Memory

The overall aim of the functional enterprise is to find out what the hippocampus does and how it does it. Identifying which tasks are hippocampus-dependent and which are not is an important part of this endeavor, particularly when they shed analytical light on the relative merits of different theories.

There are, however, a number of ways in which learning and memory tasks can be theoretically ambiguous. The first has to do with *what* an animal learns. In a simple T maze, a rat might be taught to run from a start box in the stem and then turn left to find food at the end of the arm—but has it learned the motor response of turning left? Or that food is to be found near landmarks positioned on the left? One way to find out is to rotate the maze through 180° and now start the animal from the stem of the ⊥ maze. If it has learned the motor response of turning left, it should move toward what had been the right-hand side of the maze during training. Conversely, if it has learned to approach landmarks on the left-hand side of the room, it should now turn right at the choice point. This manipulation nicely dissociates control and hippocampus-lesioned rats early in training; but, interestingly, if training continues too long, normal rats develop a "turning habit" that is inflexible to manipulations of the starting location (Packard and McGaugh, 1996). Another example of ambiguity about what has been learned concerns recognition memory. Recognition can be defined as the memory of past occurrence (Brown and Xiang, 1998), but there are several ways it can be achieved. For example, recognition of a past stimulus by a monkey may be mediated by a feeling of familiarity evoked by the stimulus itself. Alternatively, the stimulus may evoke a covert mental recollection of past experience. The monkey cannot tell us about either of these possibilities in the way that a person would through language, but its sense of familiarity or its sense of recollection is expressed as appropriate choice behavior in a memory test (performance). A current challenge is trying to find a way of distinguishing these two possibilities of what the animal has learned.

The second kind of ambiguity arises if two or more theories offer different accounts of *how* an animal has learned a particular task. In this case, there is agreement about what the mouse, monkey, or human has learned but not how it has been achieved. Allocentric spatial learning is a relevant case in point, as there is widespread agreement that animals can learn where things are and that the hippocampus is involved but disagreement about how it is done. Questions include whether there is anything special about spatial learning that might require specialized neural circuitry, or is it just an instance of a more general form of declarative memory? Are different learning rules involved for spatial learning than other types of learning? Do different brain areas have to interact for spatial learning than for other forms of declarative or relational learning?

A third ambiguity arises from the distinction between *types* of learning and memor*y processes*. The classic concept of a hippocampus-dependent learning task is one that is impaired by permanent hippocampal lesions. An unambiguous hippocampus-dependent learning task is one that is affected by such lesions but unaffected by others. However, this categorization does not capture the subtlety that neural activity in the hippocampus may be required at one stage of learning but not at another. It might, for example, be required at encoding but not at retrieval or during the initial stages of memory storage but not during consolidation. The logically orthogonal concept of a memory "process" refers to important distinctions that must be made between the distinct memory processes associated with encoding, storage, consolidation, and retrieval. It is orthogonal, as each of these processes applies to many types of learning and memory. They are distinguished experimentally through the various hemodynamic, physiological, or cell biological correlates that are seen in association with these various phases, by the impact of lesions made at different stages of training, and by the effects of reversible interventions (such as drugs) used to inactivate brain areas temporarily or to disrupt specific neural mechanisms.

Thus, the overarching task of dissociating theories of regional brain function involves zeroing in on *what*, *how*, and *when*. Many subtle variations in behavioral protocol are designed to explore the hypotheses. These variations of protocol are guided by predictions, better still by the counterintuitive predictions, of functional hypotheses about structure–function relations (Crabbe and Morris, 2004). The declarative memory, cognitive mapping, and predictive ambiguity theories outlined below often make common predictions about standardized versions of specific tasks but distinct predictions about their variants.

Cerebral Localization or Dissociation Between Mental Processes?

A frequent non sequitur in the interpretation of an interventional study is the assertion, following a positive experimental finding, that a function can somehow be "localized" to the targeted brain structure or pathway. A classic and amusing critique of this "localizational" way of thinking was presented by Gregory (1961), who pointed out that if removing a part of an old valve radio causes the radio to howl it need not mean that the "function" of this bit is to suppress howling. This overly "symptomatic" way of thinking pervaded the hippocampal field early on and indeed much of the brain sciences since the early days of experimental neurology. One early claim about hippocampal function was that it is involved in "behavioral inhibition" (Kimble, 1968). This claim rested, in part, on the observation that hippocampus-lesioned animals are very inflexible in their behavior; they often persist much longer in carrying out well learned habits in inappropriate situations than do control subjects. Analysis of behavior in runways, mazes, and operant tasks has revealed, however, a number of

reasons why behavioral inflexibility could arise from other than excision of neural machinery that had (somehow) evolved to inhibit inflexibility. For example, if the lesioned animal has a deficit in spatial memory and so cannot learn or remember that one end of a runway (A) is in a different "place" than the other end of a runway (B), it cannot acquire knowledge about their relative location. It learns only to run. Changing a spatial performance strategy is much easier for normal animals than the "slamming on the brakes" to constrain a habitual running response (Nadel et al., 1975). The debate about the relative merits of these specific views has largely subsided, although the inhibitory view still has its followers (Chan et al., 2001; Davidson and Jarrard, 2004), but the logical point remains that the overt phenotype of response stereotypy need not imply the existence of an inhibition module localized in the hippocampus or, indeed, anywhere else in the brain.

Gregory's (1961) critique should, however, not be overstated. If one were to lesion a car's exhaust system, it would be right to infer that its function is to make the engine quieter. Damaging the earphones of an iPOD limits its ability make a sound. By the same token, in a modular structure such as the brain, inferences about localization may often be correct. If the overarching aim of the enterprise is to develop a theory of what different parts of the brain do and how they do it, we must also consider how brain areas interact to realize the seamless control of all aspects of behavior. It is an article of faith in the field that different brain areas or neuromodulatory transmitter systems must have different and therefore, at least in principle, dissociable functions.

Equally, however, it is also understood that no brain area is an island; different brain areas work together in networks. In recent years, there has been growing interest in the issue of how memory systems interact—when they compete, when they complement each other, when the interruption of one enables another to learn faster or slower, and so on (White and McDonald, 2002; McDonald et al., 2004; Voermans et al., 2004). This change of emphasis is refreshing, as it counterbalances the near-exclusive stress on "dissociations" of earlier years. A desire to understand how these systems interact is taking its place as the brain sciences mature. In any event, whether the immediate aim is functional dissociation or the understanding of competition and/or complementarity, data secured using lesions and other interventions are a powerful way of testing theories.

13.2.3 Contemporary Lesion Techniques: Pharmacological and Genetic Interventions

Neurotoxic Lesions

The technique by which a lesion is made can be important because certain techniques, such as the use of excitotoxins, first introduced to study hippocampal function by Jarrard (1989), have the effect of damaging cells while leaving fibers of passage intact (Fig. 13–1). Thus, if a brain function critically

A. Topological arrangement of HPC Formation

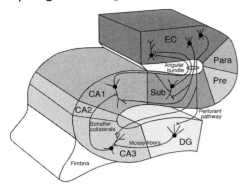

B. Selective neurotoxic and knife-cut lesions in rats

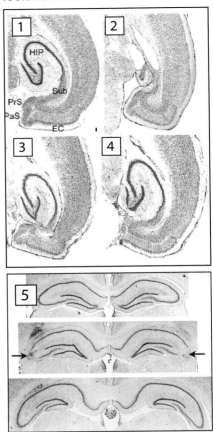

C. Quantitative assessment of partial lesion volume

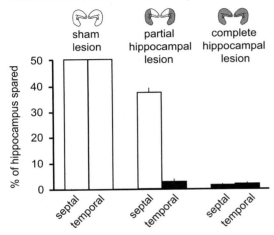

Figure 13–1. Excitotoxic and knife-cut lesions of the hippocampal formation in rats. *A.* Topological arrangement of the structures comprising the hippocampal formation (from Chapter 3, Figure 3–1). *B.* Photomicrographs of horizontal sections from a representative control rat (B1) and rats with neurotoxin lesions of hippocampus (2), subiculum (3), and presubiculum/parasubiculum (4). EC, entorhinal cortex; HIP, hippocampus; PaS, parasubiculum; PrS, presubiculum; Sub, subiculum. (*Source*: Courtesy of Len Jarrard.) *C.* Use of three-dimensional volumetric techniques to establish the quantitative extent of the cell loss associated with partial lesions placed at different points along the septotemporal axis. (*Source*: Courtesy of Livia de Hoz.) *D.* Use of a knife cut through the longitudinal-association pathway in area CA3. This cuts fibers (not shown) and damages a small number of cells in CA3 at one particular point along the axis. Animals to which the same amount of neurotoxic damage was deliberately applied without damaging the longitudinal fibers are used as controls in such a study. (*Source*: Courtesy of Hill-Aina Steffenach.)

depends on communication from area X to area Z, with fibers passing through area Y, old-fashioned lesions might lead to the false conclusion that area Y is essential for this function whereas the modern approach would not. By the same token, a positive outcome of a lesion study using an excitotoxin gives comfort to the notion that it is the targeted neurons that are functionally significant for the task under examination. Conversely, lesions that cut fibers while leaving cells intact can also be valuable, especially when the axons of a population of neurons have axon collaterals. Neurotoxic lesions can be highly localized (e.g., to distinct components of the hippocampal formation such as the dentate gyrus, subiculum, or entorhinal cortex). They may even extend to killing specific cell types in the region to which the toxin is delivered, such as the use of immunoglobulin G (IgG) saporin to ablate cholin-ergic cells afferent to the hippocampus while leaving nearby γ-aminobutyric acid (GABA)ergic neurons intact (Gallagher and Rapp, 1997). It has been claimed that lesions restricted to area CA1 but not CA3, or vice versa, can be achieved with precise stereotaxic techniques (Lee and Kesner, 2004). This precision can certainly be achieved along a small length of the longitudinal axis of the hippocampus, but it remains unclear how complete and yet still selective such lesions can be. Lesions that cut fibers while leaving cells intact can also be valuable, especially when the axons of a population of neurons have axon collaterals, but it is extremely difficult to do this in a manner that interferes with one and only one fiber pathway.

Techniques for making permanent lesions are accompanied, when testing is complete, by histological analysis of the damage caused. Was the target brain area damaged as expected? Was the lesion complete? Did it encroach on other brain areas? Did it damage cells and fibers or only cells? If the latter, was confirmation obtained through tract tracing techniques that the apparently intact fibers are capable of axonal transport? Doing this is part of the point of using animals rather than just studying people. Nissl stains, silver stains that reveal degenerating fibers, and other histochemical techniques can all be used to good effect. More ambitiously, one might enquire whether an apparently intact fiber tract at or near to a lesion site is electrophysiologically functional. Likewise, the check might be on whether the lesion has selectively affected one but not another neuromodulatory system by using in vivo neurochemistry to monitor changes of particular neurotransmitters. The use of all of these techniques for postexperiment histology is the "gold standard" to which most laboratories aspire, but a difficulty shared by all is that it is not always practical to dot every "i" and cross every "t" in every experiment. Much has to be taken on trust so research can proceed at a reasonable pace—but this trust is sometimes misplaced, which sows seeds of confusion. As will become clear, the size of a lesion can be a major factor to consider when interpreting experiments on hippocampal function in relation to recognition memory or spatial memory.

Permanent lesions are often used to realize network "disconnections" (Aggleton and Pearce, 2001). Most lesion studies in animals involve bilateral damage to a brain structure, but, in an ingenious twist, a unilateral lesion of one structure can be made in conjunction with contralateral damage to another. In right-handed people language is largely mediated by structures in the left hemisphere such that a stroke in the left brain can interfere with speech, whereas one on the right does so rarely (McCarthy and Warrington, 1990). Conversely, right-hemisphere damage to the parietal cortex is associated with the fascinating syndrome of spatial neglect (Behrmann et al., 2004; Farah, 2004). Laterality is barely present in animals (one exception being song birds), such that unilateral lesions in animals are often behaviorally benign. Thinking is shifting from a focus on localization toward a "crossed-lesion" approach to reveal the importance of functional connectivity. For example, a unilateral lesion might be made to the entorhinal cortex (on the left) and a second unilateral lesion to the fimbria-fornix (on the right) with, perhaps, section of the hippocampal commissures to prevent cross-talk of information within the hippocampus via residual interhemispheric connectivity. Such a lesion might produce a syndrome similar to that of an entire hippocampal lesion (even though the hippocampus and dentate gyrus are actually intact, and neither brain area that is lesioned has a bilateral lesion) because it has successfully disconnected cortical and subcortical structures that normally interact via the hippocampus. The "disconnection" approach is increasingly popular (Warburton et al., 2001; Gaffan, 2002; Miyashita, 2004). Disconnection of the hippocampus need not always be achieved by damaging afferent or efferent structures in opposite hemispheres. It can also be done by sectioning major interconnecting pathways, such

as the fimbria-fornix, or by selective knife cuts of intrinsic circuitry such as the longitudinal-associational pathway of area CA3 (Steffenach et al., 2002).

Pharmacological and Genetic Manipulations

Drugs and genetic manipulations are alternative ways of intervening in brain function. The turn of the twenty-first century is something of a methodological "tipping point" (Gladwell, 2002) as the major behavioral neuroscience laboratories move on from deploying classic lesions on their own to using them in conjunction with single-unit recording and tract-tracing techniques, together with reversible pharmacological and cell biological manipulations. With respect to the opportunities afforded by targeted molecular engineering Wulff and Wisden quoted Francis Crick's view that "the lesion approach needs new methods, especially as the usual ways of ablating the parts of the brain are so crude. For example, it would be useful to inactivate, preferably reversibly, a single type of neuron in a single area of the brain" (Wulff and Wisden, 2005, p. 44). As it happens, this would not be very useful for behavioral studies, as a certain minimum amount of tissue must be affected, but the point is taken nonetheless.

The use of drugs in conjunction with behavioral studies has a long scientific history (McGaugh, 2000). One aspect of this approach has been the analytical use of intracerebral infusions of microiter and nanoliter quantities of active compounds targeted to specific regions, often (although not always) given with posttraining to avoid the impact of known side effects. In relation to hippocampal function, typical drugs used include excitatory amino acid antagonists acting at α-amino-3-hydroxy-5-methyl-4-isoxazolepropionate (AMPA), N-methyl-D-aspartate (NMDA), and metabotropic glutamate (mGluR) receptors, and ligands at inhibitory synapses such as GABAergic agonists (as described in Chapter 6). These compounds interfere with (or potentiate) normal excitatory or inhibitory neurotransmission for as long as the drug remains present and active at its site of administration. Drugs interacting with the synthesis, transport, or degradation of neuromodulatory transmitters—acetylcholine (ACh), norepinephrine (NE), dopamine (DA), and serotonin (5-HT), for example—or antagonists of their target receptors are also analytically powerful. There is growing interest in drugs acting intracellularly on signal-transduction pathways downstream of postsynaptic receptors, such as CAMKII and MAPkinase (see Chapters 6, 7, and 10). Their use requires compounds capable of penetrating cell membranes to reach their site of action rather than acting extracellularly at membrane-bound receptors (Sweatt, 2003).

The exploitation of drug actions in the hippocampal formation as a tool to study learning and memory function is a relatively new departure. One aspect capitalizes on the developments in our understanding of synaptic function discussed earlier in the book. An AMPA receptor antagonist, such as CNQX, shuts down normal fast synaptic transmission for a period of time (see Chapter 6). In principle, its effects should be similar to that of a neurotoxic lesion that spares fibers of passage—with the analytical advantage of reversibility. In contrast, an NMDA antagonist such as D-AP5 has the distinct effect of blocking NMDA receptor-dependent mechanisms, such as activity-dependent synaptic plasticity (LTP and LTD), while leaving fast synaptic transmission intact. This should and does have very different effects on cognition than any permanent lesion could have, allowing previously acquired spatial memory to be displayed in performance but preventing new learning (Morris et al., 1986b). Interestingly, the effects of an NMDA antagonist such as D-AP5 are "regionally dependent" because NMDA receptors mediate different physiological functions in different brain areas. In the spinal cord, NMDA receptors help mediate suprasegmental connectivity, partly by enabling the rhythmical activation of Ca^{2+}-dependent K^+ currents (Dale and Roberts, 1985; Grillner et al., 1998), whereas in the hippocampus they serve as a trigger for certain forms of neuronal plasticity (see Chapter 10).

What virtually all drugs have in common and what makes them so useful compared to lesions is that their actions are, at least in principle, reversible. Reversibility has two main ramifications. First, the intended dysfunction lasts only a short time, and thus the chances of brain damage or compensatory changes are reduced. Second, reversibility makes it possible to dissect different phases of memory—encoding, storage, consolidation, retrieval—in a more exacting way. However, no less than lesions, the impact of drugs must be studied with care. Drugs diffuse, raising questions about variation in concentration across a target brain region. This variation may itself vary with time, particularly with acute injections. Osmotic minipumps enable drugs to be infused at a steady rate over periods ranging from 1 day to 1 month. A steady-state concentration is then achieved when the rates of infusion and diffusion of a drug match precisely—a great advance on acute infusions. Last and by no means least, it is essential to establish precisely what and where a drug has had its effect. It is astonishing how rarely this is done independently of the effects on behavior that the drug may have. The use of autoradiography to establish the local spread of action of a radiolabeled version of a drug is valuable (Steele and Morris, 1999; Attwell et al., 2001), but this is a surrogate for an independent marker of its functional effect. If an AMPA antagonist is used, physiology should be undertaken to establish the extent to which synaptic transmission has been compromised. Monitoring glucose metabolism is one way of looking at this and direct physiological recording another (Riedel et al., 1999).

The last 15 years have witnessed considerable excitement regarding the introduction of transgenic and knockout mice as in vivo methods of genetic manipulation. Their application to study the systems-level and cellular mechanisms of learning and memory has been particularly imaginative (Tonegawa et al., 1995). Beginning with pioneering studies that targeted molecules such as αCAMKII and *fyn* tyrosine kinase, which were implicated in LTP (Grant et al., 1992; Silva et al., 1992), an "industrial production line" of transgenic and mutant mice soon became available in virtually all fields of neuroscience

(Morris and Kennedy, 1992). Knockouts are now (almost) routine, with many a PhD student in well-founded molecular-genetic laboratories saying that they "would like to make a mouse" during the course of their studies. The development of these techniques has been accompanied by databases and repositories of mouse lines, such as those at the Jackson Laboratory in the United States (http://www.jax.org/lab), the development of testing facilities such as those at the Mary Lyon Centre in the United Kingdom (http://www.mlc.har. mrc.ac.uk/aboutUs.html), and meetings at which ideas and recommendations about breeding different lines of mice are debated in an open, constructive manner (Conference, 1997). Neuroinformatics expertise is having a considerable impact on the field (http://www.neuroinf.de/Members/stefan/mbl).

This molecular-genetic approach has now advanced from homologous recombination to regionally specific manipulations, using the cre-LOX procedure, enabling studies to focus on the role of genes in specific brain areas such as the hippocampus (Tsien et al., 1996). The introduction of inducible constructs, such as tetracycline, has taken the mouse knockout enterprise into a third phase of sophistication, potentially allowing the inactivation of specific genes at specific times in specific cells of specific regions of the hippocampal formation or other areas (Mayford et al., 1996). For all this enviable specificity, however, there remain formidable technical problems to be solved—not least the discovery of region-specific promoters and the apparent "leakiness" of inducible manipulations. Another problem is that most studies have to be conducted on mice. Many molecular behaviorists look on mice as "miniature rats," but this is clearly absurd. Rats are different. A rarely tested assumption in the field is that hippocampus-dependent tasks for rats may be used similarly in mice. Other technical issues have to do with running appropriate controls for knockout mice made using homologous recombination (Gerlai, 1996), pleiotropic developmental abnormalities associated with deletion of a gene throughout embryogenesis and postnatal life (Tonegawa et al., 1995), and issues associated with the genetic or pharmacological rescue of a normal phenotype by transgenic expression of a gene in a mouse with a knockout background (Ohno, 2001). Others are longstanding conceptual problems such as the need, so rarely addressed, for the double dissociations that are common in conventional lesion studies. Fortunately, these problems are being recognized, and the solutions are forthcoming. The technological innovations are remarkable; they are continuing, and the molecular-genetic approach has a great deal to offer.

13.2.4 Biological Continuity of Hippocampal Function

Virtues of a Comparative Approach

All mammals possess a brain with the same basic pattern of organization: spinal cord, hindbrain, midbrain, forebrain, and cerebral hemispheres (Swanson, 2000). The simplest view

The genetic similarity of mammals

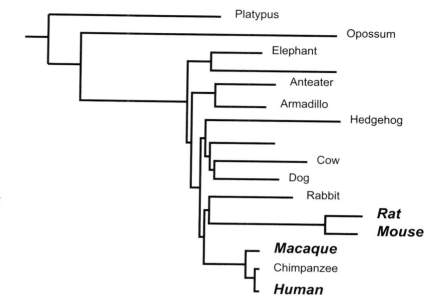

Figure 13–2. Genomic sequence similarity in mammals. Publication of the genomic sequence of the rat brain, following those of the mouse and of humans, provided an opportunity to assess the degree of sequence "similarity" across species. The outcome places rodents on a line less distant from primates and humans than that of many other mammalian species. (*Source*: Consortium, 2004.)

of this common pattern is that although there has been substantial encephalization of function in primates and humans relative to rodents the core functions of various areas of the central nervous system (CNS)—cerebellum, midbrain, neocortex—are most likely conserved across all mammalian species. Even where anatomical similarities may seem cryptic, there are striking genetic similarities that justify the use of primates and other mammals (Fig. 13–2), and there may even have been convergent evolution of certain aspects of anatomy and intelligence in avian species (Jarvis et al., 2005), as in the case of corvids (Emery and Clayton, 2004).

If this comparative assumption also applies to the hippocampus, which it surely should, the key advantage of using animals is that invasive anatomical, physiological, and behavioral studies can be carried out. Although not everyone shares the view that such work is ethically acceptable—a concern exacerbated by growing evidence of the complex emotional, cognitive, and cultural life of higher primates—most neuroscientists adopt the utilitarian perspective that such work is justified on its scientific merits and by its potential to relieve both human and animal suffering. The macaque monkey is a particularly suitable subject because Old World monkeys are closely related to humans, although the last common ancestor was about 30 million years ago (Kay et al., 1997). Its brain is remarkably similar to that of humans (see Chapter 3), and functional imaging studies are revealing striking similarities in, for example, the dynamic organization and responsiveness of the cerebral cortex (Van Essen and Drury, 1997). Rodents may seem less well justified on this account, although the topological organization of their brain is also quite similar (Whishaw, 2004b). The comparative similarity argument may

take flight with birds, but unlike rodents they are visual animals and have a number of other advantages than make them useful for certain studies.

When using animals, it is essential to be respectful of their biological needs, to use the minimum number necessary to realize the required level of statistical power, and to think carefully about how to motivate and reward them in an ethically acceptable manner. Reduction and refinement are laudable goals in animal experimentation. In general, we cannot ask animals to do something through language, but mild food deprivation creates the opportunity to "reinforce" an animal with rewards for performing a task. This is more charitable than it sounds because, as it happens, food deprivation actually lengthens the life of laboratory animals (Nelson, 1988). The use of mild electric shock to motivate animals in studies of learning and memory may seem unfortunate to some, but the neurobiological study of fear and stress is important; and there are circumstances in which the rapid learning achieved with shock cannot easily be achieved in other ways. Electric shock has the advantage of being variable and can be motivating even when quite mild, but it is artificial. It is probably no more stressful than the first day of swimming in a watermaze, although the stress of the latter habituates quickly, and escaping from water may be a more biologically meaningful form of motivation.

Limitations in the Use of Laboratory Animals to Investigate Brain Function

Animal work does have its disadvantages. In comparison with human studies, animal studies include problems associated with what the animals may be said to "know," with language and communication, and the artificiality of the physical and social environments in which animals are tested.

Can we be confident that animals possess "knowledge" in the same way humans do? As certain kinds of human knowledge come to us via language (such as semantic, or "fact," memory), some observers have questioned whether such forms of knowledge exist in animals (Macphail, 1998). An American knows that a "slam dunk" is a shot in basketball, and he can explain it to a puzzled foreigner; but how do we teach "knowledge" to animals? Do they have "semantic-like" knowledge or merely conditioned responses? Should we assume that a monkey "knows" that a particular object "means" reward simply because it has been consistently paired with reward, or that one stimulus leads to another because they are associated? The presence of pair-asssociate neurons in the temporal regions of the neocortex of monkeys is suggestive (Miyashita, 2004); and at a strictly behavioral level something akin to word learning has been demonstrated in dogs (Kaminski et al., 2004; Markman and Abelev, 2004). The primary reason for believing that animals "know" things is because they behave in relation to stimuli—food, water, shelter, danger—as if they know what these stimuli are. A monkey that has learned to use a rake to collect food that is beyond arm's length probably does "know" what a rake is and what it can be used for. Receptive fields in appropriate somatosensory areas of the cortex expand in association with learning (Maravita and Iriki, 2004).

The problem is that, although the possession of knowledge does not logically require language, communication about it to others usually does. For example, episodic and autobiographical memories are about specific events ("what") that happen in particular places ("where") at particular times ("when") (see Section 13.6). The memory that one person has of "what, where, and when" may be different from that of another person who experiences the same event; in fact, much discourse is concerned with debating such differences. It follows that it is difficult to investigate episodic memory in animals. The medium of communication is different and unlikely to be one that satisfactorily reflects that animal's personal experience. Indeed, Tulving took the view that "as far as we know, members of no other species possess quite the same ability to experience again now, in a different situation and perhaps a different form, happenings from the past, and know that the experience refers to an event that occurred in another time and in another place" (Tulving, 1983, p. 1). Regardless of whether this skepticism is justified, we should recognize that distinguishing both "episodic-like" and "semantic-like" memory from mere changes in learned behavior is far from straightforward. Several studies have suggested that animals probably can remember events as events, and there is no a priori reason why language is necessary for them to be able to do so "at another time and in another place."

The "training" (of animals) and the "asking" (of humans) may not always yield the same answer in experiments on learning and memory. The primary ways of teaching animals to perform particular behavioral tasks are, as we have seen, by engaging their curiosity and the use of reward and punishment. Such techniques are more painstaking than merely asking a person to remember something; and they run the risk of missing important subtleties. The answers you get from humans who are doing memory tasks depend critically on the way the questions are put and thus the subject's awareness of the problem at hand (Graf et al., 1984; Squire, 2004). This issue was discussed in detail in Chapter 12: recognizing the distinction between "explicit" and "implicit" memory processing. Although this distinction may also apply to animals—and the declarative memory theory argues that it does—it is difficult to get a handle on it analytically. It seems unlikely that we shall ever know whether animals are "conscious," although here again experimenters have come forward with ingenious ideas to try tackle the problem.

Finally, behavioral tasks in the laboratory are clearly artificial, but then so are cyclotrons and supercolliders and, for that matter, test tubes. Science often has to be artificial to proceed. Biomedical laboratory work generally requires that animals are kept in somewhat artificial conditions, trained when they are experimentally "naïve" rather than after they have accumulated knowledge, skill, or experience, and often trained on protocols that seem to bear little relation to "normal" behavior in the wild. Many primatologists and evolutionary psychologists see this as a major problem (Tooby and Cosmides, 2000), particularly with respect to the evolution of social behavior. In contrast, others look upon ecological factors (and species differences) as somewhat tangential to the primary task of searching for general principles of brain function (Macphail, 1982; Bolhuis and Macphail, 2001). This disagreement has provoked much debate (Healy and Braithwaite, 2000; Hampton et al., 2002). What is not always appreciated is the extent to which certain laboratory tasks are either explicitly designed to be analogous to things that animals do in the wild (e.g., recognizing a previously seen stimulus) or unexpectedly turn out to be analogous to naturalistic behavior. An example is the ability of rhesus macaques to learn arbitrary "sensory-motor mappings." These are tasks that require a monkey to perform action A to stimulus A, action B to stimulus B, and so on. In one laboratory investigation of this ability, different visual cues were presented to rhesus monkeys, with the monkeys then having to make different movements of a computer joystick (Brasted et al., 2002). Such sensorimotor mappings are learned quite slowly; and on the face of it, this may seem hardly surprising as monkey cognition did not evolve to play computer games. However, as pointed out by the authors, the different actions of vervet monkeys to different alarm calls made by troop members (Seyfarth et al., 1980) are also examples of arbitrary sensory-motor mappings. Monkeys climb trees in response to the "barking call" uttered when a leopard is nearby and look skyward followed by hiding in bushes to the "cough call" uttered when an eagle is spotted. Brasted et al. (2002) summarized evidence indicating that these different actions to distinct stimuli seem to be learned, just as the computer joystick movements have to be. An apparently abstract laboratory task may be somewhat closer to primate "cognitive ecology" than might be appreciated.

To conclude: interventional studies in animals are a powerful way of investigating brain function. When using them in conjunction with behavioral tasks, we must accept that the way in which hippocampal function is studied in animals has to be different from the approaches described in Chapter 12 because animals cannot talk, they cannot tell us of what they are aware (if anything), and they are unlikely to have a sense of their past or their future or to have, to quote Tulving (1983) again, "quite the same ability to experience the past" that humans do. It does not follow, however, that these differences of approach mean that the hippocampal formation in animals is carrying out a different memory function than exists in humans.

The enlightened possibility, reflecting the commonalities of anatomy, physiology, and cell biology, is that it carries out essentially the same information-processing algorithms but that they might *seem* to be different because the human hippocampus and the animal hippocampus are operating on different inputs and so provide different outputs to downstream targets. A metaphor may help to explain the gist of this idea. Imagine being able to transplant the hippocampus of a monkey into the brain of a human. Suppose the neurosurgeon is the wizard we know all neurosurgeons to be, and that she successfully connects up all the nerves and blood vessels to their appropriate targets. Our perspective is that the result of such an operation is that all should be well—our monkey hippocampus should work normally inside the human brain. However, because it would now be receiving different kinds of information from its cortical and subcortical inputs, the end result would be appropriate to the *human*, not the monkey. Laterality of function in the human brain is a less fanciful illustration of the same argument because it seems unlikely that the left and right hippocampi of humans are anatomically, physiologically, or biochemically very different; yet the outcomes of their processing are clearly distinct. With this "optimistic" perspective of the enterprise at hand, we now proceed to discuss the major theories of hippocampal function.

13.3 Declarative Memory Theory

13.3.1 Outline of the Theory

In 1980, Cohen and Squire suggested that the distinction between "declarative" and "procedural" information processing could be relevant to the pattern of memory deficits seen with amnesia. Drawing upon Gilbert Ryle's distinction between "knowing that" and "knowing how" (Ryle, 1949), they proposed that amnesic patients are impaired in forming conscious memories of facts and events ("remembering that") but have relatively normal learning motor and cognitive skills ("remembering how"). Following Milner's observations of successful motor learning in patient H.M. (see Chapters 2 and 12), this

distinction was prompted by their finding that amnesic patients could acquire and retain the cognitive skill of mirror-reading novel words (in which words and all their letters were printed backward) despite showing no conscious memory of the training experience itself. Control subjects learned at an identical rate and, of course, could also recall their training on the task (Cohen and Squire, 1980). Squire went on to develop and articulate the "declarative memory" theory of amnesia, implicating the hippocampal formation and other structures of the medial-temporal lobe (Squire and Cohen, 1984; Squire and Zola-Morgan, 1991; Squire, 1992; Squire et al., 2004). Four key propositions of this theory (Box 13–1) are as follows.

The first proposition—that *the hippocampus is primarily involved in memory*—is now relatively noncontroversial. It is strongly supported by work on amnesic patients and functional imaging studies (see Chapter 12). Observations on people have been extensively confirmed and elaborated in studies of the effects of experimental lesions in animals. In keeping with the overriding theme of this chapter, we accept this first proposition of the theory without further comment.

The second proposition defines "declarative memory" as *representing both facts and events* (Fig. 13–3). What fact (semantic memory) and events (episodic memory) have in common is that both are propositional and can be brought to conscious awareness. Information about facts and events can be "declared" ("Paris is the capital of France" or "I ate an almond croissant for breakfast"). and such declarations can be either true or false. By virtue of this shared property of fact and event memory, such memories can be combined inferentially with other information to yield new propositions (a point developed further in the "relational-processing" version of this theory—see Section 13.5). This inferential property is

---

Box 13–1
Declarative Memory Theory

1. *Memory:* The primary function of the hippocampal formation is in memory.
2. *Selectivity:* The role of the hippocampal formation in memory is selective. It mediates the memory of facts and events, called "declarative memory." This is the type of memory that, in humans, can be consciously recalled.
3. *Memory systems:* The hippocampal formation is one of a number of structures that comprise a "medial temporal lobe memory system." Although the components of this system may have distinct subfunctions, it operates collectively to mediate the formation and initial storage of declarative memories.
4. *Time-limited:* The role of the hippocampus in memory is time-limited. Memory is gradually reorganized as time passes after learning. The hippocampus contributes to a time-dependent systems-level consolidation process such that, once completed, long-term memory traces are stored in the cortex and neural activity in the hippocampus is no longer required for or involved in recall.

Declarative memory theory: a taxonomy of mammalian memory systems

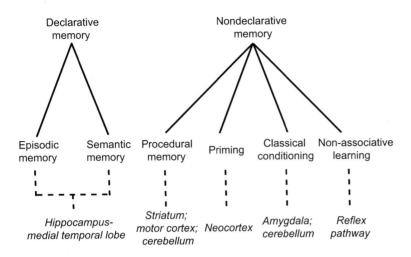

Figure 13–3. Taxonomy of mammalian memory systems. The declarative memory theory recognizes many types of "memory system" and their mediation by distinct neural brain areas. The scheme was first introduced by Squire (1987) and has been updated many times since (e.g., Squire, 2004). The relative independence and interdependence of these separate systems has not been clearly delineated.

an important point of similarity between information about facts and events, but controversy surrounds the theory's assertion that there is a common neural substrate for the formation of both episodic and semantic types of memory.

A key psychological difference is that unique events occur only once and are specific to particular contexts and moments in time, whereas factual knowledge is often gradually accumulated and (generally) nonspecific with respect to the context of learning. Certain other neuropsychological theories of human memory argue that the nervous system encodes, stores, and retrieves episodic information in a way that is qualitatively different from that for semantic information (Shallice, 1988; McCarthy and Warrington, 1990; Schacter and Tulving, 1994; Aggleton and Brown, 1999). Such theories generally embrace or, at least, start off from the concept of episodic memory as a distinct entity (Tulving, 1983) and question whether it is helpful to subsume it with semantic memory into the unitary category of declarative memory. In contrast, declarative memory theorists see the distinction between facts and events as descriptive rather than fundamental, both being initially encoded by structures in the medial temporal lobe (MTL) that collectively comprise what they believe to be a unitary "memory system." Anatomically, the MTL is positioned downstream of structures in the ventral "what" pathway of the visual system in primates (Ungerleider and Mishkin, 1982) and so is well placed to receive attended, perceptually processed information. Damage to this downstream system is therefore held as likely to cause a proportionate impairment in both fact and event processing, at least in the anterograde domain..

Whether viewed as a merely descriptive or fundamental distinction, these two forms of memory are not thought (by anyone) to operate in isolation. There is a dialectic here, such that our ability to form new event memories depends on both our general and our personal knowledge of the world (semantic knowledge) and on accumulating information from our experience of events in the world (episodic memory). As

Tulving has long argued, the input to episodic memory must be partly via semantic memory; equally, we add to that knowledge structure through our experience and memory of events, so the development of new semantic memories generally depends on episodic memory. The two forms of memory are "interdependent." However, they can also act in parallel and independently with, for example, direct input of information from perceptual-representational systems to both semantic and episodic memory (Graham et al., 2000). Investigations of developmental amnesia—focusing on a set of young people referred to a neurological clinic who had grown up being very forgetful about everyday life but able to do reasonably well in school—raised the alternative possibility that the hippocampus plays an exclusive role in the formation of episodic memory (Vargha-Khadem et al., 1997). However, rigorous assessment of this idea is hampered by uncertainties about the extent of hippocampal damage in these cases and theoretical uncertainties about the relative degree of "independence" and "interdependence" of episodic and semantic memory. We discuss these cases in the critique below.

Notwithstanding this qualification, the second proposition of the declarative memory theory implies that a central focus of the theory has to do with the information processing and neural representation of what we ordinarily think of as "memory"—the things we bring to mind as conscious recollections. For some, the term "explicit" memory is preferred to describe certain types of memory task in which the subject is consciously aware of the earlier study episode—in contrast to "implicit" memory tasks, which lack the requirement for recollective awareness (Graf and Schacter, 1985). The differences between the declarative/nondeclarative and explicit/implicit distinctions are important at some levels of analysis but are arguably little more than terminological at another. In practice, the declarative memory theory treats "explicit" and "declarative" memory as interchangeable terms (see Chapter 12). In the same vein, no strong philosophical position about consciousness is implied by the theory's supposition that declarative memories entail "awareness" or "consciousness." The theory is not tied to any particular theory of this problematic but fascinating concept (Zeman, 2004); it quite reasonably takes a "folk psychology" view of the matter.

Another issue about the second proposition of the theory is its skepticism that a categorical subdivision of memory retrieval with respect to familiarity and recollection (Yonelinas, 2001) can be mapped onto distinct MTL brain structures. Both forms of remembering involve conscious awareness, the defining attribute of declarative memory. Familiarity appears to be a phenomenological attribute that is acquired by a novel stimulus, within several sensory systems, after its first presentation. A stimulus that has been presented before may then be judged "familiar," but this can happen without the subject having any recollection of when or where that stimulus was seen, heard, or smelled previously. Recollection is more complicated, as it also involves source memory pertaining to where or when the stimulus was previously presented. Subjects may even engage in "mental time travel"—the act of moving in their mind's eye back to the time or place of prior occurrence while simultaneously remaining in the temporal present and responsive to their perceived surroundings (such as in conversations about the past with someone while simultaneously driving a car). Certain theorists look upon these two forms of memory retrieval as independent (Baddeley et al., 2002), with only recollection or "relational" memories critically dependent on processing in the hippocampal formation and diencephalon (Cohen and Eichenbaum, 1993; Aggleton and Brown, 1999; Eichenbaum and Cohen, 2001). Yonelinas (2001) has outlined quantitative techniques derived from signal detection theory to identify circumstances in which people may be using recollection rather than familiarity, arguing that recollection is a "threshold" process, whereas familiarity can be better understood in signal-detection terms; they then applied this to the analysis of selected amnesic patients (Yonelinas et al., 2002). However, this approach has been the subject of fierce criticism by Manns et al. (2003) and Wixted and Squire (2004). As some of these ideas constitute major changes to the declarative memory theory as it was originally conceived, they are presented in separate sections (see Sections 13.5 and 13.6). For the present, we accept "declarative memory" as a conceptual category on its own merits.

How are other types of long-term memory considered in the theory? Collectively called "nondeclarative memory," they are thought to reflect acquired information, habits, and learned dispositions that are expressed in behavior but cannot be "declared." Initially called "procedural" (Squire and Cohen, 1984), a term first used in the field of artificial intelligence by Winograd (1975), these types of learning are held to include the following.

- Motor skills and learned dispositions (e.g., the stimulus–stimulus associations and stimulus–response habits acquired during simple conditioning tasks) (Corkin, 1984; Cavaco et al., 2004)

- Perceptual and cognitive skills (e.g., the mirror-reading task of Cohen and Squire, 1980); priming phenomena (e.g., word-stem completion) (Graf et al., 1984), perceptual priming (Hamann and Squire, 1997), and conceptual priming (Levy et al., 2004) (see discussion in Chapter 12)
- Simple forms of nonassociative learning such as habituation (waning of responsiveness following repetition) and sensitization (augmented responsiveness) (e.g., Kandel et al., 2000)

The collective attributes of this heterogeneous group of skills is that they are not propositional (and so can be neither true nor false), are generally learned gradually (although are sometimes rapidly acquired), do not require conscious awareness of the knowledge implicit in their execution, and are simply things that people or animals learn to do. For some (Macphail, 1998), they are the sum-total of what animals can learn to do—such as the proverbial rat that presses the lever in an operant chamber because doing so in the past he has been rewarded but not because it has any expectation of securing reward. Although not what we would ordinarily regard in everyday discourse as "remembering," nondeclarative learning is important in constituting "the dispositions, habits, attitudes, and preferences that are inaccessible to conscious recollection, yet are shaped by past events, influence our behavior and our mental life, and are a fundamental part of who we are" (Kandel et al., 2000, p. 1119).

The third proposition of the theory concerns the existence of distinct *brain systems for memory*. Systems are distinguished with respect to structure as well as function. Different forms of memory are held to depend on anatomically distinct, though partially overlapping, brain regions. Different brain systems for memory probably evolved to mediate functionally incompatible purposes (Sherry and Schacter, 1987a), although the lack of a "fossil record" for memory makes it extremely difficult to draw firm conclusions about their evolution. However, that different memory systems might be mediated by anatomically different brain substrates nicely reflects Francois Jacob's idea that evolution is a tinkerer," adding qualitatively distinct circuits rather than bringing about wholescale changes to the brain.

The putative "medial temporal lobe memory system" (Squire and Zola-Morgan, 1991) is held to be one of these brain systems for memory. It comprises the hippocampal formation (as defined in Chapter 3) and both the perirhinal and parahippocampal cortices of the medial temporal lobe (Fig. 13–4). Damage to these structures in humans and nonhuman primates causes disturbances of declarative memory without necessarily affecting other types of learning or memory. Damage to homologous structures in rats causes apparently similar dissociations. In an evocative phrase, Squire wrote of the distinction between declarative and nondeclarative memory as being "honored by the nervous system." He suggested that, in addition to the *medial temporal lobe* mediating declarative memory, the *striatum* is important for stimulus-response habits, the *neocortex* is the substrate for simple perceptual

The medial-temporal lobe memory system

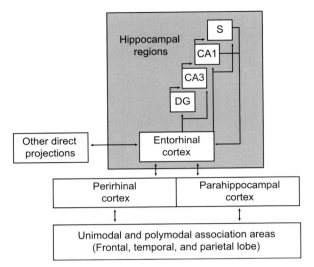

Figure 13–4. Medial temporal lobe memory system. Major components of Squire and Zola-Morgan's (1991) "medial-temporal lobe memory system" (structures with gray shading), which is believed to be the neural substrate for the formation of declarative memories (as updated in 2004). Information enters the system from neocortical association areas. It is projected via the adjacent perirhinal and parahippocampal cortices to the entorhinal cortex, which has the pivotal role of being both the point of entry of information into the hippocampal formation and a point of exit. Information passes within the hippocampal formation via a cascade of unidirectional projections before signals relevant to the encoding of new memories, or their consolidation, are fed back to the neocortex. CA1, CA3, and SUB represent areas CA1 and CA3 and the subiculum, as defined in Chapter 3; DG, dentate gyrus.

representations and priming (see Chapter 12), the *amygdala* for emotional and social learning, and the *cerebellum* for the learning of skeletal components of classic conditioning. This anatomically based taxonomy is seen as a crucial advance in understanding by those neuroscientists who hold a relatively "localizational" view of brain systems.

However, as outlined in Section 13.2, current ideas about information processing in the CNS refer to networks of interacting brain areas whose normal operation can be disrupted by disconnections rather than lesions of specific brain areas (McCarthy and Warrington, 1990; Aggleton and Brown, 1999; Gaffan, 2002; Murray and Wise, 2004). Human brain imaging work has also moved rapidly from a "localizationist" perspective to one that stresses the importance of "effective connectivity" between brain areas (Friston, 1995, 2004) and the dynamic interaction of medial temporal and frontal regions during intentional aspects of memory retrieval (Miyashita, 2004). Accordingly, the "one-to-one" mapping of memory type to brain area of the original statements of declarative memory theory is now somewhat dated.

Another complication associated with the mapping of types of memory onto brain areas, explicit in Figure 13–3, is that even the proponents of declarative memory theory recognize that brain areas outside the hippocampal formation, and

even outside the medial temporal lobe itself, are also involved in declarative memory. For example, Shimamura and Squire (1987) claimed that the frontal lobes contribute memory of the context in which information is acquired (i.e., "source memory") on the basis of what they observed in amnesic patients with additional frontal damage. As recalling the context where an event happened is a fact that one can declare and of which one is conscious, it must (by definition) be a type of declarative memory. Similarly, Squire has written of a "limbic/diencephalic" brain system that incorporates structures such as the "anterior thalamic nucleus, the mediodorsal nucleus and connections to and from the medial thalamus that lie within the internal medullary lamina" (Squire et al., 1993, p. 462). Squire and Zola asserted that declarative memory is dependent "on the integrity of medial temporal lobe and midline diencephalic structures" (Squire and Zola, 1998, p. 205). This anatomical liberalism wisely recognizes that medial temporal structures do not operate in isolation from the rest of the brain (hence the reference to direct projections in Fig. 13–4), but it leaves skeptics wondering where the anatomical boundaries of the medial temporal lobe memory system begin and end. In any event, the key point of this third proposition is clear: The declarative memory theory places the hippocampal formation at the apex of declarative memory processing supported by a network of other brain structures.

The fourth major postulate of the theory concerns *memory consolidation*. This is a particularly important aspect of the theory and a focus of much current research. The basic idea is that the hippocampal formation has a time-limited role in memory for an individual fact or event. Some interaction is held to take place between it and presumed long-term storage sites in the neocortex. Gradually, through some time-dependent "consolidation" process in which the hippocampus and neocortex interact, initially labile memory traces in the cortex become stabilized. This renders them resistant to later brain damage to the medial temporal lobe itself, although not, of course, to brain areas that are the eventual storage sites of lasting memory traces (Fig. 13–5). Implicit in this fourth proposition of the theory is the supposition that memory for remote events depends on the strength of memory traces (i.e., information encoded within ensembles of spatially dispersed neocortical neurons), where trace strength can be roughly thought of in reductionist terms as alterations in membrane excitability, the strength of synaptic connections, or other activity-dependent properties of cellular physiology. Memories with high trace strength can be recalled easily; those with lower trace strength cannot. Consolidation is thought to be a process that gradually, sometimes through the interleaving of new traces with existing traces, brings trace strength from low to high levels.

A key issue when thinking about consolidation is exactly what is temporarily stored in the hippocampal formation itself. There are several possibilities. One view is that detailed sensory/perceptual information is stored there for an intermediate period of time and then literally shuttled to the neocortex. At the start of the consolidation period, the memories would be "in" the hippocampus; by the end, they would be

Systems-level memory consolidation

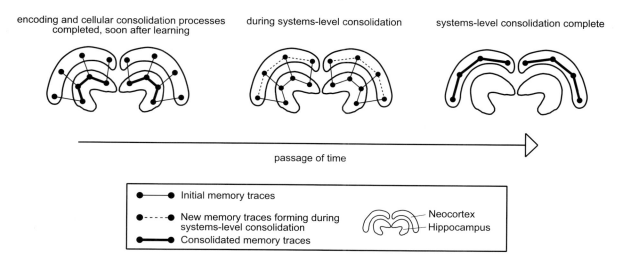

encoding and cellular consolidation processes completed, soon after learning

during systems-level consolidation

systems-level consolidation complete

passage of time

● ──── ● Initial memory traces

● ---- ● New memory traces forming during systems-level consolidation

● ━━━━ ● Consolidated memory traces

Neocortex
Hippocampus

Figure 13–5. Systems-level memory consolidation. Pathways between neocortical areas representing recent events or recently acquired facts are held to be weak initially, even after the protein synthesis-dependent cellular consolidation that sometimes follows immediately after initial encoding (left). Memory soon after learning relies on rapidly formed connections between these neocortical areas and the hippocampal formation. Over time, a consolidation signal emanating in the hippocampus is thought to strengthen neo-cortical connections (middle) to the point where hippocampal activity is no longer necessary (right). The time this consolidation process takes may be quite long—weeks, months, or even longer (Squire and Alvarez, 1995).

"in" the cortex. No one has much confidence in this possibility—as if the brain were some kind of railway shunting yard; and it was never considered seriously by Squire. Another idea, albeit a somewhat metaphorical one, is that hippocampal storage consists of "pointers" or "indices" (Teyler and DiScenna, 1986). These representations do not contain detailed information; they are more like cartoons and are thought to do two things. First, they help activate—by pointing at them—the relevant but dispersed neocortical neurons at which traces representing detailed sensory information are located (presumably through alterations in synaptic strength between interconnecting neurons—see Chapter 10). This is a lovely metaphor—neurons pointing at each other—but exactly how such an addressing mechanism would work is unclear. How does a neuron in the hippocampus "point at" one or more neurons in the cortex or, even more difficult, a subset of their synaptic interconnections? The answer, if this metaphor is on the right lines, is likely to involve diffuse activation coupled to local signals, in much the same way that in the dark a flashlight (diffuse) lights up a prowling cat's eyes (local). It is the conjunction of light and the cat that enables spatial specificity, it not being a property of either feature alone. More generally, "specificity" is one of the big issues of modern neuroscience at every level of analysis applying as much to intracellular synaptic stabilization mechanisms (Goelet et al., 1986; Frey and Morris, 1997) as to the systems-level memory consolidation processes that involve several brain structures (Dudai and Morris, 2001).

Given that areas in the neocortex are the likely sites of perceptual processing and the eventual sites of storage, we might reasonably wonder why the hippocampus is ever needed. Why bother with such apparent duplication? Moreover, even though systems-level memory consolidation is a process revealed through experiments in which the hippocampus is rendered dysfunctional, it is unlikely that the evolutionary pressure to develop a consolidation mechanism was to avoid the deleterious effects on memory of brain damage. So what is the function of consolidation and why the need for a brain area with a time-limited role in memory? One answer, from McNaughton et al. (2003), is that the numerous neocortical interconnections that exist for creating an associational framework of acquired knowledge are weak, slowly formed, and/or liable to rapid decay. It is essential to protect against "everything-becoming-connected-to-everything" during the long process of learning throughout development and adult life. More generally, consolidation is held to be a gradual, selective process precisely because it has to be—ensuring that only the relevant connections are made across ensembles in and between cortical networks to represent information about facts and events accurately (O'Reilly and Norman, 2002). We revisit the issue of whether consolidation always has to be gradual in Section 13.6.

The second thing that hippocampus indices and pointers are supposed to do is guide the consolidation process over time (Squire and Alvarez, 1995). It may take place over hours, days, weeks, months, or even years—the virtue of such slow processing being that it helps avoid catastrophic interference in distributed associative memory traces stored in the cortex (McClelland et al., 1995). This is the "teenager's bedroom" type of interference that occurs when one set of new memories (new junk) overlays earlier formed traces (old junk) in such a manner as to interfere with their subsequent retrieval ("Has anyone seen my iPOD?"). Cautious interleaving, guided by hippocampal pointers, prevents this from happening. As this consolidation process eventually comes to an end for a particular set of information, the pointers have done their job. There is therefore no need for extensive long-term memory retention in hippocampus. Like forgotten movie stars, hippocampal pointers just fade away.

Declarative memory theory therefore asserts that after consolidation is complete damage to the hippocampus should have no effect on memory. However, as consolidation takes time, the theory makes the important prediction that temporal gradients of retrograde amnesia should be obtained in both humans and animals after damage to the medial temporal lobe. This prediction is attractively counterintuitive: It states that if the hippocampus is damaged at time *t* an event experienced several weeks *before* time *t* would be remembered *better* than an event experienced only a few days earlier because the former, despite being older, would have enjoyed a longer period of consolidation. Testing this prediction has become a cottage industry in its own right within the field.

This completes our presentation of the major features of the theory. In the discussion that follows, we first present relevant interventional studies on animals (primarily primates but with some mention of other species) and then a critique. As noted earlier, the relevant human studies have been discussed in Chapter 12, and an important extension of the declarative memory theory called the "relational processing" theory (Cohen and Eichenbaum, 1993; Eichenbaum and Cohen, 2001) is considered separately (see Section 13.5). It has inspired a body of experimentation somewhat separate from Squire's version of declarative memory theory. Similarly, work on the consolidation of spatial memory is reserved for discussion in Section 13.4.

13.3.2 Development of a Primate Model of Amnesia

In the historical survey of Chapter 2, we noted that the initial efforts to model human amnesia in animals were largely unsuccessful. Monkeys given lesions of the medial temporal lobe showed deficits in certain tasks. but overall they were capable of learning tasks that one might not expect an "amnesic" monkey to learn. Similarly, rats given hippocampal lesions showed diminished exploration and striking inflexibility in their learned behavior but were quite capable of learning many quite complex tasks. The apparent discrepancy between the human and animal data did not go unnoticed, and various attempts were made to explain it (Iversen, 1976; Weiskrantz, 1982).

Development of New Tasks for Monkeys to Parallel the Types of Memory Lost in Amnesia

An important insight by Gaffan was that the tasks then used in animal studies were quite unlike those on which amnesics were seen to fail (Gaffan, 1974). He suggested that new tasks be developed to capture what he then saw as an important distinction between "recognition-memory" and "associative-memory." Recognition memory refers, at least operationally, to the ability to discriminate between stimulus items that have been seen recently and others that have not. A judgment of prior occurrence (Brown, 1996), it is generally impaired in global amnesia, as shown by a standard test such as Warrington's Recognition Memory Test; however, it is not always severely impaired in patients with more restricted hippocampal damage (Aggleton and Shaw, 1996). Associative memory, on the other hand, refers to the ability to learn that two stimulus items go together, such as a stimulus and a reward or a response and a reward, without regard to their familiarity. This is a "habit" type of learning that Gaffan argued was preserved in the presence of amnesia.

To model recognition memory, he collected a set of 300 junk objects and presented 60 of them to the monkeys each day. Each trial consisted of a "sample" phase, during which the experimenter presented one object on its own, and a "choice" phase in which two objects were presented: the one that had just been shown as a sample together with another, novel object. These objects were presented on trays inside a Wisconsin General Testing Apparatus (WGTA) (Fig. 13–6A). To motivate the monkeys to perform the task, a "sugar puff" reward could be retrieved when they displaced the object presented during the sample phase and again when they chose that same object during the choice phase. The only way the monkeys could perform correctly was if they: (1) learned and then applied the rule that a reward was available for displacing the familiar object rather than the novel one; and (2) remembered which object was familiar during the choice phase of each trial after the memory interval following sample presentation. This technique of probing recognition memory was therefore called "delayed matching to sample with trial-unique cues," where "matching-to-sample" refers to the rule for solution, "trial-unique" to the fact that an absolute judgment of familiarity of the objects is required, and "delayed" because of the memory interval between the sample and choice phases of each trial. It is usually abbreviated as DMTS. After learning using the short memory delay of 5 to 8 seconds (at which the monkeys performed extremely well), two performance challenges were added. One was to increase the memory delay up to several minutes; the other was to present a "list" of several sample objects, one after the other, and then do a seriesof choice trials. Delays and lists are widely used in modern variants of this task. Finally, to model associative memory, Gaffan used a small subset of the same junk objects but a different protocol. The monkeys had to learn which objects were consistently rewarded and which consistently unrewarded, presenting the objects time and again until they were all completely familiar. The animals indicated their knowledge of the object-reward relations correctly by reaching for rewarded objects when they were presented and toward a small brass disk placed alongside when the nonrewarded objects were presented. Correct choices were rewarded; incorrect choices were not (Box 13–2).

The monkeys given fornix lesions showed delay-dependent impairment in the recognition task (Fig. 13–6B) and list

A   Recognition memory in a WGTA

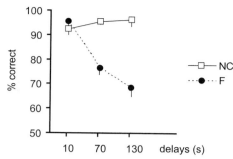

B   Delayed matching to sample (DMTS)

C   Delayed non-matching to sample (DNMTS)

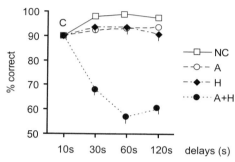

Figure 13–6. Recognition memory in the monkey. *A.* Rhesus macaque in a Wisconsin General Testing Apparatus (WGTA) reaching for and displacing objects that hide a food reward. (*Source*: Courtesy Christopher Coe, Harlow Primate Laboratory.) *B.* Fornix lesions cause delay-dependent impairment of delayed matching to sample (DMTS). (*Source*: After Gaffan, 1974.) *C.* Conjoint aspiration lesions of the hippocampus and amygdala lesions, including neocortical structures of the medial temporal lobe, cause delay-dependent (left) and list-dependent (right) impairment of delayed nonmatching to sample (DNMS) after the animals reach the initial criterion of 90% correct with single-sample objects. (*Source*: After Mishkin, 1978.)

length-dependent impairment, but their associative learning was unimpaired. As correct performance at short delays depends on successful execution of the procedural rule learned preoperatively (matching-to-sample), the deficit caused by the fornix lesion at longer delays is unlikely to have been due to the monkeys not remembering the rule. Rather, it suggested that fornix lesions have no effect on (1) short-term memory or (2) intellectual function (they had learned the rule preoperatively and could still execute it postoperatively), but (3) they prevent the formation of memories lasting much longer than about 2 minutes. This conjunction of three important characteristics of human amnesia in a single experiment represented the first apparently successful attempt to model key features of the syndrome in animals. Ironically, although explicitly introduced on the grounds that it would cause "the least extrahippocampal damage" (Gaffan, 1974, p. 1100), fornix lesions are associated with only modest amnesia in humans (see Chapter 12). This represented something of a puzzle but one that was soon solved.

Emergence of Delayed Nonmatching to Sample as the Benchmark Test of Recognition Memory in Primates

DMTS tasks had been used previously with animals, but Gaffan's innovation of trial-unique cues during each week of testing appeared to ensure that the familiarity discrimination demanded of the monkeys was effectively an absolute judgment ("Have I ever seen this object before?") rather than, as happens with pairs of cues that are repeatedly given across trials, a judgment of relative recency ("Which of these objects have I seen most recently"?). Relative recency may still be a

---

Box 13–2
Procedures for Testing Learning and Memory in Primates

Apparatus:	Wisconsin general testing apparatus
	Computerized touch screens
Procedures:	Pattern discrimination
	Spatial discrimination and reversal
	Object discrimination and reversal
	Concurrent object discrimination
	Delayed response
	Delayed matching-to-sample (DMTS)
	Delayed nonmatching-to-sample (DNMTS)
	Visual paired comparison
	Object-in-place memory
	Scene memory

factor, even with 300 junk objects, as testing requires that they be reused within a week or so (Charles et al., 2004a). In any event, this subtle procedural change successfully engaged a brain system that operated in the domain of long-term, rather than short-term, memory. Additionally, the use of lists of items appeared to make the task analogous to the list-learning tasks so widely used in human studies. It is, perhaps, a slightly unrealistic model of human list learning because the stimulus materials usually presented to people (e.g., words or word-pairs) are items with which people are already familiar. The human test is not whether the word "cat" has *ever* been seen before, but if this word appeared in the list presented by the experimenter several minutes earlier. Thus, in the human experiment, word lists are context-specific, a distinction not thought to matter at the outset but, as we shall see later, arguably critical to the anatomical mediation of different types of memory. For the monkeys, whether a judgment of absolute familiarity or relative recency is required may not matter provided a sufficiently large number of objects are used. However, it most certainly does matter if only two objects are used, as Owen and Butler (1981) were to show, because fornix lesions have no effect on remembering which of two objects has been seen most recently. This is not surprising because normal monkeys can do this well only over a few seconds, and they use short-term memory to do so; the task is impaired by a combined orbitofrontal and temporal stem lesion (Cirillo et al., 1989). Thus, fornix lesions do not interfere with short-term memory but may affect long-term memory.

Another, more important difficulty with DMTS relates to the matching rule. With such a rule, the monkey is rewarded during the sample trial for displacing a *novel* object but rewarded on the choice trial for displacing what is then the *familiar* object. This potential source of confusion can be avoided with several variants of the delayed-matching protocol, but the simplest and most influential change in procedure was the shift to tasks employing a "delayed *non*matching-to-sample" rule. With nonmatching, the monkey is rewarded for reaching for a novel object each time he reaches out: on sample trials for the single sample object and on choice trials when presented with a pair of objects. Mishkin and Delacour (1975) developed such a task and found that normal monkeys could learn nonmatching more easily than matching, probably because of their natural inquisitiveness about novelty. Being easier and being later shown to be sensitive to large lesions of the medial temporal lobe, delayed nonmatching to sample became the task of choice for many years.

In an important study, Mishkin (1978) exploited both characteristics of delayed nonmatching to sample to investigate the effects of hippocampal, amygdala, and combined hippocampal/amygdala lesions on recognition memory. He trained monkeys on the delayed nonmatching to sample task until they were performing at 90% correct or better. They were then divided into four groups, with most undergoing bilateral surgery to the medial temporal lobe; three monkeys were left as normal controls. Of the nine operated monkeys, three were

subjected to hippocampal lesioning, three to amygdala lesioning, and three to lesioning of both structures. Postoperatively, the animals that had lesions of the hippocampus (but including the caudal perirhinal cortex and parts of the parahippocampal cortex because an aspiration technique was used) and those with lesions of the amygdala (including parts of the rostral perirhinal cortex) all relearned the task quickly. Those with the combined lesion—a lesion analogous to the medial temporal lobectomy in patient H.M.—were severely impaired. Mishkin (1978) also found that once criterion levels of performance had been reached by all groups with a short memory delay the combined lesion group showed pronounced list-length and delay-dependent impairments in recognition memory (Fig. 13–6C). The other groups performed well—indistinguishably from the nonoperated controls. Thus, the group that had been subjected to lesioning similar to that applied to H.M. showed strikingly similar memory impairment. This was a great step forward, and the paper has been justly celebrated as a classic paper of twentieth-century neuroscience (Aggleton, 1999).

Both lesions involved removing cortical tissue adjacent to the target structures of the amygdala and hippocampus. At the time, this was not thought to be of particular significance by most observers (Horel, 1978), and the results were long described by Mishkin's group and by almost everyone else in the field as lesions of the "hippocampus" and of the "amygdala," respectively. The pattern in the findings suggested that these two structures played a parallel role in memory (which might yet be dissociated by other tasks), the "dual circuit" idea emerging as part of a theory of memory proposed a few years later (Mishkin, 1982).

Delayed nonmatching-to-sample (DNMTS) rapidly emerged as, in Zola's phrase, the "benchmark test" of recognition memory. It was used in numerous studies, notably by the National Institutes of Health (NIH) group led by Mishkin and colleagues Bachevalier, Murray, Saunders, and others and separately by the San Diego group of Squire, Zola-Morgan (Zola), Amaral, Suzuki, and others. A distinctive and laudable feature of their work over the 20-year period from 1978 to 1998 was partial standardization of the manual testing protocols such that comparisons could be made across studies, at least within each laboratory. With the sole but important exception that the NIH experiments typically involved extensive pretraining prior to the lesion whereas the San Diego series always involved surgery prior to training (Zola-Morgan et al., 1982), this standardization was extremely valuable. In the case of the San Diego experiments, it made possible a comparison of lesion groups with first one and later a second "standardized" group of unoperated control animals. Research using primates is not undertaken lightly because of the ethical, conservation, and financial reasons referred to earlier (see Section 13.2). Thus, establishing a set of repeatable protocols for a test that models several aspects of amnesia was an important step forward. If there was a weakness of this standardization, it was that different experimenters were inevitably involved in testing the two control groups and the various lesion groups over the years, a practice that would not ordinarily be accepted in research on rodents. The experimenter was typically not "blinded" with respect to the lesion created in the animal, whereas this also is common practice in the best laboratories working with rodents. However, the robustness of the task and the tight variability of the forgetting functions with memory delays make it unlikely that these weaknesses seriously limit its validity, even if it slightly injures their elegance.

The outcome of studies conducted throughout the 1980s and early 1990s indicate that after the combined lesion (lesions that include the underlying cortical structures of the posterior entorhinal cortex, perirhinal cortex, and parahippocampal gyrus), a DNMTS deficit is observed whose main characteristics can be summarized as follows (Box 13–3):

Working through these numbered points in turn, the following additional comments and qualifications should be noted. First, despite the use of different monkey species and different surgeons, experimenters, and WGTA designs, bilateral damage to the medial temporal lobe similar to that produced in the original study of Mishkin (1978) always causes a memory deficit in DNMTS (Squire et al., 2004). It is, however, important to stress that this does not mean that the hippocampus alone is involved in recognition memory, as the lesions that were used initially typically encompassed extrahippocampal structures. Second, performance is good at short delays but appears to decline monotonically as the time between sample and choice is lengthened (Mishkin, 1978; Zola-Morgan and Squire, 1985; Overman et al., 1990; Alvarez et al., 1994a; but see Ringo, 1991, 1993). Securing this claim involved the development of computer-automated systems for presenting stimulus material to get around the difficulty that there was always a small delay in the WGTA when the screen separating the monkey and the experimenter was raised and lowered. Notwithstanding this technological improvement in testing procedure, there was an intense if somewhat technical debate about delay-dependence, an issue we shall come to shortly. Third, a deficit occurs in the visual and tactile modalities, and by inference it is probably multimodal. For example, monkeys tested in the dark so they can only feel the sample and choice objects also show a memory deficit following medial temporal lobe lesions (Murray and Mishkin, 1983;

Suzuki et al., 1993). However, the inference about other modalities is insecure. The available data on auditory DNMTS indicates no impact of perirhinal lesions (Fritz et al., 2005), a finding also observed in dogs (Kowalska et al., 2001). The data of Fritz et al. (2005) led to the intriguing speculation that language may be unique to humans not only because it depends on speech but because it requires long-term auditory memory, although, as they pointed out, this appears to be contradicted by field studies showing their ability to recognize alarm calls that signal predators (Seyfarth et al., 1980). To our knowledge, the impact of medial temporal lesions on olfactory recognition has not been reported in primates (T. Otto and M. Munoz, personal communication), partly owing to the difficulty of making olfactory cues salient for monkeys (M. Baxter, personal communication). Fourth, the effects of distraction in DNMTS are analogous to what happens with amnesic patients. They can retain small amounts of information for extended periods when not distracted but forget more rapidly when their attention is diverted (Zola-Morgan and Squire, 1985)—although interaction between distraction and the effects of a lesion is not always present (Zola-Morgan et al., 1989). Fifth, there is no recovery of function; a deficit is still seen when memory testing is conducted up to 4 years after surgery as well as when it is carried out shortly after surgery (Zola-Morgan et al., 1986). These five characteristics of DNMTS performance after large medial temporal lobe lesions map neatly onto several features of the amnesic syndrome. It is not without reason that object recognition memory, as measured in DNMTS, was championed as an "animal model of amnesia" (Squire and Zola-Morgan, 1991) and even declared a "millennial achievement" in neuroscience (Kandel et al., 2000).

Other Tasks Used in a Comprehensive Test Battery to Explore Declarative Memory in Primates

Although DNMTS became the most widely used task, it was complemented by other tasks designed to probe different types of declarative memory. During the early years, Squire and Zola-Morgan often used a standardized "test battery" consisting of several of the tasks shown in Box 13–2. Large medial temporal lobe lesions cause a learning impairment in the *concurrent object discrimination task* involving the interleaved presentation of eight pairs of objects of which one member of each pair is consistently rewarded, and the *delayed retention of object discriminations* (Zola-Morgan and Squire, 1985). Deficits in the *delayed response* task are sometimes seen, but they are capricious. This is because lesioned monkeys have no deficit in short-term memory and even normal monkeys can tolerate only short memory delays before they become confused about whether they are remembering the present or a previous trial. This is never a problem for DNMTS because of the use of trial-unique cues.

Each of these and other tasks in the battery is held to be "declarative" in the sense that, with only slight suspension of disbelief, they can be seen as analogous to tasks given to

---

Box 13–3
Delayed Nonmatching to Sample Reveals an Important Role for the Medial Temporal Lobe in Recognition Memory

1. The deficit in DNMTS after large medial temporal lobe lesions is robust and repeatable.
2. The deficit is apparently delay-dependent.
3. The deficit may be independent of modality.
4. The deficit is exacerbated by distracting stimuli presented during the delay interval.
5. The deficit is enduring.

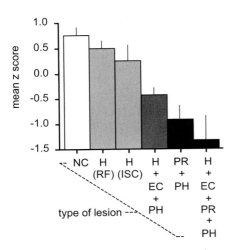

Test battery and different MTL lesions

Figure 13–7. Pooling data across the test battery. The results of several tasks of the San Diego test battery were pooled using z-scores to reveal a graded deficit proportional to the extent of the medial temporal lobe lesion and the way it was made. EC, entorhinal cortex; H, hippocampal lesions; ISC, ischemic; NC, normal control; PH, parahippocampal cortex; PR, perirhinal cortex; RF, radiofrequency. (*Source*: Zola-Morgan et al., 1994.)

people. For example, the concurrent object discrimination task can be thought of as analogous to learning a list of words, the delayed retention of object discriminations to remembering a passage of prose, and so on. Moreover, when the data from all of tasks used in the San Diego test battery are combined across experiments by averaging z-scores (reflecting relative statistical variability rather than absolute values), a clear deficit is observed after lesions of the medial temporal lobe that, with some exceptions (Baxter and Murray, 2001b), is nicely graded with respect to extent of damage (Zola-Morgan et al., 1994) (Fig. 13–7). However, the test battery has gradually fallen out of favor, partly because components of it are now thought to depend on other brain structures. For example, the deficit in the concurrent object discrimination task after large medial temporal lobe lesions is probably due to damage to area TE (Buffalo et al., 1998b), and this same task involves habit learning in humans rather than declarative memory (Bayley et al., 2005a).

Adequacy of These Tasks as Models of Declarative Memory

One qualification of this ostensibly tidy picture was an argument first posed by Ringo to the effect that the delay dependence of the DNMTS deficit may depend on the choice of numerical scale with which performance is scored (Ringo, 1991, 1993). This is an important technical point. The outcome of a single trial in DNMTS is the monkey choosing the correct or incorrect object. It is therefore usual to plot performance on a scale from 50% (chance) to 100% (perfect per-

formance) using a linear scale. Ringo argued that statistical considerations require an arcsine or other transformation for such data, particularly if scores come close to 90% correct as they often do at short memory delays. His reanalysis of several published DNMTS studies using such a transformation led him to conclude that medial temporal lesions may not, in fact, cause delay-dependent forgetting. He suggested that *apparent* delay dependence in several studies could arise because lesion-induced deficits are concealed at short memory-delay intervals through use of the linear scale. For example, controls may be scoring 92% correct and lesioned monkeys 90%—performance levels that do not differ statistically when the variability is computed using the entire data set. However, an arcsine transformation (which "stretches" the scale as values approach either 0 or 100%) may show a different picture, as Ringo's reanalysis of several data sets indicated. This is a cogent argument, although it did play down the overlap of performance by lesioned and control monkeys at short delays in some studies, as pointed out by Alvarez-Royo et al. (1992). Its importance was nevertheless taken on board. It spurred the development of, or at least the better appreciation of, automated versions of the WGTA that permit the presentation of very short sample-choice intervals. Under these conditions, no lesion-induced deficit is observed in the rate of acquisition of the DNMTS task at "zero delay," with control and lesioned animals reaching the same performance asymptote. An unambiguous delay-dependent deficit still pops out at long delays (Overman et al., 1990; Alvarez et al., 1994). Ringo's concern, however, should not be forgotten, as findings obtained more recently with neurotoxic lesions of structures *within* the hippocampal formation add a further note of caution. To claim a *differential* effect on memory rather than perception, it is essential to secure the statistical interaction between group and memory delay. This is because a lesion that impaired perception would be expected to have as large an effect at short memory delays as at long ones—the animals being just as poor at seeing the objects in front of them at both intervals. This is the gold standard for establishing that the performance of groups differs across the domain of long-term memory. Many studies have aspired to this standard; the truth is that few primate DNMTS studies have reached it.

A separate concern about the test battery is that the psychological justification for regarding tasks in the test battery as "declarative" is not always clear, and in some cases the argument borders on the circular. We have just noted that concurrent discrimination learning might be thought akin to a person learning a list of words. The trouble is that there are lists and there are lists. For example, Squire (1992) claimed that the concurrent discrimination task in which eight pairs of objects are presented a number of times during a single testing session (a task developed originally by Moss et al., 1981) is declarative, whereas a 20-pair concurrent task in which each pair of objects is presented only once per day is not (Malamut et al., 1984). The basis for these assertions was that the former was impaired by medial temporal lobe lesions, whereas the latter was not. Clearly this circularity, if that is all there is to it, is unsatisfactory. In fairness, there is more to it, namely that many behavioral tasks can be learned using different strategies—even those of ostensibly the same logical structure (task ambiguity being one of the key conceptual issues discussed in Section 13.2). Varying the pattern and temporal spacing of the trials may bias animals toward or away from using a "declarative strategy"—an example of a *quantitative* change having a *qualitative* effect. In the case of concurrent object discrimination tasks, normal monkeys might be able to remember the "fact" that a particular object was paired with reward for a period of time despite the interference produced by the other eight interposed problems with different objects. Provided another trial of the first problem comes along soon enough, they could then use their fact-based declarative memory to solve the problem. However, if the intertrial interval is long, as with the 24-hour delay task, even the normal monkey may find a declarative strategy less reliable. It might then fall back on a stimulus-response strategy, by which is meant the gradual strengthening of a disposition to reach for the rewarded object and not for the nonrewarded object, rather than explicit memory of a prior object and reward episode. Because this nondeclarative strategy, according to the theory, is also available to the lesioned monkey, no difference in performance would be expected between groups. Interestingly, people generally use a declarative strategy to learn lists, irrespective of how long the list and how many trials are presented per day, although, as already noted, people also learn the concurrent object discrimination task in a habit-like manner (Bayley et al., 2005a). Debate about the interpretation of tasks first published 20 years ago may seem like a historical sideline, but it is not. For the issue of "strategy used" versus "logical structure' is a key one and, as we shall see, has reemerged as an issue with respect to the memory strategies mediating DNMTS.

The way to avoid circularity is to come up with independent psychological evidence that a particular strategy is being used or that performance on one task correlates with that on another and allow this evidence to help guide definitive predictions from the theory. In the case of concurrent object discrimination learning, one way might be to use the "reward-devaluation" procedure as originally developed in experiments on rats (Adams and Dickinson, 1981). If the association between reaching for an object and securing reward is learned as a "fact," pairing the reward with a toxin such as lithium chloride should render it less palatable and so make the animal less inclined to reach for the object. This is because the animal would, in some sense, infer from his "propositional knowledge" that reaching for the object leads to the reward, and thus seeing the object should retrieve a memory representation of the reward and that it is now no longer worth having. However, if the animal had merely learned the habit of reaching for the object as a disposition (and learned it because it was repeatedly paired with reward during training), reward devaluation would not have any immediate effects on performance. The animal would reach for the reward because reaching for rewards is what it had been trained to do, not because it has in any sense "remembered" that doing so actually leads to anything. Murray and her colleagues at the NIH laboratory have used this reinforcer-devaluation procedure to dissociate fact and habit learning in studies that have revealed that excitotoxic damage to the amygdala disrupts the ability of animals to change their internal representations of reinforcement value (Malkova et al., 1997). Stimulus–stimulus associations can therefore be represented in a manner that might be thought of as a "fact." However, neither the hippocampus nor the rhinal cortex seems to be a brain structure mediating reinforcer devaluation (Thornton et al., 1998).

As an aside, exclusion of the amygdala from a revised medial temporal lobe memory system may also be mistaken because there are aspects of recognition memory that do seem to involve stimulus value. Seeing old friends again, such as colleagues at an annual scientific gathering, invokes great pleasure. We all witness and experience this on the first day of such a meeting—a curious pleasure as it is all too often followed by heated debate in the lecture theater with these self same people. Although this emotional characteristic of stimulus familiarity may be mediated by the hippocampus and/or the perirhinal cortex, it seems unlikely. It is tempting to speculate that there may be role for the amygdala as well.

13.3.3 Domains of Preserved Learning Following Medial Temporal Lobe Lesions in Primates

When constructing an animal model of amnesia, it is important to model *spared* memory as well as impaired memory, of which Gaffan's (1974) use of an associative task was an early example. Historically, systematic analysis of the issue of multiple types of learning and memory and their differential sensitivity to different lesions began in the rodent literature (see Sections 13.4 and 13.5). It was, however, not long before the idea was taken up in studies with primates beginning with tasks involving motor skill. For example, Zola-Morgan and Squire (1984) found that control and medial temporal lobe (MTL)-lesioned monkeys could learn to thread a "lifesaver" candy (which contains a central hole) along and then off a thin wire. Eating the candy was the monkey's reward. With experience, normal and lesioned monkeys got steadily faster, and they learned at an equivalent rate. Presumably, the lesioned monkeys did not remember doing the task from one day to the next or recognize the apparatus when it was shown to them again, but they threaded the "lifesaver" nonetheless. If only we could "ask" them about their mental experience in such a situation!

Perceptual skills have also been studied in monkeys using pattern discrimination tasks (Squire and Zola-Morgan, 1983). These are slowly learned discriminations in which two similar patterns (such as alpha-numeric characters) are differentially paired with reward. Learning typically takes place slowly, over hundreds of trials; and with one exception no deficit in learning is seen following even large MTL lesions or after hippocampus-specific lesions. The interesting exception noted by Squire is that performance is sometimes poorer over the first few trials of the day. He suggested that this difference between groups is due to controls remembering the first few trials in an explicit or declarative way prior to the build-up of within-session interference and the reliance on learned habits. However, more recent experiments, discussed in the critique later on, challenge the idea that components of the MTL memory system are not involved in learning stimulus-reward associations (Murray and Wise, 2004).

With respect to cognitive skills, that lesioned monkeys can learn tasks such as DNMTS at a normal rate at zero delay (Alvarez-Royo et al., 1992) seems to imply that they are able to abstract, from the sequence of trial events, the appropriate rule for performance. This finding is inconsistent with their having any major deficit in "intelligence." However, although the investigation of primate cognitive skills, knowledge, and "metaknowledge" (i.e., what they know they know) has been considered by those working in a more ecological context (Hauser, 2003), it has only recently been considered seriously by behavioral neuroscientists (Hampton, 2001). Monkeys have not yet been taught the subtle tasks of learning a finite grammar or to make accurate weather forecasts—tasks that have imaginatively extended the domain of preserved learning in amnesics (Knowlton and Squire, 1993), but the range of laboratory tasks of nondeclarative memory is steadily expanding.

13.3.4 Selective Lesions of Distinct Components of the Medial-temporal Lobe Reveal Heterogeneity of Function

Squire and Zola-Morgan's development of a test battery was motivated by the reasonable ambition of developing tasks that are analogues of the verbal and visual memory protocols on which MTL amnesics are impaired. Combining data from these tasks in the form of z-scores to create a single quantitative index (Fig. 13–7) revealed a monotonic effect of lesions within the MTL: the larger the lesion, the greater the deficit (Zola-Morgan et al., 1994). However, mindful of the uncertainties surrounding the classic but misleading concepts of mass action and equipotentiality (Lashley, 1950), it is not surprising that critics of declarative memory theory are wary of the notion that the entire MTL functions as a single homogeneous unit. Indeed, further research has revealed that restricted lesions of MTL structures cause little or no impairment in some declarative tasks but do affect others. This is not just a matter of graded task difficulty, as double dissociations are seen (as we shall see shortly). Particularly problematic are data suggesting that neither restricted hippocampal lesions nor damage confined to the entorhinal cortex necessarily cause an enduring deficit in DNMTS.

Absolute confidence in the "benchmark test" of DNMTS began to unravel for a number of reasons. One problem has to do with understanding what the test is really measuring psychologically; another relates to identifying the necessary and sufficient lesion that impairs it. These two issues are connected.

Mishkin's "dual-circuit" theory relating to the putative role of the "hippocampus" and "amygdala" in recognition memory prompted the question of whether different types of information processing occurred in the two routes of his dual pathway (Mishkin, 1982). One prescient idea, based in part on theorizing by Mandler (1980) was that recognition memory could be based on either a memory of the polymodal features of an object or on memory of where the object had been seen before. We may think of this as, on the one hand, distinguishing between features that are intrinsically *part* of the object and, on the other, between features that *reflect the context* in which an object is seen. Whereas the former are part of (and so would move with) an object when it is displaced, the latter might not.

Two studies began the systematic exploration of this issue. One examined cross-modal transfer of information, and the other examined memory for the place where an object had been presented. Murray and Mishkin (1985) found that "amygdala" lesions (which included damage to the perirhinal cortex) caused impaired cross-modal transfer, whereas "hippocampal" lesions (which also damaged the parahippocampal cortex) were with without effect. Monkeys were trained to sample one of a restricted set of 40 objects in complete darkness and then make a choice between the sample and another member of the set in the light. Information acquired in the tactile modality was sufficient to guide visually directed choices accurately, but performance, at even short memory delays, was selectively impaired by the "amygdala" lesions. In contrast, Parkinson et al. (1988) found that their hippocampal lesions selectively impaired both a place task and an object-in-place task, whereas the amygdala lesions had no effect. In a concurrent "place" and "object-in-place" tasks, two objects were presented during the sample trial in two of three possible locations on the tray in front of the monkey. On the choice trial, these objects were again put in front of the monkey. In the "place" choice trials, the monkey had only to choose on the basis of the locations occupied by the objects in the sample trial; whereas for the "object-in-place" choice trials, the animals had to choose on the basis of remembering the particular places occupied by particular objects. It was later established that monkeys with "hippocampal" lesions could remember one place but not two (Angeli et al., 1993).

The sufficient lesions for seeing these deficits are now known to be purely neocortical, but the historically still important point to emerge from these studies is that recognition of novelty might be mediated by either "intrinsic" or "contextual" components that are not disambiguated in the standard DNMTS test. The distinction echoes the concept of recognition being mediated either by a sense of familiarity (intrinsic) or by recollection (contextual recall) (Mandler, 1980). Recognition by familiarity would involve the monkey making its choice because of the two objects confronting him in the choice test one evokes a sense of familiarity. It could do that even if the monkey was unable to recollect the occasion when or where it had seen it before. Recognition by contextual recall, on the other hand, would involve the monkey utilizing the cues of the WGTA surrounding him to "bring back to mind" that of the two objects before him one had been presented before in this context. Although we cannot talk to the monkey about it, we can nonetheless imagine the animal having a private "recollective experience" in much the same way that we would do in a similar situation.

Unfortunately, the important line of psychological thinking embedded in these ingenious studies was largely overshadowed by preoccupation with the anatomical implications of the aspiration lesion technique. Damage to tissue lying in the entorhinal, perirhinal, and/or parahippocampal cortices might have been contributing to poor performance in the "amygdala"- and "hippocampus"-lesioned animals rather than damage to these target areas. Later studies using more selective lesions have borne this out. For example, we now know that cross-modal memory is affected principally by the perirhinal but not the amygdala component of the original lesions (Murray and Bussey, 1999). Similarly, the spatial task appears to be unaffected by neurotoxic hippocampal lesions (Malkova and Mishkin, 2003).

Studies during the late 1980s revealed, somewhat surprisingly, that neurons in the perirhinal cortex were sensitive to familiarity and relative recency (Brown et al., 1987; Brown and Xiang, 1998). In parallel, careful anatomical studies began to focus on the neocortical regions neighboring the hippocampus, such as the entorhinal cortex (Amaral et al., 1987; Insausti et al., 1987a,b) and both the perirhinal and parahippocampal cortex (Suzuki and Amaral, 1994a, b). This work was accompanied by further lesion studies. With few excep-

tions, Gaffan's laboratory in Oxford being one of them, these studies remained focused on using the old warhorse DNMTS. Lesions described as being in the "rhinal cortex" (part of the anterior perirhinal cortex) were sufficient to cause severe, enduring delay-dependent impairment of DNMTS irrespective of whether the hippocampus had also been damaged (Meunier et al., 1993; Suzuki et al., 1993; Mishkin and Murray, 1994). Following these important discoveries, Murray and Mishkin (1998) reinvestigated the role of the hippocampus and amygdala using excitotoxic lesions. Not only does this type of lesion leave the surrounding cortex unaffected, excitotoxins should not damage fibers from the anterior perirhinal cortex passing through the ventral amygdalo-fugal pathway to the medial thalamus or the posterior perirhinal efferents projecting through the fimbria-fornix and posterior thalamus to the same nucleus (see Chapter 3). The key finding was that monkeys with average lesion sizes of 88% damage to the amygdala and 73% damage to the hippocampus showed no impairment in DNMTS (Fig. 13–8A). This comprehensive study included varying list lengths and memory delays and, following the protocols set by Alvarez et al. (1995), included delays of up to 40 minutes in a subset of four monkeys. As no deficit was observed, Murray and Mishkin concluded that, in the MTL, "the rhinal cortex is not only necessary but also sufficient to sustain visual recognition ability" (Murray and Mishkin, 1998, p. 6579). This conclusion is entirely compatible with the available electrophysiological and lesion data. In passing it should be noted that these findings rescue part of the memory circuit for memory originally proposed by

Figure 13–8. Conflicting findings in studies of selective lesions of the hippocampus upon delayed nonmatching to sample (DNMTS). *A.* Murray and Mishkin (1998) found that conjoint damage of both amygdala and hippocampus without major damage to surrounding perirhinal and parahippocampal cortex had no effect on DNMTS with memory delays as long as 40 minutes. *B.* Zola et al. (2000) reported that damage restricted to the hippocampus made using ischemia, radiofrequency heating, or excitotoxins caused a delay-dependent deficit in DNMTS over the same time delays. *C.* Zola et al. (2000) observed a similar deficit in another test of recognition memory—visual paired comparison.

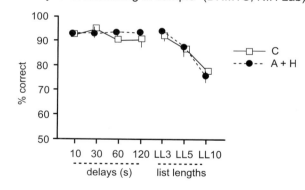

A Delayed nonmatching to sample (DNMTS; NIH Lab)

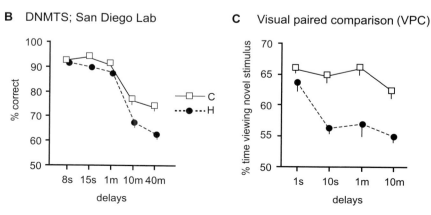

B DNMTS; San Diego Lab

C Visual paired comparison (VPC)

Mishkin (1982) by showing that the critical pathway for a judgment of familiarity emanates from the perirhinal cortex to the medial nucleus of the thalamus, bypassing the hippocampus itself.

However, in contrast and over memory delays of as short as 2 and 10 minutes, Beason-Held et al. (1999) found hippocampus lesion-induced impairment. Zola et al. (2000) also reported that restricted hippocampal damage can be sufficient to cause impairments in both DNMTS and another test of recognition memory called the visual paired-comparison (VPC) task (Fig. 13–8B,C). The latter task, like certain tasks developed by Gaffan much earlier (e.g., Gaffan et al., 1984), involves no formal training—merely exposing the monkey to pairs of black and white line drawings on a computer screen (Bachevalier et al., 1993). After looking at these drawings for about 30 seconds, monkeys spontaneously direct their eye movements to a new drawing presented on the screen beside one of the old ones (a phenomenon first observed experimentally in studies of human infant perception (Fantz, 1964). Many pairs of such stimuli can be presented, one after the other, to build up a profile of the animal's ability to detect novelty spontaneously.

Drawing together data from experiments over 10 years using a variety of lesion techniques and a large number of monkeys, Zola et al. (2000) claimed that ischemic, radiofrequency, and excitotoxic lesions of the hippocampal region all cause a modest but significant deficit in recognition memory in both DNMTS and VPC. The deficit is apparent at delays as short as 15 seconds, with larger effects seen (at least on DNMS) at longer delays of 10 and 40 minutes. Consistent with the declarative memory theory, they concluded that the integrity of the hippocampal region is essential for recognition memory. The extent of hippocampal damage varied substantially among these three studies, ranging from 33% to 62% in the San Diego animals but, paradoxically, averaging 73% in Murray and Mishkin's NIH study that found no deficit. However, Nemanic et al. (2004) came to a somewhat different conclusion after a similar comparison of DNMTS and VPC. Their data point to a substantial deficit in both tasks after perirhinal lesions but no deficit in VPC in hippocampus-lesioned monkeys until longer delays are interposed and only a slight deficit in DNMTS at a memory delay interval of 10 minutes. Bachevalier raised the important qualification about her own study (Nemanic et al., 2004) that the average lesion size in her hippocampal group was only 43.5% (this being made with ibotenic acid), but this does not appear to be substantially different from the mean lesion size prevailing in the San Diego studies that also used excitotoxins.

Comparison of Conflicting Studies Reveals Subtle Differences in Lesion Size and Methodology

How is the discrepancy between these experiments to be explained? Some reports have indicated that apparently restricted hippocampal lesions did impair recognition memory and others that they did not. There were several procedural differences. One of these was the use of extensive pretraining by the NIH laboratory. Zola et al. commented that: "Training on the rule provides the monkeys with extended practice at holding novel objects in memory across short delays, which might then make it easier to hold novel objects in memory across the longer delays from which the performance scores are derived" (Zola et al., 2000, p. 459). The implication seems to be that avoiding preoperative training makes for a more sensitive behavioral assay, a view consistent with the apparently greater sensitivity to hippocampal lesions of the VPC task in which there is no formal training at all. This may be true empirically but is unsatisfying intellectually, as there is nothing in declarative memory theory to explain this dependence. Indeed, we should be wary of a logical inconsistency with respect to mission of this enterprise, namely, modeling amnesia. Amnesic patients have extensive experience recognizing things prior to becoming amnesic but, according to Squire, have a recognition deficit even if their brain damage is restricted to the hippocampus. Why should the animal model be any different? Furthermore, why did the San Diego laboratory insist on using a protocol so different from what they were doing with their patients?

A major of focus of attention has been on the extent of damage to hippocampal and extrahippocampal regions. Growing awareness of the importance of the extent of lesion damage in individual animals led to the development of MRI-based evaluations of the locus and extent of damage (Malkova et al., 2001). Suitably calibrated, these evaluations offer the opportunity of providing accurate, noninvasive estimates of brain damage in advance of extensive postoperative testing (an ethically desirable development apart from anything else). The more usual postmortem histology has often—no doubt to the dismay of experimenters (after years of training an individual animal)—revealed wide variations in locus and size after lesions made by various techniques. There was, for example, an average of 18% extrahippocampal damage (to the parahippocampal cortex) in the monkeys trained by Zola et al. (2000), who claimed a specific hippocampus lesion-induced deficit in DNMS; but there was only 4% extrahippocampal damage in a study by Murray and Mishkin (1998), who claimed the opposite. To be fair, despite incursion into this neighboring brain area, there was no evidence of any within-group correlation between performance and the extent of parahippocampal damage in the Zola et al. (2000) study (damage ranged from 0% to 46%). Not much comfort should be drawn from this, however, as the study did not report any correlation between the extent of hippocampal damage and the recognition performance (ranging from 13% to 76% across all 14 animals tested). In contrast, Murray and Mishkin's findings indicated, paradoxically, a positive correlation between the extent of hippocampal damage and performance at the longer delays: the *greater* the hippocampal damage, the *better* the recognition performance.

Baxter and Murray (2001b) took this curious inverse relation further with a meta-analysis of these three studies of DNMTS in monkeys with restricted hippocampal lesions.

Using an optimum d′ statistic (which takes into account differences in the performance of control monkeys across studies), their analysis revealed an inverse correlation between the loss in d′ and percent damage to the hippocampus (Fig. 13–9). Zola and Squire (2001) argued that this meta-analysis was invalid because it failed to partial out the potential influence of various factors that differed across studies, other than lesion size, such as whether pretraining had been given, the way the lesions were made, and the delays used to assess memory—a caution that ironically did not prevent Zola himself from generating a z-score statistic to characterize a wide range of tasks (as in Fig. 13–7, p. 600). Baxter and Murray (2001a) conceded the weakness of pooling data across studies that used slightly different training protocols but asserted that even when factors relating to lack of task identity are partialed out a nonparametric analysis of the inverse relation between loss of d′ and lesion size remains significant. As in Ringo's earlier analysis of delay dependence, the use of a d′ statistic was helpful, though by no means critical, as the same result pertains when raw percent correct difference scores are used (M.G. Baxter, personal communication). Moreover, each of the pooled studies secured a trend or significant inverse relation on their own.

Baxter and Murray's meta-analysis is an empirical observation, not an explanation about why there might be an inverse correlation. One possibility is that residual hippocampal tissue adjacent to the lesion produces aberrant neural activity that disrupts neighboring brain regions. There is, however, another possible reason for this paradoxical correlation that deserves careful discussion. Once again, like the debate about concurrent object discrimination learning (above), it is the old problem of task ambiguity. We saw earlier that DNMTS is amenable to two distinct strategies: a "familiarity" strategy and a "recollection" strategy. If recollection is either exclusively or

Figure 13–9. Meta-analysis of DNMTS. Systematic comparison of data from several laboratories reveal the paradoxical inverse relation between DNMTS performance and hippocampal lesion size (Baxter and Murray 2001). The various symbols represent data from different studies: squares, Murray and Mishkin (1998); triangles, Beason-Held et al. (1999); circles, Zola et al. (2000).

Paradoxical relationship between DNMTS and lesion size

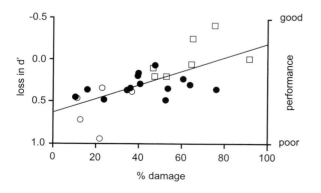

most effectively mediated by the hippocampus, animals with large hippocampal lesions would most likely use a familiarity strategy and so rely on their intact perirhinal cortex to make judgments of prior occurrence using the neuronal ensembles identified in the pioneering work of Brown and colleagues (Brown et al., 1987; Brown, 1996). Conversely, if recollection remains feasible and is ordinarily preferred, animals with small hippocampal lesions may automatically continue to use their damaged hippocampus, attempt a recollection method of solving the problem, but perform less well than control animals precisely because this structure is damaged. A negative correlation between performance and size of lesion would then emerge. It is not unreasonable to suppose that extensive pretraining may also predispose animals to use a less effortful familiarity strategy preferentially, thereby accounting, at least in part, for the persistent failure to see restricted hippocampal lesion effects on DNMTS in the NIH laboratory but their presence in the San Diego laboratory (that generally did not use preoperative training). The situation is laden with irony, as Squire and colleagues have been uncertain of any simple mapping of the recollection/familiarity distinction onto structures in the MTL (Squire et al., 2004) (a view endorsed by Stark in Chapter 12), yet it could be precisely because the unoperated monkeys in San Diego used recollection to perform DNMTS that hippocampal deficits were seen.

The available data suggests that the VPC test may be a more hippocampally sensitive test of recognition memory than DNMTS (Zola et al., 2000; Bachevalier et al., 2002; Nemanic et al., 2004). Unfortunately, we do not yet have a principled understanding of why. Manns et al. (2000b) have shown in humans that performance on VPC is predictive of subsequent recognition memory performance in a standard two-alternative forced-choice test, whereas performance in perceptual priming (a measure of perceptual fluency) is unrelated to recognition performance. This is helpful because it suggests that, in humans, VPC really is in the declarative domain. Subjects do have some "awareness" of having seen one of two stimuli before. However, this analytical study does not directly address the familiarity versus recollection issue. The problem we face is that monkeys may be using explicit recollection to direct their gaze, or they may be using stimulus familiarity (or perhaps both). If VPC is a pure "familiarity" task uncontaminated by recollection, it is unlikely to prove to be of continuing value for understanding the role of the primate hippocampus in more complex aspects of event memory in which recollection is definitively engaged (e.g., cued recall in which one stimulus brings to mind another with which it has been associated). Bachevalier suspected that it entails little more than familiarity but went on to suggest that its greater sensitivity may reflect the greater role that novelty plays with respect to all the stimuli in the task.

In VPC, animals are passively exploring two-dimensional back/white novel stimuli, not actually memorizing the sample to select a future response (i.e., incidental learning). It is presumably more ecological for monkeys (and humans) passively witnessing a new event to keep a trace (however weak it is) of the whole event, because anything can later prove to be behaviorally relevant (i.e., the stimulus, its elements, and its spatial and temporal contexts). This incidental encoding could favor the formation of conjunctive representations not only of the different elements of the sample but also of its location and contexts. (Nemanic et al., 2004, p. 2025)

We come back to this thoughtful comment in Sections 13.5 and 13.6, where the argument is presented that *incidental* encoding of stimuli does not necessarily commit an animal to being able to make only familiarity judgments about them and that the formation of conjunctive representations, even if encoded automatically, is an essential building block of recollection. Whatever the psychological basis of the VPC task, proponents of declarative memory theory do, nonetheless, like it. However, there is a lurking suspicion of circularity in this attraction; unlike DNMS, the task is reliably impaired by hippocampal lesions at reasonably short memory delays.

Again, what is needed is an information-processing analysis of specific tasks that is independent of any tests of their sensitivity to brain damage. DNMTS and VPC both suffer from the problem that there are at least two ways in which a monkey might perform the test. We need either new, less ambiguous tests of memory or new behavioral assays to establish when an animal is performing these ambiguous tasks one way or the other. Assuming that these could be developed, we could then return to the main task of mapping the cognitive process onto underlying brain systems and networks. Given that stimulus familiarity suffices to solve the DNMTS task, instances where excitotoxic hippocampal lesions have no effect (Murray and Mishkin, 1998) may be because the task has been set up to encourage no more than a judgment of familiarity (extensive pretraining?). By the same token, instances where a deficit is seen (Zola et al., 2000) may occur because the control animals enjoy the benefit, at least on some trials, of explicit recollection. In such cases, the hippocampus may provide the processing necessary for remembering the object or its image on a computer screen in its spatiotemporal context.

If this analysis is correct, a novel prediction is that context-specific recognition memory is impaired by discrete hippocampus damage in monkeys. A possible experiment might be one in which the monkey would be shown object A once in context 1 and a short while later object B in context 2. After a memory delay, it would then be presented with different types of recognition judgment. Numerous novel objects would be used across of a series of trial triads. Some tests would require no more than an *absolute* familiarity judgment: Has either of the two objects been presented before? Others would involve making a *context-specific* judgment: Can the monkey indicate that object B in context 1 (or A in context 2) is a novel condition? On the analysis just presented, discrete hippocampal lesions might affect context-specific recognition memory but

not judgments of absolute familiarity. However, such a task might only work in "incidental" mode. Deliberate training with multiple objects in the different contexts, or objects over multiple trials, may engage conditioning processes that utilize configural cues mediated by neocortical circuitry (see Section 13.5). However, if this or another appropriate protocol could be developed, disagreement about whether the hippocampus is or is not involved in "recognition" might then move forward toward discussion about qualitatively different types of recognition memory. Such experiments would start the process of fractionating "declarative" into different kinds of propositional knowledge, just as the "visual system" has been fractionated into different streams of processing. Precisely such context-specific recognition experiments are already underway using rodents (Dix and Aggleton, 1999; Eacott and Norman, 2004). In primates, context-specific discrimination tasks have been explored (Dore et al., 1998), showing deficits after neurotoxic hippocampal lesions but not yet recognition memory.

The era of primate lesion experiments on recognition memory using DNMTS has probably drawn to a close. This is partly because of the ambiguities discussed above but also because the individuals particularly interested in these issues have moved on and a new generation of primate researchers is tackling other issues. Some primate lesion experiments are underway using new tasks, and others are focusing on single-unit and multiple single-unit recording during memory tasks (Suzuki and Eichenbaum, 2000; Squire et al., 2004). One common feature of these experiments is abandoning the notion that recognition and association are likely to be fundamentally different; both may be associative processes. Buckmaster et al. (2004) have developed tests of paired-associate learning that are more sophisticated than merely pairing an object with a reward. The animal must learn that object A goes with object B. Tests of transitive inference and delayed spatial recall are also being added to the arsenal of tests with which the multiple types of memory in the primate brain will eventually be uncovered. Similarly, Suzuki and her colleagues have examined the hippocampal single-unit correlates of paired-associate learning in monkeys, for new pairs and for well-established pairs (Wirth et al., 2003; Yanike et al., 2004). We consider the application of new behavioral tests of declarative memory later in our discussion of relational-processing theory (see Section 13.5).

13.3.5 Remote Memory, Retrograde Amnesia, and the Time Course of Memory Consolidation in Primates

Given the uncertainties of testing remote memory in humans (see Chapter 12), there has been interest in examining retrograde amnesia in animals. The value of doing this is that studies can be done *prospectively*. The training experience of laboratory animals can be accurately controlled, with no ambiguity about precisely what events—and when or where—have occurred prior to a lesion. The experimenter knows and does not have to rely on the uncertain testimony of relatives. There are, however, looming difficulties in the use of animals for such studies, one being the critical episodic/semantic distinction.

Zola-Morgan and Squire (1990) sought evidence for gradual memory consolidation by first teaching monkeys a series of 100 object discrimination problems. They were divided into five sets of 20 problems scheduled at intervals of 2, 4, 8, 12, and 16 weeks prior to creating aspiration lesions in the animals' hippocampus and surrounding parahippocampal cortex. Two weeks later they were retested on each of the 100 problems by presenting pairs of discriminanda just once (to examine retention uncontaminated by new learning). The lesioned monkeys were impaired relative to controls on the problems learned shortly before surgery, but the two groups performed at a comparable, above-chance level for problems learned 12 or 16 weeks earlier (Fig. 13–10).

As just described, the results do not necessarily require reference to a concept such as memory consolidation – they could reflect no more than damage to a storage site and differential rates of forgetting in control and lesioned animals (Fig. 13–10, pattern in panel B1). Of greater significance are the within-subject comparisons. The controls did best on the most recent problems and worst on the problems learned initially, a pattern that reflects gradual forgetting over time. In contrast, the lesioned monkeys did not fail at both training-lesion intervals (Fig. 13–10, data pattern in panel B2), but actually did *worse* on problems learned 2 weeks before surgery than those learned 12 weeks earlier (Fig. 13–10, the true pattern, in panel B3). This dual pattern of performance—*forgetting* in controls but gradual *improvement* in the lesion group—is critical to the interpretation of the data. It strongly

suggests that a memory consolidation process must have been taking place in normal animals that was interrupted by the hippocampal/parahippocampal lesion.

Other primate studies failed to obtain positive evidence for consolidation (Dean and Weiskrantz, 1974; Salmon et al., 1987; Gaffan, 1993), but there are several reasons why no temporal gradient may have been observed. Inferotemporal lesions, as studied by Dean and Weiskrantz, could have damaged the actual site of memory storage in the neocortex, making it impossible to see the effect on remote memory of any putative process of consolidation orchestrated by the MTL. The study by Salmon et al. (1987), also using large MTL lesions, showed little forgetting in control animals and very poor performance in the lesioned animals—concerns about ceiling and floor effects that led directly to the design of the later experiment with more restricted lesions. Gaffan (1993) examined picture memory with various retention intervals prior to the administration of fornix lesions, but it had several curious features: First, a different number of pictures were presented in the set just before surgery than at the earlier time point; and second, a retention test was given just before surgery that could have reminded the animals of the pictures and so altered the extent to which they can be considered as exclusively belonging to the "recent" or "remote" set. Indeed, demonstrable improvement in the performance of the control group between the two retention tests strongly suggested that reminding altered the effective "age" of the memories. Although this weakens the force of Gaffan's study, the possibility that recall can induce "re-storage" of information and so alter trace strength should not to be ignored.

The study by Zola-Morgan and Squire (1990) is therefore widely considered the definitive study of gradual time-

Figure 13–10. Retrograde amnesia and declarative memory theory. *A.* Average performance during a single postsurgery probe trial for each of 100 object discrimination problems learned earlier. The data are plotted as a function of the time interval between training and the subsequent lesion. Problems learned 12 weeks before surgery are remembered better than those only 2 weeks beforehand. (*Source:* Zola-Morgan and Squire, 1990.) *B.* Data to be expected on various models of how lesions might affect storage sites or memory consolidation. *B1.* The lesion causes partial disruption of the site of storage.

Performance by the lesion group is always poorer than that of controls, although they may display a shallower gradient of forgetting. *B2.* The lesion causes disruption of retrieval. Performance is poor at all time intervals. *B3.* The lesion causes selective disruption of long-term consolidation. Performance shows an inverted-U shape, being better for problems when there has been time for consolidation prior to the lesion but, like normal controls, also forgetting over time. The exact form of the memory gradients is critical to the interpretation.

A Memory for object discriminations

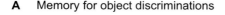
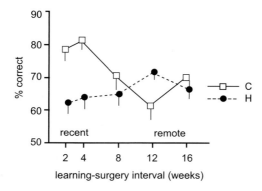

B Theoretical models

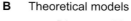
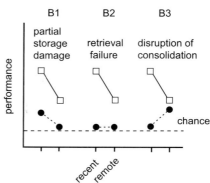

dependent memory consolidation in primates, although there are aspects of the results that are troubling. The use of lesions encompassing both the hippocampus and the parahippocampal cortex raises the question of whether damage restricted to the hippocampus would cause a retrograde effect. This is important given the lack of much retrograde amnesia in patients R.B. and G.D. (see Chapter 12). A study using monkeys in whom ischemic and/or neurotoxic lesions were created could offer a more exact model of the etiology and damage in these patients. To our knowledge, this has not been done. The use of a within-subjects design is a strength (with respect to mimicking the human syndrome and allowing modest use of animals), but it raises the question of whether the repeated act of "reminding" the animal of the testing situation preoperatively could influence the memory strength of earlier trained items. Putting a monkey back into the WGTA apparatus to learn a new set of problems 4 weeks after it has learned an earlier set could re-activate memory representations of the first trained problems even though the specific stimulus items are not presented again. This could happen because the training context may be sufficient to activate hippocampus-specific "pointers." Put simply, being in a place you have been in previously reminds you of things that happened there and may make these remembered events more memorable in the future, a process that is more akin to a cyclical "reactivation and re-storage" process than an inexorable time-dependent consolidation process. Insofar as this did happen in the within-subjects design, it would particularly affect the problems learned earliest before surgery—the very ones remembered best by the lesioned animals (a different problem from that in the Gaffan study where reminding occurred just before surgery). This argument would be more convincing had there been an improvement in memory for these same "early" problems in the control group, but the controls exhibited forgetting over time. here is also the further possibility of all animals developing a "learning-set" over the succession of discrimination problems (Murray and Bussey, 2001). What is needed to settle this issue is a systematic comparison of training conditions that involve repeated reexposure to the context and of training conditions that do not. Such a study is now most unlikely to be conducted in primates, but fortunately this issue has been followed up using rodents.

Studies of retrograde amnesia in nonprimate species have been conducted using social transmission of food preferences, cue and context fear conditioning, trace-eyeblink conditioning, spatial learning, and object discrimination learning tasks (e.g., Winocur, 1990; Kim and Fanselow, 1992; Bolhuis et al., 1994; Anagnostaras et al., 1999; see Squire et al., 2001 for review). Some studies suffer from "ceiling" or "floor" effects in the data (i.e., performance being so good or so bad across a range of intervals that not all studies have both a forgetting and a consolidation gradient). However, the general pattern is of temporal gradients of retrograde amnesia consistent with a gradual process of memory consolidation, with the sole exception being certain spatial tasks that are discussed in detail later (see Section 13.4). Data showing gradual time-

dependent changes in 2-deoxyglucose utilization in the hippocampus after learning are also consistent with the idea that increases in hippocampal activity occur for a limited period time after learning (Bontempi et al., 1999; Frankland et al., 2004; Maviel et al., 2004b). These changes may constitute a physiological and molecular signature of consolidation.

There are numerous outstanding issues concerning memory consolidation as envisaged within the declarative memory theory. A key issue is what determines whether new memories are consolidated or allowed to fade. Most event memories that humans make automatically during a typical day are lost; some passive or active selection process must come into play that determines what is retained or discarded (Morris et al., 2003). Second, once set in motion, is consolidation a gradual, inexorable, largely time-dependent process? Or is it a more "quantal" process in which short consolidation episodes occur repeatedly over a longer period of time, perhaps triggered by contextual retrieval (Dudai and Morris, 2001)? Both gradual and quantal ways of thinking about consolidation could result in gradual temporal functions of retrograde amnesia when average data are considered, but the underlying mechanism by which individual traces are strengthened might be very different. Third, how does consolidated information become integrated or interleaved with information already stored in the neocortex (McClelland et al., 1995)? Fourth, should a distinction be made between "consolidation" and "semanticization"? The former would allow the persistent memory of discrete events and enable the "recovered consciousness" and mental time travel characteristic of episodic memory (Moscovitch, 1995). The latter would involve an interleaving process through which the regularities that emerge from successive similar episodes are abstracted and so be able to add to the subject's semantic knowledge. The later recall of such information need not entail access to spatiotemporal tags (Winocur et al., 2005). Fifth, is there just one type of memory consolidation, or is there a family of distinct processes? Some have argued for a distinction between "cellular" consolidation that putatively operates rapidly within single neurons in a single brain area, and "systems-level" consolidation involving the interaction of different brain areas (Dudai and Morris, 2001). Finally, what are the indices or pointers, what do they index or point at, and how is neuronal and synaptic specificity in neocortex realized by the signals emanating from hippocampus? These and related issues constitute an important next step in the development of declarative memory theory.

13.3.6 Critique

The declarative memory theory of hippocampal function has been immensely influential and remains the most cited theory of memory in neuroscience textbooks (Kandel et al., 2000; Bear et al., 2001). Yet, although simplicity is desirable, one should always remember Einstein's dictum that scientists should "keep things as simple as possible, but no simpler." Several critics empathize with this view, two describing the theory bluntly as follows: "It is attractive, it is parsimonious, it is extraordinarily popular, and it is wrong" (Murray and Wise, 2004, p. 194). Others, notably Gaffan (2002), go further in opposing the whole concept of memory systems, particularly that of a unitary declarative memory system encapsulated entirely within the MTL. Whether these and other critiques are well founded or merely idiosyncratic is a matter of opinion.

What is clear is that several problems with declarative memory theory are now widely recognized. They range from empirical issues to do with how well the data really do fit the theory, many of which have already been discussed, to conceptual issues such as the status of the taxonomy of memory systems, the role of conscious awareness in the encoding and retrieval of declarative information in humans and animals, and problems surrounding the concept and time scale of systems-level memory consolidation.

What Is the Status of the Memory Taxonomy?

The taxonomy depicted in Figure 13–3 is easy to grasp and easy to remember. It is a joy to teach, and many a lecture in research seminars begins with this diagram—but what does it really mean? Is it meant to be an accurate depiction of evolutionary or logical distinctions between different forms of learning and their mapping onto specific structures in the human brain? Or is it actually no more than an *aide memoire*?

Taking issue with the taxonomy may seem no more than a semantic side show; but if the taxonomy is conceptually confused, it is important to reflect on this. The term "taxonomy" is used in evolutionary biology to denote "relatedness," such as between species, orders, and groups. Clearly, the use of the term here is not intended to imply that the evolution of memory proceeded first through some ancient differentiation between short-term and long-term memory and then on through all the binary divisions of the hierarchy. To the contrary, it is generally assumed that nondeclarative memory evolved earliest (Sherry and Schacter, 1987). The term "taxonomy" is being used in a different sense—one expressing ostensibly qualitative distinctions between types of memory. Nonetheless, some critics of declarative memory theory feel the need to move beyond mere taxonomy to more precise, noncircular statements of what is different (in information-processing terms) about the identified forms of memory depicted within the framework. Do the distinct nodes of the taxonomy have different "inputs" such that they operate on different types of information? Schacter and Tulving (1994), for example, argued for the flow of information into memory occurring in a serial, parallel, independent manner—the information passing first via perceptual representational systems, then through semantic memory, and on into episodic memory (Fig. 13–11). Activated subsets of semantic and episodic memory constitute the inputs to working memory, thereby creating a set of input-output relations between memory systems quite different from those envisaged in the declarative memory theory. Continuing in this vein, we may ask of the standard taxonomy (and of Schacter and Tulving's alternative), whether the memory systems in it use different learn-

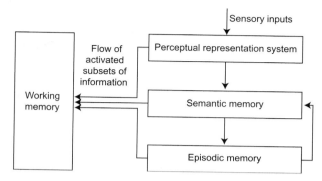

Tulvings's alternative SPI framework for propositional memory

Figure 13–11. Tulving's SPI model of propositional memory. An alternative framework for the flow of information into and between memory systems. Information flows into memory systems that operate in a serial, parallel, independent (SPI) manner (Schacter and Tulving, 1994). The flow is from a perceptual-representation system into semantic memory and then into episodic memory. Activated subsets of these systems interact with working memory (Baddeley, 2001).

ing rules. Do they encode, store, and retrieve information differently and so provide "outputs" different from those of the rest of the brain? Do their storage mechanisms express memory traces differently, with differing patterns of persistence or susceptibility to consolidation? Others are concerned that certain types of memory storage may start off in one way (e.g., declarative) but then become another (e.g., nondeclarative) through repetition in multiple contexts and/or the passage of time. That is, the ostensibly sharp boundaries of any memory taxonomy may neither be immutable nor adequately reflect dynamic changes in memory representation that occur during the course of learning. However, to be fair to the architects of declarative memory theory, these are in part issues for the future and precisely the sort of topics they have been attempting to address, notably in the many studies characterizing the nature of preserved learning in the presence of amnesia (Squire et al., 1993; Cavaco et al., 2004).

These computational- and algorithmic-level questions have to be addressed before we can proceed securely toward any mapping onto the neural substrate in which they are expressed—at the circuit, cellular, and even intracellular levels of analysis. As currently drawn, the taxonomy implies that types of learning and memory at the bottom of the hierarchy can be mapped onto specific brain areas, ranging from regions in the MTL to such structures as the striatum and cerebellum. Matters, however, are unlikely to be so simple. One controversial claim, made by Murray and Wise (2004), is that radically new concepts of the embryology and anatomical organization of major parts of the primate and rodent brain need to be taken on board by memory researchers, notably ideas most closely associated with those of Swanson (2000, 2004). One aspect of this is a shift away from thinking of brain functions as localized to discrete brain regions or to closely connected brain areas such as MTL, toward thinking in terms of "recurrent loops." It is too early to assess this idea securely. However, one lesson of the last decade of functional imaging research in humans is that distributed cerebral networks for memory involving "top-down" interactions between the medial temporal and frontal lobes need to be considered and analyzsed (Fletcher and Henson, 2001; Miyashita, 2004).

A last point about the taxonomy is the growing concern is that it does not readily capture the sense that the "seamless" control of behavior is almost certainly a matter of the coordinated regulation of numerous brain networks. When learning to drive a car for example, there is perceptual learning, motor control, knowledge of facts about road signs, and memory for previous similar traffic situations that one may have encountered. The taxonomy is suspiciously silent about how the outputs of the ostensibly independent forms of memory interact, compete, or are coordinated in the brain. Experimental work to date has been devoted largely to devising tasks that *dissociate* the psychological and anatomical components of memory processing rather than investigating how these entities compete or cooperate. As noted in Section 13.2, new developments in memory research are turning toward this more synthetic goal (Poldrack et al., 2001; White and McDonald, 2002). None of these comments and criticisms on their own definitively indicate that the standard memory taxonomy and its mapping onto brain areas is wrong, but they are grounds for caution.

Inconsistencies Between the Animal Lesion Data and the Declarative Memory Theory

Several lines of inquiry have turned up data that appear inconsistent with the declarative memory theory or, at best, are handled awkwardly. Much of this is considered later in relation to other theories of hippocampal function, notably spatial, configural, and episodic theories. Studies of the neural basis of recognition memory in rats and of other forms representational memory in primates have been conducted as explicit tests of the declarative theory and so are considered here.

Hardly unique in science, there is conflict about the data. Like the proverbial housewives living in medieval tenements who always bickered at each other across the narrow alleyways (they were always arguing from different "premises"), there is a persisting conflict about the way studies of recognition memory in rats are perceived. Mumby summarized the situation fairly as one in which "most investigators are looking outside the hippocampus" (Mumby, 2001, p. 159) to explain the neurobiological basis of recognition memory. In contrast, Squire et al. (2004) continued to defend the view that damage to the hippocampus does impair recognition memory at long memory delays.

A range of techniques have been developed to study recognition memory in rodents that complement the DNMTS and VPC paradigms for monkeys. There are several DNMTS protocols in which rats are explicitly trained to learn a matching or nonmatching rule and selectively rewarded on correct choice trials. They include a Y maze nonmatching goal-boxes procedure (Aggleton, 1985; Aggleton et al., 1986), tasks in

which rats traverse runways to displace goal objects that are either familiar or unfamiliar (Rothblat and Hayes, 1987; Mumby et al., 1990; Kesner et al., 1993), and even procedures for rats using images on computer screens (Gaffan and Eacott, 1995). A continuous delayed nonmatching paradigm, teasingly called cDNM, uses a "go/no-go" digging response for the recognition of odors (Otto and Eichenbaum, 1992). Spontaneous novel object recognition (NOR), analogous to the VPC protocol for primates, is an increasingly popular paradigm for recognition memory first developed by Ennaceur and Delacour (1988). After prior habituation to the context of testing, the animal is confronted by two objects that it investigates and explores, though never formally rewarded for doing so. The objects are generally identical in a sample phase but differ in the memory test phase. Trial-unique goal boxes, objects, or smells are used for rodent DNMS, cDNM, and NOR, with the relative probability of the choice or the extent of spontaneous investigation of the novel cue serving as the index of memory of prior occurrence. One issue of concern has been that not all of the rodent studies have routinely varied the memory delay within the protocol as has been the custom in the primate work; this is important, as use of only short memory delays can yield inappropriate conclusions (Clark and Martin, 2005). There are also subtle but important differences of protocol across ostensibly similar paradigms. For example, some studies of NOR require all subjects to accumulate some minimum period of object exploration during each trial (e.g., 30 seconds), these trials of necessity then being of indeterminate duration; others have a set trial duration but then average the normalized exploration scores across subjects. Clark et al. (2000) presented data that favor the former approach, and they thereby set new standards for these types of experiment in rats (a move by the San Diego group into rodent work that may have been prompted by a certain frustration about the way so many rodent experiments were being conducted). Mumby (2001) provided a perceptive discussion of many other differences between these and the primate tasks discussed earlier.

Most of the data reported on rats indicates that restricted hippocampal dysfunction (lesions of various kinds, fornix section, intrahippocampal drug infusions) has minimal effect on these tasks (see Table 1 in Mumby, 2001). In contrast, perirhinal and postrhinal cortex lesions, including reversible inactivation using glutamatergic ligands and disruption of cholinergic neuromodulation, cause clear deficits (Bussey et al., 1999; Warburton et al., 2003; Winters et al., 2004; Winters and Bussey, 2005). There are exceptions to this pattern, but when taken as a whole it is inconsistent with the prediction from declarative memory theory that damage *anywhere* within this group of MTL structures, including the hippocampus, should cause a proportionate deficit in recognition memory. Starting with a study by Aggleton et al. (1986) using novel and familiar goal-boxes in a Y maze, a series of analytical studies led by Rawlins resolved why hippocampal dysfunction impaired nonspatial working memory in a radial maze but appeared to have no reliable effect on DNMTS (Rawlins et al., 1993; Steele and Rawlins, 1993; Cassaday and Rawlins, 1995, 1997). It turned out that the size of the goal box is critical, with small compact goal boxes being treated by rats as discrete "objects," whereas larger boxes are treated as "spaces" and so engage spatial and relational encoding (see Sections 13.4 and 13.5). Hippocampal lesions only affect memory for large goal boxes. These findings have been complemented by concern that certain protocols for testing nonspatial recognition memory may have cryptic spatial or contextual components. For example, Nadel (1995) was the first to point out that the deficit in DNMTS at long memory delays in certain primate studies was confounded by the monkeys being, for practical reasons, removed from and then later returned to the WGTA testing apparatus at the longer but not the shorter delays. Control but not hippocampus-lesioned monkeys might then benefit from contextual cues aiding recall.

However, cryptic spatial processing is unlikely to be an issue for a different DNMTS protocol developed by Mumby et al. (1992a). They trained rats with memory delays varying from 4 to 600 seconds with the sample and choice components at opposite ends of a runway during a trial but scheduled equally often at both ends across trials. Subsequent to surgery, no impairment was seen in rats with aspiration lesions of the hippocampus, or of hippocampus and the amygdala, at any delay except the longest (10 minutes) at which the hippocampal lesion groups then performed more poorly than controls. Although sometimes cited as support for the idea that hippocampal lesions can affect recognition memory in rats, there is a caveat here also. Specifically, the within-subject comparisons showed that the control group got paradoxically *better* at the 10-minute delay rather than the lesion group getting worse. This improvement by controls was not seen in several later studies, and thus Mumby's (2001) reasonable conclusion was that this single statistical difference was the exception to the rule that hippocampal lesions have minimal if any effect on rodent DNMTS. However, using a large test battery in the manner of Zola-Morgan and Squire (1985), Mumby et al. (1995) again found a small but significant hippocampal lesion deficit in DNMTS at the longest delay tested (120 seconds) relative to both no surgery and partial parietal cortex lesion control groups. Clark et al. (2001) later also secured a deficit in rats with excitotoxic hippocampal lesions at the longest delay tested (also 120 seconds). Thus, another equally reasonable way of summarizing the data is that when hippocampal lesion-associated deficits have been seen they have tended to be at long memory delays or with long list lengths (Mumby et al., 1992b; Steele and Rawlins, 1993; Mumby et al., 1995; Wiig and Bilkey, 1995; Clark et al., 2001). This would be consistent with the declarative memory theory were it not for the much greater sensitivity of these tasks to perirhinal lesions of comparable or even smaller size. Either the hippocampus is at the "apex" of declarative memory processing or it is not.

What might be the key difference between studies that find a deficit after hippocampal lesions (Clark et al., 2000; Broadbent et al., 2004) and those that do not (Ennaceur and Aggleton, 1994; Winters et al., 2004; Forwood et al., 2005)? Lesion size or, more generally, the degree of hippocampal dysfunction is one possibility. For example, Ennaceur and Aggleton (1994) found no effect of fornix lesions on NOR at delays varying from 1 to 15 minutes but dropping to chance levels over 4 hours. Other studies using fornix lesions reported similar results, but it should be remembered that fornix lesions in monkeys have little impact on DNMTS and may leave many aspects of MTL function intact. Perirhinal lesions have consistently been observed to impair NOR (Bussey et al., 1999; Murray and Bussey, 1999). Consistent with these findings but drawing a very different conclusion, Clark et al. (2000) conducted a comprehensive study of NOR using groups of rats subjected to sham surgery, fornix lesioning, or radiofrequency and excitotoxic hippocampal lesioning. Importantly, they required the absolute accumulation of 30 seconds of total object exploration time by all subjects. Fornix-lesioned subjects did not show a deficit, consistent with earlier findings. However, rats with either type of hippocampal lesion showed impairments at a 1-hour memory delay. In a follow-up study by Broadbent et al. (2004), a deficit in NOR was observed as a function of hippocampal lesion size. Small lesions caused no impairment, whereas larger lesions did. Given the parallel, distributed nature of hippocampal processing (see Chapter 14), it is reasonable to suppose that many functions of the MTL that require hippocampal processing could continue relatively normally after partial lesions.

Finally, turning back to primates, Murray and Wise's (2004) critique of the declarative memory theory offers several other examples of instances where the two sides in the debate draw different conclusions from a common set of data. One example has to do with whether the perirhinal cortex has only memory functions (Buffalo et al., 1998a; Teng et al., 2000) or also participates in aspects of perceptual processing. For example, Teng et al. (2000) reported that rapid learning of a discrimination between simple three-dimensional objects (e.g., a red versus a green peanut shell) is only slightly impaired by hippocampal lesions, notably over the first few trials of the day (which were described as more "declarative" in nature), whereas the much slower learning of two-dimensional pattern discrimination (e.g., N versus W) is unaffected by hippocampal lesions unless they extend to include damage to the tail of the caudate nucleus. In contrast, Bussey et al. (2002) reported that discrimination of compound visual stimuli with the ambiguity between the features maximized is strikingly impaired by perirhinal lesions, whereas the discrimination of those with minimal common features is unaffected. A follow-up study by Bussey et al. (2003) used morphed images to produce a single-pair discrimination task in which the two stimuli to be discriminated had either very high or very low feature ambiguity (Fig. 13–12). The results show a clear perirhinal deficit on the slowly learned, maximal feature ambiguity task. These findings are problematic for the declarative memory theory for two reasons. First, the theory asserts that the MTL receives

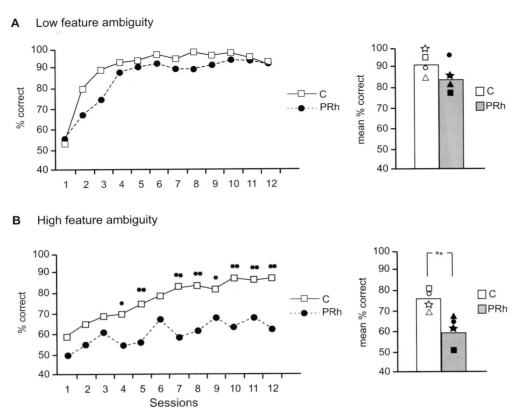

Figure 13–12. Perirhinal cortex and perception. Lesions of the perirhinal cortex, ostensibly part of a medial temporal lobe memory system, cause a deficit in the perceptual discrimination of stimuli with high-feature ambiguity (*B*) but not low-feature ambiguity (*A*). The symbols in the bar graphs on the right indicate scores of individual monkeys. (*Source*: After Bussey et al., 2003.)

perceptually processed visual inputs from the inferotemporal cortex and is not itself involved in making perceptual discriminations. Second, it asserts that rapidly learned visual discrimination tasks, other things being equal, are most likely to be learned in a declarative manner whereas slowly learned discriminations are acquired in a habit-like way, as in the Teng et al. (2000) study. Yet here it is the *slowly* learned discrimination that is most sensitive to lesions of the perirhinal cortex. Indeed, a body of data from rats, monkeys, and humans as well as relevant computational modeling support the notion that the perirhinal cortex has a role in object perception (Murray et al., 2005). Data from amnesic patients with restricted hippocampal damage or damage extending into neocortical structures of the MTL (identified radiographically) indicate that the discrimination of faces and scenes of ever greater similarity can pose a particular challenge for patients (Lee et al., 2005).

Certain Comparative Problems When Asserting that Declarative Memory Must Be Conscious

The insistence on MTL structures mediating memory that can be consciously declared is clearly problematic for a theory that seeks to encompass both humans and animals. In numerous laboratory tasks, animals have been shown to remember things that people would describe as facts (e.g., that a certain food is safe to eat) and that they can remember events (e.g., that an initially novel object has been seen before). However, will we ever know whether an animal is conscious of its memories? Moreover, even if we did, how could an animal ever "consciously declare" that it knows or remembers something from the past? Does it have a sense of its own life in the way that humans do—of the state of mental awareness that Tulving (1983) called "autonoetic consciousness"? If the answers to these questions are negative, one is tempted to wonder whether a central feature of the theory lies more in the realm of metaphysics than in empirical science. In fact, a comprehensive theory of brain and mind should identify under what circumstances animals and humans are conscious, what they are conscious of, and perhaps why consciousness is advantageous for some but not other forms of memory (Zeman, 2002).

This issue is usually finessed in what was referred to earlier as the "folk psychology" approach to consciousness that the declarative memory theory has taken to date. Nonetheless, in the context of work on "blindsight," animal experiments are making inroads into the issue of mental awareness. For example, Cowey and Stoerig (1995) devised an ingenious procedure in which monkeys that had been trained to reach accurately toward one of several targets were also required to "report" whether they were visually aware of the targets. Monkeys were placed in front of a touch screen. Each trial began with them looking at a fixation point and ended with their reaching out to touch various images presented a little while later in the left or right visual field. Operated monkeys (with large unilateral striate cortex lesions) were observed to reach as accurately in their blind hemifield as normal monkeys (Fig. 13–13A). The "reporting" of awareness was achieved in a separate training condition in which the monkeys had to touch a specific area of the screen if a target failed to occur at a time when they might have expected to see one (the possibility of a target was indicated by an auditory cue). The lesioned monkeys *correctly* reported that they could not see a target when targets were deliberately not presented on selected trials to their intact hemifield, but the monkeys *incorrectly* reported not seeing targets that were actually presented to their blind hemifield (Fig. 13–13B). These "unseen" targets were the very ones to which, in the first training condition, the animals had reached accurately. To all intents and purposes, these monkeys lack "phenomenal" vision; that is, they lacked the ability to "comment on" seeing things to which they could reach accurately (Weiskrantz, 1997).

Analogous procedures might be developed for studies of memory in primates, the point being to devise a way of dissociating between the successful performance of a memory task and the quite separate display of awareness that one is (or is not) remembering. In an important step, Hampton (2001) exploited techniques developed in parallel for pigeons (Sole et al., 2003) to examine whether rhesus monkeys know when they remember. Using computer-controlled techniques, each of two monkeys was briefly shown an image on a touchscreen (Fig. 13–14). The image then disappeared for a delay interval during which the animals may have sometimes remembered it and other times forgotten it. They were later tested for their memory of the image. What made this experiment different from conventional delayed match-to-sample testing was that the monkeys were allowed, for two-thirds of the trials, to choose between progressing to the memory test or declining to do it. Declining resulted in a guaranteed but less preferred reward than could be obtained by accepting to do the memory test and choosing correctly. For the remaining one-third of the trial sequences, the monkeys were not given a choice and were forced to take the memory test. The results showed that both monkeys performed more accurately on memory tests they had opted to take than on enforced tests. A control experiment included trial sequences that began without an image to remember during the delay interval; the monkeys routinely reacted to these sequences by declining to do the memory test when given the option to do so. Moreover, as the memory delay interval was extended (a procedure likely to promote forgetting), the monkeys showed a temporally graded reluctance to take the memory tests. Taken together, these results suggest that the monkeys' decision whether to take the memory test at the end of a trial sequence was likely to have been based on their own self-generated "awareness" of whether they could remember the image. This sort of procedure might be adapted to establish whether lesions of the hippocampal formation (or, better still, reversible inactivation) disrupt aware-

Figure 13–13. Blindsight in primates. Cowey and Stoerig's (1995) "commentary" procedure for studying visual awareness in primates. *A.* The animals watch the fixation spot (center) and then upon hearing a tone reach toward one of four peripherally located and briefly illuminated targets. Monkeys with striate cortex lesions can do this as well as control animals. *B.* The animals again watch the fixation spot and, upon hearing the auditory cue, reach for one of the five briefly illuminated lights on the left, the light on the right or, when no flash occurs, for the panel at the top left. Normal monkeys correctly identified all trial conditions. Monkeys with unilateral striate cortex lesions identified lights flashed in their good hemisphere but treated the right-hand illumination as if it had not occurred. Thus, monkeys display "blindsight" in being able to reach toward objects they "report" being unable to see. Can an analogous "reporting" procedure be developed in the domain of memory? (*Source:* Cowey and Stoerig, 1995).

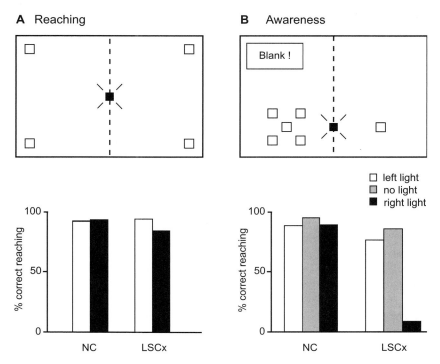

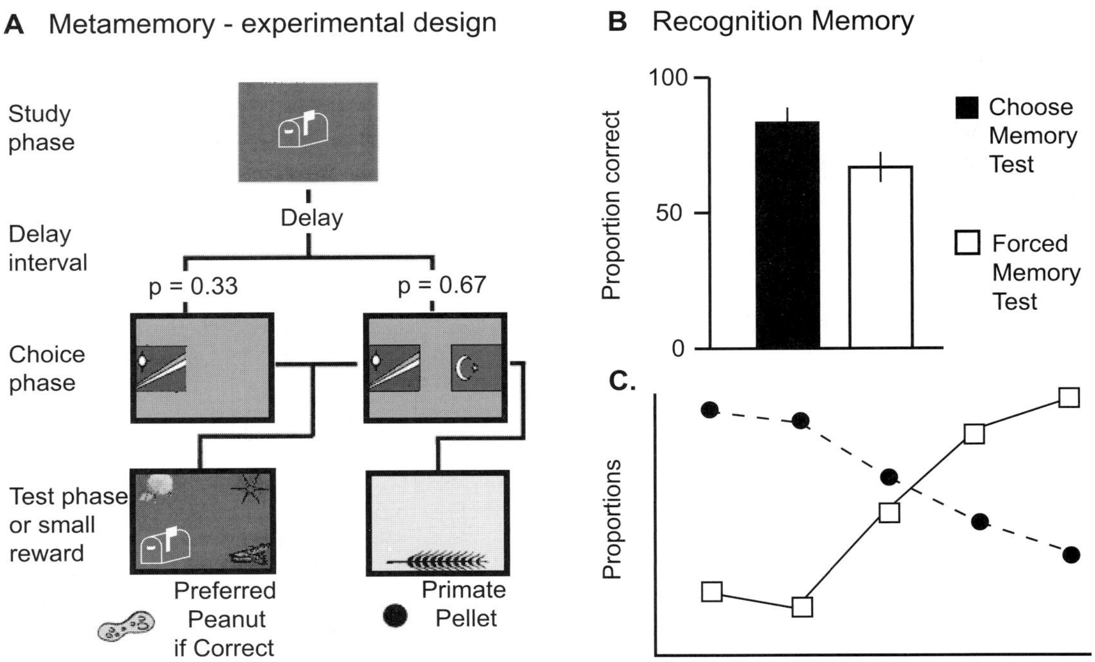

A Metamemory - experimental design

B Recognition Memory

Figure **13–14.** Metamemory. *A.* Monkeys were allowed, during two-thirds of the trials of a recognition test, to choose whether to take a memory test on the basis of their covert judgment of whether they could remember. *B.* Memory performance on trials when they chose to take the recognition test was significantly better than on the remaining one-third of trials for which they were forced to take the test. (*Source:* Cowey and Stoerig, 2001).

ness of memory to the same extent that they disrupt accurate performance. Might monkeys with hippocampal disruption show above-chance familiarity for a previously presented stimulus even though they "declare," in the optional choice test, that they would prefer not to take the test? Might they know but not remember? A human imaging study of this issue (Kao et al., 2005) suggests that such a task, even if it could be developed for monkeys, would be likely to involve an interaction between the MTL, mediating successful memory, and the ventrolateral prefrontal lobe, mediating memory awareness.

Nondeclarative Memory: Are Spared Learning Abilities Nonpropositional or Learned Tasks That Can Be Performed Without Awareness?

A critical claim of the theory is the independence of declarative and nondeclarative memory. The two key differences claimed by Squire (1992) for these superordinate categories of memory relate to the "propositional" status of the information being processed and the necessity of "awareness" during the encoding and recall of such information.

The existence of spared learning in the presence of amnesia has been the subject of comment for about a century (Claparede, 1911; Weiskrantz, 1997). It is a particularly intriguing feature of the syndrome to discuss with students or present to a public audience. How can it be that H.M. could learn to draw in a mirror yet not remember doing so? How could he and other patients have this curious disconnection in

their conscious awareness of the past? Anecdotes about spared "unconscious" memory function abound. Each new generation of neuropsychologists add their own; an excellent example is an endearingly personal article entitled "Memories of H.M." (Ogden and Corkin, 1991). Patient E.P.—one of the most profoundly amnesic patients to have been subject to detailed neuropsychological and neuroradiological examination in the San Diego neuropsychological studies—is another case in point.

> During the first 2 or 3 years in which we visited his house, he was wary and slow to accept the idea that we wished to talk with him and administer tests. After some conversation, and with encouragement from his wife, E.P. would after a number of minutes seat himself at a table for testing. During the subsequent years, the same tester has visited his house more than 150 times. Now when she arrives he greets her in a friendly manner and moves readily and promptly to the table even when his wife is not present. Yet, his pattern of greeting and acceptance occurs without any recognition of who the tester is, and he will repeatedly deny that he has seen her before. (Stefanacci et al., 2000, p. 731.)

The declarative memory theory, perhaps more than any other theory of memory, has put forward this disconnection of consciousness as a centerpiece. It makes the distinctive claim that such "nondeclarative" learning is not merely spared, as others had claimed previously, but that such learning occurs in amnesics at a normal rate and in a manner indistinguishable from that of controls. To emphasize this key point, it is not only that amnesic patients *can* display classic conditioning, as Warrington and Weizkrantz (1968) were the first to describe, it is that they do so at a *normal* rate despite a lack of awareness of the fact of learning (Gabrieli et al., 1995). However, because certain ostensibly "nondeclarative" tasks may be subject to contamination of learning using a declarative strategy, findings from patients with mild amnesia who have residual declarative memory can be misleading. The importance of drawing firm theoretical conclusions only from those rare individuals with severe amnesia was a theme of an early critique of the declarative memory theory (Weiskrantz, 1997) and, in a paradoxical twist, one now taken up by Squire et al. (2004) in their careful comparisons of performance by people and animals with partial versus complete damage to the MTL (e.g., patient R.B. versus patient E.P.).

Nondeclarative learning does not, of course, usually take place outside of consciousness. Learning to ride a bicycle, for example, is a motor skill for which most of us are acutely conscious of what we are doing as we attempt to learn. The declarative memory theory makes the radical claim, however, that although aware of the act of learning this awareness does not play any *causal* role in the encoding or expression of learned motor acts. This is a rather interesting idea but one that is difficult to test rigorously. It cannot be tested by seeing what learning capacity remains while we are unconscious—not because we cannot then ride bicycles (though that too) but because the lack of "awareness" to which the theory makes reference is not a lack of consciousness as such but an absence of awareness *of* the information relevant for learning at the moment of motor recall.

This absence of the *referent* of awareness is highly specific in the nondeclarative domain. For word-stem completion priming, for example, people are asked to think of a word—any word—that begins with the stem given as a cue. Subjects are aware they are being tested, aware that the test involves words, and attentive to the task in hand. Amnesic subjects, however, are unaware that the words they come up with are often words they were shown earlier. What they fail to "declare" is not the words themselves, but that they have the phenomenological attribute of being words they remember having seen earlier. This simultaneous sense of being tested in the present and bringing to mind events from the past is what is meant by "mental time travel" (Schacter and Tulving, 1994; Tulving and Markowitsch, 1998), and it is an attribute of mind that amnesics lack (Weiskrantz, 1997).

In a similar vein, studies of incidental learning suggest that unilateral MTL lesions can disrupt memory for information to which a person's attention is not overtly directed until the point of recall. In a famous study, Smith and Milner (1981) gave subjects a series of small toys, one by one, asking them the likely price of the real thing (e.g., a car). Their attention at encoding was directed to the value of the toys. One by one, the toys were put down by the experimenter in various places on the table in front of the subjects, without the subject's attention being drawn to the matter of location. Later, without prior warning, the experimenters asked subjects to recall where the objects had been placed. The subjects were never asked to pay attention to and, in that sense, be attentively aware of the location of the objects until the retention test. That normal subjects could do this task suggests that they may *automatically* encode attributes of a stimulus to which their attention is not directed despite paying attention to other attributes of the stimulus, such as its value. In contrast, people with large right MTL lesions were impaired. In this case, the experimental manipulation of "awareness" occurred at the point of encoding, but manifestations of this differential awareness only came to light at the point of recall. We return to the issue of differentiating "automatic" and "intentional" encoding in Sections 13.5 and 13.6.

This discussion leads us to suggest that the nondeclarative nature of nondeclarative memory may be less to do with whether the skill being performed can ever be "declared" than with whether subjects are consciously unaware of the prior occurrence of the stimulus at the time of recall. The importance of awareness rather than propositional status is particularly well revealed in studies of eyeblink conditioning, an advantageous paradigm for the present purposes as it can be studied in both humans and animals. In this form of conditioning, an initially neutral stimulus such as a tone is presented for a few hundred milliseconds before a puff of air to the eye. Through repeated pairings of these two stimuli, the subject develops a conditioned response (CR) to the tone (the conditioned stimulus, or CS). Eyeblink conditioning has been extensively studied in humans and animals and is known to obey the basis principles of classic (i.e., Pavlovian) conditioning (see Section 13.5). Learning depends on the contiguity and contingency between the CS and the puff of air (the unconditioned stimulus, or US). It is a form of conditioning for which the cerebellum was found to be essential (Clark et al., 1984). Following the observation that amnesics could acquire classic conditioning (Warrington and Weizkrantz, 1968) and that it occurs at a normal rate (Gabrieli et al., 1995), it had been widely assumed that this is not a form of learning in which the MTL is ever engaged. This turns out to be not quite right.

Two frequently studied forms of human eyeblink conditioning are named (somewhat inappropriately) the "delay" paradigm (in which, confusingly, the US follows the CS with no delay between the end of the CS and the onset of the US); the "trace" paradigm in which CS offset occurs 300 to 1000 ms prior to US onset (Fig. 13–15). As the CS and US are not contiguous in time, Pavlov suggested (and others since) that some "trace" of the CS must linger in memory if an association is to be formed with the US to allow effective conditioning (hence the name). Although no deficit is seen in amnesics using the delay paradigm, McGlinchey-Berroth et al. (1997) have shown that such patients have impaired trace eyeblink conditioning across a range of trace intervals. The contrast between these two protocols is instructive as what subjects learn to do in each case—to make automatic, appropriately timed CRs—can hardly be said to be nonpropositional in the former case but

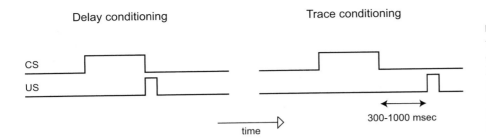

Figure 13–15. Protocols for delay and trace conditioning. Time lines showing the onset and offset of the conditional stimulus (CS) and unconditional stimulus (US) in two distinct forms of classic conditioning. Appropriately timed CRs develop in both protocols, yet only one is thought to be hippocampus-dependent.

propositional in the latter. It is therefore an important test for the theory to identify what might be "declarative" about trace conditioning.

Clark and Squire (1998) used a differential trace conditioning paradigm in which the CS+ (a tone) was followed by the air-puff US, whereas a second stimulus, the CS- (a noise), was presented on its own. Sessions consisted of multiple presentations of each stimulus to human subjects, some of whom were subject to a delay paradigm and others to a trace paradigm. All were required to watch, attend to, and try to remember a silent movie (Charlie Chaplin's "The Gold Rush") while these CS and US events were happening, thereby commanding a great deal of their conscious awareness. At the end of the experiment, in addition to being quizzed about the movie, the subjects were asked a set of questions with true/false answers designed to explore their awareness of the stimulus contingencies. The key finding was that successful trace conditioning was correlated with levels of awareness of these contingencies. A subset of control subjects who showed good awareness of the CS predicting the US after the trace delay conditioned well. Other control subjects, and all amnesic subjects tested, were less aware or even unaware of the stimulus contingencies—they conditioned poorly. Awareness was unrelated to levels of conditioning in the delay paradigm, a result that is not universally obtained (e.g., Knuttinen et al., 2001). Furthermore, to explore whether the correlation between level of awareness and degree of trace conditioning was causal, Clark and Squire (1998) manipulated awareness directly. Manipulations that facilitated awareness facilitated eyeblink conditioning; manipulations that reduced it blocked conditioning. A subsequent critique (LaBar and Disterhof, 1998) queried Clark and Squire's use of a differential conditioning protocol somewhat different from those used in many previous studies of human eyeblink conditioning; they also wondered whether a better "online" measure of awareness than a postexperimental questionnaire might be developed. Manns et al. (2000a) provided both in a study of normal subjects who showed a close predictive relation between developing awareness of the CS-US trace contingency and subsequent levels of conditioning. These investigators also showed that the critical feature of this awareness is the subject's awareness of the CS-US contingency rather than their awareness of the likelihood of blinking. Thus, it appears that what is "declarative" about trace conditioning is an awareness of the fact that the tone predicts that an air-puff will come shortly—an awareness that can be expressed propositionally. This awareness may arise

through some interaction between hippocampus and neocortex during the course of conditioning and is somehow fostered by using the trace conditoning paradigm. By virtue of this, a suitably timed signal can be sent to the cerebellum where the eyeblink response component of the conditioning takes place. The eyeblink CR, a learned but automatic defensive response, can then be executed at the appropriate time.

To summarize, what is nondeclarative about nondeclarative learning may actually be the lack of awareness of what is being remembered at the point of recall, rather than any intrinsic inflexibility in what has been learned or a lack of propositional status of the content of learning.

Are Fact-Memory and Event-Memory Processed by a Common Brain System?

Superficially, amnesics present with a deficit restricted to episodic memory. They cannot remember events for any length of time, but their factual knowledge about the world and their knowledge of language are both intact. Semantic memory shows all the appearances of being preserved. The declarative memory theory holds that this dissociation is profoundly deceptive. It asserts that there is a "unitary" process underlying the formation of both event and fact memories. The reason amnesic patients display intact semantic memory is because so much of a person's factual knowledge was acquired years earlier, extending from the years of childhood on through life. Consolidation of such memory traces would be long completed. Conversely, a patient's failure of event memory often relates to relatively recent events such as a forgotten conversation of the day before.

Although most amnesic subjects have some residual episodic memory function, a few are claimed to have little or none. In Chapter 12, we noted the striking case of patient E.P., who has essentially no measurable recent episodic memory but who, becoming amnesic when adult, displays good factual knowledge of the world acquired earlier in life and remarkably good memory for spatial and other episodic-like information acquired during childhood. However, if this interpretation is correct, people who have sustained damage to the MTL at a much younger age should also show impaired semantic memory. Data concerning the effects of bilateral hippocampal pathology sustained early in life are relevant to this issue (Vargha-Khadem et al., 1997). Three young developmental amnesics who sustained brain injuries at birth, 4 years, and 9 years of age, respectively, were aged 14, 19, and 22 at the time of first testing. The anoxic-ischemic episodes they had are likely to have affected the hippocampus preferentially. MRI measurements revealed hippocampal volumes ranging from 43% to 61% of normal. T2-weighted relaxometry measurements also revealed hippocampal abnormalities, but MR spectroscopy values were within the normal range. Additional MRI measurements in other brain areas suggested that bilateral hippocampal changes are not only the primary pathology but might be essentially the *only* pathology in all three cases (Mishkin et al., 1997).

The striking neuropsychological feature is that their amnesia is largely exclusive to episodic memory. They are temporally and spatially disoriented: forgetting the date and appointments, getting lost, mislaying their belongings. Despite severe problems of episodic memory, these children all attained levels of speech and language competence and of literacy and factual knowledge within the low average to average range. They all attended mainstream schools, and their acquisition of semantic information appears to be normal (or at least near-normal) as assessed by performance on the Wechsler Adult Intelligence Scale (WAIS) verbal intelligence tests. Their performance on a Basic Reading and Reading Comprehension subtest was normal in all three cases, as was their Spelling subtest (with the exception of one subject whose spelling is poor).

The pattern of memory preservation and memory loss shown by these children is in striking contrast to what would have been expected on the basis of the declarative memory theory. Vargha-Khadem and her colleagues argued that these three patients raise the possibility that the "basic sensory memory functions of the perirhinal and entorhinal cortices may be largely sufficient to support the formation of context-free semantic memories but not context-rich episodic memories, which must therefore require the additional processing provided by the hippocampal circuit" (Vargha-Khadem et al., 1997, p. 379). However, further research is required before such conclusions can be drawn with any certainty as later commentaries on these cases and parallel primate studies have recognized (Mishkin et al., 1998; Bachevalier and Vargha-Khadem, 2005). For one thing, the children appear to have *some* residual episodic memory, and this may have been sufficient for them to learn well in school, albeit more slowly than other children and perhaps only after frequent repetition. Moreover, although Vargha-Khadem and her colleagues interviewed the children's parents, they did not report on any discussions with the childrens' schoolteachers. It is difficult to believe that their teachers would have failed to notice their severe episodic memory difficulties and thus compensated for these problems with their teaching. The early damage to the brain may also have resulted in morphological reorganization of MTL structures in a way that does not occur when adults become amnesic. Certainly the MRI measurements do not all point to a completely destroyed hippocampus. Taken together, although fascinating cases, these concerns blunt the critical impact on declarative memory theory that they might otherwise have had.

Does it make sense to suppose that the memory of facts and events could depend on a single brain system? According to the theory, both types of information require the integrity of the hippocampal formation for their formation (encoding); and both result, after memory consolidation, in stable long-term traces in neocortex. Success in recalling either a fact or an event depends only on the "strength" of the traces established through consolidation. In contrast, Nadel and colleagues (Nadel and Moscovitch, 1997, 1998; Nadel et al., 2000) have argued that memory for an event requires access to a hippocampally based "contextual" trace (where the event happened) and a prefrontal "temporal" trace (when the event happened). Retrieval of event memory is a reconstruction based on both of these traces and other information about the event itself stored elsewhere in the neocortex. Retrieval of factual information, on the other hand, is not thought to require either a contextual or a temporal trace; it is context-independent.

In conclusion, we still do not understand the precise role of the hippocampus in episodic and semantic memory or, within the domain of episodic memory, in familiarity and recollection. The immediately preceding discussion, complementing Chapter 12, points to the need to develop new animal models of these forms of memory and of retrieval to help resolve the issues. We return to these important ideas in Section 13.6 after we have discussed the other major theories of the hippocampus: cognitive mapping and predictable ambiguity.

13.4 Hippocampus and Space: Cognitive Map Theory of Hippocampal Function

"Space," wrote O'Keefe and Nadel (1978, p. 5), "plays a role in all our behavior. We live in it, move through it, explore it, defend it . . . yet we find it extraordinarily difficult to come to grips with space." This strident rhetoric, together with discussion of the philosophical concept of space, introduced a book that outlined the then new "cognitive map" theory of hippocampal function. The theory has developed substantially over the past quarter century.

The primary stimulus for its development was the discovery of "place cells" in the hippocampus of freely moving rats (O'Keefe and Dostrovsky, 1971). These cells are neurons that, as discussed in Chapter 11, are characterized by patterns of firing that increase from a generally low level to higher rates as a freely moving animal moves through a particular region of space. As different place cells are responsive in different locations and are found throughout the septo-temporal axis of the hippocampus, it was natural to suppose that the collective firing of different place-cell ensembles in different environments might be the neural substrate of distinct "maps" of space. Observations on place cells were quickly followed by the discovery that lesions of a major fiber tract into the hippocampal formation, the fimbria/fornix, resulted in an apparently selective deficit of spatial, but not cue, learning by rats in a circular maze task (O'Keefe et al., 1975). These two findings were the trigger for a comprehensive review of the literature and one that offered an imaginative reassessment of findings hitherto explained in other ways (O'Keefe and Nadel, 1978).

The cognitive map theory was the first of several spatial theories of hippocampal function. Its authors have since outlined modifications of the theory, beginning with Nadel's work on "context" (Nadel and Willner, 1980), through ideas about multiple memory traces stored in the hippocampus (Nadel and Moscovitch, 1997), and now incorporating neuroimaging findings from humans performing virtual navigation tasks (Burgess et al., 2002). O'Keefe has also explored the relevance of the theory to the neural basis of language, in particular spatial prepositions (O'Keefe, 1996). Other spatial memory theories include the "scene memory" hypothesis of Gaffan (1991), the "fragment assembly" hypothesis (Worden, 1992), and the closely related idea of the hippocampal formation being involved in "path integration" (McNaughton et al., 1996; Whishaw, 1998; Redish, 1999). There have also been ideas about the "metrics" in which spatial information is processed (Poucet, 1993) and a "dual," or "parallel-map," theory (Jacobs and Schenk, 2003). This latest development argues for a synergistic interaction of a directional "bearing map" and an allocentric "sketch map"—each mediated by distinct but overlapping subregions of the hippocampal formation. Like the ideas about path integration, it incorporates the discovery of another category of spatially tuned cells, the head-direction units (Taube and Schwartzkroin, 1987; Taube, 1998). These are cells, described in Chapter 11, that fire when a rat's head is facing a particular direction in a familiar environment irrespective of the animal's location. In parallel with this neurobiological theorizing, there has been continuing interest in the psychological literature concerning the concept of "cognitive mapping" (Gallistel, 1980) that dates back to Tolman's classic paper (Tolman, 1948). Although the term cognitive mapping was used in a slightly different sense by Gallistel, this renewal of interest has prompted debate that, in an unexpected turn, has cast doubt on the explanatory power of the concept (Bennett, 1996; Wang and Spelke, 2002). Mackintosh has also queried its adequacy as an account of how animals get from one place to another but expressed the view that the 1978 book "deserves its status as a modern classic" (Mackintosh, 2002. p. 181). Numerous reviews have been published (Poucet, 1993; Muller, 1996; Taube, 1999), as have two comprehensive books focusing on the neurobiology of spatial, context, and episodic memory (Redish, 1999; Jeffery, 2003).

13.4.1 Outline of the Theory

The five main suppositions of the original (1978) cognitive map theory relate to representation of the environment, navigation through it, the evolution of an ostensibly specialized spatial memory system, storage of spatial information, and the relevance of a specifically spatial system in animals to the mediation of episodic and semantic memory in humans.

Box 13–4
Cognitive Map Theory

1. *Representation:* The vertebrate brain has a neural system— the "locale" system—that organizes the encoding and representation of perceived stimuli with respect to an "allocentric" spatial framework, or "cognitive map." The spatial locations of landmarks are stored in this map during exploration. This locale system is in the hippocampus.

2. *Navigation:* The locale system is used for spatial navigation. The various anatomical components of the hippocampal formation are involved in mediating different aspects of spatial information processing, with distinct classes of neurons responsive to an animal's place, head-direction, view and its movement through space.

3. *Evolution and the laws of learning:* Spatial mapping evolved as one of the multiple memory systems of the vertebrate brain with its own distinctive learning rules. Other types of learning and memory include simpler associative mechanisms and certain geometrical tasks that can be acquired using "taxon" strategies. These other systems obey laws of learning that are different from those of the locale system.

4. *Sites of storage:* Spatial maps are stored in the hippocampus. They are not consolidated or stored elsewhere in the brain, although information stored in the hippocampus does interact with information stored elsewhere for the purpose of guiding navigational behavior. An intrahippocampal consolidation mechanism may nonetheless exist.

5. *Extension of the theory to humans:* Whereas the cognitive map is purely spatial in animals, it subserves the storage and recall of linguistic and episodic memories in humans. Lateralization enables the right hippocampus to maintain a primarily spatial function, whereas the left hippocampus incorporates a temporal sense and linguistic entities that together provide the basis for mediating episodic memory.

As already noted, numerous developments of the original theory have occurred since 1978, leading to slightly different ideas about spatial memory than those in the list in Box 13–4. In the discussion that follows, there are references to these developments, as appropriate. Although distinct, they are in the same genre as the original cognitive map theory.

The first of O'Keefe and Nadel's (1978) ideas—*the concept of a "locale," or mapping, system*—implies that when forming memories of the world neural activity in the brain automatically encodes stimuli in a connected mental framework rather than as isolated stimulus traces or independent pairwise associations. This encoding happens, for example, as laboratory rats explore a novel environment (Fig. 13–16A). It occurs quickly, sometimes in one trial; and it relies on information from the place cells indicating the animal's location, particularly the distance from the boundaries of the test arena. Head-direction cells provide a representation of direction based on what are described as infinitely long vectors. This curiosity-driven exploration involves something more than perceptual learning about the identity of individual cues (objects, land-

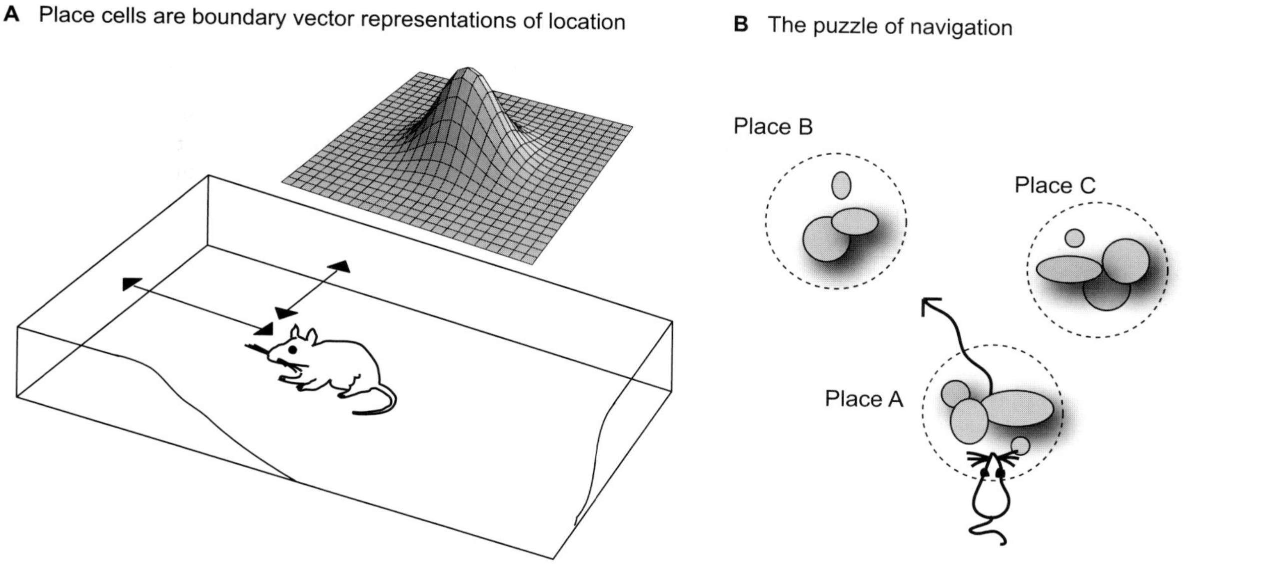

A Place cells are boundary vector representations of location

B The puzzle of navigation

Place B

Place C

Place A

Figure 13–16. Place cells, boundary vectors, and the puzzle of place cell-guided navigation. *A.* As rats explore a simple environment in a test arena, they encode information about location, such as distance from the side walls, into a map-like internal representation. Place cells emerge as the interaction of two or more Gaussians (inset) whose centers are determined by the distance from prominent features such as walls. (*Source:* After O'Keefe and Burgess, 1996.) *B.* A rat at place A wants to navigate to B but not to C. Place cells (gray circles and ellipses) have firing fields in these three areas. A subset of the cells with fields at place A fire with a certain probability with the animal there, but it is not clear how at place A the rat can activate the subset of place cells for place B but not those for place C to direct its choice behavior appropriately. Additional "goal cells" seem to be required to achieve navigation. (*Source:* After Morris, 1991.)

marks) or the development of familiarity that later enables recognition. The putative hippocampal mapping system also encodes where landmarks are located in relation to each other in some kind of geometrical framework.

The idea of an organized structure to memory is, of course, hardly unique to the cognitive map theory, as many other theories of human memory embody the same idea, including artificial intelligence-derived theories of semantic memory (Collins and Quillian, 1969) and connectionist theories of memory consolidation (McClelland et al., 1995; McClelland and Goddard, 1996; O'Reilly and Norman, 2002). Some form of memory organization would also be helpful for encoding one-time events in relation to static landmarks; and, partly for this reason, the hippocampus in humans could be helpful for encoding information into episodic memory. The recall of a specific event, such as what one did during a recent holiday, generally involves first remembering where one was before proceeding to remembering with whom one spent the holiday or what unusual things happened. Gaffan (1991) was the first to make this point explicitly, later building it into a "scene-specific" theory of episodic memory (see Section 13.6).

The second supposition is that, once stored, *locale information can be used for spatial navigation.* Whereas the first proposition was that information is *stored* in a map-like framework, the second relates to how that information is *used.* How does an animal navigate using its "cognitive map"? This question prompted the supposition that the unusual anatomical circuitry of the allocortex (see Chapters 3, 4, and 8), so unlike the

canonical local circuits of neocortex (Douglas and Martin, 2004), could be precisely what is needed to perform the geometrical computations involved in finding the way around. This might include computations for encoding the distance and direction between landmarks, rotating the map for appropriate alignment with perceived cues, identifying the location and heading direction of the animal within it, and performing various other geometrical functions essential for effective allocentric navigation through space. In short: *Where am I? Where am I going? How do I get there?*

O'Keefe and Nadel (1978) offered several speculations about how such spatial operations could be implemented in the hippocampal formation. Considering the original ideas on representation and navigation together (Box 13–4, propositions 1 and 2), they supposed that sensory information entered the hippocampal formation via the entorhinal cortex, from which it projected into the dentate gyrus and then to succeeding stages of the trisynaptic circuit as it was then understood (but see the discussion of hippocampal connectivity in Chapter 3, Section 3.7). Different pyramidal cells were thought to be driven by different proportions of excitatory or inhibitory inputs. The group with mainly excitatory inputs ("place cells") were defined as those that fired when an animal occupied a particular position in relation to a constellation of sensory cues (e.g., visual, auditory, olfactory). Because of the convergent nature of hippocampal circuitry, it was suggested that the probability (or rate) of place-cell firing should decline in a monotonic but nonlinear fashion as individual cues become obscured or are removed but be relatively insensitive to the loss of any one cue. This prediction about place cells was upheld (O'Keefe and Conway, 1978). Other pyramidal cells ("misplace cells") were presumed to have, in addition, sensory-driven inputs relayed via feedforward inhibition such that they would *increase* their rate of firing when sensory cues were removed. This increased firing was held to be the neural event that triggered exploratory behavior, perhaps via the subicular output through the fornix to the nucleus accumbens (see Chapter 3, Section 3.4.2). The original theory also stated that the firing of "theta cells" is coupled to the translational movement of the animal from one position in the map to another, an idea supported by studies in which the different frequencies of theta activity observed during jumping through space correlated directly with the distance moved rather than the force exerted (Morris, 1983). More recent neural modeling studies have modified these ideas substantially (see Chapter 14). The unfolding picture about the wide range of distinct inhibitory interneurons and their axonal connections (see Chapter 8) has also raised the specter of yet deeper subtlety at the level of local circuits.

Since 1978, there have been many technical and conceptual developments in hippocampal single-unit recording in freely moving rats. The development of multiple single-unit recording ("ensemble recording") with "stereotrodes" and "tetrodes" has shed fresh light on a range of theoretical issues: multiple place fields, local views, gating by the potential for movement, memory properties, multiple reference frames, pattern completion, and pattern separation (as discussed in Chapter 11). Numerous uncertainties have been clarified. It is now known, for example, that pyramidal cells acquire their place fields rapidly, fire in proportion to an animal's speed of motion, tend to be directionally sensitive only in directionally constrained environments (e.g., linear tracks), and show temporal precession in their phase relation to hippocampal theta as an animal moves through the cell's place field. Improved recording techniques have also established that single cells do not, in general, have place fields in different parts of a single environment, and that physically adjacent pyramidal cells may have place fields in quite different parts of the environment. A boundary vector model (BVC) has been developed (Hartley et al., 2000) according to which places can be modeled as the sum of two or more Gaussians, with the center of each Gaussian located by its distance from a specific environmental feature such as a wall (as in Fig. 13–16A). With this view, place fields represent probability distributions and do not specify precise locations. Certain theoretically unanticipated properties of CA1 place cells have also been discovered, such as their sensitivity to physical restraint, their apparent insensitivity to lesions of the dentate gyrus or CA3, and alterations in receptive field size and stability with aging (see Chapter 11). The discovery of head-direction cells in the presubiculum and thalamus (Taube et al., 1990a, b) and of "grid cells" in the dorsomedial entorhinal cortex (Fyhn et al., 2004; Hafting et al., 2005) are important additions to the idea that the hippocampal formation and interconnecting structures constitute, in animals, an essentially spatial system.

Notwithstanding these developments, we still do not fully understand how a map of space could be represented (Box 13–4, proposition 1) or used (Box 13–4, proposition 2) by means of hippocampal circuitry. The relation between location firing (in pyramidal cells of CA1 and CA3), head-directional firing (in the presubiculum and anterior thalamus), and movement firing (in the interneurons of the hippocampus and dentate gyrus) is also poorly understood. Those concerned with specific details might reasonably wonder, for example, whether the head-direction firing of presubiculum cells is a component of "locale" or "taxon" processing (or both). Various logical puzzles about the link between mapping and navigation have also been pointed out. For example, as place cells are defined as cells that fire only when an animal occupies a specific position in space, how can the mapping system access information pertaining to places other than the one presently occupied by the animal (Morris, 1991)? That is, if a rat is at place A and wants to navigate to place B but not to place C, how does it at place A access information relevant to going to B rather than going to C (Fig. 13–16B)? Place-cell firing on its own does not seem to help because the place cells corresponding to B and C cannot, *by definition*, fire until the animal gets to B or C, respectively. This kind of logical conundrum is clearly problematic for the theory, but it may not be fatal if goal cells can be identified. Perhaps these are in other brain areas (Hok et al., 2005). Other models of the neural implementation of goal representations are also being developed (Redish, 1999; Biegler, 2003). Several neural network and temporal difference learning models that grapple with these issues are outlined in Chapter 14.

The third feature of the theory is that *spatial mapping has evolved in response to specific environmental demands*, and that it *constitutes one of the multiple memory systems of the vertebrate brain* (Fig. 13-17). The emphasis on evolution, lacking prominence in the declarative memory theory, has been informed by studies of cache recovery in passerine birds, homing in pigeons, territory size and mating systems in small mammals, and other aspects of naturalistic spatial behavior (Sherry and Schacter, 1987b; Clayton and Krebs, 1995; Dyer, 1998; Healy, 1998; Shettleworth, 1998; Jacobs and Schenk, 2003). The "neuroethological" component of the thinking behind the cognitive map theory has been explicit from the outset (O'Keefe and Nadel, 1979; Nadel, 1991), fostering studies of sex and seasonal differences in spatial memory that might not have happened had all hippocampal research remained anchored solely in a paramedical context. Work in both vertebrate and invertebrate species has revealed both convergent and divergent evolution with respect to how to find food, water or sex—and then get safely back home. Studies of animal navigation have, however, revealed mechanisms that appear to have nothing to do with cognitive maps, such as ideothetic "path integration" by insects (Wehner et al., 1996) and rodents (Etienne and Jeffery, 2004) and the "snapshot" processing of landmarks by bees (Collett, 1992). The relevance of the neuroethological approach to hippocampal function and mechanisms has been the subject of cogent crit-

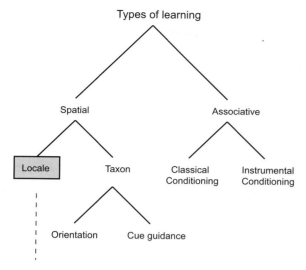

Types of learning

Spatial

Associative

Locale

Taxon

Classical
Conditioning

Instrumental
Conditioning

Orientation

Cue guidance

Hippocampal Formation

Figure 13–17. Multiple forms of memory in the cognitive map theory. Only the locale system, requiring cognitive mapping, is mediated by the hippocampus. The theory has less to say about other forms of learning and memory.

icism (Squire, 1993; Bolhuis and Macphail, 2001), but many see it as an important adjunct to the development of cognitive mapping theory.

However, the bulk of the work addressing the cognitive map theory has been conducted with the laboratory rat and, more recently, various laboratory strains of mice. A veritable "hippocampal industry" emerged, beginning with lesion/behavior studies and single-unit recording work on animals, that now finds modern expression in a variety of behavioral tasks used in conjunction with the full spectrum of contemporary neuroscience techniques. Particularly exciting are the technical innovations that complement classic lesion techniques, with the new tasks including ensemble single-unit recording from large numbers of hippocampal neurons (Wilson and McNaughton, 1993), monitoring the expression of immediate early genes (Guzowski et al., 1999; Vann et al., 2000), and reversible pharmacological interventions that are sufficiently sustained in time to investigate memory processes, such as systems-level consolidation (Riedel et al., 1999). Mice have nibbled their way onto the hippocampal stage with targeted gene deletions, hippocampus-specific deletions, and even inducible gene knockouts (Tonegawa et al., 1995; Mayford et al., 1996; Tsien et al., 1996; Abel and Lattal, 2001). The hippocampal research industry, which has seen the number of papers on rodent spatial representation and navigation rise from around 10 per year in 1980 to several hundred per year (Sutherland and Hamilton, 2004), owes a great debt to the cognitive map theory.

With respect to multiple memory systems, the scope of O'Keefe and Nadel's (1978) original analysis was narrower than that encompassed in the declarative framework discussed earlier (Figure 13.4). Their book distinguishes only

between spatial memory and nonspatial associative learning (such as classical and instrumental conditioning). Whereas allocentric "locale" learning was held to be motivated only by curiosity and to be extremely fast, associative learning was thought to be motivated by rewards related to basic motivational needs (such as food for a hungry animal) and to be slower, cumulative, and governed by quite different learning rules. However, this spatial versus associative distinction has come under close scrutiny (just as it did in connection with recognition memory in the previous section of this chapter). Certain classic phenomena in the associative domain (such as "overshadowing" and "blocking," to be explained later) have also been found to operate within the domain of spatial learning (Biegler and Morris, 1999; Chamizo, 2003) although subject to certain constraints associated with the perception and local processing of geometry (McGregor et al., 2004a). Associative learning can also be very fast, and in phenomena such as sensory preconditioning, is not obviously motivated by biological rewards. Although O'Keefe and Nadel's original dichotomy now feels incomplete, understanding the boundaries between cognitive mapping and other forms of learning and memory is proving to be a fruitful area of research. Also of interest is how spatial and nonspatial systems compete or work synergistically to ensure the seamless control of behavior; and it remains a fundamental issue (White and McDonald, 2002).

The fourth proposition of the 1978 theory is that *allocentric spatial information is stored in the hippocampus.* Unlike the time-limited role for the hippocampus in the declarative memory theory, the original version of the cognitive map theory has both initial encoding and long-term storage in the one brain structure. Nadel and Moscovitch (1997) extended this idea in a "multiple-trace theory" of episodic memory in which memory retrieval episodes can initiate re-storage. The possibility of multiple traces—even for single episodes—leads to a different account of the temporal gradients of retrograde amnesia that are sometimes seen for information acquired prior to brain damage. The key difference from the account offered by the declarative memory theory lies in the impact of partial damage. Complete lesions at various time points after training should always result in temporally extensive, or "flat gradients," of remote memory loss. In contrast, partial lesions might result in a reverse gradient if older information, recollected previously, had laid down additional traces in areas of the hippocampus spared by the lesion. The declarative memory theory makes no differential prediction as a function of lesion completeness.

Although the original cognitive map theory of hippocampal function was based largely on observations in rats, its extension and likely modification to account for primate and human hippocampal function was recognized at the outset. Proposition 5 in Box 13–4 recognizes that later chapters of O'Keefe and Nadel's monograph addressed the relevance of their ideas to human semantic memory (e.g., Chapters 14 and 15) and, specifically, the way in which spatial relations are fundamental to certain linguistic prepositions that reflect the knowledge of relations (e.g., "beside," "near," "above"). Although not originally influential in the human neuropsychology community, these ideas have nonetheless been extended to such domains as reasoning and abstract thought and are now an active area of research. For example, Gattis (2001) identified the sharp distinction between a "generalist" school of thought, in which space is merely a special case of "relational processing," and a Kantian perspective, in which space (and time) are special. Nadel and Hardt (2004) strongly reasserted the latter position, whereas O'Keefe (2005) has continued his exploration of "vector grammar" and how it might explain the essentially various meanings of spatial propositions.

Cognitive science apart, one obstacle to pursuing these lines of thought has been in securing definitive evidence for causally linking hippocampal cell activity in humans to any such processes. Hippocampal damage in humans does not obviously disrupt a person's ability to use spatial prepositions. Invasive single-unit recording in humans is rarely feasible, but some intriguing examples of "place cells" have been recorded from the human hippocampus with depth electrodes placed to monitor epileptic seizure activity (Fried et al., 1998; Ekstrom et al., 2003). Place cells have also been observed in the hippocampus of monkeys free to drive themselves around slowly in a motorized "cab" (Matsumura et al., 1999). Spatial correlates are therefore by no means unique to rodents, but securing single-unit evidence for vector grammar has not yet been achieved.

Functional brain imaging has also been used to study hemodynamic activation during human navigation. The problem here is that fMRI is a technique that does not obviously lend itself to the study of a mental process—navigation—that ostensibly requires subjects to be mobile. One solution is to use "virtual reality." Whether virtual reality in subjects lying prone in a brain scanner really engages the same neural mechanisms as "true" navigation can be debated—place cells in rats being sensitive to whether animals are restrained or allowed to move (Foster et al., 1989)—but if one accepts that a virtual reality approach might be viable, modern computing software has certainly made it possible. Numerous studies have now examined whether the hippocampus and adjacent structures of humans are activated during apparent "navigation" through imaginary towns (Maguire et al., 1998), featureless arenas, and swimming pools (Thomas et al., 2001; Parslow et al., 2004) as well as other tasks that distinguish mapping from merely following a sequential route (Morris and Mayes, 2004). Burgess et al. (2002) made a strong case that virtual reality is informative and specifically discussed patterns of activation in relation to spatial frameworks, the dimensionality of space, and both orientation and self-motion. In contrast, a more cautious stance about the findings to have emerged from functional imaging of spatial navigation is presented in Chapter 12.

Finally, by way of introduction, is there anything special about space? Declarative memory theorists think not. In their view, a memory system exists in the MTL that processes all forms of propositional knowledge, whether it comes to us via visual, tactile, olfactory, or other sensory modalities. Why, their concern continues, should space be any different? The "no different" perspective appears to look on memory processing of "space" as involving multimodal sensory information, with cues that may be familiar or unfamiliar and with the capacity to realize "declarations" of spatial knowledge such "A is near B." Given this, why would encoding or storage be any different from that of other object-orientated information that is processed via the ventral stream of the perceptual processing pathways of the neocortex terminating in the inferotemporal, perirhinal, and parahippocampal cortices (Ungerleider and Mishkin, 1982)? Indeed, so absurd may it seem to think that space could be different, a major review of the functions of the MTL considered the adequacy of the spatial theory of hippocampal function in little more than a couple of paragraphs (Squire et al., 2004).

Not surprisingly, the opposing camp is resistant to being so subsumed. For those prepared to contemplate a neural system for cognitive mapping (including critics of O'Keefe and Nadel's theory, such as the present author), thinking about space in this declarative way reflects a conceptual misunderstanding: Space is not a sensory modality. We do not have sensory organs for space or a cranial nerve devoted to it. Space is a construct of mental processing. Moreover, space has a structure that requires but is logically independent of the multimodal sensory information used to identify it. For example, many objects whose location we know are often hidden, whether it is acorns cached by a squirrel or food in a kitchen cupboard. It is precisely in this situation that spatial memory becomes so useful—the exact *opposite* of the situation that applies to normal recognition memory. Similarly, the appearance of a specific area of space can change across the seasons despite its containing inanimate or sessile living things that do not ordinarily move around. What does not change when a cupboard door is closed, a tree loses its leaves, or a rock becomes covered in snow is the location of the remembered item. There is, in short, a geometric "stability" about remembered space that is independent of the appearance of the stationary objects and landmarks that, paradoxically, define that stability (Biegler and Morris, 1993). This paradox is at the heart of why pattern separation and pattern completion are network operations at the heart of hippocampal processing (see Chapter 14). The closely related concept of "context" is also not necessarily something that is "out there" waiting for a sensory/perceptual system to process it; it is a neural construct (Jeffery, 2003). These and other features of "space" could have been major driving forces in the evolution of the distinctive cognitive systems that mediate it.

This completes the initial overview of the five key features of the cognitive map theory. A selective presentation of relevant data follows, in four successive sections, followed by a concluding critique. The relevance of the theory to humans is not considered further, and the reader referred to the very different perspective offered in Chapter 12.

13.4.2 Representing Spatial Information, Locale Processing, and the Hippocampal Formation

A key concept with respect to the representation and storage of spatial information is the distinction between egocentric and allocentric space. Egocentric space refers to the locations of objects relative to the viewer—to the left or the right—directions that necessarily alter as the viewer moves around. Representing this kind of space is not thought to require a cognitive mapping system. Allocentric space, on the other hand, is a representation of spatial relations within some kind of absolute framework. For a freely moving subject, an allocentric representation is required to identify whether an object or landmark has actually moved in relation to others. In contrast, objects are constantly "moving" in egocentric representations. The distinction between egocentric and allocentric space has not always been appreciated by critics of the cognitive map theory, with some incorrectly assuming that the theory predicts that lesions of the hippocampal formation must impair any and all spatial learning tasks (e.g., Nadel and Hardt, 2004). Many spatial tasks given to animals, such as the simple T maze task described in Section 13.2 and certain touchscreen tasks, are ambiguous because they can be solved using either an allocentric or an egocentric strategy. The study of exploratory behavior has provided a key test of this feature of the cognitive map theory together with studies examining how animals localize objects in space. Lesion studies and observations of immediate early gene activation have contributed to a detailed examination of this issue.

Lesion Studies of Exploratory Behavior Reveal the Importance of Allocentric Spatial Representation

It has long been known that rats explore spontaneously, and the phenomenon has been systematically in the laboratory for years (Berlyne, 1950, 1966; Halliday, 1968; Archer and Birke, 1983; Renner, 1990). Placed in a novel test arena, the rats remain motionless for a period of time and then start to move around, first at the periphery and then throughout the available space, where they explore objects and landmarks one by one, often returning to an object just investigated until they finally come to rest in one corner. This is not mere movement; it is exploration to gain information. For example, renewed exploration can be triggered easily after habituation by introducing a novel object into the arena, a phenomenon exploited in the visual-paired comparison task (see Section 13.3). Hippocampal lesions impair certain aspects of exploration. They tend to make animals hyperactive yet also disinclined to visit all regions of a space systematically and less likely to display habituation of activity over time (O'Keefe and Nadel, 1978; Whishaw et al., 1983). O'Keefe and Nadel (1978), Morris (1983), and Renner (1990) have repeatedly made the point that the hippocampus-dependent information-gathering function of exploratory behavior should be clearly distinguished from any motor functions to which the hippocampus

contributes (Vanderwolf and Cain, 1994). There remains, however, the question of what information is gathered.

As the cognitive map theory asserts that this curiosity-driven exploration is the basis for encoding a "map," a critical experimental prediction is that renewed exploration would be triggered by alterations in the spatial arrangement of familiar objects. Critically, hippocampus-lesioned subjects should display selective failure of renewed exploration to object displacement but not to object novelty. Using a paradigm developed by Thinus-Blanc et al. (1987), Save et al. (1992a) compared the impact of small dorsal hippocampal lesions, anterior and posterior parietal lesions, and sham lesions on exploration in a circular arena containing five objects. In a systematic series of short exploration sessions, the animals became familiar with the initial set of objects and their spatial locations, after which the critical manipulations of spatial dislocation and object novelty were introduced. The results showed renewed exploration by controls and anterior parietal cortex-lesioned animals in response to spatial dislocation; there was no detectable reaction by hippocampus- or posterior parietal-lesioned subjects. In contrast, renewed exploration was shown by all groups in response to object novelty. However, the effect was not large. In an ingenious follow-up of this dissociation, Save et al. (1992b) examined exploration at a particular point in space that was triggered by the *absence* of an expected object (Fig. 13–18). Rats that had been subject to preexperimental surgery first explored an open circular arena that was slightly unusual in that it had a transparent floor. Another rat, in a small box, was sometimes placed underneath this floor in full view of the exploring animal. In a sequential four-phase experiment, the experimental rats first explored the open but empty arena. They were then given two successive opportunities to explore the arena again with the "stimulus rat" visible at one "zone" of space, and the study ended with the final phase that, like the first, had no stimulus rat available under the floor. A neat feature of this design is that the overt visual appearance of the arena was identical in sessions 1 and 4. As expected, introduction of the stimulus rat in session 2 triggered extensive investigation centered on the zone above the stimulus rat's location, and this habituated between sessions 2 and 3. The key test was session 4 with the stimulus rat now removed. In control rats with sham lesions, exploration was focused at the zone, but this did not occur in animals with dorsal hippocampal or posterior parietal lesions. The use of a recall paradigm may have made the magnitude of the effect much larger. Taken together, these findings imply three things: (1) exploration can be triggered in normal rats by object novelty, spatial novelty, and the absence of an expected object; (2) damage to hippocampus and posterior parietal cortex selectively impairs exploration triggered by spatial novelty, including the absence of an expected object; (3) when it occurs, this exploration is not merely activated but spatially directed in an appropriate way. Such findings are consistent with the construction of a "map" of space in the manner predicted by the cognitive map theory.

A Response to spatial change in rats with HPC and parietal cortical (PPC) lesions

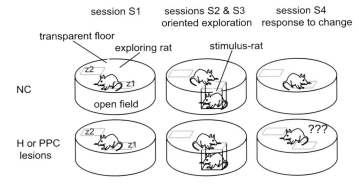

B Response to remembered places by C, HPC and PPC lesioned rats

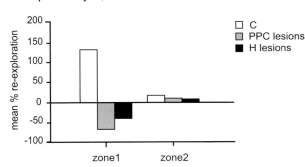

Figure 13–18. Exploration guided by the absence of an expected stimulus. *A.* In a multiple phase study, rats explored an arena with a transparent floor that sometimes revealed the presence of another rat under one zone (z1). Normal and both hippocampus- and posterior parietal cortex-lesioned rats explored differently when this second rat was removed: only control animals spent more time in z1 than z2, reflecting their recall of the now absent "cue" animal underneath. *B.* Data showing greater exploration of the area where the now absent animal had been located. See text for more details. (*Source:* After Save et al., 1992b.)

An outstanding puzzle is why similar disruption of exploration induced by spatial novelty was seen in the posterior parietal cortex-lesioned group, a finding not predicted by the theory if map storage is in the hippocampus. The absence of direct anatomical connections between this structure and the hippocampus led Parron and Save (2004) to wonder whether there may be some larger neuronal network involving the interconnected regions of the retrosplenial and entorhinal cortices. In a follow-up study using the same behavioral procedures, they observed that lesions of these cortical structures also caused disruption of renewed exploration in response to spatial novelty. This finding adds to a growing body of evidence from exploration and navigation tasks that the processing of spatial information extends beyond the hippocampus (Poucet and Benhamou, 1997; Kesner, 2000; Whishaw, 2004a; Hafting et al., 2005).

For example, although some studies have suggested that neurons in the entorhinal cortex are only weakly modulated by the position of the animal (Quirk et al., 1992; Frank et al., 2000), the dorsomedial region of the entorhinal cortex has "grid cells" whose firing shows multipeak fields that are small, stable, and directionally insensitive (Fyhn et al., 2004; Hafting et al., 2005). These firing fields are unaffected by hippocampal lesions, implying that their existence is not secondary to "upstream" hippocampal processing that might be projected back to the entorhinal cortex. Instead, they suggest that at the border between the entorhinal and postrhinal cortex (a region almost certainly lesioned in the Parron and Save, 2004, study of exploration) there is an allocentric, view-independent representation of space. This implies that steps in the computation of allocentric space can occur upstream of the hippocampus, although the multipeaked properties of entorhinal "grid" cells indicates that an individual entorhinal cortex cell provides a metric rather than a specific indication of location. Perhaps ensembles of entorhinal cells are able to "disambiguate" on their own, or they may provide a Fourier-like input to the dentate gyrus and hippocampus, where single-peaked cells are primarily observed. The discovery of the entorhinal grid cells will have a big impact on the cognitive map theory, but the full implications remain to be worked out.

Immediate Early Gene Studies Reveal Anatomical Dissociations with Respect to Environmental Representations

Instead of using lesions, visualizing the expression of immediate early genes (IEGs), such as c-*fos*, *Arc*, and *zif-268* (Morgan et al., 1987; Link et al., 1995; Lyford et al., 1995; Tischmeyer and Grimm, 1999), has been used to examine the patterns of activation in multiple brain areas during both spatial and nonspatial tasks. Some of these studies have focused on the representation of the environment, others on spatial navigation, and yet others on memory consolidation (Dragunow, 1996; Guzowski, 2002). Different IEGs are used in different studies. The choice can take advantage of the fact that some IEGs are regulatory transcription factors that influence the activity of other "downstream" genes (e.g., c-*fos*), whereas other IEGs are effector genes that directly affect cellular physiology (e.g., *Arc*).

There are several features of the IEG approach that are noteworthy. First, from a low level of basal expression in animals, experience-dependent activation of IEGs is correlated with increases in neuronal activity (Herrera and Robertson, 1996). There is, for example, a broadly similar activation profile for *c-fos, zif-268,* and *Arc* in association with spatial learning, with some indication of differential sensitivity to manipulation of task demands (Guzowski et al., 2001). Second, the imaging observations made after sacrifice are from animals whose brains are normal at the time of testing; thus, IEG mapping links behavior to physiology in a manner that complements the single-unit recording studies of Chapter 11. This does not preclude combining the lesion and IEG approaches, and studies using such a combined approach have revealed alterations in activity in areas remote from the site of the lesion (Aggleton and Pearce, 2001). Third, although the analytical focus of a given study may be on activation of a specific brain structure, the approach does not require a "prospective choice," as quantitative measures may be taken of a large number of brain structures. The drawback of the IEG approach is that, unlike single-unit recording for which the measured output is a signal that is well understood in information-processing terms, the "meaning" of an IEG signal is unclear. There has been substantial discussion about the possible functions of IEGs, ranging from metabolic replenishment to regulation of synaptic plasticity, memory consolidation, and even memory retrieval (Guzowski, 2002).

The technique was first used in relation to behavioral studies of exploration by Hess et al. (1995), who observed widespread hippocampal IEG activation in various subfields. This was a valuable first step, but it did not speak to whether the hippocampus encodes information allocentrically. IEG activation may merely occur in the hippocampus in response to novelty, stress, or the motor activity that accompanies exploration. An important step forward was made in a study using *c-fos* by Wan et al. (1999) who presented rats with computer-displayed images in which novelty was introduced as either new stimuli or novel spatial arrangements of hitherto familiar stimuli, a comparison analogous to the original lesion studies just discussed (Save et al., 1992a,b). A within-subjects protocol was used in which the images were presented bilaterally such that familiar stimuli were presented to one eye and novel stimuli (or novel rearrangements of familiar stimuli) to the other eye (Fig. 13–19). As the projections of the rat visual system are largely crossed, it was possible to compare normalized patterns of activation in the two hemispheres within individual animals. Any nonspecific *c-fos* activation associated with novelty, stress, or motor activity was effectively and elegantly "subtracted" out. The key finding was that novel rearrangements of familiar stimuli to one eye differentially activated the CA1 region of the hippocampus. Novel stimuli activated the perirhinal cortex, as previously shown by Zhu et al. (1995). Brown and Aggleton (2001) summarized a body of work using this approach.

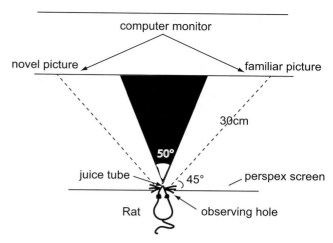

Figure 13–19. Bilateral viewing technique to image immediate early genes such as *c-fos*. Novel and familiar visual patterns are presented simultaneously to each eye. The largely crossed visual system of the rat enables the various *c-fos* patterns to be compared within individual animals and then averaged. (*Source:* Courtesy of M. Brown and J. Aggleton.)

A limitation of the bilateral viewing technique is that there is no behavioral output of the simultaneous processing of novel and familiar stimulus combinations in the two hemispheres—indeed, no way of establishing whether the animals even attend to the cues. Jenkins et al. (2004) therefore followed up the Wan et al. (1999) study by a systematic analysis of normalized *c-fos* patterns in animals running through and making choices in a radial maze task (see below for a description of this classic navigation task). Following a procedure first developed by Suzuki et al. (1980), they first trained rats with eight distinctive cue cards placed between the arms of the maze. Then, on the final day of training, the cue cards were left in their standard arrangement for half the animals (Group Familiar) or shifted to a novel spatial arrangement for the others (Group Novel) (Fig. 13–20). Spatial novelty caused *c-fos* activation in CA1, CA3, and the dentate gyrus, whereas no changes were observed in the surrounding cortical regions such as the perirhinal and parahippocampal cortex. This was not due to differential sensitivity of the imaging method between hippocampus and cortex because successful *c-fos* activation following spatial novelty was seen in the posterior parietal cortex. In addition, animals in a companion study were shown to be using the cue cards in their representation of the maze, as indexed by behavioral sensitivity to cue rotation. These findings nicely complement the lesion observations of Save et al. (1992a,b). That the hippocampal formation can detect alterations in the spatial arrangement of cues and respond by differential activation of an IEG strongly suggests that the information encoded about the familiar stimuli presented earlier must have included some representation of their spatial layout in the image or in the room. They support the notion that the hippocampus is both necessary for and involved in the representation of space. However, they also point to unexpected involvement of the posterior parietal cortex as well.

A Spatial arrangement of cues during training (left) and c-fos measurement period (right)

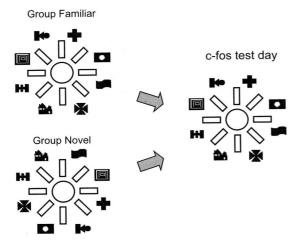

B Hippocampal (left bars) and cortical (right) c-fos patterns following spatial cue re-arrangement

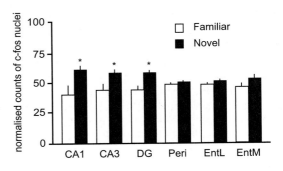

Figure 13–20. Immediate early gene activation reveals regional patterns of sensitivity to spatial novelty. *A.* The spatial arrangement of the cues placed between the ends of the arms of the maze was retained between training and the c-*fos* test session for Group Familiar but was changed for Group Novel. *B.* The normalized c-*fos* patterns show the differential sensitivity of structures in the hippocampus (CA1, CA3, DG) versus neocortical regions such as perirhinal and entorhinal cortex (medial and lateral). (*Source*: After Jenkins et al., 2004.)

Guzowski et al. (1999) introduced a highly illuminating new technique in which it is possible to identify time-locked expression of IEGs using fluorescent in situ hybridization (called catFISH after the cellular compartment in which time of expression is observed). It was first applied to the imaging of *Arc* on its own and later extended to enable simultaneous imaging of *Arc* and *Homer*. The catFISH technique enables a within-subject comparison of a different kind in which the population of neurons activated by one experience (e.g., exploring a box) can be distinguished from a second population activated by a later experience (e.g., exploring a different box). *Arc* RNA first appears as discrete small intranuclear signals within 2 to 15 minutes of the cells being activated (e.g., the activation of a place cell as an animal occupies its place field). After 20 to 45 minutes the nuclear signal disappears, and a cytoplasmic mRNA signal develops that is translocated to dendrites. As the time course of the nuclear signal is distinct from the cytoplasmic signal, the activity history of individual neurons at two time points can be inferred (see this chapter, figures in color centerpiece). Two predictions of the cognitive mapping theory were then tested. First, it was established that a common population of place cells was activated when the animals explored the same box (A) on two successive occasions, with the same population of cells expressing *Arc* mRNA in dendrites (signaling the first visit to the box) and in the soma (more recent visit). Second, they observed *Arc* RNA expression in two distinct but overlapping populations of cells on sequential visits to two different boxes (A then B). In boxes approximately 70 cm in diameter (about the same as those used in many studies of place cell firing fields), they found that approximately 38% of the CA1 pyramidal cells showed both the dendritic and the somatic IEG signals, whereas others displayed only one of the two signals. The standard c-*fos* technique would not have revealed that the activation response of the different environments was specific, whereas *Arc* catFISH provides novel information about the information content of neuronal activation.

In an extension of this work, Vazdarjanova and Guzowski (2004) have compared the sequential IEG activation patterns in CA3 and CA1 in an exploration task very like that used by the Marseille group: a box containing objects that can be moved about. Exploiting a further technical innovation, confocal images of *Homer* reflected neuronal activity that had occurred approximately 30 minutes before sacrifice, whereas nuclear images of *Arc* reflected more immediate neuronal activation. The study revealed that when confronted by two object arrangements successively (A then B), cells in area CA3 showed discontinuous activation patterns that were highly suggestive of "pattern separation." However, when confronted with either identical or very similar boxes (A then A or A'), the patterns overlapped very well, suggestive of "pattern completion." The patterns in CA1 were more continuous across these environmental manipulations. Integration of distinct CA3 and CA1 ensemble representations may provide a refined representation of spatial context reflecting intrahippocampal processing of information projected from the entorhinal cortex. The observations of Leutgeb et al. (2004) on the firing properties of CA3 and CA1 cells in various boxes and contexts are consistent with this conclusion.

Distributed Representations, Pattern Separation, and Pattern Completion

The lesion and IEG studies of exploratory behavior and reactions to novelty clearly point to a role for the hippocampus in representing spatial information, but on their own they say little about *how* spatial information is represented. Single-cell and ensemble recording is the way forward to understand and quantify the representational structure of information (see Chapter 11) guided by neural network models of how the system might work (see Chapter 14). There is also a role for behavioral studies in identifying neural network processes such as pattern separation and pattern completion that act on such representations (Rolls and Treves, 1998).

With one approach to "pattern separation," Gilbert et al. (1998) trained hungry rats to forage for food on a "cheeseboard" apparatus with a series of food wells arranged in a row such that the separation between the wells varied from 15 to 105 cm. Training took the form of pairs of trials, a sample trial followed by a choice, with as many as 16 trial-pairs per day. During each sample trial, the rats ran from a start box at the periphery of the cheeseboard to displace a single object over one of the wells to secure food. During the choice trial that followed a few seconds later, two identical copies of this same object were placed to cover two wells, with one object covering the same baited well, the other an empty one farther down the row (i.e., delayed matching to place). This task provided a way to measure how easily the rats could discriminate spatial locations in memory as a function of their distance apart. Prior to being lesioned, choice performance was very good, as high as 80% on even the smallest distance and rising to 90% at the largest separation. Large electrolytic lesions of the hippocampus caused performance at the smallest separation (15 cm) to fall to chance, but there was a graded recovery, as this distance increased reaching nearly 90% at the largest distance (105 cm). Performance was also unaffected by changing the start location by 180° between sample and choice trials. This pattern of performance indicates that one function of the hippocampus may be to "separate" patterns of spatial information, this being possible without the hippocampus for widely separated cues but not for cues close together. Findings consistent with this interpretation using a radial maze task had also been reported by McDonald and White (1995). In a follow-up study using the cheeseboard, Gilbert et al. (2001) showed that discrete neurotoxic lesions of the dentate gyrus (DG) caused a comparable pattern of impairment, whereas CA1 lesions had no effect. This dissociation is intriguing, but it raises the puzzle of how spatial information, orthogonalized at the level of the granule cells in the DG, is able to influence target structures of the hippocampus in animals that have been subjected to CA1 lesioning. The usual "output" for information, however effectively it is processed in DG, would no longer be available. An output route via the ventral hippocampus is one possibility as the CA1 lesions were restricted to the dorsal hippocampus. There may also be the possibility of output directly from the CA3 to the lateral septal nucleus, but the route to the neocortex is then indirect. It would be interesting to explore this route, as the finding hints at a radical new conception of information flow within the hippocampal formation.

Another innovative approach to pattern completion has involved molecular-genetic techniques to address what is, in effect, a systems-level issue. Nakazawa et al. (2002) engineered a mutant mouse in which the NR1 subunit of the *N*-methyl-

D-aspartate (NMDA) receptor (see Chapters 6, 7, and 10) was excised selectively in the CA3 region of the hippocampus. Using the Cre-Lox technique to realize this selective ablation, the resulting progeny (CA3-NR1 knockout mice) were shown to have normal physiology and behavior on a range of tests but certain highly specific impairments. For example, whereas LTP was normal in the mossy fiber input to CA3 and in the CA3 output to CA1, it was absent in the longitudinal association pathway of CA3. This pathway is likely to be important for building associative spatial relations between cues in an environment (McNaughton and Morris, 1987; Treves and Rolls, 1994). When trained in a watermaze (see Fig. 13–23, below, for a description of this task), the mice learned normally with all cues present but showed selective deficit in recall when tested with a subset of the training cues. Interestingly, place-specific firing of CA1 complex-spike cells was also "fuzzier" in the mutants when recording sessions took place using partial cues. Nakazawa et al. (2002) interpreted this observation as implying a role for NMDA receptors in area CA3 of the hippocampus in pattern completion, and they outlined a model of the way areas CA3 and CA1 may interact during the storage of information (Fig. 13–21). This study also nicely illustrated the power of adult-onset, cell type-restricted genetic manipulations in the integrative study of the molecular, cellular, and neuronal circuitry mechanisms underlying spatial cognition, a considerable advance on first-generation transgenic techniques (Nakazawa et al., 2004).

13.4.3 Using Spatial Information: Spatial Navigation and the Hippocampal Formation

The second key idea in cognitive map theory is that neural activity in the hippocampal formation occurs during and is required for spatial navigation. Allocentric navigation utilizes the information stored as a "map" during earlier locale processing, and reading information out of maps requires hippocampal place cells to fire. Other cognitive processes related to navigation involving the hippocampus include the ability to mentally rotate a stored representation to align it with a current view, to discover and use shortcuts, and so on. A key prediction is that the integrity of the hippocampal formation is absolutely required for locale-based navigation. This prediction led to the development of a number of novel navigational tasks for rats, the first of which was the radial maze.

Radial Maze

The radial maze is an apparatus in which rats (or mice) are given the opportunity to collect food hidden at the end of arms of the maze that radiate out from a central choice area (Olton and Samuelson, 1976). In its simplest version, a hungry rat is placed on the maze and allowed to run around until it has collected all the food. Once the food at the end of one maze arm has been eaten, it makes sense to avoid that arm, which normal rats gradually learn to do. Once mastered, the rats run to each arm without revisiting arms a second time (Fig. 13–22A). They have, in effect, solved a special case of the

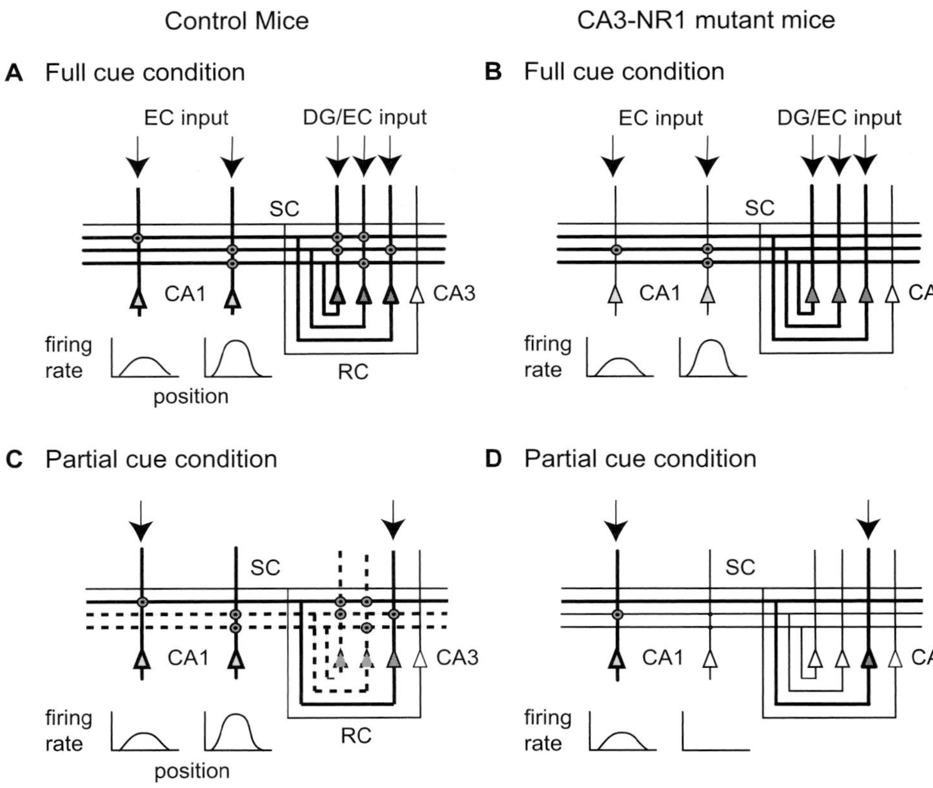

Control Mice   CA3-NR1 mutant mice

A Full cue condition   **B** Full cue condition

C Partial cue condition   **D** Partial cue condition

Figure 13–21. Pattern completion in the storage and retrieval of spatial memory using areas CA3 and CA1. Note the interconnecting circuitry of CA3 and CA1, emphasizing pathways that form NR-dependent modifiable synapses in CA3. A, B. Basic wiring of CA3 and CA1 illustrates a possible encoding mechanism for pattern completion. In normal and CA3-NR1 knockout (KO) mice (left and right columns, respectively), a full cue input (top row) is provided to CA3 from the dentate gyrus (DG) or the entorhinal cortex (EC) and to CA1 from the EC (downward-facing arrows). During learning,

the normal mice make associative changes in synaptic efficacy in the commissural-association pathway (small circles representing potentiated synapses), whereas CA3-NR1 KO mice do not. C, D. In later testing under partial cues (bottom row), a fraction of the original input is provided (fewer downward arrows) to activate any memory traces formed during training. Only control mice are able to benefit from the associative plasticity in CA3 that "completes" the pattern and so provides an output to CA1 that can then be used for spatial recognition and navigation. (*Source*: After Nakazawa et al., 2002.)

"traveling-salesman's problem" of getting everywhere with the least effort. Olton (1977) reported that rats with various lesions that deafferented or deefferented the hippocampus (e.g., fornix or entorhinal cortex lesions) were severely impaired in their initial learning. Whereas normal animals collected all available food from the ends of the maze arms with little or no retracing, those with lesions moved around the maze haphazardly, making numerous repeat entries into arms from which they had already obtained food. The initial interpretation of these data was that these surgical disconnections of the hippocampus disrupted spatial navigation and so supported the cognitive map theory.

However, Olton began to doubt his interpretation following a study suggesting that the deficit was really in trial-specific "working memory." This term was introduced into the animal literature by Honig (1978) to refer to the memory of information useful for only a single trial in a behavioral task.*

*"Working memory" has a different meaning in human memory research, where it refers to a limited capacity consisting of several subsystems such as a phonological store and visuospatial sketch pad (Baddeley, 2001).

Olton and Papas, 1979) adopted a modification of the task, originally suggested by Jarrard (1978), in which both sham-operated and fornix-lesioned rats were tested in a 17-arm radial maze in which a fixed set of arms were baited before each trial and others were never baited (Fig. 13–22B). Following pretraining as normal animals, these investigators found that fornix-lesioned rats were impaired in remembering to avoid repeat entries into arms from which they had collected the available food but were as successful as the sham-lesioned animals in avoiding the arms that were never baited. Essentially the same results were obtained whether the baited arms were arranged adjacent to each other or were mixed haphazardly with the never-baited arms. This finding conflicts with the cognitive map theory, as neither a disturbance of spatial representation nor of navigation can explain the dissociation between failure to avoid repeat entries into the initially baited arms and successful avoidance of the never-baited arms.

Olton et al. (1979) therefore argued for a distinction between the anatomical mediation of "working memory" (i.e.,

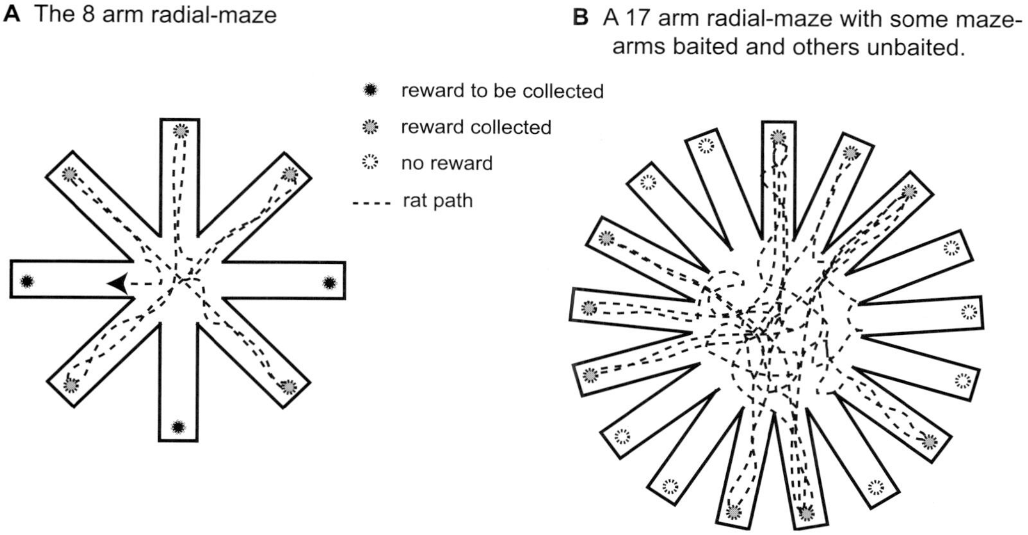

A The 8 arm radial-maze

B A 17 arm radial-maze with some maze-arms baited and others unbaited.

    ✳ reward to be collected

    ✳ reward collected

    ✳ no reward

   - - - - rat path

Figure 13–22. Radial maze. **A.** The eight-arm radial maze is a task in which rats run from a central region to collect food reward from the ends of the maze arms. The path shown is of a rat that has successfully made five choices without retracing its path and has three arms remaining where food is available (notional path data). **B.** A 17-arm radial maze with baited and unbaited arms. The path shown might be that of a fornix-lesioned rat, initially trained preoperatively, that is selectively visiting the maze arms that are always baited, making occasional repeat errors at these arms but successfully avoiding the maze arms that are never baited. (*Source*: After Olton and Papas, 1979.)

memory required for only one trial) and "reference memory" (i.e., memory used for a series of trials). They proposed that in radial maze tasks in which some arms are baited and some unbaited, the animal uses working memory to keep track of which arms it had entered as the trial proceeds and reference memory to avoid entries down arms that never contained food. Olton's insistence on thinking about reference and working memory as independent rather than interacting memory systems carries with it the implication that the animal is reading out from two memory systems simultaneously as it works its way from choice point to choice point —a prescient idea, as many behavioral tasks are likely to involve multiple memory systems. In any event, if the hippocampus is involved exclusively in working memory, not only could this account for the data it also implies that there may be a subset of allocentric spatial tasks for which the integrity of the hippocampal formation is not required—spatial reference memory tasks.

The results of the Olton et al. (1979) study were, on the face of it, damaging to the cognitive map theory; but several problems soon became apparent. First, Olton examined a variety of lesions but, strangely, never looked at discrete hippocampal lesions. Second, there is nothing to stop rats choosing adjacent arms in the standard radial maze, thereby performing perfectly without having to remember anything about the spatial layout of the maze. The path shown in Figure 13–22A indicates that our notional rat did not do this, but many radial maze studies ran into this problem. It was solved by placing doors between the central area and the maze arms that prevented successive left or right turns by allowing the experimenter to control the timing of the animals' choices. However,

even with doors, it is unclear whether a spatial map is guiding successive choices in this task (Brown, 1992; Brown et al., 1993). Third, in the Olton et al. (1979) study, the animals were initially trained as normal animals and were lesioned only after asymptotic performance had been reached. This training arrangement leaves open the possibility that the integrity of the hippocampal formation is required for the initial learning of which arms to avoid but perhaps not required for retention. Using animals that had undergone surgery prior to training, a series of studies by Jarrard (1978, 1986) established that the initial learning of place reference-memory in an eight-arm radial maze task in which four arms were never baited is consistently impaired by both complete hippocampal aspiration lesions and by more selective ibotenic acid lesions of the hippocampus and dentate gyrus. These studies were important for introducing the most selective type of hippocampal lesion that has yet been developed. In the process, the cognitive map theory was partially salvaged as the integrity of the hippocampus is required for initial learning. However, the long-term storage of information about which arms are baited or unbaited may be outside the hippocampal formation (Barnes, 1988). The theme that the hippocampal formation may be required for the initial learning of a spatial task with eventual storage in the cortex is one that recurs in many tasks, including the next one we consider.

Watermaze

Further evidence that the integrity of the hippocampal formation is essential for allocentric spatial reference memory came with the introduction of the watermaze (Morris, 1981).

Box 13–5
Watermaze

The watermaze has become one of the most widely used tasks in behavioral neuroscience. It was developed to study spatial learning and memory but is now often used as a general assay of cognitive function for testing new drugs or other treatments of the nervous system.

The basic task is simple. Animals, usually rats and mice, are required to escape from water onto a hidden platform whose location can normally be identified only using spatial memory. There are no local cues indicating where the platform is located. Conceptually, the task derives from "place cells," as these cells also identify points in space that cannot be defined in relation to local cues. This simple water escape task is then embedded into a variety of sometimes quite complicated training and testing protocols to investigate specific theoretical issues.

APPARATUS

The apparatus consists of a large circular pool, generally 1.5 to 2.0 m in diameter, containing water at around 25°C made opaque by adding milk or other substance (e.g., latex) that helps hide the submerged platform. The water in the pool is filled and drained daily via an automated filling and draining system. The choice of water temperature, around 13°C below body temperature, is sufficiently stressful to motivate the animals to escape but insufficiently stressful to inhibit learning. There is a stress reaction (corticosterone release) on day 1 of training, but this habituates over days. If the pool temperature drops to 19°C, performance improves, but when it drops to 12°C, it gets worse, reflecting the inverse U-shaped function relating stress to cognitive function. The pool is located in a laboratory room with distinctive two- and three-dimensional distal cues that aid orientation or surrounded with hanging curtains that occlude these room cues. Cues may then be hung inside the curtains so they can be rotated relative to the room when this degree of experimental control is required. A video camera is placed above the center of the pool to capture images of the swimming animal and is connected to a video or DVD recorder and an online computer system running specialized tracking software. The top surface of the hidden platform, usually about 10 to 15 cm in diameter and thus between 1/50th and 1/100th of the surface area of the pool, is 1.5 cm below the water surface (Fig.13–23A).

PROTOCOLS

"Reference memory" protocols have been widely used in which the platform is in a fixed location relative to the room cues across trials and days. The animals are placed in the water at and facing the side walls of the pool at different start positions across trials, and they quickly learn to swim to the correct location with decreasing escape latencies and more direct swim paths (Fig. 13–23B). The tracking system measures the gradually declining escape latency across trials and parameters such as path length, swim speed, directionality in relation to platform location, and so on. Observation of the animals reveals that, having climbed onto the escape platform, they often rear up and look around, as if trying to identify their location in space. Rearing habituates over trials but then dishabituates if the hidden platform is moved to a new location.

Figure 13–23. Watermaze. *A*. Axonometric drawing of a typical watermaze setup with overhead video-camera and rat swimming to find the hidden platform. *B*. Representative escape latency graph and swim paths across various stages of training: initial swimming at the side walls, then circuitous paths across the area of the pool, and finally directed path navigation. *C*. The hidden platform is removed for posttraining probe tests. Whereas normal or sham-lesioned controls swim to the target quadrant (NE, within dotted gray lines), rats with hippocampus, subiculum, or combined lesions do not. (*Source*: After Morris et al., 1990.) *D*. Overtraining of hippocampus-lesioned rats can result in quite focused search patterns during a probe test. (*Source*: After Morris et al., 1990.) *E*. Atlantis platform. The hidden platform is at the bottom of the pool where the swimming rat cannot bump into it by chance. Online automated data capture of swim paths is used to determine whether the rat swims within a virtual zone around the platform's location, raising the platform to within 1.5 cm of the water surface when a criterion is reached. This protocol trains highly focused search patterns. (*Source*: After Spooner et al., 1994.) *F*. Reversible hippocampal inactivation with a glutamate antagonist during training (encoding) or at retention (retrieval) results in poor probe test performance compared to the controls, which have the hippocampus working continuously. Analysis of the search patterns show that rats trained with the hippocampus "on" during encoding, but "off" at retrieval display searching at the wrong location in the pool, as quantified using zone analysis. (*Source*: After Riedel et al., 1999.)

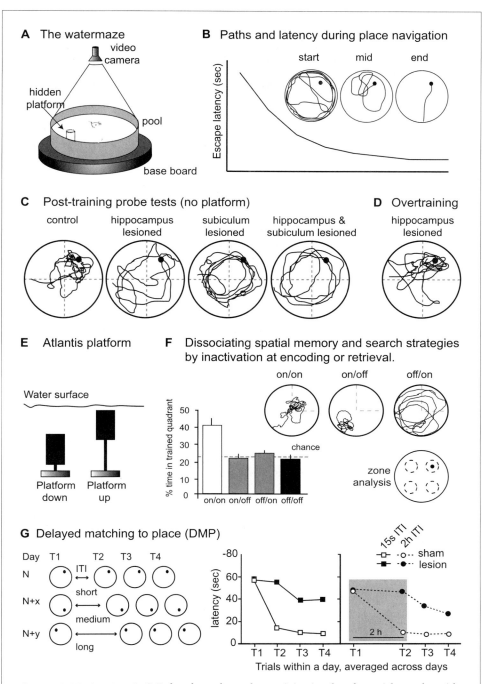

Figure 13–23. *(Continued)* *G.* Delayed match-to-place training involves four trials per day with the location of the hidden platform moved between days. Training can continue indefinitely with this protocol, enabling within-subject drug manipulations throughout the life-span and averaging across days. Acquisition typically takes 8 to 10 days. For trial 1 of each day, the animals search for the platform, typically taking 60 seconds to find it, and encode its location; they then show fast escape latencies during trials 2 to 4. Hippocampus-lesioned rats cannot learn this task irrespective of the intertrial interval (ITI) between trials 1 and 2. The shaded zone shows the ITI between T1 and T2 extended to 2 hours. (*Source:* After Steele and Morris, 1999.)

(Continued)

Box 13–5
Watermaze (Continued)

During or after training is complete, the experimenter conducts a probe trial in which the escape platform is removed from the pool, and the animal is allowed to swim for 60 seconds. Typically, a well trained rat swims to the target quadrant of the pool and repeatedly across the former location of the platform until it starts to search elsewhere (Fig. 13–23C). This spatial bias, measured in various ways, constitutes evidence for spatial memory. Rats with lesions of the hippocampus and dentate gyrus, subiculum, or combined lesions, do poorly in posttraining probe tests.

However, if rats with hippocampal lesions are given "overtraining" (typically consisting of a large number of trials over many days), performance can improve in probe tests. Even rats with hippocampal lesions can show quite localized searching (Fig. 13–23D).

Numerous other protocols have been developed to test specific hypotheses. Many involve cryptically moving the hidden platform. This might be a "reversal" procedure in which, after one location has been thoroughly trained the platform is moved to a different quadrant of the pool. Because it is hidden, it is not apparent that anything has changed until the animal fails to find the platform in its usual place. The focus is on how the animal reacts to this change and how quickly it learns the new location. The relearning that occurs with the reversal protocol has been used in a major "factor analysis" of the determinants of watermaze behavior across strains of mice.

As the animals sometimes "bump" into the submerged platform by chance, one useful innovation is an "on-demand" or "Atlantis" platform that is initially at the bottom of the pool and becomes available only when the animal swims in its vicinity for some predetermined time. An automatic release system allows the platform to rise gently to near the surface of the water (it remains hidden). This procedure results in acquisition of a highly focused searching strategy that focused on the target location during training. Reversible inactivation of the hippocampus with a drug that blocks excitatory neurotransmission after the training is completed results in animals displaying localized searching at inappropriate places in the pool. Pharmacological inactivation during training results in failure to develop this search strategy because the animals cannot learn the place at which to execute the strategy in the pool (Fig. 13–23E). The accuracy of the searching can also be measured using a zone analysis that measures time spent in a virtual zone around the place where the platform is located.

With other protocols, the platform can be moved to a new location each day, creating what is called the "delayed matching to place" (DMP) procedure (Fig. 13–23F). The animal cannot know, with this procedure, where the platform is hidden on trial 1 of each day; it can only search for it. However, if it can encode this new location in one trial, the animal finds the platform much faster during trial 2 and subsequent trials of that day. The memory delay interval between trials 1 and 2 (ITI) can then be systematically varied to explore how well one-trial spatial memory is remembered, a procedure with some similarities to delayed matching and nonmatching tasks used to examine recognition memory. Rats with complete hippocampal lesions cannot show the rapid, one-trial learning required for the DMP task and are just as poor at a short ITI between trials 1 and 2 as a long one (Fig. 13–23G). Treatment with an NMDA antagonist such as D-AP5 results in a selective deficit in memory at a long ITI, but the animals can learn with short memory intervals between trials (see Chapter 10, Section 10.9).

Other variants include alterations to the apparatus, such as constraining the path of the swimming animal to minimize navigational demands (e.g., an annular watermaze), decreasing the number of available extramaze cues between training and testing to look at pattern completion, the use of floating platforms, and yet other manipulations. A radial watermaze has also been introduced, combining the virtues of the radial maze with the ease of training to escape from water. This has proved invaluable for testing transgenic mice expressing familial Alzheimer mutations.

TREATMENTS AND CONTROLS

A wide variety of treatments have been explored including lesions, drugs, and molecular-genetic alterations. They alter watermaze "performancez" in various ways, but experimenters must be cautious, as such alterations need not be specific deficits (or improvements) in spatial learning or memory processes per se. Lesions or drugs may have a direct effect on learning mechanisms, and many seem to do so, but they may also affect an animal's ability to see the extramaze cues or their motivation to escape from the water rather than learning per se. Factor analytical studies reveal that many molecular-genetic alterations influence the probability of mice to stay at the side walls (thigmotaxis) instead of swimming into the center of the pool and that this effect is statistically independent of spatial memory.

Accordingly, treatments must be accompanied by relevant control conditions. A common protocol is to include trials in which the escape platform is made visible, the idea being that treatments that merely affect motivation to escape should impair performance in this task as well as the basic task. It is unclear how sensitive this assay is, but it does provide a first pass at detecting gross sensorimotor abnormalities. As blind rats have been claimed to do surprisingly well in the watermaze (except in probe trials), other psychophysical techniques have been introduced offering precise control of the spatial frequency of cues that are more sensitive to subtle visual deficits. The use of sham-lesioned animals, vehicle-infusion conditions, "floxed" mice, and other pertinent manipulations has also become widespread to ensure that any alterations in spatial learning in the experimental group are not an unintended by-product of achieving the treatment.

WATERMAZE AS AN ASSAY

As our understanding of the impact of various treatments has developed, the watermaze has gradually been subsumed into test batteries and assays for investigating aspects of brain function other than just hippocampal function. This is a strength of the assay but also an analytical weakness. The task is so sensitive to manipulations of normal brain function in many brain areas, not just the hippocampus, that it can be used almost like a "litmus test" of the "normality" of brain function. This is valuable, as it brings behavioral observations of function into fields of neuroscience that have historically relied exclusively on stress (corticosterone release), neuropathology (stroke research), biochemical analyses (Alzheimer's disease), or electrophysiology (development of cognitive enhancing drugs). The analytical weakness is that a task affected by such a wide variety of treatments is gradually being revealed as having less "specificity" than was once believed.

Innovation in the development of new training protocols is enabling the simplicity and speed of learning to escape from water to be retained in the arsenal of behavioral tools at the disposal of neuroscientists. Arguably, the watermaze illustrates both themes of this book: (1) a tool to study hippocampal function and (2) an illustration of how studies of hippocampal function have had a wide impact on neuroscience in general.

SELECTED REFERENCES

Morris, 1981, 1984; Sutherland and Dyck, 1984; Brandeis et al., 1989; Good and Morris, 1994; Nunn et al., 1994; Whishaw and Jarrard, 1996; Gallagher and Rapp, 1997; Lindner et al., 1997; Sandi et al., 1997; Lipp and Wolfer, 1998; Morgan et al., 2000; Prusky et al., 2000a; D'Hooge and De Deyn, 2001.

Morris et al. (1982) trained rats to find a hidden escape platform in a circular pool of opaque water. Some had been subjected to "hippocampal" aspiration lesioning (damaging the hippocampus, dentate gyrus, and subiculum), others cortical control lesioning (damaging the same small amount of cortical tissue in the region of the parietal cortex as was necessarily damaged when making the hippocampal lesion), or no surgery (unoperated control). The cortical "control" lesion was included in this and many other early rat studies (in contrast to the monkey work discussed in Section 13.3). In the watermaze, both the normal *and* the cortical tissue-lesioned groups quickly learned to swim toward the hidden platform from any starting location; only the hippocampus-lesioned group was impaired in executing directed swim-paths. Performance during a posttraining probe test showed that both control groups swam persistently across the exact spot where the platform had been located during training, a pattern of behavior that could not occur during training and was arguably reminiscent of "free recall." In contrast, the hippocampus-lesioned group swam all over the pool. The deficit in escape latency disappeared when the platform was made visible, indicating that the impaired place navigation was unlikely to be secondary to any change in motivation to escape from the water and reappeared when it was subsequently hidden again. Similar results were obtained in the first study to use neurotoxic lesions in the watermaze by Sutherland et al. (1983), investigators who were primarily responsible for popularizing the task (Box 13–5).[†]

Over the years since the watermaze was developed, there have been numerous replications of the deficit in place-navigation learning caused by hippocampal lesions. Other pertinent findings concern the impact of lesions to structures afferent or efferent to the hippocampus and of fiber pathways interconnecting these structures, as comprehensively reviewed

[†]There have been differences in opinion about the name "watermaze" for an apparatus that is not obviously a maze. Some describe it as a "water task," others as a "milk bath," and many use an acronym "MWM." The use of the term "maze" is appropriate, as it is an apparatus in which the animal has to find its way around—and that is what one does in a maze. By analogy, golfers play on a "golf course" not "golf fields."

by D'Hooge and De Deyn (2001). For example, deficits in place navigation have been reported after selective lesions of the entorhinal cortex (Schenk and Morris, 1985), perforant path (Skelton and McNamara, 1992), dentate gyrus (Sutherland et al., 1983), area CA1 (Nunn et al., 1994), medial septum (Hagan et al., 1988; Kelsey and Landry, 1988), fornix (Morris, 1983), and subiculum (Taube et al., 1992). Deficits are generally seen only after bilateral lesions. The overwhelming consensus is that the integrity of the hippocampal formation and its afferent and efferent connections is essential for the acquisition and/or consolidation of normal, appropriately directed spatial navigation.

However, as with the radial maze, further study has revealed lesion dissociations that are not predicted by the cognitive map theory and point to a functional heterogeneity that underlies normal performance. Dysfunction in a variety of structures has an impact on performance, notably damage to neocortical structures such as the retrosplenial and parietal cortices, frontal cortex, basal forebrain, striatum, and cerebellum—an issue addressed in the critique below. A problem with the watermaze is that its procedural simplicity belies an underlying complexity with respect to the numerous sensorimotor and cognitive processes that, in practice, it engages. That it has been classified as a "spatial memory task" should not lull users into believing that other sensorimotor and cognitive processes are not involved. It would be tidy if the impact of lesions or other dysfunctions of distinct brain areas or neurotransmitter systems is isomorphic to the spatial mapping or navigation processes identified within the theory, but the data point to a more complex picture in which the hippocampus engages with other brain structures to mediate effective performance.

Before considering navigation in the watermaze in detail, it should be noted that many dry-land place-finding tasks have also been developed, including the earlier Barnes arena task first developed in the context of studies linking hippocampal LTP to spatial learning (Barnes, 1979), a place preference task in which rats are systematically rewarded by intracranial brain stimulation for visiting a particular location (Fukuda et al., 1992), similar appetitive place preference tasks (Rossier et al., 2000), and a place avoidance task. These tasks are conceptually similar but, being on dry land, the animal can stop moving and is also more likely to use olfactory and somatosensory (vibrissa) cues. This is likely to make them less dependent on visual cues than the watermaze. With place avoidance, the mirror image of place navigation, animals are trained stay *away* from a location to avoid the punishment of mild footshock (Bures et al., 1998). Place avoidance has been used extensively to examine the differential role of allocentric versus ideothetic cues in location learning by allowing the circular arena to rotate slowly in relation to extramaze cues. Rats can be successfully trained to avoid a sector defined in relation to room cues or in relation to its location on the rotating arena. An interesting commercial twist on place navigation and place avoidance is incorporated into modern robot vacuum cleaners, a good example of a biologically inspired artifi-

cial navigation system (Trullier et al., 1997). These machines clean the floor as they work their way around a living space and typically incorporate two key features of spatial memory. They "remember" where in the room to go to get their battery recharged and to avoid recleaning places that they have already moved across.

Varied Training Protocols Reveal the Importance of the Dorsal Hippocampus for Spatial Navigation

A key distinction regarding the watermaze is between thinking of it as an *apparatus* and as a *task*. Sometimes described as the latter, it is really an apparatus in which a wide variety of training protocols can be carried out to address specific issues. Some modifications have come into widespread use, others not. One was a modification of the original spatial reference memory protocol (Morris et al., 1986a) that for various reasons was not taken up by other laboratories. It involves training rats to choose between two visible platforms, one of which is rigid and offers escape from the water, the other floating and so offers insufficient buoyancy for escape. Local-cue and spatial versions of this task were compared. Hippocampal lesions impair the spatial task but have no effect on the procedurally similar cue task. In many respects this is a more rigorous test of the dissociation between locale and taxon strategies proposed in the cognitive map theory than the comparison between the hidden and visible platforms of the "standard" watermaze task because it compares two tasks of comparable difficulty. It also removes the "recall" element of the standard procedure because the navigational demands are minimized and the animal need only approach either platform and then use spatial recognition to decide whether it or the other platform is associated with escape. Interestingly, the hippocampus-lesioned group displayed first-choice performance that, starting at 50%, gradually rose above chance. The effect was not large, but it was both detectable and statistically significant—a first suggestion that allocentric place navigation is possible after hippocampal dysfunction. One possibility is that it is easier in this task to bridge temporally discontiguous gaps in the processing of relevant sensory information (Rawlins, 1985).

Although a consensus emerged that the standard hidden platform reference memory version of watermaze spatial navigation is a "hippocampal task"—being easy to train and producing reliable, replicable results in different laboratories—the impact of such lesions is more variable than many may appreciate. First, the sensitivity of the "cue task" (which is unimpaired by hippocampal lesions) has been called into question following the observation that rats with experimentally reduced visual acuity display impaired place navigation but are unimpaired in the cue task (Prusky et al., 2000b). This dissociation falsely masquerades as a deficit in place learning. Although a nice "proof-of-principle," it is unlikely that hippocampal lesions cause any change in visual acuity. However, regionally nonselective transgenic manipulations and many peripherally administered drugs may affect visual acuity. Psychophysical procedures have therefore been introduced to provide a more rigorous test of sensory acuity than the cue task (Prusky et al., 2000a; Robinson et al., 2001), and it would be valuable to see these used with selected transgenic lines. Those with cell- and region-specific mutations are also unlikely to be impaired, but the important lesson that needs to be taken on board from these sensory studies is that caution must be exercised about treating the watermaze as an ostensibly selective assay of memory function. Interestingly, the cue task is impaired by dorsal striatum lesions (McDonald and White, 1994), a sensitivity that is more likely due to the role of this structure in habit learning than any sensory impairment.

Second, as in the two-platform task, some place navigation does take place in rats with hippocampal dysfunction. Using overtraining in the standard, reference-memory single platform procedure, Morris et al. (1990) found that rats with lesions in the hippocampal formation could learn to escape to the platform with short escape latencies after about 80 trials of training. Overtraining never obviated slightly elevated escape latencies relative to those of the controls; but after a mixed series of hidden and visible platform trials, probe test performance was spatially focused in the correct training quadrant and quantitatively indistinguishable from that of the controls (Fig. 13–23D). This slow, incremental spatial learning was apparent in animals with hippocampal or subiculum lesions, whereas those with combined hippocampus and subiculum lesions failed to learn despite extensive overtraining. Eichenbaum et al. (1990) also showed incremental learning in rats given fornix lesions when the animals were consistently trained from a single location. Probe test performance was, however, sensitive to the use of novel starting locations around the pool. Animals subjected to retrohippocampal lesioning that encompassed the region of the entorhinal cortex containing the entorhinal grid cells also showed gradually improving probe test performance, but analysis of the paths taken revealed accuracy in swimming across the correct platform location but little indication of "recognizing" that this was the correct place to stop and search (Schenk and Morris, 1985). However, not all studies have observed effects of entorhinal lesions on spatial reference memory in the watermaze (Bannerman et al., 2001), raising the possibility of functional heterogeneity across the medial, intermediate, and lateral regions of the entorhinal cortex. A key issue may be whether such lesions encroach on the dorsal region containing the grid cells (Hafting et al., 2005).

A third important issue, first raised by Andersen in relation to the "lamella theory" of hippocampal information processing (Andersen et al., 1971, 2000), is how much hippocampal tissue is actually required for learning or retention. This was a fresh way of looking at the impact of lesions on function—focusing less on whether a lesion causes a *deficit* than if normal performance *is still possible* with a partial lesion of a specific size. Moser et al. (1993) discovered that aspiration lesions of the ventral hippocampus that leave only small "minislabs" of dorsal hippocampus intact allow normal learning. In contrast, lesions of the dorsal hippocampus that left the ventral hippocampus apparently intact did not. They suggested that a relatively small number of lamellae in the dorsal hippocampus, if adequately connected to entorhinal cortex, the septum, and other brain regions, were sufficient for learning. A follow-up study using ibotenic acid lesions confirmed these findings (Moser et al., 1995). The second study was conducted because the aspiration lesions of the original study may have inadvertently left the ventral hippocampus deafferented, and thus the apparent dissociation between dorsal and ventral hippocampus could have been an artifact. In fact, similar results were obtained with as little as 27% of dorsal hippocampus being required for normal spatial learning that was indistinguishable from that shown by sham-lesioned controls (Fig. 13–24). In parallel, Jung et al. (1994) observed that the firing fields of place cells were less spatially selective in the ventral hippocampus. Taken together, these observations fit well with anatomical studies of the connectivity between the entorhinal cortex and hippocampus, with particular zones of the dorsomedial entorhinal cortex preferentially projecting to the dorsal (septal) hippocampus of the rat. Detailed anatomical analyses have suggested the concept of "parallel closed loops" as the substrate for both reverberation and the processing of functionally distinct sets of cortical information (Amaral and Witter, 1989; Witter et al., 2000) and of "functional differentiation" along the long axis of the hippocampus (Moser and Moser, 1998b). (For further discussion, see Chapter 3.)

Other studies using the watermaze, T maze alternation, and contextual fear conditioning are consistent with this dorsal-ventral (i.e., septo-temporal) gradation of function (Bannerman et al., 1999; Richmond et al., 1999). The search for a specific function for the ventral hippocampus has included a return to J.A. Gray's ideas about a possible role in fear and anxiety (Bannerman et al., 2004). For example, Kjelstrup et al. (2002) found that rats with selective lesions located in the ventral pole of the hippocampus were less fearful on an elevated cross maze and showed decreased neuroendocrine stress responses. These animals did, however, display normal contextual fear conditioning. Bannerman et al. (2002) have also implicated the ventral hippocampus in anxiety as ventrally lesioned animals freeze less to unsignaled foot-shock in a test chamber. They also show less neophagia (the fear of novel foods). However, the notion that the ventral hippocampus is not involved in spatial learning at all can be overstated. De Hoz et al. (2003) observed that changing the reference memory training protocol to one involving fewer trials but over a larger number of days enabled rats with large dorsal hippocampus lesions (i.e., only ventral tissue intact) to learn just as effectively as rats with only spared dorsal tissue, as measured by posttraining probe tests. Similarly, Broadbent et al. (2004) found that ventral hippocampal lesions encompassing approximately 50% of total hippocampal volume can impair spatial memory in a watermaze reference memory task. Thus, the dorsal/ventral distinction is not clear-cut.

A   Search patterns during probe tests of representative animals with partial or complete lesions

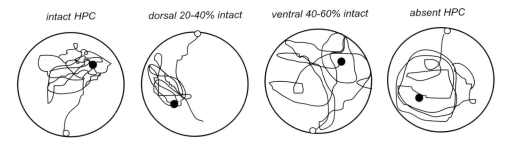

B   Relation between size of residual tissue and performance during the probe test

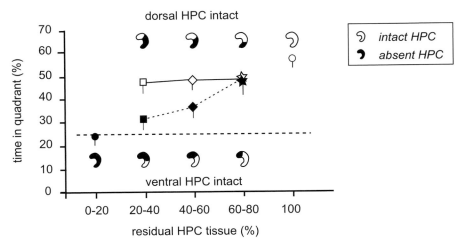

Figure 13–24. Partial lesions reveal a dissociation of function along the longitudinal axis of the hippocampus. *A.* After training by animals with spared tissue volumes of different sizes that began at different ends of the longitudinal axis of the hippocampus, posttraining probe tests (hidden platform absent) revealed a graded change in animals in which only ventrally located tissue was intact but good performance in animals with dorsal tissue. *B.* Quantitative assessment of the probe tests show near-normal performance of rats with as little as 20% to 40% of the dorsal hippocampus intact. *Inset.* Parasagittal diagrams of the hippocampus show the locations of intact (white) and lesioned (black) tissue along the longitudinal axis. (*Source*: After Moser et al., 1995.)

A fourth important issue is asymmetry in the impact of lesion size on initial acquisition versus retention. Retention is more sensitive. If normal rats are trained in the watermaze and then given small lesions of the mid- or ventral hippocampus immediately after training, memory retention is impaired. However, such lesions have no effect on learning or later retention when given before training (Moser and Moser, 1998a). This dissociation is paradoxical from the perspective of thinking about the hippocampus as a distributed associative memory system (Rolls and Treves, 1998) because such systems are generally robust in the face of partial damage. However, the finding is not necessarily incompatible with such a perspective if encoding and trace storage takes place across an extended region of the longitudinal axis in normal rats. Animals given lesions before training would use the remaining tissue, and normal learning should occur provided there was enough of it. Small lesions created after training may indeed damage only a small proportion of the synaptic storage sites but may nonetheless interrupt inputs to and outputs from such sites, even when neurotoxic lesions are used.

To test this idea more rigorously, Steffenach et al. (2002) investigated whether the integrity of the longitudinal-association pathway of CA3 pyramidal cells is critical for integrating such distributed information. In animals previously trained as normal rats in the standard reference memory task, a single transversely oriented cut of no more than 3% of the hippocampal volume was made bilaterally through the dorsal CA3 region (the lesion shown in Figure 13–1, panel 5B). Memory retention was impaired. These knife cuts inevitably damage cells as well as possibly some Schaffer collaterals coursing to CA1, but no impairment was observed in controls deliberately given small, equivalent-sized neurotoxic lesions of CA3 cells but leaving the longitudinal fibers intact. This study is unusual amongst behavioral studies in using FluoroJade tract-tracing to observe degenerating fibres on either side of the cut.

Taken together, these studies led by the Trondheim group have definitively established that the efficient acquisition and retention of spatial memory requires only a small "minislab" of hippocampal tissue, preferentially although not exclusively in the dorsal hippocampus. The integrity of longitudinally oriented, translamellar connections of CA3 pyramidal cells in this minislab is essential for normal functioning. It is not yet known if this is a deficit in memory retrieval or consolidation, but varying the interval after initial training before the longitudinal cut is made would be one way of investigating this question (see discussion of memory consolidation below).

Spatial Recognition Does Not Require CA3 Cells

If cognitive mapping involves both spatial representation and navigation, the question arises of whether different parts of the hippocampal formation are involved in recognizing a place versus navigating to it. Using a modification of the watermaze that involved changing it to no more than a circular swimming track, Brun et al. (2002) have shown that CA3 lesions can leave CA1 place cell firing fields and spatial recognition intact. Rats were intensively trained to swim in an annular watermaze for a hidden platform that could rise from the bottom of the pool at a specific location once the animals had completed two or three laps of the pool. They displayed "knowledge" of this potentially safe place in the pool by hesitating or by swimming more slowly there during the successive laps. Complete CA3 lesions leave this "spatial recognition" intact, while complete lesions of the hippocampus impair this ability (just as they impair navigation in the open pool). This finding complements the further finding that CA1 place cells can be normal in rats with CA3 lesions, which points to the importance of the direct pathway from layer III of the entorhinal cortex into CA1 (Brun et al., 2002). Taken together with the study of Steffenach et al. (2002), there is therefore a double dissociation, reflecting the importance of the longitudinal connections in CA3 for navigation and the direct perforant path input to CA1 for spatial recognition. It would, nonetheless, also be valuable to damage the cells of origin of the layer III input to investigate the impact on CA1 place cell firing and, if the lesion could made be large enough while remaining selective (a tall order), on behavior as well.

Place Cells, Head-direction Cells, and Navigation

Although these lesion studies indicate that the integrity of at least part of the hippocampus is necessary for spatial navigation, it does not require that place and head-direction units are the critical neural mediators of navigation. Indirect evidence that these cells are important has come from a number of studies in which pharmacological or genetic manipulations cause alterations in both place cell firing and spatial learning (Mizumori et al., 1994; Wilson and Tonegawa, 1997; Kentros et al., 1998; Rotenberg et al., 2000; Cooper and Mizumori, 2001). However, an alternative possibility is that these cells only provide information about current location and direction, and other still unidentified cells mediate the representation of goals and carry out the information processing responsible for navigational choices—the problem identified in Figure 13–16B. Such cells may or may not be located in the hippocampal formation.

Prompted by tantalizing observations on the relation between place cells and navigation by O'Keefe and Speakman (1987) and their dependence on the spatial reference frames used by the animals for specific tasks (Gothard et al., 1996; Zinyuk et al., 2000), Poucet and colleagues embarked on a systematic research program to identify whether the firing of place cells is critical for navigational decisions and goal identification (Lenck-Santini et al., 2001, 2002). As behavioral and cell firing had to be obtained simultaneously, they began by returning to the use of traditional mazes. The principle guiding this work was that altering place cell firing fields by rotating or otherwise changing environmental cues should also be associated with systematic changes in navigational behavior if place cell firing and navigation are causally related.

Lenck-Santini et al. (2001) trained rats in a continuous spatial alternation task on a Y maze. One arm of the maze (G) served as the goal where food could be obtained. The animal had to alternate its visits to the other arms (A, B) to secure food in G. Thus, the correct sequence would be A → G* → B → G* → A → G* → B and so on that secured reward (*) upon every visit to G, whereas an incorrect sequence might be A → G* → A → G, which did not (Fig. 13–25). This incorrect sequence was classified as an "alternation error" because the animal returned to A when it should have gone to B. A different, and initially much rarer, sequence might be A → G* → B → A in which, having correctly alternated between A and B after a visit to the goal, the animal then returned to A instead of going back to the goal. This was called an "orientation error." A prominent cue card was located on one side of the maze. Once all the animals were trained and performing well (around 80% correct choices), a total of 47 single units were recorded while the animals continued to run on the maze. Various manipulations of the cue card (rotation, removal) were systematically made to observe the impact on both place cell firing and behavior. As expected, the probability of correct alternation sequences declined during these manipulations; but more importantly, they did so in a systematic way. Pairs of recording/behavior sessions were compared. The second session of each pair was categorized as a "consistent" session when the location of a place field on the Y maze relative to the goal arm was the same as during the first session; it was categorized as "inconsistent" when the cue manipulation between the pairs of sessions caused some shift in the relative location of the place field to the goal. Behavioral choice performance was significantly poorer on inconsistent sessions. Moreover, an analysis of the kinds of errors made by the animals indicated that alternation errors occurred occasionally on consistent sessions, whereas inconsistent sessions were characterized by a striking increase in orientation errors. These findings indicate that the locations of place fields in a learned spatial navigation task are relevant to performance. Inconsistent place fields were statistically associated with disorganized spatial behavior. Similar observations were also made by Dudchenko and Taube (1997) with respect to head-direction cells.

In a follow-up study, Lenck-Santini et al. (2002) attempted to compare the value of correct place cell firing in a "locale"

The relationship between the spatial firing of CA1 cells and spatial navigation

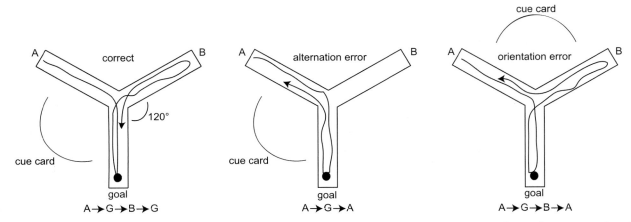

Figure 13–25. Relation between place cell firing and spatial navigation. Rats from whom CA1 cell recordings were made simultaneously were trained to alternate on a Y maze such that the correct order of arms would be A to Goal, then B, then back to Goal, and so on (A → G → B → G, and so on) (left panel). With the cue card in its training position, errors occurred rarely but when they did occur tended to be alternation errors (middle panel). However, when the cue card was rotated (as shown) or removed or the goal location was rotated, orientation errors increased in frequency. They occurred when the cells were induced to display place fields that became out of register to their standard positions. (*Source*: After Lenck-Santini et al., 2001.)

task that required spatial memory with that in a "taxon" task that did not. They reasoned, in keeping with the cognitive map theory, that inappropriate place fields induced by cue manipulations should have a greater effect on behavior in the locale task. They used a place preference task, one of the appetitive analogues of the watermaze (Rossier et al., 2000), in which rats search around a large circular arena for food they receive if they enter a virtual circular zone located at one particular position in the arena (the food drops into the zone from a hidden feeder above—a scientific version of "manna from heaven"). In animals from which place cell recordings were being taken simultaneously, this task was conducted in one of three ways: with the virtual zone defined as at a distance from a cue card at the periphery of the arena, with it placed adjacent to the cue card, and with the zone defined by a local cue explicitly outlining its area. The key finding was that certain manipulations, such as visibly rotating the cue card while the animal was in the apparatus, created shifts between the expected location of the virtual zone as defined by the animal's place fields and by the now rotated cue card. In brief situations of ambiguity (a few minutes), most rats searched in a region defined by the various place fields that were being recorded rather than as determined by the now rotated cue card. This did not occur in the taxon task when the zone was adjacent to the cue card or visibly identifiable by local cues. Poucet et al. (2003) argued that spatial searching behavior correlates well with place firing fields only when the rat is likely to be using a place navigation strategy. Data showing a correlation between the ability of an animal to find a goal on a linear track and the alignment of place fields with salient room cues is consistent with Poucet's interpretation (Rosenzweig et al., 2003). Place firing fields, however, may be maintained in a taxon task when ani-

mals alternate between locale and taxon tasks (Trullier et al., 1999).

However, as noted by Jeffery (2003), the findings of these studies are only correlational. Experiments in which neural representations of location (e.g., place fields) are manipulated directly, rather than indirectly via environmental manipulations, are required to provide a yet more rigorous test of the role of place cells in mediating behavior. It is not obvious, however, how this might be done. Dudchenko (2003) took the same view with respect to head-direction cells and suggested that selective disconnection lesions might be a way of teasing apart cause and effect.

Knowing Where, Getting There, and the Puzzle of Hippocampal Involvement in Path Integration

The term "spatial navigation" has been unpacked in various ways. The original theory made only a binary distinction between locale and taxon processing during navigation, as if there are only two ways to get from A to B. However, evolution has discovered numerous other ways to navigate, ranging from "path integration" to "local views" (Benhamou, 1997; Biegler, 2000; Rodrigo, 2002). Inspired in part by ideas relating the hippocampal theta rhythm to aspects of movement monitoring and control (Vanderwolf et al., 1973), a series of studies by Whishaw explored the possibility of functional dissociation in navigation between "getting there" and "knowing where" (Whishaw et al., 1995). They recognized that spatial learning in the watermaze involves both learning the layout of distal cues and the development of navigational strategies to use this learned information. Following the several observations that hippocampus-lesioned rats may be able to acquire spatial information slowly, Whishaw et al (1995) wondered if fimbria-fornix lesions might disrupt only the "getting there" component and not the "knowing where." This line of reasoning was to lead to unraveling the different senses of "getting there."

Although rats with fimbria-fornix lesions normally have a profound deficit in watermaze place navigation when trained to a hidden platform from several starting points, they display several indications of having learned the platform location when trained using a careful shaping procedure. They learn to head in the correct direction, slow their speed of swimming when approaching the vicinity of the platform, and search in the correct quadrant when the platform is removed. Although not as effective as control animals on all measures, there is clear evidence that fimbria/fornix-lesioned animals can learn something about location. However, a substantial deficit reappears when the animals are switched to the delayed matching-to-place (DMP) protocol in which the hidden platform is moved from one location to another between days. Whishaw et al. (1995) suggested that this profile is consistent with disruption of a process associated with getting to a hidden platform, not one of learning its location. This interpretation was backed up by a later study that, following visible platform training from three starting locations around the pool, included probe tests from a novel start location. Once again, fimbria/fornix-lesioned rats swam in the correct direction toward the now hidden platform, implying some knowledge of where it was located. Neither they nor the control rats could do this if vision was temporarily occluded (Whishaw, 1998). In both studies, section of the fimbria-fornix was complete, and the findings were in no way due to partial damage. Whishaw (1998) also drew attention to similar data demonstrating some indication of effective place navigation after prior visible cue training in the studies of Morris et al. (1982). Morris et al. (1990), in contrast, had argued that acquiring a spatial representation that encoded a single escape location might occur slowly in rats with hippocampal lesions, with the "map" stored in the neocortex, provided interference could be minimized. Visible platform training may help in this respect, particularly if many trials are undertaken. Both the "getting there" and the "slow learning" ideas can account for the failure of rapid learning in the DMP protocol in both Whishaw's and Morris's studies. Moreover, the data concerning a novel start location are ambiguous because the experimenter cannot constrain the animals' swimming patterns in the open pool during earlier training. The view from the ostensibly novel start location is likely to be familiar.

The focus by Whishaw (1998) on the "getting there" component of spatial navigation is important. One the many ways of getting from A to B is "path integration" (often called dead-reckoning), a process that has been extensively studied in a variety of animal species (Mittelstaedt and Mittelstaedt, 1982; Wehner et al., 1996; Etienne et al., 1998). Path integration was identified as the evolutionary building block of the "fragments" within the fragment-fitting extension of the cognitive mapping theory in which small parts of space (the fragments) are assembled by an annealing process into a larger map of an

entire area (Worden, 1992). Path integration operates using ideothetic cues (i.e., cues generated during the course of movement) that may be vestibular, kinesthetic, or visual flow in origin. McNaughton et al. (1991) and Bures et al. (1998) have joined Whishaw in emphasizing the importance of path integration to hippocampal function. Redish (1999) shares this view of its importance but places the path integrator outside the hippocampus.

A special case of path integration, referred to as "homing," has been extensively studied in hamsters (Etienne and Jeffery, 2004). It occurs when an animal, having left its nest site to forage for food, somehow keeps a continuous record of the distance and direction it has moved and uses this information to take a relatively direct path back to the nest. This is not a matter of retracing its steps as the paths out may be circuitous, whereas those back are direct. Field studies with desert ants have also revealed the accuracy of this form of home-base navigation and imply that it is an evolutionarily old form of navigation. It solves the problem of getting food and then getting home again without recourse to any "map." Laboratory studies of mammals using rotating arenas, movable nest boxes, and foraging trips in the dark have established that homing can function in total darkness, that it accumulates errors over both time and the circuitous movements of the animal, and that it typically returns the animal to a point near but just short of the home-base by a vector likely to intersect the initial part of the outward path. The animal can then switch to searching using local cues (e.g., olfaction) to find the exact spot of a nest or burrow entrance. As path integration accumulates errors over time, it is not surprising that the vector processor can be "reset" by visual or olfactory cues, such as familiar landmarks or territory-defining odors. In addition, as many rodents are nocturnal and live in burrow systems, a self-motion monitoring system of this kind is likely to be helpful in many situations. Etienne's view is that the neural algorithms used to yield directional and positional information in rodents remain elusive. Path integration capacity develops postnatally, presumably as specific local circuits that process the relevant sensory information become functional, and it is first observed as young pups abandon their sole use of olfactory cues to find the dam in the nest box in favor of forays in the world beyond. Right from the start, the very rapid and very direct return paths they display appear to be guided by path integration.

The idea that the hippocampal formation might be involved in path navigation has been offered by a number of investigators (Wiener, 1993; McNaughton et al., 1996; Bures et al., 1998; Whishaw, 1998). Whishaw and colleagues (Whishaw and Tomie, 1997; Whishaw et al., 2001) trained rats on an arena similar to that used by Etienne in which they spontaneously carried large food pellets back to their next box that was either visible or hidden at the edge of the arena. Search paths from the home-base were circuitous and marked by several pauses as the rats tried to find the cryptic food pellet, but the return path was much more direct. In normal animals, the return paths continued to be direct in the dark, suggesting guidance by a homing vector. However, return paths were clearly disrupted in fimbria/fornix-lesioned animals, which often took circuitous routes around the circumference of the arena and quantitative changes with respect to both direction and velocity. However, data from Alyan and McNaughton (1999) have cast doubt on this finding because rats with hippocampal lesions seem to be able to home accurately in the dark, a finding that led Redish to place the path integration machinery outside the hippocampal formation (Redish, 1999). The precise role of the hippocampus in path integration remains unclear, but the topic has been of considerable interest for neural network modeling (see Chapter 14).

13.4.4 Comparative Studies of Spatial Memory and the Distinction Between Spatial and Associative Learning

The third key feature to highlight about the cognitive map theory is the dual claim (1) that allocentric spatial mapping evolved as a distinct, independent memory system of the vertebrate brain mediated by a specific brain area and (2) that spatial learning is qualitatively distinct from associative learning in that it is rapid, flexible, and uniquely encodes information into map-like representations. These two strands of an "adaptive specialization" hypothesis of hippocampal function (Sherry and Schacter, 1987; Papini, 2002) have been investigated in two contrasting research constituencies: by students of comparative cognition (who are broadly sympathetic) and by general process learning theorists investigating possible differences between spatial and associative learning (who are not).

Comparative Studies Using Avian Species and in Naturalistic Situations

The original cognitive map theory put value on adopting a "neuroethological" as well as a neuropsychological approach to structure/function relations, an aspect reaffirmed by (Nadel, 1991. p. 224). "It is important," he wrote, "to adopt a perspective on brain and behavioral organisation that takes into account ecological, evolutionary and ethological aspects of the animal under study." The argument is that if space is important because "we live in it, move through it, explore it, defend it," there will have been selection pressures of various kinds favoring the evolution of effective cognitive mechanisms for representing and navigating through space. Since 1978, study of the hippocampus in relation to "naturalistic" spatial behavior, in both field settings and the laboratory, has thrown up some striking brain/behavior correlations in several avian and mammalian species.

One finding is that the relative volume of the hippocampus in certain species of passerine birds (e.g., tit species in Britain, chickadees in North America) is larger in the subspecies that store seeds than in those that do not (Krebs et al., 1989; Sherry et al., 1989) (Fig. 13–26A). For example, the hippocampal formation of the food-storing marsh tit is 31% larger than the

non-food-storing great tit, even though the animal and the rest of its forebrain are much smaller. The importance of this correlation between the relative size of the hippocampus and cache recovery derives from the argument of Andersson and Krebs (1978) that food-storing is an evolutionarily stable strategy provided the animal that stores seeds utilizes the privacy of memory to relocate seed caches. Not surprisingly, the alternative strategy of tagging sites with some visible marker to avoid having to use memory is vulnerable to intruders, which then steal the caches. Ingenious field studies of tits in a wood near Oxford using radiolabeled seeds to enable the relocation of nonrecovered caches provided evidence that some kind of location memory is involved (Shettleworth and Krebs, 1982; Shettleworth, 1998). Similar observations were made in corvids that cache in the autumn but do not retrieve until the winter or early spring (Balda and Kamil, 1989). Effective food caching by scatter hoarders therefore relies on memory. A nice feature of this fieldwork is the implied reminder that memory can be allied to "privacy." Like us, there are things animals do and remember and keep to themselves.

Food caching is not an isolated case. Sherry et al. (1992) pointed out that artificial selection among pigeon breeds appears to have had an effect on hippocampal volume similar to that of natural selection among passerine birds—the hippocampus of homing pigeons being larger than that of nonhoming domestic breeds. Studies of brood parasitism are also interesting: Female cowbirds that lay their eggs in the nests of other unsuspecting birds have a larger hippocampus than male cowbirds (Lee et al., 1998). Cowbirds doing this have to seek out and remember the locations of possible nests and then time their egg laying to coincide with that of the host bird. The occurrence of a common neuroanatomical feature in unrelated species ostensibly exposed to similar selection pressures raises the possibility that convergent evolution is responsible—the development of an adaptive specialization.

A potential problem with naturalistic studies is that they can be overly suggestive. As Shettleworth somewhat guardedly put it, "animals show many behaviors for which explanations in terms of human-like understanding readily come to mind: the animal has a cognitive map, a concept, a theory of mind . . . a leap of imagination may be necessary to grasp that behaviors so readily explicable by such intuitively appealing mechanisms are accomplished in completely different ways" (Shettleworth, 2001, p. 279). She and Krebs were among the first to appreciate that field studies had to be followed up, where possible, by rigorous laboratory analogues. They went on to create an avian laboratory setting in which food storing and retrieval could indeed be studied under controlled conditions, confirming the observations of the role of spatial memory in cache recovery first discovered in the wild. A typical avian food-caching laboratory is an indoor room with "trees" where seeds can be hidden (Fig. 13–26B). Such rooms are often described as "large," but they are of course much smaller than the areas over which the birds normally forage in their natural habitat, an issue always to be borne in mind when a

A Relative HPC volume in storers/non-stores

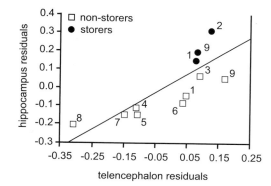

B Laboratory aviary to study food storing

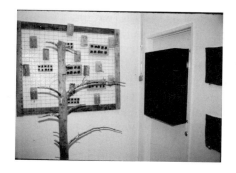

C Spatial memory error over time

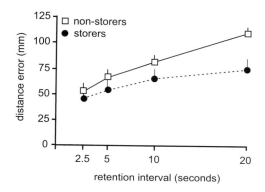

D Development of HPC size with experience

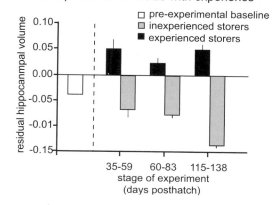

Figure 13–26. Relation between relative hippocampal size and spatial memory in birds. *A.* Study of 35 species or subspecies of passerine birds revealed that hippocampal volume, relative to the rest of the telencephalon (residuals), is larger in storing species. (*Source:* After Krebs et al (1989). *B.* Laboratory aviary used to study storing, window-shopping (see text), and other food-caching protocols in birds. (*Source:* Courtesy of Nicola Clayton.) *C.* Spatial memory is more persistent over time in coal tits (a storing species) than great tits (a nonstoring species). (*Source:* After Biegler et al., 2001). *D.* Relative hippocampal volume at different stages of development. The structure becomes larger if the young marsh tits are allowed to store sunflower seeds (black bars), but it regresses and shows more apoptotic cells if the birds are given powdered seeds that cannot be cached. (*Source:* After Clayton and Krebs, 1995.)

laboratory study yields a null result. Researchers using this kind of facility were faced with the challenge of how to compare cache memory by a species that *does* store seeds with the spatial memory displayed by a species that does *not*. Shettleworth and Krebs did this by creating a paradigm called "window shopping" in which seeds that could be retrieved later were placed "on display" behind Perspex screens in holes drilled into the trees. Thus, during the initial sampling trials, the birds were allowed to fly into the aviary without storing or retrieving—merely to see what was on offer and where. Later, the Perspex screens were removed, and the birds (presumably armed with their credit cards) could fly back and collect what they had seen earlier. In this and other one-trial associative paradigms (Clayton and Krebs, 1995), the act of caching was finessed while still allowing comparisons of spatial memory between storers and nonstorers. Other approaches include operant paradigms with "peck screens" (an avian touchscreen) to cast light on what qualitative aspects of memory might be better with a large hippocampus. In this way, Biegler et al. (2001) found that coal tits (a food-storing species) per-

form better than great tits (a nonstoring species) on a task assessing the persistence of memory over time (from 2.5 to 25 seconds) but not on tasks that assess the fine-grained resolution or, somewhat surprisingly, the capacity of memory (Fig. 13–26C). This is an important reminder that not all parameters of spatial memory are better in storers than nonstorers.

Another question that seminaturalistic studies have made possible concerns the ontogenetic development of the caching-associated difference in hippocampal size. How does experience interact with any genetic predisposition? In a classic study, Clayton (1995) reared juvenile marsh tits (a food-storing species) under conditions in which they were either allowed to store seeds or prevented from doing so (by giving them only powdered food). Tits allowed to store had the usual large hippocampal volume (Fig. 13–26D). However, birds that were prevented from storing showed a gradual decline in hippocampal size and the highest proportion of apoptotic neurons. These findings suggest that hippocampal volume, and perhaps neurogenesis also (Patel et al., 1997), may be partially regulated by activity-dependent factors such as the behavior of the animal, a concept captured by the slogan "use it or lose it." If so, it might be expected that relative volume in a species might also be seasonal. Specifically, the onset of hoarding behavior might the trigger for an increase in volume, with regression later. This has been confirmed in black-capped chickadees (Smulders et al., 1995) and appears to be due to a net increase in cell number (Smulders et al., 2000). The possibility that it is merely due to a general seasonal mechanism operating on both food-storing and nonstoring species is less likely given that seasonal changes in volume have been shown *not* to occur in at least one nonstoring species (Lee et al., 2001). Males of this same species do, however, show changes in the size of song-related nuclei, such as the higher vocal center (HVC) and archistriatum (RA) across the seasons that correlated with song stereotopy. It therefore seems reasonable to infer that changes in the relative volume of the hippocampus of food-storing avian species results from a species-specific and regionally specific form of structural plasticity that occurs in response to seasonal pressures to engage in food-caching and later retrieval. One slightly puzzling finding is that the seasonal variation in size is, in black-capped chickadees, associated with the time of year when caching occurs, but hippocampal volume regresses in the winter—the very time when caches are recovered. Why retrieval places less of a demand on the need for a large hippocampal volume than memory encoding is unclear.

Allometric brain/behavior relations in the avian brain are intriguing, but they are a "chicken and egg" problem! What causes what? Lesion studies were a first step in investigating causal relations, it being essential to check that lesions of the avian hippocampus impaired location memory, just as such lesions do in mammals. These studies confirmed this prediction (Sherry and Vaccarino, 1989). Hampton and Shettleworth (1996) went on to show specificity to location rather than color memory after hippocampal lesions, and work using reversible inactivation in chickadees has both borne out this claim and established that it operates at the time of memory encoding (Shiflett et al., 2003). These and other studies (Columbo et al., 1997) have established that the functional integrity of the avian hippocampus is required for spatial memory (Macphail, 2002), but they do not really nail down whether the variation in the size of the hippocampus is causally related to the very changes in behavior with which they are correlated. Nor is it clear to what aspect of spatial or other information processing the avian hippocampus contributes. Work on homing pigeons has shed light on the second of these issues.

Homing Pigeons Reveal Hippocampus-dependent and Hippocampus-independent Components of Navigation

Homing pigeons have a remarkable ability to fly back to their lofts over long distances from both familiar and unfamiliar release sites. The possible contribution of the hippocampus to homing behavior has been the subject of a comprehensive series of visual-sighting and radio-tracking experiments by a group based in Pisa in Italy over the past two decades. Early studies suggested that the integrity of the hippocampal formation was critical for aspects of the navigation required, particularly near the home loft, but more recent work has pointed to a more complex picture.

Pigeon homing seems to be guided by a multiplicity of strategies and mechanisms, in part because of their need to cope with differing environments and potential variation in weather conditions. When released from an unfamiliar location, experienced homing pigeons fly off with a "vanishing bearing" in the correct direction of home (this being the compass bearing that the bird takes measured from the release site to last sighting after release). To do this, it was suggested by Kramer (cited in Rodrigo, 2002) that they use a "long-range navigational map" that may, at least in Italy, be partly reliant on odors (Papi, 1990). A problem with this concept is that it is far from clear how the pigeons learn such a map. In any event, they also keep flying in the correct direction and have long been thought to have some kind of a "compass" to do it (Schmidt-Koenig, 1961, cited in Gagliardo et al., 1999). Once they approach the vicinity of the loft, they recognize the landmarks and the layout of the area they are used to flying around at home and so find their way back to their perch in the loft. It is not just the loft area that may be spatially familiar; the birds can also learn about the landmarks at familiar release sites and even the roads over which they may fly. Indeed, Italian pigeons stylishly display a classic superiority in matters navigational by following old Roman roads such as the SS Aurelia (Lipp et al., 2004).

The early lesion studies established that pigeons with telencephalic lesions, including the hippocampal formation, have vanishing bearings from an unfamiliar release site that are as accurate as controls (Bingman et al., 1984). Their long-range navigational map is therefore intact. They also reach the vicinity of the loft but sometimes have difficulty finding it—unless they have been given sufficient postoperative experience of the loft vicinity (Bingman et al., 1987). This implies that the "sun compass" can work as well, this having been learned through sightings of the sun at different times of day when outdoors at the loft site. More recent studies have confirmed that the hippocampus plays only a small role in the navigational map. Acquisition and retention is independent of the hippocampus if the birds acquire their navigational map during free flights (Ioale et al., 2000). However, young birds can also learn the navigational map when held in an outdoor aviary. Under these conditions, learning seems to be hippocampus-dependent; but perhaps surprisingly, its retention is not (Gagliardo et al., 2004). The reason for this difference is that hippocampal lesions disrupt the process by which sun compass information is used *only* in the context of new learning (Bingman and Jones, 1994). Use of this compass requires that the animals keep track of time and orient in an appropriate direction to the angle of the sun given the time of day. When "clock-shifted" by being kept on artificial light–dark schedules, the orientational bearing is shifted from the correct homeward direction. Experienced pigeons later subjected to hippocampal lesioning show the usual clock-shift effects, indicating their successful use of the sun compass. However, the hippocampus is necessary for learning to use this sun-compass information.

Landmarks they have learned about at a familiar release site can be used for homing in two distinct ways: "pilotage" in which they use the perceived layout of the landmarks to head toward the loft or "site-specific compass orientation" in which they use the landmarks to recall the sun compass direction in which to fly. Whereas pilotage requires quite a sophisticated spatial representation, site-specific compass orientation does not. Although pigeons with lesions of the hippocampal formation can learn to use familiar landmarks to navigate, it is possible that they do it in only one of these two ways. Gagliardo et al. (1999) studied experienced pigeons rendered anosmic by means of nasal zinc sulfate (a procedure that prevented the use of their navigational map) to compare the manner in which control and lesioned birds used familiar landmarks. As shown in Figure 13–27A, the birds were released on a number of occasions from La Costanza, north of Pisa, and from Livorno, situated southeast of Pisa. Prior to the critical test days, the birds were clock-shifted in their lofts by 6 hours. This should have no effect on the vanishing bearings taken from a release site if the birds use a representation of the spatial layout of the landmarks to find their way home. However, if they use site of the landmarks around each now familiar release site to work out a site-specific compass orientation, a 6-hour clock shift should result in an approximately 120° error in the initial flight direction. The results of test releases from both sites indicated a striking difference between the controls and the birds with hippocampal lesions (Fig. 13–27B). The controls headed in the correct direction, with only a small deviation of 34° in the direction expected given the clock shift; the lesioned birds showed a mean bearing error of 154° in the counterclockwise direction. Thus, the controls were using pilotage, whereas the lesioned birds were not. There is no conflict here with the earlier findings demonstrating that learning to use the sun compass requires the hippocampus because these were experienced homing pigeons that had

learned about the sun compass long before attaining hippocampal lesions. Given the multiplicity of ways that pigeons can navigate, these data represent an unambiguous demonstration of the critical role of the hippocampal formation in landmark learning in a naturalistic setting.

Although ostensibly supporting a close link between spatial memory and hippocampal function, one must recognize that the cytoarchitectonic appearance and intrinsic circuitry of the avian hippocampus is very different from that of the typical mammalian hippocampus described in Chapter 3. There are both similarities and differences between the avian and mammalian brain (Jarvis et al., 2005), but both Lee et al. (1998) and Macphail (2002) make the case—largely on embryological grounds—for the avian hippocampal formation being considered homologous to the hippocampus and dentate gyrus of mammals. Certain arguments seem unconvincing or circumstantial, such as the presence of synaptic plasticity (this also occurs outside the hippocampus) and the claimed similarity in neurotransmitters used (but similar neurotransmitters are used all over the brain in numerous orders of animals). Electrophysiological studies are also equivocal. For example, Bingman et al. (2003) reported some evidence of "space-specific" firing of hippocampal cells in homing pigeons trained in a small plus maze, but the correlate was transitory and less clearly tied to space than in recordings from rats. The possibility remains that greater spatial specificity would be observed in a task in which the pigeons were allowed to engage in homing, but this is not yet technically feasible. One prominent avian behavioral biologist, writing about the pigeon brain, noted that: "the pigeon and rat hippocampal formation reside in different forebrain environments characterized by a wulst and neocortex, respectively. Differences in the forebrain organization of pigeons and rats, and of birds and mammals in general, must be considered in making sense of the possible species differences in how the hippocampal formation participates in the representation of space" (Bingman et al., 2003, p. 117). Clearly, there are differences of opinion on the similarity of the avian and mammalian brain, and it is tempting to wonder if some of those who work on birds are making a virtue of necessity in sup-

Figure 13–27. Avian hippocampus and landmark learning. *A.* The home loft of the pigeons was near Pisa. The animals were extensively trained to fly home (to Pisa) from either of two release sites, La Costanza and Livorno. *B.* When rendered anosmic and clock-shifted by 6 hours, the controls headed in the correct direction whereas the hippocampus-lesioned birds showed greater variability around a mean, reflecting the expected shift of 120°. The reason a clock shift of 6 hours is expected to produce a deviation of 120° rather than 90° is because at around midday in summer the azimuth of the sun moves about 20° per hour. (*Source:* After Gagliardo et al., 1999.)

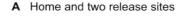 **A** Home and two release sites

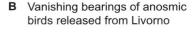 **B** Vanishing bearings of anosmic birds released from Livorno

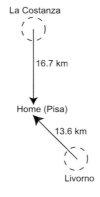

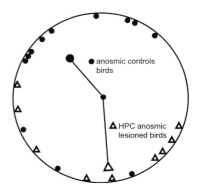

porting a claim for homology, aware of wider interest in the brains of mammals. Although understandable, the issue has to be resolved on the basis of all the evidence.

Comparative Studies of Spatial Memory in Rodents

Hippocampal-oriented neuroethology studies have been conducted in mammals as well, but the research is less well developed. One idea about mammalian hippocampal evolution is that sexual selection may have led to a relative increase in hippocampal volume of certain polygymous male rodents, an important case because sex differences evolve slowly and thus any correlated differences in cognitive function and neuroanatomy are especially strong evidence of an adaptive modification of the brain. In support of this idea, Jacobs et al. (1990) found that polygymous male meadow voles, which have an area over which they range about five times larger than that of females, show a corresponding sex difference in hippocampal volume (Fig. 13–28). In contrast, in monogamous prairie and pine voles, male and female hippocampal size is equivalent. Earlier laboratory studies revealed that males of the polygymous meadow vole are superior to females in place learning in Tolman's sunburst and other mazes (Gaulin and Fitzgerald, 1989; Gaulin et al., 1990). The interaction between natural and sexual selection has also been revealed in studies of subspecies of kangaroo rats, some of which store food and some of which do not, some polygymous and some monogamous. In comparisons across species, hippocampal size was found to be largest in males and scatter hoarding in polygymous Merriam's kangaroo rats (Sherry et al., 1992; Jacobs and Spencer, 1994).

One proposed modification of the cognitive map theory, inspired by the allometric studies, pigeon homing work and by the discovery of head-direction cells, is the parallel-map theory of Jacobs and Schenk (2003). This explicitly identifies a "bearing map" (in which olfactory gradients or distal cues are used to establish a sense of direction) and a "sketch map" (which is an allocentric representation of local landmarks). The two mapping systems are held to be mediated by and to interact at different subregions of the hippocampal formation; the primary evidence for this is the consistent patterns of distinctive search strategies seen in spatial tasks after selective lesions or other pharmacological forms of intervention. It is too early to assess the status of this proposed modification of the original cognitive map theory, but Jacobs (2003) made the case that it is pertinent to issues of evolution and ontogeny across a range of species, including other vertebrates. Jacobs and Schenk also used it to offer novel explanations of certain hitherto puzzling lesion and pharmacologically induced dissociations in task performance by laboratory rats.

The relative volume of a brain area is a limited measure. It is important to know whether this reflects variation in cell number (and, if so, of what cell type), cell proliferation or cell death, dendritic arborization, synapse number or density, or other neuronal processes. Finer grain neuroanatomical or biochemical measures could offer insights into precisely what co-varies with the type of information stored—capacity or temporal persistence. Given that neurogenesis may be under hormonal control (Galea and McEwen, 1999), there has been considerable interest in the possibility that seasonal changes in hippocampal volume reflect neurogenesis (Barnea and Nottebohm, 1994). Neurogenesis is influenced by environmental enrichment in some strains of mice (Kempermannet al., 1998) and by voluntary activity in running wheels (van Praag et al., 1999). There is evidence for seasonal changes in spatial learning ability and fine-grained aspects of hippocampal anatomy (Jacobs, 1995). However, Jacobs' own studies of possible seasonal variation in wild caught squirrels revealed no difference in cell proliferation or total neuron number in the hippocampus that co-varied with seasonal variation in demands on spatial memory (Lavenex et al., 2000). Chapter 9 discusses neurogenesis in the dentate gyrus in more detail.

Figure 13–28. Sexual selection influences hippocampal size. *A.* Space use by mammalian species with different mating systems. Under polygamy, male home ranges encompass several smaller female ranges; under monogamy, males and females share a joint home territory. (*Source*: After Jacobs, 1995.) *B.* Relative hippocampal volume in polygamous meadow voles and monogamous pine voles. The argument is that the hippocampus needs to be larger in a male meadow vole, which has to patrol a much larger territory. (*Source*: After Jacobs et al., 1990.)

A Male and female range size

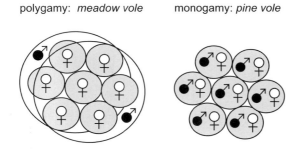

B Relative hippocampal volume

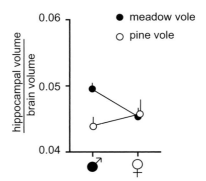

Neuroanatomical studies have nonetheless revealed consistent genetically stable variations in the intrinsic circuitry of the hippocampal formation across strains of mice (Lipp et al., 1999). Schwegler and Lipp (1981) discovered that the length of the infrapyramidal mossy fibers (IIP-MFs) is negatively correlated with two-way avoidance learning (a task impaired by hippocampal lesions) (Fig.13–29A,B), a finding that holds across a number of mouse (and rat) strains (Schwegler and Lipp, 1983). Later work showed that it is positively correlated with performance in spatial tasks, including the radial maze and reversal learning in the water-maze (Crusio et al., 1987; Bernasconi-Guastalla et al., 1994). Mouse strains, such as C57/BL6, known to be good at spatial learning have an extensive infrapyramidal mossy fiber system. Other strains, such as DBAs and BALB/C, have a limited infrapyramidal mossy fiber system. However, such correlations, although striking, should be treated cautiously not least because there may be other covariates. For example, BALB/C mice have retinal problems and limited vision; and DBA mice are reported to have deficiencies in protein kinase C (PKC), an enzyme implicated in synaptic plasticity.

To try to unravel the reported correlations and take a step toward causation, postnatal injections of thyroxine (Fig. 13–29C) have been successfully used to induce variations in infrapyramidal mossy fibers within a single strain and corresponding variations in the learning rate (Lipp et al., 1988; Schwegler et al., 1991). Still, the anatomical disquiet remains: These injections may be having other unmeasured effects. Some measure of behavioral specificity has been realized by the finding that the correlations with infrapyramidal mossy fiber length holds for spatial working memory on a radial maze but not cue working memory (Crusio et al., 1987; Schwegler et al., 1990). However, later studies revealed strain-specific covariations between the extent of the infrapyramidal mossy fiber distribution and both intermale aggression (Guillot et al., 1994) and paw preference (Lipp et al., 1996), which are clearly unrelated to spatial learning and memory; and there is a report of failure to observe the correlation with radial maze performance (Roullet and Lassalle, 1992).

Lipp et al. (1999) recognized that these "noncognitive" findings may not fit well with some prevailing theories of hippocampal function but are relevant to a "multifunctional" view in which the dorsal hippocampus mediates spatial

Figure 13–29. Avoidance learning and infrapyramidal mossy fibers. *A.* Relative location of the supra- and infrapyramidal mossy fibers (IIP-MF) projecting from the dentate gyrus (DG) to area CA3. *B.* Correlation between two-way avoidance learning and IIP-MF extent across mouse strains. *C.* Thyroxine induces alterations in both two-way avoidance learning and extent of IIP-MF. (Source: After Lipp et al., 1999.)

A Mossy fibre pathway (black) showing supra- and infra-pyramidal parts of the pathway.

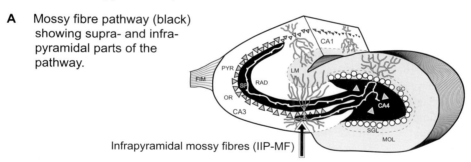

B Strain Comparisons

C DBA/2 Thyroxine Postnatal

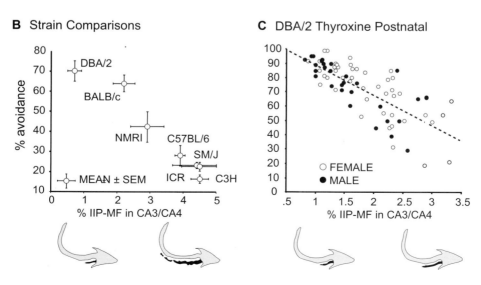

memory functions whereas the more ventral region is more relevant to emotional and aggressive behavior. They also suggested, partly on the basis of studies of the survival of various mouse strains through successive harsh winters at a Russian field station that "behavioral reactivity" rather than spatial memory may be the parameter of greatest adaptive significance in relation to the infrapyramidal mossy fibers.

To conclude this subsection, allometric brain/behavior correlations in birds and mammals have revealed several findings consistent with spatial interpretation of hippocampal function, but they have not definitively established that it is only spatial, rather than other kinds of memory, with which changes in hippocampal volume or structure are correlated. More analytical studies are required to unravel precisely what features of memory correlate with changes in hippocampal volume or circuitry. Identifying evolutionary adaptations, attributing them definitively to particular selective pressures, and then relating them to specific mosaic variations in brain size or circuitry is a slow, painstaking task (Lipp et al., 1999). The criticism has been made that studies of evolutionary function not only do not, but *cannot*, provide information about neurobiological mechanisms (Bolhuis and Macphail, 2001; Macphail and Bolhuis, 2001). However, even if this logical point were to be accepted, the implications are hotly debated (Hampton et al., 2002). Shettleworth (2003) offered a thoughtful defense of studies of the "neuroecology" of learning. She highlighted, by way of example, striking data from two populations of chickadees by Pravosudov and Clayton (2002). Instead of comparing different strains or species, they tested the "adaptive specialization" hypothesis in a single species, black-capped chickadees. One population was living in Alaska, where winters are fierce, and the other in Colorado. The different latitudes at which these distinct populations of a common species live might have resulted in a quantitative difference in the degree of selection pressure. Birds were caught in the autumn, around the time that seasonal volume changes should be maximal, and brought to a laboratory in California. Once there, the Alaska population was observed to be better at food storing and retrieval than the Colorado birds, better on spatial but not color memory (an allometric correlation analogous to earlier lesion data (Hampton and Shettleworth, 1996), and had relatively larger hippocampal volumes. It is not unreasonable to conclude that "mosaic" evolution of brain structure driven by natural selection on particular behavioral capacities (Barton and Harvey, 2000) will continue to contribute to understanding qualitative and quantitative differences in the hippocampus within and across species.

Maps, Spatial Representations, and Geometry: Is Spatial Learning Qualitatively Different from Associative Learning?

The other strand of the adaptive specialization idea is the issue of whether hippocampus-dependent spatial learning is *qualitatively* distinct from associative learning. The cognitive map theory asserts that spatial learning is different from "taxon"

learning in being rapid, flexible, and uniquely encoding information into maps. As noted above, the animal learning constituency is suspicious of this idea.

The claim that spatial learning is qualitatively different would be stronger if the psychological properties of either type of learning could be shown to be specific to that type of learning. A particular sticking point has been whether certain phenomena known to occur in classical conditioning, such as "blocking" and "overshadowing," do or do not occur in the spatial domain. Blocking refers to the ability of one stimulus to block learning about another, and overshadowing is a differential sharing of associative strength when two stimuli are conditioned together. Modern animal learning theories, discussed in more detail in Section 13.5, rely on "error-correcting" learning rules in which changes in the associative strength of a stimulus occur only when the expected outcome of that stimulus differs from the actual outcome. Although such rules enable learning to be rapid and flexible, stimuli compete with each other for associative strength rather than become linked together in anything like a "map." The conditioning phenomenon that most directly established the idea of error-correcting learning and captured everyone's attention when it was first discovered is blocking (Kamin, 1968). A stimulus, call it A, is arranged to predict reinforcement (R*). After several pairings of A and R* have occurred and the associative strength of A has reached an asymptotic value, a second stimulus is added (B). Stimulus B now also predicts R*; and one might expect, given the contiguous pairing of B and R*, that this association would be readily learned also. Often, however, little appears to be encoded about the relation between B and R*. The prior learning of the A $\rightarrow$ R* association is said to block learning about B. An important control is one in which stimuli A and B are introduced together for the first time in the second phase of a blocking experiment and arranged to predict R*. Under these conditions, both the A $\rightarrow$ R* and the B $\rightarrow$ R* associations are learned (although overshadowing sometimes occurs and is determined by such factors as stimulus salience or proximity). Many other control procedures have been conducted among a vast array of experiments investigating blocking and the processes responsible for it (Mackintosh, 1983).

One reason hippocampus-dependent learning might be thought to be qualitatively different from conventional associative conditioning is because hippocampal lesions do not reliably affect blocking. An early conditioning study indicated that there may be an effect of partial hippocampal lesions on blocking (Ross et al., 1984), but at later more definitive experiments indicated that blocking can occur normally in animals with complete hippocampal lesions (Garrud et al., 1984; Holland and Fox, 2003). Of greater concern for the cognitive map theory is whether blocking occurs between locale and taxon learning or even within the spatial domain. A comprehensive program of work led by Chamizo has shown that blocking can occur in the radial maze between intra- and extramaze cues (Chamizo et al., 1985) and entirely within the spatial domain in the watermaze (Rodrigo et al., 1997). In the later experiment, analogous to the studies using classical conditioning, the pool is surrounded by heavy black curtains and two-dimensional cues hung at specific locations within it (A, B, C, and so on). This spatial array of cues can then be rotated collectively from trial to trial; in this way, the experimenter can be confident that a rat's directed navigation in the pool is determined by this array rather than by other, experimenter-uncontrolled cues. In addition, although swimming is permitted at certain phases of the experiments (to enable learning and later testing of what has been learned), the animals can be either allowed to swim or placed on the platform during the critical blocking phase when another cue (X) is added. Blocking occurs normally. Chamizo (2003) summarized a wide range of such experiments and concluded that there is as yet no basis to suppose that spatial learning differs from conventional conditioning with respect to the use of an error-correcting learning rule. Mackintosh (2002) recognized certain tensions in the associative account between the occurrence of blocking, as required by animal learning theory, and other evidence that rats often learn about the locations of all available landmarks in simple exploratory tasks, as we saw in the work of Save et al. (1992a,b) earlier. However, he shared Chamizo's skepticism and asserted that "the behavioral evidence does not seem to have supported O'Keefe and Nadel's original hypothesis that true spatial learning or locale learning is quite distinct from associative learning" (Mackintosh, 2002, p. 165).

There remain some difficulties in accepting these conclusions without qualification. First, no lesion studies of blocking in the spatial domain have been conducted, and we must take on trust that the spatial memory seen in these studies is hippocampus-dependent. This seems likely, but we have already noted instances in which multitrial spatial reference memory tasks in the watermaze can be learned by rats with hippocampal lesions. The definitive hippocampus-dependent task in the watermaze is now recognized as being the DMP paradigm, and one-trial blocking experiments have not been conducted. Second, placement on the hidden platform may be insufficient for much learning with the kind of hanging cues used in Chamizo's laboratory. This is because two-dimensional cues at the periphery are known to be much less effective than three-dimensional cues, the animals cannot explore them proximally (e.g., using vibrissa movements), and the constellation of cues in the "blocking" phase of training (A, B, X) may be sufficiently similar to those in the earlier training phase (A,B) that the animals do not notice the difference. The outcome is then apparent rather than true blocking. Although various controls argue against this, the data measures reported are sometimes the proportion or ranking of animals showing an effect rather than absolute tracking data (such as time spent in a quadrant or zone).

Partly for these reasons, Biegler and Morris (1999) developed a food reward task in a large arena in which to explore blocking under conditions in which (1) the local cues were three-dimensional objects that could be explored by the animals in a multisensory manner, and (2) there was explicit

directional polarization provided by a specific arrangement of distal extramaze curtains. The task involved learning the location of food in relation to two identical landmarks, with a third and later fourth cue added to disambiguate two possible places where food might be found. The paths taken by the animals were tracked automatically. Blocking was again seen in the spatial domain, and this occurred despite the animals noticing and exploring the added landmark during the blocking phase (as shown by the tracking data) but then choosing not to learn about its association with reward. The use of an "instrumental" rather than a classic conditioning paradigm introduced complications, as the conditions across groups could not be exactly matched on the first trial of the blocking phase, though Biegler and Morris (1999) argued that this did not invalidate their conclusion. Unpublished lesion studies were also conducted, but performance was too poor in animals given lesions before training for any useful information to be obtained about the role of the hippocampus in blocking using this paradigm.

One point noted by Biegler and Morris (1999) concerns a potentially interesting difference between blocking in the spatial and conditional domains. With conventional conditioning, the relations learned, such as A → R*, are conditional ('if-then') associations (and not necessarily temporal although often described as such). Relations must be more than that in spatial learning because the Landmark → R* association must provide some information about the distance and direction from a landmark (L) that food is to be found. Under circumstances in which a memory representation must be formed of the *nature of the relation* between two cues, blocking may obey different rules. For example, when the relation between two spatially dispersed landmarks L1 and L2 and food has been learned, the addition of a third landmark, L3, may not always result in blocking simply because the location of R* is already predicted. The relative spatial location of the new cue L3 to the old cues L1 and L2 may be critical to its incorporation into an associative or "map-like" representation. Blocking may be more or less likely as a function of whether the vector (argument and direction) from L3 →R* is similar to or different from the vectors from L1 and L2 to R*. The conclusion of Chamizo (2002, 2003) that spatial information interacts during learning in apparently the same way as it does during conventional conditioning is probably secure, but there are issues to do with vectors and geometry that deserve further investigation.

Swimming against the tide of this developing experimental skepticism in the animal learning constituency, Cheng and Gallistel have gone farther than O'Keefe and Nadel (1978) in suggesting that the brain possesses a "geometric module" for space that operates according to distinctive learning rules (Gallistel, 1980; Cheng, 1986; Margules and Gallistel, 1988). This followed observations of the behavior of rats searching for food hidden at one corner of a rectangular enclosure. Despite the presence of disambiguating cues located at the four corners (visual or olfactory), the rats ignored them and searched systematically at *both* the correct corner and the diagonally opposite corner. These two corners are geometrically equivalent in a symmetrical rectangle. These findings seemed to imply that rats were more sensitive to environmental shape than to local features, such as the distinctive cues—hence the proposal of a geometric module. Observations and models of place cells—specifically their determination by boundary vectors—are consistent with both this and O'Keefe's preferred local feature view (O'Keefe and Burgess, 1996; Hartley et al., 2000; Lever et al., 2002).

In an ingenious test of the geometric module idea, Pearce et al. (2004) wondered if the symmetrical search patterns seen in a rectangular array reflected the operation of a specialized geometric module or something simpler. The animal learning constituency enjoys wielding Occam's razor, and this issue represented another opportunity. Might the rats have instead learned only the "rule" of searching at a corner defined by one long wall on the right and one short wall on the left? To test this, they first trained rats to search for a hidden escape platform in a rectangular watermaze and observed, in a conventional probe test with the platform absent, focused searching at both the "correct" corner and the geometrically equivalent corner (Fig. 13–30A). This result is identical to that found by Cheng and Gallistel in the food-rewarded task. The animals were then transferred to training in a kite-shaped maze (Fig.

13–30B). Training continued to the one corner with a long wall on the right and short wall on the left. In posttraining probe tests, preferential searching was now observed at the correct location but also at the apex of the maze (Fig. 13–30C). This finding makes no sense if the animals are using a geometric module representing the shape of the kite but is readily explicable if the animals have learned to search preferentially at the left-hand end of *any* long wall. Interestingly, rats with hippocampal lesions were poorer at learning to search at the correct corner unless prominent disambiguating local cues were added to walls on either side of the apex during training (Fig. 13–30D,E). Once these local cues were added, the training corner and the apex were easily distinguished visually and hippocampus-lesioned animals then learned as well as sham-lesioned controls. The implication of this ingenious study is that there need be no recourse to an abstract geometric module to learn these kinds of tasks and no need to suppose that the hippocampus mediates such a module. The data are, however, consistent with the boundary vector model of place cells in which their location is fixed by intersecting vectors from local cues.

Yet more abstract geometry is implied by the observation that rats trained to forage for food in the center of a square arena can transfer to searching at the "geometric" centre of rectangular and triangular arenas (Tommasi and Thinus-

Figure 13–30. Geometry and the shape of spatial learning to come. *A.* Rats trained to find an escape platform in one corner of a rectangular watermaze also search in the geometrically equivalent corner. *B.* The rats were then transferred to swimming in a "kite-shaped" arena, with the platform again located at the corner with a long wall on the left and a short wall on the right. *C.* During posttraining probe tests, the rats now searched at the correct location and at the apex. *D.* Hippocampus-lesioned rats (gray shading) are poorer than

sham-lesioned controls when learning to search correctly in the kite maze. *E.* When disambiguating local cues were added to the long walls of the rectangle and on either side of the apex, hippocampus-lesioned animals could learn as rapidly as controls. The bar graph data have been simplified to the long walls of the rectangle and either side aid the description of this study. (Source: After Pearce et al., 2004.)

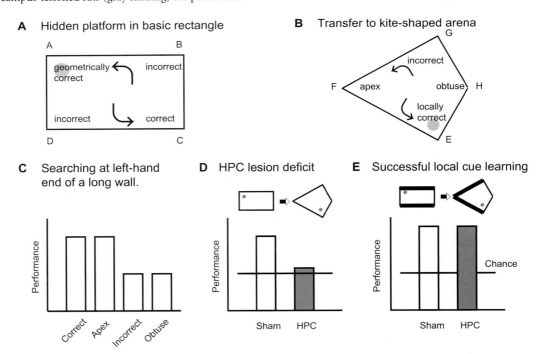

A   Hidden platform in basic rectangle

B   Transfer to kite-shaped arena

C   Searching at left-hand end of a long wall.

D   HPC lesion deficit

E   Successful local cue learning

Blanc, 2004). This result is not, however, always observed. One classic series experiments contrasted a map-like representation of space to one based on vectors (Collett et al., 1986). Vectors encode distance and direction. In a directionally polarized environment, a vector representation would be one in which object A may be represented as a vector with a specific "argument" (i.e., length) and "angle" from landmark P. Many objects (A, B, C, and so on) both visible and hidden, may be represented in such a way, but it does not require there to be any "map" of space. Specifically, there may be no encoding of the relative locations of A, B, and C to each other. To test this idea, gerbils were trained to find sunflower seeds at particular distances and directions from landmarks in a room that provided cues enabling directional polarization but not localization. The landmarks were then manipulated in various ways. In one manipulation, animals were first trained to find food hidden halfway between two identical landmarks. The two landmarks were then moved farther apart. If the animals had learned to find reward at some abstract "centre" of the array, they would be expected to search preferentially at a common point, now a bit farther from each of the landmarks. Instead, searching occurred at two locations, each at the appropriate distance from each landmark along the line between them (Fig. 13–31A). In a yet more striking example of vector-based representation, the gerbils were trained to find sunflower seeds at the center of a triangular array of three distinctive landmarks (Fig. 13–31B). The landmark array was then rotated by 60° such that the vectors representing reward location from each landmark were now *outside* the array

rather than inside. Astonishingly, a significant proportion of the search visits during a posttraining probe test with the rotated array were *outside* the landmark array. This striking pattern is not to be expected had the animals learned a "map" of space with food at the center of the landmark array. It is consistent with the encoding of three independent vectors specifying the distance and direction of food from each of the three landmarks. During training, these vectors meet at the single, central point; after rotation they do not. Collett et al. (1986) did not go on to conduct lesion studies, so we do not know the impact of the hippocampal dysfunction. However, in a conceptually similar lesion study using the watermaze, Pearce et al. (1998) found that hippocampus-lesioned rats could be trained to locate a hidden platform at a specific distance and direction from a visible landmark that moved places within the pool between days. It seems that the hippocampus is not required to encode vectors across multiple trials but may be necessary to assemble multiple vectors into a map-like representation.

With respect to multiple types of memory, there are good grounds to believe that there has been selection pressure to develop map-like spatial representation and navigation systems in vertebrates. However, the studies comparing spatial learning with conventional associative conditioning have revealed fewer differences than might have been expected on the basis of the original cognitive map theory. The possibility that spatial information is fundamentally associative, in contrast to the position adopted within cognitive mapping theory, has to be considered. Section 13.5 takes up this

Figure 13–31. Maps or vectors? *A.* Gerbils were trained to find food halfway between two landmarks (large circles). When the landmarks were moved farther apart in a posttraining probe test, the animals searched at two distinct locations (small squares denote time spent searching). *B.* Gerbils were trained to find food in the

center of an array of three distinctive landmarks in an environment in which directionally polarization is determined by other distal cues. When the landmark array was rotated by 60° in a probe test, a substantial proportion of the searching was now outside the arena. (*Source*: After Collett et al., 1986.)

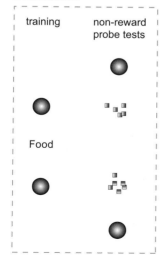

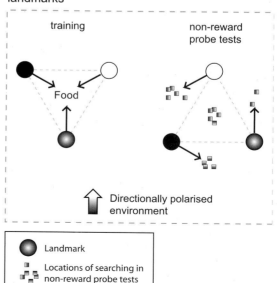

issue further; but before turning to that, we discuss the issue of where allocentric spatial information is stored in the brain.

13.4.5 Storage and Consolidation of Spatial Memory

A fourth major proposition of cognitive map theory is that the memory traces required for allocentric representations through a familiar place are stored in the hippocampal formation itself. This storage is held to be distributed, possibly along both the longitudinal and transverse axes of at least the dorsal hippocampus for even a single memory, such that damage to the structure should cause a loss of both processing capacity (encoding, retrieval, and navigation) and storage sites (local alterations in synaptic weights). Hippocampal damage should therefore cause a "flat" gradient of retrograde amnesia for spatial information, as first shown by Bolhuis et al. (1994). In contrast to the retrieval of factual information by humans or contextual fear by rats, where gradients are observed (see Section 13.3), the integrity of structures in the hippocampal formation is also claimed to be essential for successful recall of episodic memory in humans (Viskontas et al., 2000; Cipolotti et al., 2001; Maguire, 2001). Moreover, very remote episodic memories may still elicit neural activation of the hippocampus long after they were first acquired (Nadel et al., 2000), although the use of "reminders" prior to brain scanning has raised a query about the true of age of ostensibly old memories in imaging work. Given the very different perspective on these matters in declarative memory theory, it is no surprise that memory consolidation has become one of the battlefields of contemporary cognitive neuroscience.

We have seen that the "standard model" of memory persistence (see Section 13.3) is that some systems-level process of hippocampus-dependent memory consolidation takes place after learning that, by enabling an interaction of hippocampal and neocortical ensembles, secures the stabilization of memory traces outside the hippocampus (Squire and Alvarez, 1995a; Kapur and Brooks, 1999; Manns et al., 2003). The neurological function of such systems-level consolidation presumably has nothing to do with the protection of memory against brain damage. Exploiting the unfortunate occurrence of relevant brain damage in humans, or its experimental creation in animals, is just a technique for revealing this neurological process. Rather, consolidation is thought to have two functions. First, it engages mechanisms that "gate" whether memory traces are to be retained. Second, once consolidation is complete, a lasting neocortical memory site exists that would enable much faster retrieval of information than would be possible were it always necessary for there to be a neural "loop: through the hippocampus. A consolidation process might also allow retrieval of information from neocortical traces when it is required *without* recourse to consciousness, but the activation of this neural loop may be a signature of conscious awareness in the specific domain of memory (Moscovitch, 1995). One situation where conscious awareness is usually engaged is in the spatial domain, where it may be helpful in updating during navigation.

Reflecting on these putative functions of systems-level consolidation, Moscovitch wondered if memory retrieval *with* recovered consciousness might be disentangled from other features of the standard model. This led on to a series of articles in which he and Nadel proposed an alternative "multiple trace" model of memory persistence (Nadel and Moscovitch, 1997, 1998; Moscovitch and Nadel, 1998). In this model, a subset of memories is permanently mediated by corticohippocampal circuitry. Specifically, the theory holds that each reactivation of memory leads to—or at least *can* lead to—the formation of additional traces that are located at different points along the longitudinal axis of the hippocampus (anterior-posterior in humans). Temporal information is thought to be stored in the prefrontal lobe, at least in humans. Consolidation is thus a "reactivation–restorage" cycle that occurs in a punctuated manner over time, rather than as a gradual, inexorable biological process—an analogy might be drawn with the concept of "punctuated equilibrium" in evolutionary theory (Gould and Eldredge, 1977). There would then be *multiple traces* of a common past event, but these traces could entail different associations with other information that reflect their distinct provenance. Temporally graded retrograde amnesia for spatial information can then be explained by the proliferation of memory traces in the hippocampus without recourse to a neocortical consolidation process, a prediction that has been successfully modeled with a connectionist network (Nadel et al., 2000). Remote spatial memories are represented by a larger number of traces and so be more accessible than recently acquired memories. According to a later version of this model (Nadel and Bohbot, 2001; Rosenbaum et al., 2001), this multiple-trace theory applies particularly to "contextually rich" memories but not those that are context-free or semantic in character. Whether these proposals should be seen as "extensions" of the cognitive map theory or as independent ideas inspired by it is unclear. They are probably more the latter.

The declarative memory and the multiple trace theories make contrasting predictions about retrograde amnesia in the particular case of partial lesions. Unfortunately for theories of memory, the capricious nature of human brain injury results in most MTL amnesic subjects having only partial damage to the hippocampus (Rempel-Clower et al., 1996; Bayley et al., 2005b). Such patients do not discriminate the two theories. One neurological case does exist where the damage is apparently extensive yet there remains clear evidence of sparing of spatial memory from a much earlier time period in the patient's life—patient E.P. (Teng and Squire, 1999). However, we have seen that the testing of remote memory in humans and the identification of an explicit temporal gradient is fraught with difficulty (see Chapter 12). Can animal studies of spatial memory shed light on this important theoretical issue?

Studies using the watermaze have consistently shown a flat gradient of retrograde amnesia for spatial memory when it is first tested postoperatively. In such studies, rats have typically first been trained on a reference memory version of the task (i.e., to find a single hidden platform); then, at periods ranging from a few days to up to 3 months later, they have been subjected to large excitotoxic or radiofrequency lesioning of the hippocampal formation (Bolhuis et al., 1994; Mumby et al., 1999; Sutherland et al., 2001; Clark et al., 2004, 2005b). Subsequent to surgery, the animals have been retested in the watermaze either with the platform in its original training location, with it moved to a new location, or using probe tests (platform absent). Martin et al. (2005) used such a design with animals given partial hippocampal lesions (circa 35% sparing of either the dorsal or the ventral hippocampus) and others complete lesions (< 5% sparing). They used an Atlantis platform during training to encourage highly focused searching and better memory. An initial posttraining probe test provided no evidence of better retention of remote spatial memory, even in the group with a partial lesion of either the

dorsal or ventral hippocampus (Fig. 13–32A). This first finding of Martin et al.'s (2005) study is inconsistent with *both* the declarative memory and the multiple-trace theories but consistent with the original statement of the cognitive map theory, subject to the proviso of there being some threshold of intact residual tissue (> 35%) necessary to mediate effective navigation.

However, in these and other studies, the performance of sham-lesioned rats in the watermaze tends to be poor after surgery, possibly reflecting a "floor" effect that masks any consolidation or multiple trace process. To address this problem, Bolhuis et al. (1994) followed up the initial probe test with retraining to unmask cryptic spatial memory traces. If anything, their "savings" data favored better relearning by *recently* lesioned groups (made 3 days after original training) than the remote groups. Rats given subiculum lesions that left the hippocampus intact were also capable of relearning to a high

Figure 13–32. Retrograde amnesia for spatial memory. *A.* An initial "pre-reminder" probe test conducted 2 weeks after sham (white), and either partial (gray) or complete (black) hippocampal lesions revealed no evidence of spared spatial memory recall in either lesioned group. This study confirms the earlier findings of Bolhuis et al. (1994) but under conditions in which a floor effect in the sham control group did not occur. (*Source:* After Martin et al., 2005.) *B.* Reminding given in the form of successive probe tests revealed some sparing of spatial memory recall in the partially

lesioned group. The reminding procedure was shown not to induce relearning. (*Source:* After Martin et al., 2005.) *C.* Extensive training from an early age failed to reveal spared spatial memory in animals with complete hippocampal lesions. (*Source:* After Clark et al., 2005a.) *D.* Spatial recognition memory tested using an annular watermaze that obviates the need for hippocampal updating during navigation also failed to reveal spared spatial memory after complete hippocampal lesions. (*Source:* After Clark et al., 2005b.)

A Spatial recall before reminding

first probe test acts as a reminder

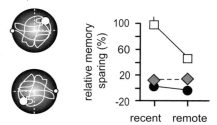

B Spatial recall with reminding

post-reminder probe test

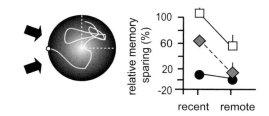

C Spatial recall with extensive training

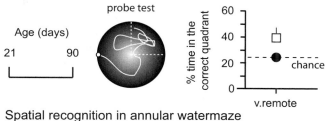

D Spatial recognition in annular watermaze

probe test

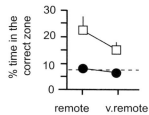

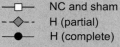

Lesion groups
—□— NC and sham
- -◇- - H (partial)
—●— H (complete)

Training-surgery intervals
recent: 0–3 days
remote: 6–9 weeks
v.remote: 14–16 weeks

degree of proficiency. This is consistent with the integrity of hippocampal circuitry being important for some aspects of spatial memory storage. Mumby et al. (1999) also used retraining and a within-subjects protocol with two watermaze tasks that were trained at different time points prior to surgery. They found little evidence of spatial memory in their complete hippocampal lesion group for either of the two tasks. Sutherland et al. (2001) used both retraining and probe tests and observed a significant trend for longer training–surgery intervals to be associated with poorer retention—once again the opposite of what is predicted by the declarative memory theory. These studies reflect a consistent pattern, but the use of retraining after surgery confounded two factors: the impact of the lesion on consolidation (the focus of interest) and its impact on new learning (a separate matter).

In their comparison of partial and complete lesions, Martin et al. (2005) used a different approach: a series of rewarded probe trials at 1-hour intervals. This gradually revealed above-chance performance by the partial hippocampus-lesioned group that had undergone surgery immediately after training (i.e., their recent group). No recovery of remote memory was observed in the group for which there was a much longer 6-week interval between the end of training and surgery (Fig. 13–32B). This apparent "unmasking" of latent spatial memory was not due to any relearning during the series of probe trials, as de Hoz et al. (2004) had separately shown that the conduct of a probe trial with an Atlantis platform serves, in animals with partial lesions, only as a reminder cue. The result vindicates the interpretation drawn by Bolhuis et al. (1994) much earlier.

Noting the same problem of weak postsurgery memory, Clark et al. (2004) extended the presurgery training to as many as 80 trials, finding that it improved the performance of the sham/control group. The point of doing this is to increase the opportunity of seeing an upward consolidation function in the data (along the lines of Fig. 13–10B3). However, using large radiofrequency lesions restricted to the hippocampus, they again observed both poor memory and a completely flat gradient of retrograde amnesia in postsurgery probe tests. Another attack on the problem was suggested by the fact that patient E.P. had learned his home neighborhood as a young man. Clark et al. (2005a) therefore trained normal rats from very early in life (21 days) for a total of 392 trials over 69 days. Hippocampal and sham lesions were made at 90 days of age, and the animals were tested 2 weeks later. Once again, the complete lesion group failed to display above-chance performance and that despite the use of a reminding procedure a few days before testing (Fig. 13–32C). Undeterred, Clark et al. (2004) wondered if there was something unusual about the standard watermaze task, as other nonspatial tasks had found evidence of a temporal gradient, albeit only using a savings or choice measure (Cho et al., 1993, 1995; Ramos, 1998; Maviel et al., 2004). Accordingly, they also trained rats in an Oasis maze, in which they have to search for water in a small well located on a "desert-like" table top, and in an annular water-maze (Hollup et al., 2001) in which the animals swim in a cir-

cular corridor until they find an escape platform. The use of the annular watermaze is interesting as the need for navigational updating is minimized; the swimming rats have only to recognize a potentially safe place along the ring and slow down when they get there. However, using a single probe test, both tasks again showed a flat gradient (Fig. 13–32D).

The animals' joy in eventually finding water in the Oasis maze cannot have been matched by any exhilaration on the part of proponents of the declarative memory theory by the outcome of this series of experiments. Clark et al. (2004) suggested that a feature that may distinguish tasks where remote spatial memory is spared (cross and radial maze tasks) compared to those where it is impaired (watermaze tasks) is that only in the latter does the expression of memory require the now-lesioned animal to recall by navigating through open space. That the hippocampus might be essential for *expressing* spatial memory, rather than storing or retrieving it, is reminiscent of Whishaw's distinction between "getting there" (impaired by lesions) and "knowing where" (which may not always be). A processing deficit of this kind conveniently predicts that any underlying hippocampal-neocortical consolidation process would remain cryptic.

There are, however, problems with this account. First, it incorrectly predicts that remote memory should be intact in the annular watermaze because its navigational demands are minimized. The animal does not have to learn or access any navigational strategies for "getting there"—it has merely to swim in a constrained circle. Second, remember that reminder cues revealed latent spatial memory in partially lesioned animals (Martin et al., 2005). Presumably. sufficient hippocampal tissue was spared for the expression of memory. However, this latent spatial memory was in the recent-memory group, not the remote. If cryptic consolidation does occur, the effects on trace strength must therefore be substantially smaller than those of forgetting. Third, remember that different results are obtained after small partial lesions as a function of whether they are made before or after training (Moser et al., 1995; Moser and Moser, 1998b). When spatial memory is acquired by normal animals and then partial lesions are made in the hippocampus, performance is seriously compromised and needs to be relearned. This makes sense if trace storage of spatial memory is *within* the hippocampus, it being fully distributed along the longitudinal axis when created in an intact hippocampus. Relearning would be possible with a partially intact hippocampus, and this would also be enough to express the memory once retrieved.

The last twist of the consolidation story comes from the use of novel techniques. Using a behavioral training protocol similar to that of Martin et al. (2005), indirect evidence for the presence of a systems level consolidation process after watermaze training was obtained using a pharmacological approach. Riedel et al. (1999) observed that chronic reversible inactivation of the hippocampus for 1 week after training through bilateral infusion of a GluR1–5 antagonist impaired spatial memory when the animals were tested 16 days later (i.e., long after the effects of the drug had worn off). The drug demonstrably blocked fast synaptic transmission in the hippocampus, implicating the necessity for hippocampal neural activity for some period after training if spatial memory was to persist. Riedel et al. (1999) explored the impact of delaying the "shut-down" by a few days and got the same results, but they did not examine a longer time course after training. This reversible but chronic inactivation approach is promising analytically; but even if hippocampal inactivation long after training was found to have minimal impact on remote memory, it would not mean that the neural activity required for memory persistence is necessarily a hippocampal-neocortical dialogue of the kind presumed with the "standard model." It could also be the creation of multiple traces in the hippocampus, or some other intrahippocampal consolidation process, that requires neural activity. Reversible inactivation may not be quite the help for distinguishing the rival theories it first promised to be. A similar ambiguity pertains to the striking evidence that sectioning the direct input from layer III of the entorhinal cortex to area CA1 of the hippocampus (the temporo-ammonic tract) is essential for memory consolidation (Remondes and Schuman, 2004). When lesions were made before 7 days of watermaze training, the animals showed good probe test performance 1 day after training but poor memory 28 days later; sham-lesioned animals showed no decline. The same result was obtained when the lesions were made 1 day after the end of training. However, if the lesions were delayed until 21 days after the end of training, both the sham and temporo-ammonic tract-lesioned animals showed a continued, albeit weaker, tendency to swim in the correct quadrant 7 days later. Collectively, these three experiments are consistent with the idea that "ongoing cortical input conveyed by the temporo-ammonic path is required to consolidate long-term spatial memory" (Remondes and Schuman, 2004, p. 702), the implication being that this pathway is necessary for the hippocampal-cortical dialogue implicated in the declarative memory theory. However, this is not absolutely required by the data. It could still be that temporo-ammonic input is essential for ongoing consolidation *in* the hippocampus.

A final expression theory, as discussed by Martin et al. (2005), relates to the role of the hippocampus in the retrieval and expression of consolidated memory traces that reside in the neocortex but for which the hippocampus plays a part in their retrieval. There are a variety of possibilities. One is that the hippocampus does store information but stores only the "indices" (Teyler and DiScenna, 1986) or the "cartoons" needed to retrieve a consolidated cortical memory trace rather than detailed sensory-perceptual information (this remains in the cortex). With this view, the hippocampus might retrieve a cortical memory in a manner analogous to conducting a keyword search on an electronic document. Partial lesions would compromise the "indices" rather than the detailed sensory-perceptual memory traces and so limit the ability to retrieve cortical memory traces when a recall process is necessary. The circumstances surrounding memory retrieval and the very character of the information retrieved (Nadel and Bohbot, 2001) may determine whether the hippocampus plays a nec-

essary role in this process. Memories are widely thought to be stored in a distributed manner (i.e., their component traces are stored across different brain areas). Retrieval of the right combination of traces might be possible under circumstances in which the retrieval cues are either particularly apposite or sufficiently rich to disambiguate cortically based traces with overlapping components. However, under circumstances in which the retrieval cues do not permit easy disambiguation or where they have to be generated indirectly through a process of recovered consciousness (Moscovitch, 1995), the processing capacity of the hippocampus and its stored indices would remain essential. Disambiguation would generally be critical for context-dependent episodic memory in which a unique combination of traces corresponds to the particular event from the past that needs to be reactivated. Consistent with this idea, the expression of human episodic memory is sometimes found to be permanently affected by hippocampal damage, as noted earlier. Notwithstanding our focus on memory retrieval processes, this account is consistent with Rosenbaum et al.'s (2001) revision of the multiple trace theory. It distinguishes between context-dependent and context-free memories and suggests that only the former remain dependent on the hippocampus for our lifetime. Winocur et al. (2005) have reported data consistent with this view in a study of rats that lived in a "rodent village" for 3 months prior to explicit training on a spatial problem in the village. Posttraining hippocampal lesions had no effect on effective navigation to the correct location in the village, which they interpreted as implying the existence of a detailed "semantic" map stored in the neocortex. Rats with less experience of the village were impaired by posttraining hippocampal lesions because they presumably lacked a context-free memory of the village. Unfortunately, the lesions used in this study were partial (around 50%), allowing some use of spared hippocampal tissue in memory retrieval. Winocur et al. (2005) argued against this being of significance on the grounds of finding no correlation between lesion size and retrieval, but this is a weak argument based on only a small number of subjects with different sized lesions.

Studies of interactions and correlations between single-unit and field-potential recordings in hippocampus and neocortex during and after sleep are highly suggestive of consolidation-like processes (Siapas and Wilson, 1998; Sirota et al., 2003). Targeted molecular studies can help resolve some of the ambiguities at the mechanistic level, although not necessarily all of them, as a daunting combination of novel behavioral protocols, lesions, and molecular interventions will probably prove necessary to unravel the complexities. Frankland et al. (2001) made the intriguing observation that heterozygous αCAMKII mutant mice show normal LTP in the hippocampus, decaying LTP in the cortex, and failure to consolidate both spatial and contextual information. They suggested that the instability of synaptic potentiation in the cortex could be the basis of the consolidation failure. This is an interesting idea, but it is equally consistent with the idea that effective retrieval relies on the synergy of different kinds of information permanently stored in both hippocampus and neocortex. Frankland and Bontempi (2005) summarized these developing new lines of research using transgenic animals and IEG markers to plot the time course and regional contributions of neocortex and hippocampus to memory consolidation.

13.4.6 Critique

The cognitive map theory has been highly influential. The role of the hippocampus in spatial learning and memory is accepted, particularly in rodents; and such learning is widely used as an "assay" for investigating the cellular and molecular mechanisms of learning and its dysfunction in models of neurodegenerative disease. "Spatial memory" has become a keyword at international meetings, such as those of the Society for Neuroscience and the Federation of European Neuroscience Societies, and there are now laboratories all over the world investigating the neurobiological basis of allocentric spatial representation and spatial navigation. Although much of this reflects a general interest in spatial learning and memory rather than commitment to one particular theory, it is perhaps not surprising that it has been criticized as the theory "that wouldn't die."

However, the theory clearly has major difficulties, both conceptual and empirical. This chapter's presentation of the theory was built around four themes—spatial representation, spatial navigation, comparative work, and studies of memory storage and consolidation—and has already included a measure of critical discussion. A few additional points should be noted in relation to these same four themes.

Spatial Representation, Maps, and the Geometric Module

With respect to representation, one set of problems center around whether the concept of a "cognitive map" is an explanation of anything or merely a beguiling metaphor (Healy, 1998). A map is an easily understood concept, but maps are things that people look at to extract information. Adopting this term for the neural activity of a region of the brain seems to carry with it the mental baggage that there must be some cryptic homunculus that is "looking at" the map to likewise. In the absence of a mechanistic account of how information is extracted from the map, the explanation it offers is incomplete. With respect to the concept of cognitive mapping itself, Bennett (1996) argued that the now widespread use of the term in many different ways by investigators in ethology, psychology, and brain science is confusing and that the concept has outlived its usefulness. This feels unpersuasive. That some people use a scientific term loosely is not grounds for castigating those who use it more precisely. As Bennett (1996) himself conceded, Tolman (1948) introduced it and O'Keefe and Nadel (1978) used it explicitly in relation to the ability to represent the environment in a viewer-independent allocentric manner and to solve such problems as novel shortcuts. This definition is concise. Time and again, O'Keefe's group

have come back to a central prediction of the theory in relation to brain activity associated with exploration and spatial novelty, most recently in showing differential activation of the human hippocampus proper when people take shortcuts in a virtual reality environment (Maguire et al., 1998; Burgess et al., 2002). Quantitative models are precise and testable, such as the boundary vector model of place cells (Hartley et al., 2000).

However, the concept of a geometric module is undergoing something of a forensic examination with experiments in rodents (Golob and Taube, 2002; McGregor et al., 2004b; Pearce et al., 2004) and humans (Wang and Spelke, 2002), raising questions about whether there is any need for a "global" representation of environmental shape, as in the study of the kite-shaped watermaze discussed earlier. Pearce's study, part of a larger series, breaks new ground because it suggests that earlier data pointing to the existence of a global geometric module centered on the hippocampus is also consistent with a different account that sees no need for such a representation. Learning may require only a perceptual system that can distinguish long barriers from short ones (i.e., perceptual features of local cues in general) and bridge the temporal delay between turning appropriately as the animal approaches the long wall and the subsequent receipt of delayed reward. It remains to be seen where this research on local features versus boundaries and geometry will lead.

Successful Spatial Navigation Without the Hippocampus

A second set of difficulties for the theory is that rodents with nearly complete cell loss in the hippocampal formation can, with certain training procedures, learn allocentric spatial tasks. This is the longstanding claim of the "working memory" theory of Olton et al. (1979), who argued that spatial reference memory tasks can be learned by lesioned rats. We have seen that this claim is correct, but the rate of learning is much slower. Regardless of whether it is slower, the inescapable implication is that extrahippocampal structures can support spatial learning. This finding that the integrity of the hippocampus, or of hippocampal synaptic plasticity, is not essential for spatial reference memory is not necessarily fatal for the cognitive map theory because recent experimental and theoretical studies have established that effective spatial navigation can be realized in many ways, including strategies other than map-guided navigation. However, certain observations, such as normal probe test performance in the watermaze by rats with complete hippocampal lesions (Morris et al., 1990) must be accepted as problematic unless the theory is to descend into irrefutability. That rapid, one-trial spatial learning in the DMP task is always impaired (Steele and Morris, 1999) suggests that the integrity of the hippocampus is essential for rapid encoding of spatial information (spatial events?), but the gradual accumulation of information about spatial regularities of an environment might be information that can, albeit slowly, be encoded, stored, and retrieved in the neocortex without recourse to the hippocampus. That retrograde amnesia is apparently always seen after both partial and complete hippocampal lesions in rats appears to be contradictory, but the initial learning in such tasks always takes place in normal animals.

In passing, it is relevant to note that knocking out the capacity to express a particular form of NMDA receptor-dependent LTP through mutation of the GluR-A receptor selectively impairs one-trial spatial working memory but not incremental spatial reference memory (Zamanillo et al., 1999; Reisel et al., 2002). The knockout is not hippocampus-specific, but a genetic rescue of the receptor mutation that appears to be largely expressed in the dorsal hippocampus (Schmitt et al., 2005) is sufficient for partially rescue of efficient spatial working memory performance. This body of work is discussed in Chapter 7. For the present, note only that it illustrates how new techniques are shedding light on what it means to classify a task as hippocampus-dependent. A mouse in which GluR-A is absent shows apparently normal fast synaptic transmission in the hippocampus but fails to show a rapidly induced form of LTP. Such an animal is like a lesioned animal in that it cannot display types of memory encoding that occur in the hippocampus; but it is more subtle than a lesioned animal, as it allows information throughput in the hippocampus, which may be essential for neocortical encoding of incremental learning.

If this is correct, one would expect that damage to certain neocortical brain areas (and not just the entorhinal cortex) would have effects on spatial navigation that are clearly not predicted by the theory. These have indeed been observed. Deficits in spatial navigation in a variety of tasks follows lesions in the posterior parietal cortex (DiMattia and Kesner, 1988a; Kesner, 1998) and the midline retrosplenial/cingulate cortex (Sutherland et al., 1988). Harker and Whishaw (2004) summarized a body of conflicting data, including strain differences, regarding involvement of the retrosplenial cortex in various spatial tasks including navigation. Aggleton and Vann (2004) concurred that retrosplenial lesions do impair allocentric spatial navigation in the watermaze, though lesion size can be a critical factor (Vann and Aggleton, 2004). Focusing on a different part of the neocortex, Kesner (2000) argued that there is parallel processing of spatial information in the hippocampus and parietal cortex, with the former more important for "spatial events" and the latter part of a neocortical "knowledge" system. This distinction echoes the episodic/semantic distinction to which we return later. It is also is relevant to the issue of whether memory storage is in the hippocampus or there is some hippocampally guided consolidation process. Kesner (1998) is not alone in regarding a strictly spatial view of hippocampal function as too narrowly drawn.

Multiple Types of Memory?

Another conceptual problem is that the simple division of learning processes into spatial versus nonspatial now appears dated. Although there have been many developments of the cognitive map theory, including its application to various aspects of human memory, its adequacy as a general theory of multiple types of memory is limited. It has little to say about the relations between propositional (declarative) and nonpropositional forms of long-term memory (e.g., skill learning), between working and long-term memory, or, more curiously, about the nature of perceptual representations. Its proponents would argue that the theory was never intended to be a general theory of memory and cognition and that Figure 13–17 reflects their primary focus. It is a theory built around the discovery of place cells and the sensitivity of spatial navigation by rodents to various kinds of brain damage. It has imaginatively extended from these beginnings, but its place as a building block of a more general neurobiological theory remains a task for the future.

However, even within the domain of the cognitive analysis of space, there are problems with respect to the claim that spatial learning is fundamentally different from associative learning. In 1978, it was valuable to make the point that associative conditioning is generally slow and inflexible, whereas place learning can occur during one trial; but strictly behavioral studies of allocentric place learning have now revealed that spatial learning displays several qualitative characteristics of associative learning, such as "blocking" (Chamizo, 2003). Spatial learning may be associative after all.

Integrity of the Hippocampus Is Required for Many Nonspatial Learning Tasks

If rats with hippocampal lesions can learn certain spatial tasks, a separate concern is that such lesions are now also known to affect a range of *nonspatial* tasks, including classic operant tasks with a temporal component, such as differential reinforcement of low rates of response (DRL). Although it has always been possible to construct a spatial account of DRL performance, a temporal one seems more reasonable (Rawlins, 1985). However, there a number of other tasks, such as nonlinear discrimination learning and socially transmitted food preferences, for which a spatial account would strain credibility. Section 13.5 is a detailed examination of such tasks in the context of the "predictable ambiguity" theories for which they are relevant.

Coda

As a last word, it is worth reflecting on the fact that the cognitive map theory—the theory that refuses to die—enjoys the security of a number of key physiological findings that are not enjoyed by the other main theory discussed so far, the declarative memory theory. The theoretical battlefield between these two theories would be very different if the discovery of other spatially responsive neurons (e.g., head-direction units, view cells, grid cells) had not occurred. All of these discoveries were made since 1978. Hippocampal neurons are not differentially active as a function of stimulus familiarity, but they clearly are responsive to an animal's location or view of the world. This is a major if somewhat neglected obstacle to the credibility of declarative memory theory. We have also seen a number of studies in which interventions in the induction and expression of LTP have an effect on spatial learning and retention (see Chapter 10), although the extent to which these effects are cognitively selective is not well understood. Some comfort for the declarative memory theory in the physiological domain can be derived from glucose uptake and IEG studies indicating greater neuronal activity in the hippocampus soon after learning than later, perhaps reflecting the dynamic process of memory consolidation. These observations are pertinent to the task of trying to build a neurobiological account of hippocampal function to which we return in Section 13.6.

13.5 Predictable Ambiguity: Configural, Relational, and Contextual Theories of Hippocampal Function

The two major theories discussed so far command strong support and continue to be refined in the light of new findings. Neither will be discarded until a cogent alternative is widely seen to account for a larger body of data. However, numerous other theories of hippocampus function have been proposed. They include hypotheses that build on modern associative learning theories whose origins, unlike the concept of multiple memory systems, lie in the phenomenon of classical and instrumental conditioning rather than human amnesia. In one way or another, their applications to thinking about hippocampus function all have to do with dealing with the problem of "predictable ambiguity." This phrase is intended to capture the sense that a stimulus can consistently mean one thing in one situation but something else in a different one.

Learning theory research is characterized by exacting training protocols that explore conditioning phenomena far removed from the classic account of learned salivation to the sound of a bell. As we touched on briefly in the preceding section, examples include protocols for examining whether learning occurs when an animal's "expectations" are violated or that it alters the "associability" of stimuli or the contexts in which they occur (Rescorla and Wagner, 1972; Pearce and Hall, 1980). Such learning could include both excitatory and inhibitory associations (i.e., that a predicted event is more or less likely to happen). Beyond simple associations, there are also experience-dependent "attentional" phenomena and "occasion-setting" paradigms in which a stimulus (or more broadly an entire context) influences the retrieval of other memories quite apart from any associations in which it may also become engaged. Such phenomena have led to the suggestion that associative conditioning, far from deserving its low-level status as a "nondeclarative" form of stimulus-response "habit" learning (within declarative memory theory) or of mere "taxon" learning (in the cognitive map theory), is more complex and might offer a conceptually economical account of a variety of ostensibly cognitive phenomena. Proponents of this approach have introduced the idea that conditioning

offers insights into the way in which animals learn about "the causal texture of their environment" (Dickinson and Mackintosh, 1978). This implies that conditioning could have to do with the acquisition of knowledge that could be used inferentially (Mackintosh, 1983; Rescorla, 1988; Pearce and Bouton, 2001; Pickens and Holland, 2004) as first discussed explicitly by Dickinson (1980). These intellectual developments are relevant here because psychological processes have been identified in modern "learning theory" for which the hippocampus is a potential anatomical substrate.

Paradoxically, it has long been known that animals with hippocampal lesions are generally normal regarding simple associative conditioning tasks. These tasks involve no more than the pairing of an initially neutral stimulus (CS) with, after a delay, the presentation of reinforcement (US). The result is the gradual development of associative strength and its expression as a conditioned response (CR). In general, simple delay conditioning depends on other brain circuits. For example, hippocampal lesions are without effect in nictitating membrane (NMR) delay conditioning in which a CS starts several hundred milliseconds before and then overlaps with the presentation of a strong puff of air to the eye (US). NMR learning was shown independently by several groups (using lesion, inactivation, and unit-recording techniques) to be mediated by circuits in the spinal cord and cerebellum (Krupa et al., 1993; Hardiman et al., 1996; Beggs et al., 1999). As noted in Chapter 11, hippocampal pyramidal cells nonetheless show firing patterns during NMR conditioning that are correlated in time with the learned response (Berger et al., 1983), but this neural activity is not usually necessary for normal performance. The exception to this is when a "trace interval" is inserted between the end of the CS and the onset of US, as we saw in the discussion of the declarative memory theory; alterations in excitability are then seen in both young animals (Moyer et al., 1996) and aged animals (Moyer et al., 2000). Simple fear conditioning to a punctate CS such as a tone (in which it is sounded for a period prior to and overlapping the delivery of an aversive stimulus such as a mild electric shock) is thought to involve storage of traces in the amygdala (Davis et al., 1993; LeDoux, 2000), although others have argued that the role of the amygdala is primarily neuromodulatory (Vazdarjanova and McGaugh, 1999; McGaugh, 2000). This alternative is important because, as we saw in the discussion of late LTP (see Chapter 10), activity in the amygdala can modulate persistence of LTP in the hippocampus. These and many other studies have broadened our understanding of the role of various brain areas in learning and memory.

The hippocampus may, however, become definitively engaged in conditioning situations in which the associations into which the initially neutral CS enters are predictably inconsistent. In Section 13.2 we saw how a specific behavioral task is said to be ambiguous if there are two or more ways to solve it. A different sense of ambiguity is when the outcome of a specific CS is sometimes one US but on other occasions either another US or the absence of the first US (often abbreviated as NoUS). For example, a light and a tone may each predict the

US when presented on their own but not when presented together. How can an organism cope with this and other forms of predictable ambiguity and so behave appropriately, as many behavioral studies have shown that they can? This class of problem is called the XOR problem in the artificial intelligence and cognitive science communities (Rumelhart and McClelland, 1986) and a nonlinear task by students of the animal learning theory. The nonlinearity arises because it had been thought that CSs acquire associative strength as a function of the reinforcement with which they are linked. However, if this were all there is to learning, the net associative strength of the combined light and tone should always be higher than that acquired by either CS on its own despite the combination of CSs always being followed by nonreward. A nonlinear solution to the problem seems to be required.

Suppose, however, that the brain has a learning device that can resolve such ambiguity. It would then be possible to learn the differential outcome of single and combined stimulus presentations and so react appropriately on every occasion. The *configural-association theory* of Sutherland and Rudy (1989b; Rudy and Sutherland, 1995b) was the first of several hypotheses about hippocampal (and cortical) function that specifically addressed this kind of problem. The *relational-processing theory* (Cohen and Eichenbaum, 1993; Eichenbaum and Cohen, 2001), a development of Squire's original declarative memory theory, also tackled the issue of ambiguity. It took things further in focusing on "relationships" being encoded between stimuli (e.g., that A is better than B and that B is better than C), rather than stimulus configurations (AB, BC). It

also emphasized the possibility that such stimulus relations can be "flexibly" retrieved in an appropriate way in novel situations (e.g., allowing inferences such as that A is better than C). Ideas about the involvement of the hippocampus in *contextual retrieval* (Hirsh, 1974; Good and Honey, 1991) are closely related. What we remember about a stimulus and its associations depends critically on the context in which it occurs, including the absence of an expected stimulus as occurs in the "extinction" of conditioning when a reinforcing US no longer follows a CS. Wide-ranging ideas about the contribution that context cues make to encoding and retrieval, including the notion that contexts "contain and predict rather than simply compete with explicit CSs" (Nadel and Willner, 1980, p. 218), helped spur the development of now widely used learning paradigms such as context fear conditioning. Although intellectually distinct and occasionally at loggerheads with each other, the configural-association, relational-processing, and contextual-retrieval theories have two common threads: They all set out to solve problems involving "predictable ambiguity," and they all argue that the hippocampal formation is central to achieving it.

One of the early theorists to recognize the problem was Hirsh (1974). He looked upon conditioning as a process in which stimulus input came to trigger motor output along a "performance line" as a function of simple CS-US associations (Fig. 13–33A). He argued that it is independent of the hippocampus. On the other hand, he also supposed that a separate "context memory" could somehow interact with the performance line, particularly during memory retrieval, and

Figure 13–33. Coping with predictable ambiguity. *A.* Hirsh's model recognized a distinction between a "performance line," which stores simple CS–US relations and expresses them as conditioned responses, and a "context memory," which modulates the performance line when a CS predicts a US in one context but something

different in another. (*Source*: After Hirsh, 1974.) *B.* Modern learning theory has developed an elaborate framework that is relevant to thinking about the ways in which the hippocampus, functioning as a context memory, could modulate internal representations of associations. See text for discussion.

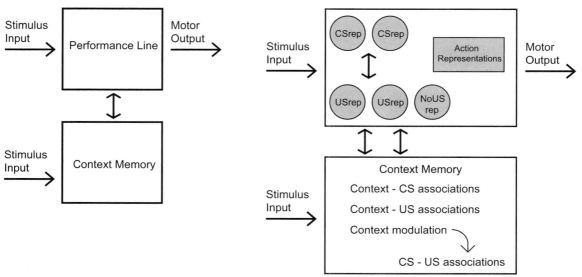

A Associative encoding and retrieval

B Contemporary representational framework for associative memory

so ensure *appropriate* motor output when a specific stimulus predicted reinforcement in one context but the absence of reinforcement in another. Both context memory and the process of contextual retrieval were identified as mediated by the hippocampus. Contemporary research has elaborated this framework in numerous ways (Fig. 13–33B). First, stimulus input is said to give rise to internal representations of CSs and USs that can enter into a variety of associative relations ranging from first-order associations (CSrep–Usrep where "rep" refers to an internal representation of these stimulus events), to second-order relations (CS1–CS2), and even predictions of the absence of a previously expected stimulus (CS–NoUS). These associative relations constitute "knowledge" and (somehow) give rise to goal-oriented action representations that constitute appropriate behavior (e.g., approach food) and then to motor output (the particular movements produced to fulfill an action). The concept of contextual modulation remains, but the manner in which contexts are represented and enter into associations is now recognized as quite complicated. The representations (lower part of Fig. 13–33B) may be "elemental" or "configural," and these in turn may become associated with specific CSs or USs that occur in their presence (context-event associations). In addition to direct associations between contexts and other stimuli, contexts may also modulate the expression of other CS-US associations, such as those expressed within the knowledge system.

Several theories addressing the problems of predictable ambiguity suppose that the hippocampus is a form of configural, relational, or context memory; but they differ with respect to the precise set of processes by which such stimuli enter into or modulate other associations. A consequence of this is that the field has become somewhat baroque and impenetrable. However, it is a serious endeavor that attempts to go beyond descriptive taxonomy to a more detailed and predictive understanding of process and mechanism. The section that follows is a selective representation of this field of research.

13.5.1 Configural Association Theory

Learning is often complicated by ambiguity. A stimulus may signify one event in one situation and another event elsewhere. It is then a "fact" that a tone predicts food in one situation and a "fact" that it does not in another—a complication that the declarative memory theory may have recognized but offered no mechanistic way of addressing. Animals can interpret ambiguous associations such as these provided they are given sufficient additional information and a learning device sophisticated enough to do it. In a series of papers, Rudy and Sutherland (Sutherland and Rudy, 1989; Rudy and Sutherland, 1995; O'Reilly and Rudy, 2001) proposed a theory of hippocampal function, building upon earlier work with animal learning theory in which the configuring of stimuli together as fused compound CSs is the way that animals solve such problems (Rescorla, 1973). The essence of Sutherland and Rudy's and later O'Reilly's proposals are as follows (Box 13–6).

Box 13–6
Configural Association Theory

1. A class of "nonlinear" associative problems can be solved by the process of stimulus "configuring."
2. The hippocampus builds and stores "configural associations" between elemental stimuli (1989), serves an enabling role in their encoding and eventual storage in neocortex (1995), or helps "pattern-separate" stimuli rapidly to aid slow cortical learning (2001).

Ambiguity, Conditioning, and the Hippocampus

Consider the case of two auditory CSs such as tones (call them A1 and A2) that, through repeated pairings, become selectively associated with two types of food (F1 and F2). The experimenter arranges matters such that when a light (L) is illuminated in the test chamber A1 signals F1 and A2 predicts F2. However, when the animals are in the dark (D), A1 is arranged to signal F2 (rather than F1) and A2 predicts F1. Rats and other animals *can* resolve this predictive ambiguity and learn "what leads to what" in each situation.

Rescorla's proposal was that animals (mentally) create stimuli that are "configural" associations between L and A1, L and A2, D and A1, and D and A2. These would be the configural cues (L+A1), (L+A2), and so on. If these configural cues are discriminable, they could enter into unambiguous associations with reinforcement without interference. Learning would otherwise obey established principles of associative learning, namely the gradual accumulation of associative strength to each configural stimulus as a function of how well the sum total of stimuli available at any one time predicts the outcome (Rescorla and Wagner, 1972; Mackintosh, 1983). The animal would have solved the problem and could express its "knowledge" of associative relations in performance.

In its original form, Sutherland and Rudy (1989) proposed that the hippocampus was the physical substrate for encoding and storing configural associations. They also proposed that the configurations could be quite arbitrary combinations of individual stimulus events (e.g., of a light and a tone) occurring together in time, one after another in sequence, or in spatial proximity. The latter aspect of this proposal neatly extended the domain of the theory to tasks such as place learning where multiple stimuli in a given context might be said to define a place. This represented something of a *volte face* for Sutherland, who had earlier argued, in keeping with cognitive map theory, that the learning of a "mapping strategy" in the watermaze was distinct from associative learning (Sutherland and Dyck, 1984). His new idea, with Rudy, was that place learning might actually be a special case of configural learning in which the individual extramaze cues around a watermaze or radial maze enter into stimulus configurations and so (somehow) guide the animal to the correct target. Data that had hitherto offered support for the spatial mapping theory could then be radically reconsidered as potentially supporting the new hypothesis instead. Similarly, the supposition that the hippocampus encodes "configurations" takes the theory into territory not considered in the original version of the declarative memory theory. With that theory, the consolidated "trace strengths" of the associations between A1 and F1 and between A1 and F2 (in the example above) would be equal, and the animal would have no way of resolving the predictive ambiguity of its factual knowledge.

An important feature of the original 1989 configural association theory was that it made a number of clear-cut predictions about when deleterious effects of hippocampal lesions would and would not be observed in associative learning. This is because Sutherland and Rudy recognized that not all kinds of associative learning require configurations to be formed (simple delay conditioning being such a case), whereas others do (nonlinear problems). In short, the theory could be tested—an attractive, widely respected but always precarious feature of any good theory.

Tests of the Original Configural Association Theory

The behavioral tasks Sutherland and Rudy considered to be valid tests are our first taste of the somewhat baroque nature of this field of research. Arguably they are problems that an animal is unlikely to face in its natural habitat, a worrying feature because it is not clear what might have been the evolutionary selection pressure to develop an "ambiguity learning module." However, the apparent artificiality of these tasks reflects a creditable desire on the part of the theory's architects for their hypothesis to be tested rigorously. Four types of task were studied intensively. They are called negative patterning, transverse patterning, biconditional discrimination, and feature-neutral discrimination learning (Fig. 13–34). An explanation of each follows, with reference to exemplar experiments.

With *negative patterning*, two stimuli are each paired individually with reinforcement, but the combination of the two stimuli is nonrewarded. This is annotated in Figure 13–34 as A+, B+, AB−, where A and B are individual stimulus elements, + refers to reward, and − is the absence of reward. As summarized by Rudy and Sutherland (1995), several studies from their laboratory from 1989 onward indicated that neurotoxic hippocampal lesions made in either of two ways (kainic acid plus colchicine or ibotenic acid alone) cause a deficit in negative patterning. These tasks included operant

lever-pressing tasks and a swimming task with cues hanging above potential escape locations (Alvarado and Rudy, 1995a).

This finding did not, however, prove replicable by others. Davidson et al. (1993) observed no deficit in negative patterning in animals with two types of hippocampal lesion. In Davidson et al.'s version of the task, the rats were required to press a lever several times during a tone (T+) or light (L+) for occasional reward (+). This requirement provided a more effective baseline against which to observe a decrease in the rate of responding during the nonreinforced TL− compound. They also used a posttraining transfer test with a novel clicker stimulus to check that learning of the original task did depend on the formation of a true TL configural cue. Although we cannot be certain why different outcomes were obtained in the two studies, Davidson et al. (1993) made the further observation that animals with the same kainic acid + colchicine lesions used by Alvarado and Rudy, but not those with ibotenic acid lesions, displayed disinhibited rates of operant responding during the intertrial interval between tone and light presentations. Both types of lesion are excitotoxic and should therefore spare fibers of passage, unlike older lesion techniques. However, kainic acid also produces lesions distant to the hippocampal formation, such as in the piriform and periamygdaloid cortex. This additional damage could have led to disinhibited responding, and its potential presence raises the possibility that altered motor performance rather than impaired learning contributed to the positive result in some of the earlier Rudy and Sutherland studies. An operant lever-pressing task used by McDonald et al. (1997) indicated that hippocampal lesions slowed down but did not ultimately prevent the rate of learning of a negative patterning task, and fornix lesions had no detectable effect on learning at all. Lesions of the avian hippocampus were also ineffective in impairing negative patterning in pigeons (Broadbent et al., 1999; Papadimitriou and Wynne, 1999). Bussey et al. (2000) found no deficit in a configural conditioning task (conditioned approach to a place where food was available) after radiofrequency fornix lesions or neurotoxic perirhinal/postrhinal (PRPH) lesions. All groups learned to approach in response to either an auditory tone or a brief period of darkness and to withhold approach when these two CSs were presented together. They also used posttraining transfer tests to establish that a configural solution had been used for the task, and "behavioral histology" that took the form of showing that the fornix-lesioned rats were impaired in T maze alternation and the PRPH-lesioned rats in object

Figure 13–34. Four tasks used to test critical predictions of the configural-association theory. The letters A, B, and so on refer to arbitrary stimuli; and the symbols + and − refer to the availability of reinforcement.

A Negative patterning	**B** Transverse patterning
A+ , B+ , AB-	**A+B- , B+C- , C+A-**
C Bidirectional discrimination	**D** Feature-neutral discrimination
AB+ , CD+ , AC- , DB-	**AC+ , C- , AB- , B+**

recognition memory. Overall, the available data from these and other studies on negative patterning represents, at best, only mixed support for the theory.

Transverse patterning fares better. It involves a series of simultaneous discrimination tasks of the form A+ versus B−, B+/C−, and C+/A− in which the stimuli A, B, and C are equally often rewarded (+) and nonrewarded (−). This set of problems, as noted by Moses and Ryan (2006) when comparing predictions of the configural and relational theories, is akin to the children's game of "rock, paper, scissors." Alvarado and Rudy 1995b) reported that rats with hippocampal lesions could readily learn to swim toward A+ and avoid B− and to learn B+/C− when either task was presented over successive trials on its own (Fig. 13–35). However, they failed to learn the full transverse pattern when all three problems were presented together. This result is beautifully consistent with the theory provided it is the AB configural stimulus that triggers approaches to stimulus A, the BC configuration to B, and the CA configuration to C. Unfortunately, it is also a task that may be amenable to solution without recourse to explicit configuring. This would be a "conditional solution" in which the animals learn that one stimulus (e.g., A) is correct given the presence of B, that B is correct given C, and that C is correct given A. The distinction between configural learning and rule learning may seem subtle, but the acquisition of an "if–then" conditional rule obviates the need to form stimulus configu-

rations and may be a form of learning that depends on other brain structures (e.g., the caudate). Conditional rules are not easy for rats to learn; but with sufficient training and provided the information with which they are provided is consistent, they can do it.

Later work on transverse patterning failed to replicate the deleterious effects of hippocampal dysfunction. For example, using an operant task that made it *less* likely that the animals would process the cues as configural "scenes, Bussey et al. (1998) found that fornix lesions significantly *facilitated* transverse patterning. An identified weakness of a first experiment was the relatively poor performance of sham-lesioned rats on the critical third phase when all three problems were trained together. This was addressed in a second study with all three phases trained concurrently. The sham-lesioned group was now above chance, but the trend toward a fornix lesion-induced facilitation remained. We come back to transverse patterning in the discussion (below) of relational processing theory.

Biconditional discrimination tasks can also be solved using configural cues, but unfortunately they may also be learned through the application of a conditional rule. Whishaw and Tomie (1991) trained rats to pull on strings of different widths (A, B) and different odors (C, D) in combinations that led to reward (e.g., AB+, CD+) or no reward (e.g., AC−, BD−). These pairings meant that any one elemental cue predicted

Figure 13–35. Transverse patterning. *A.* Rats were trained to swim toward hanging cue cards that were either placed in front of a possible escape location (e.g., A+) or merely hanging over the pool (e.g., B−). The spatial locations of A+ and B− would be randomized across trials. *B.* The stimulus patterns used for the full transverse patterning problem. *C.* Deficit in hippocampus-lesioned rats (H) compared to sham lesion controls. (Source: After Alvarado and Rudy, 1995b.)

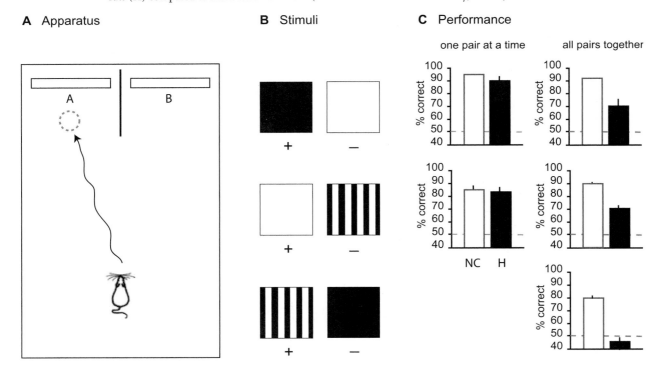

reward and nonreward equally often, but the creation of four configural cues would enable a solution. Here the configural-association theory fared less well: Rats with hippocampal damage and sham-lesioned animals were both able to learn to pull the correct string to get the reward. Similar negative results had also been found in a similar earlier study using primates (Saunders and Weiskrantz, 1989).

The fourth category of ambiguous problem that Sutherland and Rudy (1989) considered is the *feature-neutral discrimination task*. An explanation of the name for this protocol may help clarify what is being examined. The "feature" of the task is a particular stimulus; let us call it stimulus A (as in Fig. 13–34). In conjunction with stimulus C, the feature A signifies that a reward is available. Conditioning should lead to stimulus A acquiring some associative strength. However, in conjunction with stimulus B, feature A now signifies that a reward is *un*available. Stimulus A should therefore become "inhibitory." By scheduling all four types of trial, stimulus A should remain "neutral" with respect to its scheduled association with reward (it is as often paired with reward as not) while still being the critical feature that enables the rat to learn the discrimination. Hence, it is called a feature-neutral discrimination task. As in negative patterning, no combination of elementary associations between stimuli and a reward can solve the problem, and the configural association theory uniquely predicts that rats with hippocampal lesions should fail. Unfortunately, two studies using this design have both found that rats with hippocampal lesions can learn it. In fact, Gallagher and Holland (1992) found a facilitation of some aspects of feature-neutral discrimination learning by rats with neurotoxic hippocampal lesions, a result that echoes Bussey et al.'s (1998) results on transverse patterning after fornix lesions.

Taken together, this pattern of results from the four sets of tasks provided only qualified support for the configural association theory. The results of the negative and transverse patterning tasks sometimes upheld predictions of the theory, whereas the outcome of the biconditional and feature-neutral discrimination tasks did not. It is perhaps worth reflecting further on the curious paradox that whereas a normal rat can solve these problems we ostensibly smarter humans often struggle to understand them. The struggle is nonetheless worthwhile, as understanding ambiguity and its role in learning is important. All these tasks are ones in which an implicit learning device is assumed to encode a stimulus configuration that acquires associative strength through its consistent association with reward. Ostensibly, no new principles of associative learning are involved—only a configuring device. The question therefore arises of whether this device is likely to be in the hippocampal formation. One reason to be skeptical is that the anatomical and electrophysiological data discussed in Chapters 3, 4, and 8 strongly suggest that the sensory information to which the hippocampal formation has access is *already* polymodal and already highly processed. Therefore, a neurobiological concern about the theory, quite apart from the inconsistencies in the behavioral data, is not whether stimulus configurations are ever formed but that their construction is more likely to have taken place in the neocortex.

Revised Theory

In response to the mixed picture of initial results, Rudy and Sutherland presented a revised theory that wisely put the configuring part of the system outside the hippocampus in neocortex. However, they still asserted that the hippocampus plays a role in learning configural associations by "selectively enhancing the salience of configural representations" (Rudy and Sutherland, 1995, p. 382). A yet later change in the theory emphasizes, in a similar vein, the role that the hippocampus could play in rapidly separating similar patterns for effective processing in the cortex (O'Reilly and Rudy, 2001). These changes were in response to observations that ambiguous tasks that could eventually be learned by animals with hippocampal damage were often learned more slowly than by controls. It was a set of changes that would rescue aspects of the theory but at the cost of making it more difficult to test definitively. In some respects, this is unfortunate because, arguably more than other theorists, Rudy and Sutherland have been rigorously honorable in demanding explicit predictions and definitive tests.

Going down with the ship is all very well, but a key issue is whether the logical structure of tasks, such as those laid out in Figure 13–34, actually constrains the way in which an animal solves any one task. The original version of the configural association theory implied that this was the case. However, when comparing negative patterning with feature-neutral discriminations and biconditional tasks, Rudy and Sutherland (1995) noted a parametric gradation across the tasks. This gradation was from negative patterning that absolutely required animals to learn to withhold responding to a configural stimulus composed of *two* elements (i.e., AB−) that are also presented alone and reinforced (A+, B+) to biconditional tasks in which none of the elements are ever presented alone and reinforced (i.e., always X with Y and either + or −). They argued that this parametric variation is important because it relates to the extent to which individual stimuli acquire associative strength during conditioning that is likely to conflict or oppose the strength that should be shown by configural stimuli. If this gradation is significant, it might be that the task with the greatest conflict would be definitively impaired by hippocampal damage, whereas that with less conflict would be least affected. To some extent, the data available in 1995 did fit this pattern.

However, one aspect not considered was the possibility that distinct CSs may not interact only by forming configural cues but in more subtle ways as well. For example, under some circumstances, one CS may modulate or "set the occasion" for the other CS to enter into a conditioned association. A good illustration of this is the *feature negative discrimination task* in which a stimulus A is reinforced on its own A+ but not reinforced when B is presented before A (i.e., B → A−). Under these circumstances, instead of an AB configural stimulus being created (which may happen when all the stimuli are presented concurrently), B acts in a different manner, modulating whether the presentation of A retrieves a memory of the US or the absence of the US. Occasion-setting is an associative process in which one CS serves as a signal for an association between other stimuli in a hierarchical manner. Work by Holland and his colleagues indicates that hippocampal lesions can disrupt one type of negative occasion-setting (Holland et al., 1999), raising the possibility that the memory traces responsible for conditioned associations between stimuli are encoded and stored in the cortex (including configural stimuli) but can be subject to hierarchical control by stimuli processed in the hippocampus. However, an alternative interpretation remains feasible. This is that although the hippocampus is not involved in forming excitatory CS-US connections it is involved in inhibitory learning (i.e., that a particular CS does *not* lead to an otherwise expected US). Chan et al. (2001) had somewhat unfashionably defended an inhibitory view of hippocampus function. They looked on the feature negative occasion-setting task as one in which, in normal rats, a CS forms both excitatory and inhibitory associations, and the occasion-setter helps to choose between them. The disruption caused by hippocampal lesions may then be a deficit in inhibitory, rather than hierarchical, occasion-setting. The problem with this view is that there are many occasions in which hippocampal lesions have no effect on the extinction of CS-US associations—the classic test of an inhibition theory (Wilson et al., 1995).

In the further refinement of the configural framework, O'Reilly and Rudy (2001) have semantically recast the theory to refer to "conjunctive representations" rather than "configurations" and suggested that there are two kinds of conjunctive learning. One type is thought to occur incidentally or automatically, irrespective of task demands; this is the type that is rapidly learned and involves the hippocampus. The other type is slower and more deliberate, and the kind of learning that emerges as a consequence of a deliberate type of problem-solving. This new incidental versus deliberate framework is also explicit about the contribution that local circuits in the hippocampal formation make to algorithms such as "pattern separation" and "pattern completion" (in the dentate gyrus and area CA3 respectively—see Chapter 14), and to the similarities between tasks involving configurations of individual CSs with context-dependent associations. We return to issues to which these revisions of the theory are relevant in Section 13.6, together with reference to the important issue of "automaticity" in hippocampus-dependent learning.

13.5.2 Relational Processing Theory: Refinement of the Declarative Memory Theory

A significant feature of memory is the ability to recall facts and events in circumstances different from those in which the information was acquired in the first place. The inherent "flexibility" of this form of memory was particularly emphasized in a revision of the declarative memory theory advanced by Cohen and Eichenbaum (1993) and later revised by them (Eichenbaum and Cohen, 2001). It has been developed further in relation to episodic memory processing (Eichenbaum, 2004), which we address later. The theory also places emphasis on the encoding of "relations" between stimuli. This is quite different from forming configurations (as just discussed), and more akin to the idea of associations between facts, such as that one fact can remind us of another. The information processing necessary for "flexible relations" is held to occur at the time of encoding but only becomes apparent when retrieval is required in circumstances different from those of the original learning. Like the original version of the declarative memory theory, this theory holds that relational processing is within the capacity of (at least) "higher" mammals, that it depends on activity in the MTL, and that the engagement of the hippocampal formation is time-limited. "Relational processing" is held to be implemented by the hippocampal formation, whereas anatomically distinct neocortical regions of the MTL mediate the processing and storage of individual stimuli. This theory led to a number of distinctive lines of experimentation that require discussion separate from those already outlined in the discussion of the declarative memory theory but to which the configural association theory is, as we shall see, also relevant. The distinctive propositions of the theory are in Box 13–7.

"Relational representations" were defined as memory representations that are "created by and can be used for comparing and contrasting individual items in memory, and weaving new items into the existing organization of memories. This form of representation maintains the compositionality of the items, that is, the encoding of items both as perceptually distinct objects and as parts of larger scale scenes and events that capture the relevant relations between them" (Cohen and Eichenbaum, 1993).

The gist of the first proposition is that the relations that humans and animals are able to store and recall go beyond the mere fact that two stimuli were experienced together in temporal contiguity—the "CS predicts US" type of association so extensively studied in conditioning paradigms. "Comparing and contrasting" implies that relations between stimuli can be more sophisticated. They may be causal, but they may also

---

Box 13–7
Relational Processing Theory

1. Declarative memory generally involves processing the relations between different items. Relational processing at encoding enables flexible access to information in situations quite different from those of the original learning.
2. Relational processing is carried out by the hippocampal formation, but storage of individual items in intermediate memory takes place in the perirhinal and parahippocampal cortex.
3. The role of the hippocampus in memory is temporary, as in the declarative memory theory.

relate to physical relations (e.g., that A is near to, or bigger than, B; as in "Versailles is near Paris") or to abstract relations (as in "the ugly sisters were unfriendly to Cinderella"). Moreover, relations can extend beyond one-to-one pairings to elaborate networks of interconnections between facts and events—the very networks that constitute our personal understanding of the world. The theory's proponents asserted that their view echoes William James, who described memory as an elaborated network of associations that can be applied across a broad range of situations (James, 1890). Although the circumstances or conditions of learning are not well specified in the theory, in the manner of contemporary learning theory, the emphasis on relations is clearly a step beyond reference to the "facts and events" in Squire's (1992) original version of the declarative-memory theory. Cohen and Eichenbaum (1993) have put their finger on an important issue; and, indeed, Squire has now incorporated some of their ideas into his modern writings (e.g., Squire et al., 2004).

Whereas some types of factual information tend to be recalled in a rote-like fashion, as in a child's recitation of arithmetic ("two-plus-two is four, four-plus-four is eight . . ."), remembering facts and events is often deductive. They may be recalled in different contexts from those in which they were originally experienced and in a manner that permits access to other perceptual features of a current situation. Indeed, certain "facts" may not have been stored at all (such as knowing the number of windows in your house, which most people work out inferentially by mentally walking through the building and counting them). The overall network of relations does not need to be present or to be recalled to access a smaller subset of facts. Flexibility also allows deductive inference. An illustrative example is inferring geographical relations. Suppose an American schoolboy living in South Carolina has learned in school that "Paris is the capital of France," that "Madrid is the capital of Spain," and that "France is farther north than Spain." Based on these facts, the child should be able to infer the additional fact that "Paris is north of Madrid." If then told that Madrid is on the same latitude as Washington, DC, he might, assuming he knows his American geography, also draw the further inference that "Paris must be north of where I live because Madrid and Washington are on the same latitude." This illustrates how new spatial facts can be inferred even though never explicitly learned. Of course, flexibility is a hallmark of the cognitive map theory as well, but there it is held to be a specific, unique property of spatial memory. The supposition now is that flexibility includes the spatial domain but extends well beyond it to size, social relationships, and yet others. The information processing provided by the hippocampus is not domain-specific.

The second and third propositions of the theory concern the relation between the hippocampal formation and neocortex. Like Squire's theory, Cohen and Eichenbaum argued that damage to the hippocampal formation causes loss of the capacity to store new explicit memories without having an effect on implicit memory (i.e., for stimulus relations of which we are *not* consciously aware. They agreed that hippocampal lesions spare the acquisition and expression of motor, procedural, and cognitive skills. The refinement they offer is what amounts to fractionation of declarative memory into two subcomponents: (1) the processing and storage in intermediate memory (ITM) of stimulus items in isolation carried out in the perirhinal and parahippocampal gyrus; and (2) the processing of stimulus relations in such a way as to enable flexible access, carried out by the hippocampal formation (Fig. 13–36). As long-term storage is held to be in other areas of association cortex, the stimulus representations in the MTL are asserted to be "compressed." This is a metaphor taken from modern computer science; but a claim with no direct evidence to support it requires a much deeper understanding of neural representations in the hippocampal formation than we presently possess.

There are three other features to highlight. First, because spatial relations are only one of the many types of flexible relations that humans and other mammals can encode, the theory embraces some of the positive evidence hitherto held to support the cognitive map theory in an ostensibly more general theoretical position. In fact, Eichenbaum (1996) argued that spatial learning fractionates into flexible and inflexible forms, with only the former sensitive to hippocampal disruption (reminiscent of Olton's "working memory" theory in which spatial reference memory is insensitive to such lesions). This may account for successful spatial learning by hippocampus-

Figure 13–36. Three functional components of the relational processing memory system: cortical-hippocampal connections showing the three main components. The cortical areas store short-term memory (STM) and long-term memory (LTM) traces of specific items; the parahippocampal region serves as intermediate memory (ITM) for specific items and does the job of cue compression. The hippocampal formation computes relational representations in a manner that enables representational flexibility.

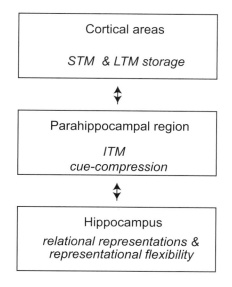

Relational processing theory - processes and anatomical mediation

lesioned rats during overtraining (Morris et al., 1990) because after extended training the animals can learn discrete approach responses from each of several starting locations in the pool. However, this finding is also consistent with the hippocampus-independent "taxon" approach strategies of the cognitive map theory. Second, the theory states that the role of the hippocampus in the formation of flexible representations is time-limited. Such representations are then consolidated in the neocortex, where they can be accessed flexibly without further hippocampal input. Thus, the machinery for creating flexibility is in the hippocampus, but (somewhat clumsily) the machinery for flexible recall is in the neocortex. Third, if the hippocampal formation is damaged, stimulus items that are presented together may become fused into configurations. Associations can still be created, but the theory supposes that they are not relational but always configural. This idea capitalizes on the same kind of data that led Rudy and Sutherland (1995a) to propose their revised theory.

Evidence for Hippocampus-dependent Relational Representations and Flexible Access

The first study directly investigating relational processing in humans involved brain imaging using positron emission tomography (PET) (Henke et al., 1997). This study required subjects to look at slides containing a person or a house and asked them to judge the gender of the person and whether an inside or outside view of the house was being displayed or to guess whether the person was likely to live in the house or be a regular visitor to it. Only the latter instructions encouraged "comparing and contrasting" of the two pictures and so triggered relational processing. Comparison of the relative brain activation in the two conditions revealed greater activation in the right MTL during the relational condition. This finding supports the relational processing account, all the more so because the associations formed were nonspatial. Other human studies, using fMRI, have partially supported the idea that relational processing can drive hippocampal activation (Cohen et al., 1999). However, in an explicit comparison of two matched spatial and social relationship tasks, Kumaran and Maguire (2005) saw activation of the human hippocampal formation only during the spatial relation task. A network of real people, some of whom were friends (or friends of friends) and all of whom lived at various places in the same city, was identified in an initial briefing session. The main tasks to be conducted in the scanner included getting a crate of wine from one person to another (together with various control tasks). In the social version of the main task, the crate could be passed from friend to friend. In the spatial version, it was passed to the nearest neighbor. Hippocampus activation was observed when subjects were required to focus on and navigate spatially (e.g., their friend's houses). A quite different network of brain areas was activated when subjects wandered mentally within their social network—retrieving knowledge about their friends and their relationships to each other—including the medial prefrontal cortex, insula, superior temporal sulcus, and other areas implicated in a proposed

circuitry for social cognition (Adolphs, 2003). In a further setback for the relational processing account of human hippocampal function, a sharp distinction between item and associative memory is also not fully supported by other contemporary fMRI studies, as reviewed in Chapter 12. Hippocampal activation can sometimes be seen with individual memory items, particularly when they are novel, though the novelty-driven nature of such activations is often the unusual spatial context in which a stimulus is presented and thus cryptically relational.

Animal studies have played a bigger part in driving the theory. Bunsey and Eichenbaum (1996) developed an odor-guided paired-associate learning task for rats to examine whether learned information could be used inferentially in novel testing situations. The animals could dig through food cups containing a mixture of ground rat chow and sand to secure a fruit-loop cereal reward. One of several odors was added to the sand/chow mixture so the rats' experience of digging was associated with the odor. The animals took to the task quickly, perhaps because digging for food is as much a part of their natural foraging strategy as remembering where they are (Fig. 13–37).

Paired-associate learning tasks are most extensively used in human cognitive psychology and typically involve presentation of the first member of each pair (the so-called cue item), followed by either free recall of the second item or a two-alternative forced-choice test between two potential associates of which only one is correct. The pairs may be word pairs, words and faces, or other combinations of stimuli. Bunsey and Eichenbaum's paired-associate training protocol for rats used the two-alternative forced-choice test. The initial training phase consisted of digging through the sample item, in which a single digging cup with a single odor was presented (e.g., cocoa = cue A), followed immediately by the two-alternative choice test in which two cups were presented and the animal's task was to dig in the cup whose odor was to be associated with the initial cue item (e.g., coffee = cue B). That is, following cue A the animal was rewarded during the choice phase if it dug through cue B but was unrewarded if it dug through the other cup (e.g., salt = cue Y). Conversely, if the animal was presented with turmeric as a first-item cue (cue X), digging in the salt cup (cue Y) in the choice phase secured reward whereas digging through cue B (coffee) did not. Having learned in this way that A goes with B and that X goes with Y (over many training trials), a second set of paired associates was then taught in which the rats learned that odor B goes with C (not Z) and that odor Y goes with Z (not C). Sham and ibotenate hippocampus-lesioned rats learned both sets of "premise" paired associates in this way quite rapidly and at the same rate (Fig. 13–37B). An ingenious feature of the experiment was inherent in the design. The two sets of paired associates deliberately contained common elements: odors B (coffee) and Y (salt). This commonality afforded the opportunity of exploring whether rats that had learned that A goes with B (and B goes with C) could access these stimulus–stimulus representations flexibly and so reveal transitive knowledge about the relation between A and C. In a probe test

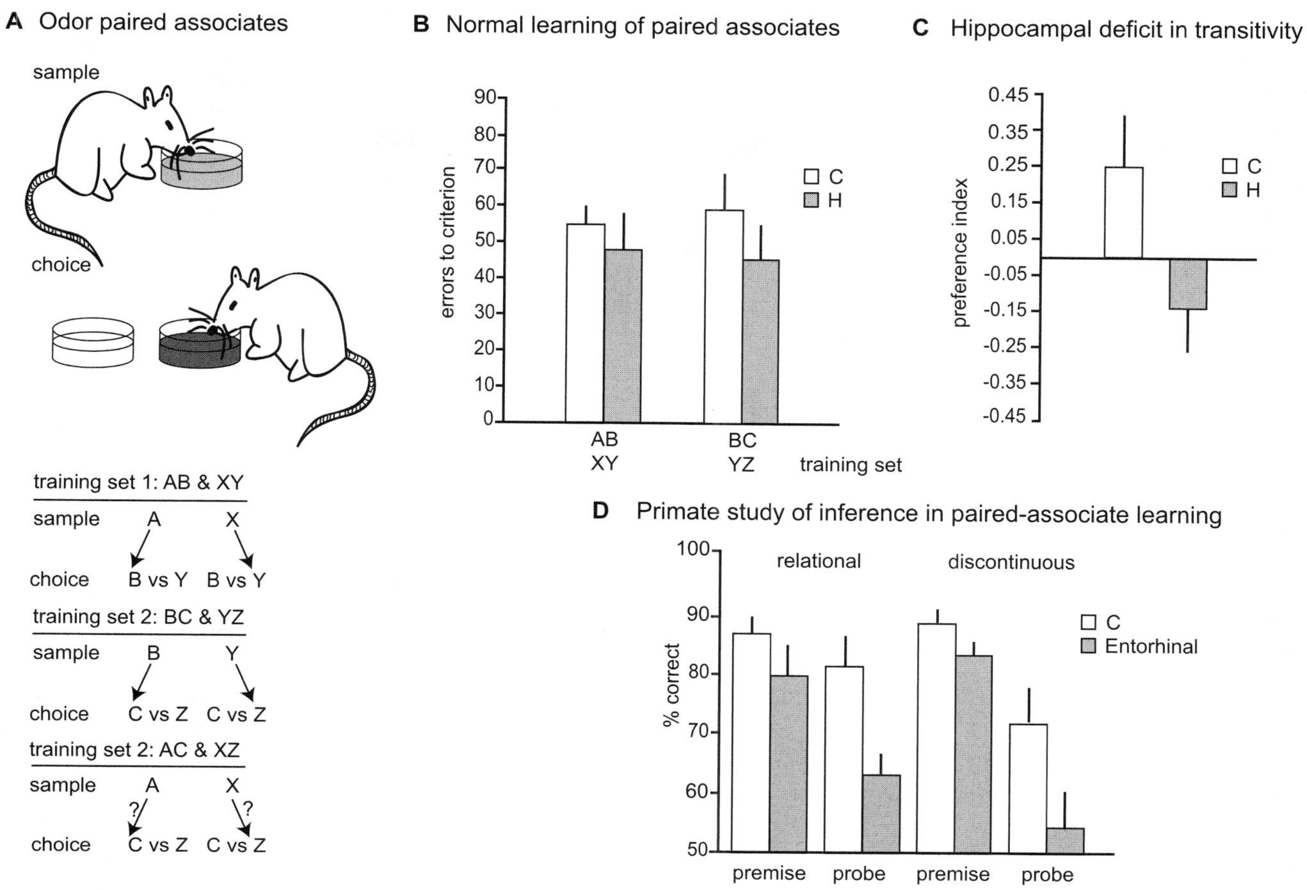

A Odor paired associates

sample

choice

training set 1: AB & XY

sample	A	X

choice   B vs Y   B vs Y

training set 2: BC & YZ

sample	B	Y

choice   C vs Z   C vs Z

training set 2: AC & XZ

sample	A	X

choice   C vs Z   C vs Z

B Normal learning of paired associates

C Hippocampal deficit in transitivity

D Primate study of inference in paired-associate learning

Figure 13–37. Flexible retrieval of learned paired-associate information. *A.* The rat approaches and digs through the scented sand/chow mixture during a "sample" trial until it gets its fruit-loop reward. A short while later, it is presented by two other scented food cups in a "two-alternative forced choice" test. The scent associated with the previous sample indicates in which of the choice cups the animal should dig to get another reward. *B.* Sham-lesioned and lesioned rats were equally capable of learning the odor-paired asso-ciations. The question at issue is the nature of the relations that were encoded during this training. *C.* The test for transitivity showed that the sham rats were above chance in choosing C given A, and Z given X, whereas the hippocampus-lesioned animals could not draw these inferences. (*Source*: After Bunsey and Eichenbaum, 1996.) *D.* Findings from an analogous primate study revealed selective impairment on the probe but not premise choice trials after entorhinal cortex lesions. (*Source*: After Buckmaster et al., 2004.)

for this, the rats were first given either odor A or X as the initial single-cup cue item and then presented with a choice between cups containing odors C and Z. The striking result was that the sham-lesioned animals chose appropriately (i.e., C after A and Z after X), but hippocampus-lesioned rats did not (Fig. 13–37C).

In further experiments also using the same sand-digging method, Dusek and Eichenbaum (1997) considered the issue of hippocampal involvement in building ordered representations using a classic Piagetian seriation paradigm. It was adapted for use in work with primates by McGonigle and Chalmers (1977). Later work established that pigeons and rats could also behave "logically," but Eichenbaum's group was the first to explore the anatomical substrate. Sham-, fornix-, and perirhinal/entorhinal-lesioned rats were trained in a "transitive inference" task to choose odor A over odor B and then B > C, C > D, and D > E using a training protocol that began with successive trials of each discrete problem and ended with the individual problems in random sequence (see Box 13–8).

After they had mastered these four problems, the animals were presented with two other novel problems: choosing between odors B and D and between A and E. Both involved a choice between odors that had never previously been presented together, but only the former pair (B > D) required knowledge of a serial order. This is because the "probe" odors B and D had each served equally often as rewarded or as nonrewarded odors during training, whereas the "end-anchor" odors, A and E, were always positive or negative odors, respectively. Sham-lesioned rats chose both B over D and A over E, whereas rats with fornix or perirhinal/entorhinal lesions could only do the A versus E comparison (Fig. 13–38).

Work in species other than the rat has revealed mixed support for the relational processing idea. A study in pigeons revealed that they could learn the paired-associate task and successfully solve the inferential probe tests, but hippocampal lesions were without effect (Strasser et al., 2004). Using objects in a WGTA, Saunders and Weiskrantz (1989) trained monkeys on a biconditional task (like those described in the previous

Transitive inference task

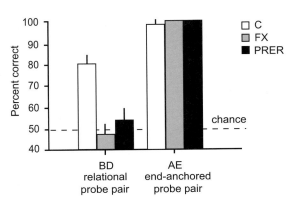

Figure 13–38. Hippocampal participation in transitive inference. Choice performance by controls and fornix-lesioned (FX) and perirhinal/entorhinal-lesioned (PRER) groups during the two choice tests after seriation training. Both lesioned groups are at chance on the B versus D comparison, but both perform as well as controls on the A versus E end-anchored choice test. (*Source*: After Dusek and Eichenbaum, 1997.)

section) followed by an interrogation of what the monkeys "knew" about which object was related to which other object. The animals were trained, through a series of stages, with pairings in which each object was equally often rewarded or non-rewarded, but specific pairings were consistently rewarded (e.g., AB+, CD+) or consistently nonrewarded (AC−, BD−). Hippocampal disruption (fornix lesions or combined fornix, hippocampal, and mammillary body damage) did not affect acquisition of the task but did impair performance in the posttraining probe test of "what goes with what." In this probe, the monkeys were confronted with three objects (A, B, C) and, having displaced A to receive a reward, got a second reward on the same trial only if they then displaced B (AB having been a rewarded pair during training). Only the con-

trols succeeded in doing this. This finding suggests that the normal controls had acquired an abstract representation of the object pairings that was more "flexible" than that acquired by the lesioned monkeys. The successful learning of the biconditional task with poor inferential probe test performance is arguably more consistent with the relational processing account than the configural-association theory.

Buckmaster et al. (2004) trained monkeys on a series of procedures intended to emphasize relational representations: a paired associate task analogous to that of the Bunsey and Eichenbaum (1996) study, a transitive inference task based on the original primate work of McGonigle and Chalmers (1977), and a novel spatial delayed recognition span procedure. They were also received training in object discrimination learning and DNMS (simple associations and recognition memory). Monkeys with large (> 90%) entorhinal lesions acquired and performed these latter tasks normally but were impaired on each of the three tasks that required relational processing. The entorhinal cortex-lesioned monkeys gradually acquired the difficult discriminations required in the paired-associate task, but acquisition was slower than normal, suggesting that a different, less flexible configural learning strategy was being used. Performance by normal monkeys in both the premise and probe trials was more than 80% correct (Buckmaster et al., 2004), but there was selective impairment on the probe trials after entorhinal cortex lesions (Fig. 13–38D). The results on the transitive inference tasks were consistent with those obtained in rats, but aberrant poor performance by one normal control monkey in this task make it difficult to draw firm conclusions. The perennial problem of the numbers of subjects used in primate studies is often quite low. The spatial span task could not be learned by the lesioned monkeys, a finding that would be consistent with the cognitive map theory were it not for the deficits in the other relational tasks that were explicitly nonspatial. These are important results, as studies of entorhinal cortex lesions had previously failed to reveal any lasting deficit in DNMTS (Leonard et al., 1995), but the commonality of the deficit here with hippocampal lesions is consistent with the proposal made in Chapter 3 that the entorhinal cortex should be viewed as a major component of the hippocampal formation.

A potential difficulty is that the transitive inference task is a classic example of a procedure in which the devil is in the detail, both conceptually and procedurally (McGonigle and Chalmers, 2003). Like other ambiguous tasks, it is a task that can be solved in several ways. Van Elzakker et al. (2003) noted at least four theoretical accounts of successful task performance and argued that a simple "excitatory stimulus value" account cannot be ruled out. This may seem surprising as, on the face of it, the novel B > D probe compares two stimuli that should be of equal excitatory stimulus value as they are equally often paired with reward and nonreward during training. However, there are some cryptic asymmetries to the training protocol that may render this assumption false. When learning D > E in the five-problem series, the pairing is with a stimulus E that is *never* reinforced. D may therefore not have

---

Box 13–8
Transitive Inference Premise Training

A > B		Individual premise problems
B > C		trained separately
C > D		
D > E		

Ordered mental representation of relations

A > B > C > D > E

Probe choice tests

B	vs.	D	Test of transitivity
A	vs.	E	Nontransitive novel pairing

to acquire a very high net excitatory stimulus value before the difference between D and E crosses the threshold necessary for criterion performance. Similarly, A is always reinforced, and thus the A > B difference might also be realized despite B actually having a fairly high associative strength. Given this, the relative values of B and D may be different despite the ostensibly equal pairing with reward and nonreward. In addition, one might then expect a B versus D probe to be easier in a four-problem series (A > B, B > C, C > D, D > E) than in a five-problem series in which an E > F problem is added. Exactly these results were found by Van Elzakker et al. (2003), who therefore queried whether relational processing and inferential memory retrieval were being used to perform the task. Computational modeling by Frank et al. (2003) has taken this further, with a detailed treatment of the impact of the "end-anchors" on the associative strength of stimuli with which they are routinely paired, the role of configural representations in the performance of normal (unlesioned) animals, and the balance between effects of "pattern separation" and "pattern completion" in the task. They also queried the adequacy of a relational processing account of transitive inference and made the interesting prediction that hippocampus or dentate gyrus lesions created after training should have no effect on performance of the BD probe, in contrast to the deleterious effect on choice when made before training. This is an important prediction because, in contrast, the relational processing theory would require the hippocampus to be intact at the time of a probe test. This valuable pretraining versus posttraining comparison of the configural and relational processing accounts has not yet been reported.

The lesion studies that have at least partially supported the relational processing theory of hippocampus function have been complemented by unit-recording data using similar paradigms (Wood et al., 1999). Multiple single-unit recordings were taken of CA1 pyramidal cells firing during a 1-second period just prior to a rat deciding whether to dig in a continuous recognition variant of the paradigms just described. Food cups containing sand were repeatedly presented to animals in different locations of an open arena. For trials in which the cups were scented with a novel odor (half the trials), the sand had a fruit-loop reward buried at the bottom; for trials in which the odor was repeated (i.e., no longer novel), no fruit loop was present. The rats quickly learned the logic of the situation: to dig when it was worth it and refrain from doing so when it was not. The unit-recording data taken during the Shakespearean "to dig or not to dig" decision period indicated that approximately one-third of the hippocampal cells had task-related *nonspatial* correlates. Place-specific firing was certainly seen in some cells (about another third). Of the nonspatial cells, some were associated with approach behavior, some with approaching a particular odor irrespective of its location in space, and some with whether the trial was with an odor that was familiar or novel (match/nonmatch)—all relations of a nonspatial character. These data indicate that the functional correlates of CA1 pyramidal cell firing may depend in part on the task a rat is being trained to perform, not just on its location in space. This is a deep idea

that requires further investigation in analytically exacting tasks. However, a follow-up study (Dudchenko et al., 2000) revealed this continuous recognition task to be insensitive to hippocampal lesions, again raising doubts about the extent to which a "relational" description of the cellular correlates is justified. The parallel to what is seen in NMR conditioning is beguiling—as if the hippocampus mischievously likes to "listen in" on things it does not have anything to do with. We later argue that this is exactly what an incidental learning system may have to do.

These experiments are taken by Eichenbaum and Cohen (2001) to indicate that: (1) rats develop a knowledge of stimulus relations that can be retrieved flexibly to guide inferences from memory; (2) hippocampal cells are responsive to such task-related attributes; and (3) the integrity of the fornix, hippocampus, and perirhinal/entorhinal cortices are essential for representing these attributes flexibly. This interpretation clearly goes beyond the domain of both the original declarative memory and cognitive map theories but leaves open whether the hippocampus is engaged in relational processing at encoding, retrieval, or both. As just noted in the contrast with a configural association account of transitive inference, making lesions before training does not distinguish these two alternatives. Reversible inactivation, using drugs that inhibit synaptic transmission cell firing, would also provide an opportunity to explore whether the hippocampus needs be active at encoding and retrieval, as it does for spatial reference memory (Riedel et al., 1999), and whether it plays a time-limited role in systems-level memory consolidation as the relational processing theory predicts. If time-limited, it would imply that "flexibility" can be displayed by neocortical circuits also, provided information is subject to both hippocampus-dependent encoding and a period of hippocampal-neocortical consolidation.

The notion of representational flexibility and its dependence on the hippocampus is also illustrated by experiments on the social transmission of food preferences using a paradigm first developed by Galef and Wigmore (1983). Two rats are put together for a short period. One of these rats, the demonstrator, is arranged to have recently eaten a novel foodstuff. The animals are then separated and, after a memory delay, the other animal, the observer, is tested with two novel foods. One novel food is the same as the one the demonstrator has eaten, and the other novel food is not. In this two-alternative forced-choice test, the observer rat shows a preference for the novel food eaten by the demonstrator over the other (Fig. 13–39A). Some social feature of the situation conquers the animal's usual neophobia. An early series of analytical studies (Galef, 1990) had established that this social transmission of food preferences is mediated by carbon disulfide (CS_2) in the breath of the demonstrator rat that acts a "carrier" of the smell of the food that the demonstrator has eaten. Although this social-transmission task is not obviously relational in quite the same way as the paired-associate task, it is flexible with respect to how the learned information is expressed. Information about the novel food is acquired by the observer on the breath of the demonstrator rather than through actual consumption, and

A Odor-guided, paired associate learning

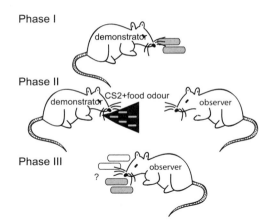

B Retrograde amnesia after hippocampal lesions

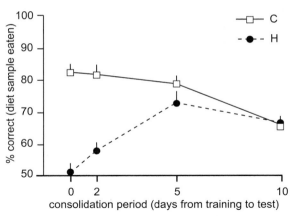

Figure 13–39. Social transmission of food preferences. *A.* Odor-guided paired associate learning in which information about a food odor that is safe to eat (gray food) is acquired by an "observer" rat smelling the breath of a "demonstrator" rat that has previously eaten that food. This acquired knowledge is later expressed in the form of a preference in a two-alternative choice test over another food (white). (*Source*: After Galef and Wigmore, 1983.) *B.* Retrograde amnesia for social transmission after hippocampal lesions. (*Source*: After Winocur, 1990.)

this "knowledge" is later expressed by the observer rat. Procedural learning systems in which knowledge is embedded in performance would not support such learning.

Winocur (1990) discovered that this task is sensitive to hippocampal lesions created either before or shortly after the demonstrator–observer interaction. Faster forgetting, over 6 days, was observed in the animals lesioned before training. In animals subjected to lesioning after the social transmission phase but before the preference test, a consolidation gradient was observed: Those with hippocampal lesions displayed retrograde amnesia 1 day after lesion creation, whereas those whose lesions were created 5 to 10 days later performed significantly better (Fig. 13–39B). Bunsey and Eichenbaum (1995) confirmed Winocur's finding of faster forgetting using rats with ibotenate lesions that encompassed the hippocampus, dentate gyrus, and subiculum. Rats with more selective hippocampus + dentate lesions showed little forgetting over 24 hours, but the longer 6-day interval used in Winocur's study was not examined and these more selective lesions were incomplete at the temporal pole. In the light of data concerning differential functions of the dorsal and ventral hippocampus, it is possible that social transmission of food preference could be one that is specifically sensitive to ventral hippocampal lesions.

Evidence for Functional Dissociations Between Anatomical Components of Declarative Memory: Role of the Hippocampus

One point of departure between this and Squire's (1992) version of declarative memory theory has to do with functional dissociations between components of the MTL memory system. Squire argued against functional distinctions, except at the input stage where some differentiation between the infor-

mation projected to the perirhinal and parahippocampal cortex is recognized (Suzuki and Amaral, 1994a,b). In contrast, the relational processing theory requires the hippocampal formation to perform a role in declarative memory distinct from that performed by the surrounding neocortical structures. The latter structures are held to be an intermediate memory store (ITM) for individual items, whereas the hippocampal formation is the "relational processor." This modification accommodates the finding that DNMTS for trial-unique cues is impaired by neocortical damage to the perirhinal and parahippocampal gyrus but is unaffected (or only very mildly affected) by hippocampal lesions. The new findings, discussed above, support the relational processing modifications of the declarative memory theory.

One point to note in passing is that, whereas most studies of DNMTS have been conducted using visual cues and objects, olfactory cues have been used extensively in Eichenbaum's rodent studies. Faster forgetting of olfactory cues after entorhinal lesions was first observed by Staubli et al. (1984). Otto and Eichenbaum (1992) confirmed this finding using a continuous delayed nonmatching task (cDNM) with odors. Fornix lesions had no effect, whereas perirhinal and parahippocampal cortex lesions caused faster forgetting. Thus, for the type of information used most extensively in the studies on which the theory has been built (odors) an intermediate memory does appear to exist in the neocortical regions of the medial temporal area.

13.5.3 Contextual Encoding and Retrieval

The original version of spatial mapping theory focused on how environmental landmarks of a specific context are explored and integrated into spatial maps for the purposes of navigation (O'Keefe and Nadel, 1978). However, "context" can be important in ways other than as a space to be moved around. Memories of discrete events could include associations between an event and its context, such as the place or time at which the event happened (Nadel and Willner, 1980). Generally, a context has also to be learned about before the representation of it can enter into other associations (Fanselow, 1990), but although this representation is often spatial it need not be (Jeffery et al., 2004). It could include temporal cues, particularly during extinction of conditioned associations (Bouton, 2004); it may include feelings associated with administered drugs (Overton, 1964) or naturally occurring motivational states such as hunger or thirst (Davidson, 1993). A context may also be "cognitive" as in the mental frameworks or schema associated with particular classes of problem (Morris, 2006). The importance of context-dependent memory is well demonstrated by occasions on which it fails, such as when we embarrassingly fail to recognize a person we have recently met in a different context. Contextual encoding is clearly an effective, often automatic associative mechanism for binding events into memory.

As shown in Figure 13–33B, the modulation of memory by contexts can be mediated by distinct associations and associative processes (Balsam and Tomie, 1985; Bouton and Moody, 2004). As with the formation of stimulus configurations or relational associations, contexts can influence the attention paid to a stimulus, "set the occasion" for a stimulus to predict one outcome or another, disambiguate stimuli and their predictive significance in other ways, or provide an incidental or deliberate way of organizing attended information. In general, the ability to form context-event associations is parasitic upon animals having previously developed a memory representation of the context if that is necessary (which may take time) and upon the occurrence of rapid one-trial learning (because unique events do not happen twice).

It turns out that some of the distinct aspects of contextual encoding, modulation, and recall depend on the hippocampus, but others do not. Accordingly, a simple formula such as "context-learning = hippocampus-dependent learning" is inadequate. Experiments on the role of the hippocampal formation in context-associated information processing have now developed a number of subtleties, and their discussion leads us on toward a more "episodic" account of hippocampal function.

Context Fear Conditioning

A learning paradigm called "context fear conditioning" is now widely used to study context-event learning. It is rapidly learned (Fanselow, 1990), generally though not always hippocampus-dependent (Winocur et al., 1987; Selden et al., 1991; Gisquet-Verrier et al., 1999), and has proved ideal as a rapid assay of lesion, drug, and forebrain-specific genetic manipulations that might differentially affect short- and long-term memory for fear and the signal-transduction mechanisms engaged in its consolidation (Aiba et al., 1994; Frankland et al., 2001; Ohno et al., 2001).

Fear conditioning to a discrete stimulus is mediated by the amygdala (Davis et al., 1993; LeDoux, 2000; Maren, 2005). Whether shown as an altered startle response or somatic immobility ("freezing"), circuits interconnecting the lateral, basolateral, and central nuclei in the amygdala have been implicated in fear conditioning using lesion, pharmacological, single-unit, and LTP studies. However, the amygdala interacts with the hippocampus in certain forms of fear conditioning. The most widely used "context-freezing" task, as developed by Fanselow, involves three conceptually separate but often overlapping phases (Fig. 13–40A). First, the rat or mouse is placed into a distinctive box with a grid floor (the context) and allowed to explore it with a view to forming an integrated representation of its shape, appearance, odor, and somatosensory characteristics. This learning takes a minute or two, a fact that points to a somewhat neglected link between this form of associative conditioning and exploratory behavior. Second, a weak or intermediate-intensity electric shock is delivered to the animal through the grid floor. This may be during the same session as the initial exploration or a later one (protocols differ slightly across laboratories). In either case, the animal's reaction to the shock may be barely detectable, it may run around for a bit, or it may immediately remain immobile. Whatever its immediate or "unconditioned" reaction to the shock, this behavior gradually gives way to sustained periods of immobility in which practically the only observable movement is breathing. This conditioned reaction (CR) is a "species-specific defense reaction" (Bolles, 1970) shown by various rodent species and is generally called "freezing." The probability of freezing varies as a function of the number and intensity of the shocks delivered. If the initial exploratory period is not included, contextual fear conditioning does not occur (Kiernan and Westbrook, 1993), a phenomenon that Fanselow (1990) referred to as the "immediate shock effect" (Fig. 13–40B). However, when sufficient exploratory time in a context is allowed, subsequent fear conditioning occurs successfully. This learning phase ends with the animal's return to its home cage. The third phase of testing involves returning the animal to the context at a prescribed memory interval after training (e.g., the next day). The experimenter monitors the level of freezing (Fig. 13–40C). Little freezing is seen during a postoperative memory test in rats subjected to hippocampal lesioning soon after context fear conditioning. However, the extent of freezing increases systematically as a function of the interval between context fear conditioning and the time when a hippocampal lesion is created (Kim and Fanselow, 1992). Animals that have conditioned well typically freeze for as much as 60% of a short testing session. This freezing response is only slowly forgotten over time (weeks or longer) and only extinguished by repeated context exposures in the absence of shock. Studies of the extinction of conditioned fear, including contextual fear, are currently a focus of considerable interest for their translational implications for the treatment of posttraumatic stress disorder (Cahill and McGaugh, 1996; Ressler et al., 2002; Nader, 2003).

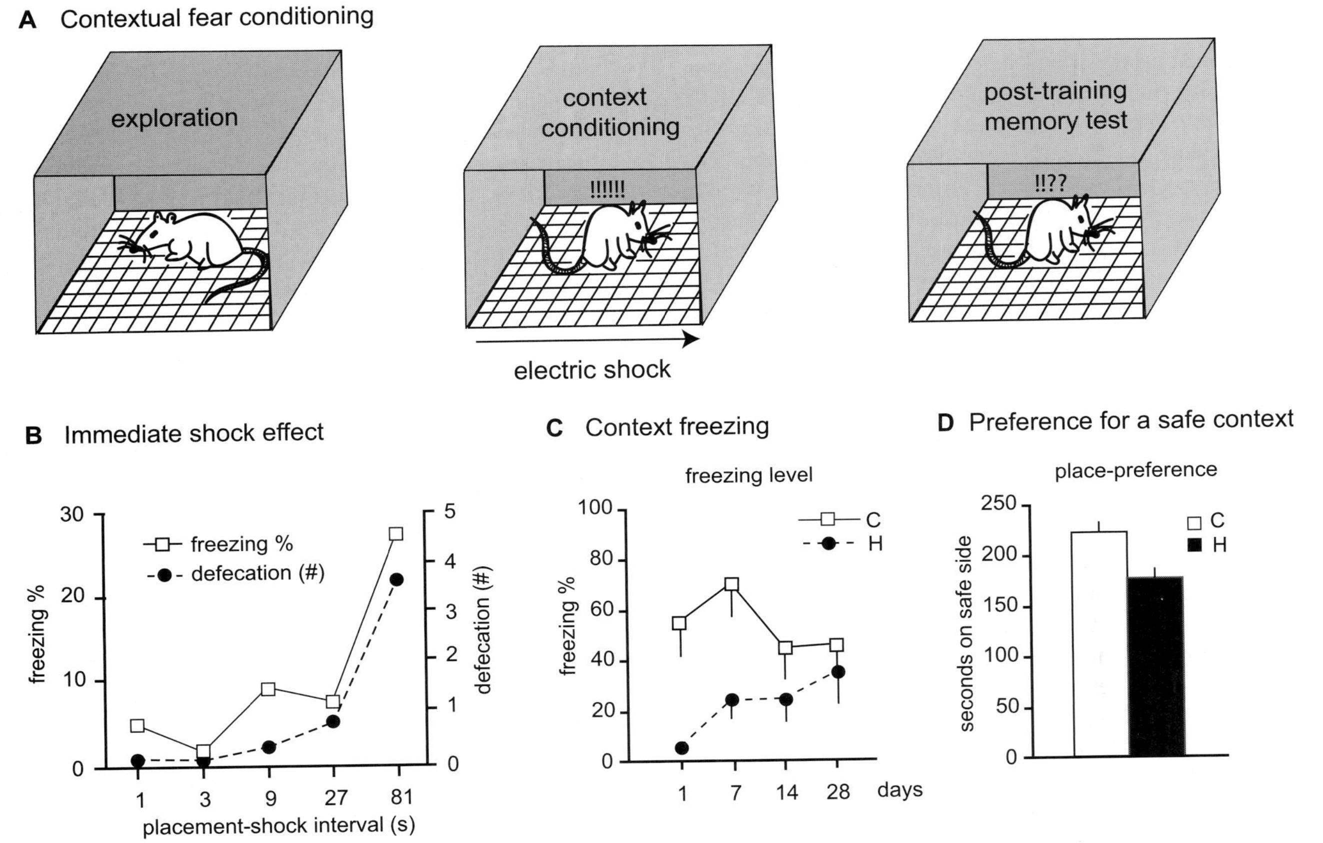

A Contextual fear conditioning

B Immediate shock effect

C Context freezing

D Preference for a safe context

Figure 13–40. Context fear conditioning. *A.* The three phases of training: context exploration, fear conditioning, and posttraining memory testing (*Source*: After Fanselow, 1990.) *B.* The "immediate shock effect" that reflects the absence of context fear conditioning unless sufficient time is allowed to explore the context (*Source*: After Fanselow, 2000.) *C.* The extent of freezing as a function of the interval after context conditioning before a hippocampal lesion is made. (*Source*: Kim and Fanselow, 1992.) *D.* The impact of hippocampal lesions on place-preference as a measure context fear. (*Source*: Selden et al., 1991.)

Although by far the most popular, freezing is not the only measure used to assess fear conditioning. Other measures used include the relative preference for a safe unshocked chamber compared to the conditioning chamber to which it is connected or the extent to which fear, conditioned to a discrete CS, inhibits appetitive or consummatory behavior. Selden et al. (1991) examined both the extent to which a clicker stimulus (the discrete CS) would evoke fear after pairings with shock and the extent to which an initially nonpreferred and brightly lit white chamber would be favored over a black one in which the clicker and shock had been presented (the safe and conditioning contexts, respectively). They observed a double dissociation between the effects of excitotoxic amygdala and hippocampal lesions on fear conditioning to explicit and contextual aversive cues. Amygdala lesions selectively impaired conditioning to the clicker measured by its capacity to reduce drinking (i.e., inhibition of consummatory behavior). Hippocampal lesions selectively impaired conditioning to the context measured by the proportion of time spent in the black and white chambers in a preference test (Fig. 13–40D). Independent work by other groups confirmed the double dissociation between the dependence of contextual freezing on the integrity of the hippocampus and of tone-elicited freezing on the amygdala (Kim and Fanselow, 1992; Phillips and LeDoux, 1992). The hippocampal dependence of contextual freezing seems to be unrelated to the level of activity the animal displays in the conditioning chamber prior to shock delivery (Gewirtz et al., 2000). This lack of correlation is important, as it is known that hippocampal lesions can sometimes cause hyperactivity (e.g., during exploration of a novel environment), and the deficit in context freezing might therefore have been no more than a secondary, nonmnemonic consequence of a lesion-induced alteration in motor behavior. Two arguments marshaled by Fanselow (2000) against this possibility include the selectivity of the hippocampal lesion deficit to context but not discrete CS-associated fear and the presence of a within-subject temporal gradient of retrograde amnesia for discriminable contexts (see below). Thus, although other measures have been developed that would not be subject to the hyperactivity objection, freezing has retained its popularity, and the research field has stuck to it.

The difference between fear conditioned to a discrete CS (amygdala-dependent) and to a context (hippocampus-dependent) reflects the prior learning of the context. Fanselow suggested that the rat must first form "an integrated mnemonic representation of the many features of the context and the rat must have this representation in active memory at the time of the shock" (Fanselow, 2000, p. 75). He likened it to a "Gestalt" memory of the environment, analogous to the spatial maps that O'Keefe and Nadel (1978) had suggested are formed during active exploration. It is therefore noteworthy that this necessary time period of exposure to a novel conditioning chamber is similar to that which Bostock et al. (1991) first reported to be necessary for rats to form a stable hippocampal firing field in a novel recording chamber. This "unified representation" of the environment then functions as an "configural" stimulus that, through classical conditioning, is associated with shock—in a manner essential identical to that implied by the configural association theory. Rudy and O'Reilly (1999) provide direct support for this view in experiments with normal rats in which they showed that preexposure to the conditioning context, but not to the individual stimulus elements that made up the context presented one after the other, facilitated later contextual fear conditioning. They also established that the extent to which fear conditioning generalizes to other contexts that had not been used for conditioning is influenced by preexposure in a manner suggestive of "pattern completion" during conditioning (see Chapter 14). Specifically, if contexts X and Y contain common elements and context Z is quite different, preexposure to context X but not to context Z facilitates generalization to context X after fear conditioning in context Y. These observations, reminiscent of Guzowski's data obtained using the immediate early gene *Arc* (see Section 13.4) suggest that contextual freezing reflects fear elicited by a "stimulus" that is a mental entity: It is a conjunctive memory representation of the environment based on polymodal sensory information. This led Rudy to an ingenious test of his context preexposure facilitation (CPF) concept. Rats were led to expect, over a series of exposure days, that being transported in a distinctive container around the laboratory would always end in them being taken to a particular test chamber (context A). On the critical conditioning day, they were transported in the container but unexpectedly put into a distinctively *different* test chamber (context B) and given an immediate shock. Remember that immediate shock does *not* ordinarily result in context fear conditioning; and, consistent with this, no contextual fear conditioning occurred to context B. However, the rats displayed freezing when placed in context A, the context they had expected to arrive at after transport in the distinctive container but not the one in which they actually received the shock. This "CPF effect" was not observed in rats with hippocampal lesions (Rudy et al., 2002)

A complication to the story that the hippocampus is critical only for contextual fear conditioning is that several studies have shown that disruption of the ventral hippocampus (with lesions or drugs) can disrupt fear conditioning to a discrete CS such as a tone (Bast et al., 2001; Zhang et al., 2001). This may, in part, be due to the presence of direct afferents from the ventral hippocampus to the amygdala (Pitkanen et al., 2000) that ordinarily mediates CS fear conditioning. Whatever the reason, a one-to-one association between hippocampal processing and context freezing is an oversimplification.

Differential Effects of Hippocampal Lesions Before and After Fear Conditioning

The importance of exploratory learning about the context is relevant to a puzzling feature of studies examining the impact of hippocampal dysfunction. Hippocampal lesions made shortly *after* conditioning are effective in blocking contextual freezing (Kim and Fanselow, 1992; Phillips and LeDoux, 1992, 1994; Maren et al., 1997; Frankland et al., 1998), whereas those made *prior to* conditioning have varied effects (Winocur et al., 1987; Maren et al., 1997; Gisquet-Verrier et al., 1999; Maren, 2001). This dissociation with respect to the relative timing of training and the lesion is not because the lesions are incomplete (although often they are). Clearly, were they incomplete, there may be sufficient spared tissue for hippocampus-dependent learning to occur when the lesion is made prior to conditioning. That this is *not* the explanation for the differential effects of lesions made pretraining versus posttraining is because if an identical incomplete lesion is made after training a substantial deficit in context fear conditioning is still observed.

The likely explanation for the differential effect, as outlined by Maren et al. (1997), Rudy and O'Reilly (1999), and Anagnostaras et al. (2001), is that an animal with a hippocampal lesion prior to conditioning is predisposed to associate the fearful shock with some "elemental" feature of the conditioning chamber (e.g., its smell) rather than the "unified representation" that because of the lesion it is unable to form. As this type of single-stimulus classical conditioning is unaffected by hippocampal lesions, less disruption of contextual freezing is to be expected in the anterograde domain. This possibility alerts us to the importance of the exact design of the chambers in which these sorts of experiments are conducted. Different contexts are sometimes readily distinguishable in terms of an elemental feature; in other cases, they may only (or more readily) be distinguished by the set of cues that forms a single unified representation. The devil is again in the detail with respect to understanding the pattern of results, particularly in relation to the impact of genetic manipulations that, unless inducible, occur long before conditioning. As inducible, region-specific mutations are rare, we do not include a discussion here of this developing and important field but do recognize its likely importance in the years ahead.

Creating lesions after training offers the opportunity to use contextual freezing as a way of investigating the temporal gradient of retrograde amnesia. Rapid learning (during a single session) and the fact that retention is extremely robust over time are features that render the task highly suitable. Kim and Fanselow (1992) produced electrolytic hippocampal lesions in rats 1, 7, 14, or 28 days after cued and context fear conditioning. As noted above (Fig. 13–40C), a graded deficit in contextual freezing is seen as a function of the training–lesion interval, with animals given lesions 28 days after training being indistinguishable from those that underwent sham surgery. This finding was interpreted in terms of a time-dependent consolidation process for contextual fear, consistent with declarative memory theory. Maren and Fanselow (1997) obtained similar results, but only over much a longer time interval, in animals with excitotoxic hippocampal lesions. An elegant within-subjects study by Anagnostaras et al. (1999) examined the effects of electrolytic hippocampal lesions on animals conditioned in two highly distinctive contexts with training scheduled 50 days apart. Conducted at UCLA, the two contexts were named after two famous streets in Hollywood. The "Sunset Room" was a darkened laboratory containing conditioning chambers that were triangular, had white plastic walls, and were scented with acetic acid. The "Wilshire Room" was a distinctive, well lit laboratory with conditioning chambers that were rectangular, made of aluminum and plexiglass, and scented with ammonium hydroxide. Previous work had indicated that there is little generalization between these two environments; the animals would have readily distinguished them during training and testing. The key finding was that lesions made shortly after context fear conditioning in the Sunset Room but 7 weeks after conditioning in the Wilshire Room (or vice versa) impaired later expression of the recent memory but not remote memory. "Location, location, location" is, not surprisingly—as important in Hollywood as anywhere else.

Contextual Control of Stimulus Significance?

There are ways in which context can affect behavior other than by entering into associations with the US as in context freezing. One way is to modulate the effectiveness of other associations. As noted long ago by Nadel and Willner (1980), contexts can be said to "contain" events that occur within them. The relation between cue and context is then "hierarchical" rather than associative in the traditional sense. Work by Moita et al. (2003) nicely illustrates the impact of contextual cues on CA1 pyramidal cell firing during auditory fear conditioning (see Chapter 11). Place fields were first observed in the conditioning chamber prior to fear conditioning. Rapid fear conditioning then took place over a few trials in which shock was presented at the end of a white-noise CS, with a control group receiving temporally random presentations of the white noise and shock. Freezing was observed in response to the CS. In parallel, there was an increase in CA1 cell responsiveness that was specific to the place fields in the chamber where a specific cell normally fired. This suggests that the spatial representation encoded and stored during the earlier exploration can incorporate elements of the task-related fear conditioning events into its representation.

Contexts can also "set the occasion" for a particular cue having a particular significance or meaning. Good and Honey (1991) developed the first satisfactory experimental design to investigate the role of the hippocampus in such a process. Their protocol ensured that subjects became familiar with two contexts (operant conditioning chambers) and two distinct cues (tones and clickers) and were equally reinforced in relation to both sets of cues. Rats were trained in an appetitive paradigm (collecting food pellets) in which one discrete stimulus (A) was reinforced in one context (X), whereas a second stimulus (B) was reinforced in Y. The critical test of the ability of either context to retrieve the appropriate significance of these cues was to present, for the first time, A in context Y and B in context X. The phenomenon of "context specificity" was displayed as a reduction in the appetitive responses elicited by A and B in their now "inappropriate" contexts. Rats subjected to electrolytic (Good and Honey, 1991) or neurotoxic (Honey and Good, 1993) hippocampal lesioning failed to show this reduction of conditioned responding. This failure was not because the subjects with lesions could not discriminate the two contexts; a separate experiment established that they had no difficulty in doing this when only one of the two contexts predicted the availability of reinforcement.

The implication appeared to be that the integrity of the hippocampus is necessary for a process associated with the contextual control of associative conditioning—associative retrieval—rather than learning a unified representation, as described by Fanselow. However, this implication is insecure for two reasons. First, remember that even the ostensibly robust deficit in contextual freezing induced by hippocampal lesions does not always occur if the lesions are produced before training as they were in the Good and Honey (1991) experiment. Second, Good and Honey's deficit in contextual retrieval has not proven easy to replicate in other laboratories. A series of experiments by Hall et al. (1996) failed to do so, and later work showed that hippocampal lesions have no effect on the rate of learning a conditional context discrimination test over a series of test sessions (McDonald et al., 1997).

Good et al. (1998) put forward the suggestion that there may be a subtle but important difference between the "incidental" processing of contextual cues (when their processing is not formally necessary to learn a task) and the "intentional" or "contingent" processing of contextual cues (when their processing is essential for learning that task). Their results indicated that when rats with hippocampal lesions were required to use context cues over several sessions to differentiate the stimulus significance of discrete cues, there was no deficit. However, when the animals were presented with a single unexpected context specificity test, with context novelty controlled, the hippocampus-lesioned group was impaired (Fig. 13–41). The possibility that there may be something critical about the hippocampus in relation to the distinction between automatic and deliberate processing is directly relevant to the conjunctive representations theory (O'Reilly and Rudy, 2001), an issue we revisit in the section of episodic memory, below.

Hunger and Thirst as Contexts

Patient H.M. is unable to report whether he is hungry. He does not ask for meals and, quite soon after eating, attempts to eat again if a plate of food is placed before him (Hebben et al., 1985). That he may have forgotten that it is a long time since

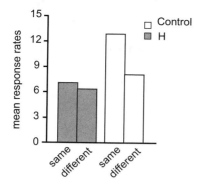

A Incidental context specificity

B Contingent context-specificity

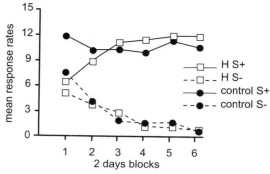

Figure 13–41. Incidental versus contingent processing of context cues. *A.* When the discrete CSs predicting the availability of food in the conditioning chamber were unexpectedly presented in the other context, controls but not hippocampus-lesioned rats showed a decrease in responding. *B.* When the discrete CSs were repeatedly

presented in both contexts and differentially rewarded in each of them, both control and hippocampus-lesioned rats readily learned to discriminate their significance appropriately. (*Source*: After Good et al., 1998.)

he last ate or that he has just had a recent meal is unsurprising—yet another indication of his memory deficit—but that he has apparently no awareness of the internal state of hunger or its absence is an additional deficit. Motivational states could contribute to the contextual control of behavior.

A number of animal experiments have addressed this question, with early studies using spatial tasks in which a rat was required to perform one spatial response when hungry and a different one when thirsty. Rats could learn this interesting contextual-dependent task, but any lesion-associated deficit could arise because of a failure to discriminate the motivational states, failure to use this information to retrieve the appropriate response, or failure of spatial memory itself. Davidson and Jarrard (1993) examined a nonspatial task in

which placement in an operant chamber was associated with footshock when the rats were hungry but not when nondeprived (or vice versa). An A/(A+B) type of discrimination ratio was used to measure the relative degree of conditioned freezing in the two situations, and the data in Figure 13–42A indicate that normal animals could learn this discrimination, whereas rats with neurotoxic lesions of the hippocampus and dentate gyrus could not. A later study by Kennedy and Shapiro (2004) sought to distinguish involvement of the hippocampus in learning such a discrimination and a role in contextual retrieval. Three visual distinct goal-boxes (shown graphically as black, gray, and white in Fig. 13–42B) were, across successive trials, randomly placed at the ends of the arms of a three-choice "pitchfork"-type maze and the animals' deprivation

Figure 13–42. Motivational states as hippocampus-dependent contextual cues. *A.* Control but not hippocampus-lesioned rats learned to discriminate whether to be afraid in a place as a function of their state of hunger. (*Source*: After Davidson and Jarrard, 1993.) *B.* After preoperative training to choose a visually distinctive goal box to secure an appropriate reward when hungry or thirsty, rats with

fornix or hippocampal lesions were no longer able to use their deprivation state to retrieve a memory of the appropriate response. They did, however, continue to avoid the never-rewarded goal box. Goal boxes were moved randomly across trials. H+, food available to a hungry rat; NoR, never-rewarded box; Th+, water available to a thirsty rat. (*Source*: After Kennedy and Shapiro, 2004.)

A Hunger as a context for fear

B Hunger and thirst as contexts for discrimination

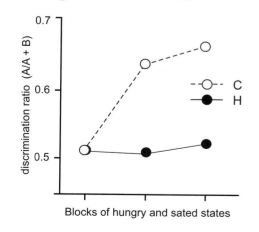

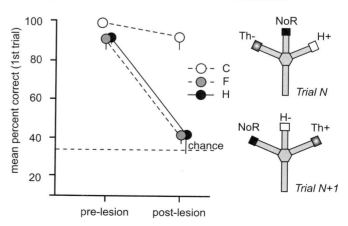

state switched between hunger and thirst on alternate days. One goal-box provided food if the animals were hungry (but not otherwise), another supplied water if they were thirsty, and the third never provided reward. Before any lesions were made, training showed that the animals could learn to make the appropriate choice as they ran the maze. After fornix lesioning or neurotoxic hippocampal lesioning, the ability to choose between the hunger and thirst boxes fell to chance, although the animals continued to avoid the goal-box that never provided reward. The sham-lesioned rats continued to perform effectively. Occasional probe trials were scheduled in which hunger was repeated across two successive days; choice behavior continued to be controlled by motivational state rather than any alternation pattern in the sham-lesioned controls. Different results in a similar task were reported by Deacon et al. (2001), but all training was postoperative and a reward was consistently available independent of motivational state. The rats with hippocampal lesions may therefore have solved the task by updating their predicted "value" of the reward (i.e., food when hungry and food when sated) using an amygdala-dependent learning process. Accordingly, it seems secure to conclude that the hippocampus is required for using internal motivational states in a contextual manner for memory retrieval.

Contextual Control of Extinction

The phenomenon of "extinction" refers to changes in learned behavior that occur when a stimulus or a response is no longer followed by the reinforcement with which it was previously associated. In the extinction of classical fear conditioning, a tone (CS) that has previously predicted the imminent arrival of shock (US) is now followed by nothing. What then happens, in terms of performance, is that the overt expression of the prior conditioning becomes weaker over successive extinction trials. An old-fashioned view of this change is that extinction is some kind of "unlearning" process, a breaking of the associative bonds between cue and consequence. However, various phenomena discovered about the determinants of extinction have led many to doubt that unlearning is what normally occurs. Extinction is more often a learning process in which contextual factors play a particularly important modulatory role—the extinction context altering what US memory is retrieved when the previously trained CS is presented (Bouton and Moody, 2004). During training the CS comes to evoke a memory representation of the US; during extinction it may acquire a memory representation of "no-US" (as in Fig. 13–33), but importantly there is no overwriting of the previous CS–US association. Which memory is retrieved in a given memory test depends on the context of testing, with the nature of the environment and how it differs from other environments, the passage of time, or other factors influencing the operative "context" as it is perceived by the animal. As Bouton and Moody put it, "the fact that extinction is more context-dependent than conditioning is consistent with the idea that the animal codes extinction as a kind of

conditional exception to the rule—one that depends on the current context" (Bouton and Moody, 2004, p. 665).

Studies by Bouton have implicated the hippocampus in certain extinction phenomena but not others. Wilson et al. (1995) using fornix lesions and Frohardt et al. (2000) using neurotoxic hippocampal lesions have provided evidence that the integrity of hippocampal function is needed for a context-processing phenomenon called "reinstatement" but is not required for another phenomenon called "renewal." The distinction between them is important. Both are instances in which an initially conditioned and then extinguished CR recovers. Reinstatement is said to occur after independent presentations of the US in the same context as original training, with memory test consisting of CS presentations in this same context (reinstatement of the CR does not occur if the US presentations occur in a different context). In renewal of the CR, the previously trained CS is extinguished in a different context and then tested in the original training context (renewal does not occur if CS extinction occurs in the same context throughout). These experiments used the classic paradigm of conditioned suppression in which rats were first trained to press a lever for food reward in each of two contexts. They were then presented with a CS (lights turning off) on a number of occasions, this stimulus being paired with weak electric shock (US). Rats reduce their rate of appetitive responding during the CS ("conditioned suppression"), and this decline in operant responding served as a quantifiable measure of fear in much the same way as freezing. Once trained in this way, the CS was then "extinguished" by being presented several times without shock over a series of lever-pressing sessions. Rates of operant responding recovered until they were as high during the CS as in its absence (this is expressed as a "suppression ratio" calculated as CSrate/(CSrate + preCSrate), a measure that tends toward 0.5 when rates of responding have equilibrated). Reinstatement was observed as the selective recovery of the fear response to the CS (i.e., somewhat confusingly, this is a return to a *low* suppression ratio) after rats had been exposed several times to the US alone in the training context. Critically, this reinstatement effect occurred in control animals but not in subjected to fornix or neurotoxic hippocampal lesioning (Fig. 13–43A). Conversely, renewal of the CR occurred just as much in control as in lesioned rats using an ABA design in which the CS was extinguished in a different context (B) from that in which it was initially conditioned and later tested (i.e., context A) (Fig. 13–43B).

Both phenomena are context-dependent, but Bouton argued that the reason reinstatement is hippocampus-dependent, but renewal is not, is because the hippocampus is important for context–US associations but not for all forms of contextual modulation of retrieval such as positive occasion-setting or conditional rules. A strong context–US association rapidly created by the unsignaled US presentations retrieves a memory representation of the shock and, consequently, reminds the animals of the original CS–US association. That is, the re-presentation of the ostensibly extinguished CS then retrieves a memory of the US (with which it was associated

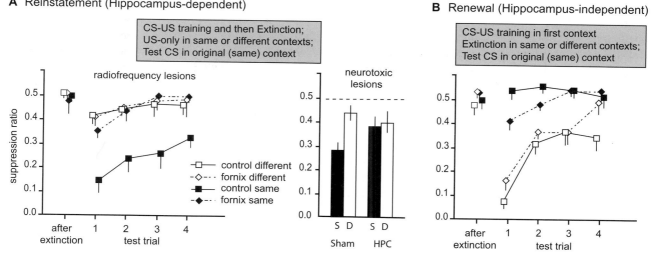

Figure 13–43. Reinstatement and renewal after the extinction of classic fear conditioning. *A.* Using conditioned suppression of operant responding as a measure of conditioning, presentation of the US only in the same context as that in which CS-US conditioning had taken place "reinstated" conditioned fear in control rats but not those that had fornix (left) or neurotoxic hippocampal (right) lesions. *B.* Renewal of fear to a conditioned CS was observed in both controls and fornix-lesioned groups after the CS was extinguished in a different context. (*Source*: After Wilson et al., 1995 and Frohardt et al., 2000.)

during training) rather than of the absence of the US (as had developed during extinction). This inferential feature of context-dependent modulation of conditioning critically involves context-US associations and thus the hippocampus. In renewal, the subject also learns a CS–US association during training and a CS–NoUS association during extinction. However, in contrast to reinstatement, there is no strong hippocampus-dependent context–US association formed. Instead, the animal's representations of the two contexts (training and extinction) modulate whether the CS–US association or the CS–noUS association is evoked, and this modulation does not require the hippocampus. It is most likely mediated by neocortical circuits on their own. Frohardt et al. (2000) offer several reasons from the animal learning literature for recognizing renewal and reinstatement as separate context effects.

This tidy picture is complicated in two ways. First, a study by Fox and Holland, (1998) that found no effects of neurotoxic hippocampus lesions on reinstatement in an appetitively motivated task. It is possible that context–US associations in appetitive conditioning are weaker than in aversive conditioning because food also occurs in the home cage, whereas shock is specific to the testing chamber. However, a clear reinstatement effect was observed in the appetitive task, the difference being that it was just as great in the rats with hippocampal lesions. An alternative and more parsimonious explanation concerns the complication, noted earlier, of elemental versus configural/conjunctive representations of contexts. In these extinction studies, the hippocampal lesions are made prior to conditioning. We have noted that contextual fear conditioning sometimes occurs normally in such animals, as they have the opportunity of representing the context with reference to

some isolated or elemental feature of the testing chamber. One way to reduce the likelihood of this happening in animals that already have lesions is to ensure that two contexts are used in the behavioral protocol and that the critical manipulations are scheduled for only a short period (e.g., one session). The Bouton studies used two contexts that differed in quite subtle ways (e.g., the orientation of the grid bars), whereas the appetitive study by Fox and Holland did not (they used the control procedure of no US reexposure). Thus, the animals in the appetitive study of reinstatement after extinction would have been able to form an "elemental" context–US association using neocortical circuitry, and this may have been sufficient to remind the animals of which CS–US association to recall as effectively in lesioned as in normal rats.

Another problem is that the "renewal" phenomenon is sensitive to muscimol-induced reversible inactivation of the hippocampus (Corcoran and Maren, 2001, 2004; Corcoran et al., 2005). In contrast to the argument just given, Maren argued that Bouton's use of pretraining lesions would have allowed "elemental" representation of the two contexts and thus a hippocampus-independent form of contextual-dependent renewal of extinction in the lesioned rats. His use of post-training muscimol infusions would have made it more likely that a configural representation, acquired normally during fear conditioning and extinction, would have been disrupted. However, this explanation does not seem to account for the dissociation between renewal and reinstatement observed in the permanent lesion studies. Another concern is that the spatial extent of the inhibition of hippocampal activity by the muscimol infusions was revealed in autoradiographic studies to be quite small and extended as much into cortex as it did along the longitudinal axis of the dorsal hippocampus

(Corcoran et al., 2005). If renewal is mediated by a form of contextual modulation controlled by extrahippocampal circuits (Bouton and Moody, 2004), these infusions may have disrupted a cortex-mediated component of that process also. As noted before, the use of reversible inactivation is analytically more powerful than permanent lesions, but there are technical problems to its use that should be recognized (Anagnostaras et al., 2002).

13.5.4 Critique

The valuable common feature of the three theories just discussed is their serious attempt to tackle the fundamental problem of dealing with ambiguity in memory. However, stepping back from the details of individual experiments, aspects of each of the ideas are problematic.

First, although it is easy to understand the selection pressure for memory systems for remembering facts and events or finding one's way around, it is not clear why mammals would have evolved a specialized neural system for solving nonlinear discrimination tasks. Ambiguity of cue significance may be a task a scientist can invent, but is it rife in nature? To be sure, there are observations indicating that monkeys execute different behavioral actions in response to distinct fear-evoking stimuli (e.g., snakes, eagles), but the stimuli from the animals and the calls then given by troop members are in no way ambiguous (Seyfarth et al., 1980). Where ambiguities do occur, they generally arise as a function of the spatiotemporal context of events and can therefore be solved without recourse to configuring. Whether an animal should freeze or flee upon hearing the sound or smell of a predator more likely depends on the relative safety of the location it presently occupies. Configuring stimuli might help solve tasks of a particular logical structure; however, for example, the occasional failure of rats with hippocampus lesions to learn transitive discrimination tasks could actually be secondary to deficits of a different kind—the inability to form relational representations or to allow a context to modulate retrieval.

Second, the relational processing theory is built around the idea that associative relations may be more abstract and more flexible than implied by traditional theories of conditioning, with their emphasis on associative strength and unlabeled associations. There are, however, aspects of the theory that seem vague. Critics such as Mackintosh (2002), prefer the precision of quantitatively precise theories of associative learning, which assert that a variety of qualitatively different associations can occur such as excitatory links, inhibitory links, and stimulus representations that set the occasion for the retrieval of others. This complexity of conditioning aside, consideration of even the simplest of associations—the pairing of a tone with shock—illustrates the problem of identifying the type of association. Is a tone–shock pairing relational or nonrelational? Can it be either depending on the training situation? In terms of the animal's phenomenal experience, the tone may come to evoke the memory representation of something painful about to happen, or it may simply assume high associative strength

that somehow triggers freezing. The speed of learning a tone–shock relationship and its ready expression in novel testing situations points to it being, by Cohen and Eichenbaum's definition, a "flexible" representation. Conversely, its slow rate of extinction suggests it is inflexible. In this and other examples, independent rules for identifying into which category an association should be classified other than observed effects of hippocampus lesions do not seem to exist. We are back to the issue that has long haunted declarative memory theories: irrefutability arising from logical circularity.

Third, both the configural and relational theories also lack detail at the level of neurobiological implementation. We are still at an early stage of thinking about how the circuitry of the hippocampal formation is used for forming or storing configural/relational associations, how it could implement the selective enhancement of the salience of configural units elsewhere in the brain, or how it could realize memory representations that would somehow afford flexibility at the time of retrieval. What are the relative roles of the dentate gyrus, CA3, and CA1 in achieving any of these tasks? How might the organization of the mossy fibers and the longitudinal associational pathway of area CA3 help implement stimulus configuring (if it does)? What role might associative LTP play in relational processing? To be fair, the relational theory has taken an important step in this direction in asserting an anatomically distinct ITM and LTM for isolated stimuli compared to relations.

Finally, fourth, ideas about contextual processing are not immune from some of the same criticisms. When is a stimulus a context and when a "discrete stimulus"? In the animal literature, a context tends to be a box. In the human literature, it is as often the color of the ink in which a word is presented. This is deeply confusing. Furthermore, how precisely can a contextual representation function in the several ways we have discussed? Why is the hippocampal formation involved in some of these aspects of contextual processing but not others? In short, how can a contextual account avoid the same charge of occasional circularity that we have leveled against the declarative memory theory? There are two strands to any answer to these questions. One is that there is a formal body of theoretical work on associative conditioning that has delineated distinct ways in which contexts can enter into associations with CSs and USs or modulate other associations, as represented in Figure 13.33B. Reinstatement and renewal are good exemplars, as their associative basis is operationally quite different, and a specific prediction could then be made about the outcome of a hippocampal lesion. Neuroscientists trying to understand mechanisms at the neural level can capitalize on this prior psychological research—as they have done with such phenomena as the immediate shock effect, the context preexposure facilitation effect, and the distinction between renewal and reinstatement.

The second strand of defense for the context ideas is the sheer plausibility and simplicity of the idea that context plays a critical role in coping with ambiguity. Events happen—at specific moments in time and space and in specific social contexts. Their meaning and significance is often context-dependent, including semantic knowledge, just as so many aspects of our behavior. In addition, events often happen unpredictably. This simple fact requires that any system whose role is to keep track of the important events of our lives must be able to respond instantly, diverting attentional resources as required and encoding information rapidly as it happens and with reference to the context in which it occurs. This is why the distinction between incidental and contingent processing of contextual information may be important. Context processing, as O'Keefe and Nadel (1978) recognized long ago, has the potential to be one building block of a true episodic memory system. It is to that issue which we now turn.

13.6 Episodic Memory, Hippocampus, and Neurobiology of Rapid Context-specific Memory

The last hippocampal theory to be considered, and one in which there is growing interest, is that the hippocampal formation participates in certain aspects of *episodic memory* (in humans) and *episodic-like memory* (in animals). This idea has emerged in an integrative manner from neuropsychological studies of developmental amnesia (Vargha-Khadem et al., 1997) and work concerning scene memory, object–scene associations, and top-down control of memory processing in monkeys (Gaffan, 1994a; Miyashita, 2004). In other animals, behavioral studies of food caching by avian species (Clayton and Dickinson, 1998), studies of sequence learning in rodents (Fortin et al., 2002), single-unit correlates of prospective and retrospective memory (Wood et al., 2000; Ferbinteanu and Shapiro, 2003), pharmacological interventions affecting the encoding and retrieval of rapid paired-associate learning (Day et al., 2003), and genetic interventions targeted conditionally at specific components of hippocampal circuitry (Nakazawa et al., 2003) are all contributing to a developing perspective. That a range of approaches are converging on the same general idea indicates that the theory may be on the right lines (Box 13–9).

13.6.1 Concept of Episodic Memory

First introduced by Tulving (1972) and elaborated in a number of ways since (Tulving, 1983, 2004; Schacter and Tulving, 1994), episodic memory refers to the memory of a unique event and/or a temporal sequence of events that collectively comprise an episode. As originally defined, the content of episodic memory is a mental representation of "what" happened during an event, "where" it happened, and "when." Writing in 1983, Tulving asserted that episodic memory "receives and stores information about temporally-dated episodes or events, and temporal-spatial relations among these events" (Tulving, 1983, p. 385). Thus, remembering what you did on holiday, where you went, and with whom would be an instance of episodic memory. It is contrasted with seman-

---

Box 13–9
Hippocampus: Episodic and Episodic-like Memory

1. *Conceptual issues:* Episodic memory is the recall, by humans, of discrete events that happened at a particular place and a particular time. Such recall entails mental time travel. Episodic-like memory in animals is the memory of "what, where, and when" with respect to events.

2. *Hippocampal involvement:* The hippocampus is one of a network of brain structures that mediate the automatic encoding and retrieval of attended events and the contexts in which they occur (episodic-like memory). Distinct brain structures, including the prefrontal lobe, mediate different and more volitional aspects of this form of memory.

3. *Differential role of subcomponents:* Components of the hippocampal formation (e.g., CA1, CA3, dentate gyrus) are differentially involved in dissociable components of episodic-like memory, such as pattern separation and pattern completion.

4. *Awareness:* Episodic memory and episodic-like memory are distinguishable, as only the former requires "autonoetic" consciousness. This cannot, at present, be studied neurobiologically. Awareness may also be an attribute of episodic-like memory in animals, but this need not be autonoetic.

---

tic memory—factual knowledge—which is not bound to any temporospatial context.

Episodic memory has several important properties. First, the encoding of attended events often occurs automatically; and by virtue of this the "temporal-spatial relations" of Tulving's definition cannot be deliberately selected or ignored. "Automaticity" implies that humans cannot normally "turn the system off" and voluntarily decide which attended events or what features of the context in which they occur are encoded (Martin et al., 1997; Morris and Frey, 1997). This paradoxically "reflexive" feature can be illustrated with reference to an example. Imagine that during a routine activity such as a shopping trip you witness a car crash. You were not expecting it to happen nor planning ahead of time to remember it. Still, what happens in front of you automatically commands your attention and it then becomes impossible *not* to encode and later remember that it happened, where it happened, and when. This inevitability of the associations formed at the time seems to be a characteristic of the brain system that processes this information. You get home and tell your family that you saw a car crash. They ask about what happened. You describe the scene of the crash, the crash itself, what happened next, and anything else that was distinctive or unusual. This is straightforward. But how strange it would be to tell your family of having seen a car crash, but then to say that you cannot remember anything about where it happened, stating only that it was "half-an-hour ago and involved two cars and a bicycle." During ordinary discourse, the "What happened?" enquiry carries with it the implicit trilogy of "what, where, and when."

This automatic "binding" of event, place, and time information is a characteristic of episodic memory that has neurobiological implications. It points to the need for a memory system that has anatomical access to highly processed information from all sensory modalities, is downstream of the attentional filters of the neocortex and the perceptual mechanisms for object-centered representations, and is downstream of but reciprocally connected with semantic memory. It must also be a system that stays online, can encode information rapidly, and is generally independent of volitional control. This last qualification of the automaticity property arises because some aspects of episodic memory can be volitional. For example, subjects in a neuropsychology experiment asked to learn a set of novel paired-associates or to remember a passage of prose are deliberately cooperating in a learning exercise. Their later memory of what happened is clearly an instance of episodic memory, but it occurs in the context of an intentional course of action, unlike the event of witnessing a car crash.

The "what-where-when" definition also captures a second important feature of episodic memory that marks it off from semantic memory, the other major category of declarative memory. This is the need for "mental time travel" as a part of our phenomenological experience of remembering. This concept may feel a bit fuzzy at first, but it is crucial. A person remembering an event, as distinct from merely declaring they know something, travels in their mind through time to that moment in the past when the event happened. Their experience is then one of being simultaneously *in the present* while also *reexperiencing the past*, a mental coexistence that transcends time. This is one of those psychological juxtapositions that may never have seemed paradoxical until it is pointed out: Mental time travel is a capacity of mind that we all take for granted, is apparently effortless, and yet is extraordinarily complex. Efforts to get a handle on this experimentally is sometimes done by asking subjects to make a subjective assessment of whether they "remember" or merely "know" something. We do not yet have the ability to pose such a question to animals in a neurobiological study.

Tulving (2004) made the strong claim that the capacity for mental time travel is unique to humans. Suddendorf and Corballis (1997) shared this view, arguing that animals are forever mentally trapped in the present or, as Roberts (2000) so nicely put it, they are "stuck in time." This is a controversial claim, as biological scientists are rarely at ease with unsupported claims of human uniqueness. Like Pinker's arguments for the uniqueness of human language (Pinker, 1994), Tulving asserted the human uniqueness of mental time travel in an arresting way. There are, he wrote, "things that bees, birds and humans all do. But there are also things that bees do but birds and humans do not. There are things that birds do that bees and humans do not. And there are things that humans do that bees and birds do not."

A third feature of episodic memory is that the event being remembered may be one in which subjects actually participated themselves (e.g., playing in a game of football) or one that was merely observed (e.g., seeing a dangerous animal). Tulving (1983) revised his earlier definition of episodic memory by adding that the observer needed to have a particular sense of self-identity. He called it "autonoetic consciousness." This form of self-consciousness is necessary for memories of the form "I remember scoring a goal" because such a memory entails a sense of self-identity. Opinion is divided, however, on the need for so sophisticated a form of awareness for all types of event memory. It is far from clear that one needs a sense of self-identity to recall having seen a dangerous animal, yet one can readily imagine evolutionary selection pressures that led to a brain system, present in nonhuman animals, for the effective memory of having seen a predator at a particular place and a specific time. Animals that stay that much safer by having such a memory system may or may not have a sense of self-identity. Tulving nonetheless insisted on his autonoetic consciousness criterion for "true" episodic memory, but this is impossible to apply to animals because we are unlikely ever to know whether animals have a sense of self-identity (Clayton et al., 2003b). Episodic memory may or may not be uniquely human and so may or may not reflect distinctive features of the human brain.

Given this somewhat metaphysical state of affairs, Griffiths et al. (1999) introduced the term "episodic-like" memory. This is something that can be defined behaviorally in terms of Tulving's older 1972 definition as memory for "what, where, and when" with the autonoetic aspect finessed for the time being. Meeting even this ostensibly more modest requirement for demonstrating episodic memory remains far from easy. Considerable ingenuity is required of behavioral scientists to invent novel memory tasks with the appropriate attributes to do it successfully (Morris, 2001). Much of what is available so far, including the many hippocampus-dependent tasks discussed in this chapter are not up to the task (Hampton and Schwartz, 2004).

However, suppose that an animal model of episodic-like memory were possible. Its value would be that we would then be able to get a handle on the neurobiology of rapid, context-specific memory formation with access to the usual range of anatomical, physiological, and biochemical data necessary for making causal inferences. It could then be classified as the class of vertebrate memory that refers to unique events and for which the representational content varies in a species-specific manner. There is nothing special about such a comparative perspective. Procedural learning is just the same—the motor skills that can be learned by a bird, bee, or human vary considerably—yet Tulving would not deny that all three species have a nonpropositional form of learning that can be classified as "sensorimotor procedural skills." By analogy, perhaps episodic-like memory may vary as a function of phylogeny with respect to both content and degree of awareness. It may have evolved in vertebrates as a "one-shot" memory because it was evolutionary adaptive to be able to encode and then later recall unique events, such as seeing an unexpected predator.

This eclectic approach opens the prospect of a neurobiological analysis provided the distinctive features of episodic-like memory can be tied down operationally. Various research groups are feeling their way toward a range of tasks that may be suitable assays. An unfortunate problem is that several such tasks are asserted to be "episodic" in character when the classification is barely deserved. In the context of the theories that have been considered in this chapter, episodic-like memory is over and beyond being merely "declarative" and something more than a "spatial memory" because, in both cases, the memory must include information about what and when something happened as well as information about a specific location. Episodic-like memory is also more than one-trial memory. Certain emotional dispositions, such as learned fear associated with a specific stimulus, can be acquired during one trial. There may be configural or relational components of episodic memory as well, yet neither of these two categories quite captures the distinctive features of the full "episodic" concept or the possible role of the hippocampus in mediating it.

13.6.2 Scene Memory as a Basis for Episodic Memory and Top-down Control by the Prefrontal Cortex

One idea about the neurobiological basis of episodic memory was Gaffan's proposal that it was a form of scene-specific encoding (Gaffan, 1991, 1994). His hypothesis included statements about the role of hippocampal formation and related structures, but the framework is anatomically more wide-ranging (Box 13–10).

These and related ideas were developed gradually through an extensive series of experiments on Old World primates, beginning with Gaffan's seminal study of recognition memory published in 1974 (see Section 13.3).

Recognition Memory, Associative Memory, and Scene Memory

The distinction between recognition and association (Gaffan, 1974) was, in certain respects, a forerunner of Mishkin's distinction between memory and habit (Mishkin, 1982). However, later work by Gaffan and his colleagues overturned

---

Box 13–10
"Scene Memory" Basis of Episodic Memory

1. *Part of a circuit*: The hippocampus is part of a circuit that includes the fornix, mammillary bodies, and anterior thalamus (the Delay-Brion circuit), which collectively encodes events with respect to the spatially organized scenes in which they occur.
2. *Spatial basis*: There is a spatial component to episodic memory ("scene-encoding") that is neuropsychologically dissociable from place memory per se and from spatial navigation.
3. *Anatomical dissociation of function*: The functions of the Delay-Brion circuit are also dissociable from the roles in memory played by the frontal lobe and the medial temporal lobe (which it connects), including the amygdala and perirhinal cortex.

---

the idea that fornix lesions leave associative memory unaffected following a series of ingenious experiments reported in somewhat impenetrable papers published during the early 1980s. The insight buried within this work was a new set of ideas about what it means to say that an animal has learned an "association." The traditional view was that associations were, to all intents and purposes, conditional reflexes or autonomous "habits," but Gaffan's studies and modern animal learning theory have considerably enriched our view of associative learning.

Inspired in part by the work of the animal learning theorist (Capaldi, 1971), Gaffan explored tasks in which an object might lead to food the first time it was seen but not the next time it was presented (Gaffan et al., 1984). That is, reward was available when the object was novel but not when it was familiar. Normal monkeys could learn this type of task, correctly reaching for the "other" object of a pair in two-alternative choice tests as quickly as in a simple association task. This novelty association task is sensitive to fornix lesions. The implication was that certain types of rapidly acquired "associations" between an object and reward are not autonomous habits at all; they are bits of stored "knowledge." Gaffan went on to suggest that the type of actions a monkey is required to perform during an association task may be critical to whether a fornix lesion that partially disconnects the hippocampus from anterior parts of the brain has a deleterious effect (Gaffan, 1983). However, this hypothesis, although supported by studies suggesting that spatially directed actions are sensitive to fornix transection (Rupniak and Gaffan, 1987), failed to attract general support.

A turning point that led to a key insight about episodic-like memory was the outcome of a study on conditional learning (Gaffan and Harrison, 1989). Monkeys were trained to reach for one of two objects (A or B), such that A was correct when the animals were facing one way in the laboratory room, but B was correct when they were facing in the other direction. This task was relatively easy for control animals to learn, but a severe deficit occurred after fornix lesioning. Interestingly, the deficit was not a general problem of conditional learning because there was no deficit if the objects were presented on trays of different colors with object A correct on an orange tray but B correct on a white tray. From a strictly logical perspective, the two tasks are identical, but they were differentially sensitive to fornix lesions. Gaffan suspected that it might have something to do with the spatial organization of the "scene" before the animal. When the monkey had to face in different directions, the scene before him changed even though many elements of it were still there (e.g., the window). When the monkey looked at objects on trays of different colors, however, the global scene was unchanged despite the minor change of a specific element in it. A third experiment contrasted "scenes" with "places." To compare them, a new set of monkeys was trained to reach for one of five objects as a function of their place in the room. The places were chosen to be as visually different from one another as possible so location rather than the spatial arrangement of the scene would differentiate the places (e.g., in front of bookshelves, by the door, by the window). Surprisingly, no fornix lesion deficit was seen. Accordingly, Gaffan argued for a distinction between places and scenes, arguing that a fornix lesion disrupts some aspect of scene encoding or the capacity of scene information to set the occasion for other stimuli to be rewarded or nonrewarded. This analysis was a forerunner of Aggleton and Brown's later description of hippocampal memory as involving the spatial organization of familiar objects (Aggleton and Brown, 1999). The elegance of Gaffan and Harrison's (1989) classic paper is marred only by a minor confounding between the selectivity of the deficit and the change from two scenes to five places, with a fornix lesion impairment in the two scenes experiment but no such effect in the five places experiment. However, subsequent work went on to establish the sensitivity of scene memory to fornix transection in monkeys that were *not* moved from place to place.

The emphasis on scenes rather than places is a subtle but important way in which Gaffan's hypothesis differs from the cognitive map theory. What is important is not *where* the monkey is itself located but *what he is looking at*. Later unit-recording work by Rolls revealing the existence of "view cells" in the hippocampus (Robertson et al., 1998) raised the possibility that fornix transection disrupts a view-specific physiological process that is implemented in or, at least projected to, the hippocampus. Gaffan, being apparently uninterested in localization of function as a scientific goal, was noncommittal about what aspect of cognitive function is mediated within the hippocampus itself—perhaps uncertain that it would map onto any psychologically defined category. His interest has generally been restricted to whether damage to area X disrupts some psychological process or, in disconnection studies, that conjoint unilateral damage to area X and contralateral damage to area Y does likewise (e.g., Easton et al., 2001). Thus, despite the extensive use of lesions as a tool to dissociate putative memory systems and a detailed specification of relevant primate neuroanatomy, the "scene-processing" theory does not identify the episodic system as located in one or more structures. The closest Gaffan's theory comes to anatomical localization is with reference to the Delay-Brion circuit, a group of structures that includes the hippocampal formation as well as the fornix, mammillary bodies, and anterior thalamus. This emphasis on the anterior connections of the hippocampal formation, not least the connectivity with the prefrontal lobe (Browning et al., 2005), is strikingly different from the perspective offered in the declarative memory theory, where the emphasis is much more on posterior neocortical connections (as in Chapter 3). Gaffan's ideas can be said to be forward-looking.

Subsequent experiments have elaborated and developed the idea of scene-specific memory as the essential basis of episodic-like memory. Before describing them, two points should be noted. First, the hypothesis captures an important phenomenological feature of episodic memory—our ability to remember the context in which an event occurred. This is relevant to many memory tasks given to humans and animals where the description provided by the experimenter can all

too easily ignore features of the surrounding scene because they do not seem relevant to the solution of the task. Recognition memory is, once again, a case in point. Although the surrounding features of the testing apparatus (the WGTA or computer touchscreen) may not help the monkey remember whether object X or image Y was seen most recently, an incidental and noncontingent memory of the context may still be important. Normal animals automatically form object–context associations, and the context may then act as a retrieval cue or as an element of the remembered visual scene. This was, it should be remembered, the basis of Nadel's concern about removing monkeys from a WGTA during long memory delays in some of the primate studies of recognition memory (Nadel, 1995).

The second point to note is methodological. The first scene-encoding study (Gaffan and Harrison, 1989) and other studies conducted around the same time involved moving the transport cage containing the monkey to change the scene around the animal. This procedural burden, coupled with the laborious nature of training monkeys by hand in WGTAs, encouraged the Oxford laboratory to be pioneers in the development of automated stimulus presentation systems. Automated testing was introduced by the National Institutes of Health (NIH) group around the same time (Murray et al., 1993), following innovative developments of T. Aigner, and later by a San Diego group to test monkeys at very short memory delays in DNMTS (Alvarez et al., 1994). Horel's group also developed systems that used slide projectors under computer control. The development of touchscreen technology was partly a matter of convenience, but it was also to have an impact on Gaffan's developing theoretical ideas. He began by using laser disks to show a large number of scenes to monkeys (e.g., scenes from a film) and later digital graphics software to generate a nearly infinite variety of abstract designs as scenes (typically of colored circles, ellipses, and typographical characters of different sizes).

Scene Memory, Place Memory, and Object-in-Place Memory Are Sensitive to Fornix Lesions

In one study, monkeys were shown scene after scene from George Lucas's film "Raiders of the Lost Ark" (Gaffan, 1992). Although we may wonder what they made of it, their task was to remember which scenes were associated with reward and which were not.* A highly significant deficit in the rate of learning was observed in fornix-lesioned monkeys. This result is important because it suggests that scene learning and object discrimination learning may be quite different. From a strictly

---

*An unpublished study by Nicholas Humphrey should be mentioned in passing. He showed cartoon movies to monkeys on a television screen. To test whether there was any understanding of what was happening, he allowed the animals to choose between seeing the film run normally or in the reverse direction. Although the scenes the animals saw were visually similar, only the normal movie "made sense." The monkeys preferred the regular film.

logical point of view, learning the reward significance of a set of scenes is identical to concurrent object discrimination learning in a WGTA. We saw earlier that concurrent discrimination tasks are sensitive to MTL lesions when multiple trials of each pair of objects are given each day but not when only one trial of each object is given per day (Malamut et al., 1984). However, somewhat paradoxically, when several hundred scenes are presented each day, each for no more than one or a few trials, a clear deficit is observed with a fornix lesion that typically produces only mild amnesia in humans and little or no deficit in many classic primate declarative memory tasks. Gaffan's finding of a positive effect of fornix lesions therefore supports his case that there may be something special about scene processing in the Delay-Brion circuit compared to merely discriminating objects.

Computer-generated abstract scenes provided another way to compare three conditions: place memory, object memory and object-in-place memory (Gaffan, 1994a). In the object-in-place task, for example, the correct response for the monkey is to reach out and touch the one object of a pair that always occupies a particular position in a unique background of abstract colors and shapes (Fig. 13–44A). The use of the term "object" is slightly misleading because, in practice, the monkeys are often required to reach toward nothing more than alpha-numeric characters on the screen. However, work by Buckley and Gaffan (1998b) showed that monkeys are very good at equating objects seen on a computer screen with real three-dimensional objects they can handle and pick up. In a series of experiments using such abstract scenes, a central finding has been that hippocampal, fornix, mammillary body, or anterior thalamic lesions each cause a deficit in recalling scenes learned preoperatively and in learning new scenes (Fig. 13–44B). The reasons for arguing that the Delay-Brion structures form a circuit responsible for this type of memory are (1) lesions to each structure individually cause a learning

impairment of comparable magnitude; and (2) adding a fornix lesion to a preexisting mammillary body lesion does not exacerbate the deficit. It therefore seems likely that these structures make their contribution to processing in a serial manner. Later studies have gone on to implicate the entorhinal and perirhinal cortex in object-in-place memory as well (Gaffan and Parker, 1996; Murray et al., 1998; Easton and Gaffan, 2000; Charles et al., 2004b).

A possible weakness is that although described as an "animal model of episodic memory" there is nothing very "event-like" in remembering which of two alpha-numeric characters is rewarded with food within particular scenes. The task could be learned semantically and stored as a "fact" rather than as an episode. There is also no "recall" element to the task. The cues are always provided on the computer screen, and the animal can recognize them rather than bring them to mind. To be sure, learning is remarkably rapid such that, in experienced monkeys, it takes only two to five trials to learn each object-in-place task. At that speed of learning—clearly much faster than traditional visual discrimination tasks—the animal is remembering correctly what to do on the basis of only one or at most a few trials. However, the episodic character of the task, like paired-associate learning in humans, is being inferred more from the sheer speed of learning than its formal logic. It does not absolutely require memory of "what, where, and when."

Memory Functions of the Temporal Lobe, Delay-Brion Circuit, and Prefrontal Cortex

The proposal that the hippocampus is part of the Delay-Brion circuit and that this circuit has a highly specialized role in memory is only one aspect of Gaffan's wider ideas about multiple types of memory mediated by circuits interconnecting the temporal and frontal lobes. His scene-specific theory of episodic memory differs from the declarative memory

Figure 13–44. Scene-encoding as a component of episodic memory. *A.* The monkey faces a computer screen that typically consists of a number of randomly placed shapes and alpha-numeric characters. The task is to reach for one object (e.g., the number 7 in the bottom-left corner) against one background and for another object

(e.g., the letter u in the right-hand side) when the presented against a different background scene (not shown). *B.* Monkeys soon learn these types of problem rapidly, whereas fornix-lesioned animals show a clear deficit. (*Source*: After Gaffan, 1994.)

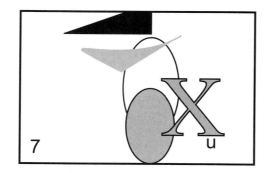

A. Greyscaled display of 'object-in-place' task

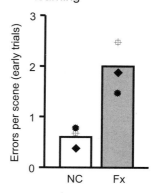

B. Mean performance during learning

theory in two major respects: First, it regards hippocampus-dependent scene memory as one of several qualitatively distinct propositional memory systems. Like the position taken by Horel a generation ago (Horel, 1978b, 1994), Gaffan therefore takes exception to the concept of a monolithic MTL memory system (Gaffan, 2002). Second, unlike both the declarative memory and relational processing theories, there is apparently no explicit consolidation mechanism. Gaffan believed that the Delay-Brion circuit is important for memory encoding and memory retrieval, even if retrieval is not required until months after original training, but it is non-committal on sites of storage. The perspective on the role of the MTL in memory is difficult to pin down. This is because the dissociations that have emerged from his experiments (using a variety of tasks and both bilateral and crossed unilateral lesion techniques) are generally described only in terms of the "necessity of a given area/pathway for a given task." No statement of what cognitive operations are carried out by each structure in the temporal lobe has been presented, nor statements about the nature of different memory systems, their rules of operation, or the type(s) of information on which they operate. Even for the best studied part of the system, the Delay-Brion circuit, there is no statement of the presumably distinct contributions to scene-specific episodic encoding and recall made by the four distinct structures of the circuit. This is puzzling because the local circuitry, numbers of cells, and extrinsic connections of the mammillary body differ radically from those of the hippocampus. Even if Gaffan is correct that they work together serially to enable a common function, it would be helpful to unpack this statement by outlining their distinct contributions to that "common function." Electrophysiological studies may be helpful here.

These points may seem unduly harsh criticisms. However, the picture that is emerging from Gaffan's seminal work is that he envisages a widespread but loose hierarchy of cortical areas involved in memory (Murray et al., 2005). The middle and inferior temporal gyri have the job of analyzing visual object features, such as shape and color. The most anterior neocortical region, the perirhinal cortex, associates these object features with nonvisual features of objects (e.g., reward significance) to form perceptual representations of unique individual objects (Buckley and Gaffan, 1998a). Information about unique objects processed in the perirhinal cortex is put together, in circuits involving the hippocampus, with spatial information to form representations of unique complex scenes (Murray et al., 2005). Finally, the entire system has important functional connections with the prefrontal lobe.

By way of a coda, it should be noted that Gaffan's emphasis on networks for memory processing has points of similarity to Miyashita's distinction between "automatic" and "active" retrieval of information (Miyashita, 2004). Although Miyashita accepted the idea of an MTL memory system, he also identified a "semantic" associational system in area 36 of the limbic cortex and the important role of "top-down" connections from the prefrontal cortex in guiding the intentional or active retrieval of information from these systems.

Miyashita's analysis extended beyond the domain of episodic memory to paired-associate learning following his identification of neocortical "pair-coding" neurons that fire differentially as a function of the association that binds two stimuli together (Sakai and Miyashita, 1991). His suggestion is that automatic retrieval of episodic or semantic information requires no more than activation in the MTL or area 36, respectively, but effortful retrieval also involves a top-down signal from the prefrontal lobe. Two main lines of evidence from animal studies support this idea. First, the latency at which unit-recording signals are observed during automatic retrieval is shortest in the most medial structures and spreads backward from the hippocampus (for episodic information) and from area 36 (for semantic information) to area TE where neurons are gradually recruited that provide a fuller representation of remembered information, be it an event or a fact. Second, during active retrieval, neurons in the inferotemporal cortex received categorical rather than stimulus-specific information from the frontal cortex to help guide the effortful process of memory searching (Tomita et al., 1999). Miyashita saw the challenge ahead as being "to understand the hierarchical interactions between multiple cortical areas" (Miyashita, 2004, p. 435) in the expression of memory. Notwithstanding differences of approach and detail, Gaffan's perspective was similar.

13.6.3 What, Where, and When: Studies of Food-caching and Sequence Learning

Food Caching by Corvids as a Model of "What, Where, and When"

A different approach to thinking about the recollection of past experience was taken by Clayton and her colleagues, who conducted a series of studies examining food caching and recovery by a corvid species, the Californian scrub-jay. Clayton and Dickinson (1998) allowed adult hand-raised scrub jays to cache food items in sand-filled ice-cube trays surrounded by trial-unique arrays of distinctive visual objects (Lego bricks). The two food items were (1) preferred but perishable wax moth larvae and (2) less-preferred but nonperishable peanuts, each of which were in plentiful supply in bowls at the time of caching. During two successive caching periods separated by an interval of 120 hours, the birds transported and then cached wax moths on one side of the caching tray and peanuts on the other, with each side being covered by a Perspex strip during the caching of the other food item (Fig. 13–45A,B). These caching periods constituted the opportunity for the animals to encode into memory what food item was being cached where and when. Recovery was permitted either 4 or 124 hours later with both sides of the ice-cube tray uncovered and available. Over a series of pretraining trials extending over several weeks, with the visual arrangement of Lego bricks and the assignment of tray sides for the two foods randomly changed on each trial, birds in the "degrade" group had the opportunity to learn that wax moths recovered after 4 hours

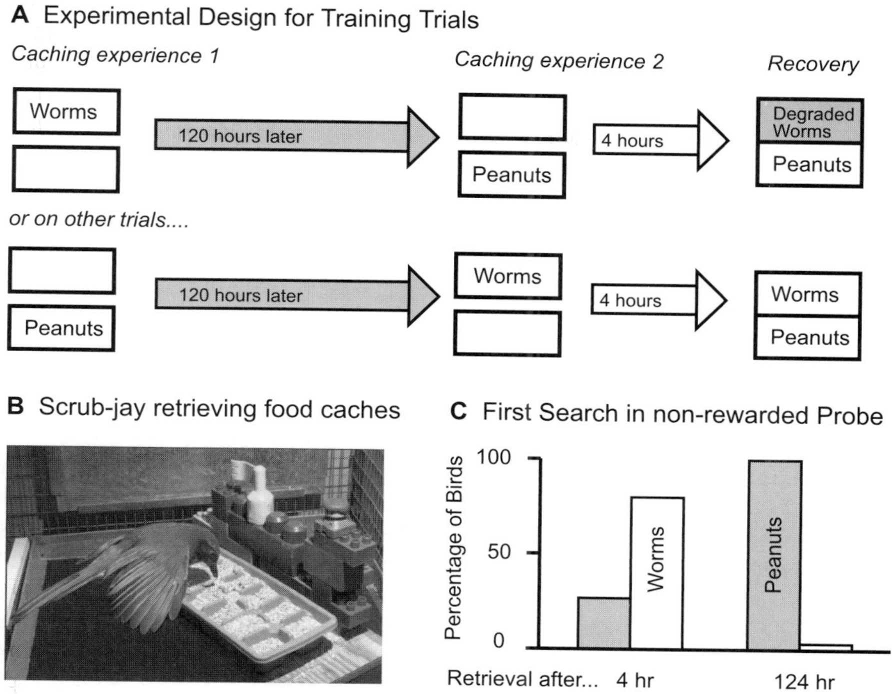

A Experimental Design for Training Trials

B Scrub-jay retrieving food caches

C First Search in non-rewarded Probe

Figure 13–45. Memory for what, where, and when in California scrub-jays. *A.* Experimental design for the training trials in which the birds in the "degrade" condition (shown) had the opportunity to learn that wax-moths become unpalatable after a period of 4 days. *B.* California scrub-jay performing the task. *C.* Results from the "degrade" group showing proportions of birds making their first pecks to the wax-moth or peanut side of the caching tray. (*Source*: After Clayton and Dickinson, 1998. Photograph courtesy of N. Clayton.)

are tasty and worth eating, whereas those retrieved after 124 hours are not. Birds assigned to a separate "replenish" control group always found fresh wax worms at recovery whether it occurred at the short or the long recovery interval. The main finding of this ingenious study was that in nonrewarded probe tests in which neither food was actually available (thereby preventing any olfactory or visual cues to guide search location) the scrub-jays in the degrade group searched preferentially for wax moths when recovery occurred 4 hours after caching but switched their search to peanuts when recovery did not occur until 124 hours had elapsed (Fig. 13–45C). This switchover was not shown by the birds in the "replenish" condition but partially shown by birds in a third, "pilfer," group in which the preferred wax worms were missing after a 124-hour delay. This pattern of results implies that, at recovery and using free recall, the birds can recollect what food item was stored where and, at least in some sense, how long ago.

In addition to careful controls, such as nonrewarded probe tests, there are several innovations in this experimental approach. The use of food caching is helpful as it ensures the animal is attentive and engaged in the task at the time of memory encoding; the act of caching is not, however, a requirement for the formation of episodic-like memory. The use of very long memory intervals over hours and days ensures that memory retrieval is outside the range over which interval timing mechanisms, mediated by short-term memory, can operate (Hampton and Schwartz, 2004). The use of

free recall at cache recovery obviates the use of a familiarity strategy that has been so problematic in studies of recognition memory. Clayton and Dickinson's claim that their initial study provides "the first conclusive behavioral evidence of 'episodic-like' memory in animals other than humans" (Clayton and Dickinson, 1998, p. 274) was vindicated by later studies in which a number of detailed issues were taken further (Clayton et al., 2001). In one of the studies, scrub-jays were allowed to cache preferred crickets (rather than wax moths) and less-preferred peanuts (Clayton et al., 2003a). After caching but before recovery, the birds were taught that the crickets, which used to remain edible for at least 3 days, now degraded rapidly and became inedible. During cache recovery, the birds now avoided the crickets and sought out the less preferred peanuts. Thus, the birds seem to be able to apply information retrospectively at the time of retrieval to guide their choice of food item. Other studies have investigated prospective aspects of food caching with the scrub-jays (Emery and Clayton, 2001) and refined the criteria for identifying mental time travel in animals (Clayton et al., 2003b).

Sequence-dependent and Context-dependent Object–Place Memory in Rats

The scrub-jays are not suitable subjects for neurobiological studies, particularly because these studies use hand-raised birds to ensure control of the caching experience. Unfortunately, efforts to demonstrate "what, where, and when" in other species, particularly laboratory animals such as rats, have not been successful so far. This has led some to question whether animals can undertake mental time travel (Roberts, 2000). Others have raised the possibility that the "when" component should be thought about in other ways, such as with reference to the context in which they occur or their sequence of occurrence. Both sequence and context sometimes act as mental surrogates for the experience of time.

With respect to context, which we have already discussed extensively (see Section 13.5), Eacott made the interesting argument that when asked about "when" an event happened people often work out where they were at the time and then use the retrieved contextual information to remember events. In this mental exercise, there is not necessarily any mental time travel as such (Eacott et al., 2005). Based on this thought, she has developed a modification of Ennaceur's novel object recognition (NOR) task for rats in which context, place, and object can be a triad of associations. That is, the rat has to remember whether a specific object was in a specific location in a particular context. Using this task, she reported that fornix lesions disrupt recollection of the what–where–where triad while, somewhat surprisingly, appearing not to affect a simpler what–where task (Eacott and Gaffan, 2005). This is a challenging result being, on the face of it, very different from the extensive results reported by Gaffan's group using object-in-place memory. However, given the importance of testing numerous memory delays in NOR tasks before claiming selectivity (Clark and Martin, 2005), it would be valuable for various memory delays to be investigated in her task. On a conceptual level also, that people sometimes cannot remember time and use the surrogate of context does not imply that they always do so, nor does it undermine the central importance of mental time travel to "true" episodic memory.

With respect to memory for the sequence of events, Honey et al. (1998) showed that rats with hippocampal lesions were less able than sham-lesioned animals to notice any change in the order of two sequentially presented stimuli during an orienting task. In another study, Fortin et al. (2002) showed that rats could remember some information about the sequence in which a series of distinctive odors was presented. Cups of sand through which rats could dig to find food (like the paired-associate and transitive inference experiments of Section 13.5) were presented at 2.5-minute intervals. Common household odors were mixed into the sand to determine its smell, with different novel sequences of odors given during each series of trials. For a given sequence, call it A-B-C-D-E, the animals were later tested for whether they could remember that sand odor A came before odor C, B before D, and so on; they were also tested for whether odors A–E were familiar compared to other novel odors. The results showed that whereas the sham-lesioned animals could perform above chance on both the sequence and recognition components of these tests, the rats with radiofrequency-induced hippocampal lesions could remember the individual odors but not the sequential information. A follow-up study by Agster et al. (2002) indicated

that rats with hippocampal lesions could eventually acquire some sequential information about repeated sequences with extended training but never well enough to disambiguate overlapping sequences. That the hippocampus could be involved in rapidly learning sequences has also been the subject of modeling studies focusing on the recurrent associative network organization of area CA3 (Jensen and Lisman, 1996; Levy, 1996). Nakazawa's observation that mice with a knockout of the NMDA receptor specific to area CA3 are poor at "one-shot" learning but successfully master a spatial reference memory task (Nakazawa et al., 2003) represents partial support for this view, but it would be interesting if such mice could also be shown to be poor at learning explicit sequences of information. Given these findings, Eichenbaum (2004) extended his relational processing theory into the episodic domain by arguing that the hippocampus is also the neural substrate for mediating the sequential organization of memory. In his view, the mediation of memory for time can often be achieved by reference to memory of the order in which items occurred rather than some absolute memory of the time at which they were initially presented.

In a complementary approach to thinking about sequential aspects of events, single-unit recording studies in rats have indicated that hippocampal pyramidal cells can sometimes mediate more than "place" information. Chapter 11 documented the extensive evidence for the spatial sensitivity of single-units in rodents, including place cells, theta units, head-direction cells, and grid cells. However, we have already seen that a growing body of evidence indicates that CA1 and CA3 pyramidal cells may have cognitive and behavioral correlates that extend beyond the domain of space (Eichenbaum et al., 1999; Wood et al., 1999; Jeffery, 2003).

Wood et al. (2000) recorded hippocampal complex-spike neurons in rats running a figure-of-eight maze in which, after moving through the common stem of the maze, the animals had to alternate between turning left or right to secure reward (Fig. 13–46). A high proportion of the cells (up to 67%) with place fields on the stem fired differentially as the rat traversed the common stem on left-turn and right-turn trials, even when potentially confounding variations in running speed and exact heading direction were taken into account. Other cells fired similarly on both trial types (i.e., were place cells), and other factors contributed to the firing determinants of the remaining cells. They argued that hippocampal representations, as represented by cell firing, encoded information about other nonspatial features of specific memory episodes. An earlier study had also found evidence of patterns of nonspatial firing correlates in an olfactory nonmatching task (Wood et al., 1999). CA1 cell firing was related consistently to perceptual, behavioral, or cognitive events, irrespective of the location where these events occurred.

Ferbinteanu and Shapiro (2003) went on to disentangle factors that could be responsible for journey sensitivity, showing that CA1 complex-spike cells certainly display "retrospective coding" and possibly also "prospective coding." They used a hippocampus-dependent plus maze task (Packard and

A   Figure-of-Eight Maze

B   Sensitivity to Memory Delay

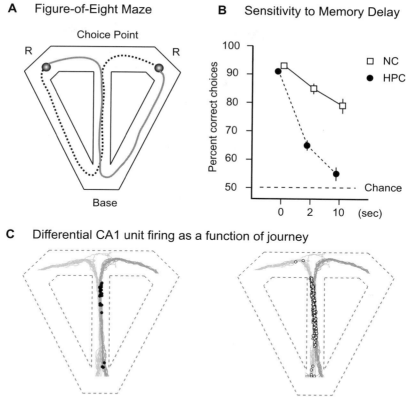

C   Differential CA1 unit firing as a function of journey

Figure 13–46. Task-dependent modulation of CA1 pyramidal cell firing. *A.* Figure-of-eight maze as used by Wood et al. (2000) to establish additional properties of complex-spike cells than just place and direction sensitivity. The dotted and continuous lines refer to alternating traverses through the central stem as the animal runs the maze, receiving a reward (R) soon after each alternating choice. *B.* Choice performance of normal and hippocampus-lesioned animals as a function of an imposed delay before entering the stem of the maze. *C.* Differential firing as a function of whether the rat has come from the left side of the maze and is about to turn right (filled symbols) or has come from the right side and is about to turn left (open symbols). (*Source*: After Wood et al., 2000 and courtesy of James Ainge.)

McGaugh, 1996) in which the start arms of the maze were switched between north and south within a block of trials, and the goal arm switched from east to west between blocks of trials. In this way, the animals could make one of four kinds of journey: from north to either east or west and from south to either east or west. Thus, in traversing the east arm up to the goal, the rats could have come either from north or from south. During recording studies, many "pure" place cells were observed, as described by Wood et al. (2000), but differential cell firing in the east and west arms was also observed, depending on whether entry was from the north or south arms, reflecting journey-sensitive "retrospective coding." "Prospective coding" is also claimed in the paper but accepting that it is slightly problematic because the recordings were then compared across blocks of trials in which the reward location had been switched. Although unlikely, this goal reversal might itself alter the firing properties of the cells, a complication that does not arise with retrospective coding in which reward location is fixed and recordings are taken from within a single block of trials in which some journeys began in the north and others in the south. One way in which this confounding might be addressed is through the use of two

rewards (e.g., different flavors of food) at the east and west arms of the plus maze, respectively. Then, through cueing of the animals with a "pre-taste" of one or other food reward in the start box, it might be possible to secure recordings within a block of trials in which the animals turned toward the east when cued with flavor 1 (from either north or south) and turned to the west when cued with flavor 2. Evidence for prospective coding uncontaminated by the use of a reversal schedule might then be obtained.

What do these unit-recording findings imply for hippocampal involvement in episodic-like memory? With respect to neurobiological mechanisms mediating the "what-where-when" trilogy, it is clearly necessary for place representations to be supplemented by temporal or sequence information (time-tagging or relative order) and by representations of objects that are to be found at each place. These new studies of the correlates of hippocampal cells raise the possibility that at least "when" and " where" might both be represented in population vectors of such cell firing. To date, the data are limited to short time periods (seconds) and to the simplest descriptors of sequence (e.g., south-before-east is encoded by cells different from those representing north-before-east).

13.6.4 Problem of Awareness

Experiments with animals that lay claim to revealing a "recollective" component of memory should somehow discriminate explicit and implicit processing. We should try to face up to the formidable problem of understanding the neurobiology of "awareness." Following Gaffan's work, "asking" a monkey if it saw a specific image on a computer screen 40 minutes ago is now routine. Another example is the seminal work on "blindsight" in monkeys (Cowey and Stoerig, 1995) that was discussed earlier (Fig. 13–13). The discovery of "mirror neurons" in primates (Rizzolatti and Craighero, 2004) further extends our appreciation of a possible neurobiology of animal awareness, as do Iriki's studies of tool use (Maravita and Iriki, 2004). These are telling examples because they are precisely the kinds of phenomenon that an honorable and scholarly skeptic who asserts the importance of language to awareness, such as Macphail (1998), might have predicted to be impossible to demonstrate in animals.

To be sure, cogent arguments have been put forward to suggest that we may never know whether any animal can ever be said to possess "autonoetic" consciousness or engage in mental time travel and that seeking true episodic memory in animals is therefore a forlorn exercise (Suddendorf and Busby, 2003). However, there is value in taking a positive view of the possibility of identifying aspects of memory awareness in animals using behavioral criteria (Clayton et al., 2003b). Language may not be central to its expression, a sense of the self may not be required, and new behavioral protocols will hopefully continue to reveal more about animal awareness and the role, if any, of the hippocampus in it. In this way, the problem of awareness is being broken down into bite-sized chunks at which experimentalists can nibble away. We have already seen (Fig. 13–14) that monkeys can reveal an awareness of whether they can remember (Hampton, 2001). Can animals also display quantitative characteristics of memory that parallel those shown by humans when they are using recollection or familiarity to solve a recognition task? Can they do one-trial cued recall? For each of these, we can go on to ask whether performance is affected by hippocampal dysfunction.

Recollection, Familiarity, and Region of Interest Curves

Studies examining the hippocampal contribution to the phenomenological experience of memory have also been inspired by developments in cognitive psychology. Fortin et al. (2004) exploited a quantitative approach for distinguishing the two components of dual-process theories of recognition memory—recollection and familiarity—that was developed during the 1990s by Yonelinas (2001). His approach, discussed in Chapter 12, involved plotting graphs called receiver operating characteristic (ROC) curves, which are an important part of the signal-detection theory (Tanner and Swets, 1954). Two sets of probability functions, usually Gaussian, are plotted that vary as a function of cost and benefit: "hits" and "false alarms."

Hits are recorded when a subject *correctly* identifies a previously presented stimulus (i.e., a signal); false alarms are recorded when the subject *incorrectly* identifies a stimulus as seen before when it had not in fact been presented earlier (i.e., noise). The range of conditions involves systematic variation of relative value, that is, the costs and benefits of correctly reporting hits and mistakenly making false alarms. If the cost of missing a correct stimulus is high and that of making a false alarm is low, subjects adjust their reporting criterion in the direction of reporting hits (i.e., to the right of the graphs in Figure 13–47A.) Conversely, if the risks associated with incorrect memory are high (as in eye-witness testimony), then subjects shift their response criterion downward (i.e., to the left in the graphs).

How can this seemingly overcomplicated way of thinking about memory performance be helpful? Yonelinas's important contribution was to recognize that the divergence from the diagonal can take two forms. It may be *symmetrical* or *asymmetrical*. In the former case, p (hit) initially rises faster than p (false alarm) until both reach 0.5, and then the increase in p (false alarm) catches up. This creates a symmetrical ROC curve and reflects the familiarity component of recognition (curved line in Fig. 13–47B). In the latter case, p (hit) rises rapidly at low values of p (false alarm), an asymmetry thought to be due to the second component of recognition memory—recollection (dotted line in Fig. 13–47B). This component operates as a threshold process in which items and their spatiotemporal context are either recollected (above threshold) or not recollected (below threshold). There is no gradation of subjective familiarity as occurs in other components of recognition memory. Like pregnancy, there are no half-measures.

Fortin et al. (2004) have now successfully established that ROC curves for recognition memory can also be plotted for rats. This was done taking advantage of their spectacular memory for odors, using a continuous recognition task in which the rats had to dig in sand wells for reward when the odor of the adulterated sand was novel and refrain from doing so when it was familiar (and then search elsewhere for reward). Wood et al. (1999) had previously shown that this is a task that displays a number of hippocampal unit correlates. Costs and benefits were manipulated by altering the height of the sand wells (making digging easier or more difficult) and the size of the reward the animals got when they dug successfully (from one-fourth of a pellet to three pellets of food reward). Their findings indicate that when normal rats were tested 30 minutes after exposure to a "list" of odors (analogous to a list of words in a human recognition experiment), the ROC curve was asymmetrical (Fig. 13–47C). When half the rats were then subjected to hippocampal lesioning, the ROC curve became symmetrical (Figure 13.47D). Together with other data in this study, it seems that recognition memory in rats complies with dual-process models of recognition memory in humans and that hippocampal lesions may remove the "recollection" component of this memory. The task of realizing a neurobiological understanding of episodic and episodic-like memory and the nature of hippocampal involve-

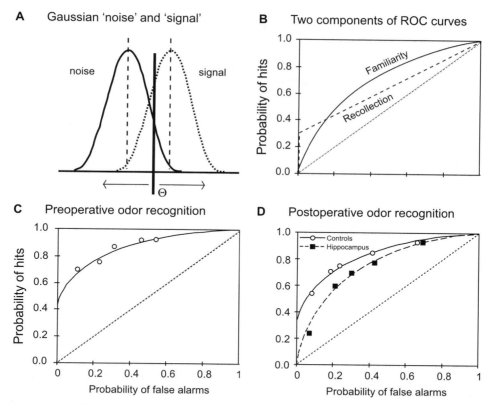

Figure 13–47. Receiver operating characteristic (ROC) analysis of recognition memory in the rat. *A.* Hypothetical Gaussian functions plotting the probability of "signal" and "noise" during memory of a prior event. The receiver operates at various points along the x-axis and can so make estimates of what constitutes a "hit" (i.e., a true signal) and what constitutes a "false-alarm" (i.e., from the noise distribution but claimed to be a memory). The threshold θ can be adjusted up or down the x-axis to enable a more conservative (to the right) or more risky (to the left) detection policy, as described in the text. *B.* Quantitative analysis of ROC functions reveals a linear recollection component and a symmetrical familiarity component of memory. The sum of the two components is a curved but asymmetrical function. *C.* Normal rats show asymmetrical function in odor recognition memory. *D.* After hippocampal lesions, rats show a symmetrical ROC function. (*Source*: After Fortin et al., 2004.)

ment in it seems no longer quite as forlorn an enterprise as once it did. It is to one developing theory of this type that we now turn.

13.6.5 Elements of a Neurobiological Theory of the Role of the Hippocampus in Episodic-like Memory

It is premature but not inappropriate to end this chapter with an attempt to tie several strands together. The focus in this chapter has been on the major historical contribution that animal lesioning studies over the past 30 years have made to our understanding of hippocampal function. Modern work has greatly expanded the levels of analysis at which neuroscientists think about function and has been converging on the idea of a role in the automatic aspects of episodic-like memory. There has been little discussion so far of the specific role hippocampal synaptic plasticity might play in this process or how the cell biological determinants of that plasticity fit with neuropsychological ideas about memory consolidation. Given the shift toward more interdisciplinary approaches in neuroscience, it is fitting to end on this note.

Automatic Recording and Retrieval of Attended Experience

One neurobiological theory of hippocampal function does attempt to specify a role for synaptic plasticity in memory formation (Morris et al., 2003). This theory supposes that hippocampal memory can, like other forms of memory, be divided into four processes: encoding, storage, consolidation, and retrieval. A key aspect of the neurobiological approach is the assertion that activity-dependent synaptic plasticity (e.g., LTP) is critical for encoding and the intermediate storage of memory traces in the hippocampus that correspond to the "indices" or "pointers" to cortical regions where detailed perceptual information is temporarily stored (as discussed in Section 13.3). These hippocampal indices are cartoons that bind event information to the context in which they occur. A novel feature of the theory is that these index memory traces decay rapidly but are sometimes rendered more persistent by the process of cellular consolidation. That is, LTP is actually something of a misnomer as many, perhaps most, memories of events captured online are soon lost. Protein synthesis-independent E-LTP is more of a system for creating the "potential" for memory with synaptic tagging at the time of E-LTP induction (see Chapter 10) playing a part in determining what traces are rendered more persistent. The rapid "snapshot" creation of a temporary event-context index involves synaptic potentiation at a large number of synapses across parts of the hippocampal network (probably in CA1 and CA3). Tags set automatically at the time of an event, irrespective of how trivial that event may be, can capture the products of the somatic or dendritic synthesis of plasticity proteins set in train by events before, during, or even after an event to be remembered. This capturing process renders the temporary indices in the hippocampus more permanent and thus allows sufficient time for systems-level consolidation to occur. This two-stage process of consolidation serves as a "protective filter" in the sense that rapidly decaying index traces do not last long enough to guide neocortical consolidation; and thus events that are *not* subject to cellular consolidation in the hippocampus do not become represented in a persistent manner in the cortex. Although hippocampal synaptic plasticity is critical for encoding and its expression subject to intrahippocampal cellular consolidation, the theory also asserts that it is not involved in memory retrieval. It is also unlikely to be involved in the widely discussed systems-level consolidation process that depends on hippocampus–neocortex interactions, although it does not preclude the possibility that neocortical synaptic plasticity is critical. More formally, the propositions of this developing theory are presented in Box 13–11.

Box 13–11
Neurobiological Theory of Hippocampal Function

1. Some animals have episodic-like memory, and the hippocampal formation is one group of brain structures that can encode and retrieve such memories.
2. Activity-dependent, associative, NMDA receptor-dependent synaptic plasticity in the hippocampus is the primary neural mechanism responsible for inducing temporary encoding and storage of hippocampal "indices" of rapidly acquired event-context memories. The detailed perceptual information associated with events is represented in the cortex.
3. An essential feature of cellular consolidation processes to which these index traces are subject is the interaction between local "synaptic tags" (set by glutamatergic activation), and diffusely targeted "plasticity proteins" (which can be triggered by heterosynaptic activation of neuromodulatory and glutamatergic inputs).
4. Systems-level consolidation requires both hippocampus and neocortical neural activity and is therefore not solely time-dependent although certainly a process that takes time. It does not require hippocampal plasticity but may engage mechanisms of neocortical plasticity.
5. The hippocampal formation is one of a number of brain regions that detects novelty, and its neural activity alters in ways that enable a representation of novel events to be encoded rapidly online.

This framework builds unashamedly on the functional/neuropsychological theories discussed earlier in the chapter, but it also makes a number of novel predictions, including some counterintuitive predictions, at other levels of analysis. Some examples of the shoulders on which it stands and these predictions are as follows. From a neuropsychological perspective, it recognizes that events happen in particular places at particular times, and their later recall generally includes the memory of where and when an event occurred (Gaffan, 1994b; Clayton et al., 2001). Thus, event encoding is necessarily associative and "contextual" in character, a point emphasized in several functional theories (e.g., cognitive mapping, configural associative, relational). Many events cannot be anticipated, occur only once, and may contain distinct features that, in sequence, form short episodes—a point about episodic memory emphasized by Eichenbaum (2004). It is vital that traces representing information about such episodes are encoded and stored in real time (as they happen), a process that Frey and Morris characterized as the "automatic recording of attended experience" (Morris and Frey, 1997). Not all events are remembered for any length of time, and to do so is not only unnecessary but might also saturate the storage capacity of relevant areas of the brain. Moser et al. (1998) exploited this feature of hippocampal memory in their contribution to studies examining the functional significance of hippocampal LTP (see Chapter 10). With respect to the level of representational detail, it is also unclear whether the hippocampus need receive, via its extrinsic afferents, detailed sensory/perceptual information pertaining to individual objects or events. The networks and local circuits for detailed perceptual processing are in the cortex. Rather, all it needs to remember events and the sequence in which they occur is binding information about the locations in the neocortex where this detail is processed and temporarily encoded—a point about hippocampus–neocortex interactions discussed in Chapter 3. Later processing, guided by these indices, determines whether the temporary neocortical encoding becomes permanent. This view of hippocampal memory processing capitalizes on the advances made in other theories; and, like them, it implies that the hippocampus is far from being an island. Realizing its functions *absolutely* requires the synergistic activity of other brain areas both upstream and downstream. This is therefore a framework that, unlike some others (McClelland et al., 1995), implies that the cortex must be able to encode information rapidly online. The view here is not only that the cortex can do this but that it loses information rapidly unless new connections are stabilized by systems-level consolidation. In this sense, consolidation is permissive rather than instructive.

The next step of this framework takes us farther into the neurobiological domain. If events are to be encoded, there must exist physiological mechanisms for capturing events as they happen and encoding traces that could later enable retrieval of event or event-associated information. A prominent candidate for the neural substrate of event memory is hippocampal NMDA receptor-dependent synaptic plasticity, so-called Hebbian plasticity. Such plasticity, as revealed by the physiological phenomenon of LTP, exhibits many properties that are suitable for a role in memory formation (Bliss and Collingridge, 1993; Martin et al., 2000), and a growing body of evidence offers support for this view (see Chapter 10). Index memory traces are achieved by an alteration in the connectivity between neurons such that retrieval cues, expressed as patterns of neural activity, are able to induce new patterns of neural activity that are one part of the substrate of "memories" of prior events.

Another strand relates to the persistence of such traces. A key supposition is that, notwithstanding the fantastic storage capacity of the brain, there is no need to store everything permanently, and the system is absolutely not evolved to do so. Indeed, most memories fade and are lost. Of those that persist, retrieval processes contribute to their accessibility such that "forgetting" is a dual function of trace decay and retrieval failure. If most automatically encoded event memories are temporary, there must be psychological processes and neural mechanisms for selecting the subset of traces that are to be rendered longer lasting or even permanent, such as the emotional significance of the event to be remembered or, more interstingly, the significance of *other* events happening close together in time or space. Experiments on "behavioral tagging" are needed to explore the predictions of the synaptic tagging framework in the context of real memory (see Chapter 10, Section 10.10). There is also evidence that the persistence of memory can also be determined by the relevance of ongoing events to the existing knowledge structures and interests of the person witnessing them (Bartlett, 1932; Bransford and Johnson, 1972; Bransford, 1979), an idea long known in educational circles but that has had curiously little impact on neuroscience until recently (Maguire et al., 1999). Mediating these psychological processes of persistence are two neuronal mechanisms of memory consolidation: (1) cellular consolidation mechanisms, which include the synthesis and synaptic capture of plasticity proteins that stabilize memory traces at the level of the individual synapse in neurons (Goelet et al., 1986; Frey and Morris, 1998; Sweatt, 2003); and (2) systems-level consolidation mechanisms, as discussed in previous sections of this chapter, which reflect a dynamic interaction between populations of neurons in the hippocampus and neocortex (Dudai and Morris, 2001). These forms of consolidation are distinct but also interdependent. This interdependence arises because cellular consolidation enables memory indices in hippocampus to last long enough for the slower systems-level consolidation process to work and thus for their time courses to dovetail.

The defining functional characteristics of associative networks such as the hippocampus are believed by several theorists to include distributed representations, interleaved storage across multiple synapses, and associative retrieval. These processes enable patterns of activity to be stored as a matrix of synaptic changes and retrieval to be "completed" from partial fragments of the original input (Marr, 1971; McNaughton and Morris, 1987; Paulsen and Moser, 1998; Nakazawa et al., 2002). Several factors determine the operating characteristics

and storage capacity of such networks. One of them, connectivity density (i.e., the number of connections per cell), provides an anatomical basis for understanding an important feature of the relation between hippocampus and neocortex (McNaughton et al., 2003). Specifically, the average connectivity in the cortex is, in general, too low to support the encoding of arbitrary associations (Rolls and Treves, 1998). The cortical mantle contains on the order of 10^{10} neurons, but each cortical principal neuron receives only about 10^4 connections. Thus, the average connection probability in cortex is only $1{:}10^6$. To overcome this apparent biological limitation, mammals seem to have evolved an arrangement whereby distributed associative memory between items represented in different sensory modalities can be accomplished through indirect associations mediated by a hierarchical organization (McNaughton et al., 2003). In such a scheme, neocortical modules at the base of the hierarchy are reciprocally connected via modifiable synapses with one or more hippocampal modules at the apex. The hippocampal modules include CA3 as well as the dentate hilus, both characterized by high internal connectivity as well as modifiable synapses. In CA3, each pyramidal cell is contacted by ~ 4% of the pyramidal cells of the same subfield (Amaral, 1990), implying that most CA3 pyramidal cells are connected via two or three synaptic steps (Rolls and Treves, 1998). This high degree of internal recurrent connectivity is probably sufficient to allow autoassociation, or association among individual elements of a patterned input (Marr, 1971). Activity patterns reflecting sensory detail in neocortical modules may generate a unique identifying index in such a network (Teyler and DiScenna, 1987). This high-level hippocampal trace index is no longer "sensory" in any strict sense but is stored associatively with other indices and the output fed back to neocortical modules via modifiable synapses. Activation of a cortical pattern (e.g., a specific flavor of food) could then result in activation of its index in the hippocampus. In turn, this enables retrieval of associated indices and thence the complementary pattern in the other cortical modules (e.g., where the food is found). Indirect associations enable memory retrieval between cortical modules that are too sparsely connected to do this directly.

This principle of indirect association in memory places high demands on the synaptic storage capacity of the hippocampus that, as noted briefly above, is otherwise in danger of becoming saturated. Once saturated, learning can no longer proceed effectively (McNaughton and Barnes, 1986; Moser et al., 1998). There are several ways in which this burden may be limited. One, as already noted, is via rapid decay of a high proportion of the traces that are automatically encoded online (a property of E-LTP). Heterosynaptic depression may also serve a normalizing function and so increase effective storage capacity (Willshaw and Dayan, 1990). A third way to limit the rate of use of storage space, also an element of the present theoretical ideas, would be to ensure that what is stored in the hippocampus is only a cartoon, with the full sensory/perceptual details encoded in the cortex. The fourth way—the process of systems-level memory consolidation itself—would be to enable hippocampal associations that are strongly and/or repeatedly recalled, such as those representing environmental regularities, to trigger the development and stabilization of low-level intermodular connections in the neocortex. It is these connections that could later enable cortical retrieval in the absence of neural activity in the hippocampus. To work, it is vital that the intermodular connections that develop are appropriate to the associations represented. This requires the gradual interleaving of appropriate connections (McClelland et al., 1995), perhaps during sleep (McNaughton et al., 2003). Interestingly, the rate of consolidation may not be strictly time-dependent. Rather, the process may be "cladistic," with the rate of consolidation affected by the frequency with which hippocampal indices are reactivated. It may also depend on an activated neocortical schema to receive the new information.

The last step to be considered relates to the detection of novelty and acting on it. If the hippocampus is critical for building context representations and encoding events in relation to them, it is likely that its neural activity reflects changes to the environment. This is not a new idea, as Gray (1982), Vinogradova (1995), and more recently Gray (2000) have extensively discussed possible "comparator" functions of the hippocampus. Novelty detection is by no means unique to the hippocampus, it being a process required in several cognitive systems; but evidence in favor of a hippocampal contribution has come from many experiments on different forms of novelty detection, including the studies of exploratory behavior in which rats examine objects and landmarks in simple arenas (see Section 13.4). The misplace cells of O'Keefe (1976) and the more recent observations of neural firing in response to the movement of a hidden escape platform in a watermaze (Fyhn et al., 2002) also suggest that the hippocampus, perhaps acting in concert with neuromodulatory systems, detects and represent changes in the conjunction of objects and their locations. Several cells fired vigorously at the new platform location, despite previously having been silent. Others that fired in different locations around the maze continued to do so after platform relocation, arguing against spatial remapping. The new activity was paralleled by reduced discharge in a subset of simultaneously recorded interneurons. The pattern of activity largely returned toward its original configuration as the rat learned the new location. However, a few of the newly recruited neurons remained active. This persistent firing may reflect facilitated synaptic plasticity during the temporary reduction in inhibition (Wigstrom and Gustafsson, 1983; Paulsen and Moser, 1998). NMDA receptor-dependent LTP may be necessary for these permanent modifications in firing patterns when novel events occur in a familiar environment.

Hippocampal Synaptic Plasticity, Neural Activity, and Rapid Paired-associate Learning

Day et al. (2003) developed a one-trial paired-associate task in which rats were trained to recall in which of two locations a particular flavor of rat chow was to be found in a large "event

arena" (Fig. 13–48). In each of two sample trials on each day a few minutes apart, rats left the start box to find a single open sand well where they could dig for a flavored food. No choices were required on this sample trial, and there was nothing in the procedure that would have required the animals to engage a contingent learning mechanism. The animals merely ran out into the arena, found a sand well, dug in it, and found food. This constituted one "event." The two sample trials did, however, use two locations and two foods. This gave the animals the opportunity of automatically encoding—in one trial for each sandell—that one flavor of chow was at one location and another flavor at another (Fig. 13–48A). They therefore had two "events" prior to the daily choice trial, which was started 5 to 20 minutes later. It began by giving the rats one of the two flavors to eat in the start box (their recall cue). A short while later, they were allowed to enter the arena where they now found two sand wells (Fig. 13–48B). On choice trials during training, going to the location associated with the flavor cue was rewarded with more of that same flavor. Nonrewarded probe trials were also run. Up to 30 locations and flavors were paired in novel combinations at the rate of two pairs per day. The results obtained with this "what–where" paradigm provided evidence that rats are capable of a limited form of episodic-like memory—and in a species more amenable to neurobiological study than the scrub-jays used by Clayton. The protocol lacks the dimension of time (the "when" element), which is a concern; but it shares with the avian food-caching paradigms that recall is required rather than recognition, and this represents a step forward from the object-in-place tasks used by Gaffan.

Day et al. (2003) also established that the one-trial encoding of such paired associates lasted no longer than 60 minutes before recall performance dropped to chance (Fig. 13–48C). Nonrewarded probe trials established that there was a preference for digging at the cued location despite the limited nature of the "event" that had uniquely taken place there that day. Encoding was sensitive to the acute intrahippocampal infusion of an NMDA receptor antagonist (D-AP5) without any effect on retrieval (Fig. 13–48D,E), whereas retrieval was insensitive to the AMPA receptor antagonist CNQX (Fig. 13–48E). These pharmacological observations were made by timing the infusions to be either just before or just after the encoding trial. That a difference between encoding and retrieval was obtained when the dorsal hippocampus was infused with D-AP5 indicates that the mere presence of the drug has no effect on memory retrieval, but it definitively blocks encoding. It seems more likely, and is in keeping with physiological studies revealing its importance for associative LTP, that an NMDA receptor-dependent mechanism in the hippocampus is involved in encoding the paired associate of an event and its location into memory in such a manner that the reactivation of one member of the pair can retrieve the memory of the other.

The "event arena" has the potential to serve as a flexible test bed for examining the neurobiology of rapid associative memory of the kind that may underlie human episodic mem-

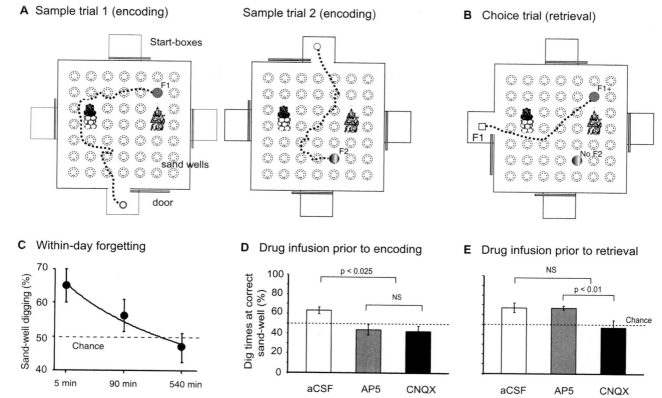

A Sample trial 1 (encoding) Sample trial 2 (encoding) **B** Choice trial (retrieval)

C Within-day forgetting **D** Drug infusion prior to encoding **E** Drug infusion prior to retrieval

Figure 13–48. Cued recall of the location of a single event. *A.* The 1.6 m² "event arena" made of plexiglass consisted of 49 sand wells, 2 intramaze landmarks, and 4 start boxes. On sample trial 1, the door to a start box is drawn back, and the rat runs out into the arena (dotted line) where it displays occasional lateral head movements to find food 1 at the single open well. Sample trial 2 is to a different food (F2) at a different location. *B.* The cued-recall choice trial begins with presentation of either of the two sample trial foods in the start box (food F1 is shown) followed by the rat being rewarded selectively for digging at the sand well containing this same food. *C.* Rapid decay of event-place memory over the course of the day. *D, E.* Nonrewarded probe trials show that the animals preferentially digs in the sand well appropriate to the cue flavor given in the start box. Memory encoding in this task is sensitive to blockade of NMDA receptors (*D*), whereas memory expression requires only fast synaptic transmission via AMPA receptors (*E*). (Source: After Day et al., 2003.)

ory (what, where, and when). However, there are several features of behavioral performance in this task that need to be clarified and improved. First, the temporal component has yet been addressed, though it may be possible to use the surrogate of contextual specificity. Second, no hippocampal lesion study has yet been reported, and there is the difficulty that the drugs used may be directly affecting only one component of the what-where-when triad, such as the spatial component. That is, the drugs' apparent impact on associative encoding or retrieval could be misleading. Studies of one-trial spatial memory in the event arena have helped clarify this point (Bast et al., 2005). Third, alterations in the protocol to look at the concurrent training of multiple places and flavors, analogous to learning a list of object–place pairs, are also underway. Conducted in the spatial domain, such a study would cast light on how multiple spatial associates could become integrated into "spatial schema" that might be constructed and stored in the neocortex. Preliminary data from such a study by Tse, Kakeyama and Langston (personal communication) indicates that such spatial schema can be gradually acquired over

several weeks; and once fully encoded and stored, new information can be added to the schema rapidly. If the schema can be shown to be neocortical, which preliminary evidence indicates they are, such a study may offer some handle on whether neocortical storage of information in a hippocampus-dependent learning task can be achieved during a single trial. This would provide vindication for the unusual prediction of this neurobiological theory that cortical learning is sometimes just as fast as hippocampal learning. Fourth, it would also be valuable to complement lesion and inactivation studies with physiological studies investigating whether there is differential *c-fos* or *Arc* activation in the hippocampus during this task, and if it is possible to identify neural representations of cued recall using ensemble single-unit recording. The latter would be a formidable undertaking but a valuable one, as it might reveal anticipatory components of place-specific unit firing driven by the task demands in which a flavor cue evokes a memory of a place. This would be a logical extension of the concepts of prospective and retrospective coding introduced by Ferbinteanu and Shapiro (2003).

Storage of Spatial/Contextual Information Outside the Hippocampus?

An important milestone in the understanding of spatial cognition was the discovery that most pyramidal cells in the hippocampus exhibit location-specific activity and that the activity of such place cells is influenced by the training history of the animal (see Chapter 11). The predominantly spatial nature of hippocampal neuronal activity led to the proposal that place cells form a distributed map-like representation of the spatial environment that an animal uses for efficient navigation (O'Keefe and Nadel, 1978). When a rat is exposed to a new environment, pyramidal cells develop distinct firing fields within a few minutes (Hill, 1978; Wilson and McNaughton, 1993b). The place fields then remain stable for weeks or more if the environment is constant (Thompson and Best, 1990; Lever et al., 2002), as predicted if these cells contribute to a particular spatial memory.

It is commonly believed that the development of hippocampal firing patterns, like hippocampal memory, might depend on LTP at hippocampal excitatory synapses. Several studies have investigated the contribution of LTP to spatial firing in hippocampal pyramidal cells. Surprisingly, interventions that abolish hippocampal LTP have only subtle effects on place fields. For example, place-specific firing fields develop normally in rats treated systemically with an NMDA receptor antagonist at a dose that prevents new LTP in the hippocampus (Kentros et al., 1998). Despite blockade of the NMDA receptor, place fields can be maintained between consecutive test sessions in the same environment for at least 1.5 hours. They do, however, show instability across days. Place fields recorded in CA1 in mice with mutations of NMDA receptors in either CA3 or CA1 are somewhat less distinct than in control mice under certain conditions; but in contrast to the pharmacological findings, firing fields remain stable across repeated tests on the same day once they have been established (McHugh et al., 1996; Nakazawa et al., 2002). Similar results were obtained when LTP was blocked by interference with Ca^{2+}/calmodulin-dependent protein kinase II (Rotenberg et al., 1996) or protein kinase A (Rotenberg et al., 1996). However, these interventions did decrease the long-term stability of the place fields, as measured 24 hours after the initial exposure to the environment. Together, these studies suggest that NMDA receptor activation may not be necessary for the development or initial maintenance of place-related activity in hippocampal neurons, although it may contribute to the fine-tuning of place fields and aspects of the long-term stabilization of spatial representations (see Chapter 11). The latter function could involve the neocortex as well as the hippocampus.

The development of place fields during NMDA receptor blockade or other forms of disruption of LTP is consistent with several lines of work suggesting that spatial information can be generated and stored upstream of the hippocampus. First, location-specific firing is already expressed in the superficial layers of the entorhinal cortex (Quirk et al., 1992; Frank et al., 2000; Fyhn et al., 2004; Hafting et al., 2005). The fact that most principal cells in entorhinal cortex exhibit view-independent spatial modulation suggests that, by this stage, a fundamental spatial computation may already have been made. It is also possible, however, that spatial firing in superficial entorhinal neurons depends on spatial input from cells in deep layers, which in turn may rely on associative computations in afferent hippocampal structures. The manner in which entorhinal cells code space remains unclear, but that they do helps to understand why pyramidal cells in CA1 exhibit spatial firing both after selective lesions of the dentate gyrus (McNaughton et al., 1989) and after disconnection of CA1 from CA3 (Brun et al., 2002). In CA3-lesioned animals, CA1 pyramidal neurons receive cortical input only via direct connections from the entorhinal cortex. The presence of place fields in these preparations suggests that direct entorhinal–hippocampal circuitry has significant capacity for transforming weak location-modulated signals from superficial layers of the entorhinal cortex into accurate spatial firing in CA1. Several simple filter mechanisms could accomplish such a transformation. For example, firing rates of perforant path fibers to CA1 could be thresholded by feedforward inhibition, such that only the highest afferent firing rates (i.e., those in the center of the entorhinal place field, are able to drive postsynaptic neurons in the hippocampus. Alternatively, single excitatory postsynaptic potentials (EPSPs) in distal pyramidal cell dendrites of CA1 may often not be sufficient to trigger somatic action potentials in these cells; reliable discharge may require summation of EPSPs (i.e., high afferent firing rates (Golding and Spruston, 1998; Golding et al., 2002).

It is important to note that the computation and storage of positional information outside the hippocampus does not preclude long-term storage of some spatial information (or the indices of such information) in the hippocampus. Indeed, the internal recurrent connectivity of hippocampal area CA3 makes the region highly suitable for storage of just these types of patterned "cartoons," at least for an intermediate period of time and perhaps longer in some cases. Other results suggest that plasticity in associational synapses of CA3 is necessary for successful "snapshot" encoding of spatial information in a manner that later allows recall with partial cues (Nakazawa et al., 2002). Longitudinal axon collaterals in CA3 may be important for successful retrieval of such information, as memory retention may be impaired by a single transversely oriented cut through the dorsal CA3 region of each hippocampus (Steffenach et al., 2002).

A Last Word

It remains to be seen how this and other neurobiological theories of episodic-like memory (Hasselmo et al., 2002; McNaughton et al., 2003; Nakazawa et al., 2004; Buzsaki, 2005; Hasselmo and Howard, 2005) will handle the growing body of data that point to a specific role for the hippocampus in at least aspects of "episodic-like" memory. The approach just described builds on the neuropsychological framework developed in this chapter. It accepts that understanding the neuroanatomical basis of recognizing a previously seen stimulus is an important foundation stone of declarative memory (see Section 13.3) but asserts that there is more to memory than this (as, indeed, declarative memory theory has long recognized). It also accepts that hippocampal cells agree that space is special but argues that they can do more than encode spatial information and calls into question the supposition that allocentric spatial memory is fundamentally different from other forms of associative memory (see Section 13.4). It tries to take on board the somewhat impenetrable developments in contemporary animal learning theory and the progress that has been made in understanding predictable ambiguity (see Section 13.5). Perhaps most difficult of all, it is part of an international effort seeking to integrate functional and mechanistic ideas about rapid, one-trial, context-specific learning. This task requires an exquisite understanding of hippocampal neuroanatomy, including that of the myriad inhibitory interneurons and the local circuits of which they are a part that surely make a major contribution to the information processing "algorithms" computed in the hippocampus. Cell biological approaches will also prove increasingly valuable when

thinking about the problems of trace stabilization and memory consolidation. A major obstacle ahead is understanding better how information is "represented" as patterns of neural activity, and progress in unraveling the physiology of hippocampal neurons will aid in that formidable task (see Chapters 5 and 6). In this research program, a wide range of behavioral tasks with animals will continue to play a key part in unraveling the functions and neural mechanisms of the hippocampal formation. This chapter has drawn on data derived from primate experiments investigating recognition memory and object-in-place memory and from rats running in radial mazes, digging in odorized sand wells for food, or swimming in watermazes; and it has touched on new behavioral techniques to investigate episodic-like memory. It is fitting to acknowledge and celebrate the contribution that laboratory animals have made to this effort (Fig. 13–49, see color insert). Progress is being made in tackling the mysteries of the hippocampal "memory machine." The challenges ahead are as formidable as have been the achievements in characterizing its role in memory over the past three decades.

Figure 13–49. Examples of common behavioral tasks used to study hippocampal function in animals. *A.* Classic Wisconsin General Testing Apparatus for macaque monkeys. *B.* Screen shot of modern "touchscreen" display. *C.* Radial maze foraging task for rats, shown with doors. *D.* Rat making a choice in a two-pot olfactory discrimination task. Only one odor is familiar or may be cued by another odor in a paired-associate manner.

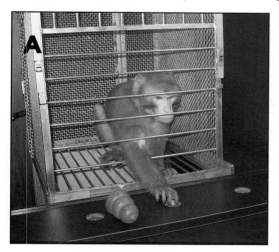
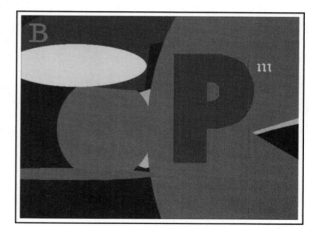
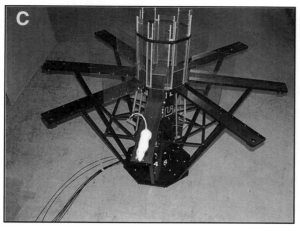
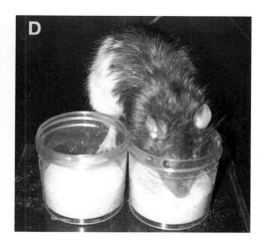

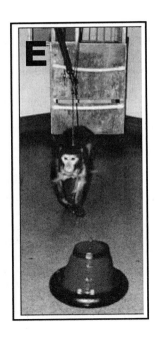

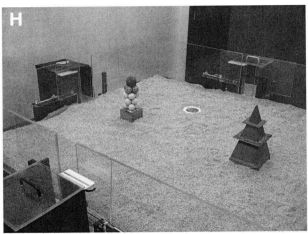

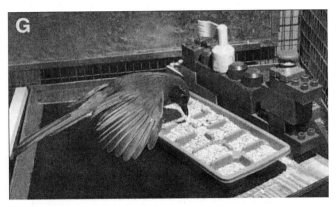

Figure 13–49. *(Continued)* *E.* Foraging monkey exploring objects in a laboratory. *F.* Watermaze. Rat swimming in a large 2-m pool trying to find a hidden escape platform under the water surface (just visible on the right). *Inset* (below). The rat is on the platform, rearing and working out his location. *G.* Scrub-jay in an episodic-like "what-where-when" memory task in which it caches various foods in an ice-cube tray and then retrieves them selectively later. *H.* Paired-associate event arena task for rats. Different foods are found at specific locations (e.g., one shown) in the apparatus.

ACKNOWLEDGMENTS

I am grateful to many people for their help in preparing this chapter. In addition to my co-editors of this book, Mark Baxter (Oxford University) read a draft of the entire manuscript and offered numerous comments and criticisms. Tobias Bast, Stephen Martin (University of Edinburgh and other members of the Laboratory for Cognitive Neuroscience), Edvard Moser and May-Britt Moser (Center for the Biology of Memory, Trondheim), and Craig Stark (Johns Hopkins) also read large parts and directed me to additional literature. I am grateful to Helen Knight, Marie Pezze, and Carolyn Smith for collecting material for and assisting with many of the figures. I am also grateful to many neuroscience colleagues around the world who provided material for the figures or advice of other kinds (including Jamie Ainge, Verner Bingman, Norbert Fortin, John Guzowski, Lucia Jacobs, Len Jarrard, Kazu Nakazawa, and Simon Rempel). Patrick Spoooner helped with many aspects of the computing. I apologize to yet others who helped but whom I have not mentioned. Finally, one institution should not be forgotten. I am eternally grateful to the UK Medical Research Council without whose support throughout my career this work would not have been possible.

REFERENCES

Abel T, Lattal KM (2001) Molecular mechanisms of memory acquisition, consolidation and retrieval. *Curr Opin Neurobiol* 11:180–187.

Adams CD, Dickinson A (1981) Instrumental responding following reinforcer devaluation. *Q J Exp Psychol* 33B:109–122.

Adolphs R (2003) Cognitive neuroscience of human social behaviour. *Nat Rev Neurosci* 4:165–178.

Aggleton JP (1985) One-trial object recognition by rats. *Q J Exp Psychol* 37B:279–294.

Aggleton JP (1999) Mapping recognition memory in the primate brain: why it's sometimes right to be wrong. *Brain Res Bull* 50:447–448.

Aggleton JP, Brown MW (1999) Episodic memory, amnesia, and the hippocampal-anterior thalamic axis. *Behav Brain Sci* 22: 425–489.

Aggleton JP, Pearce JM (2001) Neural systems underlying episodic memory: insights from animal research. *Philos Trans R Soc Lond B Biol Sci* 356:1467–1482.

Aggleton JP, Shaw C (1996) Amnesia and recognition memory: a re-analysis of psychometric data. *Neuropsychologia* 34:51–62.

Aggleton JP, Vann SD (2004) Testing the importance of the retrosplenial navigation system: lesion size but not strain matters: a reply to Harker and Whishaw. *Neurosci Biobehav Rev* 28:525–531.

Aggleton JP, Hunt PR, Rawlins JN (1986) The effects of hippocampal lesions upon spatial and non-spatial tests of working memory. *Behav Brain Res* 19:133–146.

Agster KL, Fortin NJ, Eichenbaum H (2002) The hippocampus and disambiguation of overlapping sequences. *J Neurosci* 22: 5760–5768.

Aiba A, Chen C, Herrup K, Rosenmund C, Stevens CF, Tonegawa S (1994) Reduced hippocampal long-term potentiation and context-specific deficit in associative learning in mGluR1 mutant mice. *Cell* 79:365–375.

Alvarado MC, Rudy JW (1995a) A comparison of kainic acid plus colchicine and ibotenic acid-induced hippocampal formation damage on four configural tasks in rats. *Behav Neurosci* 109:1052–1062.

Alvarado MC, Rudy JW (1995b) Rats with damage to the hippocampal-formation are impaired on the tranverse-patterning problem but not on elemental discriminations. *Behav Neurosci* 109:204–211.

Alvarez-Royo P, Zola-Morgan S, Squire LR (1992) Impairment of long-term memory and sparing of short-term memory in monkeys with medial temporal lobe lesions: a response to Ringo. *Behav Brain Res* 52:1–5.

Alvarez P, Zola-Morgan S, Squire LR (1994) The animal model of human amnesia: long-term memory impaired and short-term memory intact. *Proc Natl Acad Sci USA* 91:5637–5641.

Alvarez P, Zola-Morgan S, Squire LR (1995) Damage limited to the hippocampal region produces long-lasting memory impairment in monkeys. *J Neurosci* 15:3796–3807.

Alyan S, McNaughton BL (1999) Hippocampectomized rats are capable of homing by path integration. *Behav Neurosci* 113:19-31.

Amaral DG (1990) Neurons, numbers and the hippocampal network. *Prog Brain Res* 83:1–11.

Amaral DG, Witter MP (1989) The three-dimensional organization of the hippocampal formation: a review of anatomical data. *Neuroscience* 31:571–591.

Amaral DG, Insausti R, Cowan WM (1987) The entorhinal cortex of the monkey. I. Cytoarchitectonic organization. *J Comp Neurol* 264:326–355.

Anagnostaras SG, Maren S, Fanselow MS (1999) Temporally graded retrograde amnesia of contextual fear after hippocampal damage in rats: within-subjects examination. *J Neurosci* 19:1106–1114.

Anagnostaras SG, Gale GD, Fanselow MS (2001) Hippocampus and contextual fear conditioning: recent controversies and advances. *Hippocampus* 11:8–17.

Anagnostaras SG, Gale GD, Fanselow MS (2002) The hippocampus and pavlovian fear conditioning: reply to Bast et al. *Hippocampus* 12:561–565.

Andersen P, Bliss TVP, Skrede KK (1971) Lamellar organization of hippocampal excitatory pathways. *Exp Brain Res* 13:222–238.

Andersen P, Soleng AF, Raastad M (2000) The hippocampal lamella hypothesis revisited. *Brain Res* 886:165–171.

Andersson M, Krebs JR (1978) On the evolution of hoarding behaviour. *Anim Behav* 26:707–711.

Angeli SJ, Murray EA, Mishkin M (1993) Hippocampetized monkeys can remember one place but not two. *Neuropsychologia* 31:1021–1030.

Archer J, Birke L (1983) *Exploration in animals and humans*. London: Van Nostrand Reinhold.

Attwell PJ, Rahman S, Yeo CH (2001) Acquisition of eyeblink conditioning is critically dependent on normal function in cerebellar cortical lobule HVI. *J Neurosci* 21:5715–5722.

Bachevalier J, Brickson M, Hagger C (1993) Limbic-dependent recognition memory in monkeys develops early in infancy. *Neuroreport* 4:77–80.

Bachevalier J, Nemanic S, Alvarado MC (2002) The medial temporal lobe structures and object recognition memory in nonhuman primates. In: *Neuropsychology of memory*, 3rd ed. (Squire LR, Schacter DL, eds), pp 326–339. New York: Guildford Press.

Bachevalier J, Vargha-Khadem F (2005) The primate hippocampus: ontogeny, early insult and memory. *Curr Opin Neurobiol* 15:168–174.

Baddeley A (2001) The concept of episodic memory. *Philos Trans R Soc Lond B Biol Sci* 356:1345–1350.

Baddeley A, Conway M, Aggleton JP (2002) *Episodic memory: new directions in research*. Oxford, UK: Oxford University Press.

Balda RP, Kamil AC (1989) A comparative study of cache recovery by three corvid species. *Anim Behav* 38:486–495.

Balsam PD, Tomie A (1985) *Context and learning*. Hillsdale, NJ: Erlbaum.

Bannerman DM, Yee BK, Good MA, Heupel MJ, Iversen SD, Rawlins JN (1999) Double dissociation of function within the hippocampus: a comparison of dorsal, ventral, and complete hippocampal cytotoxic lesions. *Behav Neurosci* 113:1170–1188.

Bannerman DM, Yee BK, Lemaire M, Wilbrecht L, Jarrard L, Iversen SD, Rawlins JN, Good MA (2001) The role of the entorhinal cortex in two forms of spatial learning and memory. *Exp Brain Res* 141:281–303.

Bannerman DM, Deacon RM, Offen S, Friswell J, Grubb M, Rawlins JN (2002) Double dissociation of function within the hippocampus: spatial memory and hyponeophagia. *Behav Neurosci* 116:884–901.

Bannerman DM, Rawlins JN, McHugh SB, Deacon RM, Yee BK, Bast T, Zhang WN, Pothuizen HH, Feldon J (2004) Regional dissociations within the hippocampus—memory and anxiety. *Neurosci Biobehav Rev* 28:273–283.

Barnea A, Nottebohm F (1994) Seasonal recruitment of hippocampal neurons in adult free-ranging black-capped chickadees. *Proc Natl Acad Sci USA* 91:11217–11221.

Barnes CA (1979) Memory deficits associated with senescence: a neurophysiological and behavioral study in the rat. *J Comp Physiol Psychol* 93:74–104.

Barnes CA (1988) Spatial learning and memory processes: the search for their neurobiological mechanisms in the rat. *Trends Neurosci* 11:163–169.

Bartlett FC (1932) *Remembering*. Cambridge, UK: Cambridge University Press.

Barton RA, Harvey PH (2000) Mosaic evolution of brain structure in mammals. *Nature* 405:1055–1058.

Bast T, Zhang WN, Feldon J (2001) Hippocampus and classical fear conditioning. *Hippocampus* 11:828–831.

Bast T, da Silva BM, Morris RGM (2005) Distinct contributions of hippocampal NMDA and AMPA receptors to encoding and retrieval of one-trial place memory. *J Neurosci* 25:5845–5856.

Baxter MG, Murray EA (2001a) Effects of hippocampal lesions on delayed nonmatching-to-sample in monkeys: a reply to Zola and Squire (2001). *Hippocampus* 11:201–203.

Baxter MG, Murray EA (2001b) Opposite relationship of hippocampal and rhinal cortex damage to delayed nonmatching-to-sample deficits in monkeys. *Hippocampus* 11:61–71.

Bayley PJ, Frascino JC, Squire LR (2005a) Robust habit learning in the absence of awareness and independent of the medial temporal lobe. *Nature* 436:550–553.

Bayley PJ, Gold JJ, Hopkins RO, Squire LR (2005b) The neuroanatomy of remote memory. *Neuron* 46:799–810.

Bear MF, Connors BW, Paradiso MA (2001) *Neuroscience: exploring the brain.* Philadelphia: Lippincott.

Beason-Held LL, Rosene DL, Killiany RJ, Moss MB (1999) Hippocampal formation lesions produce memory impairment in the rhesus monkey. *Hippocampus* 9:562–574.

Beggs J, Brown T, Byrne J, Crow T, LeDoux J, LeBar K, Thompson R (1999) Learning and memory: basic mechanisms. In: *Fundamental neuroscience,* pp 1411–1454. London: Academic Press.

Behrmann M, Geng JJ, Shomstein S (2004) Parietal cortex and attention. *Curr Opin Neurobiol* 14:212–217.

Benhamou S (1997) On systems of reference involved in spatial memory. *Behav Processes* 40:149–163.

Bennett AT (1996) Do animals have cognitive maps? *J Exp Biol* 199 (Pt 1):219–224.

Berger TW, Rinaldi PC, Weisz DJ, Thompson RF (1983) Single-unit analysis of different hippocampal cell types during classical conditioning of rabbit nictitating membrane response. *J Neurophysiol* 50:1197–1219.

Berlyne DE (1950) Novelty and curiousity as determinants of exploratory behavior. *Br J Psychol* 41:68–80.

Berlyne DE (1966) Curiosity and exploration. *Science* 153:25–33.

Bernasconi-Guastalla S, Wolfer DP, Lipp HP (1994) Hippocampal mossy fibers and swimming navigation in mice: correlations with size and left-right asymmetries. *Hippocampus* 4:53–63.

Biegler R (2000) Possible uses of path integration in animal navigation. *Anim Learn Behav* 28:257–277.

Biegler R (2003) Reading cognitive and other maps: how to avoid getting buried in thought. In: *The neurobiology of spatial behaviour* (Jeffery KJ, ed), pp 259–274. New York: Oxford University Press.

Biegler R, Morris RGM (1993) Landmark stability is a prerequisite for spatial but not discrimination learning. *Nature* 361:631–633.

Biegler R, Morris RGM (1999) Blocking in the spatial domain with arrays of discrete landmarks. *J Exp Psychol Anim Behav Process* 25:334–351.

Biegler R, McGregor A, Krebs JR, Healy SD (2001) A larger hippocampus is associated with longer-lasting spatial memory. *Proc Natl Acad Sci USA* 98:6941–6944.

Bingman VP, Jones TJ (1994) Sun compass-based spatial learning impaired in homing pigeons with hippocampal lesions. *J Neurosci* 14:6687–6694.

Bingman VP, Bagnoli P, Ioale P, Casini G (1984) Homing behavior of pigeons after telencephalic ablations. *Brain Behav Evol* 24:94–108.

Bingman VP, Ioale P, Casini G, Bagnoli P (1987) Impaired retention of preoperatively acquired spatial reference memory in homing pigeons following hippocampal ablation. *Behav Brain Res* 24:147–156.

Bingman VP, Hough GE 2nd, Kahn MC, Siegel JJ (2003) The homing pigeon hippocampus and space: in search of adaptive specialization. *Brain Behav Evol* 62:117–127.

Bliss TVP, Collingridge GL (1993) A synaptic model of memory: long-term potentiation in the hippocampus. *Nature* 361:31–39.

Bliss TVP, Collingridge GL, Morris RGM (2004) *Long term potentiation: enhancing neuroscience for 30 years.* Oxford, UK: Oxford University Press.

Bolhuis JJ, Macphail EM (2001) A critique of the neuroecology of learning and memory. *Trends Cogn Sci* 5:426–433.

Bolhuis JJ, Stewart CA, Forrest EM (1994) Retrograde amnesia and memory reactivation in rats with ibotenate lesions to the hippocampus or subiculum. *Q J Exp Psychol B* 47:129–150.

Bolles RC (1970) Species-specific defense reactions and avoidance learning. *Psychol Rev* 77:32–48.

Bontempi B, Laurent-Demir C, Destrade C, Jaffard R (1999) Time-dependent reorganization of brain circuitry underlying long-term memory storage. *Nature* 400:671–675.

Bostock E, Muller RU, Kubie JL (1991) Experience-dependent modifications of hippocampal place cell firing. *Hippocampus* 1:193–205.

Bouton ME (2004) Context and behavioral processes in extinction. *Learn Mem* 11:485–494.

Bouton ME, Moody EW (2004) Memory processes in classical conditioning. *Neurosci Biobehav Rev* 28:663–674.

Brandeis R, Brandys Y, Yehuda S (1989) The use of the Morris watermaze in the study of memory and learning. *Int J Neurosci* 48:29–69.

Bransford JD (1979) *Human cognition: learning, understanding and remembering.* Belmont, CA: Wadsworth.

Bransford JD, Johnson MK (1972) Contextual prerequisites for understanding: some investigations of comprehension and recall. *J Verb Learn Verb Behav* 11:717–726.

Brasted PJ, Bussey TJ, Murray EA, Wise SP (2002) Fornix transection impairs conditional visuomotor learning in tasks involving nonspatially differentiated responses. *J Neurophysiol* 87:631–633.

Broadbent NJ, Gallagher S, Colombo M (1999) Hippocampal lesions and negative patterning in pigeons. *Psychobiology* 27:51–56.

Broadbent NJ, Squire LR, Clark RE (2004) Spatial memory, recognition memory, and the hippocampus. *Proc Natl Acad Sci USA* 101:14515–14520.

Brown MF (1992) Does a cognitive map guide choices in the radial-arm maze? *J Exp Psychol Anim Behav Process* 21:147–156.

Brown MF, Rish PA, Von Culin JE, Edberg JA (1993) Spatial guidance of choice behavior in the radial arm maze. *J Exp Psychol Anim Behav Process* 19:195–214.

Brown MW (1996) Neuronal responses and recognition memory. *Semin Neurosci* 8:23–32.

Brown MW, Aggleton JP (2001) Recognition memory: what are the roles of the perirhinal cortex and hippocampus? *Nat Rev Neurosci* 2:51–61.

Brown MW, Xiang J-Z (1998) Recognition memory: neuronal substrates of the judgement of prior occurrence. *Prog Neurobiol* 55:149–189.

Brown MW, Wilson FAW, Riches IP (1987) Neuronal evidence that inferomedial temporal cortex is more important than hippocampus in certain processes underlying recognition memory. *Brain Res* 409:158–162.

Browning PG, Easton A, Buckley MJ, Gaffan D (2005) The role of prefrontal cortex in object-in-place learning in monkeys. *Eur J Neurosci* 22:3281–3291.

Brun VH, Otnass MK, Molden S, Steffenach HA, Witter MP, Moser MB, Moser EI (2002) Place cells and place recognition maintained by direct entorhinal-hippocampal circuitry. *Science* 296:2243–2246.

Buckley MJ, Gaffan D (1998a) Perirhinal cortex ablation impairs visual object identification. *J Neurosci* 18:2268–2275.

Buckley MJ, Gaffan D (1998b) Learning and transfer of object-reward associations and the role of the perirhinal cortex. *Behav Neurosci* 112:15–23.

Buckmaster CA, Eichenbaum H, Amaral DG, Suzuki WA, Rapp PR (2004) Entorhinal cortex lesions disrupt the relational organization of memory in monkeys. *J Neurosci* 24:9811–9825.

Buffalo EA, Reber PJ, Squire LR (1998a) The human perirhinal cortex and recognition memory. *Hippocampus* 8:330–339.

Buffalo EA, Stefanacci L, Squire LR, Zola SM (1998b) A reexamination of the concurrent discrimination learning task: the importance of anterior inferotemporal cortex, area TE. *Behav Neurosci* 112:3–14.

Bunsey M, Eichenbaum H (1995) Selective damage to the hippocampal region blocks long-term retention of a natural and nonspatial stimulus-stimulus association. *Hippocampus* 5:546–556.

Bunsey M, Eichenbaum H (1996) Conservation of hippocampal memory function in rats and humans. *Nature* 379:255–257.

Bures J, Fenton AA, Kaminsky Y, Wesierska M, Zahalka A (1998) Rodent navigation after dissociation of the allocentric and idiothetic representations of space. *Neuropharmacology* 37:689–699.

Burgess N, Maguire EA, O'Keefe J (2002) The human hippocampus and spatial and episodic memory. *Neuron* 35:625–641.

Bussey TJ, Clea Warburton E, Aggleton JP, Muir JL (1998) Fornix lesions can facilitate acquisition of the transverse patterning task: a challenge for "configural" theories of hippocampal function. *J Neurosci* 18:1622–1631.

Bussey TJ, Muir JL, Aggleton JP (1999) Functionally dissociating aspects of event memory: the effects of combined perirhinal and postrhinal cortex lesions on object and place memory in the rat. *J Neurosci* 19:495–502.

Bussey TJ, Dias R, Redhead ES, Pearse JM, Muir JL, Aggleton JP (2000) Intact negative patterning in rats with fornix or combined perirhinal and postrhinal cortex lesions. *Exp Brain Res* 134:506–519.

Bussey TJ, Saksida LM, Murray EA (2002) Perirhinal cortex resolves feature ambiguity in complex visual discriminations. *Eur J Neurosci* 15:365–374.

Bussey TJ, Saksida LM, Murray EA (2003) Impairments in visual discrimination after perirhinal cortex lesions: testing 'declarative' vs. 'perceptual-mnemonic' views of perirhinal cortex function. *Eur J Neurosci* 17:649–660.

Buzsaki G (2005) Theta rhythm of navigation: link between path integration and landmark navigation, episodic and semantic memory. *Hippocampus* 15:827–840.

Cahill L, McGaugh JL (1996) Modulation of memory storage. *Curr Opin Neurobiol* 6:237–242.

Capaldi EJ (1971) Memory and learning: a sequential view. In: *Animal memory* (Honig WK, James PHR, eds), pp 111–154. San Diego: Academic Press.

Cassaday HJ, Rawlins JN (1995) Fornix-fimbria section and working memory deficits in rats: stimulus complexity and stimulus size. *Behav Neurosci* 109:594–606.

Cassaday HJ, Rawlins JN (1997) The hippocampus, objects, and their contexts. *Behav Neurosci* 111:1228–1244.

Cavaco S, Anderson SW, Allen JS, Castro-Caldas A, Damasio H (2004) The scope of preserved procedural memory in amnesia. *Brain* 127:1853–1867.

Chamizo VD (2002) Spatial learning: conditions and basic effects. *Psicologica* 23:33–57.

Chamizo VD (2003) Acquisition of knowledge about spatial location: assessing the generality of the mechanism of learning. *Q J Exp Psychol B* 56:102–113.

Chamizo VD, Sterio D, Mackintosh NJ (1985) Blocking and overshadowing between intra-maze and extra-maze cues: a test of the independence of locale and guidance learning. *Q J Exp Psychol* 37B:235–263.

Chan KH, Morell JR, Jarrard LE, Davidson TL (2001) Reconsideration of the role of the hippocampus in learned inhibition. *Behav Brain Res* 119:111–130.

Charles DP, Gaffan D, Buckley MJ (2004a) Impaired recency judgments and intact novelty judgments after fornix transection in monkeys. *J Neurosci* 24:2037–2044.

Charles DP, Browning PG, Gaffan D (2004b) Entorhinal cortex contributes to object-in-place scene memory. *Eur J Neurosci* 20:3157–3164.

Cheng K (1986) A purely geometric module in the rat's spatial representation. *Cognition* 23:149–178.

Cho YH, Beracochea D, Jaffard R (1993) Extended temporal gradi-ent for the retrograde and anterograde amnesia produced by ibotenate entorhinal cortex lesions in mice. *J Neurosci* 13:1759–1766.

Cho YH, Kesner RP, Brodale S (1995) Retrograde and anterograde amnesia for spatial discrimination in rats: role of hippocampus, entorhinal cortex, and parietal cortex. *Psychobiology* 23: 185–194.

Cipolotti L, Shallice T, Chan D, Fox N, Scahill R, Harrison G, Stevens J, Rudge P (2001) Long-term retrograde amnesia...the crucial role of the hippocampus. *Neuropsychologia* 39:151–172.

Cirillo RA, Horel JA, George PJ (1989) Lesions of the anterior temporal stem and the performance of delayed match-to-sample and visual discriminations in monkeys. *Behav Brain Res* 34:55–69.

Claparede E (1911) Recognition et moite. *Arch Psychol Geneva* 11:79–90.

Clark GA, McCormick DA, Lavond DG, Thompson RF (1984) Effects of lesions of cerebellar nuclei on conditioned behavioral and hippocampal neuronal responses. *Brain Res* 291:125–136.

Clark RE, Martin SJ (2005) Interrogating rodents regarding their object and spatial memory. *Curr Opin Neurobiol* 15:593–598.

Clark RE, Squire LR (1998) Classical conditioning and brain systems: the role of awareness. *Science* 280:77–81.

Clark RE, Zola SM, Squire LR (2000) Impaired recognition memory in rats after damage to the hippocampus. *J Neurosci* 20: 8853–8860.

Clark RE, West AN, Zola SM, Squire LR (2001) Rats with lesions of the hippocampus are impaired on the delayed nonmatching-to-sample task. *Hippocampus* 11:176–186.

Clark RE, Broadbent NJ, Squire LR (2004) Hippocampus and remote spatial memory in rats. *Hippocampus* 15:260–272.

Clark RE, Broadbent NJ, Squire LR (2005a) Impaired remote spatial memory after hippocampal lesions despite extensive training beginning early in life. *Hippocampus* 15:340–346.

Clark RE, Broadbent NJ, Squire LR (2005b) Hippocampus and remote spatial memory in rats. *Hippocampus* 15:260–272.

Clayton NS (1995) Development of memory and the hippocampus: comparison of food-storing and nonstoring birds on a one-trial associative memory task. *J Neurosci* 15:2796–2807.

Clayton NS, Dickinson A (1998) Episodic-like memory during cache recovery by scrub jays. *Nature* 395:272–274.

Clayton NS, Krebs JR (1995) Memory in food-storing birds: from behaviour to brain. *Curr Opin Neurobiol* 5:149–154.

Clayton NS, Griffiths DP, Emery N, Dickinson A (2001) Elements of episodic-like memory in animals. In: *Episodic memory: new directions in research* (Baddeley A, Conway M, Aggleton JP, eds), pp 232–248. Oxford, UK: Oxford University Press.

Clayton NS, Yu KS, Dickinson A (2003a) Interacting cache memories: evidence for flexible memory use by Western scrub-jays (Aphelocoma californica). *J Exp Psychol Anim Behav Process* 29:14–22.

Clayton NS, Bussey TJ, Emery NJ, Dickinson A (2003b) Prometheus to Proust: the case for behavioural criteria for 'mental time travel.' *Trends Cogn Sci* 7:436–437.

Cohen NJ, Eichenbaum HE (1993) *Memory, amnesia and the hippocampal system*, 1st ed. Cambridge, MA: MIT Press.

Cohen NJ, Squire LR (1980) Preserved learning and retention of pattern-analyzing skill in amnesia: dissociation of knowing how and knowing that. *Science* 210:207–210.

Cohen NJ, Ryan J, Hunt C, Romine L, Wszalek T, Nash C (1999) Hippocampal system and declarative (relational) memory: summarizing the data from functional neuroimaging studies. *Hippocampus* 9:83–98.

Collett TS (1992) Landmark learning and guidance in insects. *Philos Trans R Lond B* 337:295–303.

Collett TS, Cartwright BA, Smith BA (1986) Landmark learning and visuo-spatial memories in gerbils. *J Comp Psychol A* 158:835–851.

Collins AM, Quillian MR (1969) Retrieval time from semantic memory. *J Verbal Learn Verbal Behav* 8:240–247.

Columbo M, Cawley S, Broadbent NJ (1997) The effects of hippocampal and area parahippocampalis lesions in pigeons. II. Concurrent discrimination and spatial memory. *Q J Exp Psychol* 50B:172–189.

Conference B (1997) Mutant mice and neuroscience: recommendations concerning genetic background; Banbury conference on genetic background in mice. *Neuron* 19:755–759.

Consortium RGSP (2004) Genome sequence of the brown Norway rat yields insights into mammalian evolution. *Nature* 428:493–521.

Cooper BG, Mizumori SJ (2001) Temporary inactivation of the retrosplenial cortex causes a transient reorganization of spatial coding in the hippocampus. *J Neurosci* 21:3986–4001.

Corcoran KA, Maren S (2001) Hippocampal inactivation disrupts contextual retrieval of fear memory after extinction. *J Neurosci* 21:1720–1726.

Corcoran KA, Maren S (2004) Factors regulating the effects of hippocampal inactivation on renewal of conditional fear after extinction. *Learn Mem* 11:598–603.

Corcoran KA, Desmond TJ, Frey KA, Maren S (2005) Hippocampal inactivation disrupts the acquisition and contextual encoding of fear extinction. *J Neurosci* 25:8978–8987.

Corkin S (1984) Lasting consequences of bilateral medial temporal lobectomy: clinical course and experimental findings in H.M. *Semin Neurol* 4:249–259.

Cowey A, Stoerig P (1995) Blindsight in monkeys. *Nature* 373:247–249.

Crabbe JC, Morris RGM (2004) Festina lente: late-night thoughts on high-throughput screening of mouse behavior. *Nat Neurosci* 7:1175–1179.

Crusio WE, Schwegler H, Lipp HP (1987) Radial-maze performance and structural variation of the hippocampus in mice: a correlation with mossy fibre distribution. *Brain Res* 425:182–185.

Dale N, Roberts A (1985) Dual-component amino-acid-mediated synaptic potentials: excitatory drive for swimming in Xenopus embryos. *J Physiol* 363:35–59.

Davidson TL (1993) The nature and function of interoceptive signals to feed: toward integration of physiological and learning perspectives. *Psychol Rev* 100:640–657.

Davidson TL, Jarrard LE (1993) A role for hippocampus in the utilization of hunger signals. *Behav Neural Biol* 59:167–171.

Davidson TL, Jarrard LE (2004) The hippocampus and inhibitory learning: a 'gray' area? *Neurosci Biobehav Rev* 28:261–271.

Davidson TL, McKernan MG, Jarrard LE (1993) Hippocampal lesions do not impair negative patterning: a challenge to configural association theory. *Behav Neurosci* 107:227-234.

Davis M, Falls WA, Campeau S, Kim M (1993) Fear-potentiated startle: a neural and pharmacological analysis. *Behav Brain Res* 58:175-198.

Day M, Langston RF, Morris RGM (2003) Glutamate receptor dependent encoding and retrieval of paired associate learning. *Nature* 424:205-209.

Deacon RM, Bannerman DM, Rawlins NP (2001) Conditional discriminations based on external and internal cues in rats with cytotoxic hippocampal lesions. *Behav Neurosci* 115:43–57.

Dean P, Weiskrantz L (1974) Loss of preoperative habits in rhesus monkeys with inferotemporal lesions: recognition failure or relearning deficit? *Neuropsychologia* 12:299–311.

De Hoz L, Knox J, Morris RGM (2003) Longitudinal axis of the hippocampus: both septal and temporal poles of the hippocampus support watermaze spatial learning depending on the training protocol. *Hippocampus* 13:587–603.

De Hoz L, Martin SJ, Morris RGM (2004) Forgetting, reminding, and remembering: the retrieval of lost spatial memory. *PLoS Biol* 2:E225.

De Kloet ER, Oitzl MS, Joels M (1999) Stress and cognition: are corticosteroids good or bad guys? *Trends Neurosci* 22:422–426.

D'Hooge R, De Deyn PP (2001) Applications of the Morris watermaze in the study of learning and memory. *Brain Res Brain Res Rev* 36:60–90.

Dickinson A (1980) *Contemporary animal learning theory*. Cambridge: Cambridge University Press.

Dickinson A, Mackintosh NJ (1978) Classical conditioning in animals. *Annu Rev Psychol* 29:587–612.

DiMattia BV, Kesner RP (1988a) Role of the posterior parietal association cortex in the processing of spatial event information. *Behav Neurosci* 102:397–403.

Dix SL, Aggleton JP (1999) Extending the spontaneous preference test of recognition: evidence of object-location and object-context recognition. *Behav Brain Res* 99:191–200.

Dore FY, Thornton JA, White NM, Murray EA (1998) Selective hippocampal lesions yield nonspatial memory impairments in rhesus monkeys. *Hippocampus* 8:323–329.

Douglas RJ, Martin KA (2004) Neuronal circuits of the neocortex. *Annu Rev Neurosci* 27:419–451.

Dragunow M (1996) A role for immediate-early transcription factors in learning and memory. *Behav Genet* 26:293–299.

Dudai Y, Morris RGM (2001) To consolidate or not to consolidate: what are the questions? In: *Brain, perception and memory: advances in cognitive sciences* (Bolhuis J, ed), pp 147–162. Oxford, UK: Oxford University Press.

Dudchenko PA (2003) The head-direction system and navigation. In: *The neurobiology of spatial behaviour* (Jeffery K, ed). Oxford, UK: Oxford University Press.

Dudchenko PA, Taube JS (1997) Correlation between head direction cell activity and spatial behavior on a radial arm maze. *Behav Neurosci* 111:3–19.

Dudchenko PA, Wood ER, Eichenbaum H (2000) Neurotoxic hippocampal lesions have no effect on odor span and little effect on odor recognition memory but produce significant impairments on spatial span, recognition, and alternation. *J Neurosci* 20:2964–2977.

Dusek JA, Eichenbaum H (1997) The hippocampus and memory for orderly stimulus relations. *Proc Natl Acad Sci USA* 94:7109–7114.

Dyer F (1998) Cognitive ecology of navigation. In: *Cognitive ecology* (Dukas R, ed), pp 201–260. Chicago: University of Chicago Press.

Eacott MJ, Gaffan EA (2005) The roles of perirhinal cortex, postrhinal cortex, and the fornix in memory for objects, contexts, and events in the rat. *Q J Exp Psychol B* 58:202–217.

Eacott MJ, Norman G (2004) Integrated memory for object, place, and context in rats: a possible model of episodic-like memory? *J Neurosci* 24:1948–1953.

Eacott MJ, Easton A, Zinkivskay A (2005) Recollection in an episodic-like memory task in the rat. *Learn Mem* 12:221–223.

Easton A, Gaffan D (2000) Comparison of perirhinal cortex ablation and crossed unilateral lesions of the medial forebrain bundle from the inferior temporal cortex in the rhesus monkey: effects on learning and retrieval. *Behav Neurosci* 114:1041–1057.

Easton A, Parker A, Gaffan D (2001) Crossed unilateral lesions of medial forebrain bundle and either inferior temporal or frontal cortex impair object recognition memory in rhesus monkeys. *Behav Brain Res* 121:1–10.

Eichenbaum H (1996) Is the rodent hippocampus just for "place"? *Curr Opin Neurobiol* 6:187–195.

Eichenbaum H (2004) Hippocampus: cognitive processes and neural representations that underlie declarative memory. *Neuron* 44:109–120.

Eichenbaum H, Cohen NJ (2001) *From conditioning to conscious recollection.* New York: Oxford University Press.

Eichenbaum H, Stewart C, Morris RGM (1990) Hippocampal representation in place learning. *J Neurosci* 10:3531–3542.

Eichenbaum H, Dudchenko P, Wood E, Shapiro M, Tanila H (1999) The hippocampus, memory, and place cells: is it spatial memory or a memory space? *Neuron* 23:209–226.

Ekstrom AD, Kahana MJ, Caplan JB, Fields TA, Isham EA, Newman EL, Fried I (2003) Cellular networks underlying human spatial navigation. *Nature* 425:184–188.

Emery NJ, Clayton NS (2001) Effects of experience and social context on prospective caching strategies by scrub jays. *Nature* 414:443–446.

Emery NJ, Clayton NS (2004) The mentality of crows: convergent evolution of intelligence in corvids and apes. *Science* 306:1903–1907.

Ennaceur A, Aggleton JP (1994) Spontaneous recognition of object configurations in rats: effects of fornix lesions. *Exp Brain Res* 100:85–92.

Ennaceur A, Delacour J (1988) A new one-trial test for neurobiological studies of memory in rats. 1. Behavioral data. *Behav Brain Res* 31:47–59.

Etienne AS, Jeffery KJ (2004) Path integration in mammals. *Hippocampus* 14:180–192.

Etienne AS, Maurer R, Berlie J, Reverdin B, Rowe T, Georgakopoulos J, Seguinot V (1998) Navigation through vector addition. *Nature* 396:161–164.

Fanselow MS (1990) Factors governing one-trial contextual conditioning. *Anim Learn Behav* 18:264–270.

Fanselow MS (2000) Contextual fear, gestalt memories and the hippocampus. *Behav Brain Res* 110:73–81.

Fantz RL (1964) Visual experience in infants: decreased attention to familiar patterns relative to novel ones. *Science* 146:668–670.

Farah MJ (2004) *Visual agnosia.* Cambridge, MA: MIT Press.

Ferbinteanu J, Shapiro ML (2003) Prospective and retrospective memory coding in the hippocampus. *Neuron* 40:1227–1239.

Finger S, Koehler PJ, Jagella C (2004) The Monakow concept of diaschisis: origins and perspectives. *Arch Neurol* 61:283–288.

Fletcher PC, Henson RN (2001) Frontal lobes and human memory: insights from functional neuroimaging. *Brain* 124:849–881.

Fortin NJ, Agster KL, Eichenbaum HB (2002) Critical role of the hippocampus in memory for sequences of events. *Nat Neurosci* 5:458–462.

Fortin NJ, Wright SP, Eichenbaum H (2004) Recollection-like memory retrieval in rats is dependent on the hippocampus. *Nature* 431:188–191.

Forwood SE, Winters BD, Bussey TJ (2005) Hippocampal lesions that abolish spatial maze performance spare object recognition memory at delays of up to 48 hours. *Hippocampus* 15:347–355.

Foster TC, Castro CA, McNaughton BL (1989) Spatial selectivity of rat hippocampal neurons: dependence on preparedness for movement. *Science* 244:1580–1582.

Fox GD, Holland PC (1998) Neurotoxic hippocampal lesions fail to impair reinstatement of an appetitively conditioned response. *Behav Neurosci* 112:255–260.

Frank LM, Brown EN, Wilson M (2000) Trajectory encoding in the hippocampus and entorhinal cortex. *Neuron* 27:169–178.

Frank MJ, Rudy JW, O'Reilly RC (2003) Transitivity, flexibility, conjunctive representations and the hippocampus. II. A computational analysis. *Hippocampus* 13:299–312.

Frankland PW, Bontempi B (2005) The organization of recent and remote memories. *Nat Rev Neurosci* 6:119–130.

Frankland PW, Cestari V, Filipkowski RK, McDonald RJ, Silva AJ (1998) The dorsal hippocampus is essential for context discrimination but not for contextual conditioning. *Behav Neurosci* 112:863–874.

Frankland PW, O'Brien C, Ohno M, Kirkwood A, Silva AJ (2001) Alpha-CaMKII-dependent plasticity in the cortex is required for permanent memory. *Nature* 411:309–313.

Frankland PW, Bontempi B, Talton LE, Kaczmarek L, Silva AJ (2004) The involvement of the anterior cingulate cortex in remote contextual fear memory. *Science* 304:881–883.

Frey U, Morris RGM (1997) Synaptic tagging and long-term potentiation. *Nature* 385:533–536.

Frey U, Morris RGM (1998) Synaptic tagging: implications for late maintenance of hippocampal long-term potentiation. *Trends Neurosci* 21:181–188.

Fried I, Wilson CL, MacDonald KA, Behnke EJ (1998) Electric current stimulates laughter. *Nature* 391:650.

Friston KJ (1995) Functional and effective connectivity in neuroimaging: A synthesis. *Hum Brain Mapp* 2:56–78.

Friston KJ (2004) Models of brain function in neuroimaging. *Annu Rev Psychol* 56:57–87.

Fritz J, Mishkin M, Saunders RC (2005) In search of an auditory engram. *Proc Natl Acad Sci USA* 102:9359–9364.

Frohardt RJ, Guarraci FA, Bouton ME (2000) The effects of neurotoxic hippocampal lesions on two effects of context after fear extinction. *Behav Neurosci* 114:227–240.

Fukuda M, Kobayashi T, Bures J, Ono T (1992) Rat exploratory behavior controlled by intracranial self-stimulation improves the study of place cell activity. *J Neurosci Methods* 44:121–131.

Fyhn M, Molden S, Hollup SA, Moser M-B, Moser EI (2002) Hippocampal neurons responding to first-time dislocation of a target object. *Neuron* 35:555–566.

Fyhn M, Molden S, Witter MP, Moser EI, Moser MB (2004) Spatial representation in the entorhinal cortex. *Science* 305:1258–1264.

Gabrieli JDE, Fleischman DA, Deane MM, Reminger SL, Morrell F (1995) Double dissociation between memory systems underlying explicit and implicit memory in the human brain. *Psychol Sci* 6:76–82.

Gaffan D (1974) Recognition impaired and association intact in the memory of monkeys after transection of the fornix. *J Comp Physiol Psychol* 86:1100–1109.

Gaffan D (1983) Animal amnesia: some disconnection syndromes? In: *Neurobiology of the hippocampus* (Seifert W, ed), pp 513–528. London: Academic Press.

Gaffan D (1991) Spatial organization of episodic memory. *Hippocampus* 1:262–264.

Gaffan D (1992) Amnesia for complex naturalistic scenes and for objects following fornix transection in the rhesus monkey. *Eur J Neurosci* 4:381–388.

Gaffan D (1993) Additive effects of forgetting and fornix transection in the temporal gradient of retrograde amnesia. *Neuropsychologia* 31:1055–1066.

Gaffan D (1994) Scene-specific memory for objects: a model of episodic memory impairment in monkeys with fornix transection. *J Cogn Neurosci* 6:305–320.

Gaffan D (2002) Against memory systems. *Philos Trans R Soc Lond B Biol Sci* 357:1111–1121.

Gaffan EA, Eacott MJ (1995) A computer-controlled maze environment for testing visual memory in the rat. *J Neurosci Methods* 60:23–37.

Gaffan D, Harrison S (1989) Place memory and scene memory: effects of fornix transection in the monkey. *Exp Brain Res* 74:202–212.

Gaffan D, Parker A (1996) Interaction of perirhinal cortex with the fornix-fimbria: memory for objects and "object-in-place" memory. *J Neurosci* 16:5864–5869.

Gaffan D, Gaffan EA, Harrison S (1984) Effects of fornix transection on spontaneous and trained non-matching by monkeys. *Q J Exp Psychol* 36B:285–303.

Gagliardo A, Ioale P, Bingman VP (1999) Homing in pigeons: the role of the hippocampal formation in the representation of landmarks used for navigation. *J Neurosci* 19:311–315.

Gagliardo A, Ioale P, Odetti F, Kahn MC, Bingman VP (2004) Hippocampal lesions do not disrupt navigational map retention in homing pigeons under conditions when map acquisition is hippocampal dependent. *Behav Brain Res* 153:35–42.

Galea LA, McEwen BS (1999) Sex and seasonal differences in the rate of cell proliferation in the dentate gyrus of adult wild meadow voles. *Neuroscience* 89:955–964.

Galef BG (1990) Necessary and sufficient conditions for communication of diet preferences by Norway rats. *Anim Learn Behav* 18:347–351.

Galef BG, Wigmore SW (1983) Transfer of information concerning distant foods: a laboratory investigation of the information-centre hypothesis. *Anim Behav* 31:748–758.

Gallagher M, Holland PC (1992) Preserved configural learning and spatial learning impairment in rats with hippocampal damage. *Hippocampus* 2:81–88.

Gallagher M, Rapp PR (1997) The use of animal models to study the effects of aging on cognition. *Annu Rev Psychol* 48:339–370.

Gallistel C (1980) *The organisation of action: a new synthesis.* Hillsdale, NJ: Erlbaum.

Garrud P, Rawlins JN, Mackintosh NJ, Goodall G, Cotton MM, Feldon J (1984) Successful overshadowing and blocking in hippocampectomized rats. *Behav Brain Res* 12:39–53.

Gattis M (2001) *Spatial schemas and abstract thought.* Cambridge, MA: MIT Press.

Gaulin SJ, Fitzgerald RW (1989) Sexual selection for spatial-learning ability. *Anim Behav* 37:322–331.

Gaulin SJ, FitzGerald RW, Wartell MS (1990) Sex differences in spatial ability and activity in two vole species (Microtus ochrogaster and M. pennsylvanicus). *J Comp Psychol* 104:88–93.

Gazzaniga MS (2002) *Cognitive neuroscience: the biology of the mind.* New York: Norton.

Gerlai R (1996) Gene-targeting studies of mammalian behavior: is it the mutation or the background genotype? *Trends Neurosci* 19:177–181.

Gewirtz JC, McNish KA, Davis M (2000) Is the hippocampus necessary for contextual fear conditioning? *Behav Brain Res* 110:83–95.

Gilbert P, Kesner R, DeCoteau R (1998) Memory for spatial location: role of the hippocampus in mediating spatial pattern separation. *J Neurosci* 18:804–810.

Gilbert PE, Kesner RP, Lee I (2001) Dissociating hippocampal subregions: double dissociation between dentate gyrus and CA1. *Hippocampus* 11:626–636.

Gisquet-Verrier P, Dutrieux G, Richer P, Doyere V (1999) Effects of lesions to the hippocampus on contextual fear: evidence for a disruption of freezing and avoidance behavior but not context-conditioning. *Behav Neurosci* 113:507–522.

Gladwell M (2002) *The tipping point: how little things can make a big difference.* Boston: Back Bay Books.

Goelet P, Castellucci VF, Schacher S, Kandel ER (1986) The long and the short of long-term memory—a molecular framework. *Nature* 322:419–422.

Golding NL, Spruston N (1998) Dendritic sodium spikes are variable triggers of axonal action potentials in hippocampal CA1 pyramidal neurons. *Neuron* 21:1189–1200.

Golding NL, Staff NP, Spruston N (2002) Dendritic spikes as a mechanism for cooperative long-term potentiation. *Nature* 418:326–331.

Golob EJ, Taube JS (2002) Differences between appetitive and aversive reinforcement on reorientation in a spatial working memory task. *Behav Brain Res* 136:309–316.

Good M, Honey RC (1991) Conditioning and contextual retrieval in hippocampal rats. *Behav Neurosci* 105:499–509.

Good M, de Hoz L, Morris RGM (1998) Contingent versus incidental context processing during conditioning: dissociation after excitotoxic hippocampal plus dentate gyrus lesions. *Hippocampus* 8:147–159.

Good MA, Morris RGM (1994) A step linking memory to understanding? *Behav Brain Sci* 17:477–479.

Gothard KM, Skaggs WE, Moore KM, McNaughton BL (1996) Binding of hippocampal CA1 neural activity to multiple reference frames in a landmark-based navigation task. *J Neurosci* 16:823–835.

Gould SJ, Eldredge N (1977) Punctuated equilibria: the tempo and mode of evolution reconsidered. *Paleobiology* 3:115–151.

Graf P, Schacter DL (1985) Implicit and explicit memory for new associations in normal and amnesic subjects. *J Exp Psychol Learn Mem Cogn* 11:501–518.

Graf P, Squire LR, Mandler G (1984) The information that amnesic patients do not forget. *J Exp Psychol* 10:164–178.

Graham KS, Simons JS, Pratt KH, Patterson K, Hodges JR (2000) Insights from semantic dementia on the relationship between episodic and semantic memory. *Neuropsychologia* 38:313–324.

Grant SG, O'dell TJ, Karl KA, Stein PL, Soriano P, Kandel ER (1992) Impaired long-term potentiation, spatial learning, and hippocampal development in fyn mutant mice. *Science* 258:1903–1910.

Gray JA (1982) *The neuropsychology of anxiety: an enquiry into the functions of the septo-hippocampal system.* Oxford, UK: Oxford University Press.

Gray JA (2000) *The neuropsychology of anxiety: an enquiry into the functions of the septo-hippocampal system,* 2nd ed. Oxford: Oxford University Press.

Gregory RL (1961) The brain as an engineering problem. In: *Current problems in animal behaviour* (Thorpe WH, Zangwill OL, eds). Cambridge, UK: Cambridge University Press.

Griffiths D, Dickinson A, Clayton N (1999) Episodic memory: what can animals remember about their past? *Trends Cogn Sci* 3:74–80.

Grillner S, Ekeberg, El Manira A, Lansner A, Parker D, Tegnér J, Wallén P (1998) Intrinsic function of a neuronal network—a vertebrate central pattern generator. *Brain Res Brain Res Rev* 26:184–197.

Guillot PV, Roubertoux PL, Crusio WE (1994) Hippocampal mossy fiber distributions and intermale aggression in seven inbred mouse strains. *Brain Res* 660:167–169.

Guzowski JF (2002) Insights into immediate-early gene function in hippocampal memory consolidation using antisense oligonucleotide and fluorescent imaging approaches. *Hippocampus* 12:86–104.

Guzowski JF, McNaughton BL, Barnes CA, Worley PF (1999) Environment-specific expression of the immediate-early gene Arc in hippocampal neuronal ensembles. *Nat Neurosci* 2:1120–1124.

Guzowski JF, Setlow B, Wagner EK, McGaugh JL (2001) Experience-dependent gene expression in the rat hippocampus after spatial learning: a comparison of the immediate-early genes Arc, c-fos, and zif268. *J Neurosci* 21:5089–5098.

Hafting T, Fyhn M, Molden S, Moser MB, Moser EI (2005) Microstructure of a spatial map in the entorhinal cortex. *Nature* 436:801–806.

Hagan JJ, Salamone JD, Simpson J, Iversen SD, Morris RG (1988) Place navigation in rats is impaired by lesions of medial septum and diagonal band but not nucleus basalis magnocellularis. *Behav Brain Res* 27:9–20.

Hall G, Purves D, Bonardi C (1996) Contextual control of conditioned responding in rats with dorsal hippocampal lesions. *Behav Neurosci* 110:933–945.

Halliday MS (1968) Exploratory behaviour. In: *Analysis of behavioural change* (Weiskrantz L, ed), pp 107–126. New York: Harper & Row.

Hamann SB, Squire LR (1997) Intact perceptual memory in the absence of conscious memory. *Behav Neurosci* 111:850–854.

Hampton RR (2001) Rhesus monkeys know when they remember. *Proc Natl Acad Sci USA* 98:5359–5362.

Hampton RR, Schwartz BL (2004) Episodic memory in nonhumans: what, and where, is when? *Curr Opin Neurobiol* 14:192–197.

Hampton RR, Shettleworth SJ (1996) Hippocampal lesions impair memory for location but not color in passerine birds. *Behav Neurosci* 110:831–835.

Hampton RR, Healy SD, Shettleworth SJ, Kamil AC (2002) Neuroecologists' are not made of straw. *Trends Cogn Sci* 6: 6–7.

Hardiman MJ, Ramnani N, Yeo CH (1996) Reversible inactivities of the cerebellum with muscimol prevent the acquisition and extinction of conditioned nictitating membrane responses in the rabbit. *Exp Brain Res* 110:235–247.

Harker KT, Whishaw IQ (2004) A reaffirmation of the retrosplenial contribution to rodent navigation: reviewing the influences of lesion, strain, and task. *Neurosci Biobehav Rev* 28:485–496.

Hartley T, Burgess N, Lever C, Cacucci F, O'Keefe J (2000) Modeling place fields in terms of the cortical inputs to the hippocampus. *Hippocampus* 10:369–379.

Hasselmo ME, Howard E (2005) Hippocampal mechanisms for the context-dependent retrieval of episodes. *Neural Netw* 18:1172–1190.

Hasselmo ME, Bodelon C, Wyble BP (2002) A proposed function for hippocampal theta rhythm: separate phases of encoding and retrieval enhance reversal of prior learning. *Neural Comput* 14:793–817.

Hauser MD (2003) Knowing about knowing: dissociations between perception and action systems over evolution and during development. *Ann N Y Acad Sci* 1001:79–103.

Healy SD (1998) *Spatial representations in animals.* New York: Oxford University Press.

Healy SI, Braithwaite II (2000) Cognitive ecology: a field of substance? *Trends Ecol Evol* 15:22–26.

Hebb DO (1949) *The organization of behaviour.* New York: Wiley.

Hebben N, Corkin S, Eichenbaum H, Shedlack K (1985) Diminished ability to interpret and report internal states after bilat-eral medial temporal resection: case H.M. *Behav Neurosci* 99:1031–1039.

Henke K, Buck A, Weber B, Wieser HG (1997) Human hippocampus establishes associations in memory. *Hippocampus* 7:249–256.

Herrera DG, Robertson HA (1996) Activation of c-fos in the brain. *Prog Neurobiol* 50:83–107.

Hess US, Lynch G, Gall CM (1995) Regional patterns of c-fos mRNA expression in rat hippocampus following exploration of a novel environment versus performance of a well-learned discrimination. *J Neurosci* 15:7796–7809.

Hill AJ (1978) First occurrence of hippocampal spatial firing in a new environment. *Exp Neurol* 62:282–297.

Hirsh R (1974) The hippocampus and contextual retrieval of information from memory: a theory. *Behav Biol* 12:421–444.

Hok V, Save E, Lenck-Santini PP, Poucet B (2005) Coding for spatial goals in the prelimbic/infralimbic area of the rat frontal cortex. *Proc Natl Acad Sci USA* 102:4602–4607.

Holland PC, Fox GD (2003) Effects of hippocampal lesions in overshadowing and blocking procedures. *Behav Neurosci* 117:650–656.

Holland PC, Lamoroureux JA, Han JS, Gallagher M (1999) Hippocampal lesions interfere with negative occasion-setting. *Hippocampus* 9:143–157.

Hollup SA, Kjelstrup KG, Hoff J, Moser MB, Moser EI (2001) Impaired recognition of the goal location during spatial navigation in rats with hippocampal lesions. *J Neurosci* 21:4505–4513.

Honey RC, Good M (1993) Selective hippocampal lesions abolish the contextual specificity of latent inhibition and of conditioning. *Behav Neurosci* 107:22–33.

Honey RC, Watt A, Good M (1998) Hippocampal lesions disrupt an associative mismatch process. *J Neurosci* 18:2226–2230.

Honig WK (1978) Studies of working memory in the pigeon. In: *Cognitive aspects of animal behavior* (Hulse SH, Fowler HF, Honig WK, eds), pp 211–248. Hillside, NJ: Erlbaum.

Horel JA (1978) The neuroanatomy of amnesia: a critique of the hippocampal memory hypothesis. *Brain* 101:403–445.

Horel JA (1994) Some comments on the special cognitive functions claimed for the hippocampus. *Cortex* 30:269–280.

Insausti R, Amaral DG, Cowan WM (1987a) The entorhinal cortex of the monkey. III. Subcortical afferents. *J Comp Neurol* 264:396–408.

Insausti R, Amaral DG, Cowan WM (1987b) The entorhinal cortex of the monkey. II. Cortical afferents. *J Comp Neurol* 264:356–395.

Ioale P, Gagliardo A, Bingman VP (2000) Hippocampal participation in navigational map learning in young homing pigeons is dependent on training experience. *Eur J Neurosci* 12:742–750.

Iversen SD (1976) Do hippocampal lesions produce amnesia in animals? *Int Rev Neurobiol* 19:1–49.

Jacobs LF (1995) The ecology of spatial cognition. In: *Behavioural brain research in naturalistic and semi-naturalistic settings* (Alleva E, ed), pp 301–322. Boston: Kluwer Academic.

Jacobs LF (2003) The evolution of the cognitive map. *Brain Behav Evol* 62:128–139.

Jacobs LF, Schenk F (2003) Unpacking the cognitive map: the parallel map theory of hippocampal function. *Psychol Rev* 110:285–315.

Jacobs LF, Spencer WD (1994) Natural space-use patterns and hippocampal size in kangaroo rats. *Brain Behav Evol* 44:125–132.

Jacobs LF, Gaulin SJ, Sherry DF, Hoffman GE (1990) Evolution of spatial cognition: sex-specific patterns of spatial behavior predict hippocampal size. *Proc Natl Acad Sci USA* 87:6349–6352.

James W (1890) *The principles of psychology*, 1918 ed. New York: Dover.

Jarrard LE (1978) Selective hippocampal lesions: differential effects on performance by rats of a spatial task with preoperative versus postoperative training. *J Comp Physiol Psychol* 92:1119–1127.

Jarrard LE (1986) Selective hippocampal lesions and behavior: implications for current research and theorizing. In: *The hippocampus* (Isaacson RL, Pribram KH, eds), pp 93–126. New York: Plenum.

Jarrard LE (1989) On the use of ibotenic acid to lesion selectively different components of the hippocampal formation. *J Neurosci Methods* 29:251–259.

Jarvis ED, Gunturkun O, Bruce L, Csillag A, Karten H, Kuenzel W, Medina L, Paxinos G, Perkel DJ, Shimizu T, Striedter G, Wild JM, Ball GF, Dugas-Ford J, Durand SE, Hough GE, Husband S, Kubikova L, Lee DW, Mello CV, Powers A, Siang C, Smulders TV, Wada K, White SA, Yamamoto K, Yu J, Reiner A, Butler AB (2005) Avian brains and a new understanding of vertebrate brain evolution. *Nat Rev Neurosci* 6:151–159.

Jeffery KJ (2003) *The neurobiology of spatial behaviour*. New York: Oxford University Press.

Jeffery KJ, Anderson MI, Hayman R, Chakraborty S (2004) A proposed architecture for the neural representation of spatial context. *Neurosci Biobehav Rev* 28:201–218.

Jenkins TA, Amin E, Pearce JM, Brown MW, Aggleton JP (2004) Novel spatial arrangements of familiar visual stimuli promote activity in the rat hippocampal formation but not the parahippocampal cortices: a c-fos expression study. *Neuroscience* 124:43–52.

Jensen O, Lisman JE (1996) Theta/gamma networks with slow NMDA channels learn sequences and encode episodic memory: role of NMDA channels in recall. *Learn Mem* 3:2264–278.

Jung MW, Wiener SI, McNaughton BL (1994) Comparison of spatial firing characteristics of units in dorsal and ventral hippocampus of the rat. *J Neurosci* 14:7347–7356.

Kamin LJ (1968) Attention-like processes in classical conditioning. In: *Miami symposium on the prediction of behavior: aversive stimulation* (Jones MR, ed), pp 9–33. Miami: University of Miami Press.

Kaminski J, Call J, Fischer J (2004) Word learning in a domestic dog: evidence for "fast mapping." *Science* 304:1682–1683.

Kandel ER, Schwartz JH, Jessell TM (2000) *Principles of neural science*. New York: McGraw-Hill.

Kao YC, Davis ES, Gabrieli JD (2005) Neural correlates of actual and predicted memory formation. *Nat Neurosci* 8:1776–1783.

Kapur N, Brooks DJ (1999) Temporally-specific retrograde amnesia in two cases of discrete bilateral hippocampal pathology. *Hippocampus* 9:247–254.

Kay RF, Ross C, Blythe A, Williams BA (1997) Anthropoid origins. *Science* 275:797–804.

Kelsey BA, Landry JE (1988) Medial septal lesions disrupt spatial mapping ability in rats. *Behav Neurosci* 102:289–293.

Kempermann G, Brandon EP, Gage FH (1998) Environmental stimulation of 129/SvJ mice causes increased cell proliferation and neurogenesis in the adult dentate gyrus. *Curr Biol* 8:939–942.

Kennedy PJ, Shapiro ML (2004) Retrieving memories via internal context requires the hippocampus. *J Neurosci* 24:6979–6985.

Kentros C, Hargreaves E, Hawkins RD, Kandel ER, Shapiro M, Muller RV (1998) Abolition of long-term stability of new hippocampal place cell maps by NMDA receptor blockade. *Science* 280:2121–2126.

Kesner RP (1998) Neurobiological views of memory. In: *Neurobiology of learning and memory* (Martinez JL, Kesner RP, eds), pp 361–416. San Diego: Academic Press.

Kesner RP (2000) Behavioral analysis of the contribution of the hippocampus and parietal cortex to the processing of information: interactions and dissociations. *Hippocampus* 10:483–490.

Kesner RP, Bolland BL, Dakis M (1993) Memory for spatial locations, motor responses, and objects: triple dissociation among the hippocampus, caudate nucleus, and extrastriate visual cortex. *Exp Brain Res* 93:462–470.

Kiernan MJ, Westbrook RF (1993) Effects of exposure to a to-be-shocked environment upon the rat's freezing response: evidence for facilitation, latent inhibition and perceptual learning. *Q J Exp Psychol* 46B:271–288.

Kim JJ, Fanselow MS (1992) Modality-specific retrograde amnesia of fear. *Science* 256:675–677.

Kimble DP (1968) Hippocampus and internal inhibition. *Psychol Bull* 70:285–295.

Kjelstrup KG, Tuvnes FA, Steffenach HA, Murison R, Moser EI, Moser MB (2002) Reduced fear expression after lesions of the ventral hippocampus. *Proc Natl Acad Sci USA* 99:10825–10830.

Knowlton BJ, Squire LR (1993) The learning of categories: parallel brain systems for item memory and category knowledge. *Science* 262:1747–1749.

Knuttinen MG, Power JM, Preston AR, Disterhoft JF (2001) Awareness in classical differential eyeblink conditioning in young and aging humans. *Behav Neurosci* 115:747–757.

Kowalska DM, Kusmierek P, Kosmal A, Mishkin M (2001) Neither perirhinal/entorhinal nor hippocampal lesions impair short-term auditory recognition memory in dogs. *Neuroscience* 104:965–978.

Krebs JR, Sherry DF, Healy SD, Perry VH, Vaccarino AL (1989) Hippocampal specialization of food-storing birds. *Proc Natl Acad Sci USA* 86:1388–1392.

Krupa DJ, Thompson JK, Thompson RF (1993) Localization of a memory trace in the mammalian brain. *Science* 260:989–991.

Kumaran D, Maguire EA (2005) The human hippocampus: cognitive maps or relational memory? *J Neurosci* 25:7254–7259.

LaBar KS, Disterhof JF (1998) Conditioning, awareness, and the hippocampus. *Hippocampus* 8:620–626.

Lashley KS (1950) In search of the engram. In: *Symposia for the Society for Experimental Biology*, pp 454–482. New York: Cambridge University Press.

Lavenex P, Steele MA, Jacobs LF (2000) Sex differences, but no seasonal variations in the hippocampus of food-caching squirrels: a stereological study. *J Comp Neurol* 425:152–166.

LeDoux JE (2000) Emotion circuits in the brain. *Annu Rev Neurosci* 23:155–184.

Lee AC, Bussey TJ, Murray EA, Saksida LM, Epstein RA, Kapur N, Hodges JR, Graham KS (2005) Perceptual deficits in amnesia: challenging the medial temporal lobe 'mnemonic' view. *Neuropsychologia* 43:1–11.

Lee DW, Miyasato LE, Clayton NS (1998) Neurobiological bases of spatial learning in the natural environment: neurogenesis and growth in the avian and mammalian hippocampus. *Neuroreport* 9:R15–27.

Lee DW, Smith GT, Tramontin AD, Soma KK, Brenowitz EA, Clayton NS (2001) Hippocampal volume does not change seasonally in a non food-storing songbird. *Neuroreport* 12:1925-1928.

Lee I, Kesner RP (2004) Differential contributions of dorsal hippocampal subregions to memory acquisition and retrieval in contextual fear-conditioning. Hippocampus 14:301–310.

Lenck-Santini PP, Save E, Poucet B (2001) Evidence for a relationship between place-cell spatial firing and spatial memory performance. *Hippocampus* 11:377–390.

Lenck-Santini PP, Muller RU, Save E, Poucet B (2002) Relationships between place cell firing fields and navigational decisions by rats. *J Neurosci* 22:9035–9047.

Leonard BW, Amaral DG, Squire LR, Zola-Morgan S (1995) Transient memory impairment in monkeys with bilateral lesions of the entorhinal cortex. *J Neurosci* 15:5637–5659.

Leutgeb S, Leutgeb JK, Treves A, Moser MB, Moser EI (2004) Distinct ensemble codes in hippocampal areas CA3 and CA1. *Science* 305:1295–1298.

Lever C, Wills T, Cacucci F, Burgess N, O'Keefe J (2002) Long-term plasticity in hippocampal place-cell representation of environmental geometry. *Nature* 416:90–94.

Levy DA, Stark CE, Squire LR (2004) Intact conceptual priming in the absence of declarative memory. *Psychol Sci* 15:680–686.

Levy WB (1996) A sequence predicting CA3 is a flexible associator that learns and uses context to solve hippocampal-like tasks. *Hippocampus* 6:579–590.

Lindner MD, Plone MA, Schallert T, Emerich DF (1997) Blind rats are not profoundly impaired in the reference memory Morris watermaze and cannot be clearly discriminated from rats with cognitive deficits in the cued platform task. *Brain Res Cogn Brain Res* 5:329–333.

Link W, Konietzko U, Kauselmann G, Krug M, Schwanke B, Frey U, Kuhl D (1995) Somatodendritic expression of an immediate early gene is regulated by synaptic activity. *Proc Natl Acad Sci USA* 92:5734–5738.

Lipp HP, Wolfer DP (1998) Genetically modified mice and cognition. *Curr Opin Neurobiol* 8:272–280.

Lipp HP, Schwegler H, Heimrich B, Driscoll P (1988) Infrapyramidal mossy fibers and two-way avoidance learning: developmental modification of hippocampal circuitry and adult behavior of rats and mice. *J Neurosci* 8:1905–1921.

Lipp HP, Collins RL, Hausheer-Zarmakupi Z, Leisinger-Trigona MC, Crusio WE, Nosten-Bertrand M, Signore P, Schwegler H, Wolfer DP (1996) Paw preference and intra/infrapyramidal mossy fibers in the hippocampus of the mouse. *Behav Genet* 26:379–390.

Lipp HP, Amrein I, Slominanka L, Wolfer DP (1999) Natural genetic variation of hippocampal structures and behavior. In: *Cellular and quantitative methods in neurogenetics: methods in life sciences* (Jones BC, Mormede P, eds), pp 217–235. Boca Raton, FL: CRC Press.

Lipp HP, Vyssotski AL, Wolfer DP, Renaudineau S, Savini M, Troster G, Dell'Omo G (2004) Pigeon homing along highways and exits. *Curr Biol* 14:1239–1249.

Lisman JE, Zhabotinsky AM (2001) A model of synaptic memory: a Ca MKII/PP1 switch that potentiates transmission by organizing an AMPA receptor anchoring assembly. *Neuron* 31:191–201.

Lyford GL, Yamagata K, Kaufmann WE, Barnes CA, Sanders LK, Copeland NG, Gilbert DJ, Jenkins NA, Lanahan AA, Worley PF (1995) Arc, a growth factor and activity-regulated gene, encodes a novel cytoskeleton-associated protein that is enriched in neuronal dendrites. *Neuron* 14:433–445.

Lynch G, Deadwyler S, Cotman C (1973) Postlesion axonal rowth produces permanent functional connections. *Science* 180:1364–1366.

Mackintosh NJ (1983) *Conditioning and associative learning.* Oxford, UK: Clarendon Press.

Mackintosh NJ (2002) Do not ask whether they have a cognitive map, but how they find their way about. *Psicologica* 23:165–185.

Macphail EM (1982) *Brain and intelligence in vertebrates.* Oxford, UK: Clarendon Press.

Macphail EM (1998) *The evolution of consciousness.* Oxford, UK: Oxford University Press.

Macphail EM (2002) The role of the avian hippocampus in spatial memory. *Psicologica* 23:93–108.

Macphail EM, Bolhuis JJ (2001) The evolution of intelligence: adaptive specializations versus general process. *Biol Rev Camb Philos Soc* 76:341–364.

Maguire EA (2001) Neuroimaging studies of autobiographical event memory. *Philos Trans R Soc Lond B Biol Sci* 356:1441–1451.

Maguire EA, Burgess N, Donnett JG, Frackowiak RS, Frith CD, O'Keefe J (1998) Knowing where and getting there: a human navigation network. *Science* 280:921–924.

Maguire EA, Frith CD, Morris RGM (1999) The functional neuroanatomy of comprehension and memory: the importance of prior knowledge. *Brain* 122(Pt 10):1839–1850.

Malamut BL, Saunders RC, Mishkin M (1984) Monkeys with combined amygdalo-hippocampal lesions succeed in object discrimination learning despite 24-hour intertrial intervals. *Behav Neurosci* 98:759–769.

Malkova L, Mishkin M (2003) One-trial memory for object-place associations after separate lesions of hippocampus and posterior parahippocampal region in the monkey. *J Neurosci* 23:1956–1965.

Malkova L, Gaffan D, Murray EA (1997) Excitotoxic lesions of the amygdala fail to produce impairment in visual learning for auditory secondary reinforcement but interfere with reinforcer devaluation effects in rhesus monkeys. *J Neurosci* 17:6011–6020.

Malkova L, Lex CK, Mishkin M, Saunders RC (2001) MRI-based evaluation of locus and extent of neurotoxic lesions in monkeys. *Hippocampus* 11:361–370.

Mandler G (1980) Recognizing: the judgement of previous occurrence. *Psychol Rev* 87:252–271.

Manns JR, Clark RE, Squire LR (2000a) Parallel acquisition of awareness and trace eyeblink classical conditioning. *Learn Mem* 7:267–272.

Manns JR, Stark CE, Squire LR (2000b) The visual paired-comparison task as a measure of declarative memory. *Proc Natl Acad Sci USA* 97:12375–12379.

Manns JR, Hopkins RO, Reed JM, Kitchener EG, Squire LR (2003) Recognition memory and the human hippocampus. *Neuron* 37:171–180.

Maravita A, Iriki A (2004) Tools for the body (schema). *Trends Cogn Sci* 8:79–86.

Maren S (2001) Neurobiology of pavlovian fear conditioning. *Annu Rev Neurosci* 24:897–931.

Maren S (2005) Building and burying fear memories in the brain. *Neuroscientist* 11:89–99.

Maren S, Fanselow MS (1997) Electrolytic lesions of the fimbria/fornix, dorsal hippocampus, or entorhinal cortex produce anterograde deficits in contextual fear conditioning in rats. *Neurobiol Learn Mem* 67:142–149.

Maren S, Aharonov G, Fanselow MS (1997) Neurotoxic lesions of the dorsal hippocampus and pavlovian fear conditioning in rats. *Behav Brain Res* 88:261–274.

Margules J, Gallistel CR (1988) Heading in the rat: determination by environmental shape. *Anim Learn Behav* 16:404–410.

Markman EM, Abelev M (2004) Word learning in dogs? *Trends Cogn Sci* 8:479–481.

Marr D (1971) Simple memory: a theory for archicortex. *Philos Trans R Soc Lond B:* 262:23–81.

Martin A, Wiggs C, Weisberg J (1997) Modulation of human medial temporal lobe activity by form, meaning and experience. *Hippocampus* 7:587–593.

Martin SJ, Grimwood PD, Morris RGM (2000) Synaptic plasticity and memory: an evaluation of the hypothesis. *Annu Rev Neurosci* 23:649–711.

Martin SJ, de Hoz L, Morris RGM (2005) Retrograde amnesia: neither partial nor complete hippocampal lesions in rats result in preferential sparing of remote spatial memory, even after reminding. *Neuropsychologia* 43:609–624.

Matsumura N, Nishijo H, Tamura R, Eifuku S, Endo S, Ono T (1999) Spatial- and task-dependent neuronal responses during real and virtual translocation in the monkey hippocampal formation. *J Neurosci* 19:2381–2393.

Maviel T, Durkin TP, Menzaghi F, Bontempi B (2004) Sites of neocortical reorganization critical for remote spatial memory. *Science* 305:96–99.

Mayford M, Bach ME, Huang Y-Y, Wang L, Hawkins R, Kandel ER (1996) Control of memory formation through regulated expression of a CaMKII transgene. *Science* 274:1678–1683.

McCarthy RA, Warrington EA (1990) *Cognitive neuropsychology*. San Diego: Academic Press.

McClelland JL, Goddard NH (1996) Considerations arising from a complementary learning systems perspective on hippocampus and neocortex. *Hippocampus* 6:654–665.

McClelland JL, McNaughton BL, O'Reilly RC (1995) Why there are complementary learning systems in the hippocampus and neocortex: insights from the successes and failures of connectionist models of learning and memory. *Psychol Rev* 102:419–457.

McDonald RJ, White NM (1994) Parallel information processing in the watermaze: evidence for independent memory systems involving dorsal striatum and hippocampus. *Behav Neural Biol* 61:260–270.

McDonald RJ, White NM (1995) Hippocampal and nonhippocampal contributions to place learning in rats. *Behav Neurosci* 109:579–593.

McDonald RJ, Murphy RA, Guarraci FA, Gortler JR, White NM, Baker AG (1997) Systematic comparison of the effects of hippocampal and fornix-fimbria lesions on acquisition of three configural discriminations. *Hippocampus* 7:371–388.

McDonald RJ, Devan BD, Hong NS (2004) Multiple memory systems: the power of interactions. *Neurobiol Learn Mem* 82:333–346.

McEwen B, Sapolsky R (1995) Stress and cognitive function. *Curr Opin Neurobiol* 5:205–212.

McGaugh JL (2000) Memory-a century of consolidation. *Science* 287:258–251.

McGlinchey-Berroth R, Carrillo MC, Gabrieli JDE, Brawn CM, Disterhof JF (1997) Impaired trace eyeblink conditioning in bilateral, medial-temporal lobe amnesia. *Behav Neurosci* 111:873–882.

McGonigle BO, Chalmers M (1977) Are monkeys logical? *Nature* 267:694–696.

McGonigle BO, Chalmers M (2003) The growth of cognitive structures in monkeys and men. In: *Animal cognition and sequential behavior: behavioral, biological and computational perspectives* (Fountain SB, Bunsey MD, Danks JH, McBeath MK, eds). Boston: Kluwer Academic.

McGregor A, Good MA, Pearce JM (2004a) Absence of an interaction between navigational strategies based on local and distal landmarks. *J Exp Psychol Anim Behav Process* 30:34–44.

McGregor A, Hayward AJ, Pearce JM, Good MA (2004b) Hippocampal lesions disrupt navigation based on the shape of the environment. *Behav Neurosci* 118:1011–1021.

McHugh TJ, Blum KI, Tsien JZ, Tonegawa S, Wilson MA (1996) Impaired hippocampal representation of space in CA1-specific NMDAR1 knockout mice. *Cell* 87:1339–1349.

McNaughton BL, Barnes CA (1986) Long-term enhancement of hippocampal synaptic transmission and the acquisition of spatial information. *J Neurosci* 6:563–571.

McNaughton BL, Morris RGM (1987) Hippocampal synaptic enhancement and information storage within a distributed memory system. *TINS* 10:408–415.

McNaughton BL, Barnes CA, Meltzer J, Sutherland RJ (1989) Hippocampal granule cells are necessary for normal spatial learning but not for spatially-selective pyramidal cell discharge. *Exp Brain Res* 76:485–496.

McNaughton BL, Chen LL, Markus EJ (1991) "Dead reckoning," landmark learning, and the sense of direction: a neurophysiological and computational hypothesis. *J Cogn Neurosci* 3:190–202.

McNaughton BL, Barnes CA, Gerrard JL, Gothard K, Jung MW, Knierim JJ, Kudrimoti H, Qin Y, Skaggs WE, Suster M, Weaver KL (1996) Deciphering the hippocampal polyglot: the hippocampus as a path integration system. *J Exp Biol* 199:173–185.

McNaughton BL, Barnes CA, Battaglia FP, Bower MR, Cowen SL, Ekstrom AD, Gerrard JL, Hoffman KL, Houston FP, Karten Y, Lipa P, Pennartz CMA, Sutherland GR (2003) Off-line reprocessing of recent memory and its role in memory consolidation: a progress report. In: *Sleep and synaptic plasticity* (Smith C, Maquet P, eds), pp 225–246. New York: Oxford University Press.

Meunier M, Bachevalier J, Mishkin M, Murray EA (1993) Effects on visual recognition of combined and separate ablations of the entorhinal and perirhinal cortex in rhesus monkeys. *J Neurosci* 13:5418–5432.

Mishkin M (1978) Memory in monkeys severely impaired by combined but not by separate removal of amygdala and hippocampus. *Nature* 273:297–298.

Mishkin M (1982) A memory system in the monkey. *Philos Trans R Soc Lond B Biol Sci* 298:83–95.

Mishkin M, Delacour J (1975) An analysis of short-term visual memory in the monkey. *J Exp Psychol Anim Behav Process* 1:326–334.

Mishkin M, Murray EA (1994) Stimulus recognition. *Curr Opin Neurobiol* 4:200–206.

Mishkin M, Suzuki WA, Gadian DG, Vargha-Khadem F (1997) Hierarchical organization of cognitive memory. *Philos Trans Royal Soc Lond B Biol Sci* 352:1461–1467.

Mishkin M, Vargha-Khadem F, Gadian DG (1998) Amnesia and the organization of the hippocampal system. *Hippocampus* 8:212–216.

Mittelstaedt H, Mittelstaedt M (1982) Homing by path integration. In: *Avian navigation* (Papi F, Wallraff HG, eds), pp 290–297. Heidelberg: Springer-Verlag.

Miyashita Y (2004) Cognitive memory: cellular and network machineries and their top-down control. *Science* 306:435–440.

Mizumori SJ, Miya DY, Ward KE (1994) Reversible inactivation of the lateral dorsal thalamus disrupts hippocampal place representation and impairs spatial learning. *Brain Res* 644:168–174.

Moita MA, Rosis S, Zhou Y, LeDoux JE, Blair HT (2003) Hippocampal place cells acquire location-specific responses to the conditioned stimulus during auditory fear conditioning. *Neuron* 37:485–497.

Morgan DG, Diamond DM, Gottschall PE, Ugen KE, Dickey C, Hardy JD, Duff K, Jantzen P, DiCarlo G, Wilcock D, Connor K, Hatcher J, Hope C, Gordon MN, Arendash GW (2000) A beta peptide vaccination prevents memory loss in an animal model of Alzheimer's disease. *Nature* 482:982–986.

Morgan JI, Cohen DR, Hempstead JL, Curran T (1987) Mapping patterns of c-fos expression in the central nervous system after seizure. *Science* 237:192–197.

Morris RG, Mayes AR (2004) Long-term spatial memory: introduction and guide to the special section. *Neuropsychology* 18:403–404.

Morris RGM (1981) Spatial localisation does not depend on the presence of local cues. *Learn Motiv* 12:239–260.

Morris RGM (1983) Neural subsystems of exploration in rats. In: *Exploration in animals and humans* (Archer J, Birke L, eds), pp 117–146. London: Van Nostrand Reinhold.

Morris RGM (1984) Developments of a watermaze procedure for studying spatial learning in the rat. *J Neurosci Methods* 11:47–60.

Morris RGM (1991) Distinctive computations and relevant associative processes: hippocampal role in processing, retrieval, but not storage of allocentric spatial memory. *Hippocampus* 1:287–290.

Morris RGM (2001) Episodic-like memory in animals: psychological criteria, neural mechanisms and the value of episodic-like tasks to investigate animal models of neurodegenerative disease. *Philos Trans R Soc Lond B Biol Sci* 356:1453–1465.

Morris RGM (2006) Elements of a neurobiological theory of the hippocampus: the role of activity-dependent synaptic plasticity in episodic-like memory. *Eur J Neurosci* 23:2829–2846.

Morris RGM, Frey U (1997) Hippocampal synaptic plasticity: role in spatial learning or the automatic recording of attended experience? *Philos Trans R Soc Lond B Biol Sci* 352:1489–1503.

Morris RGM, Kennedy MB (1992) The pierian spring. *Curr Biol* 2:511–514.

Morris RGM, Garrud P, Rawlins JN, O'Keefe J (1982) Place navigation impaired in rats with hippocampal lesions. *Nature* 297:681–683.

Morris RGM, Hagan JJ, Rawlins JN (1986a) Allocentric spatial learning by hippocampectomised rats: a further test of the "spatial mapping" and "working memory" theories of hippocampal function. *Q J Exp Psychol* B 38:365–395.

Morris RGM, Anderson E, Lynch GS, Baudry M (1986b) Selective impairment of learning and blockade of long-term potentiation by an *N*-methyl-D-aspartate receptor antagonist, AP5. *Nature* 319:774–776.

Morris RGM, Schenk F, Tweedie F, Jarrard LE (1990) Ibotenate lesions of hippocampus and/or subiculum: dissociating components of allocentric spatial learning. *Eur J Neurosci* 2:1016–1028.

Morris RGM, Martin SJ, Moser EI, Riedel G, Sandin J, Day M, O'Carroll C (2003) Elements of a neurobiological theory of the hippocampus: the role of activity-dependent synaptic plasticity in memory. *Philos Trans Roy Soc Lond B* 358:773–786.

Moscovitch M (1995) Recovered consciousness: a hypothesis concerning modularity and episodic memory. *J Clin Exp Neuropsychol* 17:276–290.

Moscovitch M, Nadel L (1998) Consolidation and the hippocampal complex revisited: in defense of the multiple-trace model. *Curr Opin Neurobiol* 8:297–300.

Moser E, Moser MB, Anderson P (1993) Spatial learning impairment parallels the magnitude of dorsal hippocampal lesions, but is hardly present following ventral lesions. *J Neurosci* 13:3916–3925.

Moser EI, Krobert KA, Moser MB, Morris RGM (1998) Impaired spatial learning after saturation of long-term potentiation. *Science* 281:2038–2042.

Moser MB, Moser EI (1998a) Distributed encoding and retrieval of spatial memory in the hippocampus. *J Neurosci* 18:7535–7542.

Moser MB, Moser EI (1998b) Functional differentiation in the hippocampus. *Hippocampus* 8:608–619.

Moser MB, Moser EI, Forrest E, Andersen P, Morris RGM (1995) Spatial learning with a minislab in the dorsal hippocampus. *Proc Natl Acad Sci USA* 92:9697–9701.

Moses SN, Ryan JD (2006) A comparison and evaluation of the predictions of relational and conjunctive accounts of hippocampal function. *Hippocampus* 16:43–65.

Moss M, Mahut H, Zola-Morgan S (1981) Concurrent discrimination learning of monkeys after hippocampal, entorhinal, or fornix lesions. *J Neurosci* 1:227–240.

Moyer JR, Thompson LT, Disterhoft JF (1996) Trace eyeblink conditioning increases CA1 excitability in a transient and learning-specific manner. *J Neurosci* 16:5536–5546.

Moyer JR, Power JM, Thompson LT, Disterhoft JF (2000) Increased excitability of aged rabbit CA1 neurons after trace eyeblink conditioning. *J Neurosci* 20:5476–5482.

Muller R (1996) A quarter of a century of place cells. *Neuron* 17:813–822.

Mumby DG (2001) Perspectives on object-recognition memory following hippocampal damage: lessons from studies in rats. *Behav Brain Res* 127:159–181.

Mumby DG, Pinel JPJ, Wood ER (1990) Nonrecurring-items delayed nonmatching-to-sample in rats: a new paradigm for testing nonspatial working memory. *Psychobiology* 18:321–326.

Mumby DG, Wood ER, Pinel JP (1992a) Object-recognition memory is only mildly impaired in rats with lesions of the hippocampus and amygdala. *Psychobiology* 20:18–27.

Mumby DG, Wood ER, Pinel JPJ (1992b) Object recognition memory in rats is only mildly impaired by lesions of the hippocampus and amygdala. *Psychobiology* 20:18–27.

Mumby DG, Pinel JPJ, Kornecook TJ, Shen MJ, Redila VA (1995) Memory deficits following lesions of hippocampus or amygdala in rats: an assesment by an object-memory tets battery. *Psychobiology* 23:26–36.

Mumby DG, Astur RS, Weisend MP, Sutherland RJ (1999) Retrograde amnesia and selective damage to the hippocampal formation: memory for places and object discriminations. *Behav Brain Res* 106:97–107.

Murray EA, Bussey TJ (1999) Perceptual-mnemonic functions of the perirhinal cortex. *Trends Cogn Sci* 3:142–151.

Murray EA, Bussey TJ (2001) Consolidation and the medial temporal lobe revisited: methodological considerations. *Hippocampus* 11:1–7.

Murray EA, Mishkin M (1983) Severe tactual memory deficits in monkeys after combined removal of the amygdala and hippocampus. *Brain Res* 270:340–344.

Murray EA, Mishkin M (1985) Amygdalectomy impairs crossmodal association in monkeys. *Science* 228:604–605.

Murray EA, Mishkin M (1998) Object recognition and location memory in monkeys with excitotoxic lesions of the amygdala and hippocampus. *J Neurosci* 18:6568–6582.

Murray EA, Wise SP (2004) What, if anything, is the medial temporal lobe, and how can the amygdala be part of it if there is no such thing? *Neurobiol Learn Mem* 82:178–198.

Murray EA, Gaffan D, Mishkin M (1993) Neural substrates of visual stimulus-stimulus association in rhesus monkeys. *J Neurosci* 13:4549–4561.

Murray EA, Baxter MG, Gaffan D (1998) Monkeys with rhinal cortex damage or neurotoxic hippocampal lesions are impaired on spatial scene learning and object reversals. *Behav Neurosci* 112:1291–1303.

Murray EA, Graham KS, Gaffan D (2005) Perirhinal cortex and its neighbours in the medial temporal lobe: contributions to memory and perception. *Q J Exp Psychol* 58:378–396.

Nadel L (1991) The hippocampus and space revisited. *Hippocampus* 1:221–229.

Nadel L (1995) The role of the hippocampus in declarative memory: a comment on Zola-Morgan, Squire, and Ramus (1994). *Hippocampus* 5:232–239.

Nadel L, Bohbot V (2001) Consolidation of memory. *Hippocampus* 11:56–60.

Nadel L, Hardt O (2004) The spatial brain. *Neuropsychology* 18:473–476.

Nadel L, Moscovitch M (1997) Memory consolidation, retrograde amnesia and the hippocampal complex. *Curr Opin Neurobiol* 7:217–227.

Nadel L, Moscovitch M (1998) Hippocampal contributions to cortical plasticity. *Neuropharmacology* 37:431–439.

Nadel L, Willner J (1980) Context and conditioning: a place for space. *Physiol Psychol* 8:218–228.

Nadel L, O'Keefe J, Black AH (1975) Slam on the brakes: a critique of Altman, Brunner and Bayer's response-inhibition model of hippocampal function. *Behav Biol* 14:151–162.

Nadel L, Samsonovich A, Ryan L, Moscovitch M (2000) Multiple trace theory of human memory: computational, neuroimaging, and neuropsychological results. *Hippocampus* 10:352–368.

Nader K (2003) Memory traces unbound. *Trends Neurosci* 26:65–72.

Nakazawa K, Quirk MC, Chitwood RA, Watanabe M, Yeckel MF, Sun LD, Kato A, Carr CA, Johnston D, Wilson MA, Tonegawa S (2002) Requirement for hippocampal CA3 NMDA receptors in associative memory recall. *Science* 297:211–218.

Nakazawa K, Sun LD, Quirk MC, Rondi-Reig L, Wilson MA, Tonegawa S (2003) Hippocampal CA3 NMDA receptors are crucial for memory acquisition of one-time experience. *Neuron* 38:305–315.

Nakazawa K, McHugh TJ, Wilson MA, Tonegawa S (2004) NMDA receptors, place cells and hippocampal spatial memory. *Nat Rev Neurosci* 5:361–372.

Nelson W (1988) Food restriction, circadian disorder and longevity of rats and mice. *J Nutr* 118:286–289.

Nemanic S, Alvarado MC, Bachevalier J (2004) The hippocampal/parahippocampal regions and recognition memory: insights from visual paired comparison versus object-delayed nonmatching in monkeys. *J Neurosci* 24:2013–2026.

Nunn JA, LePeillet E, Netto CA, Hodges H, Gray JA, Meldrum BS (1994) Global ischaemia: hippocampal pathology and spatial deficits in the watermaze. *Behav Brain Res* 62:41–54.

Ogden JA, Corkin S (1991) Memories of H.M. In: *Memory mechanisms: a tribute to G.V. Goddard* (Abraham WC, Corballis M, White KG, eds), pp 195–215. Hillsdale, NJ: Erlbaum,

Ohno M, Frankland PW, Chen AP, Costa RM, Silva AJ (2001) Inducible, pharmacogenetic approaches to the study of learning and memory. *Nat Neurosci* 4:1238–1243.

O'Keefe J (1976) Place units in the hippocampus of the freely moving rat. *Exp Neurol* 51:78–109.

O'Keefe J (1996) The spatial prepositions in English, vector grammar and the cognitive map theory. In: *Language and space* (Bloom P, Peterson MA, Nadel L, Garrett MF, eds), pp 277–316. Cambridge, MA: MIT Press.

O'Keefe J (2005) Vector grammar, places, and the functional role of the spatial prepositions in English. In: *Representing direction in language and space* (van de Zee E, Slack J, eds), pp 69–85. Oxford, UK: Oxford University Press.

O'Keefe J, Burgess N (1996) Geometric determinants of the place fields of hippocampal neurons. *Nature* 381:425–428.

O'Keefe J, Conway DH (1978) Hippocampal place units in the freely moving rat: why they fire where they fire. *Exp Brain Res* 31:573–590.

O'Keefe J, Dostrovsky J (1971) The hippocampus as a spatial map: preliminary evidence from unit activity in the freely-moving rat. *Brain Res* 34:171–175.

O'Keefe J, Nadel L (1978) *The hippocampus as a cognitive map.* Oxford, UK: Clarendon Press.

O'Keefe J, Nadel L (1979) Precis of O'Keefe & Nadel's *The Hippocampus* as a cognitive map. *Behav Brain Sci* 2:487–533.

O'Keefe J, Speakman A (1987) Single unit activity in the rat hippocampus during a spatial memory task. *Exp Brain Res* 68:1–27.

O'Keefe J, Nadel L, Keightley S, Kill D (1975) Fornix lesions selectively abolish place learning in the rat. *Exp Neurol* 48:152–166.

Olton DS (1977) The function of septo-hippocampal connections in spatially organized behaviour. *Ciba Found Symp* 58:327–349.

Olton DS, Papas BC (1979) Spatial memory and hippocampal function. *Neuropsychologia* 17:669–682.

Olton DS, Samuelson RJ (1976) Remembrance of places passed: spatial memory in rats. *J Exp Psychol Anim Behav Process* 2:97–116.

Olton DS, Becker JT, Handelmann GE (1979) Hippocampus, space, and memory. *Brain Behav Sci* 2:313–365.

O'Reilly RC (1998) Six principles for biologically-based computational models of cortical cognition. *Trends Cogn Sci* 2:455–462.

O'Reilly RC, Norman KA (2002) Hippocampal and neocortical contributions to memory: advances in the complementary learning systems framework. *Trends Cogn Sci* 6:505–510.

O'Reilly RC, Rudy JW (2001) Conjunctive representations in learning and memory: principles of cortical and hippocampal function. *Psychol Rev* 108:311–345.

Otto T, Eichenbaum H (1992) Complementary roles of the orbital prefrontal cortex and the perirhinal-entorhinal cortices in an odor-guided delayed-nonmatching-to-sample task. *Behav Neurosci* 106:762–775.

Overman WH, Ormsby G, Mishkin M (1990) Picture recognition vs. picture discrimination learning in monkeys with medial temporal removals. *Exp Brain Res* 79:18–24.

Overton DA (1964) State-dependent or 'dissociation' learning produced with pentobarbital. *J Comp Physiol Psychol* 57:3–12.

Owen MJ, Butler SR (1981) Amnesia after transection of the fornix in monkeys: long-term memory impaired, short-term memory intact. *Behav Brain Res* 3:115–123.

Packard MG, McGaugh JL (1996) Inactivation of hippocampus or caudate nucleus with lidocaine differentially affects expression of place and response learning. *Neurobiol Learn Mem* 65:65–72.

Papadimitriou A, Wynne C (1999) Preserved negative patterning and impaired spatial learning in pigeons (Columba livia) with lesions of the hippocampus. *Behav Neurosci* 113:683–690.

Papi F (1990) Olfactory navigation in birds. *Experientia* 46:352–363.

Papini MR (2002) Pattern and process in the evolution of learning. *Psychol Rev* 109:186–201.

Parkinson JK, Murray EA, Mishkin M (1988) A selective mnemonic role for the hippocampus in monkeys: memory for the location of objects. *J Neurosci* 8:4159–4167.

Parron C, Save E (2004) Comparison of the effects of entorhinal and retrosplenial cortical lesions on habituation, reaction to spatial and non-spatial changes during object exploration in the rat. *Neurobiol Learn Mem* 82:1–11.

Parslow DM, Rose D, Brooks B, Fleminger S, Gray JA, Giampietro V, Brammer MJ, Williams S, Gasston D, Andrew C, Vythelingum GN, Loannou G, Simmons A, Morris RG (2004) Allocentric spatial memory activation of the hippocampal formation measured with fMRI. *Neuropsychology* 18:450–461.

Patel SN, Clayton NS, Krebs JR (1997) Spatial learning induces neurogenesis in the avian brain. *Behav Brain Res* 89:115128.

Paulsen O, Moser EI (1998) A model of hippocampal memory encoding and retrieval: GABAergic control of synaptic plasticity. *Trends Neurosci* 21:273–278.

Pearce JM, Bouton ME (2001) Theories of associative learning in animals. *Annu Rev Psychol* 52:111–139.

Pearce JM, Hall G (1980) A model for pavlovian learning: variations in the effectiveness of conditioned but not of unconditioned stimuli. *Psychol Rev* 87:532–552.

Pearce JM, Roberts AD, Good M (1998) Hippocampal lesions disrupt navigation based on cognitive maps but not heading vectors. *Nature* 396:75–77.

Pearce JM, Good MA, Jones PM, McGregor A (2004) Transfer of spatial behavior between different environments: implications for theories of spatial learning and for the role of the hippocampus in spatial learning. *J Exp Psychol Anim Behav Process* 30:135–147.

Phillips RG, LeDoux JE (1992) Differential contribution of amygdala and hippocampus to cued and contextual for conditioning. *Behav Neurosci* 106:274–285.

Phillips RG, LeDoux JE (1994) Lesions of the dorsal hippocampal formation interfere with background but not foreground contextual fear conditioning. *Learn Mem* 1:34–44.

Pickens CL, Holland PC (2004) Conditioning and cognition. *Neurosci Biobehav Rev* 28:651–661.

Pinker S (1994) *The language instinct.* New York: William Morrow.

Pitkanen A, Pikkarainen M, Nurminen N, Ylinen A (2000) Reciprocal connections between the amygdala and the hippocampal formation, perirhinal cortex, and postrhinal cortex in rat: a review. *Ann N Y Acad Sci* 911:369–391.

Poldrack RA, Clark J, Pare-Blagoev EJ, Shohamy D, Creso Moyano J, Myers C, Gluck MA (2001) Interactive memory systems in the human brain. *Nature* 414:546–550.

Poucet B (1993) Spatial cognitive maps in animals: new hypotheses on their structure and neural mechanisms. *Psychol Rev* 100:163–182.

Poucet B, Benhamou S (1997) The neuropsychology of spatial cognition in the rat. *Crit Rev Neurobiol* 11:101–120.

Poucet B, Lenck-Santini PP, Paz-Villagran V, Save E (2003) Place cells, neocortex and spatial navigation: a short review. *J Physiol Paris* 97:537546.

Pravosudov VV, Clayton NS (2002) A test of the adaptive specialization hypothesis: population differences in caching, memory, and the hippocampus in black-capped chickadees (Poecile atricapilla). *Behav Neurosci* 116:515–522.

Prusky GT, West PW, Douglas RM (2000a) Behavioral assessment of visual acuity in mice and rats. *Vision Res* 40:2201–2209.

Prusky GT, West PW, Douglas RM (2000b) Reduced visual acuity impairs place but not cued learning in the Morris water task. *Behav Brain Res* 116:135–140.

Quirk GJ, Muller RU, Kubie JL, Ranck JB (1992) The positional firing properties of medial entorhinal neurons: description and comparison with hippocampal place cells. *J Neurosci* 12:1945–1963.

Ramos JM (1998) Retrograde amnesia for spatial information: a dissociation between intra- and extramaze cues following hippocampus lesions in rats. *Eur J Neurosci* 10:3295–3301.

Rawlins JN, Lyford GL, Seferiades A, Deacon RM, Cassaday HJ (1993) Critical determinants of nonspatial working memory deficits in rats with conventional lesions of the hippocampus or fornix. *Behav Neurosci* 107:420–433.

Rawlins JNP (1985) Associations across time: the hippocampus as a temporary memory store. *Behav Brain Sci* 8:479497.

Redish AD (1999) *Beyond the cognitive map: from place cells to episodic memory.* Cambridge, MA: MIT Press.

Reisel D, Bannerman DM, Schmitt WB, Deacon RM, Flint J, Borchardt T, Seeburg PH, Rawlins JN (2002) Spatial memory dissociations in mice lacking GluR1. *Nat Neurosci* 5:868–873.

Remondes M, Schuman EM (2004) Role for a cortical input to hippocampal area CA1 in the consolidation of a long-term memory. *Nature* 431:699–703.

Rempel-Clower NL, Zola SM, Squire LR, Amaral DG (1996) Three cases of enduring memory impairment after bilateral damage limited to the hippocampal formation. *J Neurosci* 16:5233–5255.

Renner MJ (1990) Neglected aspects of exploratory and investigatory behavior. *Psychobiology* 18:16–22.

Rescorla RA (1973) Effect of US habituation following conditioning. *J Comp Physiol Psychol* 82:137–143.

Rescorla RA (1988) Pavlovian conditioning: it's not what you think it is. *Am Psychol* 43:151–160.

Rescorla RA, Wagner AR (1972) A theory of pavlovian conditioning: the effectiveness of of reinforcement and nonreinforcement. In: *Classical conditioning. II. Current research and theory* (Black AH, Prokasy WF, eds), pp 64–99. New York: Appleton-Century-Crofts.

Ressler KJ, Paschall G, Zhou X-L, Davis M (2002) Regulation of synaptic plasticity genes during consolidation of fear conditioning. *J Neurosci* 22:7892–7902.

Richmond MA, Yee BK, Pouzet B, Veenman L, Rawlins JNP, Feldon J, Bannerman DM (1999) Dissociating context and space within the hippocampus: effects of complete, dorsal, and ventral excitotoxic hippocampal lesions on conditioned freezing and spatial learning. *Behav Neurosci* 113:1189–1203.

Riedel G, Micheau J, Lam AG, Roloff E, Martin SJ, Bridge H, Hoz L, Poeschel B, McCulloch J, Morris RGM (1999) Reversible neural inactivation reveals hippocampal participation in several memory processes. *Nat Neurosci* 2:898–905.

Ringo JL (1991) Memory decays at the same rate in macaques with and without brain lesions when expressed in d' or arcsine terms. *Behav Brain Res* 42:123–134.

Ringo JL (1993) Spared short-term memory in monkeys following medial temporal lobe lesions is not yet established: a reply to Alvarez-Royo, Zola-Morgan and Squire. *Behav Brain Res* 59:65–72.

Rizzolatti G, Craighero L (2004) The mirror-neuron system. *Annu Rev Neurosci* 27:169–192.

Robbins TW, James M, Owen AM, Sahakian BJ, McInnes L, Rabbitt P (1994) Cambridge Neuropsychological Test Automated Battery (CANTAB): a factor analytic study of a large sample of normal elderly volunteers. *Dementia* 5:266–281.

Roberts WA (2000) Are animals stuck in time? *Psychol Bull* 128:473–489.

Robertson RG, Rolls ET, Georges-Francois P (1998) Spatial view cells in the primate hippocampus: effects of removal of view details. *J Neurophysiol* 79:1145–1156.

Robinson L, Bridge H, Riedel G (2001) Visual discrimination learning in the watermaze: a novel test for visual acuity. *Behav Brain Res* 119:77–84.

Rodrigo T (2002) Navigational strategies and models. *Psicologica* 23:2–32.

Rodrigo T, Chamizo VD, McLaren IPL, Mackintosh NJ (1997) Blocking in the spatial domain. *J Exp Psychol Anim Behav Process* 23:110–118.

Rolls ET, Treves A (1998) *Neural networks and brain function.* Oxford, UK: Oxford University Press.

Rosenbaum RS, Winocur G, Moscovitch M (2001) New views on old memories: re-evaluating the role of the hippocampal complex. *Behav Brain Res* 127:183–197.

Rosenzweig ES, Redish AD, McNaughton BL, Barnes CA (2003) Hippocampal map realignment and spatial learning. *Nat Neurosci* 6:609–615.

Ross RT, Orr WB, Holland PC, Berger TW (1984) Hippocampectomy disrupts acquisition and retention of learned conditional responding. *Behav Neurosci* 98:211–225.

Rossier J, Kaminsky Y, Schenk F, Bures J (2000) The place preference task: a new tool for studying the relation between behavior and place cell activity in rats. *Behav Neurosci* 114:273–284.

Rotenberg A, Mayford M, Hawkins RD, Kandel ER, Muller RU (1996) Mice expressing activated CaMKII lack low frequency LTP and do not form stable place cells in the CA1 region of the hippocampus. *Cell* 87:1351–1361.

Rotenberg A, Abel T, Hawkins RD, Kandel ER, Muller RU (2000) Parallel instabilities of long-term potentiation, place cells, and learning caused by decreased protein kinase A activity. *J Neurosci* 20:8096–8102.

Rothblat LA, Hayes LL (1987) Short-term object recognition memory in the rat: nonmatching with trial-unique junk stimuli. *Behav Neurosci* 101:587–590.

Roullet P, Lassalle JM (1992) Behavioural strategies, sensorial processes and hippocampal mossy fibre distribution in radial maze performance in mice. *Behav Brain Res* 48:77–85.

Rudy JW, Sutherland RJ (1995) Configural association theory and the hippocampal formation: an appraisal and reconfiguration. *Hippocampus* 5:375–389.

Rudy JW, O'Reilly RC (1999) Contextual fear conditioning, conjunctive representations, pattern completion, and the hippocampus. *Behav Neurosci* 113:867–880.

Rudy JW, Barrientos RM, O'Reilly RC (2002) Hippocampal formation supports conditioning to memory of a context. *Behav Neurosci* 116:530–538.

Rumelhart DE, McClelland JL (1986) *Parallel distributed processing: explorations in the microstructure of cognition.* Cambridge, MA: Bradford Books.

Rupniak NMJ, Gaffan D (1987) Monkey hippocampus and learning about spatially directed movements. *J Neurosci* 7:2331–2337.

Ryle G (1949) *The concept of mind.* London: Hutchinson.

Sahgal A (1993) *Behavioural neuroscience: a practical approach,*. Oxford: IRL Press.

Sakai K, Miyashita Y (1991) Neural organization for the long-term memory of paired associates. *Nature* 354:152–155.

Salmon DP, Zola-Morgan S, Squire LR (1987) Retrograde amnesia following combined hippocampus-amygdala lesions in monkeys. *Psychobiology* 15:37–47.

Sandi C, Loscertales M, Guaza C (1997) Experience-dependent facilitating effect of corticosterone on spatial memory formation in the watermaze. *Eur J Neurosci* 9:637–642.

Sapolsky RM (1985) A mechanism for glucocorticoid toxicity in the hippocampus: increased neuronal vulnerability to metabolic insults. *J Neurosci* 5:1228–1232.

Saunders RC, Weiskrantz L (1989) The effects of fornix transection and combined fornix transection, mammillary body lesions and hippocampal ablations on object-pair association memory in the rhesus monkey. *Behav Brain Res* 35:85–94.

Save E, Poucet B, Foreman N, Buhot MC (1992a) Object exploration and reactions to spatial and nonspatial changes in hooded rats following damage to parietal cortex or hippocampal formation. *Behav Neurosci* 106:447–456.

Save E, Buhot MC, Foreman N, Thinus-Blanc C (1992b) Exploratory activity and response to a spatial change in rats with hippocampal or posterior parietal cortical lesions. *Behav Brain Res* 47:113–127.

Schacter DE, Tulving E (1994) *Memory systems*, pp 269–310. Cambridge, MA: MIT Press.

Schenk F, Morris RGM (1985) Dissociation between components of spatial memory in rats after recovery from the effects of retro-hippocampal lesions. *Exp Brain Res* 58:11–28.

Schmajuk NA (1984) Psychological theories of hippocampal function. *Physiol Psychol* 12:166–183.

Schmitt WB, Sprengel R, Mack V, Draft RW, Seeburg PH, Deacon RM, Rawlins JN, Bannerman DM (2005) Restoration of spatial working memory by genetic rescue of GluR-A-deficient mice. *Nat Neurosci* 8:270–272.

Schwegler H, Lipp HP (1981) Is there a correlation between hippocampal mossy fiber distribution and two-way avoidance performance in mice and rats? *Neurosci Lett* 23:25–30.

Schwegler H, Lipp HP (1983) Hereditary covariations of neuronal circuitry and behavior: correlations between the proportions of hippocampal synaptic fields in the regio inferior and two-way avoidance in mice and rats. *Behav Brain Res* 7:138.

Schwegler H, Crusio WE, Brust I (1990) Hippocampal mossy fibers and radial-maze learning in the mouse: a correlation with spatial working memory but not with non-spatial reference memory. *Neuroscience* 34:293–298.

Schwegler H, Crusio WE, Lipp HP, Brust I, Mueller GG (1991) Early postnatal hyperthyroidism alters hippocampal circuitry and improves radial-maze learning in adult mice. *J Neurosci* 11:2102–2106.

Selden NRW, Everitt BJ, Jarrard LE, Robbins TW (1991) Complementary roles for the amygdala and hippocampus in aversive conditioning to explicit and contextual cues. *Neuroscience* 42:335–350.

Seyfarth RM, Cheney DL, Marler P (1980) Monkey responses to three different alarm calls: evidence of predator classification and semantic communication. *Science* 210:801–803.

Shallice T (1988) *From neuropsychology to mental structure*. New York: Cambridge University Press.

Sherry DF, Schacter DL (1987) The evolution of multiple memory systems. *Psychol Rev* 94:439–454.

Sherry DF, Vaccarino AL (1989) Hippocampus and memory for food caches in black-capped chickadees. *Behav Neurosci* 103:308–318.

Sherry DF, Vaccarino AL, Buckenham K, Herz RS (1989) The hippocampal complex of food-storing birds. *Brain Behav Evol* 34:308–317.

Sherry DF, Jacobs LF, Gaulin SJ (1992) Spatial memory and adaptive specialization of the hippocampus. *Trends Neurosci* 15:298–303.

Shettleworth SJ (1998) *Cognition, evolution, and behavior*. New York: Oxford University Press.

Shettleworth SJ (2001) Animal cognition and animal behaviour. *Anim Behav* 61:277–286.

Shettleworth SJ (2003) Memory and hippocampal specialization in food-storing birds: challenges for research on comparative cognition. *Brain Behav Evol* 62:108–116.

Shettleworth SJ, Krebs JR (1982) How marsh tits find their hoards: the roles of site preference and spatial memory. *J Exp Psychol Anim Behav Process* 8:354–375.

Shiflett MW, Smulders TV, Benedict L, DeVoogd TJ (2003) Reversible inactivation of the hippocampal formation in food-storing black-capped chickadees (Poecile atricapillus). *Hippocampus* 13:437–444.

Shimamura AP, Squire LR (1987) A neuropsychological study of fact memory and source amnesia. *J Exp Psychol* 13:464–473.

Siapas AG, Wilson MA (1998) Coordinated interactions between hippocampal ripples and cortical spindals during slow-wave sleep. *Neuron* 21:1123–1128.

Silva AJ, Paylor R, Wehner JM, Tonegawa S (1992) Impaired spatial learning in alpha-calcium-calmodulin kinase II mutant mice. *Science* 257:206–211.

Sirota A, Csicsvari J, Buhl D, Buzsaki G (2003) Communication between neocortex and hippocampus during sleep in rodents. *Proc Natl Acad Sci USA* 100:2065–2069.

Skelton RW, McNamara RK (1992) Bilateral knife cuts to the perforant path disrupt spatial learning in the Morris watermaze. *Hippocampus* 2:73–80.

Smith ML, Milner B (1981) The role of the right hippocampus in the recall of spatial location. *Neuropsychologia* 19:781–793.

Smulders TV, Sasson AD, DeVoogd TJ (1995) Seasonal variation in hippocampal volume in a food-storing bird, the black-capped chickadee. *J Neurobiol* 27:15–25.

Smulders TV, Shiflett MW, Sperling AJ, DeVoogd TJ (2000) Seasonal changes in neuron numbers in the hippocampal formation of a food-hoarding bird: the black-capped chickadee. *J Neurobiol* 44:414–422.

Sole LM, Shettleworth SJ, Bennett PJ (2003) Uncertainty in pigeons. *Psychon Bull Rev* 10:738–745.

Spooner RIW, Thomson A, Hall J, Morris RGM, Salter SH (1994) The Atlantis Platform: A new design and further developments of Buresova's on-demand platform for the watermaze. *Learn Mem* 1:203–211.

Squire LR (1992) Memory and the hippocampus: a synthesis from findings with rats, monkeys, and humans. *Psychol Rev* 99:195–231.

Squire LR (1993) The hippocampus and spatial memory. *TINS* 16:56–57.

Squire LR (2004) Memory systems of the brain: a brief history and current perspective. *Neurobiol Learn Mem* 82:171–177.

Squire LR, Alvarez P (1995) Retrograde amnesia and memory consolidation: a neurobiological perspective. *Curr Opin Neurobiol* 5:169–177.

Squire LR, Cohen NJ (1984) Human memory and amnesia. In: *Neurobiology of learning and memory* (Lynch G, McGaugh JL, Weinberger NM, eds), pp 3–64. New York: Gilford Press.

Squire LR, Zola SM (1998) Episodic memory, semantic memory and amnesia. *Hippocampus* 8:205–211.

Squire LR, Zola-Morgan S (1983) The neurology of memory: the case for correspondence between the findings for human and nonhuman primate. In: *The physiological basis of memory*, 2nd ed. (Deutsch JA, ed). San Diego: Academic Press.

Squire LR, Zola-Morgan S (1991) The medial temporal lobe memory system. *Science* 253:1380–1386.

Squire LR, Knowlton B, Musen G (1993) The structure and organization of memory. *Annu Rev Psychol* 44:453–495.

Squire LR, Clark RE, Knowlton BJ (2001) Retrograde amnesia. *Hippocampus* 11:50–55.

Squire LR, Stark CE, Clark RE (2004) The medial temporal lobe. *Annu Rev Neurosci* 27:279–306.

Staubli U, Ivy G, Lynch G (1984) Hippocampal denervation causes rapid forgetting of olfactory information in rats. *Proc Natl Acad Sci USA* 81:5885–5887.

Steele K, Rawlins JN (1993) The effects of hippocampectomy on performance by rats of a running recognition task using long lists of non-spatial items. *Behav Brain Res* 54:1–10.

Steele RJ, Morris RGM (1999) Delay-dependent impairment of a matching-to-place task with chronic and intrahippocampal infusion of the NMDA-antagonist D-AP5. *Hippocampus* 9:118–136.

Stefanacci L, Buffalo EA, Schmolck H, Squire LR (2000) Profound amnesia after damage to the medial temporal lobe: a neuroanatomical and neuropsychological profile of patient E.P. *J Neurosci* 20:7024–7036.

Steffenach HA, Sloviter RS, Moser EI, Moser MB (2002) Impaired retention of spatial memory after transection of longitudinally oriented axons of hippocampal CA3 pyramidal cells. *Proc Natl Acad Sci USA* 99:3194–3198.

Stein DG, Finger S, Hart T (1983) Brain damage and recovery: problems and perspectives. *Behav Neural Biol* 37:185–222.

Steward O, Cotman CW, Lynch GS (1974) Growth of a new fiber projection in the brain of adult rats: re-innervation of the dentate gyrus by the contralateral entorhinal cortex following ipsilateral entorhinal lesions. *Exp Brain Res* 20:45–66.

Strasser R, Ehrlinger JM, Bingman VP (2004) Transitive behavior in hippocampal-lesioned pigeons. *Brain Behav Evol* 63:181–188.

Suddendorf T, Busby J (2003) Mental time travel in animals? *Trends Cogn Sci* 7:391–396.

Suddendorf T, Corballis MC (1997) Mental time travel and the evolution of the human mind. *Genet Soc Gen Psychol Monogr* 123:133–167.

Sutherland RJ, Dyck RH (1984) Place navigation by rats in a swimming pool. *Can J Psychol* 38:322–247.

Sutherland RJ, Rudy JW (1989) Confugural association theory: the role of the hippocampal formation in learning, memory, and amnesia. *Psychobiology* 17:129–144.

Sutherland RJ, Hamilton DA (2004) Rodent spatial navigation: at the crossroads of cognition and movement. *Neurosci Biobehav Rev* 28:687–697.

Sutherland RJ, Whishaw IQ, Kolb B (1983) A behavioural analysis of spatial localization following electrolytic, kainate- or colchicine-induced damage to the hippocampal formation in the rat. *Behav Brain Res* 7:133–153.

Sutherland RJ, Whishaw IQ, Kolb B (1988) Contributions of cingulate cortex to two forms of spatial learning and memory. *J Neurosci* 8:1863–1872.

Sutherland RJ, Weisend MP, Mumby D, Astur RS, Hanlon FM, Koerner A, Thomas MJ, Wu Y, Moses SN, Cole C, Hamilton DA, Hoesing JM (2001) Retrograde amnesia after hippocampal damage: recent vs. remote memories in two tasks. *Hippocampus* 11:27–42.

Suzuki S, Augerinos G, Black AH (1980) Stimulus control of spatial behavior on the eight-arm maze in rats. *Learn Motiv* 1–8.

Suzuki WA, Amaral DG (1994a) Perirhinal and parahippocampal cortices of the macaque monkey: cortical afferents. *J Comp Neurol* 350:497–533.

Suzuki WA, Amaral DG (1994b) Topographic organization of the reciprocal connections between the monkey entorhinal cortex and the perirhinal and parahippocampal cortices. *J Neurosci* 14:1856–1877.

Suzuki WA, Clayton NS (2000) The hippocampus and memory: a comparative and ethological perspective. *Curr Opin Neurobiol* 10:768–773.

Suzuki WA, Eichenbaum H (2000) The neurophysiology of memory. *Ann NY Acad Sci* 911:175–191.

Suzuki WA, Zola-Morgan S, Squire LR, Amaral DG (1993) Lesions of the perirhinal and parahippocampal cortices in the monkey produce long-lasting memory impairment in the visual and tactual modalities. *J Neurosci* 13:2430–2451.

Swanson LW (2000) Cerebral hemisphere regulation of motivated behavior. *Brain Res* 886:113–164.

Swanson LW (2004) *Brain maps: structure of the rat brain*, 3rd ed. Amsterdam: Elsevier.

Sweatt JD (2003) *Mechanisms of memory*. London: Academic Press.

Tanner WP Jr, Swets JA (1954) A decision-making theory of visual detection. *Psychol Rev* 61:401–409.

Taube JS (1998) Head direction cells and the neurophysiological basis for a sense of direction. *Prog Neurobiol* 55:225–256.

Taube JS (1999) Some thoughts on place cells and the hippocampus. *Hippocampus* 9:452–457.

Taube JS, Schwartzkroin PA (1987) Intracellular-recording from hippocampal ca1 interneurons before and after development of long-term potentiation. *Brain Res* 419:32–38.

Taube JS, Muller RU, Ranck JB Jr (1990a) Head-direction cells recorded from the postsubiculum in freely moving rats. I. Description and quantitative analysis. *J Neurosci* 10:420–435.

Taube JS, Muller RU, Ranck JB Jr (1990b) Head-direction cells recorded from the postsubiculum in freely moving rats. II. Effects of environmental manipulations. *J Neurosci* 10:438–447.

Taube JS, Kesslak JP, Cotman CW (1992) Lesions of the rat postsubiculum impair performance on spatial tasks. *Behav Neural Biol* 57:131–143.

Teng E, Squire LR (1999) Memory for places learned long ago is intact after hippocampal damage. *Nature* 400:675–677.

Teng E, Stefanacci L, Squire LR, Zola SM (2000) Contrasting effects on discrimination learning after hippocampal lesions and conjoint hippocampal-caudate lesions in monkeys. *J Neurosci* 20:3853–3863.

Teuber HL (1955) Physiological psychology. *Annu Rev Psychol* 6:267–296.

Teyler TJ, DiScenna P (1986) The hippocampal memory indexing theory. *Behav Neurosci* 100:147–154.

Teyler TJ, DiScenna P (1987) Long-term potentiation. *Annu Rev Neurosci* 10:131–161.

Thinus-Blanc C, Bouzouba L, Chaix K, Chapuis N, Durup M, Poucet B (1987) A study of spatial parameters encoded during exploration in hamsters. *J Exp Psychol Anim Behav Process* 13:418–427.

Thomas KG, Hsu M, Laurance HE, Nadel L, Jacobs WJ (2001) Place learning in virtual space. III. Investigation of spatial navigation training procedures and their application to fMRI and clinical neuropsychology. *Behav Res Methods Instrum Comput* 33:21–37.

Thompson LT, Best PJ (1990) Long-term stability of the place-field activity of single units recorded from the dorsal hippocampus of freely behaving rats. *Brain Res* 509:299–308.

Thornton JA, Malkova L, Murray EA (1998) Rhinal cortex ablations fail to disrupt reinforcer devaluation effects in rhesus monkeys (Macaca mulatta). *Behav Neurosci* 112:1020–1025.

Tischmeyer W, Grimm R (1999) Activation of immediate early genes and memory formation. *Cell Mol Life Sci* 55:564–574.

Tolman EC (1948) Cognitive maps in rats and men. *Psychol Rev* 55:189–208.

Tomita H, Ohbayashi M, Nakahara K, Hasegawa I, Miyashita Y (1999) Top-down signal from prefrontal cortex in executive control of memory retrieval. *Nature* 401:699–703.

Tommasi L, Thinus-Blanc C (2004) Generalization in place learning and geometry knowledge in rats. *Learn Mem* 11:153–161.

Tonegawa S, Li Y, Erzurumlu RS, Jhaveri S, Chen C, Goda Y, Paylor R, Silva AJ, Kim JJ, Wehner JM (1995) The gene knockout technology for the analysis of learning and memory, and neural development. *Prog Brain Res* 105:3–14.

Tooby J, Cosmides L (2000) Toward mapping the evolved functional organisation of mind and brain. In: *The new cognitive neurosciences* (Gazzaniga M, ed). Cambridge, MA: MIT Press.

Treves A, Rolls ET (1994) Computational analysis of the role of the hippocampus in memory. *Hippocampus* 4:1–18.

Trullier O, Wiener SI, Berthoz A, Meyer JA (1997) Biologically based artificial navigation systems: review and prospects. *Prog Neurobiol* 51:483–544.

Trullier O, Shibata R, Mulder AB, Wiener SI (1999) Hippocampal neuronal position selectivity remains fixed to room cues only in rats alternating between place navigation and beacon approach tasks. *Eur J Neurosci* 11:4381–4388.

Tsien JZ, Chen DF, Gerber D, Tom C, Mercer EH, Anderson DJ, Mayford M, Kandel ER, Tonegawa S (1996) Subregion- and cell type-restricted gene knockout in mouse brain. *Cell* 87:1317–1326.

Tulving E (1972) Episodic and semantic memory. In: *Organisation of memory* (Tulving E, Donaldson W, eds), pp 381–403. San Diego: Academic Press.

Tulving E (1983) *Elements of episodic memory*. New York: Oxford University Press.

Tulving E (2004) Episodic memory and autonoesis: uniquely human? In: *The missing link in cognition: evolution of self-knowing consciousness* (Terrace H, Metcalfe J, eds). New York: Oxford University Press.

Tulving E, Markowitsch HJ (1998) Episodic and declarative memory: role of hippocampus. *Hippocampus* 8:198–204.

Ungerleider LG, Mishkin M (1982) Two cortical visual systems. In: *Analysis of visual behavior* (Ingle DJ, Goodale MA, Mansfield RJW, eds), pp 549–586. Cambridge, MA: MIT Press.

Vanderwolf CH, Cain DP (1994) The behavioral neurobiology of learning and memory: a conceptual reorientation. *Brain Res Brain Res Rev* 19:264–297.

Vanderwolf CH, Bland BH, Whishaw IQ (1973) Diencephalic hippocampal and neocortical mechanisms in voluntary movement. In: *Efferent organisation and the integration of behavior* (Masser JD, ed), pp 229–263. San Diego: Academic Press.

Van Elzakker M, O'Reilly RC, Rudy JW (2003) Transitivity, flexibility, conjunctive representations, and the hippocampus. I. An empirical analysis. *Hippocampus* 13:334–340.

Van Essen DC, Drury HA (1997) Structural and functional analyses of human cerebral cortex using a surface based atlas. *J Neurosci* 17:7079–7102.

Vann SD, Aggleton JP (2004) Testing the importance of the retrosplenial guidance system: effects of different sized retrosplenial cortex lesions on heading direction and spatial working memory. *Behav Brain Res* 155:97–108.

Vann SD, Brown MW, Erichsen JT, Aggleton JP (2000) Fos imaging reveals differential patterns of hippocampal and parahippocampal subfield activation in rats in response to different spatial memory tests. *J Neurosci* 20:2711–2718.

Van Praag H, Christie BR, Sejnowski TJ, Gage FH (1999) Running enhances neurogenesis, learning, and long-term potentiation in mice. *Proc Natl Acad Sci USA* 96:13427–13431.

Vargha-Khadem F, Gadian DG, Watkins KE, Connelly A, Van Paesschen W, Mishkin M (1997) Differential effects of early hippocampal pathology on episodic and semantic memory. *Science* 277:376–380.

Vazdarjanova A, Guzowski JF (2004) Differences in hippocampal neuronal population responses to modifications of an environmental context: evidence for distinct, yet complementary, functions of CA3 and CA1 ensembles. *J Neurosci* 24:6489–6496.

Vazdarjanova A, McGaugh JL (1999) Basolateral amygdala is involved in modulating consolidation of memory for classical fear conditioning. *J Neurosci* 19:6615–6622.

Vinogradova OS (1995) Expression, control, and probable functional significance of the neuronal theta rhythm. *Prog Neurobiol* 45:523–583.

Viskontas IV, McAndrews MP, Moscovitch M (2000) Remote episodic memory deficits in patients with unilateral temporal lobe epilepsy and excisions. *J Neurosci* 20:5853–5857.

Voermans NC, Petersson KM, Daudey L, Weber B, Van Spaendonck KP, Kremer HP, Fernandez G (2004) Interaction between the human hippocampus and the caudate nucleus during route recognition. *Neuron* 43:427–435.

Wan H, Aggleton JP, Brown MW (1999) Different contributions of the hippocampus and perirhinal cortex to recognition memory. *J Neurosci* 19:1142–1148.

Wang R, Spelke E (2002) Human spatial representation: insights from animals. *Trends Cogn Sci* 6:376.

Warburton EC, Baird A, Morgan A, Muir JL, Aggleton JP (2001) The conjoint importance of the hippocampus and anterior thalamic nuclei for allocentric spatial learning: evidence from a disconnection study in the rat. *J Neurosci* 21:7323–7330.

Warburton EC, Koder T, Cho K, Massey PV, Duguid G, Barker GR, Aggleton JP, Bashir ZI, Brown MW (2003) Cholinergic neurotransmission is essential for perirhinal cortical plasticity and recognition memory. *Neuron* 38:987–996.

Warrington EK, Weizkrantz L (1968) A study of learning and retention in amnesic patients. *Neuropsychologia* 6:283–291.

Wehner R, Lehrer M, Harvey WC (1996) Navigation: migration and homing. *J Exp Biol* 199:1–260.

Weiskrantz L (1982) Comparative aspects of studies of amnesia. *Philos Trans R Soc Lond B Biol Sci* 298:97–109.

Weiskrantz L (1997) *Consciousness lost and found*. Oxford, UK: Oxford University Press.

Whishaw IQ (1998) Place learning in hippocampal rats and the path integration hypothesis. *Neurosci Biobehav Rev* 22:209–220.

Whishaw IQ (2004a) Posterior neocortical (visual cortex) lesions in the rat impair matching-to-place navigation in a swimming pool: a reevaluation of cortical contributions to spatial behavior using a new assessment of spatial versus non-spatial behavior. *Behav Brain Res* 155:177–184.

Whishaw IQ (2004b) *The behavior of the laboratory rat: a handbook with tests.* New York: Oxford University Press.

Whishaw IQ, Jarrard LE (1996) Evidence for extrahippocampal involvement in place learning and hippocampal involvement in path integration. *Hippocampus* 6:513–524.

Whishaw IQ, Tomie JA (1991) Acquisition and retention by hippocampal rats of simple, conditional, and configural tasks using tactile and olfactory cues: implications for hippocampal function. *Behav Neurosci* 105:787–797.

Whishaw IQ, Tomie JA (1997) Perseveration on place reversals in spatial swimming pool tasks: further evidence for place learning in hippocampal rats. *Hippocampus* 7:361–370.

Whishaw IQ, Kolb B, Sutherland RJ (1983) The analysis of behavior in the laboratory rat. In: *Behavioral approaches to brain research* (Robinson TE, ed), pp 141–211. New York: Oxford University Press.

Whishaw IQ, Cassel JC, Jarrard LE (1995) Rats with fimbria-fornix lesions display a place response in a swimming pool: a dissociation between getting there and knowing where. *J Neurosci* 15:5779–5788.

Whishaw IQ, Hines DJ, Wallace DG (2001) Dead reckoning (path integration) requires the hippocampal formation: evidence from spontaneous exploration and spatial learning tasks in light (allothetic) and dark (idiothetic) tests. *Behav Brain Res* 127:49–69.

White NM, McDonald RJ (2002) Multiple parallel memory systems in the brain of the rat. *Neurobiol Learn Mem* 77:125–184.

Wiener SI (1993) Spatial and behavioral correlates of striatal neurons in rats performing a self-initiated navigation task. *J Neurosci* 13:3802–3817.

Wigstrom H, Gustafsson B (1983) Facilitated induction of hippocampal long-lasting potentiation during blockade of inhibition. *Nature* 301:603–604.

Wiig KA, Bilkey DK (1995) Lesions of rat perirhinal cortex exacerbate the memory deficit observed following damage to the fimbria-fornix. *Behav Neurosci* 109:620–630.

Willshaw D, Dayan P (1990) Optimal plasticity from matrix memories: what goes up must come down. *Neural Commun* 85–93.

Willshaw DJ, Buckingham JT (1990) An assessment of Marr's theory of the hippocampus as a temporary memory store. *Philos Trans R Soc Lond B Biol Sci* 329:205–215.

Wilson A, Brooks DC, Bouton ME (1995) The role of the rat hippocampal system in several effects of context in extinction. *Behav Neurosci* 109:828–836.

Wilson BA (1999) *Case studies in neuropsychological rehabilitation.* New York: Oxford University Press.

Wilson MA, McNaughton BL (1993) Dynamics of the hippocampal ensemble code for space. *Science* 261:1055–1058.

Wilson MA, Tonegawa S (1997) Synaptic plasticity, place cells and spatial memory: study with second generation knockouts. *Trends Neurosci* 20:102–106.

Winocur G (1990) Anterograde and retrograde amnesia in rats with dorsal hippocampal or dorsomedial thalamic lesions. *Behav Brain Res* 38:145–154.

Winocur G, Rawlins JNP, Gray JA (1987) The hippocampus and conditioning to contextual cues. *Behav Neurosci* 101:617–625.

Winocur G, Moscovitch M, Fogel S, Rosenbaum RS, Sekeres M (2005) Preserved spatial memory after hippocampal lesions: effects of extensive experience in a complex environment. *Nat Neurosci* 8:273–275.

Winograd T (1975) Frame representations and the procedural/declarative controversy. In: *Representation and understanding: studies in cognitive science* (Bobrow DG, Collins A, eds), pp 185–210. San Diego: Academic Press.

Winters BD, Bussey TJ (2005) Glutamate receptors in perirhinal cortex mediate encoding, retrieval, and consolidation of object recognition memory. *J Neurosci* 25:4243–4251.

Winters BD, Forwood SE, Cowell RA, Saksida LM, Bussey TJ (2004) Double dissociation between the effects of peri-postrhinal cortex and hippocampal lesions on tests of object recognition and spatial memory: heterogeneity of function within the temporal lobe. *J Neurosci* 24:5901–5908.

Wirth S, Yanike M, Frank LM, Smith AC, Brown EN, Suzuki WA (2003) Single neurons in the monkey hippocampus and learning of new associations. *Science* 300:1578–1581.

Witter MP, Naber PA, van Haeften T, Machielsen WC, Rombouts SA, Barkhof F, Scheltens P, Lopes da Silva FH (2000) Cortico-hippocampal communication by way of parallel parahippocampal-subicular pathways. *Hippocampus* 10:398–410.

Wixted JT, Squire LR (2004) Recall and recognition are equally impaired in patients with selective hippocampal damage. *Cogn Affect Behav Neurosci* 4:58–66.

Wood ER, Dudchenko PA, Eichenbaum H (1999) The global record of memory in hippocampal neuronal activity. *Nature* 397:613–616.

Wood ER, Dudchenko PA, Robitsek RJ, Eichenbaum H (2000) Hippocampal neurons encode information about different types of memory episodes occurring in the same location. *Neuron* 27:623–633.

Worden RP (1992) Navigation by fragment fitting: a theory of hippocampal function. *Hippocampus* 2:165–187.

Wulff P, Wisden W (2005) Dissecting neural circuitry by combining genetics and pharmacology. *Trends Neurosci* 28:44–50.

Yanike M, Wirth S, Suzuki WA (2004) Representation of well-learned information in the monkey hippocampus. *Neuron* 42:477–487.

Yonelinas AP (2001) Components of episodic memory: the contribution of recollection and familiarity. *Philos Trans R Soc Lond B Biol Sci* 356:1363–1374.

Yonelinas AP, Kroll NE, Quamme JR, Lazzara MM, Sauve MJ, Widaman KF, Knight RT (2002) Effects of extensive temporal lobe damage or mild hypoxia on recollection and familiarity. *Nat Neurosci* 5:1236–1241.

Zamanillo D, Sprengel R, Hvalby O, Jensen V, Burnashev N, Rozov A, Kaiser KM, Koster HJ, Borchardt T, Worley P, Lubke J, Frotscher M, Kelly PH, Sommer B, Andersen P, Seeburg PH, Sakmann B (1999) Importance of AMPA receptors for hippocampal synaptic plasticity but not for spatial learning. *Science* 284:1805–1811.

Zeman A (2002) *Consciousness: a user's guide.* New Haven, CT: Yale University Press.

Zhang WN, Bast T, Feldon J (2001) The ventral hippocampus and fear conditioning in rats: different anterograde amnesias of fear after infusion of N-methyl-D-aspartate or its noncompetitive antagonist MK-801 into the ventral hippocampus. *Behav Brain Res* 126:159–174.

Zhu XO, Brown MW, McCabe BJ, Aggleton JP (1995) Effects of the novelty or familiarity of visual stimuli on the expression of the immediate early gene c-fos in rat brain. *Neuroscience* 69:821–829.

Zinyuk L, Kubik S, Kaminsky Y, Fenton AA, Bures J (2000)

Understanding hippocampal activity by using purposeful behavior: place navigation induces place cell discharge in both task-relevant and task-irrelevant spatial reference frames. *Proc Natl Acad Sci USA* 97:3771–3776.

Zola SM, Squire LR (2001) Relationship between magnitude of damage to the hippocampus and impaired recognition memory in monkeys. *Hippocampus* 11:92–98.

Zola SM, Squire LR, Teng E, Stefanacci L, Buffalo EA, Clark RE (2000) Impaired recognition memory in monkeys after damage limited to the hippocampal region. *J Neurosci* 20:451–463.

Zola-Morgan S, Squire LR (1984) Preserved learning in monkeys with medial temporal lesions: sparing of motor and cognitive skills. *J Neurosci* 4:107–1085.

Zola-Morgan S, Squire LR (1985) Medial temporal lesions in monkeys impair memory on a variety of tasks sensitive to human amnesia. *Behav Neurosci* 99:22–34.

Zola-Morgan S, Squire LR (1990) The primate hippocampal forma-tion: evidence for a time-limited role in memory storage. *Science* 250:288–290.

Zola-Morgan S, Squire LR, Mishkin M (1982) The neuroanatomy of amnesia: amygdala-hippocampus versus temporal stem. *Science* 218:1337–1339.

Zola-Morgan S, Squire LR, Amaral DG (1986) Human amnesia and the medial temporal region: enduring memory impairment following a bilateral lesion limited to field CA1 of the hippocampus. *J Neurosci* 6:2950–2967.

Zola-Morgan S, Squire LR, Amaral DG (1989) Lesions of the amygdala that spare adjacent cortical regions do not impair memory or exacerbate the impairment following lesions of the hippocampal formation. *J Neurosci* 9:1922–1936.

Zola-Morgan S, Squire LR, Ramus SJ (1994) Severity of memory impairment in monkeys as a function of locus and extent of damage within the medial temporal lobe memory system. *Hippocampus* 4:483–495.

14 Neil Burgess

Computational Models of the Spatial and Mnemonic Functions of the Hippocampus

14.1 Overview

Some of the most striking data relating cognitive behavior to neuronal firing, damage, or metabolic activity in the brain concerns the hippocampus. The use of computational models has been invaluable for exploring the link between neurons and behavior, enabling hypothetical mechanisms to be defined precisely and examined quantitatively. Here I review many of these models, including models of spatial functions, models of more general associative mnemonic functions, models that stress feedforward processing through the hippocampal system, and those stressing recurrent processing within it. I review the spatial models first, as they are most firmly rooted in the known electrophysiology of the region. These models cover both the representation of the animal's spatial location and orientation and the use of this information in spatial navigation. The models of mnemonic function, specifically associative or episodic memory, follow from Marr's seminal 1971 model. I use this model as a generic framework in which to consider the various subsequent developments to it. Finally, I review those models attempting to bring together the spatial and mnemonic functions of the hippocampus.

14.2 Introduction

There have been many attempts to understand and quantify the contribution of the hippocampus to cognitive behavior. In this chapter I focus on models of the link between the cognitive ability of the animal and the action of individual cells and synapses. As reviewed in Chapter 13, lesion studies in a variety of mammals (including humans) have implicated the hippocampus in spatial navigation, whereas human neuropsychology has most notably implicated it in episodic or declarative memory (see Chapter 12). In addition to these

data a vast body of knowledge has been collected regarding the neural representation of the spatial location and orientation of freely moving rats (see Chapter 11). Hypotheses regarding the function of the hippocampus have traditionally been expressed in words. However, it is often possible to interpret verbal descriptions in more than one way, or to change their interpretation retrospectively to suit the facts. In addition, it can be difficult to tell whether the proposed explanation would actually work as described and, if so, difficult to make unambiguous quantitative predictions that can be used to test it. These problems become even more acute when hypotheses address the question of how a putative function arises from the cooperative behavior of large numbers of neurons and synapses. One way around this is to express such a hypothesis in terms of equations or computer simulations, referred to as a computational model. An advantage of this approach is that all of the parameter values and assumptions necessary to generate the behavior concerned need to be made explicit; another is that the operation of the model is unambiguously specified. These advantages mean that computational modeling has an important role to play in the progress of scientific understanding, most importantly in its interaction with experimental investigation: by predicting critical experiments, undergoing revision to reflect their results, and predicting new ones. They are not a panacea for all ills; and interpretation of a model, the way it works, and the values of its parameters can still be changed or disputed. At the most basic level a computational model can serve as an existence of proof of the behavior that can result from a proposed mechanism, but more generally it can serve to define a theoretical understanding and provide a powerful framework within which the nature of a theory relating brain to behavior can be understood.

Examples of potential insights into the function of the nervous system that would not have been fully understood, and in some cases even suspected, without computational modeling include the relation of voltage-dependent ion channels to the propagation of action potentials (Hodgkin and Huxley, 1952); the possible relation of the pattern of firing of dopamine neurons during conditioning experiments to the process of learning from trial and error (interpretable via the Rescorla-Wagner law and subsequent computational models of "reinforcement learning") (e.g., Shultz et al., 1997); the relation of partially shifting gain field responses in parietal cortex and optimal integration of multiple cues (made clear by computational understanding of the way attractor networks can perform this function) (e.g., Deneve et al., 2001); and the effect of genetic knockout of *N*-methyl-D-aspartate (NMDA) receptors in hippocampal region CA3 on the robustness of both the mouse's spatial memory and the firing of its place cells when a subset of environmental landmarks are removed (interpretable as "pattern completion" in a model of CA3 acting as an attractor network) (Marr, 1971; Nakazawa et al., 2002) (see Section 14.3.3 and 14.5.3).

Computational modeling of the hippocampus has followed two largely independent streams over the years: one seeking to explain a general role in associative memory and the other focusing on its role in spatial navigation. Models usually start from as detailed a biophysical level as is useful for the level of the hypothesis they seek to investigate. Although many models reviewed here involve detailed simulation of cellular and synaptic electrophysiology, the aim of this chapter is to explain the neural bases of spatial and mnemonic behavior—something that is made easier by focusing on the simplest level of description capturing the likely functional consequences of cellular and synaptic events (e.g., whether an action potential was fired). Thus, the activity (firing rate) of a neuron is simply viewed as a monotonic function of the amount by which the net input to it exceeds some threshold value. The net input to a neuron is the sum of the activity of each neuron connected to it weighted by the strength of the connection (occasionally inhibitory inputs are modeled as a divisive term in the net input rather than a subtractive term, see Figure 14–10, later). "Learning" corresponds to modification of the connection strengths. Most commonly learning is of a "Hebbian" nature (Hebb, 1949) such that simultaneous pre- and post-connection activity leads to increased connection strength and is often used in explicit analogy to synaptic processes such as long-term potentiation (LTP) (see Chapter 10) (see Box 14–1). Other concepts are explained as and where necessary. Readers interested in neural computation more generally should see the relevant literature (e.g., McClelland and Rumelhart, 1986; Rumelhart and McClelland, 1986; Hertz et al., 1990; Dayan and Abbott, 2002).

Because the anatomy of the region is similar in rats, primates, and humans, it seems sensible to start with the computational functions of the hippocampal region in the rat and then consider how these functions might have been adapted during evolution. This has the advantage of applying the most detailed electrophysiological constraints at the outset. Accordingly, in this chapter I concentrate initially on neural models starting from the reliable and well understood body of data regarding place cells and the neural representation of

space, drawing mostly on experimental data collected in rats. I next consider models of the use of spatial representations in guiding behavior. Together, models of the representation of location and orientation from sensory input and models of how these representations are used to guide behavior provide one of the best examples of quantitative understanding of the links between perception, cognition, and action and between cells and systems and behavior. The second half of the chapter concerns attempts to model the more general role of the human hippocampus in memory for personal experience. The chapter concludes with consideration of the models that attempt to reconcile these two streams of research (spatial and mnemonic). As we shall see, the role of the recurrent collaterals in area CA3 of the hippocampus maintains a common point of contact between these models: In both the spatial and episodic memory frameworks they are assumed to perform an associative memory function.

14.3 Hippocampus and Spatial Representation

This section addresses the representation of spatial location and orientation. Models of the representation of location embodied by the firing of place cells are considered first. These models take two often equivalent forms: those relying predominantly on feedforward connections to capture the data and those relying predominantly on the recurrent connections in CA3. It is not only the firing rates of place cells that encode location but also the time of firing relative to the ongoing theta rhythm on the electroencephalogram (EEG) (O'Keefe and Recce, 1993). Both of these aspects of firing have been the subjects of extensive computational modeling. The representation of the animal's orientation embodied by the head-direction (HD) cells is equally striking; and the nature of this signal, considered in the remainder of this section, has also been investigated by computational modeling in more recent years. Finally, the discovery of grid cells' (Hafting et al., 2005) has provided a new focus, reviewed by McNaughton et al. (2006).

14.3.1 Representing Spatial Location and Orientation: Data

A rich set of experimental data has been gathered on the neural representation of spatial behavior found in and around the hippocampus. Here I briefly summarize the results with the greatest relevance to the models described below (see Chapter 11 for more details). The firing of place cells in the hippocampi of freely moving rats encodes the location of the animal, each cell firing when the animal is within a particular portion of its environment (the "place field"). Cells with similar responses have also been observed in primates (Hori et al., 2003; Ludvig et al., 2004) including humans (Ekstrom et al., 2003). In open environments through which the rat can move freely, firing rates are not influenced by the animal's orientation, whereas in environments in which movement direction

Box 14–1
Learning via Synaptic Modification: Hebbian Learning Rules

In the simplest type of neural network model, the firing rate, or "activity," of a neuron (a) is simply a function (the "transfer function" f) of the net current coming into the neuron, which in turn is simply a weighted sum of the firing rates (u_i) of the neurons connecting to it. That is: $a = f(\Sigma_i w_i u_i)$, often written as: $a = f(\underline{w}.\underline{u})$, where $\underline{w}$ is the vector of connection "weights" modeling the strengths (e.g., net synaptic efficacy) of connections from the input neurons, and the dot is the vector dot product. With the simplest, linear, transfer function, the activation is given by:

$$a = \underline{w}.\underline{u} \tag{1}$$

In such networks, "learning" corresponds to modification of the connection weights $\underline{w}$. Below I discuss some of the Hebbian learning rules mentioned in the rest of the chapter, and their effects, following the discussion in Dayan and Abbott (2002), where further details can be found.

A learning rule directly implementing Hebb's (1949) postulate of coincident firing leading to increased coupling between neurons describes the change in connection weights in terms of the product of pre- and post-synaptic firing rates:

$$\tau \frac{dw_i}{dt} = au_i, \text{ or } \tau \frac{d\underline{w}}{dt} = a\underline{u} \tag{2}$$

where τ gives the rate of change of connection weights with time. When this rule is applied to a "training set" of n example input patterns of activity $\underline{u}^\mu$, each presented for an equal duration over a total time T, we can integrate equation 2 to see the total change in $\underline{w}$:

$$\underline{w} \rightarrow \underline{w} + \frac{T}{\tau}\sum_\mu a^\mu \underline{u}^\mu \tag{3}$$

where $a^\mu = \underline{w}.\underline{u}^\mu$ from equation 1. If the connection weights are updated only after presentation of all of the input patterns, we can say:

$$\underline{w} \rightarrow \underline{w} + \frac{T}{\tau}\sum_\mu (\underline{w}.\underline{u}^\mu)\underline{u}^\mu = w + \frac{nT}{\tau}Q.\underline{w} \tag{4}$$

where Q is the correlation matrix of the input patterns ($Q = <\underline{u}\,\underline{u}>$, where $< >$ denotes the average over input patterns, and $\underline{u}\,\underline{u}$ is the outer product of $\underline{u}$ with itself). Thus, simple Hebbian learning rules are also known as correlation-based learning rules. Inspection of equation 4 indicates that the weight vector $\underline{w}$, if plotted in the same space as the input vectors $\underline{u}^\mu$, eventually follows the principal eigenvector of the correlation matrix; that is, it will lie along the direction from the origin to the mean input pattern ($<\underline{u}>$) or, if $<\underline{u}>$ is at the origin, along the first principal component of the set of input patterns. However, this learning rule is not stable: Large weights produce large output activations, which produce large increases in weights and so on. More formally, it can be seen from the dot product of $\underline{w}$ in equation 2 that the length of the weight vector increases whenever the output neuron is active:

$$\frac{d\,|\underline{w}|^2}{dt} = 2\underline{w}.\frac{d\underline{w}}{dt} = \frac{2a\underline{w}.\underline{u}}{\tau} = \frac{2a^2}{\tau} \tag{5}$$

One way to introduce balance into the learning rule is to allow for a connection weight to increase or to decrease according to the levels of pre- and postconnection activity, by analogy with long-term potentiation and depression (LTP and LTD) (see Chapter 10). In this way equation 2 could become

$$\tau \frac{d\underline{w}}{dt} = (a - \theta)\underline{u}, \text{ or } \tau \frac{d\underline{w}}{dt} = a(\underline{u} - \varphi) \tag{6}$$

where either a postsynaptic threshold or a set of presynaptic thresholds are applied to determine the sense and size of weight changes (respectively: θ is the level postsynaptic activity must surpass for the connection to increase rather than decrease; or φ, which is the vector of activity levels each input neuron must surpass). The most obvious choice of threshold for the pre- or postsynaptic neuron is its average activity over the training set. In this case, following a similar derivation to equation 4, both versions produce the same learning rule:

$$\underline{w} \rightarrow \underline{w} + \frac{nT}{\tau}\underline{C}.\underline{w} \tag{7}$$

(Continued)

Box 14–1
Learning via Synaptic Modification: Hebbian Learning Rules (Continued)

where C is the covariance matrix of the input patterns: $C = <(\underline{u}-<\underline{u}>)^2> = <\underline{u}\,\underline{u}>-<\underline{u}>^2 = <(\underline{u}-<\underline{u}>)\,\underline{u}>$. These learning rules are also known as covariance rules. Inspection of equation 7 indicates that the weight vector will eventually follow the principal eigenvector of the covariance matrix (i.e., it will lie along the direction of the first principal component of the set of input patterns). It should be noted that these rules are also not stable; in this case $d\,w^2/dt$ is proportional to the variance ($<a^2> - <a>^2$) of the output activity over the training set.

The BCM learning rule, derived from experimental investigation of visual cortical plasticity (Bienenstock et al., 1982), proposes that:

$$\tau\frac{dw}{dt} = a\underline{u}(a-\theta(a)) \tag{8}$$

This requires both pre- and postsynaptic activity for modification of a connection weight (unlike the rules in equation 6), and also involves a sliding postsynaptic threshold ($\theta(a)$), which varies with postsynaptic activity. So long as the postsynaptic threshold increases as a power of $a > 1$ (typically following a time-averaged estimate of a^2), it can ensure stability of the learning rule: effectively increasing the threshold to an overactive output neuron so connection weights to it tend to be reduced.

The other common way in which Hebbian learning rules are stabilized—e.g., in Rumelhart and Zipser's (1986) "competitive learning" algorithm—is to use divisive normalization: explicitly constraining the length of the weight vector to remain constant during learning by dividing all weights by $|\underline{w}|$. Although this is a nonlocal operation, because synaptic strengths must be altered according to the state of other, distant synapses, a similar effect can be achieved by the local learning rule of Oja (1982):

$$\tau\frac{dw}{dt} = a\underline{u} - \beta a^2\underline{w} \tag{9}$$

An analysis similar to equation 5 shows that $|\underline{w}|^2$ tends to a value $1/\beta$ under repeated application of this rule.

As well as being stable, the BCM and normalized Hebbian learning rules involve competition between connections: Increasing some of the connection weights onto a neuron leads to a decrease in the others. Under the BCM rule, this occurs because of increased activity leading to a higher postsynaptic threshold and thus an increased incidence of LTD versus LTP. With normalization it occurs directly owing to the increase in the length of the weight vector. These learning rules tend to allow a neuron to become tuned to respond to specific patterns of input activation (see text). There is at least some evidence for competitive interaction between synapses such that increasing the strengths of one set of synapses leads to a decrease in the strengths of others so as to normalize the total synaptic strength onto the neuron (Royer and Pare, 2003). Note however, that recent evidence of the dependence of synaptic plasticity on the precise timing of pre- and postsynaptic activity (see Chapter 10) changes the likely nature of learning rules based on LTP and LTD, as in the effects of temporal asymmetry noted in Section 14.4.3.

is constrained (e.g., linear tracks, eight-arm mazes) firing is strongly modulated by the rat's direction of motion (see Chapter 11). The orientation of the place cell representation is controlled by "distal" cues at or beyond the edge of the environment (O'Keefe and Conway, 1978; Muller and Kubie, 1987) but not by those within it (Cressant et al., 1997). A place cell's spatially localized firing appears to be robust to the removal of subsets of cues and indeed removal of all of the controlling visual cues while the rat remains in the environment (Muller and Kubie, 1987; O'Keefe and Speakman, 1987), although remaining uncontrolled cues may be important in these cases (Save et al., 2000).

The complementary representation of orientation independent of location is found in "head direction cells" (HDCs) in the mammillary bodies, anterior thalamic nuclei, and dorsal presubiculum (Taube et al., 1990). The HDCs code for head direction within an environment, each firing whenever the animal's head points in a specific direction, independently of the animal's location. The orientation of the head direction representation is controlled by distal visual cues in the same way as the place cell representation. The overall orientation of both place and HDC representations may be disrupted by disorientation (rotating the rat in a covered container); and when both have been recorded simultaneously, both representations have remained in register with each other (Knierim et al., 1995). Interestingly, hints that an expanded representation of neurons responding to specific combinations of place and direction have been found in the presubiculum (Sharp, 1996; Cacucci et al., 2004). A third type of representation, "grid cells," has now been found in dorsomedial entorhinal cortex

(Hafting et al., 2005). Each grid cell fires in a set of locations which is laid out on a hexagonal grid. The intriguing properties of these cells are summarized at the end of Section 14.3.3. However, at the time of this writing they have not yet been fully incorporated into models of hippocampal function and so are not a focus of this chapter.

Beyond the clear encoding of spatial location and orientation in the firing rates of these neurons, the picture becomes slightly more complex. Initial experiments in which place cells were recorded in environments of different shape (Muller and Kubie, 1987) reported completely different patterns of firing in the two environments ("remapping"). A place cell active in one environment might fire in an unrelated location in the second environment or might be silent. In other experiments, perhaps involving less complete changes to the environment or less extensive pretraining in the various environments, parametric changes in the pattern of firing were observed (e.g., O'Keefe and Burgess, 1996). Interestingly, although the firing rate of place cells can be shown to encode the animal's location within a given environment (e.g., Wilson and McNaughton, 1993), the times at which they fire relative to the theta rhythm encodes additional information (see Chapter 11) (O'Keefe and Recce, 1993; Skaggs et al., 1996; Jensen and Lisman, 2000).

14.3.2 Representing Spatial Location: Feedforward Models

Computational modeling of place cell firing began with Zipser's (1985) model. In this model, sensory details of the environment feedforward to landmark detectors and thence to place cells. Landmark detectors are neurons specific to a specific place cell and to a specific aspect of the sensory scene (a "location parameter"). The output of these detectors is proportional to the match between the stored state of a location parameter and its currently perceived state. A place cell's activity corresponds to a thresholded sum of the strengths of the matches it receives from several landmark detectors. Interestingly, the most obvious location parameter—distance from a landmark—was rejected in favor of measures that scale with environmental size, such as the retinal angle between two landmarks, on the basis of a misinterpretation of Muller and Kubie's (1987) experiment. In this experiment, a significant but small number of place fields were shown to expand following a doubling in the linear size of the environment. However, this expansion corresponded to, at most, approximate doubling of the place field in area rather than the quadrupling predicted if everything scaled up proportionately. Furthermore, in many cells the expansion often appeared to be along only one environmental dimension rather than both. The model captures some of the motility of place fields in the presence of manipulations of environmental cues and some of their robustness to the removal of subsets of cues and (incorrectly) produces a place field that scales up proportionally with environmental expansion.

Sharp (1991) followed in the same vein of feedforward modeling of the response of place cells to sensory input from the environment but with the incorporation of an element of "competitive learning" (Rumelhart and Zipser, 1986). Briefly, this involves neurons arranged in groups dominated by lateral inhibition such that only the neuron with the greatest input can fire. Normalized Hebbian learning is then applied (i.e., increasing the strengths of connections between simultaneously active neurons while decreasing the others so the overall strength of connections to a neuron does not change (see Box 14–1). This results in specific neurons coming to represent specific patterns of input, with each neuron responding to a particular pattern or patterns similar to it. Sharp's model envisaged two types of sensory input regarding each distal cue: one representing its distance from the rat and the other representing both its distance from the rat and its direction relative to the rat's heading. This sensory input passed forward to a layer of entorhinal cortical cells and thence to a layer of place cells (Fig. 14–1). Competitive learning at each layer causes the entorhinal and place cells to learn to respond selectively to the pattern of sensory input present in a particular portion of the environment, and it produces reasonable robustness to cue removal. The successive layers of competition produce sharper tuning to position and greater robustness to cue removal in place cells than entorhinal cells. Due to the use of distance-related inputs, expansion of the environment produces results that are qualitatively similar to those of Muller and Kubie's (1987) experiment. The most interesting aspect of this model concerns the directional modulation of place cell firing. In the model, place cell firing is initially directionally modulated owing to the partially directional sensory inputs. During random exploration through an open environment, competitive learning allows a given place cell to learn to respond to the sensory inputs occurring for different orientations at the place field, producing nondirectional firing. By contrast, this does not occur during constrained motion (i.e., back and forth in a single direction). This provides a good, simple model of the directionality of place cell firing, although a more detailed look at directionality data indicates that, if anything, place fields in open environments are initially nondirectional and become directional as a result of experience. For alternative models see Blum and Abbott (1996), Brunel and Trullier (1998) and Kali and Dayan (2000), discussed below.

In an attempt to derive the form of the sensory input to the place cells, O'Keefe and Burgess (1996) systematically varied the shape and size of the rat's environment while recording from the same cells. The patterns of firing across environments included place fields that stretched or became bimodal when the environment expanded. These patterns were not consistent with those obtained in previous models of place fields depending on the relative locations of discrete landmarks from the rat (e.g., Zipser, 1985) but, rather, indicated continuous dependence on environmental boundaries. Specifically, place fields were viewed as a thresholded linear sum of inputs tuned to respond to the presence of a boundary at a given distance along a given allocentric direction (i.e., independent of the orientation of the rat and probably

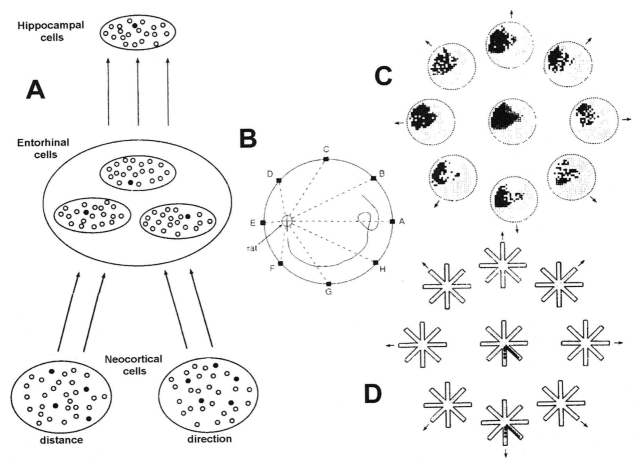

Figure 14–1. Sharp's (1991) model of place cell firing in response to sensory input. *A.* Two groups of neocortical cells respond to the distance or (egocentric) direction of specific cues as the rat moves in a cylinder (shown in *B*, cues marked by letters). Competitive learning in successive layers of entorhinal cells and place cells leads, after exploration, to spatially tuned firing that is robust to removal of subsets of cues. *C.* If exploration is unconstrained, as in an open cylinder, place cell firing is only weakly modulated by the heading direction of the animal (overall place field shown in center, firing fields at each of eight heading direction shown around the edge). *D.* If exploration is constrained to specific directions of movement, as on a radial arm maze, place cell firing is strongly modulated by the heading direction. (*Source*: Adapted from Sharp, 1991.)

determined relative to the head-direction system; see below) (Fig. 14–2). These hypothetical inputs were termed "boundary vector cells." By fitting a place cell's firing pattern across several environmental shapes, the model can predict its firing pattern in an environment of novel shape (Hartley et al., 2000). In an experiment complementary to the variation of environmental shape, Fenton et al. (2000) parametrically varied the position of two cue cards around the edge of a cylindrical environment. Although each card alone can control the overall orientation of the recorded place fields, inconsistent movement of both (i.e., moving them closer together or apart) produces inhomogeneous parametric movement of the place fields such that their movement depends on their location. The added complexity of the cue cards acting as both identifiable boundaries and directional cues can be incorporated into the boundary vector cell model by assuming that inconsistent cue-card movement warps the representation of head direction, and boundary vector cells become sensitive to variations in texture after sufficient exposure (Burgess and Hartley, 2002).

One phenomenon not addressed by the above models is the "remapping" of place cell representations across different environments. This remapping can be both partial and incremental over time (e.g., Bostock et al., 1991; Skaggs and McNaughton, 1998; Lever et al., 2002), with the eventual creation of stable but distinct patterns of firing in the two environments. The factors influencing the speed and completeness of remapping are not currently well understood, but one common change in an individual place cell is to continue to fire in the environment in which it fires most strongly and to stop firing in the other. This aspect of remapping was addressed by Fuhs and Touretzky (2000) in a model of learning in the perforant path projection from entorhinal cortex to place cells in CA3. They found that the usual learning rules relating synaptic modification to the product of pre- and postsynaptic activity (i.e.. Hebbian learning) or to its covariance were unable to reproduce this behavior. In the case of Hebbian learning, a place cell with strong firing in one environment and weak firing in the other strengthens its firing in both environments. In

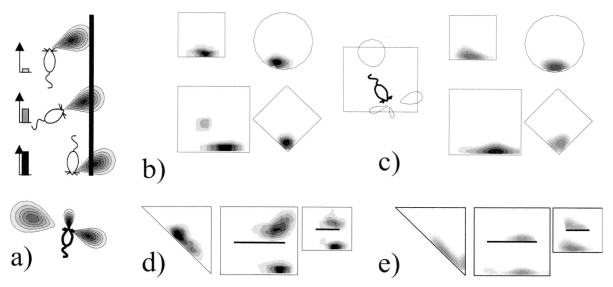

Figure 14–2. Model of the geometrical influence on place fields (Hartley et al., 2000), assuming a stable directional reference frame. Place fields are composed from thresholded linear sums of the firing rates of boundary vector cells (BVCs). *a*. Above: Each BVC has a Gaussian tuned response to the presence of a boundary at a given distance and bearing from the rat (independent of its orientation). Below: The sharpness of tuning of a BVC decreases as the distance to which it is tuned increases. The only free parameters of a BVC are the distance and direction of the peak response.

b. Place fields recorded from the same cell in four environments of different shape or orientation relative to distal cues. *c*. Simulation of the place fields in *b* by the best fitting set of four BVCs constrained to be in orthogonal directions (BVCs shown on the left, simulated fields on the right). The simulated cell can now be used to predict firing in novel situations. Real and predicted data from three novel environments are shown in *d* and *e*, respectively, showing good qualitative agreement. (*Source*: Adapted from Burgess and Hartley, 2002.)

the case of covariance learning, exposure to the second environment tends to lead to loss of the place cell representation of the first environment. By contrast, the BCM (Bienenstock-Cooper-Munro) learning rule (Bienenstock et al., 1982) (see Box 14–1), which explicitly makes the direction of synaptic modification dependent on the strength of the postsynaptic activity, did produce the desired result: strong firing remaining stable and weak firing reducing with experience. This type of learning can also capture the way place fields become more coherent with time and the temporal dynamics of their response to the introduction of a barrier into the environment (Barry et al., 2006).

Evidence of experience-dependent change in place cell firing also comes from experiments by Mehta et al. (1997, 2000). They found that, over the first few runs through a CA1 place field on a linear track, the spatial distribution of firing changes from roughly symmetrical to slightly asymmetrical, caused by additional firing at low rates earlier on the track. They suggest that this change results from the known temporal asymmetry of LTP (which is greater when presynaptic activity precedes postsynaptic activity than vice versa) acting on the CA3 to CA1 pathway (see Chapter 10). Other models have implicated the recurrent connections in CA3 as responsible for this effect. Interestingly, the phase shift seen in place cell firing (see Section 14.3.1 for data and Section 14.3.5 for models) (see also Chapter 11) acts to increase this effect of temporal asymmetry in LTP, causing place cells with fields early on the path to fire before those with fields later along the path during each theta cycle. The apparently unrelated effect of the remapping

of place cell representations across different environments has also been ascribed to the effects of the recurrent connections in CA3. Models stressing these connections are the subject of the next section.

14.3.3 Representing Spatial Location and Orientation: Feedback Models

The long-range recurrent connections between pyramidal cells in area CA3 of the hippocampus have long been interpreted as enabling this region to work as an autoassociative neural network (e.g., Marr, 1971; Hopfield, 1982; Amit, 1989). This type of network is most often used to provide a content-addressable memory, a subject explored in Section 14.5 (see Box 14–2). In this section I consider the role played by recurrent collaterals in the spatial representations of place and HD cells. Interestingly, direct experimental evidence for an associative function for CA3 has emerged recently, with indications that the NMDA receptors in this region are involved in making both the place fields and the rat's spatial memory robust to cue removal (Nakazawa et al., 2002). In parallel, attractor dynamics have been found in the place cell representation of two environments of different shape after fast remapping caused by exposure to the two environmental shapes made of different materials (Wills et al., 2005). In these representations, in contrast to those that have not fast-remapped (Leutgeb et al., 2005), the two shapes act as attractors: all place cells in intermediate shaped environments coherently returning to one or other representation.

Box 14–2
Attractors in Memory, Neural Coding, and Path Integration

POINT ATTRACTORS AND MEMORY

A network of recurrently connected neurons can be arranged so a finite number of discrete patterns of activation across the neurons are stable states, or "attractors." This means that any pattern of activation similar enough to one of these attractors will evolve into the attractor pattern under the dynamics of the network. These patterns of activation are "stored" in the network in the sense that they are "retrieved" from any similar enough initial pattern. Such networks are also referred to as "autoassociative" networks, and are an example of a "content-addressable" memory in that a pattern of activity is retrieved by a pattern of similar content, rather than, say, an unrelated index term or the address of a storage location.

In one of the simplest models (Hopfield, 1982), the activity of neuron i is modeled as $a_i = \pm 1$. Connections between neurons i and j are symmetrical, with synaptic "weight" $w_{ij} = w_{ji}$ The dynamics of the network are given by: $a_i(t+1) = \text{sign}(\Sigma_j w_{ij} a_j(t))$, such that the "energy" or Lyapunov function of the network:

$$E \propto - \sum_{ij} w_{ij} a_i a_j$$

can only reduce. If connection weights undergo a form of Hebbian learning when the to-be-stored patterns of activation ($\underline{a}^\mu$, say) are present, such that $w_{ij} \propto \sum_\mu a_i^\mu a_j^\mu$, these representations become attractors so long as the number of stored patterns is not too large (less than around $0.14N$, where N is the number of neurons, in this case). That is, a similar enough pattern of activation converges onto the stored pattern under the dynamics of the network (Cohen and Grossberg, 1983). This situation is often visualized by imagining how the "energy" of the network varies as a function of the networks' "state" $\underline{au} = (a_1, a_2, .. a_N)$—the attractor states being local minima of the energy surface to which nearby states evolve under the network's dynamics (Fig. 14–3A). Similar behavior is also shown by more biologically realistic models (Amit, 1992; Treves and Rolls, 1992; McClelland et al., 1995) (Fig. 14–10).

LINE ATTRACTORS AND NEURAL CODING

The value of a continuous variable (or "stimulus"s) often seems to be represented in the firing rates of a population of neurons, each of which is tuned to respond preferentially to a single "preferred" value. For example, head-direction cells can be thought of in this way, with s representing the rat's heading. The pattern of activation of the population is often visualized by imagining the neurons arranged so their location reflects their preferred values: showing a smooth bump of activity across the neurons peaked at the actual value of the stimulus. However, if the firing rates are noisy it is difficult to estimate the precise value of the stimulus. The presence of recurrent connections between neurons, arranged so that the weight of the connection between each pair is simply a decreasing function of the difference in their preferred values (or physical separation when arranged as above), can help by ensuring that the firing pattern takes the shape of a smooth bump[1] (Fig. 14–3B). With the appropriate choice of recurrent connections, such a network can perform optimal decoding (Latham et al., 2003), including the situation where the representation is formed from different, unreliable sources of information (Deneve et al., 2001).

The patterns of activation comprising a smooth bump can be thought of as a line in the N dimensional state space $\underline{au} = (a_1, a_2, .. a_N)$ of the network. Each point on the line corresponds to a different estimate of s (referred to as $\hat{s}$). Conversely, all of the possible noisy patterns of activation that end up producing the same $\hat{s}$ lie on an $N-1$ dimensional subspace within which the action of the recurrent connections corresponds to convergence onto the line (Fig. 14–3C). An important aspect of these networks is that, although the recurrent connections ensure that patterns of activation move onto the line attractor, movement along it, corresponding to changing $\hat{s}$, is not affected by the recurrent connections (because the connections between a pair of neurons depends only on the *difference* in their preferred values, not what those preferred values are).

LINE ATTRACTORS AND PATH INTEGRATION

Because the (symmetrical) recurrent connections provide no resistance to the motion of the bump of activity along the line attractor, its position is easily moved by asymmetrical connections from each neuron to neighbors farther along the line (Skaggs et al., 1995; Zhang, 1996).

---

[1] These patterns have low "energy" as activation is concentrated in nearby neurons, which have the strongest interconnections.

The greater the size of the asymmetrical connections—which should correspond to the spatial derivative of the symmetrical connections for the bump to move without changing shape (Zhang, 1996)—compared to the symmetrical ones, the faster the movement of the bump (Figs. 14–3 to 14–5). Thus, if the strength of the asymmetrical connections is proportional to angular velocity, the location of the bump of activity in a ring of head direction cells tracks the head direction of the animal—performing angular "path integration." For a more detailed model, see Redish et al. (1996).

As noted by Zhang (1996) and McNaughton et al. (1996), the angular path integration models of head direction cell firing can be extended to path integration models of place cell firing. In this case, the place cells are imagined as a two-dimensional array, so the location of each neuron corresponds to the location of its place field in the environment (Fig. 14–6). Again, symmetrical connections decreasing in strength with the physical separation of the pre- and postsynaptic neurons can ensure that neural activity forms a single-peaked bump over the array. Asymmetrical connections from each neuron to its neighbors along a given direction causes the bump to shift in that direction (Figs. 14–3 and 14–4). In this case, to perform path integration of position, the strength of the asymmetrical connections between a pair of neurons displaced in a given direction needs to be proportional to the velocity of the rat in that direction. See Samsonovich and McNaughton (1997) for a more detailed model and Droulez and Berthoz (1991) and Dominey and Arbib (1992) for the origins of this type of model.

Continuous Attractor Models of Head Direction Cells

The simplest examples of the use of continuous attractors (see Box 14–2) to model spatial representations come from models of the representation of head direction rather than location. In many respects the literature on head-direction cells (HDCs) is much more straightforward than that on place cells. The overall orientation of the head-direction representation can be controlled by sensory cues in a way similar to that of the place cell representation. Unlike the place cells, however, there have been no reports to date of HDCs changing their preferred orientations relative to each other. Even when the rat is disoriented or is in a symmetrical environment without polarizing cues, the preferred directions of simultaneously recorded HDCs remain in synchrony—if they rotate, all rotate together. For this reason all models of the head-direction system follow the same basic mechanism of a one-dimensional continuous attractor, or "line attractor" (Skaggs et al., 1995; Zhang, 1996) from which the two-dimensional continuous attractor models of place cells developed (Figs. 14–3 to 14–6) (see Box 14–2).

If HDCs are imagined laid out in a ring with each cell's location corresponding to its preferred direction and each is connected to its neighbors (see Box 14–2), activity is smoothly peaked at the current heading direction. Skaggs et al.'s model contains two more rings of cells, with each cell receiving connections from the corresponding HDC. One ring is composed of "left rotation" cells, which project back to the HDCs to the left (anticlockwise) of their location; the other ring is composed of "right rotation" cells, which project back to HDCs to the right (clockwise) of their location. The left rotation cells corresponding to the current heading direction are activated when the rat is turning left because of inputs from the vestibular system as well as the HDCs, causing the HDC activation to move leftward. In addition to these cells, the HDCs receive input from "sensory cells" ("visual cells" in Fig. 14–5) and so can be associated with those sensory inputs appearing at a stable bearing during exploration of a new environment. These sensory inputs subsequently prevent the cumulative errors that would otherwise occur in the integration of angular velocity.

This basic model has been implemented and extended in various ways, developing in hand with our knowledge of the operation of the head-direction system. This is now thought to involve a circuit from the mammillary bodies (MBs) to anterior thalamic nuclei (ATN) to dorsal presubiculum (PS). In this circuit, cells in the MBs code for head direction further in the future (60–70 ms) than those in the ATN (20–30 ms), whereas those in the PS code for current or past head direction (0 to −10 ms) (Blair and Sharp, 1995; Blair et al., 1998; Taube, 1998; Taube and Muller, 1998) (see Chapter 11). Various of the additional detailed properties of these systems, such as time advances and asymmetrical responses during turning, have been modeled more recently (e.g., Touretzky and Redish, 1996; Blair et al., 1997; Goodridge and Touretzky, 2000). However, here I focus on the hippocampus, and return to models of location.

Continuous Attractor Models of Place Cells

Samsonovich and McNaughton (1997) produced a detailed model of the place cell representation as a continuous attractor, following Zhang (1996). In this model, the recurrent connections in CA3 are preconfigured to provide several continuous attractor representations of location (termed "charts"). Each chart involves a different set of place cells, the relative positions of whose place fields are predetermined. The strength of the recurrent connection between two cells in a chart is set as a Gaussian function of the proximity of their place fields. The place cells connect with a "path integration" (PI) system, thought to be in the subiculum, in which neurons respond to combinations of the rat's location and orientation

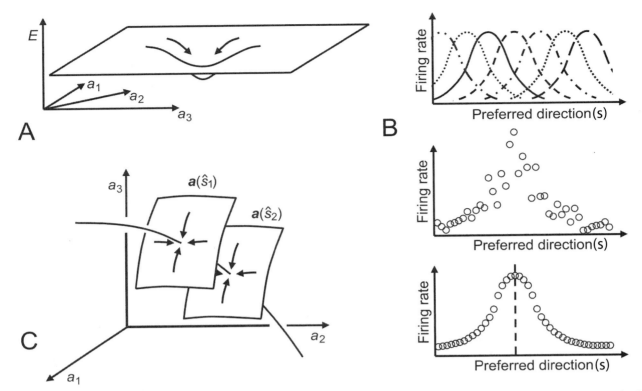

Figure 14–3. Point attractors and line attractors in neural systems (see Box 14–2). *A.* Point attractor is a pattern of activation $a = (a_1, a_2, a_3...)$ into which other nearby patterns evolve under the dynamics of the network (determined by the pattern of connection strengths, update rule, and so on). In some cases a function can be defined that can only decrease under the dynamics (a Lyanpunov function, or the energy (E) of a physical system), so that attractor states lie at local minima of this function. *B.* Population encoding and decoding. Neural populations can encode the current value of a variables, say in the pattern of activation across neurons, each of which is tuned to respond to a preferred value. These are often imagined to be laid out so that the position of each neuron on the ordinate corresponds to its preferred value. For example, a set of head-direction (HD) cells might each be tuned to a different "preferred" direction (top). If firing rates are noisy, it may be difficult to estimate the actual value of the variable (middle). Recurrent connections can be organized so all other patterns of activation evolve into smooth bump-shaped patterns of activation (below). This process can provide an optimal way of decoding the value of the variable from the population (the peak of the bump is the dashed line). *C.* The set of smooth bump-shaped patterns of activation form a "line attractor," a continuous set of patterns of activity onto which other nearby patterns evolve but along which movement is unimpeded. Locations along the line attractor can be thought of as estimates of the variable ($\hat{S}$); all of the patterns of activity that end up at a given estimate (such as $\hat{S}_1$) form a subspace $a(\hat{S})$ within which the intersection with the line is a point attractor. (*Source:* Adapted from Latham et al., 2003.)

(Sharp, 1996; Cacucci et al., 2004). Specifically, the place cells connect to PI neurons representing similar locations, and the return projections connect back to place cells representing slightly different locations shifted along the rat's direction of motion. The gain of this return projection is modulated by information relating to the rat's speed of self-motion (presumably carried by motor efference signals). This system, although demanding a highly specific set of hard-wired connections, provides a self-consistent continuous attractor representation of location that moves automatically with self-motion. Finally, the hippocampus also receives sensory input so that when the rat is placed in an environment for the first time associations between the sensory scene and the internal representation of location can be formed, which can then be used to reset the system periodically. Overall, the model can be seen as a possible implementation of O'Keefe and Nadel's (1978, pp. 220–230) view of the role of path

integration in supporting short-term continuity in a cognitive map.

The Samsonovich and McNaughton model is consistent with data showing that the stability of the place cell representation is dependent on NMDA receptors (Kentros et al., 1998) and that place field locations remain consistent with each other but slowly drift in the absence of anchoring sensory cues or if the rat is consistently disoriented before each trial (Knierim et al., 1995). In addition, the involvement of some form of path integration is suggested by the increased influence of the boundary the rat is running from compared to the one it is running toward (Gothard et al., 1996; O'Keefe and Burgess, 1996; Redish et al., 2000). Note that the important role played by path integration in this model does not, conversely, imply that the hippocampus is necessary for guiding behavior in tests of path integration (e.g., Alyan and McNaughton, 1999). The role of the CA3 recurrent collaterals

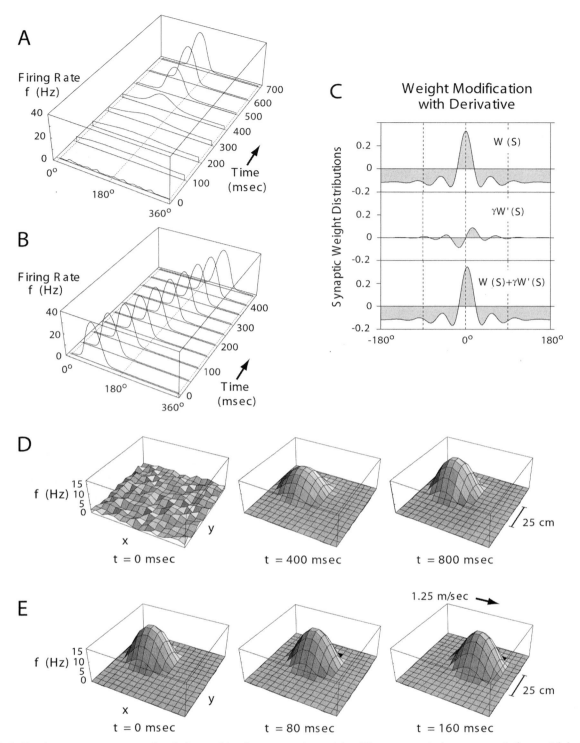

Figure 14–4. Continuous attractor networks of place and head direction cells (HDCs). *A*. Emergence of a stable firing profile from an arbitrary initial state in a network of HDCs arranged as a one-dimensional continuous attractor. The cells are indexed by their preferred firing direction and connected by weights with a symmetrical distribution (i.e., an even function of the difference between cell's tuning directions—see *C*, top row). *B*. Movement of the peak caused by an asymmetrical component in the weight distribution (see *C*, middle row). *C*. Distribution of connection weights in a one-dimensional attractor network (bottom row), showing a symmetrical component (top row) and an additional asymmetrical component (middle row). Note the slight asymmetry in the combined connec-tion weights. The asymmetrical component is the spatial derivative of the symmetrical component along the direction of drift, and its size (γ) determines the speed of drift of the represented head direction. *D*. Two-dimensional place cell network similar to the one-dimensional HDC network, showing emergence of a stereotyped stable firing profile from an arbitrary initial state, using symmetrical weight distribution (a Gaussian with constant inhibitory back-ground). *E*. As with the one-dimensional network, the addition of an asymmetrical component to the connection weights causes the represented location to drift (again, the asymmetrical component is the spatial derivative along the direction of drift, and its size deter-mines the speed of drift). (*Source*: Adapted from Zhang, 1996.)

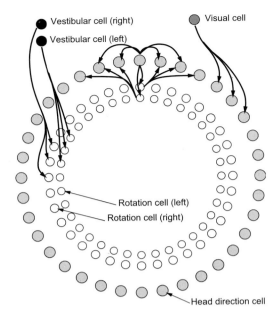

Figure 14–5. Skaggs et al.'s (1995) model of HDCs, showing the lateral connections among HDCs providing a continuous attractor and connections from left or right rotation cells, visual inputs, and vestibular inputs. The input from rotation cells serves the same purpose as the asymmetrical component of lateral connections in Figure 14–4. (Source: Adapted from Skaggs et al., 1995.)

in self-localization; forming the most accurate representation of location within a continuous attractor network given conflicting inputs was also stressed by Redish and Touretzky (1998). In addition, they elaborated the relation of this system

with other systems for path integration and for maintaining orientation (Touretzky and Redish, 1996). However, no specific mechanism has been proposed for the path integration. Because errors accumulate so rapidly in this system, it can be expected to behave very differently from a perfect system. The integration by place cells of visual inputs and inputs from a recurrently connected parietal system, and its relation to remapping, was explored further by Guazzelli et al. (2001).

Samsonovich and McNaughton suggested that remapping reflects the system switching between uncorrelated charts. This is a reasonable model of the situation after fast-remapping, which is consistent with each chart acting as an attractor (Wills et al., 2005), although in this case the charts would not be preconfigured but formed by the process of fast remapping. However, the model is not consistent with the situations in which individual place fields can move relative to each other in response to environmental change (e.g., O'Keefe and Burgess, 1996; Fenton et al., 2000). To fit these data requires feedforward inputs to dominate, replacing the model's main feature. The model is also not consistent with slow remapping (Lever et al., 2002) or partial remapping (e.g., Skaggs and McNaughton, 1998). The experimental conditions and neural mechanisms resulting in fast versus slow remapping are currently not well understood (Knierim, 2003).

Recurrent networks have also been used to model place field directionality, as modeled in a feedforward manner by Sharp (1991). In these models (Brunel and Trullier, 1998; Kali and Dayan, 2000), place cell firing is initially derived from orientation-specific sensory input at each location (referred to as the "local view" from that location), and the dynamics of the network are strongly dependent on the recurrent connec-

Figure 14–6. Place cell activity on a "chart." The activity of a population of 36 simultaneously recorded place cells shown symbolically distributed in the box (in which the rat foraged for food) each cell being placed at the center of its place field. Units on horizontal axes are centimeters. The animal is located at the center

of the square and is moving to the left and toward the viewer. The shape of the activity packet does not depend on velocity, acceleration, future trajectory of motion, or theta frequency. (*Source*: Samsonovich and McNaughton, 1997.)

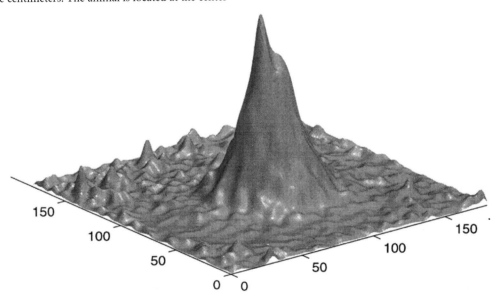

tions in CA3. If exploration is unconstrained and random, Hebbian learning in the recurrent collaterals of these models results in a continuous attractor of the sort hard-wired by Samsonovich and McNaughton and an orientation-independent place cell representation of space. One caveat to this is that the Hebbian learning must be modulated by novelty to prevent inhomogeneous exploration from causing highly nonuniform weight structures and unrealistic firing patterns (Kali and Dayan, 2000). Such novelty information has been suggested as a function of the cholinergic septal inputs to the hippocampus (Hasselmo et al., 1996; but see Hasselmo and Fehlau, 2001 and Lisman and Grace, 2005). As with Sharp (1991), in these models directionally constrained exploration results in orientation-dependent place fields.

Kali and Dayan (2000) also simulated the effects of changing the environment on the pattern of place cell firing. The model first learns a representation in one environment, as described above, and is then exposed to a second environment. If the second environment is sufficiently novel, the pattern of sensory input is assumed to be completely different and novelty-modulated learning is enabled. As a result, the system successfully learns a second, unrelated, place cell representation, corresponding to complete remapping. In simulations using two similar boxes (as in Skaggs and McNaughton, 1998), similar firing in the two boxes is imposed by similar sensory input, and the model is also shown to be capable of storing and recalling partially overlapping representations. Finally, if the second environment differs from the first only geometrically, the same sensory inputs are assumed to be used (but with different values, as the distances to boundaries have changed) and there is no new learning. This results in parametric changes to the pattern of firing. In this case, the effect of the recurrent collaterals is to preserve the relative spatial relation of the place fields and so acts to maintain the positions of fields in terms of the ratio of distances between boundaries (effectively scaling up the representation). By contrast, the sensory inputs are equivalent to the boundary vector cell model (O'Keefe and Burgess, 1996; Hartley et al., 2000) and so act to maintain the position of fields in terms of their absolute distance from boundaries. Thus, this model can account for both types of behavior. To fit the data in O'Keefe and Burgess (1996), the model should be dominated by the sensory input rather than the recurrent connections, as place fields tend to maintain a fixed distance to environmental boundaries in this experiment. By contrast, the apparently similar experiment of Muller and Kubie (1987) results in complete remapping. It is not yet clear whether models such as that of Kali and Dayan (2000), which depend on assigning different amounts of similarity to two environments, can capture the complexities of the data concerning remapping. For example, the differences between fast and slow remapping referred to above imply some learning in the feedforward connections (to model slow remapping, see, e.g., Barry et al., 2005; Fuhs and Touretzky, 2000), as well as in the recurrent connections (to model fast-remapping). Like Sharp's (1991) model, these recurrent models are also inconsistent with hints

that place cell firing in open fields is initially nondirectional but can become directional as a result of experience.

Finally, note that the recent discovery of grid cells in the dorsomedial entorhinal cortex (Hafting et al., 2005) are likely to have profound implications for ideas of hippocampal function. Each cell fires when the rat occupies multiple spatial locations laid out on a startlingly regular hexagonal grid. The orientation and scale of these grids seems to be constant in different environments and between different nearby cells. Overall, grids get larger as the recording site moves ventrolaterally. Because the grids of neighboring cells have the same orientation and scale and appear to have fixed offsets, it is possible that the recurrent connections between local sets of grid cells could be endlessly tuned to perform path integration, irrespective of the location of the animal, providing the continuous attractor envisaged in CA3 by Zhang (1996) and Samsonovich and McNaughton (1997). The stable association of each grid to the environment might occur via connections to place cells that, by virtue of generally having only a single firing location, could be associated with the environmental stimuli at that location. If this is correct, place cell firing could reflect the superposition of multiple grids that all overlap at the place field, and remapping could reflect changes in offset in these multiple inputs (O'Keefe and Burgess, 2005, see also Fuhs and Touretzky (2000) and McNaughton et al., (2006)).

14.3.4 Modeling Phase Coding in Place Cells

The origin of the intriguing phenomenon of the phase coding of place cell firing with respect to the concurrent theta rhythm of the EEG (O'Keefe and Recce, 1993) has been the subject of several computational models. Before considering these models, I briefly review the relevant experimental findings (see Chapter 11 for more details). The theta rhythm is a large-amplitude oscillation of around 6 to 10 Hz of the EEG and is present whenever the rat is moving its head through the environment. As the rat runs through a place field, the corresponding place cell tends to fire spikes with a systematic phase relation to the theta rhythm. On entering the field, spikes are fired at a "late" phase; as the rat passes through the field, spikes are fired at successively earlier phases so that on exiting the field the phase of firing may be up to 360° earlier (corresponding to an "early" phase). This effect is most pronounced when the rat runs repetitively in a directionally constrained manner (e.g., on a linear track). Interestingly, the phase of firing correlates better with the location of the rat in the place field than with other variables such as the time spent in the field or the instantaneous firing rate of the cell (Huxter et al., 2003).

The apparently tight coupling between location and phase implies that the phase of firing might depend on the sensory input driving the place cell in a simple feedforward way. Thus, O'Keefe (1990, 1991) proposed that each place cell might act as a phasor representing location relative to the centroid and eccentricity, or slope, of a subset of the sensory cues in an environment: the firing rate encoding proximity to the centroid and the phase relative to theta encoding the bearing to the centroid relative to the direction defined by the eccentricity, or slope, of the subset of cues. The advantages of the phasor representation for simple vector calculations were stressed in this model, but its easy relation to the subsequent experimental data on phase is at least as significant. Burgess et al. (1993) suggested a direct interpretation of phase of firing: that it could be used to separate place cells with fields ahead of the rat from those with fields behind the rat, which can be useful for navigation (see Section 14.4.2). This was subsequently verified experimentally (Burgess et al., 1994; Skaggs et al., 1996; Samsonovich and McNaughton, 1997). They also demonstrated that a phase shift in each individual cell is consistent with theta modulation of the net activity of the population of cells. In a simple feedforward model of place cell firing, Burgess et al. (1994) simulated the phase of firing as a function of the rat's position relative to the sensory cues that drove the cell. The input to entorhinal comes from pairs of "sensory" cells, each tuned to respond at a given distance from a particular sensory cue such that the maximum input amplitude occurs at the centroid of the two cues. The phase of firing of entorhinal cells was assumed to reflect the angle of the cue-centroid from the rat: firing at a late phase when driven by cues ahead of the rat and at an early phase when driven by cues behind the rat. This model is broadly consistent with the synchrony and oscillations seen in some sensory circuits (e.g., Nicolelis et al., 1995) but remains more qualitative than quantitative. Bose and Recce (2001) propose an alternative model that also accounts for the lack of phase shift seen in place cells when a rat runs in a running wheel (Hirase et al., 1999), involving the dynamics of the interaction of place cells and interneurons and the assumption that the frequency of the theta rhythm depends on running speed on the linear track but not in the running wheel. However, this picture became more complicated with the subsequent claim that phase shifting does occur in the running wheel at high firing rates (Harris et al., 2002).

An appealingly simple alternative feedforward model is possible (Mehta et al., 2000; Harris et al., 2002): The excitatory synaptic input to a place cell might increase as the rat runs through the place field, and the theta rhythm might reflect a sawtooth-shaped inhibitory input (i.e., inhibition decreasing through each cycle). In this model, the firing phase would advance simply because the increasing excitatory input manages to overcome the inhibitory input successively earlier in each cycle. The cause of the increasing excitatory input might reflect an exaggerated form of the asymmetry reported by Mehta et al. (1997) or an increasing then decreasing input but with lack of firing on the decreasing portion due to effects such as habituation (Harris et al., 2002). These models capture the observation that the phase shift becomes more reliable over the first few runs of a trial, as does the asymmetry of place fields (Mehta et al., 2002), and allows phase to be analyzed in terms of firing rate during nontranslational behaviors such as dreaming or wheel running (Harris et al., 2002). However, the correlation between phase and location is

stronger than that between phase and rate; and on the linear track at least, the weaker correlation is a side effect of the stronger one (O'Keefe and Burgess, 2005).

As with models of place cell firing, a second type of model of the phase shift stresses the recurrent connections in contrast to the feedforward connections. Indeed, simulations of the Samsonovich and McNaughton model, in which net activation is made to oscillate at the theta frequency, shows something qualitatively similar to the phase shift owing to path integration occurring within each cycle. That is, initially the set of active place cells settles to just those place cells with fields centered on the rat and then expands to include those with fields centered ahead of the rat. The first quantitative model of the phase shift was proposed by Tsodyks et al. (1996). In this model, the recurrent connections between place cells in CA3 are asymmetrically arranged so that each place cell projects to place cells farther along a learned path (see also Blum and Abbott, 1996, discussed below). External input to a CA3 place cell arrives at a fixed (early) phase of theta, causing place cell activity at this phase, which in turn propagates through the recurrent connections to place cells with fields farther along the path and causes them to fire. Overall activity is inhibited at the end of each theta cycle, preventing further propagation of activity into the next cycle. Thus, when the rat enters a place field, the corresponding cell starts to fire at a late phase owing to propagated activity from cells with fields earlier on the path; and it fires earlier during each cycle as the rat advances owing to activity having to propagate through fewer cells, until finally firing at the early phase is due solely to external inputs. Several similar mechanisms that depend on the association of place cells firing earlier along a learned path to those firing later along it have now been proposed (Jensen and Lisman, 1996; Touretzky and Redish, 1996; Wallenstein and Hasselmo, 1997). The Jensen and Lisman (1996) model makes interesting suggestions for the gamma rhythm, in separating the firing of cells corresponding to the current and successively farther advanced locations, and for the dynamics of NMDA channels, in separating each route retrieval into successive cycles of the theta rhythm. Wallenstein and Hasselmo (1997) emphasized the role of GABA$_B$ receptors in varying the relative influence of the inputs to CA1 from CA3 compared to those directly from entorhinal cortex (EC) over the theta cycle: allowing sensory (EC) input to dominate early and predictive input from CA3 to dominate late in the cycle.

These models fit nicely with the observations of Mehta et al. (1997, 2000): They produce a phase shift limited to 360° that is more strongly correlated with position than time, and that is greater for well learned paths than for random exploration. Interestingly, Mehta et al. (2000) suggested a similar model based on learned asymmetry in the connections from CA3 to CA1, the main testable difference here being that the phase shift should not be observed in CA3. Other aspects of these models seem less likely. First, because the initial firing of a place cell depends on both the externally driven activity of other cells and its propagation through the network, it seems likely that on cell-by-cell and run-by-run bases the initial phase of firing should be more variable than the (externally driven) final phase of firing. This is not the case in the data (Skaggs et al., 1996; Huxter et al., 2003). Second, one mechanism for producing the required asymmetrical connections is that suggested by Mehta et al., (2000). However, it has since been found that, although the development of asymmetry in place fields over the first few runs of a trial is prevented by blockade of NMDA receptors, the phase shift phenomenon is unaffected by this manipulation (Ekstrom et al., 2001).

A third type of model stresses the inherent oscillatory nature of some cellular processes, as did Jensen and Lisman (1996) for different reasons. Thus, O'Keefe and Recce (1993) pointed out that the phase and amplitude characteristics of place cell firing could be modeled as the interference pattern between an 11-Hz external input to the cell (perhaps the sensory input) and a 9-Hz external or internal oscillation corresponding to theta (perhaps driven by the septal input). This produces an oscillation of 10 Hz, corresponding to firing that shifts in phase relative to theta and a 1-Hz envelope, one-half cycle of which corresponds to the place field. This model has since been extended (Lengyel et al., 2003), identifying the first input as a voltage-controlled oscillation of the membrane potential (e.g., Hoppensteadt, 1986) in the dendrites and the second as an inhibitory input to the soma of fixed frequency. The frequency of the dendritic oscillation is assumed to increase above that of the somatic oscillation proportionally with the strength of the dendritic input, which is assumed to be zero outside the place field and proportional to the rat's running speed within it (McNaughton et al., 1983; Czurko et al., 1999; Ekstrom et al., 2001; Huxter et al., 2003). Thus, the two oscillations destructively interfere outside of the place field, whereas phase of firing relative to the somatic input within the field can shift more rapidly as the rat runs faster, preserving the relation between phase and location. In addition, the dendritic oscillation needs to be weakly driven in antiphase to the somatic input so in the absence of any dendritic input it returns to being in phase with it to ensure complete destructive interference. Recent corroborative evidence for interference models comes from the observation that the increase in place field size along the dorsoventral axis of the hippocampus parallels a corresponding decrease in the intrinsic firing frequency of place cells, reducing toward the theta frequency in more ventral regions (Maurer et al., 2005). Intriguingly, the full, repeating, interference pattern is expressed in the recently discovered entorhinal grid cells (McNaughton et al., 2006) as predicted by an inference model (O'Keefe and Burgess, 2005).

14.4 Hippocampus and Spatial Navigation

In this section we consider the contribution of hippocampal spatial representations to guiding behavior. I focus on large-scale spatial navigation, the spatial behavior most commonly associated with the hippocampus and medial temporal lobes

(see Chapter 13). This is comparable to behavior in smaller scale spaces and over shorter durations, such as visually guided reaching, which are most commonly associated with the posterior parietal lobe (e.g., Burgess et al., 1999). As with models of spatial representation, these models can be approximately divided into those stressing the role of feedforward connections and those stressing the role of recurrent connections.

14.4.1 Spatial Navigation: Data

Behavioral data indicate that rats learn about the spatial layout of their environment during exploration in the absence of explicit goals or rewards (e.g., Tolman, 1948). They can also profit from being placed at the goal location without having explored the rest of the environment (Keith and McVety, 1988). These processes are referred to as "latent learning." Rats also appear to be able to perform short cuts and detours. These abilities contributed to the idea that rats form a cognitive map of their environment rather than simply learning to associate individual stimuli with responses (Tolman, 1948; O'Keefe and Nadel, 1978). Of course, the learning of stimulus-response associations also plays an important role in spatial navigation, such as when the goal is directly visible or when a well learned turn or sequence of turns is to be performed. However, there seems to be good evidence that these types of behavior are less dependent on the hippocampus than those associated with cognitive mapping (O'Keefe and Nadel, 1978; Morris et al., 1982; Packard and McGaugh, 1996). These issues are dealt with in more detail in Chapter 13.

The other main spur to the association of the hippocampus with a cognitive map of the rat's environment was the discovery of place cells whose response is not easily described in terms of a simple response to a single stimulus. However, a gap remains between the properties of place cells and the properties required of a system for spatial navigation. Two features of place cell firing are particularly problematic. First, information about a place in an environment (i.e., firing of the corresponding place cells) can only be accessed locally (by actually visiting that place). Second, place fields appear to be no more affected by the location of the goal than by the location of any other cue. That is, place cells tell you only where you are currently and not where to go to get to your goal (Speakman and O'Keefe, 1990). A caveat to the first point may be indicated by the recording of "spatial view cells" in the macaque hippocampus (Rolls et al., 1997), which fire as a function of where the monkey is looking rather than where it is physically located.

14.4.2 Spatial Navigation: Feedforward Models

Zipser's (1986) "view field" model was built on the observation that in some circumstances place cell firing is modulated by the orientation of the rat. In this model, a set of orientation-dependent place cells, or "view-field units," become associated with a set of "goal units," which encode the direction to the goal relative to the current heading direction. So long as the appropriate cells become associated, the population vector of directions represented by the goal units guide the rat to the goal, as goal units driven by place cells representing the current location fire the most strongly. However, it is unclear how the directions to the goal would become associated with the place units if the goal were not visible. In a second model (the "beta coefficient" model), Zipser suggested that the location of the goal relative to subsets of landmarks is calculated and stored (as the coefficient of the linear sum of landmark locations that is equal to the goal location). In this model, learning at the goal location is sufficient, although the neural mechanisms required to implement the desired calculations are not explained. One possible route to enabling place cells to perform this type of computation was provided by the phasor model of O'Keefe (1991) (see above). A simplistic version of this type of model was simulated by Wilkie and Palfrey (1987), in which the distance of the goal from two landmarks is stored so that navigation back to the goal can be effected by moving so as to match these landmark distances.

Several models have followed Zipser's view field model in associating places to movements or local views. See Trullier et al. (1997) for a wider review of biologically based artificial navigation systems. McNaughton and Nadel (1990) suggested that routes might be learned as a chain of associations from a local view to an action and thence to the next local view, and so on. This model was not actually simulated, and simply storing routes is insufficient to enable spatial navigation (see Section 14.6). Even if a given route can be correctly selected in terms of the locations to which it leads, navigational abilities such as generating novel shortcuts and detours are beyond a simple route-based system. The task of accumulating route-independent spatial information faces several problems, including the "credit assignment" problem: deciding which actions along a route are critical for determining whether it eventually leads to the goal.

Brown and Sharp (1995) provided a more sophisticated model for associating locations with actions. In their model the possible actions in a place are represented by a left-turn cell and a right-turn cell (in nucleus accumbens) driven by each place cell. These "turn cells" receive modifiable connections from head-direction cells (HDCs), which support the rat's spatial learning. When the rat reaches the goal, connections between HDCs and turn cells are modified according to a recency-weighted index of their simultaneous activity. Thus, if turning left in a particular place when facing north leads immediately to the goal, the HDC representing north becomes more strongly associated with the left-turn cell driven by the corresponding place cell. The recency weighting of connection modification is designed to provide an approximate solution to the credit assignment problem (when applied over many trials) by effectively dividing credit according to the number of steps within which an action leads to finding the goal, see reinforcement learning (e.g., Dayan and Abbott, 2002) for a more principled approach. This model successfully simulates learning in the Morris watermaze but would not show latent learning; performance would not be affected by whether the rat can look around from the goal location; and navigation to

the goal would be strongly affected if stereotyped routes were used during learning.

A related way to think about spatial navigation is to imagine defining a surface over the environment such that gradient ascent on it leads to the goal. The simplest model of this sort is for the place cells to be connected to a goal cell via reward-modulated Hebb-modifiable connections such that encountering a goal causes strengthening of connections to it from the concurrently active place cells (Burgess and O'Keefe, 1996). The subsequent activity of the goal cell then increases with the proximity of the goal, as the net activity of those place cells with strengthened connections increases with the proximity to the goal (Fig. 14–7). The task for the rat in finding the goal is then to move in the direction that increases the rate of firing of the goal cell representing the desired goal (Fig. 14–7B). This type of model qualitatively captures the rapid nature of learning a goal location once place cell firing has become established and the ability to learn simply by being at the goal location rather than having to find it many times. However, finding the goal would involve the rat hunting around to determine the best direction in which to move. This behavior, known as vicarious trial and error, can be observed at choice points but is not common. A second problem raised by this model is the range over which spatial information is accessible. If there are no place cells that fire at both the goal location and the current location of the rat, there is no gradient in the firing rate of the goal cell (being locally zero). Hence, this type of model requires the population of place cells to include some cells that have nonzero firing rates at any two points in the environment, however far apart. Consideration of the population of place field shapes and sizes in the environments used so far (i.e., not more than about 2 m in diameter) indicate that this is quite probable (Hartley et al., 2000). However, whether this is true of larger environments is not known.

A more sophisticated model of navigation (Burgess et al., 1994) was proposed to make two improvements on the simple model above. The first was to be able to calculate the direction to the goal from any subsequent location after a single visit to the goal location without having to hunt around. The model made use of the fact that rats placed at the goal location like to rear up and look around and the supposition that place cells firing at a late phase relative to the theta rhythm have fields peaked ahead of the rat (see Section 14.3.4). The model posits a set of goal cells for each goal, such that each cell in a set is associated with a different head direction. The connections from place cells to a "north" goal cell are modified when the rat is at the goal and facing north and similarly for the goal cells associated with other directions. Crucially, connections are modified at "late" phases of the theta cycle so the active place cells (i.e., those from which connections are strengthened) are cells with fields ahead of the rat. Therefore, after spending at least one theta cycle at the goal facing in each direction, a north goal cell has strong connections from place cells with fields peaked to the north of the goal—and similarly for south, east, and west goal cells. As a consequence, a north goal cell's firing rate forms a surface over the environment that

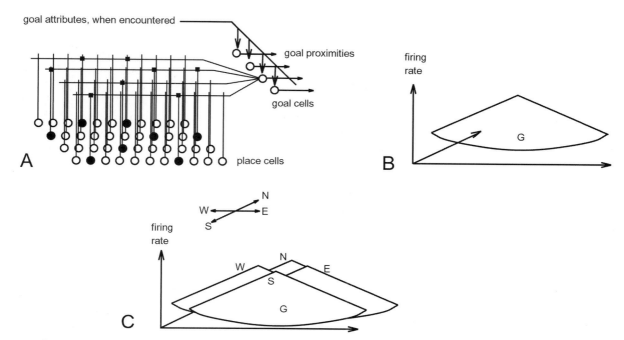

Figure 14–7. Simple model of place cells and navigation. *A.* A "goal" cell stores a goal's location by taking a snapshot of place cell activity via Hebbian synaptic modification when the goal cell is excited by the attributes of a particular goal location. Solid circles are active place cells; open circles are inactive place cells; and solid squares mark potentiated synapses between place cell axons and goal cell dendrites. *B.* Firing rate map of the goal cell (roughly an inverted cone) during subsequent movements of the rat codes for the proximity of the goal (G). *C.* Firing rate maps of four goal cells whose population vector codes for the goal location (G). Each is associated with the allocentric direction u_i in which the location of its peak firing rate is displaced from G; thus, the vector sum of the directions $\underline{u}_i$ weighted by the instantaneous firing rates f_i of the goal cells (i.e., $\Sigma_i f_i \underline{u}_i / \Sigma_i f_i$) codes for the direction of the rat from the goal, and the net firing rate of the goal cells (i.e., $\Sigma_i f_i$) codes for the goal's proximity. (*Source*: Adapted from Burgess and O'Keefe, 1996.)

is peaked to the north of the goal location—and similarly for south, east, and west goal cells (Fig. 14–7C). This is useful for subsequent navigation, as the rat can now use the relative firing rates of the various goal cells to indicate the direction of the goal. If the rat is to the north of the goal, the north goal cell has a higher firing rate than the south goal cell. More precisely, the population vector (Georgopoulos et al., 1986) of a set of goal cells successfully indicated the direction of the rat from the goal in simulations, and different sets of goal cells can be used simultaneously to indicate different locations of interest. Conversion to egocentric (e.g., left or right) movement directions was envisaged to take place in the parietal cortex or basal ganglia, given knowledge of the current head direction (Burgess et al., 2001a).

The second improvement was to ameliorate the problems of the range over which spatial information is available from place cell firing. The proposed solution was to interpose a set of subicular cells between the place cells and goal cells. Given weaker inhibitory competition between subicular cells than between place cells, competitive learning in the connections from place to subicular cells during exploration causes the subicular cells to build up larger firing fields, each effectively composed of several place fields. This learning is goal-independent and corresponds to latent learning in preparing the ground for effective one-shot learning of the location of any goals should they be encountered. Large spatial firing fields in subicular cells are consistent with experimental data

(Sharp and Green, 1994), and larger place fields have since been found in the ventral hippocampus (Jung et al., 1994) that might also serve this purpose.

To model hippocampal navigation Foster et al. (2000; see also Dayan, 1991) used "temporal difference" learning in which the "state" corresponds to the place cell representation of the rat's current location, and its value reflects the expected number of steps to reach the goal (one unit of reward is received on reaching the goal). Temporal difference learning (Sutton and Barto, 1988) can be implemented by simply connecting place cells to "actor" and "critic" units with connections that are adjusted according to a modified Hebbian rule. Activation of the critic unit is the evaluation of the current state (the expected future reward from that state, discounted by distance into the future—e.g., Dayan and Abbott, 2002), a more principled analogue of the simple goal cell above. The set of action units, only one of which can be active at a given time, represent movements North, South, and so on. At each step the connection weight from a place cell to the critic unit or to the active actor unit is adjusted by an amount proportional to the place cell's activity times the amount by which the reward exceeds that expected from the change in the activity of the critic unit (Fig. 14–8). This type of learning is consistent with a role for dopaminergic modulation of LTP (e.g., Montague et al., 1996; Schultz et al., 1997). Over many routes to the goal, ideally involving performing all actions at all locations many times, this rule causes (1) the critic to provide an accurate esti-

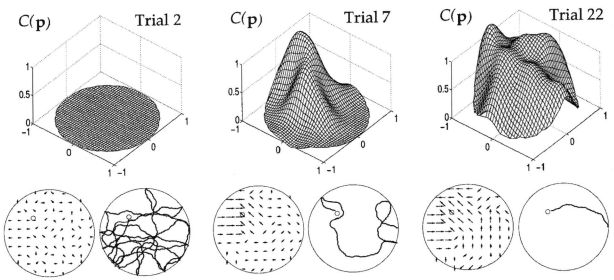

Figure 14–8. Learning in the actor-critic system in a watermaze. The plots for each trial show the critic's value function C(p) (above), the preferred actions at various locations (below left; the length of each arrow is related to the probability that the particular action shown is taken), and a sample path (below right). Trial 2: After a timed-out first trial, the critic's value function remains zero everywhere, the actions point randomly in different directions, and a long and tortuous path is taken to the platform. Trial 7: The critic's value function having peaked in the northeast quadrant of the pool, the preferred actions are correct for locations close to the platform but not for locations further away. Trial 22: The critic's value function has spread across the whole pool and the preferred actions are close to correct in most locations, so the actor takes a direct route to the platform. (Source: Foster et al., 2000.)

mation of value and (2) the appropriate actions to be associated with each state (Fig. 14–8). For a given configuration of goal and environment, this can provide the optimal strategy, which is not the case with the approximate recency weighting (see Brown and Sharp, 1995, above; Blum and Abbott, 1996, below) or, if obstacles are present, with goal cells simply indicating the physical proximity of the goal (Burgess et al., 1994). However, learning is both experience-dependent and goal-dependent (e.g., to know to head north from a given place results from this combination having previously led to the goal) and so perhaps does not capture the characteristics of the *hippocampal* contribution to spatial learning.

To simulate goal independent learning over many trials in which the location of the goal changes, Foster et al. (2000) proposed that a second system learns to form a coordinate representation of the rat's position by using the rat's locally accurate ability to estimate self-motion. The place cells are connected to two units that learn to estimate the x and y coordinates of the rat, again using temporal difference learning to adjust connection weights. In this system, the change in a connection weight to the x unit is proportional to the place cell activation times the amount by which the change in x, as estimated by self-motion, exceeds that estimated by the change in the activity of the x unit. The explicit representation of x and y coordinates enables accurate navigation after one exposure to the goal and so corresponds well with latent learning. However, it is not clear if such a representation actually exists in the brain, or if it would necessarily be more useful than a place field-like representation that covered the appropriate length scales (e.g., Burgess et al., 1994).

14.4.3 Spatial Navigation: Feedback Models

As well as being linked with spatial representation and associative memory (see Box 14–2), the CA3 recurrent collaterals have also been proposed to play a role in spatial navigation. The first model to formalize such a role was suggested by Muller et al. (1991, 1996) and focused on the Hebb-associative effects of LTP on the recurrent collaterals. If pre- and postsynaptic firing within a short time interval leads to a small increase in synaptic strength, the firing of place cells as the rat moves around an environment leads to the strength of a connection between two place cells depending on the proximity of their place fields. This occurs simply because the greater the overlap between place fields the more often they fire near-coincidentally during random exploration. Muller et al. (1996) showed that after extensive exploration the synaptic strengths represent a "cognitive graph," each approximately representing the minimum path length between the centers of the place fields of the cells it connects. Their model proposes that the rat navigates by moving through the place fields of the cells most strongly connected to the cells with fields at the current and destination positions. This mechanism, reminiscent of a resistive grid (Connelly et al., 1990), works well but relies on a graph search. It is not easy to imagine how such a process could be implemented in a biologically plausible fashion, given the apparent lack of influence of the goal location on the firing of place cells (Speakman and O'Keefe, 1990). One suggestion (Gorchetchnikov and Hasselmo, 2002) is that activation corresponding to the goal location occurs in entorhinal cortex while activation corresponding to the current location occurs in CA3. Activation in each region spreads along the available paths (although more slowly in CA3 than entorhinal cortex) until a commonly activated location is detected in CA1. This location represents the next immediate destination for the rat, although how this information is interpreted in terms of whether to turn left or right is not described.

In a related model, Blum and Abbott (1996) make use of the temporal asymmetry of LTP to strengthen recurrent connections from CA3 place cells that fire early on the rat's path to those that fire later along it. This causes the activation of place cells to spread backward along the path (see also Mehta et al., 1997, 2000 and models of spatial representation, above). If the firing of place cells is interpreted by systems downstream of CA3 as representing the location of the rat, this shift in firing (backward along the path) would be interpreted as a shift in the location of the rat forward along the path. Blum and Abbott suggested that navigation along a previously performed route could be undertaken by moving from the current location (e.g., read from CA1) to the shifted location represented in CA3, although how this could be implemented was not described. To enable navigation to a goal location, the rules for synaptic change were modified to be proportional to the amount of pre- and postsynaptic activation weighted by how recently it occurred prior encountering the goal (i.e., modification similar to that suggested by Brown and Sharp, 1995, above).

It is interesting to note that the symmetrical pattern of connection strengths learned in Muller et al.'s model resembles that used in continuous attractor models of place cell firing and so also serves to produce a consistent pattern of activity to represent each location (see above). By contrast, the additional asymmetry in connection strengths learned in Blum and Abbott's model serve to shift the represented location along the learned route. Indeed, the latter property has been shown to allow the represented location to move smoothly along the route over time, suggested as a model for mental replay during sleep (Redish and Touretzky, 1998). The goal-independent encoding of spatial proximity (as in the symmetrical connections of Muller et al.'s cognitive graph) or of previously traveled routes (as in the asymmetrical connection of the later models) correspond to latent learning. However, the way these models incorporate a new goal location necessarily requires many trips to the goal and thus probably falls short of a rat's abilities. Another drawback associated with these models is that none makes clear the details of how the rat's brain might deduce the direction it should move in or if it would be able to generate a short-cut or detour. They also assume place fields of fixed relative location but might still make some interesting predictions regarding the locus of search in environments that had changed in shape or size. To build up a true distance metric in complex environments would take a long time, in common with the reinforcement learning approaches (see Foster et al., 2000, above).

These models can be viewed in the context of a more general set of higher-level algorithms for navigation based on directed graphs. Lieblich and Arbib (1982) described a "world graph" in which locations are represented as nodes connected by (asymmetrical) edges that represent the movement necessary to get from one node to the next. In terms of the navigation of autonomous agents, Scholkopf and Mallot (1995) described a "view graph" in which the local view or sensory perception at given locations form the nodes and the actions required to get from one view to the next form the edges. See also McNaughton and Nadel (1990) for a description of how a view graph might be implemented in the hippocampus. Mallot and Gillner (2000) argued that such view graphs are a good model for human navigation despite their simplicity. One key requirement for building a world graph is to be able to decide whether to assign a new node to a location. This can be done on the basis of its familiarity (see Touretzky and Redish, 1996; Kali and Dayan, 2000, for models relating to this) or possibly on the basis of the sequence of actions that lead back to a location. Lieblich and Arbib further suggested that the nodes of a world graph might also represent a location's motivational valence and thus become a general model for goal-directed behavior, even though its creation might correspond to latent learning.

14.5 Hippocampus and Associative or Episodic Memory

In contrast to the vast amount of animal work linking hippocampal damage to deficits in spatial memory, the major impairment noted in humans following bilateral damage to the hippocampus is amnesia: a much more general impairment in memory. The extent of this impairment into various subdivisions of memory and into information acquired prior to the damage is a contentious issue (see Chapter 12). Here I briefly review the data on human hippocampal function in memory, introduce the generic model for it derived from Marr's seminal paper in 1971, and discuss various details and developments of this model over the years.

14.5.1 Hippocampus and Memory: Data

Substantial bilateral damage to the hippocampus and medial temporal lobes almost invariably leads to amnesia, characterized as a drop in the memory component of the intelligence quotient (MIQ) of at least 20 points relative to full-scale IQ. Because only a relatively small number of cases of damage restricted to the hippocampus have been studied, it is difficult to draw general conclusions regarding its role in memory, in contrast to the roles of the surrounding cortical areas. However, some general points can be made (see Spiers et al., 2001 and Chapter 12 for details). They include a ubiquitous deficit in memory for personally experienced events that occur after the lesion (i.e., an "anterograde" deficit in "episodic" memory) and spared procedural and working memory. The extent of retrograde amnesia (loss of memory for information acquired prior to the lesion) appears to vary across patients and possibly across types of information (Nadel and Moscovitch, 1997). Memory loss can extend over the entire lifetime or can be restricted to shorter periods prior to the damage; but it does seem to be relatively limited in the case of lesions to the fornix. More controversial findings include relative sparing of semantic memory (memory for facts) and of familiarity-based recognition in some cases of focal hippocampal damage. Relative sparing of recognition memory is consistent with findings in monkeys showing that this type of memory is perhaps more strongly dependent on nearby cortical areas (e.g., Gaffan, 1994; Zola-Morgan et al., 1994; Aggleton and Brown, 1999; Baxter and Murray, 2001). Finally, it should be noted that the human hippocampus, particularly in the right hemisphere, is also involved in spatial navigation (Burgess et al., 2002).

14.5.2 Marr's Hippocampo-neocortical Model of Long-term Memory

Most modeling work on the role of the hippocampus in memory can be considered part of a long tradition reaching back to Marr (1971). In this section I sketch the main components of Marr's model, which provide a common framework for all of the subsequent models, and indicate how these components correspond to various aspects of the data on human memory (see also Willshaw and Buckingham, 1990; Burgess et al., 2001a). I refer to this as the generic hippocampo-neocortical model (Fig. 14–9).

In Marr's (1971) model, events in the outside world are represented by patterns of activity in neocortical areas. The role of the hippocampus is to store these representations over the short term so relevant events can be categorized and stored for the long term in neocortex (see Marr's 1970 model of the cerebral neocortex). This is achieved by mapping the

Figure 14–9. Generic hippocampo-neocortical model of long-term memory. Strong connections and active cells are shown in black. Relatively dense recurrent connections and sparse representations in the hippocampus enable efficient pattern completion. Connections between neocortex and hippocampus allow the hippocampal representation of an event to be associated with its sensory details, including reactivation of the representations in various neocortical areas dealing with different sensory modalities. Abstracted semantic representations may also be learned over time in the neocortex. The recurrent connections in each neocortical area allow unimodal recognition. (Source: Burgess et al., 2001a.)

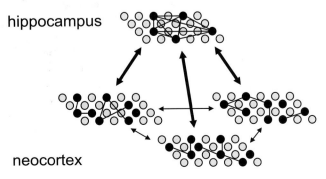

neocortical representation of an event into a "simple representation" in hippocampus, with modifiable connections to and from the hippocampus storing the mappings between the full representation and the simple representation. The CA3 recurrent collaterals are modified to store the simple representation as an associative memory—so if a simple representation is incompletely activated, the "collateral effect" results in the full representation being recovered. Thus, partial activation of the neocortical representation of an event can lead to complete reactivation of its simple representation in the hippocampus, which in turn can reactivate the entire neocortical representation. In Marr's view, the capacity of the hippocampal system should be enough to store a day's events so the process of categorization and long-term storage in neocortex can take place during the following night's sleep. Note that this now seems at odds with the much larger extent of retrograde amnesia following hippocampal lesions, and the possibility that some types of information (e.g., episodic, in contrast to semantic) remain forever dependent on the hippocampus (Nadel and Moscovitch, 1997). Marr further suggested that the simple representations need reflect only those parts of the event through which they are addressed, and that they should be sparsely encoded to reduce possible interference between representations. The sparseness of a representation refers to the fraction of neurons that are active: If this fraction is low, the chance of the same neuron being active in the representation of different events is small, and interference between representations is minimized.

It should be noted that the proposed capacity of the hippocampus has varied widely in subsequent models, as memories remain hippocampus-dependent for more than 1 day and possibly never become fully independent of it (see below). The issue of "capacity" itself is also confounded by the need to specify how to divide continuous experience into discrete binary patterns. Another confusing issue is the correspondence between Marr's rather abstract generic model of memory and the processes of retrieval in human memory. For example, it is not clear whether the model refers to recognition or recollection, where the incomplete retrieval cue comes from, or whether the model applies more to memory for some kinds of information than others. With regard to retrieval cues, the prefrontal cortex probably plays an important role in the strategic organization of retrieval, taking this issue beyond the scope of this chapter (e.g., Roberts et al., 1998). By the end of Section 14.5 some of the other issues are resolved, and others are discussed further in Section 14.6.

14.5.3 Associative Memory and the Hippocampus

Much of the development and analysis of the generic model has followed from basic research on the associative properties of feedforward networks (e.g., Willshaw et al., 1969) and recurrent networks (Kohonen, 1972; Gardner-Medwin, 1976; Hopfield, 1982) based on Hebbian learning (Fig. 14–10). Much of the initial development of the model concentrated on matching the major anatomical properties of the hippocam-

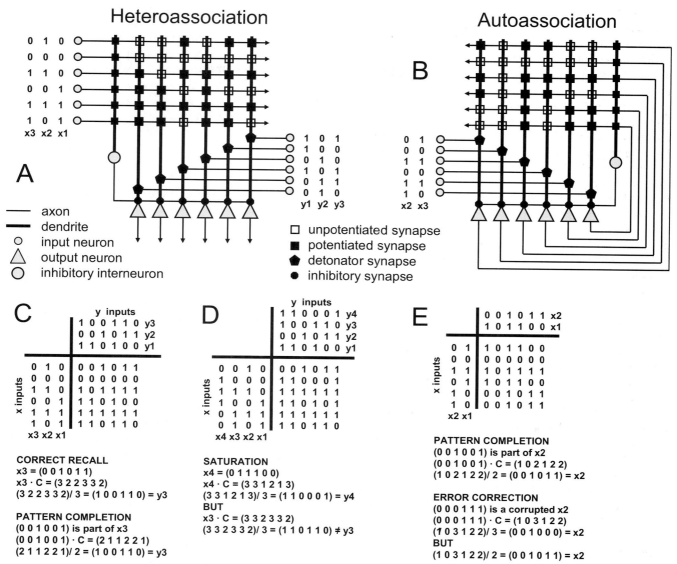

Figure 14–10. Biological implementation of associative memory in the hippocampus. *A.* Heteroassociative network associates pattern of activity y1 with input x1, and y2 with x2, and so on to form an associative memory. (The matrix of connection weights shown in *A* is the result of successive presentations of input pattern x1 and output pattern y1, x2 and y2, x3 and y3 to an initially blank matrix.) This enables input x1 to reproduce activation y1. Even an incomplete or corrupted version of x1 can reproduce y1 (see *C*). Storing too much information leads to "saturation" of the system and retrieval failures (see *D*). *B.* Autoassociative network associates pattern x1 with itself, x2 with itself, and so on to form an autoassociative memory. This enables an incomplete or corrupted pattern to be cleaned up (see *E*). The essential functional components of these networks are a set of powerful "detonator" synapses that can impose the pattern of activity to be stored, a set of extensively connected inputs with modifiable synapses, and a set of inhibitory interneurons whose role is to set a divisive threshold for the activity of the cells. *C–E.* Details of associative memory using the correlation matrix formalism (Willshaw et al., 1969; Kohonen, 1972). Pairs of binary vectors (e.g., x1, y1) are presented to the system for storage. A Hebbian learning rule is used: A synaptic connection is strengthened (set to 1 from 0) given pre- and postsynaptic activity (i.e., both inputs set to 1). Because the net input to a cell is the sum of inputs multiplied by the strength of the connection mediating it, the net input to a cell corresponds to the number of active inputs arriving via strengthened connections. To fire, the net input to a cell must equal the number of currently active inputs. Thus, retrieval of a vector given its corresponding paired associate is achieved by matrix-vector multiplication (e.g., pattern y3 in *A* is extracted by multiplying the matrix rows by corresponding elements of vector x3 and summing the columns) followed by integer division by the number of active bits in the input vector. Provided not too many patterns have been stored, any unique subset of an x vector can recall the correct y vector. The autoassociative cases (*B* and *E*) work as the heteroassociative cases (*A*, *C*, *D*), with output y1 = input x1, y2 = x2, and so on. (*Source:* Adapted from McNaughton and Nadel, 1990.)

pus (see Chapter 3), with constraints on the representations and learning mechanisms indicated by functional analysis of associative memory (see Figs. 14–10 to 14–12). The first major attempt of this sort (McNaughton and Morris, 1987) highlighted the potential contribution of the dentate gyrus (DG).

First, the much larger number of projection cells in the DG (around one million granule cells in the rat) than in either the entorhinal cortex (EC) (around 200,000 layer II cells project into the hippocampus) or region CA3 (around 300,000 pyramidal cells) indicate that it could be used for "pattern separation" (Amaral et al., 1990). This means that distinct (i.e., nonoverlapping) patterns of activation are created in the DG despite similarity in patterns of EC activation representing similar events. This process is also referred to as orthogonalization. Thus pattern completion in CA3, so important for retrieving the representation of a familiar event, does not lead to a similar novel event also causing retrieval of the representation of the familiar event. Of course, one cannot have perfect pattern completion of the representation of an event from partial cues *and* perfect pattern separation of it from the representations of similar events in the same system. One mechanism must fail once the partial cue is less similar to the old event than the new event.

Second, the specific nature of the various synaptic inputs to CA3 pyramidal cells suggests different functions for them. The input from DG comes from a small number (around 46) of very large synapses around the soma. A much large number of connections are received farther up the dendrites from within CA3 (up to 12,000), and up to 3750 connections are received from the EC onto the distal apical dendrites. It was suggested (McNaughton and Morris, 1987) that the powerful input from DG (via "detonator synapses") serve to impose a new pattern of activity to be learned. A strong input is required to impose a new pattern of activity in CA3 in the face of the interference due to feedback via the recurrent connections, which tend to cause the system to return to a previously stored pattern of activity. Once the representation of a new event has been imposed, the Hebbian modification of both the recurrent connections and the connections from EC can

Figure 14–11. Anatomy of the inputs to CA3 pyramidal cells, showing the approximate number of synapses onto each cell in the rat. (Adapted from Treves and Rolls, 1992.)

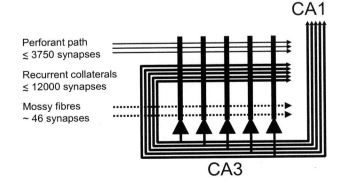

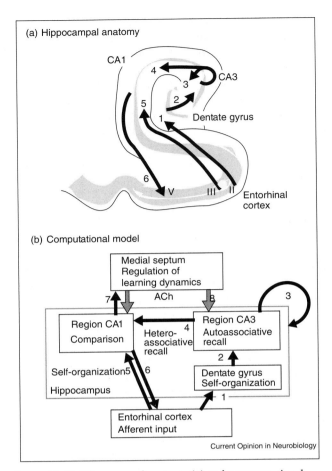

Figure 14–12. Hippocampal anatomy (*a*) and a computational model of hippocampal episodic memory function (*b*). Numbers label synaptic connections mediating various functions in the model. 1: Synapses of the perforant path fibers projecting from entorhinal cortex layer II to the dentate gyrus undergo sequential self-organization to form sparse, less overlapping representations of entorhinal activity patterns. 2: Mossy fibers projecting from dentate gyrus to region CA3 transfer dentate gyrus activity to CA3. 3: Excitatory recurrent connections in region CA3 mediate autoassociative encoding and retrieval of the features of episodic memories. 4: Schaffer collaterals from region CA3 to CA1 encode and retrieve associations between CA3 activity and activity patterns induced by entorhinal input to region CA1. 5: Perforant path input to region CA1 undergoes self-organization, forming new representations of entorhinal cortex input for comparison with recall from CA3. 6: Projections from region CA1 to deep layers of the entorhinal cortex store associations between CA1 activity and entorhinal cortex activity, allowing representations in CA1 to activate the associated patterns in entorhinal cortex. 7: Output from region CA1 to the medial septum regulates cholinergic modulation. 8: Cholinergic modulation from the medial septum sets appropriate dynamics for encoding in hippocampus. (*Source*: Hasselmo and McClelland, 1999.)

occur. The large number of recurrent synapses per cell allow large autoassociative memory capacity, and the large number of synapses in the input from EC allow large heteroassociative memory capacity in associating the EC representation to the CA3 representation (Treves and Rolls, 1992) (Fig. 14–11).

Third, the requirements of Hebbian learning in the CA3 recurrent connections and the connections from EC to CA3, but not in the connections from the DG, are consistent with the physiology of these various connections. The synapses in the former two pathways are thought to be capable of NMDA receptor-dependent LTP, whereas the mossy fiber connections from DG show only non-Hebbian modification (see Chapter 10). Equally, the divisive normalization required by associative nets (Willshaw et al., 1969) (see Box 14–2) is consistent with the action of interneurons providing inhibition by opening ion channels near the soma-to shunt input current in the dendrites (Fig. 14–10). Further analysis of autoassociative memory indicates that "progessive recall" improves performance (Gardner-Medwin, 1976). With this model, inhibition is slowly reduced during retrieval so the first few cells that become active are the most likely to be correct, and feedback from their activation decreases the chances of subsequent erroneous activation. Such periodic fluctuation of inhibition (or, equivalently, the cells' firing threshold) may provide a functional interpretation for the theta rhythm.

In Marr's model an incomplete or incorrect neocortical representation feeds into the hippocampus, where the correct hippocampal representation is retrieved and feeds back to complete or correct the neocortical representation. This simple picture has been elaborated to include separate input and output representations in the entorhinal cortex (in the superficial layers and deep layers, respectively). The processes of storage and retrieval obviously do not start and end at the entorhinal cortex. The processes of feedforward cueing of a representation, its pattern completion and feedback can be modeled as occurring sequentially in the cortical areas between sensory cortex and entorhinal cortex (Rolls, 1996). The principal difference between the processes in the hippocampus and EC and those in lower cortical areas are the additional pattern separation provided by the DG and the greater autoassociative power of the much longer-range recurrent collaterals in CA3 compared to cortex. The long-range recurrent collaterals in CA3 also provide the best opportunity to associate information from different sensory modalities. Many of the above ideas are reviewed or developed further in the literature (e.g., Amit, 1989; McClelland et al., 1995; Rolls and Treves, 1997; Hasselmo and McClelland, 1999; Redish, 1999).

14.5.4 Hippocampal Representation, Context, and Novelty

The above considerations of sparseness and pattern separation regarding the hippocampal representation of an event raise the issue of how these representations relate to the various elements of its content and context. First note that the conflicting processes of pattern separation and pattern completion serve to define the similarity space of retrieval (i.e., which dimensions a retrieval cue can vary along but still retrieve the event and which dimensions serve to discriminate events). In the limit of complete orthogonalization in the dentate gyrus, the hippocampal representations are independent of the details of the events and can be thought of as simply an index for them (Teyler and DiScenna, 1986). However, as the hippocampal representation must initially be activated by the neocortical representation, the overall memory system is still "content addressable" and its behavior (e.g., pattern separation or pattern completion) depends on how different aspects of an event and its context contribute to the activation of its hippocampal representation. This relates to Marr's observation that the hippocampal representation should include those aspects of an event used for its retrieval.

In a simple associative memory, all elements of the representation of the event are equally associated with all other elements. However, as implied by Marr, it seems plausible that some aspects of an event are better able to cue associative retrieval than others, and other aspects of an event can be associatively retrieved more easily than others. Thus, the "simple representations" envisaged for the hippocampus would reflect some aspects more than others. A related suggestion is that the hippocampal representation reflects efficient compression of the neocortical representations—extracting the distinguishing features of each event (Gluck and Myers, 1996). For example, the name of someone you met only once is often a good cue to recalling the meeting but can be difficult to retrieve, whereas the location of the meeting is often both a good cue and relatively easy to retrieve. Similar to someone's name, the sequential position of an item in a list is easier to use as a cue than it is to retrieve (Jones, 1976). Thus, even the simplest associative model of memory should include asymmetrical associations between the elements of an event.

One of the distinguishing features of episodic memory is the ability to retrieve the ongoing context within which the event occurs (Gardiner and Java, 1993; Tulving, 1993; Knowlton and Squire, 1995), and one suggestion for the role of the human hippocampus is that it provides the spatiotemporal context for episodic memory (O'Keefe and Nadel, 1978). Theoretical analyses of associative memory have also made the distinction between the content of the event and its context (e.g., Raaijmakers and Shiffrin, 1981) or between the record of the event and the "header" or index term used to reference it (e.g., Morton et al., 1985). One possibility is that the hippocampus serves to associate the content of the event with its context (e.g., Wallenstein and Hasselmo, 1997) (see Section 14.6). A related possibility is that the role of the hippocampus is to generate a representation of temporal context itself (e.g., slowly varying patterns of activity generated by its own recurrent dynamics) (Levy, 1996). This type of model coincides with a considerable psychological literature of models of memory in which retrieval of stored items is held to depend, at least in part, on their association with a representation of context that changes slowly with time or experience. In some of these models the context representation changes independently of the to-be-remembered items (Mensink and Raaijmakers, 1988; Burgess and Hitch, 1992; Davelaar et al., 2005), whereas in others the context representation is derived from the items themselves (Howard and Kahana, 2001).

Retrieval corresponds to finding the item most strongly associated with a re-presented context.

I briefly describe the operation of one of these models, the temporal context model, as I return to it in the section on models attempting to draw links between the medial temporal roles in spatial and episodic memory. As the with other models of episodic memory described above, item representations are associated with context representations such that a given item is retrieved according to the similarity between the context at retrieval and that associated with the item. However, in this model the context representation is derived from the presented or retrieved items themselves, becoming a recency-weighted sum of the context arising from each item. After presentation of the list, the context vector is most similar to the most recent items, producing the well known recency effect. In addition, when an item is presented, it affects the context vector with which subsequent items are associated. Thus, recall of a given item changes the context vector so that retrieval of immediately subsequent items in the list is more likely (by making the context vector more similar to how it was when those items were presented). This leads to an asymmetry such that forward associations in the list are stronger than backward associations, as is often found with free recall.

Consideration of the different requirements of encoding and retrieval also raises some interesting questions. Notwithstanding McNaughton and Morris's suggestion that "detonator synapses" from the dentate gyrus can impose a new pattern of activation on CA3 despite the retrieval-related feedback from recurrent connections, there must be some mechanism to determine whether the system should be in encoding or retrieval mode (McNaughton and Morris, 1987). One proposal is that the supply of acetylcholine (ACh) from the medial septum switches the hippocampus between encoding and retrieval modes (Hasselmo et al., 1995; Murre, 1996; Wallenstein and Hasselmo, 1997). In this model, increased ACh increases the rate of synaptic modification of the recurrent connections in CA3 and suppresses the synaptic transmission of intrinsic activity (within CA3 and from CA3 to CA1), enabling new patterns of activity to be stored. The level of delivery of ACh is determined by the novelty of the neocortical input, as represented by direct activation of CA1 from EC, compared to the most similar previously stored event, as represented by the input to CA1 from CA3 after it settles to a stored state. Specifically, if both CA3 and entorhinal cortex inputs to CA1 are matching (as with a familiar stimulus), strong activation of CA1 activates interneurons in the medial septum, which decrease the activity of the cholinergic cells projecting to the hippocampus (Fig. 14–12).

Two types of evidence support this model. First, by emphasizing the connections between the hippocampus and the medial septum, the model begins to address data showing the importance of the fornix, the large fiber bundle connecting the hippocampus with the medial septum and other subcortical structures. In the model, sectioning the fornix prevents the learning of new memories due to lack of ACh, which corresponds well to reviews of the effects of damage to the fornix in neuropsychological patients (e.g., Spiers et al., 2001) (see Chapter 12). Second, blocking the ACh receptors prior to encoding (by injecting scopolamine) seems to impair recall more strongly than recognition (Hasselmo and Wyble, 1997). This is also the case in the model, assuming that CA3 serves to associate events and their contexts because recall is more reliant on these associations than recognition. However, disruption of the hippocampus might also impair recall more than recognition in many other models (e.g., due to disrupting associations with context) (see Section 14.6). In addition, more recent work has begun to include the role of dopamine in novelty and encoding (Lisman and Grace, 2005).

14.5.5 Consolidation and Cross-modal Binding of Events in Memory

Ever since the initial reports of dense anterograde amnesia but weaker or temporally graded retrograde amnesia after bilateral medial temporal lobectomy (Scoville and Milner, 1957) (see Chapter 12 and the caveats in Section 14.5.2), researchers have considered how the hippocampus contributes to the long-term consolidation of memories. One mechanism for consolidation, consistent with the preservation of information acquired prior to hippocampal damage, is that the hippocampus enables information to be stored elsewhere in the brain after which it is no longer needed for retrieval. Marr's (1971) model follows this view, suggesting that the day's events are stored in the hippocampus and that this information is used to allow long-term categorization and storage in the neocortex. Note that processes of temporal consolidation might also occur in the hippocampus (i.e., without transfer of information from one region to another).

The experimental data regarding the gradient of retrograde amnesia (i.e., the sparing of memories acquired sufficiently long enough before the damage) is inconsistent and remains controversial in animals (see Chapter 13) and humans (see Chapter is 12) (Spiers et al., 2001). One problem in the human data is that the amnesia often extends back to childhood, implying that the hippocampus stores several decades worth of information. Several computational arguments have also been put forward for the transfer of information out of the hippocampus for consolidation in the neocortex. Marr (1971) suggested that a short-term buffer is needed to store information online (i.e., the hippocampus), whereas only information deemed relevant to the animal's future needs to be incorporated into the animal's long-term store of knowledge and must be first appropriately categorized with respect to it. The hippocampal store of unprocessed experience necessarily has a limited capacity, and the process of abstracting relevant information from this experience to expand a long-term database requires extensive offline processing, perhaps during sleep (see also McClelland et al., 1995).

A second argument concerns the anatomical convergence of information from difference sensory modalities at the hippocampus. Thus, in the absence of long-range connections between different sensory cortical areas, associations between the elements of an event, such as its sight, sound, and smell, cannot be formed in the lower-level cortices. Damasio (1989) suggested that "convergence zones" must exist where these associations could be formed. Several models have extended this idea to include rapid learning of a hippocampal, or medial temporal lobe, representation reciprocally connected to all the unimodal cortical representations of the event which allows them to be associated with each other (Alvarez and Squire, 1994; Murre, 1996; Moll and Miikkulainen, 1997). These models also suggest that, after multiple rehearsals of a memory driven by the hippocampus, long-range associations can be learned directly between the unimodal representations, finally making the stored information independent of the hippocampus.

The arguments regarding data abstraction and anatomical convergence are represented in a model by Kali and Dayan (2004). In this model the hippocampus serves to aid the learning of a hierarchical semantic system by being able to reinstate the top-level (i.e., entorhinal/ perirhinal/ parahippocampal) representation of events during sleep. The semantic system contains reciprocal connections between higher cortical areas and those immediately below them in the hierarchy but no direct connections between areas at the same level. Aided by the hippocampus, the neocortical system learns to form an associative representation of patterns of activation in lower cortical areas. This is achieved by the higher level representations learning a "generative model" of representations lower in the hierarchy (e.g., Hinton and Sejnowski, 1999). Thus higher-level representations can be cued by input from a subset of lower cortical areas and can then cause pattern completion in all lower areas via the reciprocal connections. During further simulations, Kali and Dayan (2004) noted that regular reactivation of episodic hippocampal representations is required to maintain them in register with the slowly changing semantic representations.

A third argument for consolidation refers to the effects of interference. In some learning systems—such as using a fixed feedforward structure and the error back-propagation learning rule (Rumelhart et al., 1986) to form associations consistent with a set of examples—new information can interfere with previously stored information, sometimes "catastrophically" such that all information is lost. This problem can also occur with associative memories (Fig. 14–10). McClelland et al. (1995) proposed a solution to this in which long-term neocortical learning involves random interleaved re-presentation of all previous knowledge along with newly acquired knowledge to produce a single integrated neocortical representation of semantic knowledge. Note, however, that this mechanism requires the temporary store to have capacity for the entire data set. Other solutions include associative memories with continuous but bounded connection weights (Hopfield, 1982) and "constructive" algorithms in which the addition of new information is accompanied by the addition of new processing units (Gallant, 1986; Mezard and Nadal, 1989; Fahlman and Lebiere, 1990; Frean, 1990). The latter algorithms may relate to the recent observation of neurogenesis in the adult dentate gyrus that is related to learning (Shors et al., 2001).

A reinterpretation of the experimental data regarding the gradient of retrograde amnesia associated with medial temporal lobe damage led Nadel and Moscovitch (1997) to a different conclusion regarding consolidation. Noticing that in many instances retrograde amnesia extends back over a much longer time than that envisaged by Marr, they proposed that the hippocampus remains necessary for the retrieval of detailed episodic or spatial information (but for evidence that early spatial memories become hippocampus-independent see Teng and Squire, 1999; Rosenbaum et al., 2000). They proposed a new model to account for both the common occurrence of a temporal gradient in memory for other types of information and the possibility of partial damage to the hippocampus in some cases. In this model, whenever a memory is rehearsed or reactivated, a new hippocampal representation is formed, again connected to all of the neocortical representations. The result is that although a complete lesion of the medial temporal lobe impairs retrieval of all memories, the older the memory, the more robust it is to partial damage by virtue of being represented in multiple locations. Some evidence for the reactivation of specific memories comes from the recently revived study of reconsolidation (Nader et al., 2000). In these experiments re-presentation of the context of an event (usually application of an electric shock) appears to render the memory for the event labile in the sense that protein synthesis is again required for long-term storage of the memory, as is the case when the event is first experienced.

14.5.6 Hippocampal Contributions to Various Types of Memory and Retrieval

A distinction has been made between retrieval of episodic information, retrieval of semantic information, and familiarity-based recognition (see Chapter 12). Episodic retrieval is characterized by the ability to retrieve detailed information about the event and its context. Semantic retrieval is characterized by factual knowledge without retrieval of the individual events and contexts in which it was acquired. Familiarity-based recognition depends purely on an unattributable feeling of familiarity associated with a stimulus in the absence of detailed information about the event and context in which it was encountered. Of these three processes, the hippocampus is claimed to be primarily involved in episodic retrieval (e.g., Aggleton and Brown, 1999) (see Chapter 12).

The hippocampo-neocortical model suggests that semantic knowledge is abstracted from combinations of hippocampal memories of unique events, but eventually becomes independent of the hippocampus. This is consistent with memory for the unique content and context of a specific event (episodic memory) depending on the hippocampus but semantic memory depending on other areas of the temporal lobe (e.g., Graham and Hodges, 1997). It is also consistent with the suggestion of Nadel and Moscovich (1997) that semantic memories show a temporal gradient of retrograde amnesia, whereas detailed episodic memories do not. The model is less obviously consistent with the observation that semantic information can be acquired despite early bilateral hippocampal pathology (Vargha-Khadem et al., 1997). However, the possibility of partial sparing of the hippocampus (Squire and Zola, 1998) or the use of external rehearsal of information (Baddeley et al., 2001) might provide explanations for these developmental cases within the framework of the model.

The distinction between episodic retrieval and familiarity-based recognition also has interesting parallels in the hippocampo-neocortical model. It has been argued that the hippocampus is required to provide associations between representations in disparate cortical areas, whereas associations within each area can be formed locally. Thus, effects mediated by the familiarity of single stimuli might be supported by the association of elements within each of the neocortical areas, independent of the hippocampus. By contrast, correct recognition of a pair of cross-modal associates among equally familiar distractors would require the hippocampus. Evidence indicates that simple recognition memory does not depend on the hippocampus but on nearby neocortical areas (Zhu et al., 1996; Baxendale et al., 1997; Vargha-Khadem et al., 1997; Murray and Mishkin, 1998; Aggleton and Brown, 1999; Wan et al., 1999; Holdstock et al., 2000; Baddeley et al., 2001: but see also Manns and Squire, 1999; Zola et al., 2000). In contrast, there is some evidence that recognition of cross-modal associations is impaired by bilateral damage restricted to the hippocampus (Vargha-Khadem et al., 1997; Holdstock et al., 2000). More extensive unilateral damage may also impair the binding of elements within the same modality (Kroll et al., 1996). The logical extension of this idea is that episodic memory requires full recollection of an event and its context in all of its multimodal detail and so requires an intact hippocampus.

Much of the analysis of the differential role of the hippocampus in episodic retrieval (or "recollection"), and familiarity-based recognition has focused on the idea that these two processes contribute independently to the performance of recognition memory tests (e.g., Yonelinas, 2002). In forced choice and yes–no recognition paradigms, the recollective component is assumed to be "all or nothing" and "high-threshold." That is, the stimulus is recalled in great detail or not at all, and a novel foil is never falsely recalled. By contrast, the familiarity-based process is more like a signal detection problem: The subject guesses whether the item is familiar, informed by a noisy measure of familiarity (see Chapter 13). The hippocampus has been associated with the recollective component (Aggleton and Brown, 1999; Yonelinas et al., 2002) and so should provide a high-threshold, all-or-nothing mechanism in recognition memory tests. One method for detecting this component involves the receiver-operator characteristic (ROC) curve: the plot of the proportion of previously seen items that are correctly identified ("hits") versus the proportion of new items incorrectly identified ("false alarms") as a function of the subject's confidence in their response. Recollection is marked by high-confidence hits in the absence of high-confidence false alarms, producing a positive intercept in the ROC curve. See Chapter 13 and Rugg and Yonelinas (2003) for a review.

The hippocampal contribution to recognition memory (via "recollection") can be modeled by using the stimulus-driven medial temporal neocortical representation as the cue to retrieval of a stored pattern of activation in CA3 and comparing the retrieved activation to the stimulus-driven activation in the entorhinal cortex (Norman and O'Reilly, 2003). By explicitly retrieving an entire stored pattern, the process is all-or-nothing, and even foils that resemble presented patterns and are not falsely recognized because the retrieval product still differs from the stimulus-driven activation. The use of sparse hippocampal representations, orthogonalized via the dentate gyrus, serves to prevent interference between different stored events. By contrast, familiarity-based recognition is modeled in terms of "sharpening" of the neocortical representation. With this model, although a new item is represented by weak activation of a large number of neocortical neurons, repeated presentation of the item results in strong activation of a smaller number of neocortical neurons via a competitive learning mechanism. Activation of the neocortical neurons that fire in response to a given stimulus can then be used as a measure of familiarity-based recognition. One advantage of this scheme is that repeated presentations of some items in a list does not impair recognition of the other items in the list, as seen experimentally (Ratcliff, 1990), which is not true of some other psychological models of recognition memory (Norman, 2003). A characteristic of this model is that hippocampal damage specifically impairs recognition memory when related lures (novel items that resemble previously seen items) are included in the test. The familiarity-based recognition mechanism would produce false alarms to these stimuli, whereas the hippocampal recollection mechanism would not. Some evidence consistent with this hypothesis has been found (Holdstock et al., 2002).

14.6 Reconciling the Hippocampal Roles in Memory and Space

In this section I discuss some of the models that have attempted to draw together the common strands present in the plethora of hippocampal models reviewed above. One feature common to most of the spatial and nonspatial models is use of the autoassociative properties of the recurrent network in CA3. Even feedforward models of spatial representation (see Section 14.3.2) usually note that the various sets of cells used to represent different environments might be stored in this way (e.g., McNaughton and Nadel, 1990; Burgess et al., 1994; Kali and Dayan, 2000).

Many other models concern the common functional requirement of storing and retrieving a *sequence* of patterns of activation. For example, Redish and Touretzky (1998) used replay of a spatial route as a demonstration of episodic recall. In Levy's (1996) model, the slowly varying patterns of activity (resulting from the presence of asymmetrical connections in CA3) (see Section 14.3.3) might be used as a context representation, associations to which could store sequences of memories. In a rat moving through its environment, it is argued that they might also resemble place fields, although it is not clear that this would be the case for a trajectory that crosses itself. Jensen and Lisman's (1996, 2005) model of long-term memory and working memory, involving association of one item to the next and preservation of serial order during each theta cycle, is also applied to model the storage of routes as sequences of place fields.

However, spatial navigation is not just a subset of episodic memory; simply storing routes and sequences of places would not enable accurate navigation, detours, or shortcuts. These require a metric or at least a representation of proximity (see Section 14.4.2). Put another way, specific constraints apply to spatial information that are not necessarily required of a more general memory system. What then is the relation between the constraints involved in spatial and episodic memory such that a unique structure, the hippocampus, might support both? O'Keefe and Nadel (1978) argued that the spatial function seen in the rat hippocampus is augmented by a linear sense of time in humans, which allows the human hippocampus to supply the spatiotemporal context of events required by episodic memory. This idea has been taken up by two types of model: one investigating the provision of temporal context and the other the provision of spatial context.

Following the models of Levy (1996) and Jensen and Lisman (1996) described above, Wallenstein et al. (1998) investigated the idea that the hippocampus could provide a signal representing temporal context as a solution to the need to form associations between temporarily discontiguous events. Associating events that occur much farther apart in time than the time scale required for pre- and postsynaptic activity to induce LTP (i.e., around 100 ms) (see Chapter 10) obviously requires some kind of bridging mechanism. One indication that the hippocampus is involved in this process comes from "trace conditioning," in which the animal must learn to respond at a fixed delay after the disappearance of a cue, because the timing of the response is disrupted by hippocampal lesions. This contrasts with "delay conditioning" in which the cue does not disappear, for which there is no hippocampal lesion effect (see Chapter 13). In Wallenstein et al. (1998), as with Levy (1996), unsupervised learning in the hippocampus in the presence of temporally correlated inputs creates patterns of activity that vary more slowly in time than the original stimuli (Fig. 14–13). Associations between the various states of this temporal context signal can allow the original stimuli to be reproduced in order. Indeed, this type of mechanism provides a good model for short-term serial recall (Burgess and Hitch, 2005). This model can be extended to spatial navigation in terms of associations between spatially discontiguous events, but note that, as with storing temporal sequences to aid navigation, temporal contiguity alone is insufficient to generate metric information.

Howard et al. (2005) attempted to draw parallels between the roles of the hippocampal region in both spatial and episodic memory by extending the "temporal context model"

(TCM) of free recall (Howard and Kahana, 2001), described above, to model the noisy place-specific firing of some cells in entorhinal cortex (Quirk et al., 1992; Frank et al., 2000; Fyhn et al., 2004). To model free recall, the TCM forms a context representation derived from a recency-weighted sum of the contributions to context from the nature of the list items themselves. Howard et al. proposed that, in terms of spatial memory, these context contributions might be encoded by neurons with firing rates reflecting running speed in particular head directions. If each context neuron performed a recency-weighted sum of one of these inputs, they would be effectively supporting an approximate route memory, or "path integration." In simulations, these cells show noisy place-specific firing, rather like some cells in the entorhinal cortex, as they fire most following a series of movements along their preferred direction (e.g., a cell with a west head direction input fires most along the west edge of the environment). They also show "retrospective coding": that is, modulation of firing by the recent history of movements, as found by Frank et al. (2000). In addition, cells whose firing rate reflects the time integral of their input have been found in entorhinal cortex (Egorov et al., 2002), and systematic errors in path integration have been found that are consistent with recency weighting (Etienne et al., 1996). However, the model predicts that entorhinal cell firing is directionally selective and always peaks at the edge of the environment, which may not be the case (Fyhn et al., 2004). This idea of entorhinal processing may also have to be reviewed in the light of the discovery of grid cells (Hafting et al., 2005) (see Section 14.3.3).

The idea of using spatial context to index memory was combined with Marr's hippocampo-neocortical model to produce a simple navigation system (Recce and Harris, 1996). In this model, perceptual representations of the environment are stored in parietal cortex and retrieved via an index representation in the hippocampus corresponding to the location of the animal. This allows retrieval of the correct perceptual map for a given location. Navigation additionally requires that the location of an encountered goal be added to the perceptual maps (the mechanism for this is not specified). A more detailed model of long-term memory and retrieval of a spatial environment (Becker and Burgess, 2001) also serves as a model of memory for the spatial context of an event (Burgess et al., 2001a) (Fig. 14–14). This model explicitly makes use of the constraints associated with spatial information, and our detailed knowledge of how it is represented in the brain. The representations of spatial layout in long-term memory are assumed to be allocentric (e.g., independent of the orientation of the person) in contrast to the egocentric short-term representations involved in perception, action, and working memory (Goodale and Milner, 1992; Burgess et al., 1999; Milner et al., 1999). By extension from spatial models of the hippocampus (Hartley et al., 2000), the geometry of the environment is encoded in (parahippocampal) boundary vector cells bidirectionally connected to (hippocampal) place cells. The place cells are connected up to form a continuous attractor. This

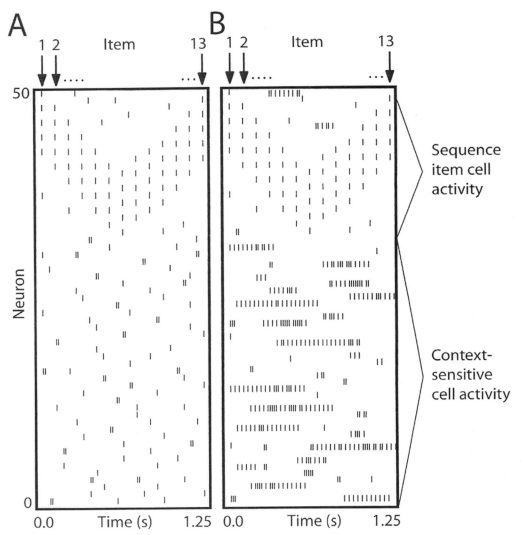

Figure 14–13. Context field development. Each rectangle shows a subset of 50 simulated pyramidal cells firing across time, each action potential represented by a vertical line. A unique group of five cells firing at the same time encodes a single item in a 13-item sequence (see the top portion of each rectangle). This can be thought of as afferent activation of CA3 pyramidal cells due to a specific pattern of sensory events. *A.* Note the background firing during the first learning trial that does not encode sequence items directly. This stems from activity at recurrent excitatory synapses. Repeated exposure to the same sequence can lead to enhanced synaptic potentiation between cells firing in the background and cells that encode sequence items owing to a simple Hebbian learning rule. *B.* After the fourth learning trial, this repeated potentiation leads to a condition where background cells begin to respond to the appearance of contiguous segments of the entire sequence. The portion of the full sequence to which the cell responds is called the "context field" of the cell. Because the context fields overlap, the entire sequence can be reconstructed by interdigitating them in the proper order. (*Source*: Wallenstein et al., 1998.)

acts as a spatial memory system in that partial activation of boundary vector cells (representing the occurrence of particular large objects at particular distances and bearings) causes activation of the corresponding place cells, which then activate the boundary vector cells representing the remaining landmarks in the environment. The location of a specific event is represented by a goal cell, as in the simple model of navigation (Burgess and O'Keefe, 1996) (see Section 14.4.2). Bidirectional connections between place cells and these "event" cells allows for both navigation to the location (via the feedforward connections) and retrieval of its spatial context (via the feedback connections).

Retrieval of allocentric spatial information into a format appropriate for visual imagery requires that it be translated into an egocentric reference frame. Accordingly, in the model, the parahippocampal boundary vector cell representation (arranged in terms of distances and bearings) is translated successively into trunk-centered then head-centered representations by networks designed for this purpose to model posterior parietal cortex (e.g., Pouget and Sejnowski, 1997).

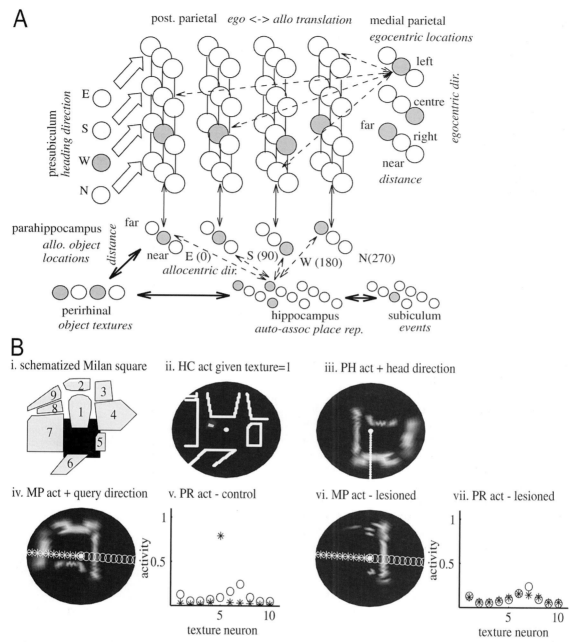

Figure 14–14. *A.* Functional architecture of the model for encoding and retrieving the spatial context of an event. Neurons shown in gray illustrate a possible pattern of activation corresponding to an imagined location with extended landmarks nearby to the west, far away to the north, and at intermediate distances east and south; the imagined westerly heading direction means that these landmarks are imagined as far to the right, near straight ahead, and at an intermediate distance to the left (and behind, but this is not in view). (*Source*: Burgess et al., 2001a.) *B.* Simulation of retrieving spatial information in the Milan square experiment of Bisiach and Luzzatti (1978). i: Training consists of simulated exploration of the square (shaded area, north is up). The system is cued to imagine being near the cathedral (i.e., the perirhinal cell for the texture of building 1 and parahippocampal cell for a building at a short distance north are activated), and the hippocampal-parahippocampal-perirhinal system settles. ii: The hippocampus settles to a location in the northwest corner of the square (hippocampal cell activity shown as the brightness of the pixel corresponding to the location of each cell's place field). iii: The parahippocampus correctly retrieves the locations of the other buildings (parahippocampal cell activity shown as the brightness of the pixel for the location encoded by each cell, relative to the subject at the center). The line indicates that the imagined head direction is south. iv: Medial parietal (MP) cell activity. The parahippocampal map has been correctly rotated given head direction south (straight ahead is up); stars indicate a direction of inspection to the left, circles to the right. v: Perirhinal (PR) cell activations correctly showing building 5 to the left and building 7 to the right. vi: Effect of a right parietal lesion on the medial parietal representation (note lack of activation on the left) and perirhinal activations (vii). Note the decrease in activation of building 5 when inspection is to the left. (*Source*: Adapted from Becker and Burgess, 2001.)

Likewise, forming an allocentric representation from egocentric perception requires translation in the reverse direction. Visual imagery occurs in medial parietal areas using the final head-centered representation with the intermediate representations buffered in retrosplenial cortex. This model is consistent with the observation of hemispatial neglect in imagery following parietal damage (e.g., Bisiach and Luzzatti, 1978) and functional imaging of the retrieval of spatial context (Burgess et al., 2001b). It also provides an explanation for the involvement of Papez's circuit (see Chapter 3) in supporting both episodic memory (see Chapter 12) and the representation of head direction (see Chapter 11). Finally it implies a strong link between episodic recollection (and its neural bases) and mental imagery.

14.7 Conclusions

As in other areas of neuroscience, the ability to specify a proposed mechanism of hippocampal function in terms of a computational model has been invaluable in many ways. First, it reduces ambiguity and "hypothesis drift." Second, it enables quantitative simulation of the resulting behavior. At the very least this can serve as a demonstration of the viability of a given proposal. Beyond this, it enables quantitative predictions to be made at the levels of cells, systems, and behavior regarding the effects of experimental manipulations. Some of the models reviewed here have been used to make such predictions and have also contributed to the design of experiments to test them. Many questions for future research are prompted by these models, not least the possibility of comparing or combining the influences of spatial and temporal contexts as retrieval cues. Because any worthwhile theory must make potentially falsifiable predictions, computational modeling has a crucial role to play in the development of the field. Investigating the link between the properties of cells interacting in a complex system such as the brain to the resulting behavior of the animal would become almost impossible without the aid of computational models.

ACKNOWLEDGMENTS

I am pleased to acknowledge useful discussions with Peter Latham and John O'Keefe, and the support of the Medical Research Council, UK.

REFERENCES

Aggleton JP, Brown MW (1999) Episodic memory, amnesia, and the hippocampal-anterior thalamic axis. *Behav Brain Sci* 22:425–490.

Alvarez P, Squire LR (1994) Memory consolidation and the medial temporal lobe: a simple network model. *Proc Natl Acad Sci USA* 91:7041–7045.

Alyan S, McNaughton BL (1999) Hippocampectomized rats are capable of homing by path integration. *Behav Neurosci* 113:19–31.

Amaral DG, Ishizuka N, Claiborne B (1990) Neurons, numbers and the hippocampal network. *Prog Brain Res* 83:1–11.

Amit DH (1989) *Modelling brain function.* Cambridge, UK: Cambridge University Press.

Amit DJ (1992) *Modeling brain function: the world of attractor neural networks.* Cambridge, UK: Cambridge University Press.

Baddeley AD, Vargha-Khadem F, Mishkin M (2001) Preserved recognition in a case of developmental amnesia: implications for the acquisition of semantic memory? *J Cogn Neurosci* 13:357–369.

Barry C, Lever C, Hayman R, Hartley T, Burton S, O'Keefe J, Jeffery KJ, Burgess N (2006) The boundary vector cell model of place cell firing and spatial memory. *Rev Neurosci* 17:71–97.

Baxendale SA, Van Paesschen W, Thompson PJ, Duncan JS, Shorvon SD, Connelly A (1997) The relation between quantitative MRI measures of hippocampal structure and the intracarotid amobarbital test. *Epilepsia* 38:998–1007.

Baxter MG, Murray EA (2001) Opposite relationship of hippocampal and rhinal cortex damage to delayed nonmatching-to-sample deficits in monkeys. *Hippocampus* 11:61–71.

Becker S, Burgess N (2001) A model of spatial recall, mental imagery and neglect. *Adv Neural Inform Proc Syst* 13:96–102.

Bienenstock EL, Cooper LN, Munro PW (1982) Theory for the development of neuron selectivity: orientation specificity and binocular interaction in visual cortex. *J Neurosci* 2:32–48.

Bisiach E, Luzzatti C (1978) Unilateral neglect of representational space. *Cortex* 14:129–133.

Blair HT, Sharp PE (1995) Anticipatory head direction signals in anterior thalamus: evidence for a thalamocortical circuit that integrates angular head motion to compute head direction. *J Neurosci* 15:6260–6270.

Blair HT, Lipscomb BW, Sharp PE (1997) Anticipatory time intervals of head-direction cells in the anterior thalamus of the rat: implications for path integration in the head-direction circuit. *J Neurophysiol* 78:145–159.

Blair HT, Cho J, Sharp PE (1998) Role of the lateral mammillary nucleus in the rat head direction circuit: a combined single unit recording and lesion study. *Neuron* 21:1387–1397.

Blum KI, Abbott LF (1996) A model of spatial map formation in the hippocampus of the rat. *Neural Comput* 8:85–93.

Bose A, Recce M (2001) Phase precession and phase locking of hippocampal pyramidal cells. *Hippocampus* 11:204–215.

Bostock E, Muller RU, Kubie JL (1991) Experience-dependent modifications of hippocampal place cell firing. *Hippocampus* 1:193–205.

Brown MA, Sharp PE (1995) Simulation of spatial learning in the Morris watermaze by a neural network model of the hippocampal formation and nucleus accumbens. *Hippocampus* 5:171–188.

Brunel N, Trullier O (1998) Plasticity of directional place fields in a model of rodent CA3. *Hippocampus* 8:651–665.

Burgess N, Hartley T (2002) Orientational and geometric determinants of place and head-direction. In: *Neural information processing systems 14*, pp 165–172. Cambridge, MA: MIT Press.

Burgess N, Hitch GJ (1992) Toward a network model of the articulatory loop. *J Mem Language* 31:429–460.

Burgess N, Hitch GJ (2005) Computational models of working memory: putting long term memory into context. *Trends Cogn Sci* 9:535–541.

Burgess N, O'Keefe J (1996) Neuronal computations underlying the firing of place cells and their role in navigation. *Hippocampus* 6:749–762.

Burgess N, O'Keefe J, Recce M (1993) Using hippocampal 'place cells' for navigation, exploiting phase coding. In: *Neural information processing systems 5* (Hanson SE, Cowan JD, Giles CL, eds), pp 929–936. San Francisco: Morgan Kaufmann.

Burgess N, Recce M, O'Keefe J (1994) A model of hippocampal function. *Neural Netw* 7:1065–1081.

Burgess N, Jeffery KJ, O'Keefe J (1999) Integrating hippocampal and parietal functions: a spatial point of view. In: *The hippocampal and parietal foundations of spatial cognition* (Burgess N, Jeffery KJ, O'Keefe J, eds), pp 3–29. Oxford, UK: Oxford University Press.

Burgess N, Maguire E, O'Keefe J (2002) The human hippocampus and spatial and episodic memory. *Neuron* 35:625–641.

Burgess N, Becker S, King JA, O'Keefe J (2001a) Memory for events and their spatial context: models and experiments. *Philos Trans R Soc Lond B Biol Sci* 356:1493–1503.

Burgess N, Maguire EA, Spiers HJ, O'Keefe J (2001b) A temporoparietal and prefrontal network for retrieving the spatial context of lifelike events. *Neuroimage* 14:439–453.

Cacucci F, Lever C, Wills TJ, Burgess N, O'Keefe J (2004) Theta-modulated place-by-direction cells in the hippocampal formation in the rat. *J Neurosci* 24:8265–8277.

Cohen MA, Grossberg S (1983) Absolute stability of global pattern formation and parallel memory storage by competitive neural networks. *IEEE Trans Syst Man Cybern* 13:815–821.

Connelly CI, Burns JB, Weiss R (1990) Path planning using Laplace's equation. In: *Proceedings of the 1990 IEEE international conference on robotics and automation*, pp 2102–2106.

Cressant A, Muller RU, Poucet B (1997) Failure of centrally placed objects to control the firing fields of hippocampal place cells. *J Neurosci* 17:2531–2542.

Czurko A, Hirase H, Csicsvari J, Buzsaki G (1999) Sustained activation of hippocampal pyramidal cells by 'space clamping' in a running wheel. *Eur J Neurosci* 11:344–352.

Damasio AR (1989) The brain binds entities and events by multiregional activation from convergence zones. *Neural Comput* 1:123–132.

Davelaar EJ, Goshen-Gottstein Y, Ashkenazi A, Usher M (2005) A context activation model of list memory: dissociating short-term from long-term recency effects. *Psychol Rev* 112:34–53.

Dayan P (1991) Navigating through temporal difference. In: *Neural information processing systems 3* (Lippman RP, Moody JE, Touretzky DS, eds), pp 464–470. San Mateo, CA: Morgan Kaufmann.

Dayan P, Abbott LF (2002) Computational neuroscience. Cambridge, MA: MIT Press.

Deneve S, Latham PE, Pouget A (2001) Efficient computation and cue integration with noisy population codes. *Nat Neurosci* 4:826–831.

Dominey PF, Arbib MA (1992) A cortico-subcortical model for generation of spatially accurate sequential saccades. *Cereb Cortex* 2:153–175.

Droulez J, Berthoz A (1991) A neural network model of sensoritopic maps with predictive short-term memory properties. *Proc Natl Acad Sci USA* 88:9653–9657.

Egorov AV, Hamam BN, Fransen E, Hasselmo ME, Alonso AA (2002) Graded persistent activity in entorhinal cortex neurons. *Nature* 420:173–178.

Ekstrom AD, Meltzer J, McNaughton BL, Barnes CA (2001) NMDA receptor antagonism blocks experience-dependent expansion of hippocampal "place fields." *Neuron* 31:631–638.

Ekstrom AD, Kahana MJ, Caplan JB, Fields TA, Isham EA, Newman EL, Fried I (2003) Cellular networks underlying human spatial navigation. *Nature* 425:184–188.

Etienne AS, Maurer R, Seguinot V (1996) Path integration in mammals and its interaction with visual landmarks. *J Exp Biol* 199:201–209.

Fahlman S, Lebiere C (1990) The cascade-correlation learning architecture. In: *Neural information processing systems 2* (Touretzky DS, ed), pp 524–532. San Francisco: Morgan Kaufmann.

Fenton AA, Csizmadia G, Muller RU (2000) Conjoint control of hippocampal place cell firing by two visual stimuli. I. The effects of moving the stimuli on firing field positions. *J Gen Physiol* 116:191–209.

Foster DJ, Morris RG, Dayan P (2000) A model of hippocampally dependent navigation, using the temporal difference learning rule. *Hippocampus* 10:1–16.

Frank LM, Brown EN, Wilson M (2000) Trajectory encoding in the hippocampus and entorhinal cortex. *Neuron* 27:169–178.

Frean MR (1990) The Upstart algorithm: a method for constructing and training feedforward neural networks. *Neural Comput* 2:198–209.

Fuhs MC, Touretzky DS (2000) Synaptic learning models of map separation in the hippocampus. *Neurocomputing* 32:379–384.

Fuhs MC, Touretzky DS (2006) A spin glass model of path integration in rat medial entorhinal cortex. *J Neurosci* 26:4266–4276.

Fyhn M, Molden S, Witter MP, Moser EI, Moser MB (2004) Spatial representation in the entorhinal cortex. *Science* 305:1258–1264.

Gaffan D (1994) Dissociated effects of perirhinal cortex ablation, fornix transection and amygdalectomy: evidence for multiple memory systems in the primate temporal lobe. *Exp Brain Res* 99:411–422.

Gallant SI (1986) Three constructive algorithms for network learning. In: *Proceedings of the 8th annual conference of the Cognitive Science Society*, pp 652–660.

Gardiner JM, Java RI (1993) In: *Theories of memory* (Collins A, Gathercole S, Morris P, eds), pp 168–188. Hillsdale, NJ: Erlbaum.

Gardner-Medwin AR (1976) The recall of events through the learning of associations between their parts. *Proc R Soc Lond B Biol Sci* 194:375–402.

Georgopoulos AP, Schwartz AB, Kettner RE (1986) Neuronal population coding of movement direction. *Science* 233:1416–1419.

Gluck MA, Myers CE (1996) Integrating behavioral and physiological models of hippocampal function. *Hippocampus* 6:643–653.

Goodale MA, Milner AD (1992) Separate visual pathways for perception and action. *Trends Neurosci* 15:20–25.

Goodridge JP, Touretzky DS (2000) Modeling attractor deformation in the rodent head-direction system. *J Neurophysiol* 83:3402–3410.

Gorchetchnikov A, Hasselmo ME (2002) A model of hippocampal circuitry mediating goal-driven navigation in a familiar environment. *Neurocomputing* 44–46:423–427.

Gothard KM, Skaggs WE, McNaughton BL (1996) Dynamics of mismatch correction in the hippocampal ensemble code for space: interaction between path integration and environmental cues. *J Neurosci* 16:8027–8040.

Graham KS, Hodges JR (1997) Differentiating the roles of the hippocampus complex and the neocortex in long-term memory storage: evidence from the study of semantic dementia and Alzheimer's disease. *Neuropsychology* 11:77–89.

Guazzelli A, Bota M, Arbib MA (2001) Competitive Hebbian learning and the hippocampal place cell system: modeling the interaction of visual and path integration cues. *Hippocampus* 11:216–239.

Hafting T, Fyhn M, Molden S, Moser MB, Moser EI (2005) Microstructure of a spatial map in the entorhinal cortex. *Nature* 436:801–806.

Harris KD, Henze DA, Hirase H, Leinekugel X, Dragoi G, Czurko A, Buzsaki G (2002) Spike train dynamics predicts theta-related phase precession in hippocampal pyramidal cells. *Nature* 417:738–741.

Hartley T, Burgess N, Lever C, Cacucci F, O'Keefe J (2000) Modeling place fields in terms of the cortical inputs to the hippocampus. *Hippocampus* 10:369–379.

Hasselmo ME, Fehlau BP (2001) Differences in time course of ACh and GABA modulation of excitatory synaptic potentials in slices of rat hippocampus. *J Neurophysiol* 86:1792–1802.

Hasselmo ME, McClelland JL (1999) Neural models of memory. *Curr Opin Neurobiol* 9:184–188.

Hasselmo ME, Schnell E, Barkai E (1995) Dynamics of learning and recall at excitatory recurrent synapses and cholinergic modulation in rat hippocampal region CA3. *J Neurosci* 15:5249–5262.

Hasselmo ME, Wyble BP (1997) Free recall and recognition in a network model of the hippocampus: simulating effects of scopolamine on human memory function. *Behav Brain Res* 89:1–34.

Hasselmo ME, Wyble BP, Wallenstein GV (1996) Encoding and retrieval of episodic memories: role of cholinergic and GABAergic modulation in the hippocampus. *Hippocampus* 6:693–708.

Hebb DO (1949) *The organisation of behavior*. New York: Wiley.

Hertz J, Krogh A, Palmer R (1990) *Introduction to the theory of neural computation*. New York: Perseus Books.

Hinton GE, Sejnowski TJ (1999) *Unsupervised learning*. Cambridge, MA: MIT Press.

Hirase H, Czurko HH, Csicsvari J, Buzsaki G (1999) Firing rate and theta-phase coding by hippocampal pyramidal neurons during 'space clamping.' *Eur J Neurosci* 11:4373–4380.

Hodgkin AL, Huxley AF (1952) A quantitative description of membrane current and its application to conduction and excitation in nerve. *J Physiol* 117:500–544.

Holdstock JS, Mayes AR, Cezayirli E, Isaac CL, Aggleton JP, Roberts N (2000) A comparison of egocentric and allocentric spatial memory in a patient with selective hippocampal damage. *Neuropsychologia* 38:410–425.

Holdstock JS, Mayes AR, Roberts N, Cezayirli E, Isaac CL, O'Reilly RC, Norman KA (2002) Under what conditions is recognition spared relative to recall after selective hippocampal damage in humans? *Hippocampus* 12:341–351.

Hopfield JJ (1982) Neural networks and physical systems with emergent collective computational abilities. *Proc Natl Acad Sci USA* 79:2554–2558.

Hoppensteadt FC (1986) *An introduction to the mathematical properties of neurons*. Cambridge, UK: Cambridge University Press.

Hori E, Tabuchi E, Matsumura N, Tamura R, Eifuku S, Endo S, Nishijo H, Ono T (2003) Representation of place by monkey hippocampal neurons in real and virtual translocation. *Hippocampus* 13:190–196.

Howard M, Kahana MJ (2001) A distributed representation of temporal context. *J Math Psychol* 46:269–299.

Howard MW, Fotedar MS, Datey AV, Hasselmo ME (2005) The temporal context model in spatial navigation and relational learning: toward a common explanation of medial temporal lobe function across domains. *Psychol Rev* 112:75–116.

Huxter J, Burgess N, O'Keefe J (2003) Independent rate and temporal coding in hippocampal pyramidal cells. *Nature* 425:828–832.

Jensen O, Lisman JE (1996) Hippocampal CA3 region predicts memory sequences: accounting for the phase precession of place cells. *Learn Mem* 3:279–287.

Jensen O, Lisman JE (2000) Position reconstruction from an ensemble of hippocampal place cells: contribution of theta phase coding. *J Neurophysiol* 83:2602–2609.

Jensen O, Lisman JE (2005) Hippocampal sequence-encoding driven by a cortical multi-item working memory buffer. *Trends Neurosci* 28:67–72.

Jones VJ (1976) A fragmentation hypothesis of memory: cued recall of pictures and of sequential position. *J Exp Psychol Gen* 105:277–293.

Jung MW, Wiener SI, McNaughton BL (1994) Comparison of spatial firing characteristics of units in dorsal and ventral hippocampus of the rat. *J Neurosci* 14:7347–7356.

Kali S, Dayan P (2000) The involvement of recurrent connections in area CA3 in establishing the properties of place fields: a model. *J Neurosci* 20:7463–7477.

Kali S, Dayan P (2004) Off-line replay maintains declarative memories in a model of hippocampal-neocortical interactions. *Nat Neurosci* 7:286—294.

Keith JR, McVety KM (1988) Latent place learning in a novel environment and the influence of prior training in rats. *Psychobiology* 16:146–151.

Kentros C, Hargreaves E, Hawkins RD, Kandel ER, Shapiro M, Muller RV (1998) Abolition of long-term stability of new hippocampal place cell maps by NMDA receptor blockade. *Science* 280:2121–2126.

Knierim JJ (2003) Hippocampal remapping: implications for spatial learning and navigation. In: *The neurobiology of spatial behaviour* (Jeffery KJ, ed), pp 226–239. Oxford, UK: Oxford University Press.

Knierim JJ, Kudrimoti HS, McNaughton BL (1995) Place cells, head direction cells, and the learning of landmark stability. *J Neurosci* 15:1648–1659.

Knowlton BJ, Squire LR (1995) Remembering and knowing: two different expressions of declarative memory. *J Exp Psychol Learn Mem Cogn* 21:699–710.

Kohonen T (1972) Correlation matrix memories. IEEE Trans Comp C-21:353–359.

Kroll NE, Knight RT, Metcalfe J, Wolf ES, Tulving E (1996) Cohesion failure as a source of memory illusions. *J Mem Language* 35:176–196.

Latham PE, Deneve S, Pouget A (2003) Optimal computation with attractor networks. *J Physiol Paris* 97:683–694.

Lengyel M, Szatmary Z, Erdi P (2003) Dynamically detuned oscillations account for the coupled rate and temporal code of place cell firing. *Hippocampus* 13:700–714.

Leutgeb JK, Leutgeb S, Treves A, Meyer R, Barnes CA, McNaughton BL, Moser MB, Moser EI (2005) Progressive transformation of hippocampal neuronal representations in "morphed" environments. *Neuron* 48:345–358.

Lever C, Wills T, Cacucci F, Burgess N, O'Keefe J (2002) Long-term plasticity in the hippocampal place cell representation of environmental geometry. *Nature* 416:90–94.

Levy WB (1996) A sequence predicting CA3 is a flexible associator that learns and uses context to solve hippocampal-like tasks. *Hippocampus* 6:579–590.

Lieblich I, Arbib MA (1982) Multiple representations of space iunderlying behavior. *Behav Brain Sci* 5:627–659.

Lisman JE, Grace AA (2005) The hippocampal-VIA Loop: controlling the entry of information into long-term memory. *Neuron* 46:703–713.

Ludvig N, Tang HM, Gohil BC, Botero JM (2004) Detecting location-specific neuronal firing rate increases in the hippocampus of freely-moving monkeys. *Brain Res* 1014:97–109.

Mallot HA, Gillner S (2000) Route navigating without place recognition: what is recognised in recognition-triggered responses? *Perception* 29:43–55.

Manns JR, Squire LR (1999) Impaired recognition memory on the doors and people test after damage limited to the hippocampal region. *Hippocampus* 9:495–499.

Marr D (1970) A theory for cerebral cortex. Proc R Soc Lond B Biol Sci 176:161–234.

Marr D (1971) Simple memory: a theory for archicortex. *Philos Trans R Soc Lond B Biol Sci* 262:23–81.

Maurer AP, Van Rhoads SR, Sutherland GR, Lipa P, McNaughton BL (2005) Self-motion and the origin of differential spatial scaling along the septo-temporal axis of the hippocampus. *Hippocampus* 15:841–852.

McClelland JL, McNaughton BL, O'Reilly RC (1995) Why there are complementary learning systems in the hippocampus and neocortex: insights from the successes and failures of connectionist models of learning and memory. *Psychol Rev* 102:419–457.

McClelland JL, Rumelhart DE (1986) *Parallel distributed processing: explorations in the microstructure of cognition.* Vol 2. *Psychological and biological models.* Cambridge, MA: MIT Press.

McNaughton BL, Barnes CA, O'Keefe J (1983) The contributions of position, direction, and velocity to single unit activity in the hippocampus of freely-moving rats. *Exp Brain Res* 52:41–49.

McNaughton BL, Barnes CA, Gerrard JL, Gothard K, Jung MW, Knierim JJ, Kudrimoti H, Qin Y, Skaggs WE, Suster M, Weaver KL (1996) Deciphering the hippocampal polyglot: the hippocampus as a path integration system. *J Exp Biol* 199:173–185.

McNaughton BL, Battaglia FP, Jensen O, Moser EI, Moser MB (2006). Path integration and the neural basis of the 'cognitive map'. *Nat Rev Neurosci* 7:663–678.

McNaughton BL, Morris RG (1987) Hippocampal synaptic enhancement and information storage within a distributed memory system. *Trends Neurosci* 10:408–415.

McNaughton BL, Nadel L (1990) Hebb-Marr networks and the neurobiological representation of action in space. In: *Neuroscience and connectionist theory* (Gluck MA, Rumelhart DE, eds), pp 1–63. Hillsdale, NJ: Lawrence Erlbaum.

Mehta MR, Barnes CA, McNaughton BL (1997) Experience-dependent, asymmetric expansion of hippocampal place fields. *Proc Natl Acad Sci USA* 94:8918–8921.

Mehta MR, Quirk MC, Wilson MA (2000) Experience-dependent asymmetric shape of hippocampal receptive fields. *Neuron* 25:707–715.

Mehta MR, Lee AK, Wilson MA (2002) Role of experience and oscillations in transforming a rate code into a temporal code. *Nature* 417:741–746.

Mensink GJ, Raaijmakers JG (1988) A model for interference and forgetting. *Psychol Rev* 95:434–455.

Mezard M, Nadal J-P (1989) Learning in feedforward layered networks: the Tiling algorithm. *J Physics A* 22:2191–2203.

Milner AD, Dijkerman HC, Carey DP (1999) Visuospatial processing in a case of visual form agnosia. In: *The hippocampal and parietal foundations of spatial cognition* (Burgess N, Jeffery KJ, O'Keefe J, eds), pp 443–466. Oxford, UK: Oxford University Press.

Moll M, Miikkulainen R (1997) Convergence-zone episodic memory: analysis and simulations. *Neural Networks* 10:1017–1036.

Montague PR, Dayan P, Sejnowski TJ (1996) A framework for mesencephalic dopamine systems based on predictive Hebbian learning. *J Neurosci* 16:1936–1947.

Morris RGM, Garrud P, Rawlins JN, O'Keefe J (1982) Place navigation impaired in rats with hippocampal lesions. *Nature* 297:681–683.

Morton J, Hammersley RH, Bekerian DA (1985) Headed records: a model for memory and its failure. *Cognition* 20:1–23.

Muller RU, Kubie JL (1987) The effects of changes in the environment on the spatial firing of hippocampal complex-spike cells. *J Neurosci* 7:1951–1968.

Muller RU, Kubie JL, Saypoff R (1991) The hippocampus as a cognitive graph (abridged version). *Hippocampus* 1:243–246.

Muller RU, Stead M, Pach J (1996) The hippocampus as a cognitive graph. *J Gen Physiol* 107:663–694.

Murray EA, Mishkin M (1998) Object recognition and location memory in monkeys with excitotoxic lesions of the amygdala and hippocampus. *J Neurosci* 18:6568–6582.

Murre JM (1996) TraceLink: a model of amnesia and consolidation of memory. *Hippocampus* 6:675–684.

Nadel L, Moscovitch M (1997) Memory consolidation, retrograde amnesia and the hippocampal complex. *Curr Opin Neurobiol* 7:217–227.

Nader K, Schafe GE, LeDoux JE (2000) The labile nature of consolidation theory. *Nat Rev Neurosci* 1:216–219.

Nakazawa K, Quirk MC, Chitwood RA, Watanabe M, Yeckel MF, Sun LD, Kato A, Carr CA, Johnston D, Wilson MA, Tonegawa S (2002) Requirement for hippocampal CA3 NMDA receptors in associative memory recall. *Science* 297:211–218.

Nicolelis MA, Baccala LA, Lin RC, Chapin JK (1995) Sensorimotor encoding by synchronous neural ensemble activity at multiple levels of the somatosensory system. *Science* 268:1353–1358.

Norman KA (2003) Episodic memory, computational models of. In: *Encyclopedia of cognitive science* (Nadel L, ed), pp 15–23. London: Nature Publishing.

Norman KA, O'Reilly RC (2003) Modeling hippocampal and neocortical contributions to recognition memory: a complementary-learning-systems approach. *Psychol Rev* 110:611–646.

O'Keefe J (1990) A computational theory of the hippocampal cognitive map. *Prog Brain Res* 83:301–312.

O'Keefe J (1991) The hippocampal cognitive map and navigational strategies. In: *Brain and Space* (Paillard J, ed), pp 273–295. Oxford, UK: Oxford University Press.

O'Keefe J, Burgess N (1996) Geometric determinants of the place fields of hippocampal neurons. *Nature* 381:425–428.

O'Keefe J, Burgess N (2005) Dual phase and rate coding in hippocampal place cells: theoretical significance and relationship to entorhinal grid cells. *Hippocampus* 15:853–866.

O'Keefe J, Conway DH (1978) Hippocampal place units in the freely moving rat: why they fire where they fire. *Exp Brain Res* 31:573–590.

O'Keefe J, Nadel L (1978) *The hippocampus as a cognitive map.* Oxford, UK: Oxford University Press.

O'Keefe J, Recce ML (1993) Phase relationship between hippocampal place units and the EEG theta rhythm. *Hippocampus* 3:317–330.

O'Keefe J, Speakman A (1987) Single unit activity in the rat hippocampus during a spatial memory task. *Exp Brain Res* 68:1–27.

Oja E (1982) A simplified neuron model as a principal component analyzer. J Math Biol 15:267–273.

Packard MG, McGaugh JL (1996) Inactivation of hippocampus or caudate nucleus with lidocaine differentially affects expression of place and response learning. *Neurobiol Learn Mem* 65:65–72.

Pouget A, Sejnowski TJ (1997) A new view of hemineglect based on the response properties of parietal neurones. *Philos Trans R Soc Lond B Biol Sci* 352:1449–1459.

Quirk GJ, Muller RU, Kubie JL, Ranck JB Jr (1992) The positional firing properties of medial entorhinal neurons: description and comparison with hippocampal place cells. *J Neurosci* 12:1945–1963.

Raaijmakers JG, Shiffrin RM (1981) Search of associative memory. *Psychol Rev* 88:93–134.

Ratcliff R (1990) Connectionist models of recognition memory: constraints imposed by learning and forgetting functions. *Psychol Rev* 97:285–308.

Recce M, Harris KD (1996) Memory for places: a navigational model in support of Marr's theory of hippocampal function. *Hippocampus* 6:735–748.

Redish AD (1999) *Beyond the cognitive map: from place cells to episodic memory.* Cambridge, MA: MIT Press.

Redish AD, Elga AN, Touretzky DS (1996) A coupled attractor model of the rodent head direction system. *Network* 7:671–685.

Redish AD, Rosenzweig ES, Bohanick JD, McNaughton BL, Barnes CA (2000) Dynamics of hippocampal ensemble activity realignment: time versus space. *J Neurosci* 20:9298–9309.

Redish AD, Touretzky DS (1998) The role of the hippocampus in solving the Morris watermaze. *Neural Comput* 10:73–111.

Roberts AC, Robbins TW, Weiskrantz L (1998) *The prefrontal cortex.* Oxford, UK: Oxford University Press.

Rolls ET (1996) A theory of hippocampal function in memory. *Hippocampus* 6:601–620.

Rolls ET, Treves A (1997) *Neural networks and brain function.* Oxford, UK: Oxford University Press.

Rolls ET, Robertson RG, Georges-Francois P (1997) Spatial view cells in the primate hippocampus. *Eur J Neurosci* 9:1789–1794.

Rosenbaum RS, Priselac S, Kohler S, Black SE, Gao F, Nadel L, Moscovitch M (2000) Remote spatial memory in an amnesic person with extensive bilateral hippocampal lesions. *Nat Neurosci* 3:1044–1048.

Royer S, Pare D (2003) Conservation of total synaptic weight through balanced synaptic depression and potentiation. *Nature* 422:518–522.

Rugg MD, Yonelinas AP (2003) Human recognition memory: a cognitive neuroscience perspective. *Trends Cogn Sci* 7:313–319.

Rumelhart DE, McClelland JL (1986) *Parallel distributed processing: explorations in the microstructure of cognition.* Vol 1. *Foundations.* Cambridge, MA: MIT Press.

Rumelhart DE, Hinton GE, Williams RJ (1986) Learning internal representations by error propagation. In: *Parallel distributed programming.* Vol 1. *Foundations* (Rumelhart DE, McClelland JL, eds), pp 318–364. Cambridge, MA: MIT Press.

Rumelhart DE, Zipser D (1986) Feature discovery by competitive learning. In: *Parallel distributed programming* Vol. 1.

Foundations (Rumelhart DE, McClelland JL, eds), pp 151–193. MIT Press.

Samsonovich A, McNaughton BL (1997) Path integration and cognitive mapping in a continuous attractor neural network model. *J Neurosci* 17:5900–5920.

Save E, Nerad L, Poucet B (2000) Contribution of multiple sensory information to place field stability in hippocampal place cells. *Hippocampus* 10:64–76.

Scholkopf B, Mallot HA (1995) View-based cognitive mapping and path planning. *Adaptive Behav* 3:311–348.

Schultz W, Dayan P, Montague PR (1997) A neural substrate of prediction and reward. *Science* 275:1593–1599.

Scoville WB, Milner B (1957) Loss of recent memory after bilateral hippocampal lesions. *J Neurol Neurosurg Psychiatry* 20:11–21.

Sharp PE (1991) Computer simulation of hippocampal place cells. *Psychobiology* 19:103–115.

Sharp PE (1996) Multiple spatial/behavioral correlates for cells in the rat postsubiculum: multiple regression analysis and comparison to other hippocampal areas. *Cereb Cortex* 6:238–259.

Sharp PE, Green C (1994) Spatial correlates of firing patterns of single cells in the subiculum of the freely moving rat. *J Neurosci* 14:2339–2356.

Shors TJ, Miesagaes G, Beylin A, Zhao M, Rydel T, Gould E (2001) Neurogenesis in the adult is involved in the formation of trace memories. *Nature* 410:372–376.

Skaggs WE, Knierim JJ, Kudrimoti H, McNaughton BL (1995) A model of the neural basis of the rat's sense of direction. In: *Neural information processing systems 7* (Hanson SJ, Cowan JD, Giles CL, eds), pp 173–180. Cambridge, MA: MIT Press.

Skaggs WE, McNaughton BL, Wilson MA, Barnes CA (1996) Theta phase precession in hippocampal neuronal populations and the compression of temporal sequences. *Hippocampus* 6:149–172.

Skaggs WE, McNaughton BL (1998) Spatial firing properties of hippocampal CA1 populations in an environment containing two visually identical regions. *J Neurosci* 18:8455–8466.

Speakman A, O'Keefe J (1990) Hippocampal complex spike cells do not change their place fields if the goal is moved within a cue controlled environment. *Eur J Neurosci* 7:544–555.

Spiers HJ, Maguire EA, Burgess N (2001) Hippocampal amnesia. *Neurocase* 7:357–382.

Squire LR, Zola SM (1998) Episodic memory, semantic memory, and amnesia. *Hippocampus* 8:205–211.

Sutton RS, Barto AG (1988) *Reinforcement learning: an introduction.* Cambridge, MA: MIT Press.

Taube JS (1998) Head direction cells and the neuropsychological basis for a sense of direction. *Prog Neurobiol* 55:225–256.

Taube JS, Muller RU (1998) Comparisons of head direction cell activity in the postsubiculum and anterior thalamus of freely moving rats. *Hippocampus* 8:87–108.

Taube JS, Muller RU, Ranck JB Jr (1990) Head-direction cells recorded from the postsubiculum in freely moving rats. II. Effects of environmental manipulations. *J Neurosci* 10:436–447.

Teng E, Squire LR (1999) Memory for places learned long ago is intact after hippocampal damage. *Nature* 400:675–677.

Teyler TJ, DiScenna P (1986) The hippocampal memory indexing theory. *Behav Neurosci* 100:147–154.

Tolman EC (1948) Cognitive maps in rats and men. *Psychol Rev* 55:189–208.

Touretzky DS, Redish AD (1996) Theory of rodent navigation based on interacting representations of space. *Hippocampus* 6:247–270.

Treves A, Rolls ET (1992) Computational constraints suggest the need for two distinct input systems to the hippocampal CA3 network. *Hippocampus* 2:189–199.

Trullier O, Wiener SI, Berthoz A, Meyer JA (1997) Biologically based artificial navigation systems: review and prospects. *Prog Neurobiol* 51:483–544.

Tsodyks MV, Skaggs WE, Sejnowski TJ, McNaughton BL (1996) Population dynamics and theta rhythm phase precession of hippocampal place cell firing: a spiking neuron model. *Hippocampus* 6:271–280.

Tulving E (1993) What is episodic memory? *Curr Perspect Psychol Sci* 2:67–70.

Vargha-Khadem F, Gadian DG, Watkins KE, Connelly A, Van Paesschen W, Mishkin M (1997) Differential effects of early hippocampal pathology on episodic and semantic memory. *Science* 277:376–380.

Wallenstein GV, Eichenbaum H, Hasselmo ME (1998) The hippocampus as an associator of discontiguous events. *Trends Neurosci* 21:317–323.

Wallenstein GV, Hasselmo ME (1997) GABAergic modulation of hippocampal population activity: sequence learning, place field development, and the phase precession effect. *J Neurophysiol* 78:393–408.

Wan H, Aggleton JP, Brown MW (1999) Different contributions of the hippocampus and perirhinal cortex to recognition memory. *J Neurosci* 19:1142–1148.

Wilkie DM, Palfrey R (1987) A computer simulation model of rat's place navigation in the Morris watermaze. *Behav Res Meth Instrum Comput* 19:400–403.

Wills T, Lever C, Cacucci F, Burgess N, O'Keefe J (2005) Attractor dynamics in the hippocampal representation of the local environment. *Science* 308:873–876.

Willshaw DJ, Buckingham JT (1990) An assessment of Marr's theory of the hippocampus as a temporary memory store. *Philos Trans R Soc Lond B Biol Sci* 329:205–215.

Willshaw DJ, Buneman OP, Longuet-Higgins HC (1969) Non-holographic associative memory. *Nature* 222:960–962.

Wilson MA, McNaughton BL (1993) Dynamics of the hippocampal ensemble code for space. *Science* 261:1055–1058.

Yonelinas AP (2002) The nature of recollection and familiarity: a review of 30 years of research. *J Mem Language* 46:441–517.

Yonelinas AP, Kroll NE, Quamme JR, Lazzara MM, Sauve MJ, Widaman KF, Knight RT (2002) Effects of extensive temporal lobe damage or mild hypoxia on recollection and familiarity. *Nat Neurosci* 5:1236–1241.

Zhang K (1996) Representation of spatial orientation by the intrinsic dynamics of the head-direction cell ensemble: a theory. *J Neurosci* 16:2112–2126.

Zhu XO, McCabe BJ, Aggleton JP, Brown MW (1996) Mapping visual recognition memory through expression of the immediate early gene c-fos. *Neuroreport* 7:1871–1875.

Zipser D (1985) A computational model of hippocampal place fields. *Behav Neurosci* 99:1006–1018.

Zipser D (1986) Place recognition. In: *Parallel distributed programming. Vol 2. Psychological and biological models* (McClelland JL, Rumelhart DE, eds), pp 432–470. Cambridge, MA: MIT Press.

Zola SM, Squire LR, Teng E, Stefanacci L, Buffalo EA, Clark RE (2000) Impaired recognition memory in monkeys after damage limited to the hippocampal region. *J Neurosci* 20:451–463.

Zola-Morgan S, Squire LR, Ramus SJ (1994) Severity of memory impairment in monkeys as a function of locus and extent of damage within the medial temporal lobe memory system. *Hippocampus* 4:483–495.

15 ▦ Richard Morris

Stress and the Hippocampus

15.1 Overview

Anxiety, fear and stress are, on the face of it, very different entities from memory, and it may therefore come as a surprise that the hippocampus has also been implicated in these processes. This chapter focuses primarily on the role of the hippocampal formation and other "higher" structures, such as the amygdala and prefrontal cortex, in the negative feedback regulation of the hypothalamic-pituitary-adrenal (HPA) axis—the major system involved in orchestrating the body's reactions to both acute and chronic stress. There are two main aspects to consider. The first concerns how hippocampal memory processing and synaptic plasticity is modulated by stress hormones, with particular reference to an inverted U-shaped function relating stress to optimal performance. The second is how the hippocampus interconnects with structures that, in turn, innervate the paraventricular nucleus of the hypothalamus to "complete the loop" of HPA axis regulation. The larger part of the chapter is concerned with the first of these topics, about which much more is known, but we also touch on the second.

Before outlining these subjects, it is important to note that an early proponent of the idea that fear and anxiety were mediated by the hippocampus was Gray (1982) with his "septo-hippocampal" theory. It was based on the notion of hippocampal processing of signals of reward and punishment and the specific role the hippocampal theta rhythm, at frequencies of around 7 Hz, might play in mediating the inhibition of prepotent behavioral responses that lead to punishment or frustrating nonreward One experimental phenomenon—increased resistance to extinction after partial reinforcement for running in a simple runway—was a cornerstone of the original theory. Over the years modifications became necessary, and it was been updated and elaborated by Gray in 2000. Not alone in maintaining that the brain has a behavioral inhibition system (BIS) of which the hippocampal

formation is a part, others also have suggested that inhibitory processing should not be ignored (as it tends to be in the memory theories discussed in Chapter 13) because hippocampal lesions also cause deficits in various forms of nonspatial-context extinction, negative-occasion settings, and discrimination reversal (Chan et al., 2001; Davidson and Jarrard, 2004). Acceptance of the earliest version of the septo-hippocampal theory of anxiety suffered from exclusion of the amygdala from the BIS despite growing evidence of the role of the amygdala in learned fear and the modulation of memory in emotional situations. This exclusion has been remedied in the updated theory that now extends the envelope of the putative BIS to a number of brain structures that are held to mediate the neural processing involved in coordinating behavior in conflict situations, such as those involving fear and anxiety. McNaughton and Corr (2004) have taken this further by incorporating the Blanchards' idea of a categorical distinction between fear and anxiety and by extending their intriguing concept of "defensive distance" (Blanchard et al., 1997). Fear, according to this view, is a set of behaviors elicited by a predator that includes fight, flight, and freezing. What behavior is chosen depends, in part, on the perceived "distance" of the prey from the predator. Anxiety, in contrast, is a process of risk assessment associated with the potential presence of a predator that is expressed as the inhibition of whatever behavior in which the prey animal is then engaged. Anxiety—but not fear—is thought to be sensitive to anxiolytic drugs and only learned anxiety mediated by the amygdala/septo-hippocampal system. Fear is in the province of the amygdala. The main empirical basis for implicating the hippocampus in anxiety is the perceived similarity between the pattern of effects of a wide range of anxiolytic drugs on hippocampus-dependent tasks and that of the frank lesions that define such tasks (Gray, 2000). Certain studies pointing to differential functions of the dorsal (septal) and ventral (temporal) regions of the hippocampal formation provide partial support for this idea, as lesions of the ventral hippocampus do impair tasks involving both unconditioned fear (Kjelstrup et al., 2002) and some anxiety-related behaviors (Bannerman et al., 2004). However, the theory's treatment of amnesia as "hypermnesia" rather than true memory loss does not command much support.

An ostensibly related idea, but of distinct provenance, is that the hippocampus has a key role in the regulation of the HPA axis. The discovery by McEwen in 1968 that the hippocampus contains a high density of corticosteroid receptors opened up a field of research that had hitherto focused largely on the HPA axis alone (McEwen et al., 1968). This field has enabled classic concepts, such as the "general adaptation syndrome" of Seyle (1936) and the inverted U-shaped function relating stress to alterations in many aspects of performance, to be tackled at a more mechanistic level. Modern molecular and cell-biological research coupled to behavioral studies is also helping us toward an understanding of why low levels of stress are good for cognitive flexibility and memory formation but higher levels are not. Indeed, sustained high levels of stress cause deleterious structural changes to specific regions of the hippocampal formation. On this view, two strands of thinking about the hippocampus are linked: its role in stress and in memory. Thinking about this issue is also a preliminary to the topic of the final chapter of this book, which deals with the hippocampus and neurological disease (see Chapter 16).

Following his pioneering work, further studies by McEwen and his colleagues revealed that the highest concentrations of mineralocorticoid receptors in the brain are found in the hippocampus (McEwen et al., 1980). As increased release of corticosterone from the adrenals occurs during stressful situations, these observations linked the hippocampus directly with bodily responses to stress, a concept that is extremely difficult to define precisely because it can refer to both distress and exhilaration (Goldstein and McEwen, 2002). McEwen's seminal observations on corticosterone led to the birth of the stress–hippocampus link (Lupien and Lepage, 2001). There has since been a great deal of research evaluating the participation of the hippocampus in the many facets of Selye's general adaptation syndrome. Five key lines of evidence implicate the hippocampus in stress (see Box 15–1).

On perception of a "stressor," be it physical or cognitive, the central nervous system (CNS) mediates the synergistic activation of the neuroendocrine, immune, and autonomic nervous systems. In so doing, it optimizes physiological parameters that help subserve short-term coping needs (e.g., gluconeogenesis, enhanced oxygen delivery, increased heart rate, effective vigilance). The most commonly studied physiological systems—the sympathetic-adrenal medullary system (SAM) and the HPA axis—coordinate a two-phase cascade of events. First, emotional arousal triggers rapid sympathetic adrenergic activity, inducing the release of catecholamines from the adrenal medulla into the bloodstream. This SAM activation mediates the rapid phases of the "fight or flight" response to a threat, with adrenaline modulating the memory for events triggering this arousal via an action within the amygdala (McGaugh, 1973; Davis et al., 1993). The second wave—HPA

> **Box 15–1**
> **Evidence Linking the Hippocampus and Stress**
>
> 1. The presence of mineralocorticoid and glucocorticoid receptors in the animal and human hippocampus.
> 2. An inverted U-shaped function between level of acute stress and memory.
> 3. Stress modulation of intrinsic hippocampus excitability and activity-dependent synaptic plasticity associated with learning and memory.
> 4. Chronic exposure to high levels of stress or stress hormones is associated with structural changes in area CA3 of the hippocampus and, during pregnancy, fetal reprogramming of the HPA axis that lasts into adulthood.
> 5. Stress or stress hormones can impair neurogenesis in the dentate gyrus.

axis activity itself—has multiple effects, including the cascade of corticotrophin-releasing hormone (CRH) release from the paraventricular nucleus (PVN) of the hypothalamus, leading to ACTH secretion in the anterior pituitary and consequently glucocorticoid (GC) release from the adrenal cortex into the circulatory system. The cortisol (humans) or corticosterone (rodents) so released then feeds back onto both hypothalamic and higher brain structures, including the hippocampus. The HPA axis also functions in constitutive "housekeeping" mode by regulating the secretion of GCs in response to the diurnal cycle of rest and activity, primarily through "reflexive" feedback routes rather than via higher brain structures mediating planning and memory. Under basal conditions, GCs exhibit a 24-hour circadian rhythm during which maximum steroid concentrations (cortisol in humans, corticosterone in rats and mice) are associated with awakening and minimum levels with nocturnal sleeping periods. A rhythm is also observed in nocturnal species but with a different pattern of entrainment.

The term "allostasis" was introduced by Sterling and Eyer (1988) to characterize how blood pressure and heart rate responses vary with experience and throughout the day and how the "set-point" for these can be changed. McEwen (2002) argued for a broader definition in which allostasis refers to a process, including activation of the SAM and HPA axes, whose essential function is to actively maintain homeostasis. Allostasis is thus a process of "stability through change" (somewhat analogous to the shock absorbers and suspension of a car), and it applies not only to protective internal physiological responses but also to overt, ostensibly paradoxical alterations in cognition or behavior that favor future survival (McEwen, 2002). It may, for example, include enhanced memory for significant aspects of a stressful experience coupled with poorer consolidation of other unrelated information. This shift in the pattern of information processing is to be distinguished from merely asserting that, for example, memory has gotten better or worse. Stress has a further downside if it is sustained. The separate concept of "allostatic load" (McEwen, 2000) refers to the pathological cost of prolonged or overactive allostatic stress that can, over time, induce tissue damage and maladaptive functioning.

This chapter considers findings relevant to the stress–hippocampus link beginning with a model of HPA axis regulation; it then turns to allostatic modulation of hippocampal processing and, next, to the problems that arise with allostatic load. This is followed by discussion of the interaction between the hippocampus and other brain structures in regulating stress and, finally, the mechanistic issue of how the hippocampus orchestrates certain cognitive sequelae of arousing aversive experiences.

15.2 Glucocorticoid Receptors and Hippocampal Function

15.2.1 Glucocorticoid Receptors Are Present in the Animal and Human Hippocampus

The discovery that glucocorticoid receptors are highly expressed in the rodent hippocampus led to the conjecture that they might regulate aspects of the HPA axis. A number of early studies led to the supposition that the hippocampus has an inhibitory action (i.e., negative feedback) on circulating levels of glucocorticoids (Feldman and Conforti, 1980; Fischette et al., 1980; Wilson et al., 1980; Sapolsky et al., 1984, 1990; Lupien and Lepage, 2001). The primary observation was a sustained corticosteroid response to various stressors in animals given hippocampus or fornix lesions. However, this result

is not always obtained. Whereas neurotoxic lesions of area CA3 of the hippocampus do cause stress-induced hypersecretion of corticosterone in rats (Roozendaal et al., 2001), large selective neurotoxic lesions of the entire hippocampus have, paradoxically, been observed to cause no changes in corticosterone levels at rest or under stress (Tuvnes et al., 2003). Moreover, work during the 1970s revealed inconsistencies in the patterns of regional retention of naturally occurring corticosterone and synthetic corticosteroids, raising the possibility of there being more than one adrenal steroid recognition system (de Kloet et al., 1975; McEwen et al., 1976). These questions are now resolved in favor of models such as that shown in Figure 15–1 in which the HPA axis itself (shown in gray) is regulated reflexively by input from, for example, the subfornical organ and more "cognitively" by a composite of higher brainstructures.

Following the development of selective "pure" glucocorticoid compounds (Veldhuis et al., 1982) confirmed that corticosterone binds to two separate glucocorticoid receptor types in the rat hippocampus. These receptors are transcription factors and now commonly referred to as the high-affinity mineralocorticoid (MR), or type I, receptor and the lower-affinity glucocorticoid (GR), or type II, receptor. They display differential binding properties, distribution, and intracellular mechanisms (Joels, 2001). MRs are highly expressed in the hippocampus and amygdala, and they have an approximately 10-fold higher affinity for corticosterone than GRs. In contrast, GRs are widely expressed in most brain tissues and are detected, among other regions, in limbic structures, the cerebral cortex, and brain stem monoaminergic nuclei (Reul and de Kloet, 1985; de Kloet et al., 1999; Helm et al., 2002; de

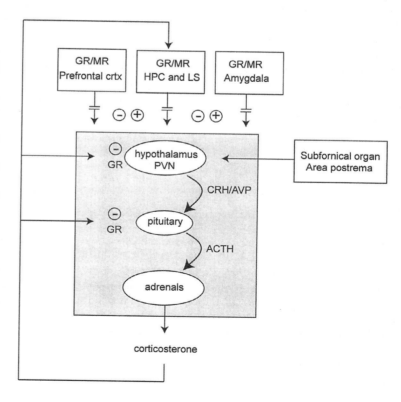

Figure 15–1. Neural afferents, corticosteroids, and hypothalamo-pituitary-adrenal (HPA) control. The HPA axis (gray shading) consists of the paraventricular nuclei (PVN) of the hypothalamus that is activated (+) and inhibited (-) via descending pathways from the prefrontal cortex, the hippocampus and lateral septum, and the amygdala. It is also regulated reflexively by corticosteroid signals entrained to the diurnal circadian rhythm and by neural input from the subfornical organ and area postrema. The PVN releases cortico-releasing hormone (CRH) and vasopression (AVP) via the portal blood vessels to activate the pituitary, which, in turn, releases adrenocorticotropic hormone (ACTH) into the bloodstream, which activates the adrenal gland. The corticosterone then released into the bloodstream finds its way to the "higher" brain structures involved in its feedback regulation. Binding of corticosteroid to mineralocorticoid (type I) receptors (MRs) and glucocorticoid (type II) receptors (GRs) triggers genomic and nongenomic mechanisms with one eventual result being negative feedback (-) from the hippocampus onto the PVN. (*Source*: After Welberg and Seckl, 2001 and Herman et al., 2003.)

Kloet, 2004). It is now recognized that corticosteroid actions in the brain are, at least in part, mediated by both MRs and GRs, with the ratio of receptor activation at these two sites being critical to the modulatory effects observed on cellular activity, neural excitability, and network function (de Kloet et al., 1999; Joels, 1999). We shall see that other parameters, such as the context in which a stressor is perceived, also influence the dynamics of the HPA axis response.

The various routes by which these higher brain structures might affect the PVN are gradually being unraveled (Herman et al., 2003). A key idea is the contrast between a "reflexive" and an "anticipatory" route by which the PVN is activated or inhibited. With the former, sensory information reflecting actual homeostatic challenges (e.g., nociception) promotes the activity of the PVN and thus the appropriate release of stress hormones. With the latter, signals associated with planning and decision-making (prefrontal lobe), memory of stressful or potentially stressful experiences (hippocampus), and learned fear (amygdala) can all activate pathways leading to hypothalamic nuclei in the neighborhood of the PVN. In this way, stress hormone release anticipates the circumstances in which it may be needed. For example, lesions of the ventral subiculum reduce the corticosterone response to novelty (Herman et al., 1998). Conversely, binding of corticosterone to MRs and GRs in the hippocampus can also inhibit PVN activity upon termination of the stressor or the risk associated with it and so limit the duration of a stress response. As we have seen, it was the extended duration of the stress response in hippocampus-lesioned animals that indicated that this structure participated in regulation of the HPA axis. That this response is not always seen suggests that multiple brain systems are capable of exerting independent tonic inhibition of the HPA axis.

Risold and Swanson (1996) suggested that there may be two routes by which the hippocampus mediates such memory-associated effects. One is via the orderly CA3 output to the lateral septum (LS) and thence, via the precommissural fornix, as a tripartite projection to the hypothalamus. The other route is via the postcommissural fornix, which arises in the subiculum and ends in the mammillary body and anterior thalamus. Interestingly, there do not appear to be any direct, monosynaptic inputs from the hippocampal formation to the PVN. The sophisticated summary by Herman et al. (2003) of the relevant neuroanatomy suggests that central stress regulation "relies heavily on hierarchical rather than dichotomous pathways" (p. 169) with the overall output of the stress response (+ or −) being dependent on the overall set of both reflexive and anticipatory inputs. Forebrain influences on the PVN are polysynaptic, with the hippocampus having interactions with the bed nucleus of the stria terminalis (BST) and the hypothalamus, whereas the prefrontal lobe projects to the BST and nucleus of the solitary tract. Notwithstanding numerous important anatomical studies, it is still unclear how activity in the hippocampus can both trigger corticosterone release and limit its duration.

15.2.2 There Is an Inverted U-Shape Function Between Level of Stress and Memory

It is commonplace for parents and schoolteachers to assert that a small amount of stress is good for you while also recognizing that too much can be harmful. This folk wisdom is now on a firmer scientific footing (Fig. 15–2), with a large scientific literature attesting to an inverted U-shaped function between severity of acute stress and cognitive function in animals—the so-called Yerkes-Dodson law. This now classic idea emerged from studies showing the initially synergistic but later deleterious effects of increasing stress on learning in mice (Yerkes and Dodson, 1908). Experimentally, this is often investigated with surrogate indices, such as "stress" being administration of a particular dose of adrenal steroids and "cognitive function" being performance in a watermaze or other learning/memory task. For example, mild stress and low concentrations of administered steroids can facilitate spatial memory (Sandi et al., 1997; Akirav et al., 2004), passive avoidance learning in chicks (Sandi and Rose, 1994, 1997; Liu et al., 1999), contextual fear conditioning (Cordero et al., 2003), and classic eyeblink conditioning (Shors, 2001). Conversely, moderate to high levels of stress or exogenous steroid have been reported to impair spatial memory (Diamond et al., 1996; de Quervain et al., 1998; Stillman et al., 1998; Conrad et al., 1999; Diamond and Park, 2000), recognition memory (Baker and Kim, 2002), and contextual fear conditioning (Pugh et al., 1997; Rudy et al., 1999). These data fall neatly across the putative inverted U-shaped function linking levels of stress to learning ability, the first part of the function being the improvements that mild stress can bring about, and the later parts of the curve being the impairments (Fig. 15–2). Although the criticism can be

Figure 15–2. Yerkes-Dodson law. Cognitive function, including learning, has a biphasic relation to levels of stress. As stress increases, learning first improves and then declines to levels below baseline.

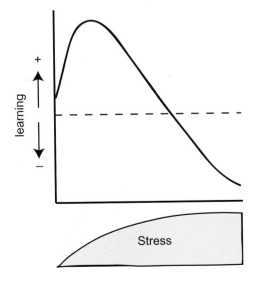

made that the full inverted-U function has been witnessed in few if any behavioral studies, this interpretation of the data is still reasonably secure.

Two illustrative examples of behavioral studies of the inverted U-shaped function are the work of Sandi et al. (1997), in which mild stress improved the performance of rats in a conventional watermaze, and that of Diamond et al. (1999) in which exposure to a predator impaired performance in a working-memory version of a radial-arm watermaze. In Sandi et al.'s (1997) study, rats trained over 3 days with the water temperature at 19°C showed a faster rate of acquisition and better retention 1 week later than those trained at 25°C (Fig. 15–3A). When trained at 25°C and given injections of either vehicle or corticosterone immediately after each training session, retention in the corticosterone-treated group was comparable to that of the 19°C trained animals from the first experiment. In the third study of the series, the corticosterone-induced improvement did not occur when it was given to animals being trained in 19°C water. These data reflect the left-hand side of the inverted U-shaped function. In Diamond et al.'s study (Fig. 15–3B), the rats were trained for

four trials per day in a hippocampus-dependent radial-arm watermaze (with the water at 24°C), which contained either four or six arms, and then given a retention trial 30 minutes later as their fifth exposure to the maze. Training continued across days with a new start and goal location (hidden platforms) on each day. This is a working-memory task in which the animals must acquire new information daily and flexibly retrieve information acquired that day, rather than a previous day, during the retention trial. As shown in Figure 15–3B, exposure of the animals to a cat predator during the memory delay interval between training and retention, which demonstrably increased stress in the rats exposed to the cat, resulted in an elevation of the number of errors in the six-arm maze and in one of two training protocols for the four-arm maze. These data reflect the right-hand side of the inverted U-shaped function, with the stress-induced impairment being more prominent on a more a difficult learning task.

In keeping with this body of work, the performance of adrenalectomized (ADX) rats is impaired in a variety of behavioral tasks but is restored by administration of steroids in a dose-dependent manner (Vaher et al., 1994; Conrad et al.,

Figure 15–3. The inverted U-shaped impact of stress on spatial learning. *A*. Mean escape latencies during a retention test 1 week after training in a wate rmaze at two temperatures. Training at the colder temperature produced better performance (lower escape latency). This response was mimicked after administration of corti-

costerone at the higher but not the lower water temperature during training. (*Source:* After Sandi et al., 1997.) *B*. Exposure to a cat predator after daily training trials caused disruption of performance (increased errors) in a difficult radial-arm watermaze but not an easier one. HC, home cage. (*Source:* After Diamond et al., 1999.)

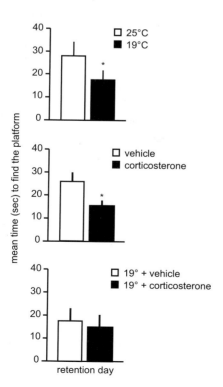

A. Mild stress improves retention of spatial memory

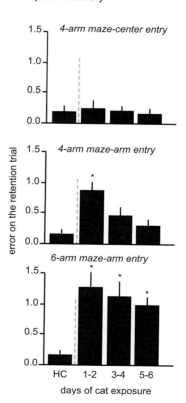

B. More severe stress impairs retention of spatial memory

1997; McCormick et al., 1997). In a striking report, it has been claimed that steroids can even reverse the deficit in memory in a watermaze task that is induced by neurotoxic CA3 lesions, though it is unclear how they can compensate for the interrupted intrahippocampal communication that would necessarily occur with such lesions (Roozendaal et al., 2001). Indeed, with respect to the freezing response that reflects conditioned fear and is often used in studies of contextual fear conditioning, the reestablishment of control levels of performance by steroid administration in ADX rats is reported to occur only when the hippocampus is intact (Takahashi, 1995).

There are several outstanding puzzles with respect to these ideas and data. First, the definition of "severity" of stress differs across research groups and behavioral paradigms. For example, lowering water temperature during watermaze training by 6°C has been described as moderate to high stress (Akirav et al., 2004), whereas repeated foot shocks given over 5 days has been reported as mild (Xiong et al., 2003). The basis of these assignations is unclear. There is also circularity of the attempts to identify "severity" because comparisons of exposure to foot shock, placement in a watermaze, or confrontation with a potential predator are not easily made in procedural terms but can be quantified by resorting to the surrogate measure of circulating corticosteroid levels. This is probably reasonable but clearly assumes the very relation that the experiments are in part intended to help establish. Although many studies have shown a correlation between presumed severity of stress and circulating corticosterone levels, elevations in serum concentrations also accompany nonaversive "arousing" experiences such as the presentation of a sexually receptive female to a male rat. Spatial working memory was unimpaired by the exposure to a sexually receptive female rat, a stimulus that was novel and arousing but not aversive. There was, nonetheless, an equivalent increase in serum corticosterone levels in the male rats exposed to a cat or to the female rat, but only the cat-exposed rats exhibited a significant correlation between corticosterone levels and impaired memory (Woodson et al., 2003).

Second, defining stress for animals used in experimental work can also be problematic. In humans, specific arousing or aversive situations may be perceived and then declared stressful by some but not others, an opportunity for distinguishing differing potential stressors that we do not have with animals. Even in humans, stress really is an interaction between disposition or personality on the one hand and a range of different physical or cognitive "potential" stressors on the other. As animals cannot make overt declarations of what is stressful to them, there is no alternative but to resort to assumptions or surrogate markers. The likely cognitive outcome of stress after a training experience, such as facilitated or impaired memory consolidation, seems to depend on the aversive qualities of the stress experience and stressor-specific pathways activated (i.e., sensory or psychological) and even the sex of the animal (de Kloet, 2003; Shors, 2004).

A third concern about some research on stress using animals is that it sometimes seems needlessly cruel, such as procedures in which rodents are exposed to long periods of enforced immobility and unavoidable electric shock. That these procedures work is not in doubt, but it is unclear that such extreme conditions are really necessary to investigate the biological mechanisms of stress. Opinions change over time, and the techniques used by Seyle (1936), for example, would not be regarded as ethical today. Mindful of the "neuroethological strategy" discussed in relation to the cognitive map theory (see Chapter 13), the assumption that the delivery of electric shock is a biologically "valid" stressor is less clear than researchers on stress may appreciate. Appearances may, however, be deceptive as exposure to the first day of swimming in the more "ecologically" natural situation of a watermaze can yield changes in corticosterone levels comparable to those seen after delivery of electric shock. This habituates rapidly such that a watermaze probe test as early as day 3 of training is associated with minimal corticosterone release (Tuvnes et al., 2003). The use of predator stress, introduced by Diamond (Diamond et al., 1999; Mesches et al., 1999), appears to be a useful step forward and one that avoids using a stimulus that, like shock, can cause overt tissue damage.

Research on the inverted U-shaped function in humans has, for the most part, substantiated the dose-dependent effect of GCs on cognitive function. Supraphysiological stress (or administration of cortisol) impairs declarative memory (Kirschbaum et al., 1996; Newcomer et al., 1999; de Quervain et al., 2000). In contrast, acute low doses of cortisol administered 1 hour before memory encoding has been shown to facilitate word recall performance (Becker and Olton, 1980). It also improves the long-term recall of emotionally arousing pictures compared to neutral stimuli (Buchanan and Lovallo, 2001). Not all such effects are likely to be due to the actions of GCs alone, however, with a well known study by (Cahill et al., 1994) showing that the enhanced memory of an emotionally laden prose passage compared to that of a more neutral story can be blocked by the β-adrenergic receptor antagonist propranolol. When focusing on hippocampal regulation of the HPA axis, it is vital not to ignore the key role that the SAM plays in immediate reactions to anxiety- and stress-provoking stimuli. Discrepancies in published findings also exist and have been explained as being a consequence of differential time of steroid administration during the natural circadian rhythm (Lupien and Lepage, 2001). These disquieting items aside, a body of work using a plethora of methodologies and behavioral paradigms in both humans and animals has provided solid evidence that varying corticosteroid levels may account for many aspects of the inverted U-shaped function with respect to the hippocampus and, indeed, other brain structures.

15.2.3 Stress Modulates Intrinsic Hippocampal Excitability and Activity-dependent Synaptic Plasticity Associated with Learning and Memory

When thinking about the mechanisms by which stress has its impact on hippocampal function, the time course is critical. Some effects are fast. Immediate effects of a stressor, such as those mediated by the sympathetic system, may occur via the action of adrenaline on the amygdala, which then affects the hippocampus through their mutual anatomical connections. Corticosteroid receptor activation can also induce immediate responses through reaggregation and molecular remodeling of receptor molecules in the cytoplasm (de Kloet, 2003). The modulatory effects on glutamate and γ-aminobutyric acid (GABA)-mediated transmission, apparent after as short a period as 20 minutes, are two examples of responses now thought to be mediated by fast nongenomic mechanisms. For example, Karst et al. (2005) have shown very rapid increases in the frequency of miniature excitatory postsynaptic currents (EPSCs) in CA1 pyramidal cells in vitro that are blocked by an MR antagonist and absent in MR knockout mice. They suggested that such effects are likely due to MRs that have shuttled from the nucleus/cytoplasm to cell membranes.

However, the delayed effects of corticosteroids are now widely agreed to involve gene transcription. Intracellular studies in vitro by Joels and her colleagues have examined the consequences of delayed GC transcriptional regulation (Joels, 2001). Although no striking effects on hippocampal electrical activity are observed following MR occupation, there are a number of clear effects: reduced turnover of dentate granule cells, reduced after-hyperpolarization (AHP), weaker responses to serotonin (5-HT), and smaller Ca^{2+} currents. Moreover, induced alterations in membrane potential have revealed effects of GR activation on Ca^{2+} currents through voltage-dependent Ca^{2+} channels. The increased influx of Ca^{2+} may, for example, activate Ca^{2+}-dependent K^+ currents that help limit excitability. As this then limits the fast transfer of excitatory information, it causes subtle alterations in hippocampal network activity that may be the basis of the impaired memory seen in the presence of a strong stressor.

As discussed in Chapter 10, long-term potentiation (LTP) and long-term depression (LTD) are physiological models of activity-dependent synaptic plasticity and memory formation. Extensive observations obtained using in vitro and in vivo electrophysiological techniques and a variety of physical and psychosocial stressors have revealed that high levels of stress impair both LTP and primed burst potentiation (PBP), a lower threshold form of LTP, whereas they enhance LTD induction in the dentate gyrus and CA1 regions of the hippocampal formation (Foy et al., 1987; Diamond et al., 1992; Kim et al., 1996; Garcia et al., 1997; Xu et al., 1997; Mesches et al., 1999; Diamond and Park, 2000). Furthermore, low corticosteroid serum levels and acute, low doses of glucocorticoid receptor agonists are positively correlated with facilitated induction of both PBP and LTP (Bennett et al., 1991; Pavlides et al., 1994). PBP appears to be particularly sensitive (Diamond et al., 1992). These findings indicate that adrenal steroids and acute stress reversibly and biphasically modulate synaptic plasticity in the hippocampal formation (Fig. 15–4A), leading to the suggestion that stress and associated steroids might also induce "metaplasticity" (i.e., alter the physiological range of endogenous plasticity without necessarily inducing either LTP or LTD directly) (Abraham, 1996, 2004;

de Kloet et al., 1999; Kim and Diamond, 2002). The parallel effects of varying levels of stress on synaptic plasticity and on certain forms of memory is tantalizing and can be taken as indirect support for the "synaptic plasticity and memory" hypothesis outlined in Chapter 10.

How stress engenders such dose-dependent biphasic effects on hippocampal plasticity and memory performance has been explained in terms of differential concomitant corticosteroid receptor mediated action—a theory known as the "binary hormone response" (Evans and Arriza, 1989) or the "MR/GR balance" (Oitzl et al., 1995) hypothesis. Owing to the high affinity of MRs to bind GCs, MRs are thought to be predominantly, though not entirely, occupied at basal circulatory levels of corticosteroids (observed during the circadian trough and nonstress periods). As corticosterone levels increase, GRs become progressively occupied until both MRs and GRs are extensively activated. The action of GRs has a higher capacity to be modulated through this progressive increase in occupancy. In contrast, MR actions can be regulated through a change in receptor number more than by ligand occupation per se. For example, acute swim stress, which leads to upregulation of MR expression in the hippocampus (Gesing et al., 2001), can result in prolongation of LTP in the dentate gyrus when given after the induction of early LTP (Korz and Frey, 2003). Similarly, rats treated with the antidepressant amitriptyline resulted in increased MR mRNA expression in the hippocampus, and this increase correlated positively with their improved spatial memory performance in a watermaze (Yau et al., 1995). These effects are shown in Figure 15–5. MR activation and partial GR occupancy is associated, through cell-biological mechanisms that are still unclear, with stable or even enhanced glutamatergic receptor transmission. This promotes the maintenance of hippocampal information flow and a tonic influence on the HPA system (de Kloet et al., 1999; Joels, 2001). In contrast, strong stress and consequent GR saturation attenuate excitatory input, a state thought to underlie the negative effects on plasticity mechanisms. These opposing effects are also schematically represented in the model linking synaptic plasticity to the classic inverted U-shaped function shown in Figure 15–4B.

In parallel with these differential effects on neural plasticity, MR and GR activation are thought to modulate distinct components of information processing. Pharmacological intervention using selective receptor antagonists administered at specific stages of information processing indicate that MR activation can influence processes involved in the attention to and interpretation of environmental stimuli and the consequent selection of appropriate behavioral responses in animals (Oitzl and de Kloet, 1992; Sandi and Rose, 1994), a process akin to "selective attention" in humans. For example, Oitzl and de Kloet (1992) showed that blocking MR receptors can alter the search strategies of rats in a watermaze. In contrast, activation of GRs is thought to regulate the acquisition and consolidation processes of memory (Oitzl and de Kloet, 1992; Conrad et al., 1999). For example, in an elegant study using a Y maze, Conrad et al. (1999) investigated the effects of

A. Primed burst potentiation with increasing corticosterone

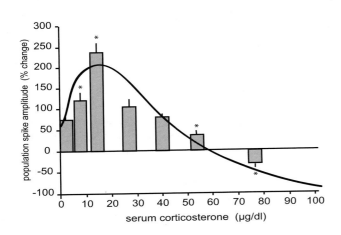

B. MR/GR regulation of synaptic plasticity

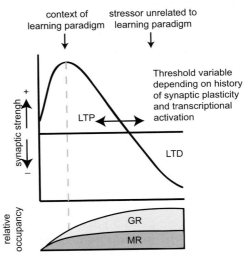

Figure 15–4. The inverted U-shaped relation between stress, synaptic plasticity, and cognitive function. *A*. The magnitude of primed burst potentiation (PBP) as a function of corticosterone levels. (*Source*: After Diamond et al., 1992). *B*. Stress is plotted on the x-axis as the endogenous corticosteroid level induced by a stressor or as the surrogate of an artificial exogenous corticosteroid dose.

As it increases, it differentially occupies MRs and GRs. The y-axis depicts the potential for altering synaptic plasticity (+ or −) and/or cognitive performance. The diagram depicts a model of how the pattern of activation of the hippocampal corticosteroid receptors could affect both plasticity and memory. (*Source*: After de Kloet et al., 1999.)

MR/GR agonists and antagonists on both ADX and unoperated rats. They found that spatial memory was impaired during both complete blockade of GRs (left-hand side of inverted U) and high occupation (right-hand side) but was normal for all other treatments. In a similar protocol, Oitzl and de Kloet (1992) had earlier shown that GR, but not MR, blockade interfered with the consolidation of spatial information. Taken together, this suggests that GRs may, paradoxically, be responsible for both the upward and downward slopes of the

U-shaped function, whereas the positive action of MRs and GRs acting in concert on attentional and consolidation processes may account for the peak in the inverted curve.

The molecular mechanisms underlying the delayed modulatory effects of corticosterone on hippocampal cell properties are known to be transcription-dependent (de Kloet et al., 1998; Joels, 2001). Current understanding of the mode by which transcription is regulated is predominantly based on investigations of GR processes in CA1 pyramidal and dentate

Figure 15–5. Parallels between the persistence of long-term potentiation (LTP) and spatial memory induced by exposure to stress. *A*. Induction of LTP by a weak tetanus results in decaying E-LTP unless followed by a 2-minute period of swimming in cold water. This exposure increases serum corticosterone. The persistence of

LTP over 24 hours is sensitive to an MR antagonist but not a GR antagonist. (*Source*: After Korz and Frey, 2003.) *B*. Rats treated with the antidepressant amitriptyline showed an increase in MR mRNA. The extent of the increase correlated positively with spatial memory. (*Source*: After Yau et al., 1995.)

A. Post-induction stress can transform E-LTP into L-LTP

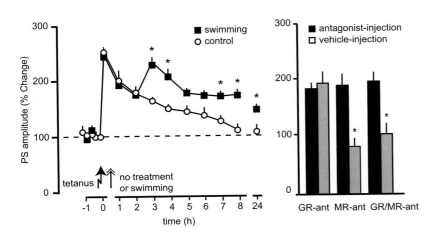

B. Mineralocorticoid mRNA and spatial learning

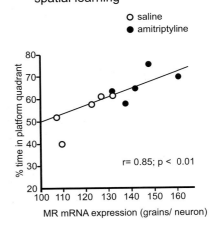

granule cells of the hippocampal formation. However, there is some indication that these molecular processes may differ between receptor types. The long-established view was that GR complexes translocate to the nucleus, where they bind as homodimers to glucocorticoid response elements (GRE) in DNA of target genes, such as *N*-methyl-D-aspartate (NMDA) receptors (Weiland et al., 1997) and *sgk* (rat serum- and glucocorticoid-inducible kinase), one of the genes proposed to be involved in memory consolidation of spatial learning in rats (Tsai et al., 2002). In addition, however, GR complexes have also been reported to regulate gene expression through trans-activation or protein–protein interaction with transcription factors such as AP1, NFKB, and CREB (Auphan et al., 1995). This finding indicates that steroid receptor-mediated and transcription-dependent events in the hippocampus potentially operate through the same signaling pathways. Given this, if cross-talk between signaling cascades were to occur, the timing and nature of the inputs would be critical for determining whether gene transcription was enhanced or repressed. It is important to emphasize, however, that MR/GR gene-mediated processes that alter neuronal activity do so conditionally, such as only when the membrane potential is shifted from its resting level (de Kloet, 2003). Thus, there is considerable potential for dynamic interaction between the strictly neural and strictly neuroendocrine modes of cellular communication.

Glucocorticoid receptor action is only part of the story: Stress-induced alterations in electrophysiological function are likely to involve multiple mechanisms and pathways over various time courses. Several endogenous neurotransmitter/modulators (e.g., catecholamines, GABA, serotonin, opioids, and tissue mediators such as glucose and neurotrophins to name but a few) can modulate intrinsic properties and cellular activity in the hippocampus and elsewhere in the forebrain (McEwen and Sapolsky, 1995; McEwen, 2000; Joels, 2001). Whether these mechanisms act independently in parallel or are "downstream" of adrenal steroid action is yet to be elucidated. Nevertheless, progress in this field has provided valuable insight into the neurobiological processes underlying acute allostatic responses as well as the chronic maladaptive stress consequences that may contribute to conditions such as depression and neurodegenerative diseases such as Alzheimer's that have been associated with aberrant HPA axis activity and hippocampus-dependent cognitive deficit (Holsboer and Barden, 1996; Welberg and Seckl, 2001; Muller et al., 2004).

15.3 Stress and Hippocampal Structure

15.3.1 Chronic Exposure to High Levels of Stress or Stress Hormones Is Associated with Structural Changes in the Hippocampus

Evidence that adrenal steroids have a role in neuronal aging in the hippocampus was first provided by Landfield et al. (1978) and Sapolsky et al. (1984). This led Sapolsky to formulate the "glucocorticosteroid cascade hypothesis" (Sapolsky et al.,

1986), a theory relating the effects of chronic stress to hippocampal damage and dysfunction. As McEwen described it: "The hypothesis states that glucocorticoids participate in a feed-forward cascade of effects on the brain and body, in which progressive GC-induced damage to the hippocampus promotes progressive elevations of adrenal steroids and dysregulation of the HPA axis" (McEwen, 1999). Subsequent research has generally provided support for this hypothesis, the key observation being that prolonged stress and chronically elevated HPA activity results in microscopic and even gross structural changes in the hippocampus in a variety of species.

There are several lines of evidence for different types of structural change in the hippocampal formation (Fig 15–6). First, moderate durations of stress and high GC exposure in rats (and tree shrews) cause reversible atrophy of apical dentrites of CA3 pyramidal cells and dentate gyrus neurons (Woolley et al., 1990; Magarinos and McEwen, 1995; Magarinos et al., 1996) and alteration in synaptic terminal structure (Magarinos et al., 1997). Not surprisingly, such dendritic remodeling is accompanied by reversible impairment of the initial learning of a spatial reference memory task (Luine et al., 1994). Second, chronic longer-term physical and psychosocial stress was reported to result in overt loss of hippocampal CA1 and CA3 neurons in rats and primates (Sapolsky et al., 1985; Kerr et al., 1991; Mizoguchi et al., 1992). However, these findings have not been replicated using improved stereological methodology (West and Gundersen, 1990; West, 1993), and whether cell death occurs in response to stress is now an issue of debate. Third, MRI studies of individuals suffering from Cushing's disease—a syndrome associated with chronic endogenously induced elevated levels in cortisol—show atrophy of the hippocampus. Specifically, significant correlations have been found between the severity of the hypercortisolemia, the extent of atrophy, and the magnitude of cognitive impairment in a verbal learning and recall test (Starkman et al., 1992).

Stress-induced changes in hippocampal morphology can be attributed to reduced dendritic branching (in CA3) or possibly to apoptosis (in the dentate gyrus). However, a third factor has recently been considered as an additional contender: suppression of adult neurogenesis in the dentate gyrus.

15.3.2 Stress or Stress Hormones Can Impair Neurogenesis in the Hippocampus

Neurogenesis, the generation of new neurons in the adult brain (see Chapter 9), is now known to occur in (at least) two regions of the CNS: the lateral ventricle and the subgranular zone in the dentate gyrus (DG) of the hippocampus. It has been reported in a range of species, including rodents, monkeys and humans, as discussed in detail in Chapter 9. Extensive studies using both acute and chronic stress/steroid protocols have also revealed that corticosteroids can inhibit postnatal and adult granule cell proliferation (Cameron and Gould, 1994; Gould et al., 1997). As granule cell precursors do not express MR and GR, this implies an indirect glucocorti-

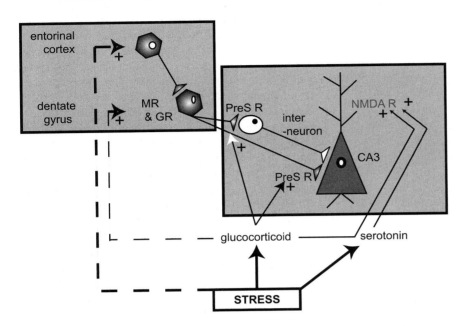

Inhibition of neurogenesis   Dendritic atrophy

Figure 15–6. Chronic stress causes structural changes in the hippocampal formation. A model of the mechanisms by which stress alters neurogenesis and cell death (left), and the integrity of the dendrites of area CA3 of the hippocampal formation. (*Source:* After McEwen, 1999.)

coid mechanism, which Kim and Diamond (2002) suggested may occur through NMDA receptor activation.

McEwen argued that short-term structural plasticity (dendritic pruning in CA3) and inhibition of neurogenesis (Fig. 15–6) are examples of adaptive "protective" mechanisms (allostasis) that could reduce the impact of glutamate and glucocorticoids causing more permanent damage. However, stress is also known to exacerbate the effects of neurological insults such as hypoxia, ischemia, and seizures, increasing the susceptibility of hippocampal cell death putatively through both GC-induced inhibition of glucose transport and enhanced Ca^{2+} influx. Why such a maladaptive response occurs after neurological injury is puzzling. An intriguing idea proposed by Sapolsky, supported by evidence that the HPA glucocorticosteroid cascade is an evolutionary conserved phenomenon, is that "the body simply has not evolved the capacity or tendency to not secrete glucocorticoids during a crisis" (Sapolsky, 2004). In effect, evolution has only gotten so far.

With this view, during protracted periods of intermittent stress the hippocampus may become impeded in its role in "shutting off" HPA axis stress activity. This results in increased secretion of GCs and, in a positive feedback cycle with negative consequences, ends up damaging the hippocampus itself, thereby further reducing the ability of the hippocampus to regulate the HPA axis. The observations by Lupien et al. (1998) of reduced hippocampal volume and poorer memory in humans in association with chronically high levels of cortisol is an apparently striking example of such an effect (Fig. 15–7). Whether hippocampal atrophy and inhibition of neurogenesis are the causes or consequences of elevated GCs is therefore a "chicken or egg" question. What is apparent is that this brain structure is both centrally involved in the neural reaction to aspects of prolonged stress and itself a target of chronic stress.

15.3.3 Fetal Programming of GC Regulation

Adverse events during early life can influence prenatal development and may cause structural and functional changes in the brain that persist for the life-span, a phenomenon known as "early-life programming" (Seckl and Meaney, 2004). Fetal exposure to GCs has been proposed as a likely programming factor. Although GCs are clearly necessary for normal development, excess exposure has deleterious effects: inhibiting fetal growth and altering the trajectory of tissue maturation. For example, exposure of pregnant rats to exogenous or endogenous GCs not only reduces the birth weight of their progeny, it produces permanent hypertension, hyperglycemia, and hyperinsulinemia in the offspring, continuing through to adult life.

Figure 15–7. Stress and hippocampal size in humans. A longitudinal study of the correlation between sustained cortisol levels and hippocampal volume in humans. Higher cortisol levels are associated with a smaller volume, providing evidence for the atrophy predicted in the model. (*Source:* Lupien et al., 1998.)

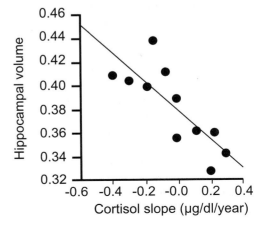

Given that MRs and GRs are highly expressed in the developing brain (Fuxe et al., 1985; Kitraki et al., 1997), it is not surprising that the brain is particularly sensitive to early environmental manipulations. The fetus is normally protected from the relatively high levels of maternal physiological GCs by an enzyme called 11β-HSD2, which catalyzes the conversion of active GCs to inert forms; this enzyme is highly expressed in the placenta. There is also abundant 11β-HSD2 in the CNS at mid-gestation that presumably "protects" vulnerable developing cells from the premature action of GCs (Brown et al., 1996). Expression of this enzyme is then dramatically switched off at the end of mid-gestation in the rat and mouse brain, and similarly in the human fetal brain between gestational weeks 19 and 26 (Stewart et al., 1994), thereby allowing exposure of the developing brain regions to circulating GCs during the later stages of pregnancy.

In animal studies, stress and late prenatal GC exposure permanently increase HPA axis activity and impair cognitive function in adults. This is likely, in part, because of reduced MR and GR expression in the adult hippocampus. Interestingly, postnatal events such as "neonatal handling" or adoption can reverse the effects of prenatal stress (Maccari et al., 1995; Vallee et al., 1999). Thus, there appear to be several distinct time windows during which GC exposure has minimal (early) or maximal (late) effects in rodents. The human HPA axis also appears to be programmed by the early life environment. Maternal stress during pregnancy in humans reduces birth weight, just as it does in rats. Mutations of the 11β-HSD2 gene that alter its effectiveness to protect the developing fetus also cause low birth weight, and low birth weight in humans has been shown to correlate with increased basal and stimulated cortisol levels during adult life. Interestingly, the glucocorticoid agonist dexamethasone (DEX) is often given in obstetric practice, such as when preterm labor threatens during the last trimester. However, DEX readily crosses the placenta, but its effects on cognition and behavior in humans have not yet been investigated in detail. This point is important to investigate as human neonates exposed to DEX may be at risk of later disturbances of the HPA axis.

Insight into the molecular mechanisms by which early life environmental factors may program offspring physiology have come from studies dissecting the processes that underpin postnatal environmental programming of the HPA axis in the "neonatal handling" paradigm (Meaney et al., 2000). A short period of daily handling of rat pups during the first 2 weeks of life (around 15 min/day) results in enhanced maternal care-related behaviors and permanently increased hippocampus GR levels. This potentiates the HPA axis sensitivity to GC-negative feedback and lowers plasma GC levels throughout life—a programmatic resetting of the axis. The "daily handling" model is of physiological relevance because natural variation in such maternal behavior correlates similarly with offspring HPA physiology and hippocampal GR expression (Liu et al., 1997). The altered maternal care-related behaviors elevate thyroid hormones, which then induces 5-HT to increase GR gene expression in the hippocampus via 5-HT7

receptors, increase cAMP generation, and the induction of specific transcription factors, most notably NGFI-A and AP-2. These then bind to the GR gene promoter, inducing a specific GR transcript in the hippocampus (McCormick et al., 2000).

However, a key question that remains is how perinatal environmental events (e.g., stress) can *permanently* alter gene expression. Some evidence is emerging for methylation/demethylation of specific promoters of the GR gene. This may change histone structure (acetylation/deacetylation), permanently opening or hiding specific transcription features for the life-span. Preliminary data suggest that the putative NGFI-A site on the GR promoter (around exon 1_7—one of the six alternate first exons/promoters of the GR gene that is utilized in the hippocampus) is subject to differential and permanent methylation and/or demethylation in association with variations in maternal care (Weaver et al., 2004).

To summarize this section, chronic exposure to GCs can cause structural changes in the hippocampus, can alter neurogenesis, and during pregnancy can program cardiovascular, metabolic, and neuroendocrine disturbances that persist into adult life. The molecular mechanisms may reflect permanent changes in the expression of specific transcription factors including GR itself.

15.4 Other Higher Brain Structures Implicated in Stress and Their Interaction with the Hippocampus

In a book focusing on the hippocampus, it is important to recognize once again that it cannot be considered alone and, specifically, to appreciate the synergistic role that other brain structures play in hippocampus-mediated aspects of stress. For example, electrophysiological and lesion studies provide strong evidence that activation of the amygdala plays a critical role in the rapid mediation of the effects of emotionally arousing events on memory consolidation (McGaugh, 2000; McGaugh and Roozendaal, 2002). Adrenaline, like glucocorticoid, is known to modulate long-term memory consolidation for fear-related or emotionally arousing events. Gold and Van Buskirk (1975) were the first to demonstrate that systematic injections of adrenaline (epinephrine) administered after inhibitory avoidance training produced dose-dependent enhancement of long-term retention. Subsequent research has indicated dose- and time-dependent effects of epinephrine the consolidation of a variety of aversion- and appetite-motivated tasks (Cahill and McGaugh, 1998). Many effects of amygdala activation are entirely separate from hippocampal function, but not all.

An accumulating body of evidence suggests that the amygdala, particularly the basolateral nucleus, is involved in modulating memory storage processes in the hippocampus. For instance, the integrity of the basolateral nucleus is essential for the memory-modulatory effects induced by intrahippocampal infusion of GR agonists and antagonists (Roozendaal,

2002). Amygdala lesions also prevent the stress-induced suppression of hippocampal LTP (Kim et al., 2001, 2005), and amygdala stimulation potentiates the long-term persistence of hippocampal LTP (Frey et al., 2001). Moreover, intra-basolateral amygdala (BLA) infusions of a GR antagonist impair retention of spatial memory in the watermaze (Roozendaal and McGaugh, 1997). Such findings have been interpreted as support for the concept of "emotional tagging," which refers to the idea that, "emotional arousing events mark an experience as important" (Richter-Levin and Akirav, 2003). More specifically they suggest that full expression of the effects of stress on the persistence of hippocampus-dependent memory requires the co-activation of the amygdala, acting via reciprocal hippocampus-amygdala circuitry (Majak and Pitkanen, 2003). Furthermore, in a study using event-related functional magnetic resonance imaging (MRI) to measure neural activity in young healthy female adults during the retrieval of emotional and neutral pictures after a 1-year retention period, it was found that emotion selectively enhanced activity that indexed retrieval success in both the amygdala and the hippocampus (Dolcos et al., 2005). As Dolcos put it: "One way of explaining their co-activation during emotional recollection is that emotion enhances recollection-related activity in the hippocampus, whereas recollection enhances emotion-related activity in the amygdala." The two brain structures are acting in synergy. Emotional tagging and the related idea of synaptic tagging (see Chapter 10) both provide ways of thinking about how activity in an afferent brain structure can modulate the persistence of synaptic potentiation in the hippocampus. A detailed discussion of the impact of adrenal stress hormones on the amygdala and its contribution to the modulation of memory is beyond the scope of this book but is discussed by McGaugh and Roozendaal (2002).

Another brain area implicated in regulation of the HPA axis is the prefrontal cortex (Diorio et al., 1993). In humans, an individual's perception of an experience, intricately tied to past experience of similar events, strongly influences whether a specific arousing event has a positive or negative effect on performance. For example, the impact of a specific physical stressor on animals may depend on whether they can perform any adaptable response to escape it or must merely endure it. Such psychologically driven factors are thought to involve planning and decision-making in higher brain structures (e.g., frontal cortex) that then positively triggers "top down" stressor specific pathways resulting in decreased HPA axis activity (de Kloet, 2003). In this and other ways, the frontal cortex has now been elevated to the status of being part of the regulatory HPA feedback circuitry (Lupien and Lepage, 2001), an additional anatomical component, as shown in Figure 15–1.

The role of the frontal cortex during short-term and chronic stress has also received attention. Interest has arisen, in part, by the discovery that the GR distribution in humans and nonhuman primates differs from rodent expression patterns (Sarrieau et al., 1986; Patel et al., 2000; Sanchez et al., 2000). For instance, in monkeys GRs are reported to be preferentially distributed in cortical areas particularly the pre-

frontal cortex but are detected only weakly in the hippocampal formation (Sanchez et al., 2000). Lupien and Lepage (2001) have also drawn attention to studies indicating that frontal lobe processing, (e.g., executive and working memory tasks) can be more sensitive than hippocampus-dependent processing to acute and short-term increases in corticosteroids. In short, although research of stress-induced frontal lobe dysfunction is in its relative infancy, it is now recognized that other higher brain structures than the hippocampus play a role in engendering changes in cognitive function associated with stress states. Stress is thus partially "emancipated" from the grip of pituitary control.

There is a wider context in which to understand the changing role of higher brain structures, such as the hippocampus and prefrontal cortex, over the course of evolution. As discussed by Keverne et al. (1996), much behavior in small-brained mammals is part of physiological homeostasis and strongly determined by endocrine state. Thus, maternal behavior never occurs outside the context of pregnancy and parturition; sexual behavior is inevitably reproductive and generally restricted to periods of fertility; and forging and feeding frequently occur in response to signals from the gut and fat reserves. In contrast, in large-brained mammals such as primates and humans, most sexual activity is nonreproductive; feeding occurs to avoid, rather than react to, hunger; and females do not necessarily have to undertake pregnancy and parturition to be maternal. Decision-making has switched from hormonal to cognitive determinants (Keverne, 2004). The mediation of stress by the HPA axis can be considered another example of how the evolution of the mammalian brain has provided increased executive control of behavior and a degree of emancipation from hormonal determinants (Herman et al., 2003). In the case of human stress, cortisol is still released from the adrenals, but the entire HPA axis is regulated, both positively and negatively, by cognitive processing in areas of the brain involved in planning, decision-making, and memory.

15.5 How the Hippocampus Orchestrates Behavioral Responses to Arousing Aversive Experiences

To conclude, several lines of evidence support the idea of an allostasis–hippocampus link. They point to likely mechanisms by which stress steroids generate changes in hippocampal excitability and synaptic plasticity and how the hippocampus (with other higher brain structures) is involved in stress feedback circuitry. The final topic for discussion is the nature, or character, of hippocampal processing during stress and the impact that cognitive changes induced by it may have on behavior during such experiences.

First, acute stress induces an adaptive response that not only involves internal physiological mechanisms serving short-term coping needs but also changes in behavior that favor future survival. Which action is taken—fight, flight, freeze—is determined in part by information acquired during the stress episode or recalled from previous episodes. Focused attention to and encoding of salient features of an individual stress experience is therefore critical to the "adaptiveness" of the response. That emotionally arousing experiences tend to be well and long remembered could be one selection pressure that may have helped the various body and brain mechanisms mediating stress to evolve (Cahill and McGaugh, 1996; Schafe et al., 2001; McGaugh and Roozendaal, 2002).

Why does stress have both positive and negative effects on hippocampus-dependent memory? Severity of stress is one factor influencing the outcome—the system may have evolved to cope constructively with mild stress, but the mechanisms involved play the dangerous price of interacting with important entities such as Ca^{2+} channels. Another possibility is that retrograde amnesia induced by unrelated (i.e., "out of context") stress, whereas ostensibly a "negative" outcome is actually a positive adaptive response that helps to ensure greater priority to the storage of information relevant to enhancing survival. Spatial memory in rats is impaired when learning is followed by a variety of unrelated stressors, including inhibitory avoidance training, contextual fear conditioning, and forced exposure to an unfamiliar environment or predator (Diamond et al., 2004). Diamond suggested that unrelated stressors cause alterations in synaptic weight (owing to LTP-like plasticity in the hippocampus caused by stress), which results in neural representations of the stressful experience itself having the effect of "overwriting" any original and unrelated learning going on at the time.

Emotionally charged experiences "within the context" of a learning task have been the focus of much research by Sandi. With others, she has recognized that strong context-related aversive stimuli can also give rise to poor memory of very demanding learning tasks. However, her data also indicate that moderate cold-water stress elicited during training can result in better acquisition even though the corticosteroid levels then induced are actually equivalent to those seen in stressful situations that are deleterious to memory (Sandi et al., 1997; Akirav et al., 2001, 2004). A possible explanation relates to the in-context nature of the stressor and an apparent rightward shift in the inverted U-shaped function; that is, high corticosterone levels are now within the optimum performance zone.

Facilitation of memory induced by mild within-context stress has also been explained in terms of the enhanced attention and reactivity to stimuli and improved consolidation of information (de Kloet et al., 1999; Akirav et al., 2004; Joels et al., 2006). These factors may also contribute to a striking human memory phenomenon—flashbulb memory—in which the vivid and persistent memories for the context of an emotionally arousing public event are also associated with surprisingly good memory for otherwise innocuous details of the circumstances in which they were witnessed. Different generations have different exemplars of this phenomenon, such as remembering when and where one heard the news of the death of President John Kennedy (November 1963) or the unfolding events of the 9/11 tragedy (September 2001). Importantly, it is not only the stressor itself that is marked as important material to be remembered but also certain trivial details of the day on which it happened. Simultaneous hippocampal and amygdala memory processing is likely to be involved in the encoding, storage, and consolidation of any potentially relevant information that may then aid adaptive action another time (McGaugh et al., 1993; Nadel and Jacobs, 1996; Frey and Morris, 1998).

Another connection between HPA "housekeeping" activity and the hippocampus is in relation to the processing of novel contextual information. Humans with unilateral or bilateral hippocampal damage do not show the normal peak cortisol response to awakening even though the remainder of the diurnal cycle is unaffected (Buchanan et al., 2004; Wolf et al., 2004). The psychological significance of the cortisol awakening response is unclear. However, one explanation is that it is part of the process of detecting change such as the transition from the sleeping state to the waking state. It would be interesting to know if this response is larger when a person awakens in an unusual or unexpected place (e.g., a different place from that in which they went to sleep).

Finally, the experience of unique, acute, life-threatening traumatic events (e.g., being unexpectedly involved in military action) can give rise to a persistent clinical condition called posttraumatic stress disorder (PTSD). Evidence from extensive studies investigating the neurobiology and cognitive characteristics of PTSD implicate GR receptor mechanisms in the hippocampus. Three lines of evidence support this assertion. First, blood samples from PTSD subjects indicate lymphocyte GC receptors are more numerous and have increased sensitivity (Yehuda et al., 1995). Second, enhanced cortisol suppression in response to administration of exogenous corticosteroids (i.e., "sensitization" of the HPA axis) is consistent with the clinical presentation of hyperreactivity (Yehuda, 2001). Third, brain imaging studies point to hippocampal atrophy and lack of the activation sometimes seen in the hippocampus during declarative memory tasks (Bremner et al., 1995; Gurvits et al., 1996; Bremner, 2001; Villarreal et al., 2002), and deficits in attention and short-term verbal memory are commonly reported (Elzinga and Bremner, 2002; Sala et al., 2004).

From a psychological perspective, individuals suffering from PTSD display repetitive reliving of the stress experience and evident amplification of memory for the traumatic stimulus with, in contrast to flashbulb memory, poor memory for the surrounding contextual material (Layton and Krikorian, 2002). This failure to consolidate material proximate to the trauma could be due to strong activation of the amygdala and a negative impact of GCs on hippocampal function. This would then be expected to give rise to the memory of the trauma lacking any spatial and temporal frame of reference (Nadel and Jacobs, 1996). Instead of the events being firmly bound in the past, the memory takes on a quality of the here and now, leading individuals to believe they are literally reexperiencing the event.

The themes of this chapter have been that stress mediates certain of its effects via the hippocampus, which provides feedback regulation of the HPA axis. Acute stress has a biphasic effect on synaptic plasticity and cognition. Chronic stress is, however, maladaptive and destructive—one of a number of ways in which the hippocampal formation can become damaged through life. Other pathological changes that affect the hippocampal formation include the onset of specific neurological diseases, such as epilepsy and neurodegenerative conditions such as Alzheimer's disease. It is to these topics that we turn in Chapter 16.

■ ACKNOWLEDGMENTS

R.G.M.M. acknowledges the advice and help of Helen Knight, Marie Pezze, Carmen Sandi, and Joyce Yau on preparation of the chapter and the critical comments of Marian Joels and Joyce Yau on the text.

■ REFERENCES

Abraham WC (1996) Activity-dependent regulation of synaptic plasticity (metaplasticity) in the hippocampus. In: *The hippocampus: functions and clinical relevance* (Kato N, ed), pp 15–26. Amsterdam: Elsevier Science.

Abraham WC (2004) Stress-related phenomena. *Hippocampus* 14:675–676.

Akirav I, Sandi C, Richter-Levin G (2001) Differential activation of hippocampus and amygdala following spatial learning under stress. *Eur J Neurosci* 14:719–725.

Akirav I, Kozenicky M, Tal D, Sandi C, Venero C, Richter-Levin G (2004) A facilitative role for corticosterone in the acquisition of a spatial task under moderate stress. *Learn Mem* 11:188–195.

Auphan N, DiDonato JA, Rosette C, Helmberg A, Karin M (1995) Immunosuppression by glucocorticoids: inhibition of NF-kappa B activity through induction of I kappa B synthesis. *Science* 270:286–290.

Baker KB, Kim JJ (2002) Effects of stress and hippocampal NMDA receptor antagonism on recognition memory in rats. *Learn Mem* 9:58–65.

Bannerman DM, Rawlins JN, McHugh SB, Deacon RM, Yee BK, Bast T, Zhang WN, Pothuizen HH, Feldon J (2004) Regional dissociations within the hippocampus—memory and anxiety. *Neurosci Biobehav Rev* 28:273–283.

Becker JT, Olton DS (1980) Object discrimination by rats: the role of frontal and hippocampal systems in retention and reversal. *Physiol Behav* 24:33–38.

Bennett MC, Diamond DM, Fleshner M, Rose GM (1991) Serum corticosterone level predicts the magnitude of hippocampal primed burst potentiation and depression in urethane-anesthetized rats. *Psychobiology* 19:301–307.

Blanchard RJ, Griebel G, Henrie JA, Blanchard DC (1997) Differentiation of anxiolytic and panicolytic drugs by effects on rat and mouse defense test batteries. *Neurosci Biobehav* Rev 21:783–789.

Bremner JD, Randall P, Scott TM, Bronen RA, Seibyl JP, Southwick SM, Delaney RC, McCarthy G, Charney DS, Innis RB (1995) MRI-based measurement of hippocampal volume in patients with combat-related posttraumatic stress disorder. *Am J Psychiatry* 152:973–981.

Bremner JD (2001) Hypotheses and controversies related to effects of stress on the hippocampus: an argument for stress-induced damage to the hippocampus in patients with posttraumatic stress disorder. *Hippocampus* 11:75–84.

Brown RW, Diaz R, Robson AC, Kotelevtsev YV, Mullins JJ, Kaufman MH, Seckl JR (1996) The ontogeny of 11 beta-hydroxysteroid dehydrogenase type 2 and mineralocorticoid receptor gene expression reveal intricate control of glucocorticoid action in development. *Endocrinology* 137:794–797.

Buchanan TW, Lovallo WR (2001) Enhanced memory for emotional material following stress-level cortisol treatment in humans. *Psychoneuroendocrinology* 26:307–317.

Buchanan TW, Kern S, Allen JS, Tranel D, Kirschbaum C (2004) Circadian regulation of cortisol after hippocampal damage in humans. *Biol Psychiatry* 56:651–656.

Cahill L, McGaugh JL (1996) Modulation of memory storage. *Curr Opin Neurobiol* 6:237–242.

Cahill L, McGaugh JL (1998) Mechanisms of emotional arousal and lasting declarative memory. *Trends Neurosci* 21:294–299.

Cahill L, Prins B, Weber M, McGaugh JL (1994) Beta-adrenergic activation and memory for emotional events. *Nature* 371:702–704.

Cameron HA, Gould E (1994) Adult neurogenesis is regulated by adrenal steroids in the dentate gyrus. *Neuroscience* 61:203–209.

Chan KH, Morell JR, Jarrard LE, Davidson TL (2001) Reconsideration of the role of the hippocampus in learned inhibition. *Behav Brain Res* 119:111–130.

Conrad CD, Lupien SJ, Thanasoulis LC, McEwen BS (1997) The effects of type I and type II corticosteroid receptor agonists on exploratory behavior and spatial memory in the Y-maze. *Brain Res* 759:76–83.

Conrad CD, Lupien SJ, McEwen BS (1999) Support for a bimodal role for type II adrenal steroid receptors in spatial memory. *Neurobiol Learn Mem* 72:39–46.

Cordero MI, Venero C, Kruyt ND, Sandi C (2003) Prior exposure to a single stress session facilitates subsequent contextual fear conditioning in rats: evidence for a role of corticosterone. *Horm Behav* 44:338–345.

Davidson TL, Jarrard LE (2004) The hippocampus and inhibitory learning: a 'gray' area? *Neurosci Biobehav Rev* 28:261–271.

Davis M, Falls WA, Campeau S, Kim M (1993) Fear-potentiated startle: a neural and pharmacological analysis. *Behav Brain Res* 58:175–198.

De Kloet ER (2003) Hormones, brain and stress. *Endocr Regul* 37:51–68.

De Kloet ER (2004) Hormones and the stressed brain. *Ann N Y Acad Sci* 1018:1–15.

De Kloet R, Wallach G, McEwen BS (1975) Differences in corticosterone and dexamethasone binding to rat brain and pituitary. *Endocrinology* 96:598–609.

De Kloet ER, Vreugdenhil E, Oitzl MS, Joels M (1998) Brain corticosteroid receptor balance in health and disease. *Endocr Rev* 19:269–301.

De Kloet ER, Oitzl MS, Joels M (1999) Stress and cognition: are corticosteroids good or bad guys? *Trends Neurosci* 22:422–426.

De Quervain DJ-F, Roozendaal B, McGaugh JL (1998) Stress and glucocorticoids impair retrieval of long-term spatial memory. *Nature* 394:787–790.

De Quervain DJ, Roozendaal B, Nitsch RM, McGaugh JL, Hock C

(2000) Acute cortisone administration impairs retrieval of long-term declarative memory in humans. *Nat Neurosci* 3:313–314.

Diamond DM, Park CR (2000) Predator exposure produces retrograde amnesia and blocks synaptic plasticity: progress toward understanding how the hippocampus is affected by stress. *Ann N Y Acad Sci* 911:453–455.

Diamond DM, Bennett MC, Fleshner M, Rose GM (1992) Inverted-U relationship between the level of peripheral corticosterone and the magnitude of hippocampal primed burst potentiation. *Hippocampus* 2:421–430.

Diamond DM, Fleshner M, Ingersoll N, Rose GM (1996) Psychological stress impairs spatial working memory: relevance to electrophysiological studies of hippocampal function. *Behav Neurosci* 110:661–672.

Diamond DM, Park CR, Heman KL, Rose GM (1999) Exposing rats to a predator impairs spatial working memory in the radial arm watermaze. *Hippocampus* 9:542–552.

Diamond DM, Park CR, Woodson JC (2004) Stress generates emotional memories and retrograde amnesia by inducing an endogenous form of hippocampal LTP. *Hippocampus* 14:281–291.

Diorio D, Viau V, Meaney MJ (1993) The role of the medial prefrontal cortex (cingulate gyrus) in the regulation of hypothalamic-pituitary-adrenal responses to stress. *J Neurosci* 13:3839–3847.

Dolcos F, LaBar KS, Cabeza R (2005) Remembering one year later: role of the amygdala and the medial temporal lobe memory system in retrieving emotional memories. *Proc Natl Acad Sci USA* 102:2626–2631.

Elzinga BM, Bremner JD (2002) Are the neural substrates of memory the final common pathway in posttraumatic stress disorder (PTSD)? *J Affect Disord* 70:1–17.

Evans RM, Arriza JL (1989) A molecular framework for the actions of glucocorticoid hormones in the nervous system. *Neuron* 2:1105–1112.

Feldman S, Conforti N (1980) Participation of the dorsal hippocampus in the glucocorticoid feedback effect on adrenocortical activity. *Neuroendocrinology* 30:52–55.

Fischette CT, Komisaruk BR, Edinger HM, Feder HH, Siegel A (1980) Differential fornix ablations and the circadian rhythmicity of adrenal corticosteroid secretion. *Brain Res* 195:373–387.

Foy MR, Stanton ME, Levine S, Thompson RF (1987) Behavioral stress impairs long-term potentiation in rodent hippocampus. *Behav Neural Biol* 48:138–149.

Frey S, Bergado-Rosado J, Seidenbecher T, Pape HC, Frey JU (2001) Reinforcement of early long-term potentiation (early-LTP) in dentate gyrus by stimulation of the basolateral amygdala: heterosynaptic induction mechanisms of late-LTP. *J Neurosci* 21:3697–3703.

Frey U, Morris RGM (1998b) Synaptic tagging: implications for late maintenance of hippocampal long-term potentiation. *Trends Neurosci* 21:181–188.

Fuxe K, Wikstrom AC, Okret S, Agnati LF, Harfstrand A, Yu ZY, Granholm L, Zoli M, Vale W, Gustafsson JA (1985) Mapping of glucocorticoid receptor immunoreactive neurons in the rat tel- and diencephalon using a monoclonal antibody against rat liver glucocorticoid receptor. *Endocrinology* 117:1803–1812.

Garcia R, Musleh W, Tocco G, Thompson RF, Baudry M (1997) Time-dependent blockade of STP and LTP in hippocampal slices following acute stress in mice. *Neurosci Lett* 233:41–44.

Gesing A, Bilang-Bleuel A, Droste SK, Linthorst AC, Holsboer F, Reul JM (2001) Psychological stress increases hippocampal mineralocorticoid receptor levels: involvement of corticotropin-releasing hormone. *J Neurosci* 21:4822–4829.

Gold PE, Van Buskirk RB (1975) Facilitation of time-dependent memory processes with posttrial epinephrine injections. *Behav Biol* 13:145–153.

Goldstein DS, McEwen B (2002) Allostasis, homeostats, and the nature of stress. *Stress* 5:55–58.

Gould E, McEwen BS, Tanapat P, Galea LA, Fuchs E (1997) Neurogenesis in the dentate gyrus of the adult tree shrew is regulated by psychosocial stress and NMDA receptor activation. *J Neurosci* 17:2492–2498.

Gray JA (1982) *The neuropsychology of anxiety: an enquiry into the functions of the septo-hippocampal system.* Oxford, UK: Oxford University Press.

Gray JA (2000) *The neuropsychology of anxiety: an enquiry into the functions of the septo-hippocampal system,* 2nd ed. Oxford, UK: Oxford University Press.

Gurvits TV, Shenton ME, Hokama H, Ohta H, Lasko NB, Gilbertson MW, Orr SP, Kikinis R, Jolesz FA, McCarley RW, Pitman RK (1996) Magnetic resonance imaging study of hippocampal volume in chronic, combat-related posttraumatic stress disorder. *Biol Psychiatry* 40:1091–1099.

Helm KA, Han JS, Gallagher M (2002) Effects of cholinergic lesions produced by infusions of 192 IgG-saporin on glucocorticoid receptor mRNA expression in hippocampus and medial prefrontal cortex of the rat. *Neuroscience* 115:765–774.

Herman JP, Dolgas CM, Carlson SL (1998) Ventral subiculum regulates hypothalamo-pituitary-adrenocortical and behavioural responses to cognitive stressors. *Neuroscience* 86:449–459.

Herman JP, Figueiredo H, Mueller NK, Ulrich-Lai Y, Ostrander MM, Choi DC, Cullinan WE (2003) Central mechanisms of stress integration: hierarchical circuitry controlling hypothalamo-pituitary-adrenocortical responsiveness. *Front Neuroendocrinol* 24:151–180.

Holsboer F, Barden N (1996) Antidepressants and hypothalamic-pituitary-adrenocortical regulation. *Endocr Rev* 17:187–205.

Joels M (1999) Effects of corticosteroid hormones in the hippocampus. *Acta Physiol Scand* 167:A3.

Joels M (2001) Corticosteroid actions in the hippocampus. *J Neuroendocrinol* 13:657–669.

Joels M, Pu Z, Wiegert O, Oitzl MS, Krugers HJ (2006) Learning under stress: how does it work? *Trends Cogn Sci* 10:152–158.

Karst H, Berger S, Turiault M, Tronche F, Schutz G, Joels M (2005) Mineralocorticoid receptors are indispensable for nongenomic modulation of hippocampal glutamate nongenomic modulation of hippocampal glutamate transmission by corticosterone. *Proc Natl Acad Sci USA* 102:19204–19207.

Kerr DS, Campbell LW, Applegate MD, Brodish A, Landfield PW (1991) Chronic stress-induced acceleration of electrophysiologic and morphometric biomarkers of hippocampal aging. *J Neurosci* 11:1316–1324.

Keverne EB, Martel FL, Nevison CM (1996) Primate brain evolution: genetic and functional considerations. *Proc Biol Sci* 263:689–696.

Keverne EB (2004) Understanding well-being in the evolutionary context of brain development. *Philos Trans R Soc Lond B Biol* Sci 359:1349–1358.

Kim JJ, Diamond DM (2002) The stressed hippocampus, synaptic plasticity and lost memories. *Nat Rev Neurosci* 3:453–462.

Kim JJ, Foy MR, Thompson RF (1996) Behavioral stress modifies hippocampal plasticity through *N*-methyl-D-aspartate receptor activation. *Proc Natl Acad Sci USA* 93:4750–4753.

Kim JJ, Lee HJ, Han JS, Packard MG (2001) Amygdala is critical for stress-induced modulation of hippocampal long-term potentiation and learning. *J Neurosci* 21:5222–5228.

Kim JJ, Koo JW, Lee HJ, Han JS (2005) Amygdalar inactivation blocks stress-induced impairments in hippocampal long-term potentiation and spatial memory. *J Neurosci* 25:1532–1539.

Kirschbaum C, Wolf OT, May M, Wippich W, Hellhammer DH (1996) Stress- and treatment-induced elevations of cortisol levels associated with impaired declarative memory in healthy adults. *Life Sci* 58:1475–1483.

Kitraki E, Kittas C, Stylianopoulou F (1997) Glucocorticoid receptor gene expression during rat embryogenesis: an in situ hybridization study. *Differentiation* 62:21–31.

Kjelstrup KG, Tuvnes FA, Steffenach HA, Murison R, Moser EI, Moser MB (2002) Reduced fear expression after lesions of the ventral hippocampus. *Proc Natl Acad Sci USA* 99:10825–10830.

Korz V, Frey JU (2003) Stress-related modulation of hippocampal long-term potentiation in rats: involvement of adrenal steroid receptors. *J Neurosci* 23:7281–7287.

Landfield PW, Waymire JC, Lynch G (1978) Hippocampal aging and adrenocorticoids: quantitative correlations. *Science* 202:1098–1102.

Layton B, Krikorian R (2002) Memory mechanisms in posttraumatic stress disorder. J *Neuropsychiatry Clin Neurosci* 14:254–261.

Liu D, Diorio J, Tannenbaum B, Caldji C, Francis D, Freedman A, Sharma S, Pearson D, Plotsky PM, Meaney MJ (1997) Maternal care, hippocampal glucocorticoid receptors, and hypothalamic-pituitary-adrenal responses to stress. *Science* 277:1659–1662.

Liu L, Tsuji M, Takeda H, Takada K, Matsumiya T (1999) Adrenocortical suppression blocks the enhancement of memory storage produced by exposure to psychological stress in rats. *Brain Res* 821:134–140.

Luine V, Villegas M, Martinez C, McEwen BS (1994) Repeated stress causes reversible impairments of spatial memory performance. *Brain Res* 639:167–170.

Lupien SJ, Lepage M (2001) Stress, memory, and the hippocampus: can't live with it, can't live without it. *Behav Brain Res* 127:137–158.

Lupien SJ, de Leon M, de Santi S, Convit A, Tarshish C, Nair NP, Thakur M, McEwen BS, Hauger RL, Meaney MJ (1998) Cortisol levels during human aging predict hippocampal atrophy and memory deficits. *Nat Neurosci* 1:69–73.

Maccari S, Piazza PV, Kabbaj M, Barbazanges A, Simon H, Le Moal M (1995) Adoption reverses the long-term impairment in glucocorticoid feedback induced by prenatal stress. *J Neurosci* 15:110–116.

Magarinos AM, McEwen BS (1995) Stress-induced atrophy of apical dendrites of hippocampal CA3c neurons: involvement of glucocorticoid secretion and excitatory amino acid receptors. *Neuroscience* 69:89–98.

Magarinos AM, McEwen BS, Flugge G, Fuchs E (1996) Chronic psychosocial stress causes apical dendritic atrophy of hippocampal CA3 pyramidal neurons in subordinate tree shrews. *J Neurosci* 16:3534–3540.

Magarinos AM, Verdugo JM, McEwen BS (1997) Chronic stress alters synaptic terminal structure in hippocampus. *Proc Natl Acad Sci USA* 94:14002–14008.

Majak K, Pitkanen A (2003) Projections from the periamygdaloid cortex to the amygdaloid complex, the hippocampal formation, and the parahippocampal region: a PHA-L study in the rat. *Hippocampus* 13:922–942. 929.

McCormick CM, McNamara M, Mukhopadhyay S, Kelsey JE (1997) Acute corticosterone replacement reinstates performance on spatial and nonspatial memory tasks 3 months after adrenalectomy despite degeneration in the dentate gyrus. *Behav Neurosci* 111:518–531.

McCormick JA, Lyons V, Jacobson MD, Noble J, Diorio J, Nyirenda M, Weaver S, Ester W, Yau JL, Meaney MJ, Seckl JR, Chapman KE (2000) 5'-Heterogeneity of glucocorticoid receptor messenger RNA is tissue specific: differential regulation of variant transcripts by early-life events. *Mol Endocrinol* 14:506–517.

McEwen BS (1999) Stress and the aging hippocampus. *Front Neuroendocrinol* 20:49–70.

McEwen BS (2000) The neurobiology of stress: from serendipity to clinical relevance. *Brain Res* 886:172–189.

McEwen BS (2002) Sex, stress and the hippocampus: allostasis, allostatic load and the aging process. *Neurobiol Aging* 23:921–939.

McEwen BS, Sapolsky RM (1995) Stress and cognitive function. *Curr Opin Biol* 5:205–216.

McEwen BS, Weiss JM, Schwartz LS (1968) Selective retention of corticosterone by limbic structures in rat brain. *Nature* 220:911–912.

McEwen BS, de Kloet R, Wallach G (1976) Interactions in vivo and in vitro of corticoids and progesterone with cell nuclei and soluble macromolecules from rat brain regions and pituitary. *Brain Res* 105:129–136.

McEwen BS, Stephenson BS, Krey LC (1980) Radioimmunoassay of brian tissue and cell nuclear corticosterone. *J Neurosci Methods* 3:57–65.

McGaugh JL (1973) Drug facilitation of learning and memory. *Annu Rev Pharmacol* 13:229–241.

McGaugh JL (2000) Memory—a century of consolidation. *Science* 287:258–251.

McGaugh JL, Roozendaal B (2002) Role of adrenal stress hormones in forming lasting memories in the brain. *Curr Opin Neurobiol* 12:205–210.

McGaugh JL, Introini-Collison IB, Cahill LF, Castellano C, Dalmaz C, Parent MB, Williams CL (1993) Neuromodulatory systems and memory storage: role of the amygdala. *Behav Brain* Res 58:81–90.

McNaughton N, Corr PJ (2004) A two-dimensional neuropsychology of defense: fear/anxiety and defensive distance. *Neurosci Biobehav Rev* 28:285–305.

Meaney MJ, Diorio J, Francis D, Weaver S, Yau J, Chapman K, Seckl JR (2000) Postnatal handling increases the expression of cAMP-inducible transcription factors in the rat hippocampus: the effects of thyroid hormones and serotonin. *J Neurosci* 20:3926–3935.

Mesches MH, Fleshner M, Heman KL, Rose GM, Diamond DM (1999) Exposing rats to a predator blocks primed burst potentiation in the hippocampus in vitro. *J Neurosci* 19:RC18.

Mizoguchi K, Kunishita T, Chui DH, Tabira T (1992) Stress induces neuronal death in the hippocampus of castrated rats. *Neurosci Lett* 138:157–160.

Muller MB, Uhr M, Holsboer F, Keck ME (2004) Hypothalamic-pituitary-adrenocortical system and mood disorders: highlights from mutant mice. *Neuroendocrinology* 79:1–12.

Nadel L, Jacobs WJ (1996) The role of the hippocampus in PTSD, panic and phobia. In: *The hippocampus: functions and clinical relevance* (Kato N, ed). Amsterdam: Elsevier.

Newcomer JW, Selke G, Melson AK, Hershey T, Craft S, Richards K, Alderson AL (1999) Decreased memory performance in healthy humans induced by stress-level cortisol treatment. *Arch Gen Psychiatry* 56:527–533.

Oitzl MS, de Kloet ER (1992) Selective corticosteroid antagonists modulate specific aspects of spatial orientation learning. *Behav Neurosci* 106:62–71.

Oitzl MS, van Haarst AD, Sutanto W, de Kloet ER (1995) Corticosterone, brain mineralocorticoid receptors (MRs) and the activity of the hypothalamic-pituitary-adrenal (HPA) axis: the Lewis rat as an example of increased central MR capacity and a hyporesponsive HPA axis. *Psychoneuroendocrinology* 20:655–675.

Patel PD, Lopez JF, Lyons DM, Burke S, Wallace M, Schatzberg AF (2000) Glucocorticoid and mineralocorticoid receptor mRNA expression in squirrel monkey brain. *J Psychiatr Res* 34:383–392.

Pavlides C, Kimura A, Magarinos AM, McEwen BS (1994) Type I adrenal steroid receptors prolong hippocampal long-term potentiation. *Neuroreport* 5:2673–2677.

Pugh CR, Tremblay D, Fleshner M, Rudy JW (1997) A selective role for corticosterone in contextual-fear conditioning. *Behav Neurosci* 111:503–511.

Reul JM, de Kloet ER (1985) Two receptor systems for corticosterone in rat brain: microdistribution and differential occupation. *Endocrinology* 117:2505–2511.

Richter-Levin G, Akirav I (2003) Emotional tagging of memory formation—in the search for neural mechanisms. *Brain Res Brain Res Rev* 43:247–256.

Risold PY, Swanson LW (1996) Structural evidence for functional domains in the rat hippocampus. *Science* 272:1484–1486.

Roozendaal B (2002) Stress and memory: opposing effects of glucocorticoids on memory consolidation and memory retrieval. *Neurobiol Learn Mem* 78:578–595.

Roozendaal B, McGaugh JL (1997) Basolateral amygdala lesions block the memory-enhancing effect of glucocorticoid administration in the dorsal hippocampus of rats. *Eur J Neurosci* 9:76–83.

Roozendaal B, Phillips RG, Power AE, Brooke SM, Sapolsky RM, McGaugh JL (2001) Memory retrieval impairment induced by hippocampal CA3 lesions is blocked by adrenocortical suppression. *Nat Neurosci* 4:1169–1171.

Rudy JW, Kuwagama K, Pugh CR (1999) Isolation reduces contextual but not auditory-cue fear conditioning: a role for endogenous opioids. *Behav Neurosci* 113:316–323.

Sala M, Perez J, Soloff P, Ucelli di Nemi S, Caverzasi E, Soares JC, Brambilla P (2004) Stress and hippocampal abnormalities in psychiatric disorders. *Eur Neuropsychopharmacol* 14:393–405.

Sanchez MM, Young LJ, Plotsky PM, Insel TR (2000) Distribution of corticosteroid receptors in the rhesus brain: relative absence of glucocorticoid receptors in the hippocampal formation. *J Neurosci* 20:4657–4668.

Sandi C, Rose SP (1994) Corticosterone enhances long-term retention in one-day-old chicks trained in a weak passive avoidance learning paradigm. *Brain Res* 647:106–112.

Sandi C, Rose SP (1997) Training-dependent biphasic effects of corticosterone in memory formation for a passive avoidance task in chicks. *Psychopharmacology (Berl)* 133:152–160.

Sandi C, Loscertales M, Guaza C (1997) Experience-dependent facilitating effect of corticosterone on spatial memory formation in the watermaze. *Eur J Neurosci* 9:637–642.

Sapolsky RM (2004) Stressed-out memories. *Sci Am Mind* 14:28–33.

Sapolsky RM, Krey LC, McEwen BS (1984) Glucocorticoid-sensitive hippocampal neurons are involved in terminating the adrenocortical stress response. *Proc Natl Acad Sci USA* 81:6174–6177.

Sapolsky RM, Krey LC, McEwen BS (1985) Prolonged glucocorticoid exposure reduces hippocampal neuron number: implications for aging. *J Neurosci* 5:1222–1227.

Sapolsky RM, Krey LC, McEwen BS (1986) The neuroendocrinology of stress and aging: the glucocorticoid cascade hypothesis. *Endocr Rev* 7:284–301.

Sapolsky RM, Armanini MP, Packan DR, Sutton SW, Plotsky PM (1990) Glucocorticoid feedback inhibition of adrenocorticotropic hormone secretagogue release: relationship to corticosteroid receptor occupancy in various limbic sites. *Neuroendocrinology* 51:328–336.

Sarrieau A, Dussaillant M, Agid F, Philibert D, Agid Y, Rostene W (1986) Autoradiographic localization of glucocorticosteroid and progesterone binding sites in the human post-mortem brain. *J Steroid Biochem* 25:717–721.

Schafe GE, Nader K, Blair HT, LeDoux JE (2001) Memory consolidation of Pavlovian fear conditioning: a cellular and molecular perspective. *Trends Neurosci* 24:540–546.

Seckl JR, Meaney MJ (2004) Glucocorticoid programming. *Ann N Y Acad Sci* 1032:63–84.

Seyle H (1936) A syndrome produced by diverse nocuous agents. *Nature* 138:32.

Shors TJ (2001) Acute stress rapidly and persistently enhances memory formation in the male rat. *Neurobiol Learn Mem* 75:10–29.

Shors TJ (2004) Learning during stressful times. *Learn Mem* 11:137–144.

Starkman MN, Gebarski SS, Berent S, Schteingart DE (1992) Hippocampal formation volume, memory dysfunction, and cortisol levels in patients with Cushing's syndrome. *Biol Psychiatry* 32:756–765.

Sterling P, Eyer J (1988) Allostasis: a new paradigm to explain arousal pathology. In: *Handbook of life stress, cognition and health* (Fisher S, Reason J, eds), pp 629–649. New York: Wiley.

Stewart PM, Murry BA, Mason JI (1994) Type 2 11 beta-hydroxysteroid dehydrogenase in human fetal tissues. *J Clin Endocrinol Metab* 78:1529–1532.

Stillman MJ, Shukitt-Hale B, Levy A, Lieberman HR (1998) Spatial memory under acute cold and restraint stress. *Physiol Behav* 64:605–609.

Takahashi LK (1995) Glucocorticoids, the hippocampus, and behavioral inhibition in the preweanling rat. *J Neurosci* 15:6023–6034.

Tsai KJ, Chen SK, Ma YL, Hsu WL, Lee EH (2002) sgk, a primary glucocorticoid-induced gene, facilitates memory consolidation of spatial learning in rats. *Proc Natl Acad Sci USA* 99:3990–3995.

Tuvnes FA, Steffenach HA, Murison R, Moser MB, Moser EI (2003) Selective hippocampal lesions do not increase adrenocortical activity. *J Neurosci* 23:4345–4354.

Vaher PR, Luine VN, Gould E, McEwen BS (1994) Effects of adrenalectomy on spatial memory performance and dentate gyrus morphology. *Brain Res* 656:71–78.

Vallee M, MacCari S, Dellu F, Simon H, Le Moal M, Mayo W (1999) Long-term effects of prenatal stress and postnatal handling on age-related glucocorticoid secretion and cognitive performance: a longitudinal study in the rat. *Eur J Neurosci* 11:2906–2916.

Veldhuis HD, Van Koppen C, Van Ittersum M, De Kloet ER (1982) Specificity of the adrenal steroid receptor system in rat hippocampus. *Endocrinology* 110:2044–2051.

Villarreal G, Hamilton DA, Petropoulos H, Driscoll I, Rowland LM, Griego JA, Kodituwakku PW, Hart BL, Escalona R, Brooks WM (2002) Reduced hippocampal volume and total white matter volume in posttraumatic stress disorder. *Biol Psychiatry* 52:119–125.

Weaver IC, Cervoni N, Champagne FA, D'Alessio AC, Sharma S, Seckl JR, Dymov S, Szyf M, Meaney MJ (2004) Epigenetic programming by maternal behavior. *Nat Neurosci* 7:847–854.

Weiland NG, Orchinik M, Tanapat P (1997) Chronic corticosterone treatment induces parallel changes in *N*-methyl-D-aspartate receptor subunit messenger RNA levels and antagonist binding sites in the hippocampus. *Neuroscience* 78:653–662.

Welberg LA, Seckl JR (2001) Prenatal stress, glucocorticoids and the programming of the brain. *J Neuroendocrinol* 13:113–128.

West MJ (1993) New stereological methods for counting neurons. Neurobiol Aging 14:275–285.

West MJ, Gundersen HJG (1990) Unbiased stereological estimation of the number of neurons in the human hippocampus. *J Comp Neurol* 296:1–22.

Wilson MM, Greer SE, Greer MA, Roberts L (1980) Hippocampal inhibition of pituitary-adrenocortical function in female rats. *Brain Res* 197:433–441.

Wolf OT, Kuhlmann S, Buss C, Hellhammer DH, Kirschbaum C (2004) Cortisol and memory retrieval in humans: influence of emotional valence. *Ann N Y Acad Sci* 1032:195–197.

Woodson JC, Macintosh D, Fleshner M, Diamond DM (2003) Emotion-induced amnesia in rats: working memory-specific impairment, corticosterone–memory correlation, and fear versus arousal effects on memory. *Learn Mem* 10:326–336.

Woolley CS, Gould E, McEwen BS (1990) Exposure to excess glucocorticoids alters dendritic morphology of adult hippocampal pyramidal neurons. *Brain Res* 531:225–231.

Xiong W, Yang Y, Cao J, Wei H, Liang C, Yang S, Xu L (2003) The stress experience dependent long-term depression disassociated with stress effect on spatial memory task. *Neurosci Res* 46:415–421.

Xu L, Anwyl R, Rowan MJ (1997) Behavioural stress facilitates the induction of long-term depression in the hippocampus. *Nature* 387:497–500.

Yau JL, Olsson T, Morris RG, Meaney MJ, Seckl JR (1995) Glucocorticoids, hippocampal corticosteroid receptor gene expression and antidepressant treatment: relationship with spatial learning in young and aged rats. *Neuroscience* 66:571–581.

Yehuda R (2001) Biology of posttraumatic stress disorder. J Clin Psychiatry 62(Suppl 17):41–46.

Yehuda R, Boisoneau D, Lowy MT, Giller EL Jr (1995) Dose-response changes in plasma cortisol and lymphocyte glucocorticoid receptors following dexamethasone administration in combat veterans with and without posttraumatic stress disorder. *Arch Gen Psychiatry* 52:583–593.

Yerkes RM, Dodson JD (1908) The relation of strength of stimulus to rapidity of habit-formation. *J Comp Neurol Psychol* 18:459–482.

16 Matthew Walker, Dennis Chan, and Maria Thom

Hippocampus and Human Disease

16.1 Overview

The hippocampus is involved in many disparate disease processes, but only in rare instances is the hippocampus the sole site of pathological damage. It is subject to the same pathologies that can affect other cortical areas, such as tumors, vascular malformations, and cortical dysgenesis; but in addition the hippocampus is also notable for its particular vulnerability to damage as a consequence of ischemia/hypoxia, trauma, and hypoglycemia. There are also instances in which involvement of the hippocampal formation is critical to the manifestation of the disease; foremost among them are Alzheimer's disease and temporal lobe epilepsy, representing approximately 60% of all partial epilepsies. Alzheimer's disease and epilepsy are among the most prevalent of all neurological diseases, with 20 million and 50 million people affected, respectively. Damage to the hippocampus is also the central component of a variety of rare conditions, such as limbic encephalitis and dementia with isolated hippocampal sclerosis. In addition, involvement of the hippocampus is being increasingly recognized in schizophrenia, another common neuropsychiatric disorder.

Acute encephalitis due to herpes simplex virus shows a predilection for limbic structures, and infection can result in selective damage to the hippocampus, amygdala, and associated structures, resulting in acute limbic encephalitis. Subacute limbic encephalitis has also been described in which the pathology more specifically affects the limbic system (Corsellis et al., 1968). The clinical presentation is characterized by behavioral and psychiatric problems (usually aggression and depression), disorientation, short-term memory deficits, hallucinations, seizures, and sleep disturbances (Corsellis et al., 1968; Gultekin et al., 2000). The pathological finding is aggregation of lymphocytes around blood vessels (perivascular lymphocytic cuffing), neuronal cell loss, and gliosis particularly affecting the hippocampus, dentate gyrus, amygdala, cingulate, and parahippocampal structures. There

is also often coincidental involvement of the brain stem and cerebellum. Limbic encephalitis can occur in response to certain cancers such as small-cell lung carcinomas, lymphomas, thymomas, and testicular tumors, as an immune-mediated syndrome (one of a number of so-called paraneoplastic syndromes). A similar syndrome has, however, been described in association with Wernicke's encephalopathy, systemic lupus erythematosus, and herpes simplex encephalitis. In these cases, there is a strong association with anti-neuronal antibodies directed against intracellular antigens, but the pathological role of these antibodies remains uncertain. Treatment of the underlying malignancy can alleviate the symptoms.

Hippocampal sclerosis has been observed in a proportion of elderly patients presenting with cognitive impairment. In one study (Dickson et al., 1994), hippocampal sclerosis was observed in 26% of demented patients over the age of 80 years and in 16% of all patients aged over 80. In all cases there was neuronal loss and gliosis affecting CA1, the subiculum, and dentate granule cells, with additional neuronal loss in the entohinal cortex in a proportion of cases. However, concomitant pathology, such as ischemic vascular damage or Alzheimer pathology, was noted in most of the cases in this study; "pure" hippocampal sclerosis is much rarer, affecting only 0.4% of patients with dementia (Ala et al., 2000). These rare instances of pure hippocampal sclerosis are not associated with any increase in risk factors for cerebrovascular disease, and in none of the cases was there a history of a hypoxic episode preceding the onset of cognitive impairment. The relation between hippocampal sclerosis, as a rare cause of dementia in the elderly, and mesial temporal sclerosis, as a substrate for epilepsy affecting a younger age group, remains undetermined, but it is possible that the two diseases arise as a consequence of differing etiologies, with pure hippocampal sclerosis occurring as a consequence of a primary degenerative process rather than secondary to a systemic insult such as hypoxia or fever.

Schizophrenia is thought to involve primarily the prefrontal cortex (Grossberg, 2000), but there is accumulating evidence for involvement of mesial temporal lobe structures in its pathophysiology. Indeed, there is evidence accumulating that schizophrenia may be a result of fronto-hippocampal integration. Some patients with temporal lobe epilepsy exhibit a psychosis indistinguishable from schizophrenia. Structural neuroimaging studies have shown a subtle but definite reduction in hippocampal volume (Nelson et al., 1998), which in some cases is present early in the disease; and functional imaging studies using magnetic resonance spectroscopy have documented a reduction in levels of the metabolite *N*-acetyl-D-aspartate, a marker of neuronal viability, in patients with schizophrenia (Maier et al., 1995). Neuropathological studies indicate that the loss of hippocampal volume correlates with a reduction in the size of hippocampal neurons rather than neuronal loss (Arnold et al., 1995). A reduction in neuronal density in certain hippocampal regions, with the CA2 interneurons particularly affected, is also observed in schizophrenia, as well as in manic depression (Benes et al., 1998). Loss of synaptic proteins in the hippocampus (Eastwood and Harrison, 1995) and abnormal MAP2 expression in subicular neuron dendrites also indicate abnormalities of connectivity in patients with schizophrenia (Cotter et al., 2000). The lack of demonstrable gliosis in those with schizophrenia has been argued to support a neurodevelopmental rather than degenerative disease process; the demonstration in schizophrenia of cytoarchitectural abnormalities of pre-alpha cells in the entorhinal cortex and of abnormal orientation of hippocampal pyramidal neurons (Conrad et al., 1991) also support a maldevelopmental disorder.

The human hippocampus is the beneficiary of a generous arterial supply originating from a number of major arteries, including the anterior choroidal artery and branches of the posterior cerebral artery (Erdem et al., 1993). Despite this, the vascular supply to the hippocampus may be interrupted as a result of embolic disease, as well as by prolonged anoxic insults. Ischemic damage to the hippocampus can occur in isolation or as part of a more widespread cerebrovascular disease process. In addition, animal experiments have shown that hippocampal damage, particularly affecting the CA1 subfield, can occur as a result of chronic nonembolic vascular insufficiency (de la Torre et al., 1992). Despite the known vulnerability of CA1 to ischemic damage (an observation dating back to the observations made by Sommer in 1898) and evidence from animal studies that the hippocampus is particularly sensitive to ischemic insult (Schmidt-Kastner and Freund, 1991), there exist in the clinical literature very few cases in which selective damage to the hippocampus has been observed. Hypoglycemia results in a pattern of damage different from that of ischemia, as it causes necrosis of predominantly the dentate granule cells (Auer and Siesjo, 1988); the clinical significance of such damage is not clear. Lastly, mesial temporal structures are particularly vulnerable to traumatic brain injury; this is partly because of their location in the middle cranial fossa, leaving them susceptible to contusion and vascular injury, but it may also be due to direct excitotoxic effects (Tate and Bigler, 2000).

The characterization of hippocampal involvement in human disease has been of great value to neuroscientists and clinicians. For instance, the unilateral nature of hippocampal sclerosis in temporal lobe epilepsy has provided the opportunity to analyze the individual functions of the left and right hippocampi. Also, the identification of hippocampal sclerosis by high-resolution magnetic resonance imaging (MRI) in epilepsy patients has stimulated the use of curative epilepsy neurosurgery. The hippocampal atrophy that occurs as a result of the pathological changes of Alzheimer's disease can be detected and quantified using in vivo neuroimaging techniques. As a biomarker of disease, the presence of hippocampal atrophy provides important corroborative information at the time of the clinical diagnosis, and the demonstration of progressive hippocampal volume loss is valuable for tracking disease progression. Finally, case studies documenting the nature of cognitive impairments in those rare patients with selective hippocampal pathology have provided important insights into the functions of the human hippocampus (see Chapter 13).

This chapter focuses on two disorders in which the role of the hippocampus has been extensively investigated: Alzheimer's disease and temporal lobe epilepsy. Although in Alzheimer's disease the disease process results eventually in widespread destruction of the cerebral cortex, the damage in the earliest stages of disease is restricted to the entorhinal cortex and the hippocampus, and the memory impairment that results from this disruption of the hippocampal formation represents one of the common characteristics of Alzheimer's disease. In temporal lobe epilepsy, the pathological damage is often restricted to the hippocampus in the form of hippocampal sclerosis. However, unlike Alzheimer's disease, in which the hippocampal damage is secondary to the underlying pathological process, the hippocampus in temporal lobe epilepsy is not only sensitive to damage by seizure activity but can also act as the substrate for epileptic seizure generation.

16.2 Mesial Temporal Lobe Epilepsy and Hippocampal Sclerosis

16.2.1 Introduction

Epilepsy is the propensity to have seizures and is one of the most common serious neurological conditions, affecting 0.4% to 1.0% of the world's population (Sander and Shorvon, 1996). There are approximately 20 to 70/100,000 new cases per year, and the lifetime chance of seizures is 3% to 5% (Sander and Shorvon, 1996). Seizure types can be divided into partial seizures, arising from one part of the brain, and generalized seizures, arising simultaneously throughout the cortex; respectively, these constitute approximately 40% and 50% of seizures in newly diagnosed epilepsy (10% of seizures are unclassifiable) (Sander and Shorvon, 1996). Epilepsy itself can be divided into a number of syndromes determined by seizure type, electroencephalographic (EEG) abnormalities and concomitant neurological deficits. Although all epilepsies are the result of an underlying brain abnormality (e.g., tumor or scar tissue in partial epilepsies, and a metabolic or genetic basis in generalized epilepsies), a convincing cause is identified in only approximately 30% of patients with epilepsy (Sander and Shorvon, 1996). The clinical manifestation of a seizure depends not only on where the seizure starts but also on the speed and pattern of seizure spread. Differing epilepsy syndromes have different pathophysiologies and mechanisms; in this chapter we are concerned solely with temporal lobe epilepsy.

Temporal lobe epilepsy represents approximately 60% of all partial epilepsies. The commonest neuropathological lesion identified in temporal lobectomy series in patients with mesial temporal lobe epilepsy (TLE) is hippocampal sclerosis, or Ammon's horn sclerosis, which is seen in approximately half of the cases (Bruton, 1988). Other major pathologies can be grouped under "lesion-associated TLE" and include vascular malformations, malformations of cortical development, and glioneuronal tumors (Wolf et al., 1993). Of those patients with drug-resistant epilepsy, hippocampal sclerosis is the commonest aetiology.

In 1825, Bouchet and Cazauvielh presented their findings on 18 autopsied patients in a thesis that attempted to establish the relation between epilepsy, "l'épilepsie," and insanity, "l'aliénation mentale" (Bouchet and Cazauvielh, 1825). They noted that in five cases where there were changes in the cornu ammonis four were characterized by induration and one had softening. Sommer (1880) further described in detail the neuropathological finding of hippocampal sclerosis in the brains of patients with chronic epilepsy. He noted gliosis and pyramidal cell loss in predominantly the CA1 region of the hippocampus, and he proposed that these lesions were the cause of the epilepsy. That same year, Pfleger described hemorrhagic lesions in the mesial temporal lobe of a patient dying in status epilepticus and concluded that neuronal necrosis was the result of impaired blood flow or metabolic disturbances that occurred during the seizure (Pfleger, 1880). Since that time the debate as to whether hippocampal sclerosis is the cause or result of epilepsy has continued.

Three lines of evidence indicate that seizures originate in the sclerosed hippocampus. First, hippocampal sclerosis is closely associated with a particular seizure semiology, the psychomotor seizure—a seizure type first recognized by John Hughlings Jackson. Second, EEG evidence points to seizure onset in the sclerosed hippocampus. Lastly, surgical resection of the sclerosed hippocampus results in seizure remission.

16.2.2 Clinical Features

The typical history of a patient with hippocampal sclerosis is contained in Figure 16–1, see color insert. There is often an antecedent history of an insult (usually febrile seizures) followed by a gap before seizures begin many years later. These seizures often prove resistant to treatment. There is an increased co-morbidity including psychiatric problems (depression, psychosis), increased mortality and neuropsychological deficits that relate to the side of the hippocampal sclerosis: verbal memory deficits with dominant (usually left) temporal lobe involvement and nonverbal memory deficits with nondominant lobe involvement.

Seizure Semiology

Mesial temporal lobe seizures usually take the form of complex partial seizures, in which consciousness is disturbed, and less commonly simple partial seizures, in which consciousness is preserved (Walker and Shorvon, 1997). The seizure usually has a gradual evolution over 1 to 2 minutes (substantially longer than extratemporal seizures) and lasts longer (2–10 minutes) than complex partial seizures originating in extratemporal sites. The commonest warning (often termed aura, literally "breeze") is that of a rising sensation from the stomach. Other gastrointestinal auras can occur, especially nausea, stomach rumbling, and belching. Auras can also consist of olfactory-gustatory hallucinations, autonomic symptoms, affective symptoms, disturbances of memory, or visual hallucinations and illusions (especially with seizures involving the temporal neocortex). Autonomic symptoms include changes in heart rate and blood pressure, pallor or flushing of the face, pupillary dilatation, and piloerection. Affective symptoms typically take the form of fear (the most common and often extremely intense), depression, anger, and irritability. Euphoria and erotic thoughts have also been described. Dreamy states and feelings of depersonalization commonly occur. Déjà vu, déjà entendu, and other abnormalities of memory such as recollections of childhood or even former lives can also be present with this form of epilepsy.

After the aura and in the early stages, motor arrest and absence are prominent. Typically, this is followed by marked automatisms. The automatisms of mesiobasal TLE can be prolonged and are characteristically oroalimentary (e.g., lips-macking, chewing) and/or gestural (e.g., fidgeting, undressing, walking). Typically, the automatisms are more marked ipsilaterally and may be associated with contralateral posturing. There may be some apparent responsiveness, and "conscious behavior" can occur during nondominant temporal lobe seizures. During the seizure, speech with recognizable words lateralizes the focus to the nondominant temporal lobe. Secondary generalization is less common than in extratemporal lobe epilepsy. Postictal confusion is typical, and postictal dysphasia can occur following dominant temporal lobe seizures. Postictal headache and postictal psychosis have also been described. There is profound amnesia for the absence and automatism (Walker and Shorvon, 1997).

EEG Characteristics

Scalp EEG recordings usually demonstrate interictal epileptiform abnormalities (spikes, sharp waves) over the mid/anterior temporal region, but it is common for these epileptiform

A

A 32-year old man presented with refractory partial epilepsy. He had a prolonged febrile seizure at the age of 18 months, and spontaneous seizures began at the age of 8 years. These seizures have continued despite trying all available antiepileptic drugs. The seizures take the form of simple partial seizures in which he perceives a sense of fear rising from his stomach, and complex partial seizures in which he has an aura as above and then loses touch with his surroundings. During the complex partial seizure he is described as making chewing movements, his right hand is postured and he fiddles with his clothes with his left hand. The seizure lasts a couple of minutes, and he is then confused and dysphasic afterward for approximately 5 minutes.

B

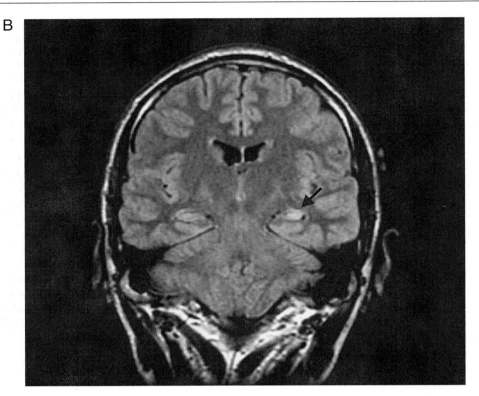

C

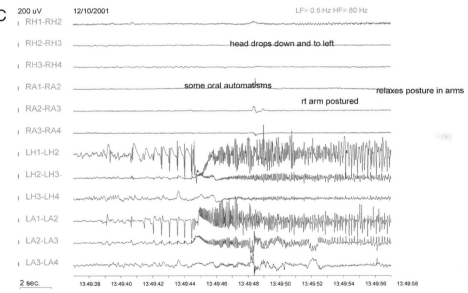

Figure 16–1. Clinical features of mesial temporal lobe epilepsy. *A.* Typical history. *B.* Magnetic resonance imaging (MRI) findings of left hippocampal sclerosis with high T2 signal in shrunken hippocampus (arrow). *C.* Intracranial recordings from left (LH) and right (RH) hippocampus and left (LA) and right (RA) amydala demonstrate well localized 1- to 2-Hz spikes in left hippocampus and amygdala that evolve to low-amplitude fast activity at seizure onset.

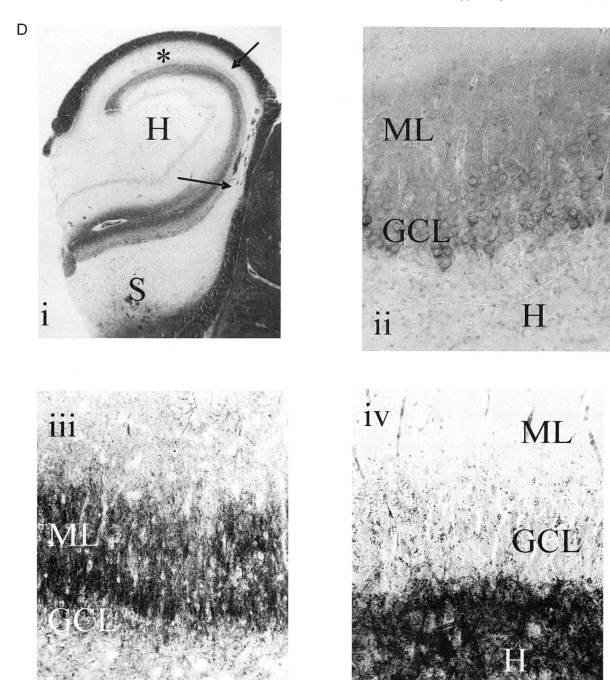

Figure 16–1. *(Continued) D.* Histology of left hippocampal sclerosis. i. Loss of cells in hilus (H) and CA1 (arrows) with preservation of CA2 (star) and subiculum (S); ii. Dynorphin staining demonstrating many fiber sprouting in granule cell layer (GCL) and molecular layer (ML); iii. Mossy fiber sprouting illustrated with Timm's stain; iv. Hippocampus with minimal mossy fiber sprouting for comparison with iii.

abnormalities to occur bilaterally or independently over both temporal regions (reasons why this may be so are discussed below) (Williamson et al., 1993). Ictal scalp recordings usually demonstrate a build-up of 5- to 10-Hz sharp activity localized to the mid/anterior temporal region. This activity may remain localized or commonly spreads to involve a wider field including the contralateral temporal lobe.

Depth electrode studies have further confirmed the electrographic origin of these seizures in the hippocampal formation (King and Spencer, 1995). Although interictal spikes may occur independently from either the hippocampus or extrahippocampal sites (see below), the ictal discharges are usually relatively well localized. Preictal abnormalities can occur with well localized 1- to 2-Hz spikes that recur over seconds or minutes (Fig. 16–1C, see color insert). With clinical seizure onset, there is a 10- to 15-Hz low-amplitude discharge that is initially confined to hippocampal electrodes (Fig.–16 1C, see color insert) but grows in amplitude and then spreads to other regions (King and Spencer, 1995). A second pattern has also been described in which the seizure begins as a low-amplitude, high-frequency discharge without the preictal spiking. These two types of onset can occur in the same patient. The exact location for seizure onset can vary not only from patient to patient but also within the same patient. This suggests that seizure onset and generation is not from a single area in mesial temporal structures but from a distributed network.

Hippocampal Resection

Surgery has provided the most compelling evidence of hippocampal sclerosis as the substrate for the epilepsy. Surgical outcome for intractable TLE is most successful when mesial temporal structures are included in the resection. In patients with drug-resistant epilepsy in whom there is concordance between neuroimaging, electroclinical characteristics of the seizure, and neuropsychological tests, there is a better than 80% chance of "curing" the epilepsy with temporal lobe resection (Arruda et al., 1996). Furthermore, over 80% of patients without tumors rendered seizure-free by temporal lobectomy have hippocampal sclerosis as their main pathology (French et al., 1993). In these patients depth electrode recordings also localized the seizure onset to the sclerosed hippocampus. There is thus a strong correlation between resection of a sclerosed hippocampus and cure of the epilepsy. Temporal lobe surgery, however, also involves removal of or damage to structures outside the hippocampus, including the amygdala and parahippocampal structures and temporal neocortex. Furthermore, many patients, despite successful surgery, remain dependent on antiepileptic drugs. These observations argue that structures beyond the hippocampus are involved in the epileptic network.

16.2.3 Etiology

Pathogenesis of Hippocampal Sclerosis and Developmental Aspects

There are predictable patterns of cell loss and alterations to the intrinsic circuitry of hippocampal sclerosis. However, the factors critical to the initiation of the cell loss and hippocampal reorganization are still debated, and the precise etiology of hippocampal sclerosis remains elusive.

A significant cerebral insult (or initial precipitating injury) occurring early in life, such as a febrile or prolonged seizure, is often reported (30–50% of cases—but up to 80% in one surgical series) in retrospective studies of patients with hip-

pocampal sclerosis (French et al., 1993). The "injury" hypothesis implies that this insult irreversibly damages or alters the hippocampus, resulting in a template for the progression to hippocampal sclerosis following a "latent" interval. There appears to be age-specific sensitivity for this injury, with more severe neuronal loss demonstrated with earlier onset of epilepsy (Davies et al., 1996). The most direct evidence of the association is the observation with serial neuroimaging that hippocampal sclerosis occurs following prolonged febrile convulsions (Van Landingham et al., 1998). Febrile seizures have been modeled in animals by inducing hyperthermic seizures in rats by blasts of hot air or water. The similarities between the animal model and the human condition are that seizures occur in response to high body temperature and that increasing age confers resistance to these seizures (Baram et al., 1997; Walker and Kullmann, 1999). Although fever in humans is associated with other physiological changes, reducing the body temperature is an effective way to reduce the likelihood of seizures; thus, hyperpyrexia is probably the main trigger. There are, however, major differences between hyperthermic seizures in rats and febrile convulsions in humans. Inducing hyperthermia in young Sprague-Dawley rats apparently results in seizures in most of these animals (Baram et al., 1997), but convulsions are relatively rare in children with fever. In experimental models, prolonged hyperthermic seizures in immature rats did not cause spontaneous seizures during adulthood but did increase seizure susceptibility following administration of a convulsant (a "second hit") (Dube et al., 2000). However only 2% to 7% of children with a history of febrile convulsions go on to develop epilepsy (i.e., unprovoked seizures) later in life (Annegers et al., 1987). Because many children with febrile convulsions may have a predisposing susceptibility to seizures, the low incidence of subsequent epilepsy could be explained by a protective effect of febrile seizures. Alternatively, febrile seizures alone are not sufficient to result in development of epilepsy. (Walker and Kullmann, 1999).

Other insults can result in hippocampal sclerosis including neonatal hypoxia and head injuries. In rat models, fluid percussion injury to the dura results in hilar interneuron loss in the hippocampus (Lowenstein et al., 1992). The mechanism by which this occurs is unknown. The neuronal loss is accompanied by enhanced excitability of the hippocampus but again no spontaneous seizures (Lowenstein et al., 1992). These experimental and human studies do not, however, address two fundamental questions: (1) Why is hippocampal sclerosis predominantly a unilateral disease process in humans (see below) following a "global" cerebral insult? (2) What is the nature of the "second hit" that results in the expression of epilepsy?

The second hit does not necessarily have to be environmental but could be the coexistence of various genetic factors or concomitant developmental abnormalities. Temporal lobe epilepsy is generally regarded as an acquired disorder with only a small genetic contribution. There are familial cases of febrile seizures, which are associated with ion channel mutations: sodium channel subunit and γ-aminobutyric acid ionotropic receptor family A (GABA$_A$) subunit mutations) (Table 16–1) (Kullmann, 2002). However, these families usually present with a hetererogeneous group of epilepsies that are distinct from the typical history of hippocampal epilepsy. More recently, the leucine-rich, glioma-inactivated 1 gene has been associated with familial neocortical temporal lobe epilepsies, although the mechanisms by which this mutation results in epilepsy are unknown (Kullmann, 2002). We are at present ignorant of the genetic mutations underlying most of the genetically determined epilepsies, let alone those that contribute to other epilepsies. Genetic predisposition to some forms of temporal lobe epilepsy and febrile convulsions have been described, and there are familial cases of febrile convulsions and TLE but without hippocampal sclerosis (Baulac et al., 2001).

More recent attention has focused on an underlying maldevelopment of the hippocampus as a primary abnormality predisposing to hippocampal sclerosis and to febrile seizures. In an MRI study of families with familial febrile convulsions, a subtle preexisting hippocampal abnormality was detected (Fernandez et al., 1998), and hippocampal sclerosis has also been reported in patients in association with isolated malformations of the hippocampus (Baulac et al., 1998). In addition, an abnormal persistence of calretinin positive Cajal-Retzius cells in the hippocampus has been reported in hippocampal sclerosis specimens (Blumcke et al., 1999b). Cajal Retzius cells, through secretion of the reelin protein, play a critical role in neuronal organization in the developing brain. Higher numbers of Cajal-Retzius cells were particularly prominent in patients with hippocampal sclerosis and a history of febrile seizures. It is plausible that such an injury occurring early in life disrupts normal hippocampal development and maturation (one manifestation of which is an excess of Cajal-Retzius cells), which in turn predisposes to hippocampal sclerosis. As it has been suggested that reelin in the adult cortex has a role in plasticity and axonal remodeling, an increased number of these cells may also be important for the reorganization of circuitry occurring in hippocampal sclerosis (described below).

The final argument supporting a maldevelopmental basis for hippocampal sclerosis comes from the observation that hippocampal sclerosis is often observed in association with subtle cytoarchitactural malformations in the neocortex, also termed microdysgenesis (Hardiman et al., 1988). This may be indicative of a more widespread maldevelopmental process involving both mesial and lateral temporal lobe structures. One cytoarchitectural feature observed in microdysgenesis is also an excess of Cajal Retzius cells in the molecular layer (Garbelli et al., 2001), which interestingly seems to parallel findings in hippocampal sclerosis.

Table 16–1.
Monogenic Epilepsies and Ion Channels Implicated in Human Epilepsy

Syndrome	Gene	Locus	Protein
Autosomal Dominant Inheritance			
Autosomal dominant nocturnal frontal lobe epilepsy (ADNFLE)	CHRNA4	20q13.2-q13.3	Nicotinic ACh receptor subunit
	CHRNB2	1p21	Nicotinic ACh receptor subunit
Benign familial neonatal convulsions (BFNC)*	KCNQ2	20q13.3	Potassium channel subunit
	KCNQ3	8q24	Potassium channel subunit
Generalized epilepsy with febrile seizures plus (GEFS†)	SCN1A	2q24	Sodium channel subunit
	SCN1B	19q13.1	Sodium channel subunit
	GABRG2	5q33.1-q33.1	GABA$_A$ receptor subunit†
Juvenile myoclonic epilepsy (JME)	GABRA1	5q34	GABA$_A$ receptor subunit
Autosomal dominant partial epilepsy with auditory features [ADPEAF]‡	LGI1	10q24	Leucine-rich, glioma-inactivated 1 [unknown function—not an Ion channel]
Sporadic			
Severe myoclonic epilepsy of Infancy (SMEI)	SCN1A	2q24	Sodium channel subunit
Other Ion Channel Genes Implicated in Epilepsy§			
Febrile and afebrile seizures	SCN2A	2q23-q24.3	Sodium channel subunit
Episodic ataxia type 1 with partial epilepsy	KCNA1	12p13	Potassium channel subunit
Episodic ataxia type 2 with spike-wave epilepsy	CACNA1A	19p13	Calcium channel subunit
JME	CACNB4	2q22-23	Calcium channel subunit¶

Source: After Kullmann (2002), with permission.
ACh, acetylcholine; GABA$_A$, γ-aminobutyric acid ionotropic receptor family A; GABA$_B$, GABA ionotropic receptor family B.
*A 15% risk of epilepsy continuing beyond infancy.
†Also associated with febrile seizures and absences.
‡Also known as autosomal dominant lateral temporal epilepsy.
§Mutations identified in small number of patients, so role in epilepsy is less clear.
¶Also associated with generalized epilepsy with praxis-induced seizures.

Hippocampal sclerosis is also well recognized to occur in association with more severe cortical malformations, vascular malformations, and low-grade glioneuronal tumors (Cendes et al., 1995; Li et al., 1999). It possible that in these cases the epileptogenic extrahippocampal lesion "kindles" the hippocampal neuronal loss (i.e., the hippocampal sclerosis in these cases is a secondary event) (see below). It has been shown, however, that in patients with dual pathologies removal of both the lesion and the abnormal hippocampus has the best outcome in terms of seizure control (Li et al., 1999), emphasizing the role of the hippocampus in temporal lobe seizures even when there is a second pathology.

Animal Models of Mesial Temporal Lobe Epilepsy

The interpretation of many of the pathological findings and the electrophysiologic studies in human postsurgical specimens is confounded by: (1) the influence of treatment; (2) the difficulty differentiating cause from effect (i.e., it is possible that the changes are the result, not the cause, of the seizures); and (3) the lack of adequate control tissue for comparison. To overcome these handicaps, animal models of mesial TLE are used. The two most studied are the kindling model and the poststatus epilepticus model. Intrahippocampal injection of tetanus toxin also results in spontaneous seizures even after clearance of the toxin, and this model has also contributed to our understanding of the pathophysiology of mesial TLE (Mellanby et al., 1977). This model does not result in hippocampal sclerosis (Jefferys et al., 1992), and the seizures usually abate, in contrast to the human condition. We discuss the kindling and the poststatus epilepticus models in more detail, as these models possibly have human correlates.

Kindling. Kindling is the repetition of tetanic (trains of) stimuli that initially evoke after-discharges but not seizures (Goddard, 1967; McNamara et al., 1993). Repetition of the same trains of stimuli results in gradual lengthening of the after-discharges, eventually leading to progressively more severe seizures. Once an animal has been kindled, the heightened response to the stimulus seems to be permanent, and spontaneous seizures can occur (McNamara et al., 1993). The hippocampus and amygdala are easily kindled, resulting in a well described progression of limbic seizures. Kindling shares several characteristics with NMDA-dependent long-term potentiation (LTP) of excitatory synaptic transmission. This has led to the suggestion that kindling and LTP have similar underlying mechanisms. In support of this, the rate at which kindling occurs is retarded in rodents treated with NMDA receptor antagonists. There are, however, several differences between kindling and LTP. Although NMDA receptor antagonists can completely block the induction of LTP, they are unable to block kindling completely (Cain et al., 1992). Perhaps a more fundamental difference is that the kindling process requires after-discharges; the repeated induction of LTP without after-discharges does not induce kindling. LTP of

glutamatergic synaptic transmission may contribute to kindling by increasing the excitatory synaptic drive and the likelihood of evoking after-discharges but is alone insufficient to explain the cellular mechanisms of kindling (Cain, 1989; Cain et al., 1992).

Kindling alone is unlikely to explain the occurrence of hippocampal sclerosis in association with other pathology because kindling itself usually results in no or minimal hippocampal damage and sclerosis (Tuunänen and Pitkänen, 2000). Kindling could, however, explain the progression of mesial temporal epilepsy. Eventually spontaneous seizures in the kindling model result in progressive neuronal loss in the hippocampus (Cavazos et al., 1994). Indeed, even following single seizures there is evidence of both apoptotic cell death and neurogenesis in the dentate granule cell layer (Bengzon et al., 1997). This suggests that recurrent seizures may cause further structural and functional changes in the hippocampus. Human evidence for this has mainly been indirect. Epilepsy duration correlates with hippocampal volume loss and progressive neuronal loss and dysfunction (Theodore et al., 1999). There has also been a case reported of hippocampal volumes decreasing with time in hippocampal sclerosis (Van Paesschen et al., 1998) and the appearance of hippocampal sclerosis de novo following secondary generalized brief tonic-clonic seizures (Briellmann et al., 2001).

Poststatus Epilepticus. Seizures are usually self-terminating and brief. Occasionally seizures persist unabated, or repeated seizures can occur without recovery; this situation is termed status epilepticus. Although status epilepticus may occur in individuals with preexisting epilepsy, more than half of patients who present with status epilepticus have no history of seizures (DeLorenzo et al., 1996). In these patients, the status epilepticus is often acutely precipitated by a central nervous system (CNS) infection, cerebral vascular accident, hypoxia, or alcohol. The probability of then developing epilepsy (unprecipitated seizures) is 41% within 2 years compared with 13% for those with acute symptomatic seizures but no status epilepticus (Hesdorffer et al., 1998). This suggests a relation between the prolonged seizures of status epilepticus and subsequent epileptogenesis, although a relation between the length of the seizure and the nature and severity of the precipitant cannot be discounted. In humans, status epilepticus has been shown to result in hippocampal damage and subsequent hippocampal sclerosis. The hippocampus thus has a dichotomous role: as the substrate for epilepsy and as the structure susceptible to damage by prolonged seizures. Animal models of generalized convulsive as well as limbic status epilepticus have supported these findings. Limbic status epilepticus has been induced by the systemic or local administration of kainic acid, systemic administration of pilocarpine (a muscarinic receptor agonist), or protocols using electrical stimulation of limbic areas (Walker et al., 2002). Status epilepticus in these models in adult animals results in hippocampal damage similar to that observed in humans. Following these acute episodes of limbic status epilepticus, many of the animals go on to develop spontaneous limbic seizures after a latent period lasting days to weeks (Walker et al., 2002).

16.2.4 Pathophysiology

One of the major points of confusion in understanding the pathophysiology of epilepsy is the differentiation of a seizure (ictus) from interictal discharges and, indeed, from epilepsy itself. Although obviously linked, they are separate entities. An epileptic seizure is a transient paroxysm of excessive discharges of neurons in the cerebral cortex causing a clinically discernible event. Brief synchronous activity of a group of neurons leads to the interictal spike, and as we discuss, this shares some mechanisms with seizure generation; spikes should, however, be recognized as a distinct phenomenon (de Curtis and Avanzini, 2001). Epilepsy, on the other hand, is the propensity to have seizures; and epileptogenesis is the development of a neuronal network in which spontaneous seizures occur.

Interictal Spike

Epileptiform interictal EEG abnormalities include spikes, which are fast electrographic transients lasting less than 80 ms, and sharp waves, which last 80 to 120 ms (de Curtis and Avanzini, 2001). That these abnormalities are pathological is supported by their rare occurrence ($< 1\%$) in healthy individuals (Gregory et al., 1993) and their strong association with epilepsy (Ajmone-Marsan and Zivin, 1970). Spikes and sharp waves are often followed by a slow wave lasting hundreds of milliseconds. As discussed below, this slow wave probably represents a period of relative refractoriness. It has been established from concomitant field potential and intracellular recordings that the intracellular correlate of the interictal spike is the paroxysmal depolarizing shift (PDS) (Matsumoto and Ajmone-Marsan, 1964), a slow depolarizing potential with a high-frequency (> 200 Hz) burst of action potentials.

In hippocampal slices from healthy animals, PDSs can be observed if GABA$_A$ inhibition is reduced or if "excitability" is increased by increasing potassium, reducing magnesium, reducing calcium, or blocking potassium channels with 4-aminopyridine (de Curtis and Avanzini, 2001). The PDS is characterized by an early phase that is maintained by intrinsic properties of the neuron followed by a later phase that is secondary to recurrent excitation. Thus, the generation of interictal spikes is dependent on two phenomena: the intrinsic burst properties of neurons and the synchronization of neuronal populations. Within the hippocampus, pyramidal cells in area CA3 and some in area CA1 demonstrate burst properties (see Chapter 5). The mechanisms underlying this are different for neurons from these two subfields. The bursting in CA3 pyramidal cells appears to be dependent on regenerative dendritic potentials secondary to activation of calcium and sodium channels (Traub and Jefferys, 1994), whereas the burst properties of some CA1 pyramidal cells is probably due to

persistent sodium currents (Su et al., 2001). The effect of a burst of action potentials is to increase synaptic reliability; within the excitatory network of the CA3 pyramidal cells, burst firing in a single CA3 pyramidal cell can generate a synchronized burst throughout the whole network (Miles and Wong, 1983). Because of the propensity for the CA3 pyramidal cells to generate this synchronized burst, this region has often been considered the "pacemaker" for seizure activity. Synchronized bursts can, however, also occur in the CA1 subfield (Karnup and Stelzer, 2001). In some situations the synchronization of CA1 pyramidal cells is secondary to a CA3 generated burst, but synchronization can also occur through a combination of nonsynaptic mechanisms including gap junctions, ephaptic transmission, and changes in the extracellular milieu. The importance of these nonsynaptic mechanisms in neuronal synchronization has been emphasized by the "zero" calcium model of ictal discharges, in which reducing extracellular calcium in a hippocampal slice preparation below that necessary for synaptic transmission results in synchronized epileptiform discharges due to increased axonal excitability and ephaptic transmission (Jefferys, 1995). Furthermore, decreasing extracellular space (indirectly increasing ephaptic transmission) can promote bursting (Roper et al., 1992), whereas intracellular acidification with sodium propionate—indirectly decreasing electrotonic coupling (Perez and Carlen, 2000)—inhibits epileptiform bursts (Xiong et al., 2000). Synchronization of principal cells can occur secondary to oscillations in the inhibitory interneuron network; indeed, single basket cells have been shown to synchronize the discharges of pyramidal cells through synchronized somatic inhibition (Cobb et al., 1995). Although the precise mechanisms of neuronal synchronization in the hippocampus are still unclear, the observation of high-frequency oscillations superimposed on spike discharges has led to the hypothesis that the same physiological mechanisms that subtend fast oscillations in the hippocampus are also responsible for pathological synchronization (Perez and Carlen, 2000; Traub et al., 2001).

The interictal spike is terminated by activation of hyperpolarizing GABA$_A$ and GABA$_B$ receptor-mediated currents and calcium-dependent potassium currents (Alger and Nicoll, 1980; Domann et al., 1994; Scanziani et al., 1994). There is also some evidence of a contribution by other potassium currents, such as the sodium-dependent potassium current (Schwindt et al., 1989). Blocking the after-hyperpolarization, however, only results in moderate prolongation of the burst in CA3; and exhaustion of the immediately releasable pool of glutamate has also been proposed to be a critical process in burst termination (Staley et al., 1998). Furthermore, large depolarizations (rather than hyperpolarizations) herald the termination of brief epileptic after-discharges (Bragin et al., 1997). This depolarization can be replicated by focal microinjection of potassium, and it has been hypothesized that potassium ions released by discharging neurons result in propagating waves of depolarization, which block spike generation in neurons akin to spreading depression (Bragin et al., 1997).

Nevertheless, interictal spikes activate hyperpolarizing currents resulting in a postspike refractory period, during which neuronal activity is inhibited (de Curtis and Avanzini, 2001). The effective activation of these currents by the interictal spike thus raises the possibility that spikes can be anti-ictogenic. There is evidence that this may be the case or at least that spikes are intrinsically different from a seizure. Depth EEG recordings in humans suggest that the interictal spike can originate from a much wider field than the ictal zone (see above). Therefore, it is not uncommon to find spikes originating in either hippocampus, whereas seizure activity is confined to one hippocampus.

A seizure is not the evolution of spike discharges but can begin as a distinct high-frequency rhythm (see above). Spike discharges can precede the seizure with progressively less effective after-hyperpolarizations, but ictal activity remains a distinct phenomenon. Furthermore, activation of interictal spikes occurs after the seizure, raising the possibility that this is a compensatory antiepileptic response (de Curtis and Avanzini, 2001). Critical experiments in entorhinal cortex-

hippocampal slice preparations, in which there is partial preservation of the trisynaptic loop, have confirmed the antiepileptic potential of spikes. Spike discharges generated in CA3 inhibited epileptic activity in the entorhinal cortex, so sectioning of the Schaffer collaterals led to potentiation of entorhinal cortex seizure activity (Fig. 16–2) (Barbarosie and Avoli, 1997).

Most of the ictal activity described thus far in the hippocampal slice preparation has been brief and difficult to relate to seizures in vivo that last tens of seconds. Can such prolonged activity be mimicked in the slice, and does it differ from briefer discharges? Prolonged ictal activity (seizure-like activity) has been induced in the slice with high extracellular potassium (Traynelis and Dingledine, 1988). In this preparation, the CA3 subfield generates regular interictal spikes, which "drive" the generation of prolonged rhythmic "seizure" activity in the CA1 region; interestingly, the CA3 region in this preparation is resistant to generating this ictal activity (Traynelis and Dingledine, 1988). Inducing seizure-like activity in brain slices by other means (e.g., the lowering magne-

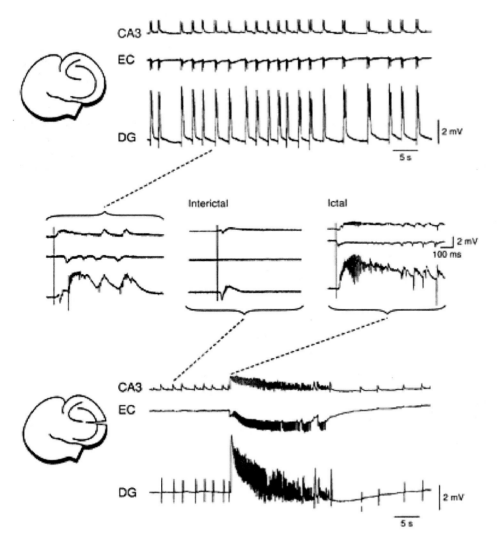

Figure 16–2. Interictal spikes inhibit seizure activity. Spontaneous epileptiform activity induced by Mg^{+2}-free artificial cerebrospinal fluid (ACSF) before and after a Schaffer collateral cut. Before the lesion (*top*), synchronized interictal discharges are recorded in the CA3, entorhinal cortex (EC), and dentate gyrus (DG). Sectioning the Schaffer collaterals (*bottom*) abolishes interictal discharges in the EC and discloses ictal epileptiform activity that is recorded in the three areas. Expanded traces of the experiment shown in the *top* and *bottom* are illustrated in the *middle*. Note that before the Schaffer collateral cut Mg^{+2}-free-induced interictal discharges consist of multiple components, whereas after the cut (Interictal) they are markedly reduced in duration and number of events. (*Source:* Adapted from Barbarosie and Avoli, 1997.)

sium level or GABA$_A$ receptor blockade) can result in the generation of such activity in other regions in the hippocampal/parahippocampal formation such as the subiculum (Behr and Heinemann, 1996), area CA3 (Borck and Jefferys, 1999), and the entorhinal cortex (Jones, 1989). That small areas can generate seizure-like activity in the slice supports the hypothesis that a network of only a few thousand neurons is necessary to sustain seizure activity (Borck and Jefferys, 1999). That the maintenance of seizure-like activity is different from the mechanisms underlying briefer epileptiform discharges is suggested by their differing pharmacology; NMDA receptor antagonists can terminate brief epileptiform discharge but are ineffective during the "maintenance phase" of seizure-like activity (Borck and Jefferys, 1999).

So how do spontaneous seizures (epilepsy) occur in vivo? The brain slice studies can give us an insight into specific questions concerning the generation of epileptiform discharges. The interpretation and the in vivo extrapolation of such studies are, however, complicated by certain observations: Seizure-like activity can be generated in vitro by quite disparate means, and the mechanisms and structures involved in the generation of such activity can differ from study to study. Seizure activity relies on oscillatory synchronization; thus, mechanisms similar to those described in Chapter 8 undoubtedly contribute to the emergence of in vivo seizure activity. Furthermore, it is likely that mechanisms similar (but not necessarily identical) to those that underlie spike discharges and longer "epileptic after-discharges" promote in vivo seizure activity. The transition from normal, physiological oscillatory behavior to epileptiform behavior is likely to be due to greater spread and neuronal recruitment secondary to enhanced connectivity, enhanced excitatory transmission, or a failure of inhibitory mechanisms. Indeed, in human studies,

the EEG becomes less chaotic in large areas of cortex at the start of an ictus, suggesting that widespread synchronization is occurring (Martinerie et al., 1998). To understand how a network that usually maintains oscillatory behavior becomes "epileptic," it is paramount to consider the changes that occur in the hippocampus during epileptogenesis.

One problem with much that has been described is that it is associational (i.e., changes are observed and are assumed to contribute to the epileptogenic process). This may not hold true for many of the changes, which could be compensatory (i.e., protecting against the epileptogenic process). Unfortunately, it has been difficult to distinguish between these possibilities, and we are far from a comprehensive model of epileptogenesis. The changes that occur can be divided into structural change (neuronal loss, reorganization, synaptic reorganization, changes in glia and extracellular space), changes in neurotransmission, and lastly changes in neuronal properties. We discuss how each of these changes may contribute to the epileptogenic process (Fig. 16–3).

Structural Change

Neuronal Loss. Hippocampal sclerosis is typically a unilateral process, affecting either hemisphere equally, with involvement of the whole length of the hippocampus. In some cases more focal damage may be observed (Babb et al., 1984). and in others there is bilateral sclerosis (Van-Paesschen et al., 1997a). In so-called classic hippocampal sclerosis, selective loss of pyramidal cells is seen in the CA1 subfield and in the hilar region with accompanying astrocytic gliosis. In some patients neuronal loss is restricted to the CA1 subfield (de Lanerolle et al., 2003). Pyramidal cells of CA2 and dentate granule cells appear more resistant (Bruton, 1988). In severe hippocampal

Figure 16–3. Structural changes, changes in neurotransmission, and changes in the intrinsic properties of neurons all contribute to the development of epilepsy.

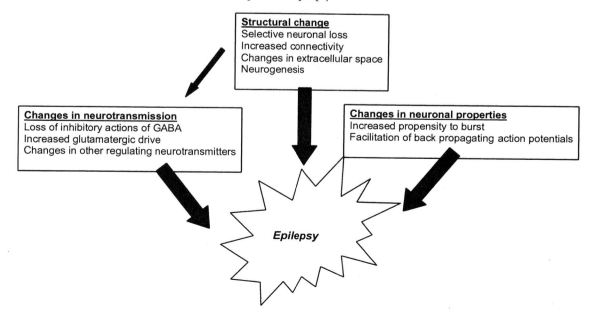

sclerosis almost total neuronal loss is seen in all hippocampal subfields and may be accompanied by marked deposition of corpora amylacea. In the pattern of hippocampal sclerosis termed "end folium gliosis," encountered in 3% to 4% of surgical cases (Bruton, 1988), the neuronal cell loss appears confined to the hilus and includes loss of both principal cells and interneurons. This pattern of hippocampal atrophy is less easily detected on preoperative MRI and is associated with a later onset of epilepsy than classic hippocampal sclerosis and a worse postoperative seizure outcome (Van Paesschen et al., 1997b).

Quantitative histological studies have been carried out in hippocampal sclerosis series, and pathological grading systems have been proposed to categorize the severity of neuronal loss in hippocampal sclerosis; for example, in one system, grade I hippocampal sclerosis correlates with less than 10% of neuronal dropout in CA1 up to grade IV hippocampal sclerosis, which shows more than 50% neuronal loss in all subfields (Wyler et al., 1992). This is based on a semiquantitative assessment of neuronal loss in histological sections. Such analyses have proved useful as they allow pathological correlation with clinical parameters (e.g., the age of the patient at epilepsy onset and the duration of seizures) (Davies et al., 1996) and with neuroimaging features. These grades may also reflect a progressive evolution of hippocampal sclerosis from grades I to IV, mirroring ongoing hippocampal atrophy that has been occasionally reported in sequential neuroimaging studies.

Marked cytological alterations have been observed in surviving neurons in hippocampal sclerosis using immunohistochemistry, electron microscopy, and confocal imaging techniques (Blumcke et al., 1999a). These changes include enlargement and accumulation of neurofilaments in end folial neurons, abnormal dendritic nodular swellings, and ramifications of these cells. These features more likely represent secondary or adaptive cellular changes due to the altered connectivity in the reorganized hippocampus rather than a primary cellular abnormality.

Neuronal loss and gliosis may also be present in adjacent limbic structures, including the amygdala (Yilmazer-Hanke et al., 2000) and parahippocampal gyrus, which along with hippocampal sclerosis are collectively referred to as mesial temporal sclerosis. Neuronal loss may also involve the entorhinal cortex, and volume loss has been demonstrated in the entorhinal cortex with quantitative MRI studies (Salmenpera et al., 2000). Neuropathological studies of this cortical region in patients with hippocampal sclerosis have suggested significant loss of layer III cells (Du et al., 1993), although other studies have suggested a more variable pattern of cell loss involving all layers, including loss of pre-alpha cells (Yilmazer-Hanke et al., 2000). The observed loss of entorhinal neurons could indicate either primary or secondary involvement of this region in the pathophysiology of temporal lobe seizures. An important observation, however, has been the demonstration of entorhinal cortex neuronal loss in the absence of hippocampal sclerosis (Yilmazer-Hanke et al., 2000; Bernasconi et al., 2001).

This and the observation that the entorhinal cortex can alone maintain seizure-like activity (Jones, 1989) perhaps implicate a more specific role for this region in seizure generation.

The extent of any temporal neocortex neuronal loss does seem to correlate with the severity of hippocampal damage (Bruton, 1988). Neocortical neuronal loss also appears to be layer-specific, with cortical layers II and III more severely affected.

Mechanisms of Neuronal Death in Status Epilepticus. The pattern of neuronal death in hippocampal sclerosis is mirrored by neuronal death seen in postmortem specimens following status epilepticus (DeGiorgio et al., 1992). Imaging studies have demonstrated the occurrence of hippocampal sclerosis following status epilepticus and prolonged seizures, further emphasizing the vulnerability of the hippocampus to neuronal damage. Insights into the mechanisms underlying this damage have largely been derived from animal models of status epilepticus (Meldrum, 1991). They have shown that although a certain amount of neuronal damage is secondary to physiological compromise that occurs during status epilepticus (e.g., hypoxia, hypoglycemia, hypotension) a large proportion of the damage is independent of these factors. This neuronal damage is due to excitotoxicity in which the presence of epileptic activity mediates neuronal death through the activation of glutamate receptors. Excessive influx of calcium (and zinc at mossy fiber synapses) through primarily NMDA receptors, but also through α-amino-3-hydroxy-5-methyl-4-isoxazolepropionate (AMPA) receptors lacking the GluR2 subunit, results in a cascade of reactions leading to cell death (Weiss et al., 2000; Lipton and Rosenberg, 1994; Tanaka et al., 2000).

Specific Neuronal Vulnerability in Hippocampal Sclerosis. Loss of the principal pyramidal cells in hippocampal sclerosis is established, but it is difficult conceptually to conceive how removal of principal excitatory neurons can contribute to a state of hyperexcitability. Undoubtedly, neuronal loss may contribute to synaptic rearrangements and perhaps increased connectivity, but more important perhaps is the vulnerability of specific subsets of interneurons in the hippocampal formation, which may influence the intrinsic circuitry of the hippocampus and seizure propagation. Most interneurons contain the neurotransmitter GABA but can be further subdivided according to their connectivity, calcium-binding protein content, and neurotransmitter receptor status (Freund and Buzsaki, 1996).

Neuropeptide Y (NPY)- and somatostatin-containing inhibitory interneurons are normally numerous in the hilus and form a dense plexus of fibers in the outer molecular layer of the dentate gyrus which co-localizes with glutamic acid decarboxylase (GAD) (Amaral and Campbell, 1986). Loss of these interneuronal subtypes in the hilus was noted in hippocampal sclerosis (deLanerolle et al., 1989; Mathern et al., 1995a). NPY-containing axons also appeared to be reorganized in the dentate molecular layer in hippocampal sclerosis, and ectopic expression of NPY in granule cells has been observed following seizures (Vezzani et al., 1999). This is likely to represent plasticity in NPY inhibitory mechanisms in the epileptogenic hippocampus. A more recent quantitative study using in situ hybridization however, has suggested that NPY and somatostatin neurons in the fascia dentata are lost in proportion to the overall cell loss and are not specifically "targeted" in the disease process (Sundstrom et al., 2001).

The calcium-binding proteins calbindin D-28-K, parvalbumin, and calretinin label different, nonoverlapping subsets of inhibitory hippocampal interneurons, and the resistance or susceptibility of these cell populations in hippocampal sclerosis may directly affect hippocampal epileptogenesis. The normal distribution of calbindin is not restricted to interneurons but is also present in the dentate gyrus granule cells, mossy fibers, and CA2 pyramidal cells; parvalbumin and calretinin are present only in interneurons. Calbindin-positive interneurons are mainly involved in the inhibition of principal cells in the dendritic region, whereas calretinin-positive interneurons probably selectively innervate other interneurons (Magloczky et al., 2000). An early study had suggested preferential survival of calbindin and parvalbumin immunoreactive neurons in hippocampal sclerosis (Sloviter, 1991). Furthermore, increased complexity of the terminal processes of powerful inhibitory interneurons, the chandelier cell (which may be parvalbumin- or calbindin-positive) has also been demonstrated in hippocampal sclerosis (Arellano et al 2004). More recent quantitative studies, however, have shown selective loss of parvalbumin-immunoreactive neurons in the hilus disproportionate to the overall cell loss (Zhu et al., 1997). The distribution of calbindin-positive interneurons in the dentate gyrus in hippocampal sclerosis was shown not to differ from controls in one study but striking enlargement of their cell bodies with enhanced expression of calbindin and modification of the dendritic trees and synapses of these cells was noted (Magloczky et al., 2000). Marked plasticity and reorganization of calbindin-positive interneurons in the CA1 subfield in the hippocampus has also been shown, which may predate the pyramidal cell loss (Wittner et al., 2002). The findings support a complex set of changes in interneural anatomy with changes in interneuron targets. Calretinin cells do not appear to show abnormal distribution in hippocampal sclerosis (Blumcke et al., 1996); but increased numbers of a subset of calretinin-positive neurons, the Cajal-Retzius cells, occurs in hippocampal sclerosis in some patients (Blumcke et al., 1999b). Studies have demonstrated an expansion of calretinin-positive axonal networks in the molecular layer of the dentate gyrus in hippocampal sclerosis (Blumcke et al., 1996, 1999b; Magloczky et al., 2000). These fibers are likely to represent those of the excitatory supramammillary pathway terminating on granule cells rather than local axons. This observation may indicate enhanced excitation of granule cells by this pathway (Magloczky et al., 2000).

The observed relative resistance of certain calbindin-containing neurons to neuronal damage has led to the suggestion that calbindin itself may be neuroprotective (Leranth and Ribak, 1991). However, in calcium-binding protein knockout mice, the absence of these proteins does not appear to affect the numbers of interneurons or excitotoxic-mediated cell loss in epilepsy (Bouilleret et al., 2000). Furthermore, in hippocampal sclerosis there is loss of calbindin expression by granule cells (Magloczky et al., 2000). Granule cells are typically more resistant to damage in hippocampal sclerosis than other principal neurons and it has controversially been proposed that the calbindin loss actually protects these cells from Ca^{2+}-mediated neuronal damage (Nagerl et al., 2000). The proposed mechanism underlying this proposal is that lack of calbindin results in larger intracellular free calcium transients that inactivate calcium channels, thus limiting intracellular calcium accumulation; on the other hand, buffering of free calcium transients with calcium-binding proteins permits greater accumulation of intracellular calcium. Thus, although these calcium-binding proteins may identify neurons that are resistant to damage, the calcium-binding protein itself is probably not neuroprotective.

Selective loss of hilar mossy cells, an excitatory interneuron with distinctive dendritic arborizations, has been described in hippocampal sclerosis cases compared to patients with generalized seizures (Blumcke et al., 2000b). These excitatory interneurons project to inhibitory basket cells, and their loss may result in reduced feedforward granule cell inhibition supporting the experimental "dormant basket cell hypothesis" (Sloviter, 1991). However it is recognized in animal models that basket cells also receive direct excitatory input from the granule cells and perforant path fibers, thus bypassing the mossy cells (Kneisler and Dingledine, 1995).

Pathophysiological Role of Neuronal Damage. Are epileptogenesis and neuronal damage directly related? Following status epilepticus, those animals that develop spontaneous seizures have greater hilar interneuronal loss, perhaps resulting in decreased inhibitory drive (Gorter et al., 2001). It has also been suggested that damage to CA3 and the Schaffer collaterals may prevent spikes generated in CA3 from inhibiting epileptic activity in the limbic system (see above). Selective neuronal death can also result in a change in the nature of inhibition. Dendritically expressed inhibitory postsynaptic potentials (IPSPs) modify the transmission of excitatory postsynaptic potentials (EPSPs) to the soma, whereas somatic and perisomatic IPSPs depress the excitability of the neuron (Cossart et al., 2001). Basket cells, which make multiple perisomatic and somatic synapses, have extensive axonal arborizsations leading to connection of one basket cell with many pyramidal cells. By synchronously modulating the excitability of a group of pyramidal neurons, one basket cell can synchronize pyramidal cell activity (Cobb et al., 1995). The loss of oriens/lacunosum-moleculare interneurons in CA1 results in loss of distal dendritic inhibition, whereas the preservation and increased connectivity of basket cells may result in greater pyramidal cell synchronization (Fig. 16–4) (Cossart et al., 2001). The selective loss of certain interneuronal populations in hippocampal sclerosis is thus probably pro-epileptogenic; but is neuronal loss necessary for epileptogenesis? That there is a distinction

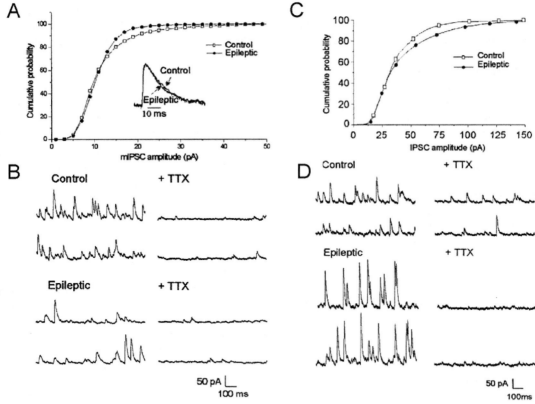

Figure 16–4. Inhibition is decreased in dendrites but increased at the soma. *A, B.* Recordings from the apical dendrites of CA1 pyramidal cells. *A.* The cumulative probability plot of the amplitudes of miniature events was shifted to the left, indicating decreased frequency of amplitudes larger than 15 pA in epileptic animals. The kinetics of miniature events (normalized averages) did not seem modified (*inset*). *B.* Whole-cell recordings of spontaneous (control) and miniature (TTX, 1 μM) inhibitory postsynaptic currents obtained at the reversal potential of glutamatergic events in a control and a kainate-treated animal. Continuous 4-s recordings are shown. The frequency of spontaneous events is lower in the epilep- tic tissue. *C, D.* Somatic recordings from CA1 pyramidal cells. *C.* The cumulative probability plot of the amplitudes of spontaneous IPSCs was shifted to the right, indicating an increased frequency of large-amplitude events in experimental animals (n = 6 cells) as compared to controls (n = 6 cells). *D.* Whole-cell recordings of spontaneous (control) and miniature (TTX, 1 μM) inhibitory postsynaptic currents obtained at the reversal potential of glutamatergic events. The frequency of spontaneous events was similar in control and epileptic neurons, but the number of large-amplitude events seemed to be increased in the epileptic neuron. (*Source*: Adapted from Cossart et al., 2001, with permission.)

between neuronal damage and epileptogenesis is indicated by kindling, in which epileptogenesis occurs in the setting of no or minimal neuronal damage, and similarly in the intrahippocampal tetanus toxin model (see above). Indeed, kindling may protect against neuronal damage induced by kainic acid (Kelly and McIntyre, 1994), raising the intriguing possibility that epilepsy itself can be neuroprotective.

Granule Cell Dispersion. The observation of disorganization or dispersion of granule cells into the molecular layer of the dentate gyrus in hippocampal sclerosis was first described in detail by Houser (Houser, 1990; Houser et al., 1992). Dispersed granule cells appear separated from the normally compact cell layer, which gives the impression of an undulated irregular border with the molecular layer. In some cases the deep (hilar border) of the granule cell layer is also ill-defined. As a result, in hippocampal sclerosis the cell layer appears broadened with a mean width of 180 μm in TLE patients

compared to 100 μm in control subjects (Houser, 1990). The dispersed cells often appear elongated or fusiform in shape, reminiscent of migrating neurons. Less often a bilaminar arrangement of granule cells is observed (Houser et al., 1992; Thom et al., 2001) or nests of GCs are present in the hilus (Houser, 1990; Thom et al., 2001). The incidence of granule cell dispersion in hippocampal sclerosis surgical series is of the order of 40% (Houser, 1990; Thom et al., 2001).

It has been suggested that granule cell dispersion represents a primary abnormality of neuronal migration or an underlying hippocampal malformation (Houser et al., 1992). There are occasional reports of granule cell dispersion in association with cortical malformations in the absence of a history of seizures and with bilateral hippocampal involvement (Harding and Thom, 2001). Disorganization of the granule cell layer and ectopic localization of neurons have also been noted in several animal models with cortical malformations such as the reeler, and *p35* mutant mice. The presence of granule cell dispersion in human hippocampal sclerosis has also been correlated with epileptic events occurring early in life, including febrile seizures (Houser, 1990), suggesting a vulnerability of these neurons during this time period. It has further been shown that the presence of granule cell dispersion correlates well with the severity of hippocampal neuronal loss (Thom et al., 2001). This suggests that granule cell dispersion represents an epiphenomenon of hippocampal sclerosis rather than a primary abnormality, the migration of granule cells perhaps being influenced by neurotrophin secretion during seizures or other cellular signals. Interestingly, an inverse correlation between the levels of reelin protein and the extent of granule cell dispersion in the hippocampus has been shown, suggesting a possible functional role for Cajal Retzius cells in this process (Frotscher et al., 2003).

In animal models of epilepsy, such as the pilocarpine model, there is evidence to suggest that abnormally migrated granule cells are newly generated cells, neurogenesis being stimulated by the seizures (Parent et al., 1997) (see Chapter 9). Rapid dispersion of granule cells has been demonstrated following injury (Omar et al., 2000) and it has been shown that newly generated cells can migrate as far as CA3 and integrate into the CA3 neuronal network (Scharfman et al., 2000). Abnormal connections formed by new cells may contribute to seizure development (Parent et al., 1997), although experimental inhibition of neurogenesis does not prevent granule cell axon reorganization (see below) in epilepsy models (Parent et al., 1999). Studies have confirmed that neurogenesis also occurs in adult human dentate gyrus (Eriksson et al., 1998), and neuronal progenitor cells have been isolated from the dentate gyrus (Roy et al., 2000). This pool of precursor cells may have important physiological roles, but it is conceivable that in human epilepsy, stimulated by seizures, an increased rate of granule cell neurogenesis occurs, leading to the abnormal cell localization and reorganization observed in hippocampal sclerosis. There is also evidence emerging that radial glial cells in this region could act as neuronal precursors, and neurogenesis may be stimulated by NPY (Howell et al., 2003).

Another study has demonstrated the stem cell intermediate filament protein nestin in granule cell neuronal precursors in young patients with mesial TLE and surgery before the age of 2 years (Blumcke et al., 2001). Similar cells were not found in adults with hippocampal sclerosis; whether the nestin-positive cells represent newly generated cells or a delay in hippocampal development in these younger patients is not clear. Studies of cell cycle proteins, including Ki67, showed low expression in the dentate gyrus subgranular layer in adult hippocampi from patients with epilepsy (Del Bigio, 1999). Although this is an insensitive technique for measuring cells with a low turnover rate, it does imply that neurogensis in hippocampal sclerosis is a rare event and likely to be dependent on age.

Even if migrated granule cells do represent newly generated cells, it is unknown whether there are any differences in the physiological properties of these less mature cells. Electrophysiological studies in human hippocampal sclerosis

have already demonstrated the existence of distinct populations of granule cells, with one group showing abnormal excitability (Dietrich et al., 1999). We also know from animal studies that there is considerable potential for adaptability and plasticity of granule cells, such as increased basal expression of GAD (Sloviter et al., 1996), NPY induction (Vezzani et al., 1999), loss of calbindin expression (Magloczky et al., 1997), and altered ionotropic and metabotropic glutamate and GABA neurotransmitter receptor profiles on granule cells (Loup et al., 2000). It is plausible that such plasticity could be enhanced in newly generated granule cells and that it could contribute to seizure propensity.

Mossy Fiber Sprouting. In 1974, using Golgi techniques, Scheibel and colleagues identified aberrant axons from granule cell neurons ascending into the molecular layer of the dentate gyrus in hippocampal specimens from patients with epilepsy (Scheibel et al., 1974). It has long been considered that reorganization of the excitatory glutamatergic mossy fiber pathway is a key event in the development of chronic seizures (Sutula et al., 1989). Mossy fiber sprouting in human hippocampal sclerosis specimens results in aberrant innervations of other granule cells and also of CA3 pyramidal neurons, resulting in both feedback and feedforward excitation (Babb et al., 1991; Mathern et al., 1995b). In addition, aberrant mossy fibers in animal models innervate interneurons, suggesting that new inhibitory circuits are established (Kotti et al., 1997).

Mossy fiber sprouting in the supragranular layer of the dentate gyrus can be demonstrated using the Timms histochemical method, which highlights the zinc-rich mossy fiber synaptic terminals (Babb et al., 1991), or with dynorphin immunohistochemistry (Houser et al., 1990). Increased expression of growth-associated protein GAP-43 in the supragranular layer is thought to be indicative of active mossy fiber sprouting in hippocampal sclerosis specimens (Proper et al., 2000). Similarly increased syanaptogenesis in this region has been demonstrated by studying the distribution of 5′nucleotidase activity, which localizes in regions with more active synaptic turnover (Lie et al., 1999). Overall reorganization of synaptic terminals in hippocampal sclerosis has also been demonstrated in human specimens using immunohistochemistry for synaptic antigens such as synaptophysin, which shows a loss in the hilus and increased labeling in the dentate gyrus molecular layer (Honer et al., 1994; Davies et al., 1998; Proper et al., 2000). Similarly, prominent immunolabeling for chromogranins (neuropeptide precursors that can be co-released with catecholamines and peptides) in the inner molecular layer of the dentate gyrus has been shown to correspond with reorganized mossy fibers in patients with epilepsy (Kandlhofer et al., 2000). In parallel with increased synaptogenesis, elaboration and increased complexity of granule cells dendrites in the inner molecular layer has been demonstrated in hippocampal sclerosis patients (von Campe et al., 1997). The hypothesis that mossy fiber collaterals form granule cell–granule cell synapses has been confirmed by visualizing dentate granule cells and their mossy fibers after terminal uptake and retrograde transport of biocytin in epileptic rats secondary to status epilepticus (Okazaki et al., 1995).

Sprouting of mossy fibers is thought to result from epilepsy-induced loss of target cells (e.g., hilar mossy cells). However, in animal models it may be an early event, occurring within 4 weeks following the start of kindling (Elmer et al., 1996) and independent of hippocampal cell loss, possibly regulated by neurotrophic factors (Adams et al., 1997). Preliminary studies also indicate that mossy fiber sprouting is likely to be independent of any granule cell neurogenesis (Parent et al., 1997).

Pathological Role of Mossy Fiber Sprouting. It has long been considered that reorganization of the excitatory glutamatergic mossy fiber pathway is a key event in the development of chronic seizures. The dentate granule cells of the hippocampus probably act as a brake against seizure propagation through limbic circuitry (Perlin et al., 1992; Lothman and Bertram, 1993). This is mediated by the relative inexcitability of dentate granule cells through strong tonic GABAergic inhibition and relatively hyperpolarized membrane potentials. Dentate granule cells do not show the burst properties characteristic of hippocampal pyramidal cells in response to reduced GABAergic inhibition. Furthermore, dentate granule cell synchronization is difficult to achieve because of the low rate of connectivity between the granule cells.

Epileptogenesis may change the properties of dentate granule cell receptors (see below); but, importantly, mossy fiber sprouting greatly increases their connectivity. Even with sprouting, it is difficult to recruit dentate granule cells into epileptiform activity perhaps because of the extensive and increased synaptic input from GABAergic interneurons. Epileptiform activity can be induced in the dentate granule cells when mossy fiber sprouting is present by increasing extracellular potassium or by reducing $GABA_A$ receptor-mediated inhibition (Cronin et al., 1992; Wuarin and Dudek, 1996). This has led to the compelling hypothesis that epileptogenesis results in a potentially hyperexcitable granule cell layer that can be recruited into epileptic activity either by a rise in extracellular potassium, which could occur secondary to a sustained discharge from the entorhinal cortex, or through breakdown of inhibition (see below).

Is mossy fiber sprouting necessary for epileptogenesis? Blocking mossy fiber sprouting with the protein synthesis inhibitor cycloheximide does not prevent epileptogenesis (Longo and Mello, 1998). The interpretation of these experiments is confounded, however, by the likelihood that inhibiting protein synthesis inhibits other antiepileptogenic processes. In a recent study, the presence (or not) of dynorphin-positive mossy fiber sprouting in hippocampal sclerosis correlated with the postsurgical outcome; those with sprouting more often having a seizure-free outcome (de Lanenerolle et al., 2003). It is also becoming increasingly apparent that there is sprouting of axons from other neuronal populations, including sprouting of CA1 pyramidal cell axons, resulting in an increase in interconnectivity that results in increased excitability of the CA1 subfield (Esclapez et al., 1999). Sprouting of excitatory axons leading to increased interconnectivity may be a powerful means of generating hyperexcitable circuits that can maintain and propagate epileptic activity.

Dormant Basket Cell Hypothesis. Immediately following 24 hours of perforant path stimulation, there is loss of paired-pulse inhibition to perforant path stimulation in the dentate granule cell layer (Sloviter, 1987). The mechanism underlying this change was proposed to be the loss of excitatory input onto basket cells due to excitotoxic loss of mossy cells (Sloviter, 1987). However, application of NBQX, an AMPA receptor antagonist, was shown to inhibit the loss of mossy cells but to have no effect on the loss of paired-pulse inhibition (Penix and Wasterlain, 1994). Similarly, in the tetanus toxin model, disinhibition occurs in the absence of hilar cell loss (Whittington and Jefferys, 1994). Other factors are therefore likely to be responsible for the loss of paired-pulse inhibition, such as loss of affinity and activity of $GABA_A$ receptors in the hippocampus or a shift in the chloride reversal potential to more positive values (Kapur et al., 1994). These changes may be due in part to altered phosphorylation of $GABA_A$ receptors (Kapur et al., 1994) but could also be due to altered $GABA_A$ receptor subunit composition and expression (Sperk et al., 1998). Perhaps one of the main mechanisms is decreased recruitment of basket cells by excitatory inputs from dentate granule cells, the perforant path, and CA3 pyramidal cells through upregulation of presynaptic metabotropic glutamate receptor activity (Doherty and Dingledine, 2001).

Loss of paired-pulse inhibition was proposed to be an epileptogenic phenomenon, but subsequent studies have shown that paired-pulse inhibition becomes increased during the latent period (i.e., with epileptogenesis) and that epileptogenesis is associated with increased recruitment of basket cells (Milgram et al., 1991; Sloviter, 1992).

Synaptic rearrangement also occurs in CA1; and the hyperexcitability in CA1 with epileptogenesis has been proposed to be secondary to reduced recruitment of inhibitory interneurons (Bekenstein and Lothman, 1993). The main evidence for this is the loss of the IPSP from the EPSP–IPSP sequence on distant stimulation of the Schaffer collaterals. This evidence is perhaps flawed because this study does not adequately differentiate loss of the IPSP from prolongation of the EPSP. Subsequent data have shown increased excitability of CA1 interneurons following epileptogenesis (Sanabria et al., 2001). There are, however, other mechanisms underlying possible disinhibition in the CA1 region including changes in the pattern of inhibition (see above) and postsynaptic changes (see below).

Glial Cells and Extracellular Space. There are alterations in astrocytic function in the gliotic hippocampus. Astrocytes show physiological changes characteristic of immature astrocytes, including prolonged depolarization, that may contribute to seizure generation (Hinterkeuser et al., 2000; Schroder et al., 2000). Indeed, there is altered expression of ionotropic glutamate receptors on astrocytes in hippocampal sclerosis which may facilitate seizure spread (Seifert et al., 2004). In another study of rat and human hippocampi in TLE, the proliferation of glial cells in areas of neuronal loss were associated with alterations in extracellular potassium, which also may affect conduction of seizure activity (Heinemann et al., 2000). Altered levels of glial glutamate transporters (e.g., EAAT2), which has been shown in hippocampal sclerosis (Proper et al., 2002), may also influence the extracellular pool of glutamate. Furthermore, calcium oscillations in astrocytes can result in glutamate release, which may contribute to epileptic activity (Tian et al., 2005).

During seizures there is considerable shrinkage of the extracellular space due to intracellular accumulation of sodium chloride; indeed, a single seizure can result in a 10% to 30% decrease in extracellular space (Lux et al., 1986). This may result in increased nonsynaptic transmission through ephaptic and ionic mechanisms. Indeed, decreased extracellular space during seizures has been indirectly shown to have a role in seizure maintenance and spread; hypotonic extracellular solutions that decrease extracellular space are proconvulsant, whereas hypertonic solutions (increasing the extracellular space) can terminate seizure discharges (Roper et al., 1992). Although overall there is an expansion of the extracellular space in hippocampal sclerosis (Hugg et al., 1999; Wieshmann et al., 1999), how this relates to local changes in extracellular space and neurotransmission are unknown.

Neurotransmitter Systems

GABAergic Mechanisms. Alteration in the distribution of neurotransmitter receptors has been extensively investigated as a pathogenic mechanism in the hyperexitability of the hippocampus in TLE. The "GABA" hypothesis proposes that a deficit in inhibitory GABAergic transmission is implicated in seizures. GABA$_A$ and to a lesser extent GABA$_B$ receptor subtype expression (Barnard et al., 1998) and reuptake mechanisms have been studied in human hippocampal sclerosis tissues. Many alterations in GABA transmission may represent an adaptive mechanism in the brain in response to repetitive seizures, and increased expression of GABA$_A$ receptors has been documented in animal models of epilepsy as a compensatory mechanism (Fritschy et al., 1999). There is also upregulation of GAD, the main GABA-synthesizing enzyme, in interneurons following acute seizures. GABA and GAD are also upregulated in the mossy fibers and dentate granule cells (Sloviter et al., 1996). The finding of a mossy fiber-like GABAergic signal has raised the possibility that mossy fibers co-release glutamate and GABA (Walker et al., 2001); seizures may upregulate the GABAergic component (Gutierrez and Heinemann, 2001). In human hippocampal sclerosis, selective upregulation of GABA$_A\alpha2$ subunit in granule cells has been

observed, highlighting the plasticity of this neurotransmitter system in hippocampal sclerosis (Loup et al., 2000). The changes that are observed differ with time and between regions. Thus, specific GABA$_A$ receptor changes occur during acute seizures. As acute seizures continue they can become less responsive to benzodiazepines, which is mirrored by decreased potency of benzodiazepines on GABA-mediated synaptic currents in dentate granule cells (Kapur and Macdonald, 1997). In contrast, the potency of GABA itself and pentobarbitone remained unaltered, suggesting that rapid changes in GABA receptor properties occur during seizures. Although the pathophysiological consequences of these changes are difficult to predict, they have implications for the treatment of acute, prolonged seizures. During epileptogenesis the GABA$_A$ receptor changes are more complex and are region-specific. In the dentate granule cells, there is an increase in the number of GABA$_A$ receptors per synapse, leading to increased quantal size (Nusser et al., 1998). An especially interesting finding is that the increased GABA receptor-mediated signaling to dentate granule cells becomes more sensitive to zinc (Buhl et al., 1996; Brooks et al., 1998). To understand the potential involvement of zinc in epilepsy, it is necessary to consider the role of the sprouted mossy fibers. Mossy fiber terminals contain zinc and release it during synaptic activity (Assaf and Chung, 1984; Howell et al., 1984). Thus, it is conceivable that in the epileptic hippocampus zinc released from mossy fibers results in disinhibition, unmasking the potentiated excitatory dentate granule cell circuits (Buhl et al., 1996). This hypothesis is confounded by the observation that the zinc released from sprouted mossy fibers failed to affect GABA$_A$ receptor-mediated currents induced by local release of caged GABA (Molnar and Nadler, 2001). Furthermore, mice that lack the zinc transporter (ZnT3) and so lack synaptically available zinc have an exaggerated response to a convulsant; this observation does not, however, preclude a role for zinc in epileptogenesis (Cole et al., 2000).

Decreased sensitivity of GABA$_A$ receptor-mediated signals to zolpidem (a selective benzodiazepine agonist) has also been noted (Brooks et al., 1998). Using a combination of patch-clamp recording and single-cell mRNA amplification, it was found that the increased zinc sensitivity and decreased benzodiazepine sensitivity of the GABA$_A$ receptor was associated with (and possibly explained by) decreased expression of the $\alpha1$ subunit and increased expression of the $\alpha4$ subunit (Brooks et al., 1998). In addition, there were changes in β subunit expression that may affect benzodiazepine efficacy and the efficacy of barbiturates, steroids, zinc, and loreclezole, a new antiepileptic drug (Brooks et al., 1998). These changes were seen during the latent period that predated the onset of epilepsy, suggesting a role in the epileptogenic process. GABA$_A$ receptor-mediated transmission in CA1 undergoes different changes. In contrast to dentate granule cells, GABA$_A$ receptors on CA1 pyramidal cells are less responsive to applied GABA following epileptogenesis (Gibbs et al., 1997). There are also changes that suggest there may be a decrease in the presynaptic GABA reserve, although the synaptic consequences of this are unknown (Hirsch et al., 1999).

The effects of GABA$_A$ receptor activation on membrane potential depend on the chloride reversal potential. High internal chloride such as occurs developmentally can result in depolarizing GABA$_A$ receptor-mediated potentials. Could such depolarizing GABA$_A$ receptor-mediated potentials occur in epileptic tissue and contribute to epileptogenesis? Evidence from a study of hippocampal slices from patients who underwent temporal lobectomy suggest that this is so (Cohen et al., 2002). Synchronous rhythmic activity was found to be generated in the subiculum of slices of temporal lobe from patients with temporal lobe epilepsy, and this synchronous rhythmic activity was abolished by the GABA$_A$ receptor antagonist bicu-

culline and by glutamate receptor antagonists, suggesting that both excitatory and inhibitory signaling contributed to the spontaneous interictal-like events. Further studies in these cells demonstrated that the GABAergic synaptic events reversed at depolarized potentials (Fig. 16–5). Thus, depolarizing GABAergic responses potentially contributed to human ictal activity in the subiculum. The mechanism by which such depolarizing GABA$_A$ receptor-mediated potentials occur is unknown, but might be downregulation of the K$^+$/Cl$^-$ co-transporter KCC2 that maintains the low intracellular chloride.

GABA$_B$ receptor changes have also been demonstrated in human hippocampal sclerosis tissue. GABA$_B$ receptors inhibit neurotransmitter release from presynaptic terminals and

Figure 16–5. Depolarizing γ-aminobutyric acid-A (GABA$_A$) receptor-mediated potentials may contribute to seizure generation. Pyramidal cells active during interictal-like events showed excitatory GABAergic transmission. A. Discharges in pacemaker cells were triggered by orthodromic stimulation (right, upper trace). Depolarizing synaptic potentials persisted when glutamatergic transmission was suppressed (middle trace). They were suppressed by blocking GABA$_A$ receptors (lower trace). BIC, bicuculline. B, C. Reversal potential for GABAergic transmission in cells that fired during interictal events was more depolarized than at rest (B, left; C, squares). Reversal in inhibited cells was hyperpolarized from rest (B, right; C, circles). Records were obtained in NBQX and APV. Linear fits are indicated. PSP, postsynaptic potential. (Source: Adapted from Cohen et al., 2002, with permission.)

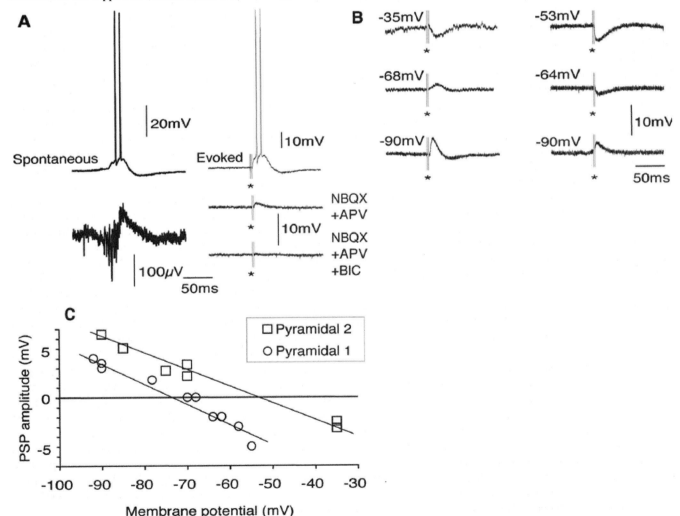

cause late inhibitory synaptic potentials (Barnard et al., 1998). Increased expression of GABA$_B$1 receptor has been shown in the subiculum of hippocampal sclerosis cases and in surviving CA1 neurons and granule cells with augmented receptor binding in CA3 (Billinton et al., 2001), although functional interpretation of these findings is difficult. The upregulation could represent a greater number of inhibitory synapses, increased postsynaptic GABA$_B$ receptors, or increased presynaptic GABA$_B$ receptor number, leading to decreased neurotransmitter release mainly from inhibitory axonal terminals. More recently, downregulation of mossy fiber presynaptic GABA$_B$ receptors has been found in tissue from epileptic animals. It resulted in decreased mossy fiber heterosynaptic depression, and may contribute to increased signal flow through the hippocampus (Chandler et al., 2003). Decreased presynaptic GABA$_B$ receptor activity on interneurons has also been proposed to underlie the enhanced inhibition that occurs in the dentate gyrus during epileptogenesis (Haas et al., 1996).

Changes in GABA uptake have also been described in the dentate gyrus (During et al., 1995; Patrylo et al., 2001). Both animal and human data support a decrease in clearance of synaptically released extracellular GABA, perhaps owing to decreased expression or impairment of GABA transporters (During et al., 1995; Mathern et al., 1999; Patrylo et al., 2001). This has been speculated to lead to increased interictal inhibitory "efficacy." Because the rises in extracellular potassium that occur during seizures may result in reversal of GABA uptake, decreased GABA transporter function results in impairment of extracellular GABA rises during seizure activity, possibly resulting in impaired inhibition during seizure activity. The change in GABA$_A$ receptor subunits resulting in a greater response to endogenously applied GABA (Brooks et al., 1998) could compensate for decreased extracellular GABA rises. Nevertheless, these data raise the possibility that decreased GABA transporter function could be proepileptogenic during times of seizure activity but promote inhibitory transmission during the interictal period.

Glutamatergic Mechanisms. Upregulation of excitatory metabotropic glutamate receptors (mGluR1 subunit) has been observed in the dentate gyrus in both human and animal models of hippocampal sclerosis, and it could contribute to the development of chronic seizures through increased excitatory transmission (Blumcke et al., 2000a). In addition, upregulation of the presynaptic inhibitory metabotropic receptor subunit mGluR4 in the dentate gyrus and granule cells in hippocampal specimens was also observed, which may contribute to the dampening of seizure activity (Lie et al., 2000). In studies employing in situ hybridization techniques, increases in pyramidal and granule cell AMPA receptor mRNA (Mathern et al., 1997) and in granule cell NMDAR1 and NMDAR2 subunit mRNA have been shown, results that are supported by autoradiographic studies (Brines et al., 1997). Studies in kindled models have supported the hypothesis that during epileptogenesis there is enhanced transmission from the entorhinal cortex to dentate granule cells (Behr et al., 2001).

One of the major mechanisms underlying this is undoubtedly an increase in NMDA receptor-mediated neurotransmission (Mody and Heinemann, 1987). Kindling results in fast, long-lasting posttranslational modifications in the function of dentate granule cell NMDA receptor channels, leading to increases in the mean open time and burst and cluster duration and to decreases in the channel-blocking effect by magnesium (Kohr et al., 1993). Similar changes in NMDA channels have been reported in human epileptic tissue (Lieberman and Mody, 1999). Modification of the NMDA receptor channels probably results from a decrease in the activity of intracellular phosphatases, leading to increased phosphorylation of the receptors (Kohr et al., 1993; Lieberman and Mody, 1994).

There is more uncertainty concerning changes in AMPA receptor neurotransmission. Certainly, changes in AMPA receptor subunit composition are seen in animal models prior to neurodegeneration; there is a decrease in the expression of the GluR2 subunit in vulnerable cells (Grooms et al., 2000). This evidence supports a role for calcium flux through GluR2 lacking AMPA receptors in mediating neuronal death (Grooms et al., 2000). Conversely, there appears to be upregulation of GluR2 in less vulnerable neurons such as the dentate granule cells (de Lanerolle et al., 1998).

Changes in glutamate uptake during epileptogenesis could also have an important role. There is burgeoning evidence that glutamate may escape from the synaptic cleft to activate extrasynaptic receptors, or even receptors at neighboring synapses (Kullmann and Asztely, 1998). Glutamate "spillover" can activate presynaptic glutamate receptors on GABAergic terminals, resulting in decreased inhibitory drive, and can increase NMDA receptor-mediated signaling (Min et al., 1999; Semyanov and Kullmann, 2000). Extrasynaptic accumulation of glutamate may play a role in epilepsy: Rodents lacking the gene coding for the glial glutamate transporter GLT-1 (EAAT2) show lethal spontaneous seizures (Tanaka et al., 1997). Rather surprisingly, chronic administration of antisense oligonucleotide to knock down the same transporter produces a different phenotype, characterized by neurodegeneration rather than seizures (Rothstein et al., 1996). Reduction of expression of the neuronal transporter EAAC1 (EAAT3), however, also causes seizures in rats. Subtle alterations in transporter levels have been reported in hippocampal tissue taken from patients with TLE (Mathern et al., 1999), although it is difficult to determine to what extent this reflects selective neurodegeneration. In an animal model of hippocampal sclerosis there was downregulation of the glial glutamate transporter that could contribute to glutamate spillover but upregulation of the neuronal glutamate transporter, which has been hypothesized to play a dominant role in reversed glutamate uptake (Ueda et al., 2001). Furthermore, marked extracellular glutamate rises have been recorded in humans using in vivo microdialysis prior to seizure onset, leading to the suggestion that these glutamate rises are an initiating factor in spontaneous seizures (During and Spencer, 1993).

Other Neurotransmitters. Alterations of many other transmitter systems have been described in association with acute limbic seizures and with hippocampal sclerosis. Perhaps one of the most intriguing roles for many of these transmitters is in seizure termination, and acute alterations have been implicated in the progression of seizures to status epilepticus. Adenosine, opioids, NPY, and galanin have all been proposed to play an important role in seizure termination (Young and Dragunow, 1994; Mazarati et al., 1998, 1999; Vezzani et al., 1999), whereas accumulation of substance P has a proepileptogenic effect (Mazarati et al., 1999).

Adenosine is a potent inhibitor of neurotransmitter release and has been shown to be effective for terminating brief seizures. Indeed, accumulation of adenosine seems to be a credible contender for a prominent role in seizure termination, as seizures promote adenosine release (Berman et al., 2000). Adenosine antagonists shorten the stimulation protocol or lessen the chemoconvulsant dose necessary to induce status epilepticus (Young and Dragunow, 1994). Also, adenosine agonists are effective at stopping both the induction and maintenance of status epilepticus (Handforth and Treiman, 1994). To what degree changes in adenosine anticonvulsant activity contribute to epileptogenesis or to the failure of seizure termination (status epilepticus) is unknown. Although regional changes in adenosine receptor density have been described during epileptogenesis (Ekonomou et al., 2000), it may reflect cell loss and synaptic rearrrangement.

Opioid release has also been suggested as a major mechanism underlying the termination of seizures. The observed loss of dynorphin-like immunoreactivity in the hippocampus during sustained seizure activity is consistent with loss of a potent endogenous antiepileptic (Mazarati et al., 1999). Opioid antagonists facilitate the establishment of status epilepticus, and agonists inhibit both the induction and maintenance of status epilepticus.

In addition to opioids, a variety of other modulatory neuropeptides exist. NPY is such a peptide that has potent effects on neurotransmission. Cloning has revealed five NPY receptors, Y1–Y5 (Vezzani et al., 1999). In human hippocampal sclerosis, there is increased NPY, upregulated presynaptic Y2 receptors that inhibit neurotransmitter release, and downregulated Y1 receptors that are expressed postsynaptically and are excitatory (Furtinger et al., 2001). Furthermore, Y5 receptor knockout mice and NPY knockout mice have an exaggerated response to kainic acid with prolonged seizures (Baraban et al., 1997; Marsh et al., 1999).

Galanin is another bioactive peptide that is widely distributed throughout the CNS. Galanin in the hippocampus is predominantly inhibitory, decreasing the release of excitatory amino acids. In the hippocampus, galanin immunoreactivity is confined to axons, the bulk of which are the axons of medial septal neurons (Mazarati et al., 1998). Status epilepticus in two models—perforant path stimulation and lithium pilocarpine—resulted in the disappearance of galanin immunoreactive fibers in the hippocampus; this may have resulted from loss of medial septal neurons or through exhaustion of galanin

stores (Mazarati et al., 1998). This would have a disinhibitory effect. Soon after the status epilepticus, however, galanin immunoreactive-positive neurons appeared in the hilus; they increased in number after the first day but gradually declined a few days later. This increase in galanin-immunoreactive neurons in the hippocampus is possibly a compensatory response to prolonged ictal activity and depletion of galanin from septal afferents. Galanin injected into the hilus prevented the induction of status epilepticus and also stopped established status epilepticus. Conversely, antagonists of galanin receptors facilitated the development of status epilepticus (Mazarati et al., 1998). Further confirmatory evidence of the importance of galanin comes from studies of transgenic mice in which overexpression of galanin had an antiepileptic effect, and galanin knockouts were more susceptible to the induction of status epilepticus (Mazarati et al., 2000).

Changes in Neuronal Properties

Although most recent research into epileptogenesis and seizure generation has concentrated on changes in the neuronal network, alterations in intrinsic neuronal properties could also contribute to this process. Importantly, ion channel mutations in which there may be only subtle changes to the kinetics of ion channels can result in epilepsy.

As discussed in the section on the interictal spike, CA3 pyramidal cells can generate burst firing, whereas few pyramidal cells in CA1 demonstrate such firing properties. Alterations in intrinsic membrane properties can dramatically affect the firing properties of such neurons and could promote burst firing. Such burst firing in a dense excitatory network has the potential to generate synchronized bursts and may thus promote epileptic activity. In the pilocarpine model of epileptogenesis, the proportion of bursting CA1 pyramidal cells increases dramatically, such that more than half demonstrate bursting properties (Fig. 16–6) (Su et al., 2002). This may be due to upregulation of a T-type calcium channel that can produce a significant calcium tail current following an action potential, resulting in significant afterdepolarization (Su et al., 2002). Persistent sodium currents may also contribute to this propensity for bursting.

More recently, downregulation of dendritic A-type potassium channels has been found in the pilocarpine epilepsy model (Bernard et al., 2004). This downregulation is partly due to increased channel phosphorylation by extracellular signal-regulated kinase but also to decreased transcription. These potassium channels limit the back-propagation of action potentials from the soma into the distal dendrites. The functional consequence of back-propagating action potentials is likely to be an amplificatioin of EPSPs and thus increased excitation. The effect of downregulation of A-type potassium channels on dendritic calcium spikes and burst firing is unknown.

Epileptogenesis can thus lead to an acquired channelopathy in neurons that may promote burst firing and hyperexcitability.

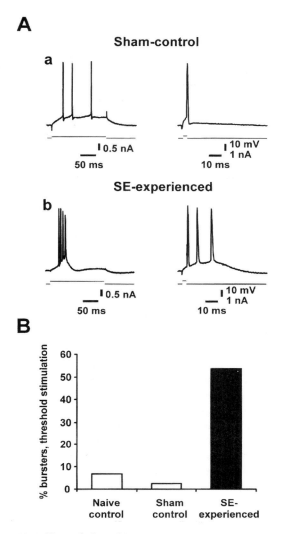

A

Sham-control

a

$\vert$ 0.5 nA

50 ms

$\vert$ 10 mV
1 nA

10 ms

SE-experienced

b

$\vert$ 0.5 nA

50 ms

$\vert$ 10 mV
1 nA

10 ms

B

% bursters, threshold stimulation

60
50
40
30
20
10
0

Naive control | Sham control | SE-experienced

\Figure 16–6. Upregulation of intrinsic burst-firing in CA1 pyramidal cells from SE-experienced versus control animals. *A.* Representative responses of CA1 pyramidal cells from sham-control (a) and SE-experienced animals (b) 30 days after pilocarpine treatment. In each panel, the responses of CA1 pyramidal cells to long (leftmost traces) and brief (rightmost traces) depolarizing current pulses (injected through the recording microelectrode) are shown. Top and bottom traces depict the neuronal response and the current stimulus, respectively. *B.* Most of the CA1 pyramidal cells in the sham-control group ($n = 42$) and in the naive-control group ($n = 15$) were regular firing cells, with only a small fraction displaying burst discharges to threshold stimulation (white bars). In contrast, CA1 pyramidal cells in the SE-experienced group showed a high incidence of intrinsic bursting (54%, $n = 97$), with bursting neurons displaying all-or-none bursts of three to four clustered spikes in response to either brief or long current injection (Ab). (*Source*: Adapted from Su et al., 2002. with permission.)

16.2.5 Conclusion

The hippocampus through its physiological role can initiate and maintain oscillatory behavior. It is this property along with the plasticity of the hippocampus and its vulnerability to neuronal damage that contribute to the pathological role of the hippocampus in epileptic activity. In association with neuronal damage associated with hippocampal sclerosis, there is a vast array of changes in organization, connectivity, receptors, intrinsic neuronal properties, and astrocyte function that can contribute to epileptogenicity. The great challenges are to differentiate pro-epileptogenic changes from antiepileptogenic, compensatory changes, and to determine which are the critical processes. It is likely that epileptogenesis is not a single process but that many diverse processes can result in the expression of epilepsy.

16.3 Alzheimer's Disease

16.3.1 Introduction

Alzheimer's disease (AD) is the most common cause of dementia worldwide. AD is a neurodegenerative disorder in which the accumulation of amyloid plaques and neurofibrillary tangles represents the pathological hallmark of the disease. Five million people in the United States and 400,000 in the United Kingdom are estimated to have AD, with a disease onset typically occurring early in the eighth decade of life. Disease prevalence increases with age: 1 in 2000 people aged below 60 years are affected and 1 in 200 aged over 60 years. In the elderly population the prevalence rises dramatically, with AD occurring in 20% of those aged $\geq$ 80 years and in 50% of those $\geq$ 90 years of age.

Memory loss is the predominant feature of AD. Impairment of episodic memory occurs early during the course of the disease and is usually the most prominent symptom throughout the disease course. Progressive dysfunction of other cognitive domains is also observed in AD, and the final stages of the disease are characterized by severe global impairment of cognitive function.

The neuropathological changes in AD are thought to be manifest initially in the entorhinal cortex (EC), progressing from there to the hippocampus, with increasing involvement of the neocortex as the disease progresses (Braak and Braak, 1991). However, significant neocortical pathology is already present by the time dementia is clinically diagnosed, which has prompted efforts to identify the clinical manifestations of AD in its earliest stages, when the pathological changes are primarily restricted to the medial temporal lobe structures. This has resulted in the introduction of the concept of "mild cognitive impairment" (MCI), representing the predementia stage of AD. Within the broad overview of AD provided in this chapter, particular attention is devoted to the involvement of the hippocampal formation in AD and MCI and on the implications that improved identification of this involvement has for earlier diagnosis and treatment of AD.

16.3.2 Clinical Features

Memory impairment of insidious onset typifies the initial stages of AD. Patients exhibit poor memory for autobiographical events, current affairs, and the names and faces of acquaintances. Frequently they exhibit difficulty remembering familiar routes, and "getting lost" is a commonly experienced symptom early in the disease. These early symptoms may be attributed initially to cognitive decline as a consequence of normal aging; but as the disease progresses the memory impairment becomes severe enough to disrupt activities of daily living, and patients begin to lose their functional independence. The central nature of the memory problem in AD is reflected in the National Institute of Neurological and Communicative Diseases and Stroke/Alzheimer's Disease and Related Disorders Association (NINCDS-ADRDA) criteria (McKhann et al., 1984) for the diagnosis of probable AD, which state that the presence of progressive memory impairment and impairment of at least one other cognitive function are required for a clinical diagnosis of AD. However, atypical forms of AD are well recognized, in which the prevailing symptomatology reflects dysfunction of nonmemory cognitive domains, such as speech or visuoperceptual function, but these are much less common than the classic amnestic presentation.

Impairment of other cognitive functions becomes increasingly prominent during the course of the disease. Word-finding difficulty is a relatively frequent early symptom, and speech output is often diminished. Executive functions, such as problem solving and abstract reasoning, decline progressively. Later in the disease there is impairment of word comprehension, reflecting a breakdown in semantic memory function. Other characteristic early symptoms include limb apraxias (higher order motor disorders affecting the execution of skilled or learned limb movements), impaired calculation skills, and disorders of visuospatial and visuoperceptual function. The progressive involvement of multiple cognitive domains in AD reflects the accumulation of pathological changes predominantly in the frontal, temporal, and parietal lobes; the occipital lobes are usually relatively spared in the early stages of AD.

The disorders of cognitive function are accompanied by a variety of neuropsychiatric symptoms, which include depression, changes in personality, delusions, and hallucinations, with depression often preceding diagnosis. Behavioral disturbances such as aggression, agitation, and nocturnal wandering increase with disease severity. Loss of insight is common. In the late stages of the disease, parkinsonian signs (e.g., limb rigidity, motor slowing) and various involuntary limb movements are observed, and seizures may also be observed in severe AD. Finally, patients become bedbound and entirely dependent on caretakers, and in this state they are vulnerable to intercurrent medical complications such as sepsis.

From the time that AD is diagnosed initially, the disease runs approximately 5 to 10 years until the time of death, with a mean survival of 8 years.

Mild Cognitive Impairment

There is increasing awareness that AD may be associated with a prolonged prodromal or "preclinical" phase, during which the cognitive dysfunction is relatively subtle and circum-scribed and insufficiently severe to warrant a diagnosis of dementia. The introduction of drug treatments for AD, in the form of the acetylcholinesterase inhibitors, has helped stimulate efforts to identify this prodromal phase in AD, culminating in the introduction of the concept of mild cognitive impairment (MCI) (Smith et al., 1996). Although there exists a degree of debate about the defining criteria for MCI, the most widely accepted criteria for the diagnosis of MCI are based on the presence of significant objective memory decline in the context of normal activities of daily living and intact function in other cognitive domains.

Figures for the prevalence of MCI in the population vary considerably, ranging from 3.0% to 16.8% depending on definitions (DeCarli 2003). Epidemiological data support the notion that MCI represents a precursor state of AD: Patients with MCI "convert" to AD at a rate of approximately 12% per annum, compared with an annual rate of 1% to 2% in the normal elderly population.

The current definition of MCI is predicated on impaired memory. However, the heterogeneity in the clinical presentation of AD suggests "amnestic MCI" that may represent a particular precursor state of AD. Future efforts to categorize the initial clinical phases of AD will include the identification of equivalent MCI states affecting other cognitive domains and will aim to differentiate MCI (due to AD) from cognitive impairment as a consequence of other cognitive disorders, as well as from the memory decline that accompanies the normal aging process. In this context, the fact that the pathological damage in the earliest phases of AD is largely restricted to the entorhinal cortex and hippocampus may be used to direct diagnostic investigations, including structural and functional neuroimaging techniques and clinical neuropsychological assessments of memory.

Pattern of Cognitive Deficits in AD

The deficit in memory that characterizes early AD is primarily impaired episodic memory. Patients are unable to learn new material and have difficulty recalling recent events. A number of factors contribute to this disruption of episodic memory, including deficiencies in encoding and storing new information and heightened sensitivity to the disruptive effects of proactive interference. AD patients also exhibit impaired priming performance (facilitated performance by prior exposure to stimuli); patients with AD, Huntington's disease, and Korsakoff syndrome are equally impaired on tests of verbal recognition and recall, but only AD patients show additional impairment of verbal priming, indicating that AD is also associated with a deficit of implicit memory.

Studies on the rate of long-term forgetting, or the rate of loss of memory after successful learning, have yielded conflicting results. Some studies have shown that AD patients have faster forgetting rates than either controls or patients with depression or Korsakoff syndrome (Hart et al., 1987), but others have failed to demonstrate accelerated forgetting in AD (Becker et al., 1987). Studies of retrograde amnesia in AD have revealed that recent memories are more affected than remote memories.

The diagnostic utility of memory tests in AD varies according to the severity of cognitive impairment. In the presymptomatic phase of the disease, the tests currently considered to predict with greatest accuracy the progression to AD are tests of verbal learning and immediate visual recall. By contrast, for established AD, tests of delayed recall are most sensitive at differentiating between early AD and normal controls but are of limited value in tracking disease severity in AD because performance on these tests often declines rapidly to a plateau. Recognition memory tests, involving verbal and visual subtests, are less sensitive than recall tasks for detecting early AD but are more useful for staging disease severity.

Disorders of speech and language also occur early in the course of AD. Word-finding difficulty is often the first problem to become manifest, and it is associated with compensatory circumlocution. Naming is initially preserved but becomes progressively more impaired during the course of the disease. Neologisms, verbal and literal paraphasias, also become more prominent and are accompanied by loss of word comprehension, reflecting a breakdown of verbal semantic knowledge. Severe AD may be associated with palilalia (the repetition of words and phrases) and logoclonia (repetition of the final syllable of a word), and speech may deteriorate into unintelligibility. Ultimately, some patients may become entirely mute.

Topographical disorientation is another characteristic early feature of AD. Patients complain of "getting lost," initially only in unfamiliar environments, but subsequently they experience difficulty finding their way around familiar places, including their own homes. The presence of topographical disorientation may help differentiate early AD from other dementias; for instance, patients with frontotemporal lobe degeneration, typified by focal atrophy of the frontal and anterior temporal lobes, typically do not get lost. This topographical disorientation in AD has been variously ascribed to impaired visuospatial function as a result of damage to the parieto-occipital region; to topographical agnosia, representing an impairment of the ability to recognize those cues or landmarks that are required to permit successful navigation through an environment; and to an impaired memory for places as a consequence of damage to the hippocampus or parahippocampal regions. The last possibility is consistent with the observation that the medial temporal lobe structures are preferentially affected in the earliest stages of the AD disease process.

Apraxia (impairment of sensorimotor integration due to disorders of higher cerebral function) is observed in most patients with mild to moderate AD. Ideational apraxia, in which there is an inability to construct the idea of a purposeful movement, such that patients are unable to perform these movements (e.g., using a manual tool), may occur as a result of damage to the parietal and frontal associations areas, particularly in the left hemisphere. Ideomotor apraxia, in which the construct of a purposeful movement is intact but the execution of the movement is faulty, is associated more with damage to the parietal association areas as well as damage to the premotor cortex and the supplementary motor areas.

Visual agnosia (inability to recognize objects) is a common feature of AD in its more advanced stages and results from damage to the visual association areas. Subtypes of visual agnosia include apperceptive agnosia, in which the disorder of object perception is exemplified by difficulty recognizing unusual views of common objects; it is typically associated with damage to the right parietal lobe. In associative agnosia, there is no perceptual deficit but, instead, inability to assign the correct semantic meaning to the perceived objects, resulting again in misidentification of objects. In this instance, the cortical damage most frequently involves the left occipitotemporal region. More specific forms of agnosia include prosopagnosia, in which there is impairment of familiar face recognition, typically associated with damage to the right temporal lobe.

Together, amnesia, aphasia, apraxia, and agnosia form the core disorders of cognitive function in AD. However, the global nature of the cortical involvement in established AD is reflected in a multitude of additional cognitive deficits, prominent among which are disorders of attention and calculation. The involvement of the frontal lobes in the pathological process results in "neurological" symptoms such as impaired executive function and reduced problem-solving ability, as well as a variety of "neuropsychiatric" symptoms including changes in personality and disturbances of social conduct.

Structural Imaging

Generalized cerebral atrophy is a characteristic gross pathological feature of AD. The utility of cerebral atrophy as a biomarker of disease is reflected in the NINCDS-ADRDA diagnostic criteria (McKhann et al., 1984), which state that the diagnosis of probable AD is supported by "evidence of cerebral atrophy on CT or MRI and progression documented by serial observation." The presence of cerebral atrophy in AD may be determined using a variety of techniques. Qualitative assessment of brain atrophy (visual inspection of brain scans) has the benefit of general applicability but the disadvantage of wide interobserver variability. Of the various quantitative techniques currently in use, volumetric analyses have been shown to have greater diagnostic specificity and sensitivity than linear measurements of atrophy. Analyses may be cross-sectional (i.e., based on a single scan) or longitudinal (repeated measurements performed over serial scans). The diagnostic utility of data obtained from cross-sectional imaging studies is limited by the variability in brain size among individuals, reflecting differences in head size in the normal population, and by the reduction in total brain volume that occurs as a consequence of normal aging. Longitudinal studies have greater diagnostic specificity and sensitivity than cross-sectional studies but are necessarily disadvantaged by the need for at least two scans and as a consequence cannot provide corroborative information at the time of the initial diagnostic inquiry.

Most volumetric MRI studies have relied on manual segmentation of brain regions of interest. Information on the structural brain changes in AD can also been obtained using semiautomated, increasingly sophisticated techniques such as voxel-based morphometry, in which the distribution of atrophy in the AD brain is determined by comparison with a nonatrophied "template" brain (Good et al., 2002), and fluid registration MRI, in which longitudinal patterns of atrophy throughout the brain can be observed by tracking the brain changes over time on a voxel-by-voxel basis (Fox et al., 2001) (Fig. 16–7, see color insert).

Prior understanding of the pattern of pathological involvement of the cerebral cortex has prompted the assessment of regional brain volume measurements in AD as an alternative to measurements of whole-brain volume. Most studies have concentrated on the medial temporal lobe, but other researchers have investigated structures such as the frontal lobes, the cingulate gyrus, the superior temporal gyrus, and the corpus callosum. As with the measurement of whole-brain atrophy, there are several methods for assessing atrophy of the medial temporal lobe structures. They include the use of a visual rating scale for medial temporal lobe atrophy, in which

the degree of atrophy is classified according to a five-point grading scale following visual inspection of MRI scans (Wahlund et al., 2000). Linear measures of atrophy include measuring the height of the hippocampus and parahippocampal gyrus, the interuncal distance, and the width of the temporal horn of the lateral ventricles. Area measurements include changes in the cross-sectional area through the hippocampus and in the surface area of the entorhinal cortex. Of these various measurement techniques, perhaps the most useful in the clinical domain is that based on visual rating of medial temporal lobe atrophy, which has benefits in terms of ease of use and widespread applicability and compares favorably with quantitative volumtric analysis in the diagnostic differentation of patients with AD.

Hippocampus. In recent years increasing emphasis has been devoted to volumetric analyses of structural change derived using quantitative MRI techniques, with the hippocampus representing the primary region of interest in most instances. The use of volumetric MRI measures of hippocampal atrophy as surrogate markers of disease in AD is validated by the demonstration of a strong correlation between MRI-determined hippocampal volumes and neuronal numbers in the hippocampus in AD (Bobinski et al., 1999). A number of

Figure 16–7. Coronal MRI at the mid-hippocampal level using voxel-compression mapping overlay to show the change in brain volume over 12 months in a patient with Alzheimer's disease (AD). Particular features to note are the marked involvement of the temporal lobes including the hippocampi, the relative symmetry of the structural changes, and the diffuse involvement of both gray and white matter.

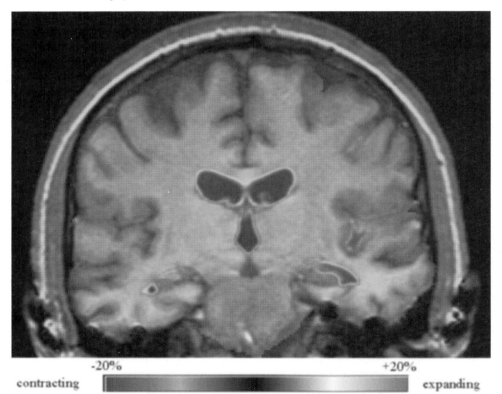

studies have demonstrated that AD is associated with significant hippocampal volume loss. Data from cross-sectional studies are complemented by longitudinal data indicating that AD is associated with an increased rate of hippocampal atrophy (Jack et al., 1998). Although most of these studies have concentrated on the structural changes in patients with established dementia, hippocampal atrophy has also been found to be present in the presymptomatic stage of AD, as determined by scan data acquired on familial AD (FAD) patients prior to symptom onset (Convit et al., 1997).

Determination of hippocampal atrophy can distinguish AD from normal aging with a high degree of specificity and sensitivity. At a fixed specificity of 80%, the sensitivity of hippocampal volumetric measurements for differentiating patients with mild-to-moderate AD is approximately 88% (Jack et al., 1997).

Several imaging techniques have been applied to the hippocampus in recent years. MRI-based high-dimensional brain mapping (Csernansky et al., 2000) is a technique in which a control MRI template is transformed onto individual scans in such a way that changes in the shape of the hippocampus are detectable. Using this technique, AD was found to be associated with a symmetrical deformity of hippocampal shape that differentiated it from the morphological changes seen with normal aging. The particular deformities affecting the head of the hippocampus and along the lateral aspect of the body of the hippocampus are consistent with pathological changes affecting the CA1 field in AD. A similar technique was subsequently used by the same authors to demonstrate hippocampal deformations in patients with mesial TLE (Hogan et al., 2004).

A technique has also been developed for visualizing neuritic plaques in autopsy-acquired human brain tissue using magnetic resonance (MR) microscopy, which provides greater spatial resolution than MRI (Benveniste et al., 1999). Technical limitations currently militate against in vivo application, but advances in scan technology may permit the future use of a similar technique in the antemortem diagnosis of AD.

Entorhinal Cortex.

In view of the early, severe involvement of the EC in the AD pathological process, it has been argued that EC atrophy may be a more sensitive marker of AD than hippocampal atrophy. However, the theoretical benefits of assessing EC volume changes in AD are partially offset by the difficulty of determining with confidence the boundaries of the EC on MRI scans, which have led some to undertake measurements of the parahippocampal gyrus (which contains the EC in its entirety) instead, with the presence of atrophy in this structure taken as a surrogate marker of EC atrophy. Despite these perceived difficulties, a technique for delineating the EC from volumetric MRI scans was developed (Insausti et al., 1998) using the cytoarchitectonic boundaries of the EC as the guidelines for segmentation of the EC volume. In various modified forms (modifications in segmentation protocol resulting primarily from the difficulty of establishing the medial border of the EC at the junction with the perirhinal

cortex along the medial lip of the collateral sulcus), this technique has been used to demonstrate significant bilateral EC atrophy in established AD (Fig. 16–7, see color insert). Longitudinal studies on AD patients, with volume measurements of the EC and the hippocampus performed on scans with an average scan interval of 21 months, reveal a significantly greater rate of atrophy affecting the EC (mean annual volume loss 7.1% per annum) than the hippocampus (mean annual volume loss 5.9%), which would support the idea that the pathological changes in AD are more severe in the EC than in the hippocampus.

Structural Imaging in MCI.

Neuroimaging studies reveal that MCI is also associated with atrophy of the EC and the hippocampus. Volumetric MRI analysis indicates that there is a progression of atrophy of these structures from normal aging through MCI to AD; the degree of atrophy in these structures is sufficiently great to differentiate effectively between MCI patients and age-matched controls and between MCI and AD patients, with significantly greater atrophy observed in the latter group. The etiological relation between MCI and AD is underlined further by the observation that the presence of hippocampal atrophy in MCI patients is predictive of future conversion to AD (Jack et al., 1999).

A comparison of hippocampal and EC volumes in normal control subjects, patients with MCI, and patients with early AD revealed that assessment of EC volumes is most effective for discriminating between control subjects and MCI patients, whereas measurement of hippocampal volumes provided better discrimination between patients with MCI and those with AD, which suggests that atrophy of the EC precedes that of the hippocampus and is more pronounced in the initial stages of AD (Pennanen et al., 2004).

Medial Temporal Lobe Atrophy in Non-Alzheimer Dementias.

Atrophy of medial temporal lobe structures discriminates effectively between AD and age-matched controls but is less effective at differentiating between AD and other diseases that cause dementia. Hippocampal atrophy has been found in other neurodegenerative disorders such as dementia with Lewy bodies and frontotemporal lobar degeneration (FTLD), as well as in vascular dementia. With regard to the latter, the determination of hippocampal atrophy to differentiate between different dementias is complicated further by the frequent coexistence of AD and vascular pathology. With regard to other temporal lobe structures, atrophy of the EC has also been observed in FTLD and, in particular the clinical subtype of FTLD described as semantic dementia (SD). In this instance, the severity of EC atrophy exceeds that noted in AD patients of comparable disease severity, although the atrophy is predominantly left-sided, in keeping with the language dominance of the left hemisphere (Chan et al., 2001).

The fact that the presence of hippocampal or EC atrophy alone is insufficiently specific to discriminate effectively between these disorders suggests that greater diagnostic differentiation may require evaluation of the particular distribution of atrophy in these regions. One example of this is provided by the left/right asymmetry of medial temporal lobe atrophy in SD, which contrasts with the symmetrical atrophy that is typical of AD. An alternative approach is to examine the distribution of atrophy in regions of interest. For instance, in AD there is an even distribution of atrophy along the rostrocaudal length of the hippocampus, whereas in SD there is asymmetrical atrophy affecting primarily the rostral portion of the left hippocampus.

Memory Impairment and Medial Temporal Lobe Atrophy in Alzheimer's Disease.

Deficits of episodic memory correlate with atrophy of the hippocampus but not with atrophy of structures outside the medial temporal lobe, such as the caudate nucleus and the lateral temporal cortex. Although differing results have been observed across a number of studies, partly as a consequence of differences in methodology and in data interpretation, most studies have revealed that performance on tests of memory correlate with hippocampal volume but not with the volumes of the amygdala or of the whole temporal lobe. Hemispheric differences are also found; the volume of the left hippocampus has been found to correlate with verbal recall, whereas the volume of the right hippocampus correlates with performance on tests of visual or spatial recall. Studies of the relation between hippocampal volume and immediate and delayed recall have yielded differing results: In one study, hippocampal volumes correlated with both recall tasks (de Toledo-Morrell et al., 2000), whereas in another a positive correlation was observed between the volumes of the hippocampus and parahippocampal gyrus with delayed, but not immediate, recall (Kohler et al., 1998). The volume of the right parahippocampal gyrus was positively associated with delayed visual recall. Hippocampal and parahippocampal gyrus volumes have also been found to correlate with a different verbal learning task (Libon et al., 1995).

In summary, most studies attempting to correlate the memory deficits in AD with atrophy of specific brain regions have implicated the hippocampus as the main region of interest. The difficulty of establishing the nature of the memory task that provides the best correlation with hippocampal volume in AD are reminiscent of the problems experienced in the clinical setting with identifying the memory tests that are most able to detect early AD.

Functional Imaging

The neuronal death and the dysfunction of surviving neurons in affected brain regions in AD results in a reduction in neuronal activity, which in turn produces an alteration in metabolic demands, with a lowering of glucose metabolism and oxygen uptake. Cerebral blood flow (CBF) to affected brain regions is likewise reduced. Cerebral hypometabolism and hypoperfusion are detectable using various functional imaging techniques, and the information derived from functional imaging complements the structural data obtained from computed tomography (CT) and MRI. To date, most of the functional imaging studies in AD have compared patients with AD with age-matched normal control subjects rather than with patients with other neurodegenerative disorders.

Positron Emission Tomography.

Cerebral glucose metabolism can be measured by positron emission tomography (PET) imaging of the radioactive tracer ^{18}F-fluorodeoxyglucose (^{18}F-FDG). PET can also be used to measure oxygen metabolism or CBF using $^{15}O_2$- or $^{15}O_2$-labeled water. Statistical parametric mapping (SPM) (Friston et al., 1995) is commonly used to analyze scan data on a voxel-by-voxel basis.

Positron emission tomography (PET) scans in AD demonstrate bilateral temporoparietal hypometabolism and hypoperfusion. The reductions in CBF and oxygen uptake have been found to correlate with the severity of the dementia. A number of studies have demonstrated correlations between memory scores and metabolism or blood flow in AD, and an association between hippocampal atrophy and regional glucose metabolism has also been demonstrated. In advanced AD, hypoperfusion changes are more widespread and additional reductions in CBF are seen in the frontal lobes.

The efforts to identify the earliest structural abnormality in AD using MRI are mirrored by studies performed using functional imaging paradigms. These have shown that hypoperfusion of the EC in cognitive normal elderly subjects is predictive of progression to MCI (de Leon et al., 2001), indicating that abnormalities of brain function may be detected at the very earliest stages of the disease.

The relation between the functional imaging data obtained from PET studies and data from structural imaging studies remains unclear. Although both imaging modalities have identified abnormalities involving the EC in the earliest stages of AD, PET studies have also shown hypofunctioning of the temporoparietal regions and the posterior cingulate cortex in early AD, whereas structural scans have revealed atrophy predominantly affecting the medial temporal lobe regions at this stage of the disease process. Given that these regions receive significant inputs from the hippocampal formation, it is possible that the PET data reflect a disconnection syndrome, in which deficits are observed in regions with disturbed activity due to reduced afferent input from damaged regions upstream in the projection. An alternative explanation for this apparent discrepancy might rest with methodological considerations. With regard to the structural imaging data, reproducible and easily validated protocols for the measurement of brain volumes are primarily restricted to the temporal lobe structures, within which atrophy is also readily detected on visual inspection. By contrast, the anatomical landmarks of regions such as the posterior cingulate gyrus are less easily identified on MRI, as a consequence of which volume loss in these regions is more difficult to detect and may therefore be underreported. In terms of the PET data, the absence of observed hypometabolism in the hippocampus and parahippocampal regions in early AD may reflect in part the low spatial resolution of the current generation of PET scans. Finally, the nature of the relation between regional brain atrophy and detection of regional hypofunction has yet to be established fully for progressive degenerative disorders such as AD.

In one study, Klunk et al. (2004) employed PET imaging using a novel tracer, named Pittsburgh compound-B (PIB), designed as a marker for brain amyloid. In patients with early AD, PET scans demonstrated increased retention of PIB (compared with control subjects) in regions of association cortex that are known to contain significant numbers of amyloid deposits. By contrast, there was no significant difference in PIB retention between AD patients and controls in those brain regions largely devoid of amyloid deposition, such as the cerebellum. The evidence from this study that PET, in conjunction with targeted tracer compounds, may be used to provide quantification of the pathological changes in AD raises the possibility that PET may be used in the future to detect, and possibly to track over time, the key pathological changes in AD.

Single Photon Emission Computed Tomography. Single photon emission computed tomography (SPECT) has an advantage over PET in that it is less expensive and more widely available, but it is less informative in that it provides only semiquantitative perfusion images and has poorer spatial resolution. CBF is measured by detection of radioactive tracers such as the lipophilic technetium ^{99m}Tc-hexamethyl propyleneamine oxamine (^{99m}Tc-HMPAO). There is a reduction in CBF in the temporoparietal regions of patients with mild-to-moderate AD (Battistin et al., 1990), with a correlation between the reduction in blood flow and hippocampal atrophy. However, the low diagnostic sensitivity and relatively poor spatial resolution of SPECT has limited its use as a diagnostic tool.

Functional MRI. The different magnetic properties of oxygenated and deoxygenated blood can be measured using the technique of blood oxygen level-dependent (BOLD) functional MRI (fMRI), with increased levels of blood oxygenation resulting in greater signal intensity. As with PET, fMRI scan data can be analyzed using SPM.

During a verbal episodic memory task patients with mild AD showed reduced activation of anterior prefrontal cortex when compared with control subjects and, instead, exhibited increased activation in a number of other brain regions, with the latter believed to represent compensatory reallocation of brain resources in response to the frontal lobe dysfunction. In a cued recall task, AD patients failed to demonstrate any increased activity in the left hippocampus—a phenomenon observed in control subjects—but, instead, were found to have increased activity in other cortical regions. These observations of increased functional activation during cognitive tasks as compensation for dysfunction of brain regions normally associated with those tasks raises the possibility that fMRI may be used in the diagnosis of AD. Functional brain changes have also been detected prior to the clinical onset of AD; subjects at

risk for AD exhibit different patterns of brain activation in the absence of any clear cognitive impairment.

Particular attention has been devoted to the regional activation patterns with the hippocampal formation in view of the early pathological involvement of the hippocampus in AD. A comparison of the fMRI activation patterns in patients with AD and patients with isolated memory decline reveals that AD patients exhibit reduced activation in all hippocampal regions. By contrast, patients with selective memory impairment either exhibited diminished activation in all hippocampal regions (similar to the pattern observed in AD) or reduced activation affecting only the subiculum. In the latter cases, the preferential involvement of the subiculum in these cases may reflect neuronal loss in the subiculum or loss of input to the subiculum in patients at risk of developing AD.

The observation that regional BOLD fMRI activation correlates with excitatory input, as manifested by the EPSP, rather than the regional output (spiking activity), suggests that reductions in regional fMRI activation patterns in AD may reflect damage in upstream neuronal populations providing excitatory inputs to the region in question (Logothetis et al., 2001). However, several outstanding issues remain with regard to the association of abnormal fMRI activation and structural pathology in AD. Specifically, the relation between fMRI activation and cerebral atrophy, as demonstrated on structural MRI, remains unclear, particularly in terms of the potential confounding effect of atrophy on fMRI activation patterns. In addition, the presence of vascular pathology in AD may represent another confounding factor in fMRI analysis in that changes in activation may be attributable to alterations in hemodynamic response as well as to changes in neural activity.

Magnetic Resonance Spectroscopy. Detection of changes in the concentration of brain metabolites using magnetic resonance spectroscopy (MRS) represents an alternative imaging modality that can be applied to disease states affecting the brain. Two metabolites that are of greatest interest are *N*-acetyl aspartate (NAA) and myoinositol (MI), which are markers of neuronal and glial cell metabolism, respectively. MRS has demonstrated levels of NAA that are reduced by 10% to 15% in AD, with the magnitude of metabolite reduction correlating with disease severity. Other studies (Jessen et al., 2000) have shown a 15% to 20% increase in MI, and a combination of NAA and MI measurements increases the ability of MRS to differentiate AD from normal aging. At present, MRS is less useful for distinguishing AD from other neurodegenerative diseases, and the utility of this imaging technique beyond the research domain has yet to be established.

16.3.3 Genetics

Most AD cases occur in sporadic form, with familial AD (FAD) accounting for less than 5% of all cases. Apart from the earlier age at onset (typically before the age of 65 years) no consistent differences in the clinical features of sporadic and familial AD have been identified. This similarity in clinical presentation has underpinned the belief that greater understanding of the defects occurring as a result of the genetic mutations associated with FAD will, in turn, yield key insights into the mechanisms of disease in AD.

Amyloid Precursor Protein

Most cases in which the patients have early-onset AD (aged ≤ 50 years) are attributable to familial forms of AD. Causative genetic mutations have been identified in these cases. The first reported FAD-associated mutations were those in the amyloid precursor protein (APP) on chromosome 21 (Chartier Harlin et al., 1991). The exact function of APP remains undetermined, with a role in growth promotion, signaling mechanisms, and cell adhesion having been variously suggested (Breen et al., 1991; Milward et al, 1992; De Strooper and Annaert, 2000). APP is cleaved at its N- and C-termini by β- and γ-secretases, respectively, to produce the peptide Aβ, comprising 40 to 42 amino acids, which is the main constituent of the amyloid plaques in AD. Despite the uncertainty over the role of APP, its role in the pathogenesis of AD appears unequivocal; all currently identified mutations of the APP gene result in an increased amount of Aβ or an increased proportion of Aβ containing 41 or 42 amino acids, which are more amyloidogenic and therefore predispose to the formation of amyloid plaques.

Presenilins

·The APP mutations account only for a small proportion of early-onset FAD. Most of these cases are caused by mutations of the *PS1* gene on chromosome 14, coding for the protein presenilin 1 (PS1). In all, *PS1* mutations are responsible for 30% to 50% of all cases of familial AD. Shortly after the discovery of the *PS1* gene, a second presenilin gene, *PS2*, on chromosome 1 was identified (Li et al., 1995). Known *PS2* mutations account for less than 10% of all FAD cases. More than 50 different mutations of *PS1* have been described, but to date only two causative *PS2* mutations have been identified.

The presenilins are transmembrane domain proteins. As with APP, the function of the presenilins remains unclear, although some clues can be derived from understanding the function of the homologous proteins SEL-12 and SPE-4 in *Caenorhabditis elegans*. SEL-12 is involved in receptor trafficking and localization, mediated via the *lin-12/Notch* pathway, and SPE-4 plays a role in intracellular protein sorting during spermatogenesis. The demonstration of a relation between PS1 and γ-secretase function (De Strooper et al., 1999) has fueled speculation that PS1 represents γ-secretase or that PS1 and γ-secretase form part of a macromolecular complex that mediates the cleavage of APP. Accordingly, presenilin mutations may alter the membrane conformation of APP, resulting in a different position of cleavage by γ-secretase; and thus generation of the more amyloidogenic forms of Aβ. The

observation that mice underexpressing PS1 exhibit a reduction in LTP following repeated tetanic stimulation of the CA1 region (Morton et al., 2002) suggests that PS1 is also implicated in the maintenance of LTP.

Apolipoprotein E

Linkage to chromosome 19 was observed in families with late-onset FAD (Pericak-Vance et al., 1991). The responsible susceptibility gene was found to encode for apolipoprotein E (ApoE), a 299-amino-acid lipid transport protein that mediates the intracellular uptake of lipids through binding to the low density lipoprotein (LDL) receptor. Three alleles for the ApoE gene exist: *APOE-ε2*, *APOE-ε3* (the common form), and *APOE-ε4*. The likelihood of developing AD has been found to correlate with the number of *APOE-ε4* genes (Saunders et al., 1993); ε4 heterozygotes had a greater risk and earlier disease onset than non-ε4 individuals, and ε4 homozygotes had the greatest risk of all. Homozygous ε4 patients were also found to have a greater number of amyloid plaques than patients homozygous for the ε3 allele. When compared with age-matched normal controls (in whom the ε4 allele is found in 16% of cases), the presence of the ε4 allele is more frequent in both late-onset AD with a positive family history (52% of all cases) and sporadic AD (40% of all cases).

One theory concerning the role of ApoE4 in the pathogenesis of AD proposes that ApoE4 binds more easily to Aβ than ApoE3, resulting in increased deposition of amyloid in plaques. Another theory is based on the observation that ApoE4 binds less well to the microtubule-associated protein tau than ApoE3 or ApoE2. This has the effect of destabilizing microtubules, which in turn results in the formation of neurofibrillary tangles.

16.3.4 Pathophysiology

Neuropathology

On macroscopic examination, the AD brain can vary in appearance from normal to severely atrophic, with cases of early-onset AD often exhibiting the most marked atrophy. Typically, the AD brain features widening of the sulci and ventricular enlargement, which is most prominent in the lateral ventricles. There is generalized atrophy of the cerebral cortex, but closer inspection of the temporal lobes may reveal a greater degree of atrophy affecting the amygdala, hippocampus, and parahippocampal gyrus.

The definitive diagnosis of AD relies on the demonstration of histological features that were first described around the turn of the twentieth century. Most prominent among them are the amyloid plaques and neurofibrillary tangles, and their significance is reflected in the various published criteria for the pathological diagnosis of AD, which are based on an evaluation of the frequency of neuritic plaques, on quantitative assessment of both plaques and tangles, and most recently on the number of tangles and neuropil threads in the cerebral cortex. Other pathological changes in AD include granulovacuolar degeneration and Hirano bodies, both of which primarily affect the hippocampus, as well as amyloid angiopathy and in severe AD mild spongiosis. Little is known about the pathogenesis of granulovacuolar degeneration or Hirano bodies or their relation to the natural history of AD, but the predominance of hippocampal involvement in both instances may provide another explanation for the prominence in AD of symptoms of hippocampal dysfunction.

Amyloid Plaques. Extracellular amyloid plaques (APs) are visualized best using silver stains or immunohistochemical techniques using an antibody to Aβ. APs are divided into two main types: diffuse plaques and neuritic plaques. Diffuse plaques are composed of homogeneous deposits of fibrillary material but contain only scant numbers of amyloid fibrils and do not stain with the Congo red stain for amyloid. Neuritic plaques are more heterogeneous in composition, with a central dense core of amyloid fibrils surrounded by glial and abnormally swollen neuritic processes, occasionally containing paired helical filaments. Neuritic plaques stain with Congo red. The two types of plaque differ crucially in that the Aβ in neuritic plaques occurs in the form of insoluble, possibly neurotoxic β-pleated sheets. APs are observed mainly in the neocortex, with only small numbers seen in the hippocampal formation during the early stages of AD; plaque density in the cortex increases with disease severity, although the progression of AP deposition does not follow a clear hierarchical pattern (Arriagada et al., 1992).

Neurofibrillary Tangles. Neurofibrillary tangles (NFTs) are found in the perikarya of neurons. They are stained with the Bielschowsky silver stain (a stain for thioflavine S) and by immunohistochemistry using an antibody to the tau protein. They are commonly flame-shaped in appearance and occupy the cell body and proximal portion of the apical dendrite of the affected neuron. NFTs are usually intraneuronal but occasionally extracellular and represent the insoluble remains of a dead neuron (the "ghost tangle"). Ultrastructural examination reveals that NFTs are primarily comprised of paired helical filaments, which are composed of a number of proteins including tau, β-amyloid, ubiquitin, and neurofilament proteins such as actin.

A hierarchical staging system for the neuropathological changes in AD has been elaborated based on the distribution of NFTs in the cerebral cortex (Braak and Braak, 1991). The first neurons to exhibit NFTs and neuropil threads (NTs)—straight and paired helical filaments composed of abnormally phosphorylated tau protein—are the pre-alpha projection neurons in the transentorhinal cortex, a transition zone between the entorhinal cortex and the adjacent isocortex. Other areas with early development of NFTs are the entorhinal cortex (EC) and field CA1 of the hippocampus. In stages I and II (the "transentorhinal stages") these minor pathological changes are restricted to the EC and hippocampus. Stages III and IV (the "limbic stages") are characterized by moderate

numbers of NFTs and NTs in the transentorhinal cortex, EC, and CA1, with additional scant numbers of NFTs in CA4, the subiculum, and the parasubiculum. Small numbers of NFTs and NTs are also found in association cortices. In stages V and VI (the "isocortical stages") all hippocampal subfields and isocortical association areas are severely affected. The progression of these pathological changes is depicted in Figure 16–8, see color insert.

Granulovacuolar Degeneration. In marked contrast to the widespread distribution of APs and NFTs, granulovacuolar degeneration is restricted primarily to one neuronal population: the pyramidal cells of the hippocampus. This pathological change is observed in up to 50% of AD cases. Vacuoles (3–5 μm diameter) are found in the cytoplasm of the pyramidal neurons, either singly or in combination. Within each vacuole is an electron-dense granular core. These features can be seen on light microscopy using either silver staining or hematoxylin and eosin (H&E) preparations.

Granulovacuolar degeneration is not specific to AD. It is also a pathological feature of other neurodegenerative disorders such as amyotrophic lateral sclerosis (ALS) and the Parkinson-dementia–ALS complex of Guam and has been found in young adults with Down's syndrome.

Hirano Bodies. Hirano bodies are ovoid eosinophilic inclusions about 10 to 30 μm in length. They can be visualized using the H&E stain. They are most commonly observed adjacent to the hippocampal pyramidal cells, when they indent the neuronal perikaryon, although they can also be found in isolation in the stratum lacunosum. Electron microscopy reveals that Hirano bodies are comprised of parallel filaments 60 to 100 nm in length.

Hirano bodies have been observed in many disorders as well as in the aged normal brain. Although they are most commonly seen in the hippocampus, Hirano bodies have been observed in most other structures of the CNS.

Medial Temporal Lobe Pathology in Alzheimer's Disease. *Entorhinal cortex:* Within the EC, the stellate cells of layer II are the first to exhibit NFTs and NTs. These cells are consistently involved in AD. In one study of patients with pathological diagnoses of definite AD, severe infiltration of stellate cells by NFTs was observed in 100% of cases (Hyman et al., 1990). These degenerative changes are accompanied by neuronal loss, which is prominent even in the early stages of AD. By late AD, severe loss of layer II cells in observed. Examination of the perforant path reveals a number of associated changes. Myelin cuffing and argyrophilic degenerative changes are seen throughout the course of the perforant path as well as in its termination zone in the outer two-thirds of the molecular layer of the dentate gyrus. Increased acetylcholinesterase staining in the outer two-thirds of the dentate molecular layer suggests that there is partial cholinergic reinnervation of the hippocampus in response to the deafferentation of the dentate gyrus.

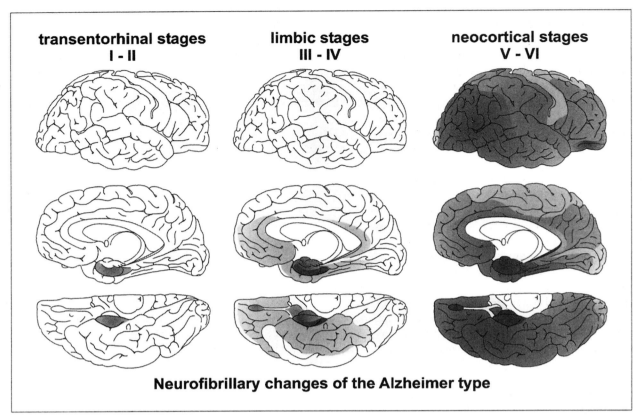

Neurofibrillary changes of the Alzheimer type

Figure 16–8. Distribution patterns of neurofibrillary changes in AD, including both neurofibrillary tangles and neuropil threads. In stages I and II the pathological changes are largely restricted to the transentorhinal region (tangles may also be found in CA1). Stages III and IV are characterized by severe involvement of the transentorhinal and entorhinal regions, with additional changes in CA1 and the subiculum. The isocortex is minimally affected. In stages V and VI the entire hippocampal formation is involved, with severe neuronal loss in CA1. The temporal lobes and cortical association areas are severely affected, but typically there is relative sparing of the primary sensory cortices. (*Source*: Courtesy of Dr. Heiko Braak.)

Of the other layers of the EC, NFT formation is observed in most of the pyramidal cells of layer IV. By contrast, significantly fewer NFTs are observed in layers III, V, and VI, although in layer III the superficial layer of neurons is more severely affected, compounding the disruption of perforant path input to the hippocampus. Assessment of neuritic plaque density reveals a different pattern of laminar involvement, with most plaques observed in layer III. Layers IV, V, and VI are associated with similar plaque density, but relatively few plaques are seen in layer II. Neither NFTs nor neuritic plaques have been demonstrated in layer I.

Hippocampus: Of the hippocampal subfields, NFT and AP density is greatest in CA1 and the subiculum. The CA1/subiculum interface zone is particularly affected, with large number of plaques and tangles observed in all cases. In CA3 and CA4, only small numbers of plaques and tangles are observed. The outer two-thirds of the molecular layer of the dentate gyrus is heavily infiltrated by NFTs and neuritic plaques, and NFTs are also seen in the dentate granule cells. Pathological changes in the mossy fiber zone are negligible. In stark contrast to the subiculum, NFTs and plaques are largely absent from the presubiculum. In terms of the hierar-

chical staging of AD pathology, the CA1 pyramidal cells are the first hippocampal neurons to exhibit changes and, in fact, represent the second neuronal population to be affected in AD, after the stellate cells of the EC. The nonpyramidal cells of CA4 and the subicular neurons are next to be affected; the granule cell layer of the dentate gyrus, CA3, and the presubiculum are involved only in the late stages of AD. Interestingly, NFTs are observed in the inner third of the dentate molecular layer in the most severely affected AD cases, which suggests that in the late disease stages there is additional deafferentation of the input to the dentate gyrus from the hilar cells. Although the hippocampus is affected throughout its extent, morphometric studies have found that there is a proportional increase in the number of neurons exhibiting NFTs and granulovacuolar degeneration in the posterior hippocampus when compared with the distribution of changes observed in the hippocampi of age-matched control subjects (Ball, 1987).

The degree of overall hippocampal pyramidal cell loss in AD has been estimated to be around 43% to 47%, with an increase in neuronal loss correlating with disease severity. Some disagreement exists with regard to the distribution of neuronal loss affecting the hippocampus proper; some observers have reported that the greatest proportion of neuronal loss occurs in CA1, with additional neuronal loss observed in CA4, the subiculum, and the prosubiculum and relative sparing of the dentate granule cells and neurons in CA3 and CA2 (Doebler et al., 1987; West et al., 1994). In a later study, no significant difference was noted in the amount of cell loss in CA1 in AD and normal aging; instead, the greatest differences in neuronal numbers were observed in the granule cell layer and the subiculum (Simic et al., 1997). An inverse correlation exists between hippocampal neuronal density and the number of neurons with NFT infiltration or granulovacuolar degeneration. In terms of the clinical significance of the severity of hippocampal involvement, the degree of neuronal loss in CA1, CA4, and the subiculum is found to correlate with the duration and severity of AD.

Amygdala: In the amygdala, NFT density is highest in the accessory basal and cortical nuclei and lowest in the medial, lateral, and central nuclei. APs were most prominent in the accessory basal and medial basal nuclei and least numerous in the medial, lateral, lateral basal, and central nuclei. Neuronal loss is greatest in the medial group of nuclei. The projections between the amygdala and the hippocampal formation are severely disrupted in AD: There is a prominent afferent projection from the accessory basal nucleus both to the hippocampus and to layer III of the EC. The return projection to the amygdala arises primarily from CA1, the subiculum, and layer IV of the EC, all of which exhibit marked pathological damage.

Pathological Changes in MCI.

Postmortem analysis reveals that the pathological changes associated with MCI primarily affect the EC and the hippocampus. Patients with very mild dementia at the time of death exhibit severe neuronal loss primarily affecting layer II, with neuronal numbers being reduced by almost 60% (Gomez-Isla et al., 1996). In layer IV, there is a 40% reduction in neuronal numbers, whereas layers I, III, and V are less affected. The degree of neuronal loss is greater in cases of severe dementia, with the drop in neuronal counts in layers II and IV rising to about 90% and 70%, respectively. These reductions in neuronal numbers are accompanied by increased deposition of NFTs and neuritic plaques. A comparison of the severity of EC pathology in MCI and AD reveals that AD is associated with greater volume loss affecting layer II, but the absence of any corresponding decrease in the number of layer II neurons indicates that the development of frank dementia may be associated with other structural changes, such as alterations in the extent of dendritic arborization.

The distribution of pathological damage in the EC in MCI patients bears comparison with the initial stages of pathology described in AD (Braak stages I and II). Given that the onset of frank dementia in AD is associated with more advanced pathological involvement, equivalent to Braak stages III and IV, it might reasonably be assumed that the syndrome of MCI represents the clinical correlate of the earliest pathological ("transentorhinal") stages of the AD disease process.

Comparison with the Pathological Changes of Normal Aging.

The APs and NFTs are also observed in the brains of nondemented aged individuals. Diffuse plaques are found throughout the cerebral cortex, with additional plaques in the amygdala, EC, and CA1. Smaller numbers of neuritic plaques are also found in these regions but with proportionally greater quantities in the medial temporal lobe structures. NFTs are commonly present in the nondemented elderly brain and are most prominent in the hippocampus and parahippocampal regions (including the EC), with NFT numbers in CA1 correlating with age.

These AD-like changes have led to the suggestion that some "normal" elderly subjects may in fact have covert, or preclinical, AD. However, the observation that normal aging and AD are associated with different patterns of neuronal loss in the hippocampus suggest, instead, that the two do not share a common pathological substrate. The demonstration of Alzheimer-type pathology in "normal" elderly individuals and the concomitant difficulty distinguishing these changes from those observed in the earliest stages of AD mirrors the problem in clinical practice with respect to the differentiation between individuals exhibiting minor cognitive decline in keeping with increasing age, and patients manifesting the earliest symptoms of AD.

Cholinergic Deficit in AD

The cholinergic innervation to the hippocampal formation arises from various components of the basal forebrain. The medial septal nucleus and the nucleus of the diagonal band provide most of the inputs, with a smaller afferent projection originating from the basalis of Meynert. By comparison, the cerebral cortex receives its major cholinergic input from the basalis of Meynert, with additional lesser projections from the pedunculopontine and lateral dorsal nuclei. Cholinergic afferents are distributed to all cortical regions, but the limbic and paralimbic cortices (including the parahippocampal areas) are the recipients of a particularly strong projection. As a consequence, lesions of the basal forebrain in monkeys result in widespread behavioral abnormalities, within which disruption of memory functions are particularly prominent (Berger-Sweeney et al., 1994).

In AD, NPs and NFTs are observed in the basalis of Meynert, the nucleus of the diagonal band, and the medial septal nuclei. There is marked neuronal loss in the nucleus basalis and the nucleus of the diagonal band. The severity of the neuropathological changes in the basalis of Meynert have been found to correlate with clinical disease severity. The concomitant depletion of cortical cholinergic axons results in a reduction in the activity of choline acetyltransferase (ChAT) in the cortex and diminished choline uptake in AD. ChAT activity is reduced by 60% in cortical biopsies obtained from patients with AD.

The observation that in AD the basal forebrain nuclei are affected by plaques and tangles, in conjunction with the reduction in cortical cholinergic innervation and the demonstration that disruption of the cholinergic system causes impaired learning and memory underpin the "cholinergic hypothesis of AD." The hypothesis proposes that the cognitive dysfunction associated with AD is at least partly attributable to impairment of cholinergic neurotransmission. Support for the hypothesis comes from studies demonstrating that the reductions in ChAT activity and acetylcholine (ACh) synthesis correlate with dementia severity in AD (Wilcock et al., 1982). However, the primary role of the cholinergic system in the pathogenesis of AD is cast into question by the observation that there is relative preservation of the cholinergic neurons of the nucleus basalis in MCI and early AD (Gilmor et al., 1999). Furthermore, the cholinergic system is not selectively affected in AD; pathological changes are also observed in a number of brain stem nuclei, including the locus coeruleus, the ventral tegmental area, and the rostral raphe nuclei. These nuclei, in turn, provide major components of the noradrenergic, dopaminergic, and serotoninergic innervation of the cerebral cortex, and it is likely that their involvement contributes to the cognitive dysfunction observed in AD.

Impairment of Synaptic Function in AD

Synaptic density microdensitometry performed on pathological specimens obtained from the frontal and temporal lobes has revealed significant reductions in the density of presynaptic boutons in AD (approximately 60% of that observed in control brains). The antemortem Mini Mental State Examination score, employed as a global measure of dementia severity, was more closely correlated with synaptic density than with amyloid plaque density or ChAT activity. Consistent with the known involvement of the entorhinal cortex in AD, there is a reduction in the markers for synaptic vesicle proteins in the termination zone of the perforant path in the outer molecular layer of the dentate gyrus. This is accompanied by a reduction in synaptic density in the inner molecular layer, although this is associated with an expansion in the size of the remaining synapses, resulting in the maintenance of the total synaptic contact area in this region (Scheff et al, 1996).

Abnormalities of synaptic transmission in early AD have been demonstrated using in vitro and in vivo preparations. In vitro studies using hippocampal slices prepared from PDAPP transgenic mice overexpressing human mutant amyloid precursor protein have demonstrated alterations in synaptic transmission and LTP (Larson et al., 1999). Enhanced paired-pulse facilitation of synaptic transmission was observed in slice preparations taken from young PDAPP mice. In addition, there was a small (about 10%) reduction in the size of the CA1 dendritic EPSPs following stimulation of the Schaffer collaterals and commissural fibers. By contrast, slice experiments performed on slices taken from aged mice revealed diminution, rather than enhancement, of paired-pulse facilitation and a marked (around 55%) reduction in CA1 field EPSPs. LTP could be induced in both young and aged prepa-

rations, but this was associated with an abnormally rapid decay function. In vivo studies using PDAPP mice have demonstrated impaired induction and maintenance of LTP in CA1 following high-frequency stimulation (Giacchino et al., 2000). PDAPP mice also exhibited attenuation of paired-pulse facilitation, indicating impaired presynaptic function in these animals. Although these changes were most prominent in aged transgenic mice, the demonstration of abnormalities in young transgenic mice prior to the development of AD-related pathological changes indicates that defects of hippocampal synaptic transmission may precede the onset of gross neurodegenerative changes.

Mouse Models of AD

The discovery of the pathogenic APP mutation in 1991 stimulated efforts to create a mouse model in which the characteristic cognitive and pathological features were expressed. Gene-targeted knockout models provide information on the possible actions of the proteins coded by the mutant genes, whereas studies using transgenic mice explore the consequences of the overexpression of mutant AD genes.

Knockout Models. APP knockout mice with functionally inactivated alleles of APP are observed to have mild impairment of forelimb grip strength and decreased locomotor activity associated with reactive gliosis. PS1 knockout mice were found to have disrupted development of the axial skeleton as a result of impaired somitogenesis. Examination of the brains of these mice reveals thinning of the ventricular zone and severe regional neuronal loss. Cerebral hemorrhages were seen in all mouse embryos. PS2 knockout mice were found to have mild pulmonary fibrosis and hemorrhage but no pathological brain changes. Absence of PS2 did not affect APP processing. However, the double homozygous PS1/PS2 knockout mice are more severely affected than the PS1 mice, suggesting that PS1 and PS2 have partially overlapping functions.

Transgenic Models. Several lines of transgenic mice are currently in existence. The PDAPP mice overexpressing V717F β-APP (an FAD-associated mutation) exhibit amyloid plaques with dystrophic neurites surrounding β-amyloid cores. Transgenic mice with overexpression of human APP_{695} (a 695-amino-acid length APP isoform representing one of the more abundant APP isoforms in the AD brain and a potential source of the Aβ peptide) have abnormally high levels of Aβ and β-amyloid deposits in the amygdala, hippocampus, and cortex between 6 and 12 months of age. Neither of these two lines of mice was found to have significant neuronal loss. None of the APP transgenic mice developed NFTs, although abnormally phosphorylated tau immunoreactivity has been observed. Deficits of spatial memory are noted by 9 to 10 months of age, and APP transgenic mice also exhibit impaired LTP (Chapman et al., 1999). PDAPP mice have been found to exhibit an age-related deficit in learning a succession of spatial locations in the watermaze (Chen et al., 2000). By contrast, object recognition was normal. In these mice, impaired performance on the watermaze task was found to correlate with amyloid plaque density.

The PS1 transgenic mice have elevated levels of $A\beta_{1-42}$. In view of the fact that patients with familial AD due to PS1 mutations have amyloid plaques comprised primarily of this longer $A\beta$ peptide, these observations provide further evidence that PS1 is involved in this aspect of plaque deposition.

Earlier studies involving APP and PS1 transgenic mice were able to provide reliable models of amyloid deposition, but the absence of any significant tau pathology meant that these studies were of limited value as realistic models of the human AD disease process. However, subsequent research has now provided evidence of a causal association between amyloid and tau pathology. The observation that bigenic mice expressing both mutant APP and mutant tau are found to have significantly greater quantities of intracytoplasmic tau tangles in the limbic system and olfactory cortex than similarly aged mice expressing the mutant tau gene alone can be taken as evidence that that the formation of NFTs is influenced by amyloid protein (Lewis et al., 2001). Furthermore, injection of $A\beta_{1-42}$ fibrils into the hippocampi of transgenic mice expressing the mutant P301L tau gene results in a fivefold increase in the number of NFTs in the amygdala (Gotz et al., 2001), which suggests that NFT deposition may be driven by $A\beta_{1-42}$. These data represent a significant advance in our understanding of the underlying nature of the neurodegeneration of AD, particularly in terms of the link between the two key aspects of AD pathology: β-amyloid deposition and tangle formation.

16.3.5 Treatment Options

The introduction of pharmacological treatments for AD during the last decade has resulted in a fundamental change in the approach to the clinical management of a condition previously considered to be associated with an inexorable and unalterable decline. At present, cholinesterase inhibitors are licensed for use in Europe and the United States, and the NMDA antagonist memantine is currently licensed for use in certain European countries. Both treatment options represent symptomatic therapy aimed at attenuating the rate of cognitive and functional decline by enhancing synaptic function. However, neither of these licensed treatments has been demonstrated to exert any effect on the underlying pathological process and so neither is likely to affect the natural history of the disease. As a consequence, efforts have been directed toward the development of treatments that may interrupt the disease process, in the anticipation that any disease-modifying drug may prove successful in altering the natural history of AD.

Enhancement of Cholinergic Function

Therapeutic strategies aimed at redressing the cholinergic deficit have led to the development of AChE inhibitors, which block the breakdown of ACh, thereby increasing ACh concen-

trations in the synaptic cleft. Clinical trials have demonstrated that usage of these drugs results in improved cognitive function. AChE inhibitors are currently licensed for the treatment of mild to moderate AD. There is accumulating evidence that they also attenuate the progression of noncognitive symptoms in AD, such as agitation and aggression, and may serve to maintain activities of daily living. However, meta-analyses of randomized clinical trials relating to the use of AChE inhibitors indicate that these drugs provide only a modest benefit in AD (Doody et al, 2001; Kaduszkiewicz et al., 2005), and to date there is little evidence that these drugs have the capacity to alter the natural history of the disease.

AChE inhibitors are at present the only drugs licensed for the treatment of mild to moderate AD. However, other drugs are being developed that are designed to enhance the cholinergic system by alternative means. They include ACh agonists, m1 muscarinic receptor agonists, and stimulators of ACh release. There have been some reports that cigarette smoking may have a protective effect in AD, which may relate to the effect on nicotinic receptors, but these findings have yet to be fully substantiated. In addition, any potentially beneficial effect on cholinergic transmission is at least partly offset by the increased risk of cerebrovascular disease associated with smoking, which increases not only the risk of AD per se but also the risk of developing concomitant vascular dementia.

NMDA Receptor Antagonists

Enhancement of glutamate-mediated synaptic function has been implicated in the pathophysiology of several neurodegenerative disorders including AD, Huntington's disease, and Parkinson's disease. The aminoadamantane compounds amantadine and memantine have been found to confer neuroprotection by noncompetitive inhibition of glutamate activity at NMDA receptor. The low affinity of both compounds for the NMDA receptor and their fast voltage-dependent channel unblocking kinetics have been cited as the explanation for their low toxicity and good clinical tolerance. This contrasts with the neurotoxicity and psychotogenicity associated with compounds that are more potent NMDA receptor antagonists, such as MK-801 and phencyclidine. A clinical trial involving the use of memantine in patients with severe AD has demonstrated a good safety profile and clinical improvement as measured using cognitive and functional assessment scores (Winblad and Poritis, 1999). As a consequence, memantine has been licensed for use in patients with moderately severe to severe AD.

Antiamyloid Immunotherapy

PDAPP mice immunized with $A\beta_{1-42}$ at 6 weeks of age, prior to the development of pathological damage, developed anti-$A\beta_{1-42}$ antibodies and were observed to have significant reductions in amyloid deposition and plaque formation (Fig. 16–9) (Schenk et al., 1999). Injections of $A\beta_{1-42}$ into older mice, in whom AD pathological changes were established, resulted in

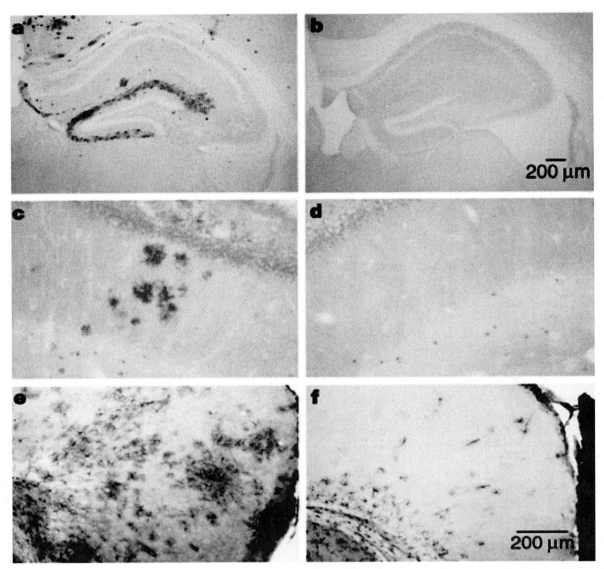

Figure 16–9. Hippocampal Aβ deposition, neuritic plaque formation, and astrocytosis in 13-month-old mice injected with phosphate-buffered saline (PBS) and Aβ$_{42}$. There is marked Aβ deposition in the outer molecular layer of the dentate gyrus of the PBS-injected mice (*a*), which contrasts with the absence of Aβ observed in the Aβ$_{42}$-injected mice (*b*). Dystrophic neurites labeled with the APP-specific monoclonal antibody 8ES were found in the hippocampal sections of the PBS-injected (*c*) but not the Aβ$_{42}$-injected mice (*d*). Plaque-associated astrocytosis is abundant in the retrosplenial cortex of the PBS-injected (*e*) but not the Aβ$_{42}$-injected (*f*) mice. (*Source*: Schenk et al., 1999, with the permission of Dr. Dale Schenk and Nature Publishing Group.)

reduced neuritic plaque burden and associated neuritic dystrophy and gliosis compared with nonimmunized mice. The pattern of amyloid pathology in the hippocampus was strikingly different in the treated mice, with an absence of diffuse deposits and an altered pattern of Aβ immunoreactivity.

Transgenic mice expressing the mutant human APP$_{695}$ transgene that were vaccinated with the Aβ$_{1-42}$ peptide exhibited a reduction of impairment when tested ozn a reference memory version of the watermaze task over a number of weeks subsequent to immunization (Janus et al., 2000). However, immunized transgenic mice remained impaired compared with nontransgenic control mice. As with the PDAPP mice, Aβ$_{1-42}$ immunization was associated with reduced amyloid plaque density when compared with nonimmunized mice.

Although initial safety trials of antiamyloid immunization indicated that the treatment could be used in human subjects, a subsequent Phase II safety trial was terminated following the development of subacute meningoencephalitis in 5% of the study population. Interestingly, a pathological study of the brain of the first immunized patient to come to postmortem (Nicoll et al., 2003) revealed large areas of cerebral cortex containing very few amyloid plaques and plaque-associated dystrophic neurites, although quantities of NFTs and neuropil threads were comparable to those observed in nonimmunized cases. Microglial cells were also found to be associated with immunoreactivity to Aβ, indicating that the immunization had been successful in generating an appropriate immune response, which in turn resulted in clearance of amyloid plaques.

Secretase Inhibitors

Whereas the vaccination approach is designed to clear amyloid from the brain, an alternative approach is to prevent formation of amyloid plaques by interfering with the production of $A\beta_{1-42}$ from its precursor protein. With this aim in mind, attention has been focused on the discovery of potential inhibitors of the β- and γ-secretase enzymes that cleave APP to form $A\beta_{1-42}$. Despite extensive animal studies, at present no secretase inhibitor has been put forward openly for clinical trials.

Other Therapeutic Options

Information derived from epidemiological observations and from research into factors influencing the development of AD pathological changes have stimulated trials with a number of treatments with potentially disease-modifying effects. Following the initial report in 1990 of a reduced incidence of AD in patients with arthritis taking nonsteroidal antiinflammatory drugs (NSAIDs), a number of other reports have drawn attention to the apparent protective effect of long-term NSAID use (in t'Veld et al, 2001). The underlying mechanism for this neuroprotection has not been established, but the observation that amyloid plaques are surrounded by immune cells (e.g., microglia) suggests that NSAIDs may serve to reduce the degree of immune-mediated neuronal destruction. An alternative explanation relates to the suppression by NSAIDs of oxygen free radical-mediated cellular damage. Finally, there may also be a direct effect on the key underlying pathological processes in AD; some NSAIDs have been demonstrated to suppress $A\beta_{1-42}$ formation. Although the epidemiological data are convincing, conclusions arising from clinical trials assessing the value of these drugs in AD must be tempered by the known profile of adverse effects associated with these drugs, particularly the risk of peptic ulceration and gastrointestinal bleeding.

Other long-term studies have documented the beneficial effects of compounds with antioxidant properties; most prominent among them are gingko biloba and vitamins C and E. Preliminary studies have indicated that all three preparations may delay the progression of AD. Similar benefits have been shown for estrogen preparations, but progress in clinical trials has been delayed following the demonstration of an increased risk of breast cancer, stroke, and myocardial infarction in a large study using hormone replacement therapy (Rapp et al, 2003).

The observation that individuals with high serum cholesterol levels are more likely to develop AD, coupled with the results from some studies suggesting that cholesterol promotes the formation of β amyloid, has led to clinical trials involving the use of statins (cholesterol-lowering agents) in patients with mild AD. The first published reports have indicated that patients on statin therapy experience a small, but not significant, reduction in the rate of cognitive decline over a 6-month period.

Certain metals have been implicated in the AD disease process. Zinc and copper cations play a critical role in the aggregation of β amyloid; in addition, the combination of these cations with β amyloid results in oxidative damage as a consequence of the generation of hydrogen peroxide. Clinical trials involving the use of metal chelators (agents that bind to metal ions) are currently under consideration (Scarpini et al, 2003).

Ultimately, any drug with true disease-modifying potential must fulfill a number of core criteria. First, a reduction in the rate of clinical decline must be demonstrated over several years, in view of the duration of the disease. Second, treatment benefits would have to be observed beyond the period of dosing to exclude the possibility of a symptomatic effect only. Ideally, benefits would be noted not only in memory and other cognitive functions but also in terms of more global measures such as activities of daily living. Finally, it would be desirable to supplement these clinical improvements with some evidence of attenuation of disease progression. In the absence of the ability to monitor directly the effect of treatments on the pathological brain changes, various surrogate markers of disease progression have been proposed, including structural (regional and global cerebral atrophy) and functional (cerebral hypometabolism) markers. Significant, consistent alterations in the longitudinal measurement of these surrogate markers of disease, observed over meaningful time spans, would provide convincing evidence of disease modification.

The discovery of multiple potential treatment avenues has markedly altered the clinical approach to AD. The anticipated development of genetic models of disease that more accurately reflect the core aspects of the AD disease process in conjunction with advances in our understanding of the pathophysiology of the disease are likely to give rise in the future to treatments that have the potential not only for effecting symptomatic alleviation but also for slowing down—perhaps even arresting—the pathological progression of Alzheimer's disease.

ACKNOWLEDGMENTS

We thank the editors for their help in preparing this chapter. We also thank Eberhard Buhl and Dimitri Kullmann for their helpful comments and criticisms on an earlier version.

REFERENCES

Adams B, Sazgar M, Osehobo P, Van der Zee CE, Diamond J, Fahnestock M, Racine RJ (1997) Nerve growth factor accelerates seizure development, enhances mossy fiber sprouting, and attenuates seizure-induced decreases in neuronal density in the kindling model of epilepsy. *J Neurosci* 17:5288–5296.

Ajmone-Marsan C, Zivin LS (1970) Factors related to the occurrence of typical paroxysmal abnormalities in the EEG records of epileptic patients. *Epilepsia* 11:361–381.

Ala TA, Beh GO, Frey WH (2000) Pure hippocampal sclerosis: a rare cause of dementia mimicking Alzheimer's disease. *Neurology* 54:843–848.

Alger BE, Nicoll RA (1980) Epileptiform burst afterhyperpolarization: calcium-dependent potassium potential in hippocampal CA1 pyramidal cells. *Science* 210:1122–1124.

Amaral DG, Campbell MJ (1986) Transmitter systems in the primate dentate gyrus. *Hum Neurobiol* 5:169–180.

Annegers JF, Hauser WA, Shirts SB, Kurland LT (1987) Factors prognostic of unprovoked seizures after febrile convulsions. *N Engl J Med* 316:493–498.

Arellano JI, Munoz A, Ballesteros-Yanez I, Sola RG, DeFelipe J (2004) Histopathology and reorganisation of chandelier cells in the human epileptic sclerotic hippocampus. *Brain* 127:45–64.

Arnold SE, Franz BR, Gur RC, Gur RE, Shapiro RM, Moberg PJ, Trojanowski JQ (1995) Smaller neuron size in schizophrenia in hippocampal subfields that mediate cortical-hippocampal interactions. *Am J Psychiatry* 152:738–748.

Arriagada PV, Growdon JH, Hedley Whyte T, Hyman BT (1992) Neurofibrillary tangles but not senile plaques parallel duration and severity of Alzheimer's disease. *Neurology* 42:631–639.

Arruda F, Cendes F, Andermann F, Dubeau F, Villemure JG, Jones-Gotman M, Poulin N, Arnold DL, Olivier A (1996) Mesial atrophy and outcome after amygdalohippocampectomy or temporal lobe removal. *Ann Neurol* 40:446–450.

Assaf SY, Chung SH (1984) Release of endogenous Zn^{2+} from brain tissue during activity. *Nature* 308:734–736.

Auer RN, Siesjo BK (1988) Biological differences between ischemia, hypoglycemia, and epilepsy. *Ann Neurol* 24:699–707.

Babb TL, Brown WJ, Pretorius J, Davenport C, Lieb JP, Crandall PH (1984) Temporal-lobe volumetric cell densities in temporal-lobe epilepsy. *Epilepsia* 25:729–740.

Babb TL, Kupfer WR, Pretorius JK, Crandall PH, Levesque MF (1991) Synaptic reorganization by mossy fibers in human epileptic fascia dentata. *Neuroscience* 42:351–363.

Ball MJ (1978) Topographical distribution of neurofibrillary tangles and granulovacuolar degeneration in hippocampal cortex of aging and demented patients: a quantitative study. *Acta Neuropathol (Berl)* 42:73–80.

Baraban SC, Hollopeter G, Erickson JC, Schwartzkroin PA, Palmiter RD (1997) Knock-out mice reveal a critical antiepileptic role for neuropeptide Y. *J Neurosci* 17:8927–8936.

Baram TZ, Gerth A, Schultz L (1997) Febrile seizures: an appropriate-aged model suitable for long-term studies. *Brain Res Dev Brain Res* 98:265–270.

Barbarosie M, Avoli M (1997) CA3-driven hippocampal-entorhinal loop controls rather than sustains in vitro limbic seizures. *J Neurosci* 17:9308–9314.

Barnard EA, Skolnick P, Olsen RW, Mohler H, Sieghart W, Biggio G, Braestrup C, Bateson AN, Langer SZ (1998) International Union of Pharmacology. XV. Subtypes of gamma-aminobutyric acid(A) receptors: classification on the basis of subunit structure and receptor function. *Pharmacol Rev* 50:291–313.

Battistin L, Pizzolato G, Dam M, Ponza I, Borsato N, Zanco PL, Ferlin G (1990) Regional cerebral blood flow study with ^{99m}Tc-hexamethyl-propyleneamine oxime single photon emission computed tomography in Alzheimer's and multi-infarct dementia. *Eur Neurol* 30:296–301.

Baulac M, De Grissac N, Hasboun D, Oppenheim C, Adam C, Arzimanoglou A, Semah F, Lehericy S, Clemenceau S, Berger B (1998) Hippocampal developmental changes in patients with partial epilepsy: magnetic resonance imaging and clinical aspects. *Ann Neurol* 44:223–233.

Baulac S, Picard F, Herman A, Feingold J, Genin E, Hirsch E, Prud'homme JF, Baulac M, Brice A, LeGuern E (2001) Evidence for digenic inheritance in a family with both febrile convulsions and temporal lobe epilepsy implicating chromosomes 18qter and 1q25-q31. *Ann Neurol* 49:786–792.

Becker JT, Boller F, Saxton J, McGonigle-Gibson KL (1987) Normal rates of forgetting of verbal and non-verbal material in Alzheimer's disease. *Cortex* 23:59–72.

Behr J, Heinemann U (1996) Low Mg^{2+} induced epileptiform activity in the subiculum before and after disconnection from rat hippocampal and entorhinal cortex slices. *Neurosci Lett* 205:25–28.

Behr J, Heinemann U, Mody I (2001) Kindling induces transient NMDA receptor-mediated facilitation of high-frequency input in the rat dentate gyrus. *J Neurophysiol* 85:2195–2202.

Bekenstein JW, Lothman EW (1993) Dormancy of inhibitory interneurons in a model of temporal lobe epilepsy. *Science* 259:97–100.

Benes FM, Kwok EW, Vincent SL, Todtenkopf MS (1998) A reduction of nonpyramidal cells in sector CA2 of schizophrenics and manic depressives. *Biol Psychiatry* 44:88–97.

Bengzon J, Kokaia Z, Elmer E, Nanobashvili A, Kokaia M, Lindvall O (1997) Apoptosis and proliferation of dentate gyrus neurons after single and intermittent limbic seizures. *Proc Natl Acad Sci USA* 94:10432–10437.

Benveniste H, Einstein G, Kim KR, Hulette C, Johnson GA (1999) Detection of neuritic plaques in Alzheimer's disease by magnetic resonance microscopy. *Proc Natl Acad Sci USA* 96:14079–14084.

Berger-Sweeney J, Heckers S, Mesulam MM, Wiley RG, Lappi DA, Sharma M (1994) Differential effects on spatial navigation of immunotoxin-induced cholinergic lesions of the medial septal area and nucleus basalis magnocellularis. *J Neurosci* 14:4507–4519.

Berman RF, Fredholm BB, Aden U, O'Connor WT (2000) Evidence for increased dorsal hippocampal adenosine release and metabolism during pharmacologically induced seizures in rats. *Brain Res* 872:44–53.

Bernard C, Anderson A, Becker A, Poolos NP, Beck H, Johnston D (2004) Acquired dendritic channelopathy in temporal lobe epilepsy. *Science* 305:532–535.

Bernasconi N, Bernasconi A, Caramanos Z, Dubeau F, Richardson J, Andermann F, Arnold DL (2001) Entorhinal cortex atrophy in epilepsy patients exhibiting normal hippocampal volumes. *Neurology* 56:1335–1339.

Billinton A, Baird VH, Thom M, Duncan JS, Upton N, Bowery NG (2001) GABA(B) receptor autoradiography in hippocampal sclerosis associated with human temporal lobe epilepsy. *Br J Pharmacol* 132:475–480.

Blumcke I, Beck H, Nitsch R, Eickhoff C, Scheffler B, Celio MR, Schramm J, Elger CE, Wolf HK, Wiestler OD (1996) Preservation of calretinin-immunoreactive neurons in the hippocampus of epilepsy patients with Ammon's horn sclerosis. *J Neuropathol Exp Neurol* 55:329–341.

Blumcke I, Zuschratter W, Schewe JC, Suter B, Lie AA, Riederer BM, Meyer B, Schramm J, Elger CE, Wiestler OD (1999a) Cellular pathology of hilar neurons in Ammon's horn sclerosis. *J Comp Neurol* 414:437–453.

Blumcke I, Beck H, Suter B, Hoffmann D, Fodisch HJ, Wolf HK, Schramm J, Elger CE, Wiestler OD (1999b) An increase of hippocampal calretinin-immunoreactive neurons correlates with early febrile seizures in temporal lobe epilepsy. *Acta Neuropathol (Berl)* 97:31–39.

Blumcke I, Becker AJ, Klein C, Scheiwe C, Lie AA, Beck H, Waha A, Friedl MG, Kuhn R, Emson P, Elger C, Wiestler OD (2000a) Temporal lobe epilepsy associated up-regulation of metabotropic glutamate receptors: correlated changes in mGluR1 mRNA and protein expression in experimental animals and human patients. *J Neuropathol Exp Neurol* 59:1–10.

Blumcke I, Suter B, Behle K, Kuhn R, Schramm J, Elger CE, Wiestler OD (2000b) Loss of hilar mossy cells in Ammon's horn sclerosis. *Epilepsia* 41:S174–S180.

Blumcke I, Schewe JC, Normann S, Brustle O, Schramm J, Elger CE, Wiestler OD (2001) Increase of nestin-immunoreactive neural precursor cells in the dentate gyrus of pediatric patients with early-onset temporal lobe epilepsy. *Hippocampus* 11:311–321.

Bobinski M, de Leon MJ, Wegiel J, De Santi S, Convit A, Wisniewski HM (1999) The histologic validation of MRI hippocampal volume measurements in Alzheimer's disease. *Neuroscience* 95:721–725.

Borck C, Jefferys JG (1999) Seizure-like events in disinhibited ventral slices of adult rat hippocampus. *J Neurophysiol* 82:2130–2142.

Bouchet, Cazauvieilh (1825) De l'épilepsie considéréé dans ses rapports avec l'aliénation mentale: recherches sur la nature et le siège de ces deux maladies. *Arch Gen Med* 9:510–542.

Bouilleret V, Schwaller B, Schurmans S, Celio MR, Fritschy JM (2000) Neurodegenerative and morphogenic changes in a mouse model of temporal lobe epilepsy do not depend on the expression of the calcium-binding proteins parvalbumin, calbindin, or calretinin. *Neuroscience* 97:47–58.

Braak H, Braak E (1991) Neuropathological staging of Alzheimer-related changes. *Acta Neuropathol (Berl)* 82:239–259.

Bragin A, Penttonen M, Buzsaki G (1997) Termination of epileptic afterdischarge in the hippocampus. *J Neurosci* 17:2567–2579.

Breen KC, Bruce M, Anderton BH (1991) Beta amyloid precursor protein mediates neuronal cell-cell and cell-surface adhesion. *J Neurosci Res* 28:90–100

Briellmann RS, Newton MR, Wellard RM, Jackson GD (2001) Hippocampal sclerosis following brief generalized seizures in adulthood. *Neurology* 57:315–317.

Brines ML, Sundaresan S, Spencer DD, deLanerolle NC (1997) Quantitative autoradiographic analysis of ionotropic glutamate receptor subtypes in human temporal lobe epilepsy: up-regulation in reorganized epileptogenic hippocampus. *Eur J Neurosci* 9:2035–2044.

Brooks KA, Shumate MD, Jin H, Rikhter TY, Coulter DA (1998) Selective changes in single cell GABA(A) receptor subunit expression and function in temporal lobe epilepsy. *Nat Med* 4:1166–1172.

Bruton CJ (1988) *The neuropathology of temporal lobe epilepsy.* Oxford, UK: Oxford University Press (Maudsley Monographs).

Buhl EH, Otis TS, Mody I (1996) Zinc-induced collapse of augmented inhibition by GABA in a temporal lobe epilepsy model. *Science* 271:369–373.

Cain DP (1989) Long-term potentiation and kindling: how similar are the mechanisms? *Trends Neurosci* 12:6–10.

Cain DP, Boon F, Hargreaves EL (1992) Evidence for different neurochemical contributions to long-term potentiation and to kindling and kindling-induced potentiation: role of NMDA and urethane-sensitive mechanisms. *Exp Neurol* 116:330–338.

Cavazos JE, Das I, Sutula TP (1994) Neuronal loss induced in limbic pathways by kindling: evidence for induction of hippocampal sclerosis by repeated brief seizures. *J Neurosci* 14:3106–3121.

Cendes F, Cook MJ, Watson C, Andermann F, Fish DR, Shorvon SD, Bergin P, Free S, Dubeau F, Arnold DL (1995) Frequency and characteristics of dual pathology in patients with lesional epilepsy. *Neurology* 45:2058–2064.

Chan D, Fox NC, Scahill RI, Crum WR, Whitwell JL, Leschziner G, Rossor AM, Stevens JM, Cipolotti L, Rossor MN (2001) Patterns of temporal lobe atrophy in semantic dementia and Alzheimer's disease. *Ann Neurol* 49:433–442.

Chandler KE, Princivalle AP, Fabian-Fine R, Bowery NG, Kullmann DM, Walker MC (2003) Plasticity of GABA(B) receptor-mediated heterosynaptic interactions at mossy fibers after status epilepticus. *J Neurosci* 23:11382–11391.

Chapman PF, White GL, Jones MW, Cooper-Blacketer D, Marshall VJ, Irizarry M, Younkin L, Good MA, Bliss TV, Hyman BT, Younkin SG, Hsiao KK (1999) Impaired synaptic plasticity and learning in aged amyloid precursor protein transgenic mice. *Nat Neurosci* 2:271–276.

Chartier Harlin M-C, Crawford F, Houlden H, Warren A, Hughes D, Fidani L, Goate A, Rossor M, Roques P, Hardy J, Mullan M (1991) Early onset Alzheimer's disease caused by mutations at codon 717 of the beta amyloid precursor gene. *Nature* 353:844–846.

Chen G, Chen KS, Knox J, Inglis J, Bernard A, Martin SJ, Justice A, McConlogue L, Games D, Freedman SB, Morris RGM (2000) A learning deficit related to age and β-amyloid plaques in a mouse model of Alzheimer's disease. *Nature* 408:975–979.

Cobb SR, Buhl EH, Halasy K, Paulsen O, Somogyi P (1995) Synchronization of neuronal activity in hippocampus by individual GABAergic interneurons. *Nature* 378:75–78.

Cohen I, Navarro V, Clemenceau S, Baulac M, Miles R (2002) On the origin of interictal activity in human temporal lobe epilepsy in vitro. *Science* 298:1418–1421.

Cole TB, Robbins CA, Wenzel HJ, Schwartzkroin PA, Palmiter RD (2000) Seizures and neuronal damage in mice lacking vesicular zinc. *Epilepsy Res* 39:153–169.

Conrad AJ, Abebe T, Austin R, Forsythe S, Scheibel AB (1991) Hippocampal pyramidal cell disarray in schizophrenia as a bilateral phenomenon. *Arch Gen Psychiatry* 48:413–417.

Convit A, De LM, Tarshish C, De SS, Tsui W, Rusinek H, George A (1997) Specific hippocampal volume reductions in individuals at risk for Alzheimer's disease. *Neurobiol Aging* 18:131–138.

Corsellis JA, Goldberg GJ, Norton AR (1968) "Limbic encephalitis" and its association with carcinoma. *Brain* 91:481–496.

Cossart R, Dinocourt C, Hirsch JC, Merchan-Perez A, De Felipe J, Ben-Ari Y, Esclapez M, Bernard C (2001) Dendritic but not somatic GABAergic inhibition is decreased in experimental epilepsy. *Nat Neurosci* 4:52–62.

Cotter D, Wilson S, Roberts E, Kerwin R, Everall IP (2000) Increased dendritic MAP2 expression in the hippocampus in schizophrenia. *Schizophr Res* 41:313–323.

Cronin J, Obenaus A, Houser CR, Dudek FE (1992) Electrophysiology of dentate granule cells after kainate-induced synaptic reorganization of the mossy fibers. *Brain Res* 573:305–310.

Csernansky JG, Wang L, Joshi S, Miller JP, Gado M, Kido D, McKeel D, Morris JC, Miller MI (2000) Early DAT is distinguished from aging by high-dimensional mapping of the hippocampus. *Neurology* 55:1636–1643.

Davies KG, Hermann BP, Dohan FC, Foley KT, Bush AJ, Wyler AR (1996) Relationship of hippocampal sclerosis to duration and age of onset of epilepsy, and childhood febrile seizures in temporal lobectomy patients. *Epilepsy Res* 24:119–126.

Davies KG, Schweitzer JB, Looney MR, Bush AJ, Dohan FC, Hermann BP (1998) Synaptophysin immunohistochemistry densitometry measurement in resected human hippocampus: implication for the etiology of hippocampal sclerosis. *Epilepsy Res* 32:335–344.

DeCarli C (2003) Mild cognitive impairment: prevalence, prognosis, aetiology, and treatment. *Lancet Neurol* 2:15–21

De Curtis M, Avanzini G (2001) Interictal spikes in focal epileptogenesis. *Prog Neurobiol* 63:541–567.

DeGiorgio CM, Tomiyasu U, Gott PS, Treiman DM (1992) Hippocampal pyramidal cell loss in human status epilepticus. *Epilepsia* 33:23–27.

De la Torre JC, Fortin T, Park GA, Butler KS, Kozlowski P, Pappas BA, de Socarraz H, Saunders JK, Richard MT (1992) Chronic cerebrovascular insufficiency induces dementia-like deficits in aged rats. *Brain Res* 582:186–195.

De Lanerolle NC, Kim JH, Robbins RJ, Spencer DD (1989) Hippocampal interneuron loss and plasticity in human temporal-lobe epilepsy. *Brain Res* 495:387–395.

De Lanerolle NC, Eid T, von Campe G, Kovacs I, Spencer DD, Brines M (1998) Glutamate receptor subunits GluR1 and GluR2/3 distribution shows reorganization in the human epileptogenic hippocampus. *Eur J Neurosci* 10:1687–1703.

De Lanerolle NC, Kim JH, Williamson A, Spencer SS, Zaveri HP, Eid T, Spencer DD, Eid T (2003) A retrospective analysis of hippocampal pathology in human temporal lobe epilepsy: evidence for distinctive patient subcategories. *Epilepsia* 44:677–687.

Del Bigio MR (1999) Proliferative status of cells in adult human dentate gyrus. *Microsc Res Tech* 45:353–358.

De Leon MJ, Convit A, Wolf OT, Tarshish CY, DeSanti S, Rusinek H, Tsui W, Kandil E, Scherer AJ, Roche A, Imossi A, Thorn E, Bobinski M, Caraos C, Lesbre P, Schlyer D, Poirier J, Reisberg B, Fowler J (2001) Prediction of cobjects with cognitive decline in normal elderly subjects with 2-[^{18}F]fluoro-2-deoxy-D-glucose/positron emission tomography (FDG/PET). *Proc Natl Acad Sci USA* 98:10966–10971.

DeLorenzo RJ, Hauser WA, Towne AR, Boggs JG, Pellock JM, Penberthy L, Garnett L, Fortner CA, Ko D (1996) A prospective, population-based epidemiologic study of status epilepticus in Richmond, Virginia. *Neurology* 46:1029–1035.

De Strooper B, Annaert W, Cupers P, Saftig P, Craessaerts K, Mumm JS, Schroeter EH, Schrijvers V, Wolfe MS, Ray WJ, Goate A, Kopan R (1999) A presenilin-1-dependent gamma-secretase-like protease mediates release of Notch intracellular domain. *Nature* 398:518–522.

De Strooper B, Annaert W (2000) Proteolytic processing and cell biological functions of the amyloid precursor protein. *J Cell Sci* 113:1857–1870

De Toledo-Morrell L, Dickerson B, Sullivan MP, Spanovic C, Wilson R, Bennett DA (2000) Hemispheric differences in hippocampal volume predict verbal and spatial memory performance in patients with Alzheimer's disease. *Hippocampus* 10:136–142.

Dickson DW, Davies P, Bevona C, Van Hoeven KH, Factor SM, Grober E, Aronson MK, Crystal HA (1994) Hippocampal sclerosis: a common pathological feature of dementia in very old (> or = 80 years of age) humans. *Acta Neuropathol (Berl)* 88:212–221.

Dietrich D, Clusmann H, Kral T, Steinhauser C, Blumcke I, Heinemann U, Schramm J (1999) Two electrophysiologically distinct types of granule cells in epileptic human hippocampus. *Neuroscience* 90:1197–1206.

Doebler JA, Markesbery WR, Anthony A, Rhoads RE (1987) Neuronal RNA in relation to neuronal loss and neurofibrillary pathology in the hippocampus in Alzheimer's disease. *J Neuropathol Exp Neurol* 46:28–39.

Doherty J, Dingledine R (2001) Reduced excitatory drive onto interneurons in the dentate gyrus after status epilepticus. *J Neurosci* 21:2048–2057.

Domann R, Westerhoff CH, Witte OW (1994) Inhibitory mechanisms terminating paroxysmal depolarization shifts in hippocampal neurons of rats. *Neurosci Lett* 176:71–74.

Doody RS, Stevens JC, Beck C, Dubinsky RM, Kaye JA, Gwyther L, Mohs RC, Thal LJ, Whitehouse PJ, DeKosky ST, Cummings JL (2001) Practice parameter: management of dementia (an evidence-based review): report of the Quality Standards Subcommittee of the American Academy of Neurology. *Neurology* 56:1154–1166

Du F, Whetsell WO, Aboukhalil B, Blumenkopf B, Lothman EW, Schwarcz R (1993) Preferential neuronal loss in layer III of the entorhinal cortex in patients with temporal-lobe epilepsy. *Epilepsy Res* 16:223–233.

Dube C, Chen K, Eghbal-Ahmadi M, Brunson K, Soltesz I, Baram TZ (2000) Prolonged febrile seizures in the immature rat model enhance hippocampal excitability long term. *Ann Neurol* 47:336–344.

During MJ, Spencer DD (1993) Extracellular hippocampal glutamate and spontaneous seizure in the conscious human brain. *Lancet* 341:1607–1610.

During MJ, Ryder KM, Spencer DD (1995) Hippocampal GABA transporter function in temporal-lobe epilepsy. *Nature* 376:174–177.

Eastwood SL, Harrison PJ (1995) Decreased synaptophysin in the medial temporal lobe in schizophrenia demonstrated using immunoautoradiography. *Neuroscience* 69:339–343.

Ekonomou A, Sperk G, Kostopoulos G, Angelatou F (2000) Reduction of A1 adenosine receptors in rat hippocampus after kainic acid-induced limbic seizures. *Neurosci Lett* 284:4952.

Elmer E, Kokaia M, Kokaia Z, Ferencz I, Lindvall O (1996) Delayed kindling development after rapidly recurring seizures: relation to mossy fiber sprouting and neurotrophin, GAP-43 and dynorphin gene expression. *Brain Res* 712:19–34.

Erdem A, Yasargil G, Roth P (1993) Microsurgical anatomy of the hippocampal arteries. *J Neurosurg* 79:256–265.

Eriksson PS, Perfilieva E, Bjork-Eriksson T, Alborn AM, Nordborg C, Peterson DA, Gage FH (1998) Neurogenesis in the adult human hippocampus. *Nat Med* 4:1313–1317.

Esclapez M, Hirsch JC, Ben-Ari Y, Bernard C (1999) Newly formed excitatory pathways provide a substrate for hyperexcitability in experimental temporal lobe epilepsy. *J Comp Neurol* 408:449–460.

Fernandez G, Effenberger O, Vinz B, Steinlein O, Elger CE, Dohring W, Heinze HJ (1998) Hippocampal malformation as a cause of familial febrile convulsions and subsequent hippocampal sclerosis. *Neurology* 50:909–917.

Fox NC, Crum WR, Scahill RI, Stevens JM, Janssen JC, Rossor MN (2001) Imaging of onset and progression of Alzheimer's disease with voxel-compression mapping of serial magnetic resonance images. Lancet 358:201–205.

French JA, Williamson PD, Thadani VM, Darcey TM, Mattson RH, Spencer SS, Spencer DD (1993) Characteristics of medial temporal lobe epilepsy. I. Results of history and physical examination. *Ann Neurol* 34:774–780.

Freund TF, Buzsaki G (1996) Interneurons of the hippocampus. *Hippocampus* 6:347–470.

Friston KJ, Holmes AP, Worsley KJ, Poline J-P, Frith CD, Frackowiak RSJ (1995) Statistical parametric maps in functional imaging: a general linear approach. *Hum Brain Mapp* 2:189–210.

Fritschy JM, Kiener T, Bouilleret V, Loup F (1999) GABAergic neurons and GABA(A)-receptors in temporal lobe epilepsy. *Neurochem Int* 34:435–445.

Frotscher M, Haas CA, Forster E (2003) Reelin controls granule cell migration in the dentate gyrus by acting on the radial glial scaffold. *Cereb Cortex* 13:634–640.

Furtinger S, Pirker S, Czech T, Baumgartner C, Ransmayr G, Sperk G (2001) Plasticity of Y1 and Y2 receptors and neuropeptide Y fibers in patients with temporal lobe epilepsy. *J Neurosci* 21:5804–5812.

Garbelli R, Frassoni C, Ferrario A, Tassi L, Bramerio M, Spreafico R (2001) Cajal-Retzius cell density as marker of type of focal cortical dysplasia. *Neuroreport* 12:2767–2771.

Giacchino J, Criado JR, Games D, Henriksen S (2000) In vivo synaptic transmission in young and aged amyloid precursor protein transgenic mice. *Brain Res* 876:185–190.

Gibbs JW, Shumate MD, Coulter DA (1997) Differential epilepsy-associated alterations in postsynaptic GABA(A) receptor function in dentate granule and CA1 neurons. *J Neurophysiol* 77:1924–1938.

Gilmor ML, Erickson JD, Varoqui H, Hersh LB, Bennett DA, Cochran EJ, Mufson EJ, Levey AI (1999) Preservation of nucleus basalis neurons containing choline acetyltransferase and the vesicular acetylcholine transporter in the elderly with mild cognitive impairment and early Alzheimer's disease. *J Comp Neurol* 411:693–704.

Goddard GV (1967) Development of epileptic seizures through brain stimulation at low intensity. *Nature* 214:1020–1021.

Gomez-Isla T, Price JL, McKeel-DW J, Morris JC, Growdon JH, Hyman BT (1996) Profound loss of layer II entorhinal cortex neurons occurs in very mild Alzheimer's disease. *J Neurosci* 16:4491–4500.

Good CD, Scahill RI, Fox NC, Ashburner J, Friston KJ, Chan D, Crum WR, Rossor MN, Frackowiak RSJ (2002) Automated differentiation of anatomical patterns in the human brain: validation with studies of degenerative dementias. *Neuroimage* 17:29–46.

Gorter JA, van Vliet EA, Aronica E, Lopes dSF (2001) Progression of spontaneous seizures after status epilepticus is associated with mossy fiber sprouting and extensive bilateral loss of hilar parvalbumin and somatostatin-immunoreactive neurons. *Eur J Neurosci* 13:657–669.

Gotz J, Chen F, van Dorpe J, Nitsch RM (2001) Formation of neurofibrillary tangles in P301L tau transgenic mice induced by Aβ42 fibrils. *Science* 293:1491–1495.

Gregory RP, Oates T, Merry RT (1993) Electroencephalogram epileptiform abnormalities in candidates for aircrew training. *Electroencephalogr Clin Neurophysiol* 86:75–77.

Grooms SY, Opitz T, Bennett MVL, Zukin RS (2000) Status epilepticus decreases glutamate receptor 2 mRNA and protein expression in hippocampal pyramidal cells before neuronal death. *Proc Natl Acad Sci USA* 97:3631–3636.

Grossberg S (2000) The imbalanced brain: from normal behavior to schizophrenia. *Biol Psychiatry* 48:81–98.

Gultekin SH, Rosenfeld MR, Voltz R, Eichen J, Posner JB, Dalmau J (2000) Paraneoplastic limbic encephalitis: neurological symptoms, immunological findings and tumour association in 50 patients. *Brain* 123(Pt 7):1481–1494.

Gutierrez R, Heinemann U (2001) Kindling induces transient fast inhibition in the dentate gyrus–CA3 projection. *Eur J Neurosci* 13:1371–1379.

Haas KZ, Sperber EF, Moshe SL, Stanton PK (1996) Kainic acid-induced seizures enhance dentate gyrus inhibition by downregulation of GABA(B) receptors. *J Neurosci* 16:4250–4260.

Handforth A, Treiman DM (1994) Effect of an adenosine antagonist and an adenosine agonist on status entry and severity in a model of limbic status epilepticus. *Epilepsy Res* 18:29–42.

Hardiman O, Burke T, Phillips J, Murphy S, O'Moore B, Staunton H, Farrell MA (1988) Microdysgenesis in resected temporal neocortex: incidence and clinical significance in focal epilepsy. *Neurology* 38:1041–1047.

Harding B, Thom M (2001) Bilateral hippocampal granule cell dispersion: autopsy study of 3 infants. *Neuropathol Appl Neurobiol* 27:245–251.

Hart RP, Kwentus JA, Taylor JR, Harkins SW (1987) Rate of forgetting in dementia and depression. *J Consult Clin Psychol* 55:101–105.

Heinemann U, Gabriel S, Jauch R, Schulze K, Kivi A, Eilers A, Kovacs R, Lehmann TN (2000) Alterations of glial cell function in temporal lobe epilepsy. *Epilepsia* 41(Suppl 6):S185–S189.

Hesdorffer DC, Logroscino G, Cascino G, Annegers JF, Hauser WA (1998) Risk of unprovoked seizure after acute symptomatic seizure: effect of status epilepticus. *Ann Neurol* 44:908–912.

Hinterkeuser S, Schroder W, Hager G, Seifert G, Blumcke I, Elger CE, Schramm J, Steinhauser C (2000) Astrocytes in the hippocampus of patients with temporal lobe epilepsy display changes in potassium conductances. *Eur J Neurosci* 12:2087–2096.

Hirsch JC, Agassandian C, Merchan-Perez A, Ben-Ari Y, DeFelipe J, Esclapez M, Bernard C (1999) Deficit of quantal release of GABA in experimental models of temporal lobe epilepsy. *Nat Neurosci* 2:499–500.

Hogan RE, Wang L, Bertrand ME, Willmore J, Bucholz RD, Nassif AS, Csernansky JG (2004) MRI-based high-dimensional hippocampal mapping in mesial temporal lobe epilepsy. *Brain* 127:1731–1740.

Honer WG, Beach TG, Hu L, Berry K, Dorovini-Zis K, Moore GR, Woodhurst B (1994) Hippocampal synaptic pathology in patients with temporal lobe epilepsy. *Acta Neuropathol (Berl)* 87:202–210.

Houser CR (1990) Granule cell dispersion in the dentate gyrus of humans with temporal lobe epilepsy. *Brain Res* 535:195–204.

Houser CR, Miyashiro JE, Swartz BE, Walsh GO, Rich JR, Delgado-Escueta AV (1990) Altered patterns of dynorphin immunoreactivity suggest mossy fiber reorganization in human hippocampal epilepsy. *J Neurosci* 10:267–282.

Houser CR, Swartz BE, Walsh GO, Delgado-Escueta AV (1992) Granule cell disorganization in the dentate gyrus: possible alterations of neuronal migration in human temporal lobe epilepsy. *Epilepsy Res Suppl* 9:41–48.

Howell GA, Welch MG, Frederickson CJ (1984) Stimulation-induced uptake and release of zinc in hippocampal slices. *Nature* 308:736–738.

Howell OW, Scharfman HE, Herzog H, Sundstrom LE, Beck-Sickinger A, Gray WP (2003) Neuropeptide Y is neuroproliferative for post-natal hippocampal precursor cells. *J Neurochem* 86:646–659.

Hugg JW, Butterworth EJ, Kuzniecky RI (1999) Diffusion mapping applied to mesial temporal lobe epilepsy: preliminary observations. *Neurology* 53:173–176.

Hyman BT, Van Hoesen GW, Damasio AR (1990) Memory-related neural systems in Alzheimer's disease: an anatomic study. *Neurology* 40:1721–1730.

Insausti R, Juottonen K, Soininen H, Insausti AM, Partanen K, Vainio P, Laakso MP, Pitkanen A (1998) MR volumetric analysis of the human entorhinal, perirhinal, and temporopolar cortices. *Am J Neuroradiol* 19:659–671.

in t' Veld BA, Ruitenberg A, Hofman A, Launer JJ, van Duijn CM, Stijnen T, Breteler MM, Stricker BH (2001) Nonsteroidal antiinflammatory drugs and the risk of Alzheimer's disease. *N Engl J Med* 345:1515–1521.

Jack CR, Petersen RC, Xu YC, Waring SC, O'Brien PC, Tangalos EG, Smith GE, Ivnik RJ, Kokmen E (1997) Medial temporal atrophy on MRI in normal aging and very mild Alzheimer's disease. *Neurology* 49:786–794.

Jack CR, Petersen RC, Xu Y, O'Brien PC, Smith GE, Ivnik RJ, Tangalos EG, Kokmen E (1998) Rate of medial temporal lobe atrophy in typical aging and Alzheimer's disease. *Neurology* 51:993–999.

Jack CR, Petersen RC, Xu YC, Obrien PC, Smith GE, Ivnik RJ, Boeve BF, Waring SC, Tangalos EG, Kokmen E (1999) Prediction of AD with MRI-based hippocampal volume in mild cognitive impairment. *Neurology* 52:1397–1403.

Janus C, Pearson J, McLaurin J, Mathews PM, Jiang Y, Schmidt SD, Chishti MA, Horne P, Heslin D, French J, Mount HTJ, Nixon RA, Mercken M, Bergeron C, Fraser PE, St George-Hyslop P, Westaway D (2000) A beta peptide immunization reduces behavioural impairment and plaques in a model of Alzheimer's disease. *Nature* 408:979–982.

Jefferys JG (1995) Nonsynaptic modulation of neuronal activity in the brain: electric currents and extracellular ions. *Physiol Rev* 75:689–723.

Jefferys JG, Evans BJ, Hughes SA, Williams SF (1992) Neuropathology of the chronic epileptic syndrome induced by intrahippocampal tetanus toxin in rat: preservation of pyramidal cells and incidence of dark cells. *Neuropathol Appl Neurobiol* 18:53–70.

Jessen F, Block W, Traber F, Keller E, Flacke S, Papassotiropoulos A, Lamerichs R, Heun R, Schild HH (2000). Proton MR spectroscopy detects a relative decrease of *N*-acetylaspartate in the medial temporal lobe of patients with AD. *Neurology* 55:684–688.

Jones RS (1989) Ictal epileptiform events induced by removal of extracellular magnesium in slices of entorhinal cortex are blocked by baclofen. *Exp Neurol* 104:155–161.

Kaduszkiewicz H, Zimmermann T, Bent-Bornholdt HP, van den Bussche H (2005) Cholinesterase inhibitors for patients with Alzheimer's disease: a systematic review a randomised clinical trials. *BMJ* 331:321–337.

Kandlhofer S, Hoertnagl B, Czech T, Baumgartner C, Maier H, Novak K, Sperk G (2000) Chromogranins in temporal lobe epilepsy. *Epilepsia* 41(Suppl 6):S111–S114.

Kapur J, Macdonald RL (1997) Rapid seizure-induced reduction of benzodiazepine and Zn^{2+} sensitivity of hippocampal dentate granule cell GABA$_A$ receptors. *J Neurosci* 17:7532–7540.

Kapur J, Lothman EW, DeLorenzo RJ (1994) Loss of GABA$_A$ receptors during partial status epilepticus. *Neurology* 44:2407–2408.

Karnup S, Stelzer A (2001) Seizure-like activity in the disinhibited CA1 minislice of adult guinea-pigs. *J Physiol* 532:713–730.

Kelly ME, McIntyre DC (1994) Hippocampal kindling protects several structures from the neuronal damage resulting from kainic acid-induced status epilepticus. *Brain Res* 634:245–256.

King D, Spencer S (1995) Invasive electroencephalography in mesial temporal lobe epilepsy. *J Clin Neurophysiol* 12:32–45.

Klunk WE, Engler H, Nordberg A, Wang Y, Blomqvist G, Holt DP, Bergstrom M, Savitcheva I, Huang GF, Estrada S, Ausen B, Debnath ML, Barletta J, Price JC, Sandell J, Lopresti BJ, Wall A, Koivisto P, Antoni G, Mathis CA, Langstrom B (2004) Imaging brain amyloid in Alzheimer's disease with Pittsburgh compound-B. *Ann Neurol* 55:303–305.

Kneisler TB, Dingledine R (1995) Spontaneous and synaptic input from granule cells and the perforant path to dentate basket cells in the rat hippocampus. *Hippocampus* 5:151–164.

Kohler S, Black SE, Sinden M, Szekely C, Kidron D, Parker JL, Foster JK, Moscovitch M, Winocour G, Szalai JP, Bronskill MJ (1998) Memory impairments associated with hippocampal versus parahippocampal gyrus atrophy: an MR volumetry study in Alzheimer's disease. *Neuropsychologia* 36:901–914.

Kohr G, De Koninck Y, Mody I (1993) Properties of NMDA receptor channels in neurons acutely isolated from epileptic (kindled) rats. *J Neurosci* 13:3612–3627.

Kotti T, Riekkinen PJ, Miettinen R (1997) Characterization of target cells for aberrant mossy fiber collaterals in the dentate gyrus of epileptic rat. *Exp Neurol* 146:323–330.

Kullmann DM (2002) Genetics of epilepsy. *J Neurol Neurosurg Psychiatry* 73(Suppl 2):II32–II35.

Kullmann DM, Asztely F (1998) Extrasynaptic glutamate spillover in the hippocampus: evidence and implications. *Trends Neurosci* 21:8–14.

Larson J, Lynch G, Games D, Seubert P (1999) Alterations in synaptic transmission and long-term potentiation in hippocampal slices from young and aged PDAPP mice. *Brain Res* 840:23–35.

Leranth C, Ribak CE (1991) Calcium-binding proteins are concentrated in the CA2 field of the monkey hippocampus: a possible key to this region's resistance to epileptic damage. *Exp Brain Res* 85:129–136.

Lewis J, Dickson DW, Lin WL, Chisholm L, Corral A, Jones G, Yen SH, Sahara N, Skipper L, Yager D, Eckman C, Hardy J, Hutton M, McGowan E (2001) Enhanced neurofibrillary degeneration in transgenic mice expressing mutant tau and APP. *Science* 293:1487–1491.

Li J, Ma J, Potter H (1995) Identification and expression analysis of a potential familial Alzheimer disease gene on chromosome 1 related to AD3. *Proc Natl Acad Sci USA* 92:12180–12184.

Li LM, Cendes F, Andermann F, Watson C, Fish DR, Cook MJ, Dubeau F, Duncan JS, Shorvon SD, Berkovic SF, Free S, Olivier A, Harkness W, Arnold DL (1999) Surgical outcome in patients with epilepsy and dual pathology. *Brain* 122(Pt 5):799–805.

Lie AA, Blumcke I, Beck H, Wiestler OD, Elger CE, Schoen SW (1999) 5'-Nucleotidase activity indicates sites of synaptic plasticity and reactive synaptogenesis in the human brain. *J Neuropathol* Exp Neurol 58:451–458.

Lie AA, Becker A, Behle K, Beck H, Malitschek B, Conn PJ, Kuhn R, Nitsch R, Plaschke M, Schramm J, Elger CE, Wiestler OD, Blumcke I (2000) Up-regulation of the metabotropic glutamate receptor mGluR4 in hippocampal neurons with reduced seizure vulnerability. *Ann Neurol* 47:26–35.

Lieberman DN, Mody I (1994) Regulation of NMDA channel function by endogenous Ca(2+)-dependent phosphatase. *Nature* 369:235–239.

Lieberman DN, Mody I (1999) Properties of single NMDA receptor channels in human dentate gyrus granule cells. *J Physiol (Lond)* 518:5570.

Libon DJ, Bogdanoff B, Cloud BS, Skalina S, Giovannetti T, Gitlin HL, Bonavita J (1998) Declarative and procedural learning, quantitative measures of the hippocampus, and subcortical white matter alterations in Alzheimer's disease and ischaemic vascular dementia. *J Clin Exp* Neuropsychol 20:30–41.

Lipton SA, Rosenberg PA (1994) Excitatory amino acids as a final common pathway for neurologic disorders. *N Engl J Med* 330:613–622.

Logothetis NK, Pauls J, Augath M, Trinath T, Oeltermann A (2001) Neurophysiological investigation of the basis of the fMRI signal. *Nature* 412:150–157.

Longo BM, Mello LE (1998) Supragranular mossy fiber sprouting is not necessary for spontaneous seizures in the intrahippocampal kainate model of epilepsy in the rat. *Epilepsy Res* 32:172–182.

Lothman EW, Bertram EH (1993) Epileptogenic effects of status epilepticus. *Epilepsia* 34(Suppl 1):S59–S70.

Loup F, Wieser HG, Yonekawa Y, Aguzzi A, Fritschy JM (2000) Selective alterations in GABA$_A$ receptor subtypes in human temporal lobe epilepsy. *J Neurosci* 20:5401–5419.

Lowenstein DH, Thomas MJ, Smith DH, McIntosh TK (1992) Selective vulnerability of dentate hilar neurons following traumatic brain injury: a potential mechanistic link between head trauma and disorders of the hippocampus. *J Neurosci* 12:4846–4853.

Lux HD, Heinemann U, Dietzel I (1986) Ionic changes and alterations in the size of the extracellular space during epileptic activity. *Adv Neurol* 44:619–639.

Magloczky Z, Halasz P, Vajda J, Czirjak S, Freund TF (1997) Loss of calbindin-D28K immunoreactivity from dentate granule cells in human temporal lobe epilepsy. *Neuroscience* 76:377–385.

Magloczky Z, Wittner L, Borhegyi Z, Halasz P, Vajda J, Czirjak S, Freund TF (2000) Changes in the distribution and connectivity of interneurons in the epileptic human dentate gyrus. *Neuroscience* 96:7–25.

Maier M, Ron MA, Barker GJ, Tofts PS (1995) Proton magnetic resonance spectroscopy: an in vivo method of estimating hippocampal neuronal depletion in schizophrenia. *Psychol Med* 25:1201–1209.

Marsh DJ, Baraban SC, Hollopeter G, Palmiter RD (1999) Role of the Y5 neuropeptide Y receptor in limbic seizures. *Proc Natl Acad Sci USA* 96:13518–13523.

Martinerie J, Adam C, Le Van Quyen M, Baulac M, Clemenceau S, Renault B, Varela FJ (1998) Epileptic seizures can be anticipated by non-linear analysis. *Nat Med* 4:1173–1176.

Mathern GW, Babb TL, Pretorius JK, Leite JP (1995a) Reactive synaptogenesis and neuron densities for neuropeptide Y, somatostatin, and glutamate decarboxylase immunoreactivity in the epileptogenic human fascia dentata. *J Neurosci* 15:3990–4004.

Mathern GW, Pretorius JK, Babb TL (1995b) Quantified patterns of mossy fiber sprouting and neuron densities in hippocampal and lesional seizures. *J Neurosurg* 82:211–219.

Mathern GW, Pretorius JK, Kornblum HI, Mendoza D, Lozada A, Leite JP, Chimelli LM, Fried I, Sakamoto AC, Assirati JA, Levesque MF, Adelson PD, Peacock WJ (1997) Human hippocampal AMPA and NMDA mRNA levels in temporal lobe epilepsy patients. *Brain* 120(Pt 11):1937–1959.

Mathern GW, Mendoza D, Lozada A, Pretorius JK, Dehnes Y, Danbolt NC, Nelson N, Leite JP, Chimelli L, Born DE, Sakamoto AC, Assirati JA, Fried I, Peacock WJ, Ojemann GA, Adelson PD (1999) Hippocampal GABA and glutamate transporter immunoreactivity in patients with temporal lobe epilepsy. *Neurology* 52:453.

Matsumoto H, Ajmone-Marsan C (1964) Cortical cellular phenomena in experimental epilepsy: interictal manifestations. *Exp Neurol* 9:286–304.

Mazarati AM, Liu H, Soomets U, Sankar R, Shin D, Katsumori H, Langel L, Wasterlain CG (1998) Galanin modulation of seizures and seizure modulation of hippocampal galanin in animal models of status epilepticus. *J Neurosci* 18:10070–10077.

Mazarati A, Liu H, Wasterlain C (1999) Opioid peptide pharmacology and immunocytochemistry in an animal model of self-sustaining status epilepticus. *Neuroscience* 89:167–173.

Mazarati AM, Hohmann JG, Bacon A, Liu H, Sankar R, Steiner RA, Wynick D, Wasterlain CG (2000) Modulation of hip-pocampal excitability and seizures by galanin. *J Neurosci* 20:6276–6281.

McKhann G, Drachman D, Folstein M, Katzman R, Price D, Stadlan EM (1984) Clinical diagnosis of Alzheimer's disease: report of the NINCDS-ADRDA work group under the auspices of Department of Health and Human Services Task Force on Alzheimer's disease. *Neurology* 34:939–944.

McNamara JO, Bonhaus W, Shin C (1993) The kindling model of epilepsy. In: *Epilepsy: models, mechanisms, and concepts*. (Schwartzkroin PA, ed), pp 21–47. Cambridge, UK: Cambridge University Press.

Meldrum B (1991) Excitotoxicity and epileptic brain damage. *Epilepsy Res* 10:55–61.

Mellanby J, George G, Robinson A, Thompson P (1977) Epileptiform syndrome in rats produced by injecting tetanus toxin into the hippocampus. *J Neurol Neurosurg Psychiatry* 40:404–414.

Miles R, Wong RK (1983) Single neurones can initiate synchronized population discharge in the hippocampus. *Nature* 306:371–373.

Milgram NW, Yearwood T, Khurgel M, Ivy GO, Racine R (1991) Changes in inhibitory processes in the hippocampus following recurrent seizures induced by systemic administration of kainic acid. *Brain Res* 551:236–246.

Milward EA, Papadopoulos R, Fuller SJ, Moir RD, Small D, Beyreuther K, Masters CL (1992) The amyloid protein precursor of Alzheimer's disease is a mediator of the effects of nerve growth factor on neurite outgrowth. *Neuron* 9:129–137.

Min MY, Melyan Z, Kullmann DM (1999) Synaptically released glutamate reduces gamma-aminobutyric acid (GABA)ergic inhibition in the hippocampus via kainate receptors. *Proc Natl Acad Sci USA* 96:9932–9937.

Mody I, Heinemann U (1987) NMDA receptors of dentate gyrus granule cells participate in synaptic transmission following kindling. *Nature* 326:701–704.

Molnar P, Nadler JV (2001) Lack of effect of mossy fiber-released zinc on granule cell GABA(A) receptors in the pilocarpine model of epilepsy. *J Neurophysiol* 85:1932–1940.

Morton RA, Kuenzi FM, Fitzjohn SM, Rosahl TW, Smith D, Zheng H, Shearman M, Collingridge GL, Seabrook GR (2002)

Impairment in hippocampal long-term potentiation in mice under-expressing the Alzheimer's disease related gene presenilin-1. *Neurosci Lett* 319:37–40.

Nagerl UV, Mody I, Jeub M, Lie AA, Elger CE, Beck H (2000) Surviving granule cells of the sclerotic human hippocampus have reduced Ca(2+) influx because of a loss of calbindin-D(28k) in temporal lobe epilepsy. *J Neurosci* 20:1831–1836.

Nelson MD, Saykin AJ, Flashman LA, Riordan HJ (1998) Hippocampal volume reduction in schizophrenia as assessed by magnetic resonance imaging: a meta-analytic study. *Arch Gen Psychiatry* 55:433–440.

Nicoll JA, Wilkinson D, Holmes C, Steart P, Markham H, Weller RO (2003) Neuropathology of human Alzheimer disease after immunization with amyloid-beta peptide: a case report. *Nat Med* 9:448–452.

Nusser Z, Hajos N, Somogyi P, Mody I (1998) Increased number of synaptic GABA(A) receptors underlies potentiation at hippocampal inhibitory synapses. *Nature* 395:172–177.

Okazaki MM, Evenson DA, Nadler JV (1995) Hippocampal mossy fiber sprouting and synapse formation after status epilepticus in rats: visualization after retrograde transport of biocytin. *J Comp Neurol* 352:515–534.

Omar AI, Senatorov VV, Hu B (2000) Ethidium bromide staining reveals rapid cell dispersion in the rat dentate gyrus following ouabain-induced injury. *Neuroscience* 95:73–80.

Parent JM, Yu TW, Leibowitz RT, Geschwind DH, Sloviter RS, Lowenstein DH (1997) Dentate granule cell neurogenesis is increased by seizures and contributes to aberrant network reorganization in the adult rat hippocampus. *J Neurosci* 17:3727–3738.

Parent JM, Tada E, Fike JR, Lowenstein DH (1999) Inhibition of dentate granule cell neurogenesis with brain irradiation does not prevent seizure-induced mossy fiber synaptic reorganization in the rat. *J Neurosci* 19:4508–4519.

Patrylo PR, Spencer DD, Williamson A (2001) GABA uptake and heterotransport are impaired in the dentate gyrus of epileptic rats and humans with temporal lobe sclerosis. *J Neurophysiol* 85:1533–1542.

Penix LP, Wasterlain CG (1994) Selective protection of neuropeptide containing dentate hilar interneurons by non-NMDA receptor blockade in an animal model of status epilepticus. *Brain Res* 644:19–24.

Pennanen C, Kivipelto M, Tuomainen S, Hartikainen P, Hanninen T, Laakso MP, Hallikainen M, Vanhanen M, Nissinen A, Helkala EL, Vainio P, Vanninen R, Partanen K, Soininen H (2004) Hippocampal and entorhinal cortex in mild cognitive impairment and early AD. *Neurobiol Aging* 25:303–310.

Perez VJ, Carlen PL (2000) Gap junctions, synchrony and seizures. Trends Neurosci 23:68–74.

Pericak-Vance MA, Bebout JL, Gaskell PC, Yamaoka LH, Hung W-Y, Alberts MJ, Walker AP, Bartlett RJ, Haynes CA, Welsh KA, Earl NL, Heyman A, Clark CM, Roses AD (1991) Linkage studies in familial Alzheimer's disease: evidence for chromosome 19 linkage. *Am J Hum Genet* 48:1034–1050.

Perlin JB, Churn SB, Lothman EW, DeLorenzo RJ (1992) Loss of type II calcium/calmodulin-dependent kinase activity correlates with stages of development of electrographic seizures in status epilepticus in rat. *Epilepsy Res* 11:111–118.

Pfleger L (1880) Beobachtungen uber schrumpfung und Sclerose des Ammonshornes bei Epilepsie. *Allg Z Psychiatr* 36:359–365.

Proper EA, Oestreicher AB, Jansen GH, Veelen CW, van-Rijen PC, Gispen WH, de-Graan PN (2000) Immunohistochemical char-

acterization of mossy fiber sprouting in the hippocampus of patients with pharmaco-resistant temporal lobe epilepsy. *Brain* 123:19–30.

Proper EA, Hoogland G, Kappen SM, Jansen GH, Rensen MG, Schrama LH, van Veelen CW, van Rijen PC, van Nieuwenhuizen O, Gispen WH, de Graan PN (2002) Distribution of glutamate transporters in the hippocampus of patients with pharmaco-resistant temporal lobe epilepsy. *Brain* 125:32–43.

Rapp SR, Espeland MA, Shumaker SA, Henderson VW, Brunner RL, Manson JE, Gass ML, Stefanick ML, Lane DS, Hays J, Johnson KC, Coker LH, Dailey M, Bowen D (2003) Effect of estrogen plus progestin on global cognitive function in postmenopausal women: the Women's Health Initiative Memory Study: a randomized controlled trial. *JAMA* 289:2717–2719.

Roper SN, Obenaus A, Dudek FE (1992) Osmolality and nonsynaptic epileptiform bursts in rat CA1 and dentate gyrus. *Ann Neurol* 31:81–85.

Rothstein JD, Dykes-Hoberg M, Pardo CA, Bristol LA, Jin L, Kuncl RW, Kanai Y, Hediger MA, Wang Y, Schielke JP, Welty DF (1996) Knockout of glutamate transporters reveals a major role for astroglial transport in excitotoxicity and clearance of glutamate. *Neuron* 16:675–686.

Roy NS, Wang S, Jiang L, Kang J, Benraiss A, Harrison-Restelli C, Fraser RA, Couldwell WT, Kawaguchi A, Okano H, Nedergaard M, Goldman SA (2000) In vitro neurogenesis by progenitor cells isolated from the adult human hippocampus. *Nat Med* 6:271–277.

Salmenpera T, Kalviainen R, Partanen K, Pitkanen A (2000) Quantitative MRI volumetry of the entorhinal cortex in temporal lobe epilepsy. *Seizure* 9:208–215.

Sanabria ER, Su H, Yaari Y (2001) Initiation of network bursts by Ca^{2+}-dependent intrinsic bursting in the rat pilocarpine model of temporal lobe epilepsy. *J Physiol* 532:205–216.

Sander JW, Shorvon SD (1996) Epidemiology of the epilepsies. *J Neurol Neurosurg Psychiatry* 61:433–443.

Saunders AM, Strittmatter WJ, Schmechel D, Georgehyslop PHS, Pericakvance MA, Joo SH, Rosi BL, Gusella JF, Crapper-MacLachlan DR, Alberts MJ (1993) Association of apolipoprotein-E allele epsilon-4 with late-onset familial and sporadic Alzheimers disease. *Neurology* 43:1467–1472.

Scanziani M, Debanne D, Muller M, Gahwiler BH, Thompson SM (1994) Role of excitatory amino acid and GABA$_B$ receptors in the generation of epileptiform activity in disinhibited hippocampal slice cultures. *Neuroscience* 61:823–832.

Scarpini E, Scheltens P, Feldman H (2003) Treatment of Alzheimer's disease: current status and new perspectives. *Lancet Neurol* 2:539–547.

Scharfman HE, Goodman JH, Sollas AL (2000) Granule-like neurons at the hilar/CA3 border after status epilepticus and their synchrony with area CA3 pyramidal cells: functional implications of seizure-induced neurogenesis. *J Neurosci* 20:6144–6158.

Scheibel ME, Crandall PH, Scheibel AB (1974) The hippocampal-dentate complex in temporal lobe epilepsy: a Golgi study. *Epilepsia* 15:55–80.

Scheff SW, Sparks DL, Price DA (1996) Quantitative assessment of synaptic density in the outer molecular layer of the hippocampal dentate gyrus in Alzheimer's disease. *Dementia* 7:226–232.

Schenk D, Barbour R, Dunn W, Gordon G, Grajeda H, Guido T, Hu K, Huang JP, Johnsonwood K, Khan K, Kholodenko D, Lee M, Liao ZM, Lieberburg I, Motter R, Mutter L, Soriano F, Shopp G, Vasquez N, Vandevert C, Walker S, Wogulis M, Yednock T,

Games D, Seubert P (1999) Immunization with amyloid-beta attenuates Alzheimer disease-like pathology in the PDAPP mouse. *Nature* 400:173–177.

Schmidt-Kastner R, Freund TF (1991) Selective vulnerability of the hippocampus in brain ischemia. *Neuroscience* 40:599–636.

Schroder W, Hinterkeuser S, Seifert G, Schramm J, Jabs R, Wilkin GP, Steinhauser C (2000) Functional and molecular properties of human astrocytes in acute hippocampal slices obtained from patients with temporal lobe epilepsy. *Epilepsia* 41 (Suppl 6):S181–S184.

Schwindt PC, Spain WJ, Crill WE (1989) Long-lasting reduction of excitability by a sodium-dependent potassium current in cat neocortical neurons. *J Neurophysiol* 61:233–244.

Semyanov A, Kullmann DM (2000) Modulation of GABAergic signaling among interneurons by metabotropic glutamate receptors. *Neuron* 25:663–672.

Seifert G, Huttmann K, Schramm J, Steinhauser C (2004) Enhanced relative expression of glutumate receptor 1 flip AMPA receptor subunits in hippocampal astrocytes of epilepsy patients with Ammon's horn sclerosis. *J Neurosci* 24:1996–2003.

Simic G, Kostovic I, Winblad B, Bogdanovic N (1997) Volume and number of neurons of the human hippocampal formation in normal aging and alzheimer's disease. *J Comp Neurol* 379:482–494.

Sloviter RS (1987) Decreased hippocampal inhibition and a selective loss of interneurons in experimental epilepsy. *Science* 235:73–76.

Sloviter RS (1991) Permanently altered hippocampal structure, excitability, and inhibition after experimental status epilepticus in the rat: the "dormant basket cell" hypothesis and its possible relevance to temporal lobe epilepsy. *Hippocampus* 1:41–66.

Sloviter RS (1992) Possible functional consequences of synaptic reorganization in the dentate gyrus of kainate-treated rats. *Neurosci Lett* 137:91–96.

Sloviter RS, Dichter MA, Rachinsky TL, Dean E, Goodman JH, Sollas AL, Martin DL (1996) Basal expression and induction of glutamate decarboxylase and GABA in excitatory granule cells of the rat and monkey hippocampal dentate gyrus. *J Comp Neurol* 373:593–618.

Smith GE, Petersen RC, Parisi JE, Ivnik RJ, Kokmen E, Tangalos EG, Waring S (1996) Definition, course, and outcome of mild cognitive impairment. *Aging Neuropsychol Cogn* 3:141–147.

Sommer W (1880) Erkrankung des Ammonshornes als aetiologisches Moment der Epilepsie. *Arch Psychiatr Nervenkr* 10:631–675.

Sperk G, Schwarzer C, Tsunashima K, Kandlhofer S (1998) Expression of GABA(A) receptor subunits in the hippocampus of the rat after kainic acid-induced seizures. *Epilepsy Res* 32:129–139.

Staley KJ, Longacher M, Bains JS, Yee A (1998) Presynaptic modulation of CA3 network activity. *Nat Neurosci* 1:20209.

Su H, Alroy G, Kirson ED, Yaari Y (2001) Extracellular calcium modulates persistent sodium current-dependent burst-firing in hippocampal pyramidal neurons. *J Neurosci* 21:4173–4182.

Su H, Sochivko D, Becker A, Chen J, Jiang Y, Yaari Y, Beck H (2002) Upregulation of a T-type Ca^{2+} channel causes a long-lasting modification of neuronal firing mode after status epilepticus. *J Neurosci* 22:3645–3655.

Sundstrom LE, Brana C, Gatherer M, Mepham J, Rougier A (2001) Somatostatin- and neuropeptide Y-synthesizing neurones in the fascia dentata of humans with temporal lobe epilepsy. *Brain* 124:688–697.

Sutula T, Cascino G, Cavazos J, Parada I, Ramirez L (1989) Mossy fiber synaptic reorganization in the epileptic human temporal lobe. *Ann Neurol* 26:321–330.

Tanaka H, Grooms SY, Bennett MV, Zukin RS (2000) The AMPAR subunit GluR2: still front and center-stage. *Brain Res* 886:190–207.

Tanaka K, Watase K, Manabe T, Yamada K, Watanabe M, Takahashi K, Iwama H, Nishikawa T, Ichihara N, Kikuchi T, Okuyama S, Kawashima N, Hori S, Takimoto M, Wada K (1997) Epilepsy and exacerbation of brain injury in mice lacking the glutamate transporter GLT-1. *Science* 276:1699–1702.

Tate DF, Bigler ED (2000) Fornix and hippocampal atrophy in traumatic brain injury. *Learn Mem* 7: 442–446.

Theodore WH, Bhatia S, Hatta J, Fazilat S, DeCarli C, Bookheimer SY, Gaillard WD (1999) Hippocampal atrophy, epilepsy duration, and febrile seizures in patients with partial seizures. *Neurology* 52: 132–136.

Thom M, Lin WR, Harkness W, Sisodiya S (2001) Patterns of hippocampal sclerosis in a temporal lobectomy series at National Hospital for Neurology and Neurosurgery [abstract]. *Neuropathol Appl Neurobiol* 27:147–148.

Tian GF, Azmi H, Takano T, Xu Q, Peng W, Lin J, Oberheim N, Lou N, Wang X, Zielke HR, Kang J, Nedergaard M (2005) An astrocytic basis of epilepsy. *Nat Med* 11:973–981.

Traub RD, Jefferys JG (1994) Simulations of epileptiform activity in the hippocampal CA3 region in vitro. *Hippocampus* 4:281–285.

Traub RD, Whittington MA, Buhl EH, LeBeau FE, Bibbig A, Boyd S, Cross H, Baldeweg T (2001) A possible role for gap junctions in generation of very fast EEG oscillations preceding the onset of, and perhaps initiating, seizures. *Epilepsia* 42:153–170.

Traynelis SF, Dingledine R (1988) Potassium-induced spontaneous electrographic seizures in the rat hippocampal slice. *J Neurophysiol* 59:259–276.

Tuunanen J, Pitkanen A (2000) Do seizures cause neuronal damage in rat amygdala kindling? *Epilepsy Res* 39:171–176.

Ueda Y, Doi T, Tokumaru J, Yokoyama H, Nakajima A, Mitsuyama Y, Ohya-Nishiguchi H, Kamada H, Willmore LJ (2001) Collapse of extracellular glutamate regulation during epileptogenesis: down-regulation and functional failure of glutamate transporter function in rats with chronic seizures induced by kainic acid. *J Neurochem* 76:892–900.

Van Landingham KE, Heinz ER, Cavazos JE, Lewis DV (1998) Magnetic resonance imaging evidence of hippocampal injury after prolonged focal febrile convulsions. *Ann Neurol* 43:413–426.

Van Paesschen W, Connelly A, King MD, Jackson GD, Duncan JS (1997a) The spectrum of hippocampal sclerosis: a quantitative magnetic resonance imaging study. *Ann Neurol* 41:41–51.

Van Paesschen W, Revesz T, Duncan JS, King MD, Connelly A (1997b) Quantitative neuropathology and quantitative magnetic resonance imaging of the hippocampus in temporal lobe epilepsy. *Ann Neurol* 42:756–766.

Van Paesschen W, Duncan JS, Stevens JM, Connelly A (1998) Longitudinal quantitative hippocampal magnetic resonance imaging study of adults with newly diagnosed partial seizures: one-year follow-up results. *Epilepsia* 39:633–639.

Vezzani A, Sperk G, Colmers WF (1999) Neuropeptide Y: emerging evidence for a functional role in seizure modulation. *Trends Neurosci* 22:25–30.

Von Campe G, Spencer DD, de-Lanerolle NC (1997) Morphology of dentate granule cells in the human epileptogenic hippocampus. *Hippocampus* 7:472–488.

Wahlund L-O, Julin P, Johansson S-E, Scheltens P (2000) Visual rating and volumetry of the medial temporal lobe on magnetic resonance imaging in dementia: a comparative study. *J Neurol Neurosurg Psychiatry* 69:630–635.

Walker MC, Kullmann DM (1999) Febrile convulsions: a 'benign' condition? *Nat Med* 5:871–872.

Walker MC, Ruiz A, Kullmann DM (2001) Monosynaptic gabaergic signaling from dentate to CA3 with a pharmacological and physiological profile typical of mossy fiber synapses. *Neuron* 29:703–715.

Walker MC, Shorvon SD (1997) Partial epilepsy syndromes in adults. In: *The epilepsies 2* (Porter RJ, Chadwick D, eds), pp 141–156. Boston: Butterworth-Heinemann.

Walker MC, White HS, Sander JW (2002) Disease modification in partial epilepsy. *Brain* 125:1937–1950.

Weiss JH, Sensi SL, Koh JY (2000) Zn(2+): a novel ionic mediator of neural injury in brain disease. *Trends Pharmacol Sci* 21:395–401.

West MJ, Coleman PD, Flood DG, Troncoso JC (1994) Differences in the pattern of hippocampal neuronal loss in normal ageing and Alzheimer's disease. *Lancet* 344:769–772.

Whittington MA, Jefferys JG (1994) Epileptic activity outlasts disinhibition after intrahippocampal tetanus toxin in the rat. *J Physiol* 481(Pt 3):593–604.

Wieshmann UC, Clark CA, Symms MR, Barker GJ, Birnie KD, Shorvon SD (1999) Water diffusion in the human hippocampus in epilepsy. *Magn Reson Imaging* 17:29–36.

Wilcock GK, Esiri MM, Bowen DM, Smith CCT (1982) Alzheimer's disease: correlations of cortical choline acetyltransferase activity withe the severity of dementia and histological abnormalities. *J Neurol Sci* 57:407–417.

Williamson PD, French JA, Thadani VM, KIM JH, Novelly RA, Spencer SS, Spencer DD, Mattson RH (1993) Characteristics of medial temporal lobe epilepsy: II. Interictal and ictal scalp electroencephalography, neuropsychological testing, neuroimaging, surgical results, and pathology. *Ann Neurol* 34:781–787.

Winblad B, Poritis N (1999) Memantine in severe dementia: results of the 9M-Best Study (Benefit and Efficacy in Severely demented patients during Treatment with memantine). *Int J Geriatr Psychiatry* 14:135–146.

Wittner L, Eross L, Szabo Z, Toth S, Czirjak S, Halasz P, Freund TF, Magloczky ZS (2002) Synaptic reorganization of calbinin-positive neurons in the human hippocampal CA1 region in temporal lobe epilepsy. *Neuroscience* 115:961–978.

Wolf HK, Campos MG, Zentner J, Hufnagel A, Schramm J, Elger CE, Wiestler OD (1993) Surgical pathology of temporal lobe epilepsy: experience with 216 cases. *J Neuropathol Exp Neurol* 52:499–506.

Wuarin JP, Dudek FE (1996) Electrographic seizures and new recurrent excitatory circuits in the dentate gyrus of hippocampal slices from kainate-treated epileptic rats. *J Neurosci* 16:4438–4448.

Wyler AR, Dohan FC, Schweitzer JB, Berry AD (1992) A grading system for mesial temporal pathology (hippocampal sclerosis) from anterior temporal lobectomy. *J Epilepsy* 5:220–225.

Xiong ZQ, Saggau P, Stringer JL (2000) Activity-dependent intracellular acidification correlates with the duration of seizure activity. *J Neurosci* 20:1290–1296.

Yilmazer-Hanke DM, Wolf HK, Schramm J, Elger CE, Wiestler OD, Blumcke I (2000) Subregional pathology of the amygdala complex and entorhinal region in surgical specimens from patients with pharmacoresistant temporal lobe epilepsy. *J Neuropathol Exp Neurol* 59:907–920.

Young D, Dragunow M (1994) Status epilepticus may be caused by loss of adenosine anticonvulsant mechanisms. *Neuroscience* 58:245–261.

Zhu ZQ, Armstrong DL, Hamilton WJ, Grossman RG (1997) Disproportionate loss of CA4 parvalbumin-immunoreactive interneurons in patients with Ammon's horn sclerosis. *J Neuropathol Exp Neurol* 56:988–998.

Index

Note: Page numbers followed by f refer to figures; page numbers followed by t refer to tables; page numbers followed by b refer to boxes.